Neocortical Neurogenesis in Development and Evolution

Neocortical Neurogenesis in Development and Evolution

Edited by

Wieland B. Huttner
Max Planck Institute of Molecular Cell Biology and Genetics
Dresden, Germany

WILEY

This edition first published 2023

Registered Offices
John Wiley & Sons, Inc., 111 River Street, Hoboken, NJ 07030, USA
John Wiley & Sons Ltd, The Atrium, Southern Gate, Chichester, West Sussex, PO19 8SQ, UK

For details of our global editorial offices, customer services, and more information about Wiley products visit us at www.wiley.com.

Wiley also publishes its books in a variety of electronic formats and by print-on-demand. Some content that appears in standard print versions of this book may not be available in other formats.

A catalogue record for this book is available from the Library of Congress

Hardback ISBN: 9781119860808; ePub ISBN: 9781119860822; ePDF ISBN: 9781119860815; Obook ISBN: 9781119860914

Cover Design: Wiley
Cover Image: © PIXOLOGICSTUDIO/SCIENCE PHOTO LIBRARY/Getty Images; EreborMountain/Shutterstock

Set in 9.5/12.5pt STIXTwoText by Integra Software Services Pvt. Ltd, Pondicherry, India

To Gisela

Contents

Foreword

Understanding the human brain is a fundamental challenge. Key to this challenge is gaining insight into the development of the brain and how it changed during human evolution. This book *Neocortical Neurogenesis in Development and Evolution*, edited by Wieland B. Huttner, a pioneer in the cell biology of brain development, focuses on neurons, the crucial cell type of the brain, and the neocortex, the seat of higher-order brain functions. Its 33 chapters, contributed by leading researchers, provide a state-of-the-art overview of how the various types of cortical neurons are generated from cortical stem and progenitor cells. They also cover related topics such as the folding of the neocortex to accommodate larger numbers of neurons in the skull, and disorders of cortical development and their clinical implications. The book provides a unique blend of insight into neocortex development and its evolution that will be useful for both students and researchers in this fascinating field.

Svante Pääbo
2022 Nobel Prize in Physiology or Medicine
Max Planck Institute for Evolutionary Anthropology, Leipzig, Germany

Preface

The evolution of mammalian brains, notably that of the human brain, has fascinated researchers for a long time. Inseparably linked to this evolution is the process of the development of mammalian brains. In this context, a mammalian-specific part of the brain that is of particular interest is the neocortex, the phylogenetically youngest part of the cerebral cortex. The neocortex is the seat of: sensory perception, generation of motor commands, and higher-order brain functions such as cognition and – in humans – language. An essential foundation underlying neocortex function is neurogenesis, a complex process in which the generation of neurons from cortical stem and progenitor cells (cSPCs) has a central role, but which also comprises subsequent steps such as the migration of new-born neurons to the appropriate neuronal layer of the six-layered neocortex. Topics inherent in or related to neocortical neurogenesis include (i) cell lineages within the various cSPCs and from cSPCs to neurons, (ii) the generation of diverse types of neurons, (iii) the specification of cortical regions, (iv) cortical folding, and (v) cortical malformations. It is precisely these issues that this book addresses.

I am grateful, and indeed feel honored, that of the leading researchers – and in fact pioneers – in the field whom I approached, the overwhelming majority agreed to become contributors to this book. Thanks to the wonderful efforts and major discoveries of these many colleagues and their associates, the 33 chapters of this book together provide a near-comprehensive up-to-date overview of neurogenesis in the developing neocortex and its evolutionary adaptations.

Before describing the various sections and chapters of this book, a brief introduction to the germinal zones, classes and types of cSPCs, and their terminology may be helpful. The wall of the developing neocortex with its various zones and layers arises from the neuroepithelium and retains a fundamental feature of the latter – apical–basal polarity. Thus, the ventricular surface corresponds to the apical side of the developing cortical wall, and the pial surface to its basal side. There are two principal germinal zones. First, the ventricular zone (VZ); it is the primary germinal zone, is the apical-most zone of the developing cortical wall, borders the ventricle, and is the zone most closely related to the neuroepithelium. Second, the subventricular zone (SVZ); it is a secondary germinal zone arising from the VZ and is located adjacent to the basal side of the VZ. In many mammalian species, notably those developing a relatively large and folded (gyrencephalic) neocortex such as the human, the SVZ is divided into two subzones, called the inner SVZ (iSVZ), which is located basally to the VZ, and the outer SVZ (oSVZ), which is located basally to the iSVZ. In line with this localization of the germinal zones along the apical–basal axis of the developing cortical wall, the cSPCs whose cell bodies reside in the VZ constitute one cSPC class and are collectively referred to as apical progenitors (APs), and the cSPCs whose cell bodies reside in the SVZ constitute the other cSPC class and are collectively referred to as basal progenitors (BPs). The major types of APs are the neuroepithelial cells, which transform into radial glia and are called either apical or ventricular radial glia; in turn these transform into the truncated radial glia. Additional types of

APs are discussed in the respective chapters. The major types of BPs are the basal intermediate progenitors, sometimes simply referred to as intermediate progenitors, and the delaminated radial glia called either basal or outer radial glia.

The first section of the book focuses on cSPCs and the germinal zones in which they reside. Magdalena Götz and Florencia Merino open this section with their chapter describing the discovery and role of radial glial cells as neural stem cells. Arnold Kriegstein and Alex Pollen then review the diversity of cSPCs in the developing human neocortex and discuss how the contribution of progenitor cells to the structure of the neocortex underwent changes in the course of human evolution. This is followed by Robert Hevner's chapter, which focuses on the role of one type of BP, the intermediate progenitors, in the development and evolution of the neocortex. Colette Dehay and Henry Kennedy then concentrate on a germinal zone first described in the developing macaque neocortex, the oSVZ, whose BPs have a key role in shaping the cytoarchitecture, in particular, of the primate neocortex. Víctor Borrell and Virginia Fernández subsequently broaden the evolutionary aspects of the role of cSPCs in neocortex development by comparing the cSPC-based neurogenesis in mammalian brains to the neurogenesis and progenitor cells in the developing brains of reptiles and birds. The following two chapters address two specific features of cSPCs. Ryoichiro Kageyama and Hiromi Shimojo concentrate on the role of basic helix-loop-helix transcription factors in the regulation of the proliferation and differentiation of neuroepithelial cells and radial glial cells. Takaki Miyata discusses biophysical issues, notably the mechanical forces that are relevant for the APs in the VZ, in particular the forces associated with the interkinetic nuclear migration of these cSPCs. Finally, my colleagues Lei Xing, Anneline Pinson, Felipe Mora-Bermúdez, and I discuss the role of human-specific genes and amino-acid substitutions that affect cSPC behavior and thereby influence human neocortex development in crucial ways, with relevance for neocortex expansion and modern human vs. Neanderthal differences in neocortical neurogenesis.

Linked to this discussion of the various classes and types of cSPCs and their key features, the following section of the book addresses, in two chapters, the topic of cell lineages within the various cSPCs and from cSPCs to neurons in the developing neocortex. Fumio Matsuzaki, Quan Wu, Merve Bilgic, and Yuji Tsunekawa first discuss the diversity of APs in the VZ and then report on the heterogeneity of radial glial cell lineages in the developing neocortex of the ferret, a gyrencephalic carnivore. This leads these authors to raise the issue of the temporal scaling of neocortex development, in the context of cSPC diversity, across three frequently studied mammalian species, the lissencephalic mouse, the gyrencephalic ferret and the highly gyrencephalic human. The second chapter in this section by Simon Hippenmeyer, Ana Villalba, and Nicole Amberg concentrates on the topic of radial glial cell lineage progression in the developing neocortex all the way to neurons and, eventually, to glial cells, and discusses cell-autonomous vs. non-cell-autonomous cues that affect this progression. In this context, the authors describe the MADM technology for the study of radial glial cell lineage progression and address specific genes that control this progression.

Following these two sections on cSPCs, the next section of the book addresses the generation of the various types of cortical neurons. Paola Arlotta and Ana Uzquiano open this section by discussing the mechanisms underlying projection neuron diversification and the use of human brain organoids to investigate human-specific features of neuron diversification. Tarik Haydar, Zhen Li, and William Tyler then link the topic of projection neuron diversity to the heterogeneity of cSPCs and discuss human developmental disorders resulting in alterations of cortical neurogenesis that affect neuron diversity. Nenad Sestan and his associates Navjot Kaur, Rothem Kovner, and Kevin T. Gobeske further broaden these discussions not only by addressing the topics of laminar and areal identity of cortical projection neurons, but also by introducing the subjects of human specializations of cortical projection neurons and their circuitry, and of human neuropsychiatric disorders. Denis Jabaudon, Esther Klingler, and Sergi Roig Puiggros then focus on cell-intrinsic and cell-extrinsic mechanisms that are involved in the emergence of cortical areas, and address the topic of input-dependent differentiation of the various types of cortical neurons, including the inhibitory interneurons. A different facet is introduced in the chapter by Jürgen Knoblich and Catarina Martins-Costa, who dissect the evolution and development of the corpus callosum, a key structure for the transfer of information between the brain hemispheres. Finally, Zoltán Molnár, Thomas Henning, and Sara Bandiera close this section of the book by focusing on a subpopulation of subplate neurons that persists through development into adulthood as layer 6b in mouse and interstitial white matter cells in human, and by discussing a transcriptionally based classification of these cells.

Complementing this section, the following section of the book with its two chapters focuses on the migration of the new-born neurons to the appropriate position within the six-layered neocortex. Laurent Nguyen and Míriam Javier-Torrent first discuss the modes of cell migration of the excitatory projection neurons and the inhibitory interneurons and dissect the differences between these two classes of cortical neurons that exist in mammals ranging from rodents to primates. The authors then concentrate on impairments of neuron migration that result in prototypic neuronal migration disorders, and discuss molecular mechanisms that regulate neuron migration and whose disturbances underlie these cortical malformations. Orly Reiner and Aditya Kshirsagar focus on *LIS1*, the first human gene identified and reported to be involved in neuron migration. The authors provide an in-depth analysis of the mechanisms underlying LIS1 function, its regulation, and its role in the pathophysiology of various CNS diseases.

The next section of the book addresses neural patterning and the specification of cortical regions. Madeline Lancaster and Magdalena Sutcliffe focus on early forebrain morphogenesis, specifically the patterning of the rostral neural tube and the expansion of the early forebrain neuroepithelium. They describe the role of various neural organoid models to study these processes and discuss human-specific features and their implications for microcephalic and macrocephalic disorders. The chapter by Flora Vaccarino, Soraya Scuderi, and Alexandre Jourdon covers the highly related topics of the formation of brain regions, signaling centers involved in patterning, patterning of the cortical plate and cell diversity, and the modeling of disorders of cortical development using organoids. John Rubenstein and Athéna Ypsilanti then provide an in-depth discussion of the role of transcriptional regulators in the specification of the mammalian cortex into its constituent regions and areas. They dissect how the control of gene expression that underlies cortical patterning involves a complex interplay between transcription factors, enhancers, chromatin modifiers, and epigenetics. The final chapter in this section by Elizabeth Grove on the development of the neocortical area map broadens the theme by discussing not only the mechanisms of area patterning intrinsic to the neocortex but also thalamic mechanisms of area development, as well as the conservation of patterning mechanisms among different mammalian species.

A hallmark of neocortex development and evolution is cortical folding, which occurs in many mammalian species as brain size increases, notably in the human brain. The two chapters in this section of the book address this topic. Pasko Rakic, who must be regarded as the father of the entire field covered in this book, and his colleague Jon Arellano, after providing a historical perspective, describe the main characteristics of gyrification, critically review some of the mechanisms proposed to explain cortical folding, and present their favored view on what underlies cortical folding. The second chapter by Hiroshi Kawasaki and Yohei Shinmyo focuses on the ferret as a gyrencephalic animal model of cortical folding. The authors discuss recent findings obtained in this animal model on the mechanisms underlying the development of the cerebral cortex, with an emphasis on cortical folding, and put this discussion into the broader context of common vs. species-specific mechanisms of cortical folding.

The penultimate section of the book addresses variations, disorders, and malformations of cortical development. Eva Anton, Madison Rose Glass, and Jason Stein focus on genetic variation that impacts cortical progenitor function and thereby affects human neocortex size and/or structure.

The following chapter by Chris Walsh and Robert Sean Hill dissects the roles of specific genes, including *SRGAP2C*, *ASPM*, *NOTCH2NL*, and *GPR56*, in the evolution of the human neocortex and in disorders of human brain development, neurological function, and cognition. The authors also highlight the medical relevance of these types of studies. The last chapter in this section, by Silvia Cappello, Veronica Pravata, and Pierre Gressens, provides an overview of the molecular causes underlying specific cortical malformations and of their clinical features. The authors dissect at which cellular level the various cortical malformations arise.

The final section of the book deals with topics that are relevant for many of the processes discussed in the previous sections and that are therefore referred to as overarching topics. Debra Silver, Camila Manso Musso, and Bianca Lupan provide a broad overview of the major posttranscriptional mechanisms implicated in neocortical development and evolution. The authors also discuss the dysregulation of posttranscriptional processes that contributes to neurodevelopmental diseases. Highly related to this, the chapter by Noriko Osumi, Takako Kikkawa, and Sharmin Naher addresses the regulation of mRNA localization and translation in neocortex development, evolution, and pathogenesis. The authors focus on the RNA binding protein called fragile X mental retardation protein, and on the transport of the cyclin D2 mRNA within radial glial cells. Zhiheng Xu, Dan Xu, and Yiqiang Zhi then dissect the roles of the major signal transduction pathways during cortical neurogenesis. The authors also discuss the consequences for neocortex development when specific components of these signaling pathways are mutated or deleted. The following chapter by Song-Hai Shi and Xuan Xie focuses on a key cellular organelle, the centrosome. The authors provide an in-depth discussion of the regulation and function of the centrosome during neocortical development and of the pathophysiology of centrosome-related neurological diseases. Yet another key player in cerebral cortex development, the cerebrospinal fluid, is addressed by Maria Lehtinen, Tiara Lacey, and Ryann Fame. The authors describe the various facets, and discuss concepts, connected to how the cerebrospinal fluid participates in the development of the cerebral cortex. Finally, in the last chapter of this section and – in fact – the entire book, Jon Kaas, Hui-Xin Qi, and Iwona Stepniewska address what can be regarded as a major outcome of neocortical neurogenesis in development and evolution – cognition. The authors discuss central aspects of this complex topic, including the cognition in apes and humans, language, speech and reading, and primate memory.

Of course, not all potential topics in the broad field of neocortical neurogenesis in development and evolution can be covered in a single book. Nonetheless, I hope that this brief description of the contents of the 33 chapters of this book will raise enough curiosity to actually read all of these chapters. I further hope that reading this book will not only be found informative but also will open up avenues towards novel insights into what makes us human.

January 15, 2023

Wieland B. Huttner

Part 1

Cortical Progenitors and Germinal Zones

1

Neural Stem Cells as Glia

Florencia Merino and Magdalena Götz

Biomedical Center, Ludwig-Maximilians University and Institute of Stem Cell Research, Helmholtz Center Munich, Planegg-Martinsried, Germany

1.1 Introduction and Definitions

In order to determine if and when cells act as neural stem cells and glial cells, we need to define both terms. Even though the definition of stem cells is notoriously difficult, glia is even more difficult to define. We shall discuss and explain why this is the case and why these terms are highly relevant in the ontogeny and phylogeny of the cerebral cortex and of nervous systems more broadly.

1.1.1 Neural Stem Cell Definition

As the word encompasses, a stem cell is at the root of a lineage. It has two generic hallmarks – self-renewal and generation of a range of progeny, typically more than one cell type. *Self-renewal* is well defined, namely that the mother cell generates a copy of itself. This allows the maintenance of stem cells at least for a while in development, and some even into adulthood. The difficulty of defining the term lies in the uncertainty of the length of this self-renewal, that is, for how many cell divisions, and how identical the daughter cell has to be. A stem cell needs to self-renew, otherwise it depletes when it divides and generates two differentiating progenitors in a so-called consumptive or differentiative division. Thus, neural stem cells generate at least one, sometimes two neural stem cells thereby maintaining the neural stem cell pool – but for how long? In the developing murine cerebral cortex, clonal analysis has shown that a neural stem cell typically divides and self-renews for about 11 cell cycles (Gao et al. 2014) before it differentiates at the end of neurogenesis in differentiative neuronal divisions. It can also generate postmitotic ependymal cells or glia-restricted progenitors at the end of neurogenesis. This discriminates neural stem cells in the embryo from adult neural stem cells that continue to divide, even though they exhibit heterogeneity with some dividing only for a few rounds, while others self-renew for longer (Basak et al. 2018; Bottes et al. 2021). Thus, self-renewal of neural stem cells is often limited and far from the long-term self-renewal of embryonic stem cells or adult hematopoietic stem cells that can self-renew for longer than the life of the organism they are derived from.

In regard to the other uncertainty, namely how identical to the mother cell the daughter cell should be, it is important to realize that neural stem cells often progress in development and hence do not always generate an exact copy of themselves. For example, neural stem cells generate

Neocortical Neurogenesis in Development and Evolution, First Edition. Edited by Wieland B. Huttner.

different daughter cells over time, such as in the cerebral cortex first neurons of deep layers and then of upper layers (see Chapter 11). Thus, they change in their gene expression and behavior and are hence not identical to their ancestor cells.

This brings us to the *progeny*, the other hallmark of a stem cell. The term "potency" is typically used for the stem cell's capacity to generate different cell types. The fertilized oocyte is totipotent as it can generate all cells of an organism including extraembryonic tissue. *Pluripotency* describes the ability to generate all cells of the embryo except the extraembryonic tissue, and *multipotency*, most relevant here, typically refers to the generation of all cells of a given organ. Neural stem cells should hence be able to generate all cells of the nervous system. However, this is not the case due to a rather unique hallmark of the nervous system – its patterning. Neural stem cells at the front of the brain, most relevant here, in the telencephalon, generate different types of neurons and glia than those at the back of the brain or the spinal cord. This is the fundamental principle of the brain and central nervous system (CNS) function that generates neuronal and glial cell diversity endowing different brain regions with the circuits suited for distinct information processing tasks. This principle continues within one region, such as the cerebral cortex, where distinct neuronal subtypes are generated rostrally and caudally, referred to as arealization, with rostral cortex regions devoted to different tasks than caudal regions of the cerebral cortex (see Chapter 11). This functional arealization is generated in development by expression gradients of first signaling molecules and later transcription factors that specify stem cells in the rostral and caudal regions of the cortex differently (see Chapter 11). Thus, neural stem cells generate different cell types in development, different types of neurons (e.g., of the different layers in the cortex), and different glial cells (astrocytes, ependymal cells, and oligodendrocytes), but only those appropriate for their regional position. Indeed, transplantation experiments showed that stem cells transplanted from one cortex area to another retain some information from their region of origin and their neuronal progeny does not fully adapt to the host area networks (Gaillard et al. 2003). Regarding multipotency, it is important to note that adult neural stem cells exhibit an even more limited range of progeny with often only one neuronal subtype, such as in the dentate gyrus where neural stem cells generate dentate granule neurons only (Denoth-Lippuner and Jessberger 2021). However, they would still be referred to as multipotent, as revealed in vitro, where they can also generate different glial cells, which they hardly do in vivo. This highlights the difference between what cells do in their normal environment in vivo (their lineage) and what they do in a different environment, either upon transplantation or in vitro (their potential). Thus, neural stem cells are multipotent in development and adulthood, but cannot generate ALL neurons or glia of the CNS.

1.1.2 Glial Cell Definition

As is evident in the definition of neural stem cells, cells are often defined by their function. The typical glial cell function is the support of neurons consistent with their earliest appearance in the animal kingdom as cells next to neurons (see later). Indeed, glial cells originally comprised all non-neuronal cells of the nervous system, and this very broad category was refined at some point by excluding endothelial cells (Götz 2013a). Interestingly, the phylogenetically earliest glial cells could be progenitors or stem cells as in the Cnidaria Hydra, or they could be non-proliferating support cells as in the amphid organ in *C. elegans* (Götz 2013a). The typical functions of glial cells throughout the animal kingdom are phagocytosis, that is, removing debris, formation of neuronal connections, like axon or dendrite growth, synapse development and function, and homeostasis of nutrients, neurotransmitters, or ions in the brain. A hallmark of glial cells is their diversification correlated to the increasingly complexity of the nervous systems in line with their function in supporting neurons and participating in neural network function.

1.2 Radial Glia as Neural Stem Cells

In regard to the previous definition of glial cells with a progenitor function appearing first in phylogeny, it is intriguing to note that also in ontogeny, the first glial cells to appear are stem/progenitor cells that appear when neurons are generated: the radial glial cells. The first radial glial cell function discovered was their function as supporting structures for neurons, namely as guidance structures for radially migrating neurons (Rakic 1971b, 1971a). Radial glial cells typically extend a single radial process from the inner brain surface, facing the ventricle containing the cerebrospinal fluid, to the outer surface of the brain, the pial surface where the meninges enwrap the brain (Figure 1.1). At the ventricular side, radial glial cells are anchored by junctional complexes, typically adherens junctions and gap junctions, that delineate the apical membrane domain accessing the ventricular fluid, where the stem cell associated protein prominin is localized (Figure 1.1), from the basal membrane domain that is located basally of the junctional complexes (Götz and Huttner 2005). At the pial surface, the radial glial endfeet are anchored e.g. by integrins to the basement membrane. Thus, radial glial cells are true epithelial cells with an apico-basal polarity, similar to their ancestors, the neuroepithelial cells (Götz and Huttner 2005). Due to the long radial process spanning the entire thickness of the developing cortex, they are referred to as "radial" and as "glia" based on their neuronal support function. In addition, some glial hallmarks were discovered in radial glia, such as the presence of glycogen granules in ultrastructural images and the expression of glia-fibrillary acidic protein (GFAP) in the primate cortex (Levitt and Rakic 1980; Peters and Feldman 1973).

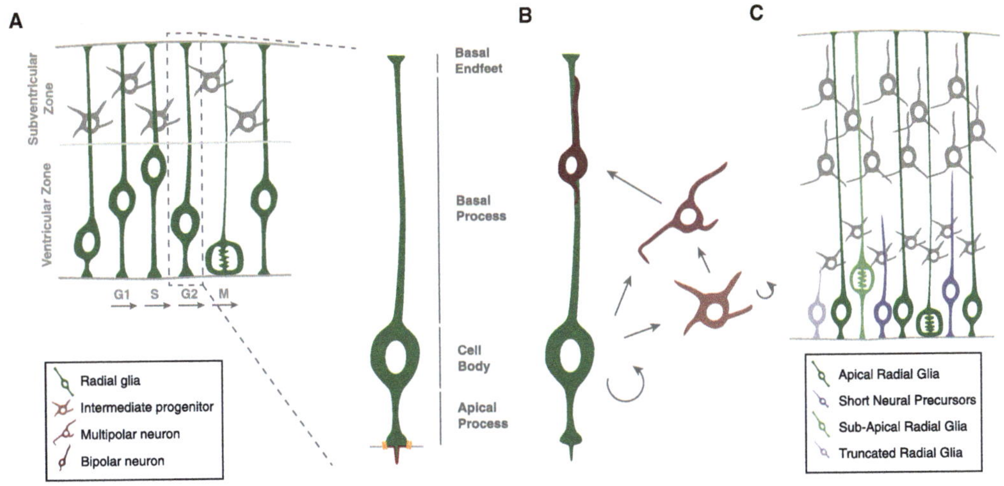

Figure 1.1 Radial glia cell features and neuronal differentiation. (A) Radial glial cells (RGC) present a characteristic movement of their cell soma during the cell cycle named interkinetic nuclear migration (INM). During INM, the nucleus moves basally from the ventricular surface during G1, undergoes the S phase at the basal part of the ventricular zone, and moves apically in the G2 phase, with mitosis occurring at the apical surface. The extent of this movement defines the ventricular zone (VZ) of the developing cortex. RGC possess a long basal radial process reaching the inner brain basal surface to which they attach via their basal endfeet. At the ventricular side, radial glial cells are anchored by junctional complexes, typically adherens junctions and gap junctions, having direct contact with the ventricle lumen. The membrane domain at the apical side is marked by the expression of Prominin (marked in red) while adherens junctions are highlighted in orange. (B) Radial glial cells can self-renew as well as differentiate into intermediate progenitors or young neurons. Intermediate progenitors, which present a multipolar morphology, can subsequently generate young neurons that migrate radially along RGC basal processes towards the cortical plate, where they mature. (C) While apical radial glial cells are the most abundant type of progenitor present in the VZ of the developing cortex, there are diverse cell types present in this region. In this scheme of the developing murine cortex, the different types of progenitors residing in the VZ are illustrated.

The definition of pure support cells was challenged when radial glial cells were identified as neural stem cells (Malatesta et al. 2000; Miyata et al. 2001; Noctor et al. 2001) as this was not included as a support function and radial glia was considered not to divide and not to generate neurons. The former was based on the fact that many cells retract their processes when they divide. The later was based on the proposal by His (1889) of two subtypes of cells in the zone lining of the ventricle, the ventricular zone (VZ), one exhibiting glial hallmarks referred to as "spongiocytes" and the other devoid of such hallmarks and hence referred to as "neuronal progenitors" (Götz 2013b). However, this apparent heterogeneity was challenged by the matrix theory of Fujita in 1963 who realized that the VZ is "pseudostratified," that is, not composed of distinct cell types but of cells that had the somata in different positions (Figure 1.1). The somata in different positions is due to a nuclear migration, known as interkinetic nuclear migration, with nuclei moving basally for S-phase and apically for M-phase (Figure 1.1A). Notably, this implies that the ventricular surface limits the number of mitoses that can occur at any given time (Smart et al. 2002) and further expansion of progenitor numbers requires the absence of interkinetic nuclear migration or basal cell divisions – both of which we discuss later. Importantly, most of the cells in the VZ have "glial" hallmarks (proteins, gene expression, etc., see later) appearing at the onset of neurogenesis, even though there is some degree of heterogeneity (Hartfuss et al. 2001). Indeed, it was the absence of any radial processes without proteins typical for glial cells that sparked the original discovery of radial glial cells as neural stem cells (Götz et al. 1998).

1.2.1 Neuronal Progeny and Multipotency

In mice, the first evidence for radial glial cells generating neurons has been achieved by fluorescence-activated cell sorting (FACS) of cells expressing the green fluorescent protein (GFP) driven by a human GFAP regulatory element and culturing them in vitro (Malatesta et al. 2000; Pinto et al. 2008). This revealed clones, that is, clusters of cells generated from a single FACS-isolated cell, of different sizes and fates, with some containing only neurons and others containing neurons and glia. FACS was later complemented by antibodies against the apical membrane protein prominin and refined regarding the GFP intensity (Pinto et al. 2008). This allowed selectively enriching radial glial cells that self-renew versus those that differentiate directly or indirectly into the neuronal lineage (Pinto et al. 2008). Unbiased transcriptome analysis of these functional subtypes has led to the discovery of several key molecular players promoting radial glia *self-renewal* (Esgleas et al. 2020; Stahl et al. 2013) or other proteins, that were found to be enriched in neural stem cells differentiating into neurons and basal or intermediate progenitors (Camargo Ortega et al. 2019) that are located in the zone above the VZ, the subventricular zone (SVZ) (Figure 1.1A).

With this progeny, the evidence of *multipotency* was obtained, namely the generation of neurons and glia in vitro in primary cultures without the addition of any growth factors. The generation of neurons was also confirmed by live imaging in acute slice preparations of the murine cerebral cortex showing that cells with a radial process divide during neurogenesis and generate young neuroblasts migrating out of the VZ (Miyata et al. 2001; Noctor et al. 2001). Finally, the generation of neurons was also shown in vivo by genetic fate mapping. For this, the Cre recombinase is expressed under glia-specific promoter elements, such as GFAP or the brain lipid-binding protein (BLBP) (Anthony et al. 2004; Malatesta et al. 2003), which excises a stop cassette in front of a ubiquitous promoter element driving a reporter gene, such as beta-galactosidase or GFP. As the expression of this reporter is not cell-type specific, but the Cre expression is, this technique allows mediating recombination in glial cells (that are all radial during development) and labeling their entire progeny. This showed that the progeny of radial glia includes most neurons and glial cells in the cerebral cortex.

1.2.2 Cell Division and Self-renewal

The evidence for self-renewal is based on imaging in acute slice preparations showing examples of consecutive divisions of radial glial cells always generating one radial glia daughter cell (Miyata et al. 2001; Noctor et al. 2001; Pilz et al. 2013). Indeed, in the murine cortex, radial glial cells are the only cells that self-renew, generating further radial glial cells, as all other cells differentiate or generate further differentiated daughter cells (see also heterogeneity Section 1.3). Live imaging in acute slice preparations of the murine cerebral cortex also revealed how cells with such a long radial process divide (Miyata et al. 2001; Noctor et al. 2001). During the M-phase the long radial process either (1) completely retracts or thins considerably with most cytoplasm going into the cell soma, (2) or is retained and inherited by one daughter cell, which is typically the one continuing to proliferate (Shitamukai et al. 2011). In more rare cases, the radial process can split along its radial length thereby symmetrically inheriting the mother radial glia process to both daughter cells (Kosodo et al. 2008). Notably, there is no strict correlation between the inheritance of the process and subsequent fate, because radial glia daughter cells not inheriting a process can regrow one and hence also become a radial glial cell. Indeed, growth cones at the tip of radial processes were found by DiI-labelling in fixed cortices during neurogenesis (Hartfuss et al. 2003). Accordingly, neither inheritance of the basal, nor the apical process is a firm predictor of fate, suggesting several mechanisms, including some yet unknown, determining this process. For example, in zebrafish, radial glial cells inheriting the apical process have been observed to differentiate into neurons, while those inheriting the basal process reestablish an apical contact and retain their proliferative activity (Alexandre et al. 2010). Indeed, the mammalian cortex radial glial cells can also regenerate their apical endfoot (Fujita et al. 2020). Accordingly, several signaling factors contribute to promote proliferation and hence self-renewal in radial glial cells: Notch signaling, cyclin D2 RNA (Tsunekawa et al. 2012) in cerebral cortex radial glia basal processes, and the integrin signaling shown to act via the basal endfoot attachment to the basement membrane (Haubst et al. 2006) all promote proliferation of cortical radial glia.

1.2.3 Glial Aspects of Radial Glia

As mentioned earlier, radial glial cells share their epithelial nature and morphology with the earlier neuroepithelial cells upregulating glial hallmarks at the onset of neurogenesis. These are many proteins shared with later astrocytes, in particular reactive astrocytes (Götz 2013b; Götz et al. 2015), such as glutamate transporter 1 (GLT-1; Slc1a2) and the astrocyte-specific glutamate transporter (GLAST; Slc1a3), glutamine synthase (GS), the Aldolase Aldh1l1, the Ca-binding protein S100β, Tenascin C, and later astrocyte-specific transcription factors, such as Sox9. Many of these proteins as well as the ultrastructural hallmark of glycogen granules reflect the "support" function of astrocytes, such as the glutamate–glutamine shuttle with astrocytes or radial glia taking up glutamate by the glia-specific glutamate transporters Slc1a2 and Slc1a3, converting it via GS into glutamine and delivering this to neurons. Like astrocytes, radial glial cells have prominent glycolysis and store glycogen and can hence also support young neurons in the developing brain by the lactate shuttle (Götz 2013a).

Their gap-junction coupling avoids ion accumulation in the extracellular milieu, such as K ions, and their secretion of factors guides neurite growth and synapse formation (Allen and Lyons 2018). Thus, beyond providing a substrate for neuronal migration, radial glial cells are involved in typical astrocyte-mediated support functions. Indeed, in many vertebrates, radial glial cells persist into adulthood and perform exactly these functions, such as in the adult zebrafish forebrain.

Thus, radial glial cells contain a multitude of glial proteins and perform typical glial support functions. Beyond this, global, unbiased transcriptome analysis also reveals clear similarities between radial glial cells and astrocytes (Götz et al. 2015). This is particularly evident after brain injury, when reactive astrocytes of the cerebral cortex up-regulate gene expression hallmarks of radial glial cells, such as Tenascin C, Vimentin, and others (Götz et al. 2015). Also, single-cell RNA-sequencing shows the alignment of radial glial cells with reactive astrocytes from stab-wound injured cortex when overlayed (Bocchi et al. pers. comm.), supporting the similarity of gene expression between radial glial cells and reactive astrocytes well beyond a handful of genes and proteins. Thus, radial glial cells are indeed glial cells that act as neural stem cells in the developing mammalian cerebral cortex.

1.3 Heterogeneity of Apical Radial Glial Cells

Besides the radial glial cells described earlier, as the vast majority of cells in the VZ during neurogenesis, other progenitor cell types have also been identified in the VZ. Importantly, the VZ is defined by the extent of the interkinetic nuclear movements with the most basal position of the nuclei in S-phase defining the basal border (Figure 1.1A). While early in development these nuclear movements reach the pial/basal surface of the brain, with cells leaving the VZ and accumulating on top, such as neurons, the basal movements become more restricted and form the basal border of the VZ (Götz and Huttner 2005).

1.3.1 Short Neural Precursors

A cell type found in the VZ first identified in the mouse developing cortex is the *short neural precursors* (Figure 1.1C) (Gal et al. 2006). Short neural precursors are characterized by having a very short basal process, and the expression of neuronal markers, including expression driven by the tubulin-alpha1 promoter, while they lack or reduce the expression of radial glial markers, such as GLAST (Gal et al. 2006; Stancik et al. 2010). Given their short basal process, short neural precursors lack the contact with the basement membrane, but otherwise have epithelial properties with their apical processes anchored by junctional complexes, and the soma undergoing interkinetic nuclear migration with mitosis occurring at the apical ventricular surface (Figure 1.1). In the cortex, these cells have a prolonged G1 phase and may differentiate directly into neurons. Their progeny predominantly resides in layer IV, while the radial glial cells labeled at this later stage of neurogenesis largely generate neurons in layers II and III (Stancik et al. 2010). Short neural precursors have also been identified in the ventral telencephalon where they can divide more than once and proliferate faster than the radial glial cells (Pilz et al. 2013). This is why they have been named "short neural progenitor cells" in this region, as "precursors" are typically nondividing stages in a lineage undergoing differentiation. Taken together, short neural precursor/progenitor cells are apically dividing VZ cells that have no glial hallmarks and seem to differ fundamentally in different brain regions. Further molecular analysis will be required for a better understanding of their identity and function.

1.3.2 Truncated Radial Glia

While short neural precursors were originally described in mice, Nowakowski et al. (2016) also identified radial glial cells with basal processes that do not extend beyond VZ in the developing human cortex at later developmental stages (GW 18–23) and named them *truncated radial glia* (Figure 1.1C). Given the thickness of the human cortex, it may be possible that truncated radial glia just fail to reach further with their radial processes, but otherwise they could resemble the apical radial glial cells. This seems, however, not to be the case as they differ in expression and lineage from apical radial glial cells. Truncated radial glial cells specifically express, for example, CRYAB and NR4A1 (Nowakowski et al. 2016), while they share other typical apical radial glia proteins, such as the transcription factors PAX6 and SOX2, as well as the Glutamate transporter, GLAST. Recent single-cell sequencing data from the developing ferret cerebral cortex where truncated radial glia have also been detected in larger numbers at the end of neurogenesis, show that they share expression hallmarks with ependymal cells and astrocytes (Bilgic et al. 2022). These data suggest that truncated radial glia assume a more gliogenic role at later stages, when neurogenesis and gliogenesis overlap, for example, in the human cortex development (Allen et al. 2022; Malik et al. 2013).

1.3.3 Subapical Radial Glia

While radial glial cells with a basal process that does not extend beyond the progenitor's zones were originally identified in the cortex, cells with the same characteristics have also been found in other brain structures such as the murine ventral telencephalon (Falk et al. 2017; Pilz et al. 2013). This region has the highest output in neuron numbers in the murine telencephalon, as it supplies all the other regions with interneurons. In this regard, it is interesting that its high apical progenitor diversity is also reflected in cortices with a high gyrification, that is, folding index (Pilz et al. 2013). Besides short neural progenitors and truncated radial glia (see earlier), detailed analysis of this region has led to the discovery of a novel subtype of radial glial cells, the "*subapical radial glia*" (Figure 1.1C). They are located within the VZ, but do not undergo interkinetic nuclear migration and hence do not divide at the apical surface. They have full radial glia morphology with a long radial process and an apical process contacting the ventricle and also express glial marker proteins, such as RC2, GLAST, and Vimentin (Pilz et al. 2013). Live imaging showed that their nucleus remains stable and undergoes division at the upper part of the VZ without any apically directed movements. Comparative analysis of these cells detected by phospho-Vimentin staining in different species revealed their highest frequency in developing cerebral cortices of mammals with a high gyrification index, such as sheep (Pilz et al. 2013). Moreover, upon manipulating the murine cerebral cortex towards folding, subapical radial glial cells become more frequent (Stahl et al., 2013). Live imaging further revealed that their progeny are often the basal radial glial cells that are particularly frequent in folded cerebral cortices (see later and Chapter 5). This occurs through a division with a cleavage furrow parallel to the surface of the brain resulting in a daughter cell retaining the apical process, but losing the basal process, and an (upper/basal) daughter cell losing the apical process but retaining the basal one, the typical morphology of a basal radial glia (Figure 1.2). Taken together, subapical radial glial cells appear to be an amplifying lineage that can increase the output from radial glia divisions by not having to move to the apical ventricular surface and are one of the ancestors of basal radial glia.

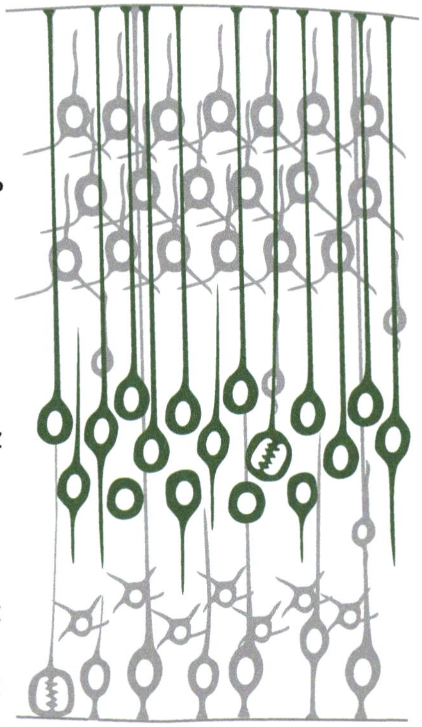

Figure 1.2 Basal radial glia heterogeneity. Scheme of a coronal section of the developing neocortex from a representative gyrencephalic species depicting the heterogeneity that basal radial glia can present in terms of morphology. CP: cortical plate; oSVZ: outer subventricular zone; iSVZ: inner subventricular zone; VZ: ventricular zone.

1.4 Basal Radial Glial Cells and their Heterogeneity

During the development of larger and increasingly folded cortices, the region above the VZ, that is, at a more basal position, the SVZ, expands more and more, consistent with the apical surface being too limited and the need to accommodate further amplifying progenitor lineages (Figure 1.2). In carnivores and primates, for example, this zone becomes so huge that it is subdivided into an inner (iSVZ) and an outer (oSVZ) subventricular zone (see Chapter 5). The presence of radial glial cells at the oSVZ was first hypothesized by the observation of the strong radial organization of this region that resembled the one present at the VZ in the developing cortex of cynomolgus monkeys (Smart et al. 2002). It was later shown by means of immunostainings and live imaging of cortical slices that the oSVZ contains indeed a vast number of progenitors, many of which possess radial fibers and express proteins typical of radial glia. Thus, a new type of radial glial cells with relevance for evolution has been identified, *the basal (or outer) radial glia* (Fietz et al. 2010; Hansen et al. 2010; Reillo et al. 2021) (Figure 1.2).

Basal radial glial cells differ from apical radial glia in many aspects. First, they differ in their morphology as they contain a basal fiber that ascends toward the pial surface, but does not contain an apical process anchored at the ventricular surface. Thus, basal radial glia neither have apico-basal epithelial features nor possess apically localized membrane components such as PAR3 and CD133 (Fietz et al. 2010). Another important difference is their cellular behavior during cell division. Although both cell types present nuclear movements prior to mitosis, the nucleus of apical radial glial cells undergoes interkinetic nuclear migration, as described in section 1.2 (Götz and Huttner 2005) (Figure 1.1A). On the other hand, the basal radial glia soma ascends a short distance along the basal radial process prior to cell division – a process known as mitotic somal translocation – and then divides within the oSVZ, that is, in basal positions (Hansen et al. 2010). Notably, other progenitor cell types in the SVZ, the multipolar basal progenitors or intermediate progenitors, do not undergo any nuclear movement prior to division. Thus, while almost all radial glia and non-radial glia in the VZ undergo nuclear movement prior to division (with only the subapical radial glia as an exception), most radial glia and non-radial glia in the SVZ undergo little to no movement prior to division.

Importantly, basal radial glia also express characteristic glial proteins, such as BLBP, GFAP, vimentin, and GLAST (Fietz et al. 2010; Nowakowski et al. 2017), even though there is some species variation (Reillo et al. 2011; Voigt 1989) – similar to the findings for apical progenitors. For example, in ferrets, neither apical nor basal radial glia express GFAP (Voigt, 1989), while this is present in both cell types in the developing human cortex. Basal and apical radial glial cells also share other hallmarks, like the expression of similar fate determinants involved in regulating self-renewal and neurogenesis, such as the transcription factors PAX6 and SOX2. However, they present differences in their gene expression, with basal radial glia expressing the transcription factor HOPX and a different integrin ITGB5 (Nowakowski et al. 2017) than the integrin ITGB1 expressed in apical radial glia (Haubst et al. 2006; Loulier et al. 2009).

Apart from the glial nature of these cells, basal radial glia also share their stem cell capacity with apical radial glia, as basal radial glial cells can self-renew and have a considerable proliferative potential (Betizeau et al. 2013; Hansen et al. 2010). Live imaging of GFP-labelled cells in human fetal cortical slices showed that the maintenance of the basal process was correlated to the maintenance of its proliferative capacity (Hansen et al. 2010), even though a greater heterogeneity in process retraction and division behavior was described later in nonhuman primate oSVZ cells (Betizeau et al. 2013). In addition to the original morphology described for basal radial glia (that is, those with a basal process composing 40 percent of all basal radial glia in the macaque mid-neurogenesis oSVZ), basal radial glia can also have a bipolar morphology with an apical process extending towards the apical side although not reaching the ventricular surface. These bipolar radial glia compose 50 percent of the basal radial glial cells in the oSVZ (Figure 1.2). Surprisingly, there were also a few (10%) basal radial glia with a short apical process but lacking a basal process (Betizeau et al. 2013) (Figure 1.2). Importantly, those with no basal process could generate some with a basal process, showing a high degree of dynamic change and demonstrating that these morphologies are not stable and may hence not be useful for identifying subtypes. Accordingly, some basal radial glia have been observed to alternate between the presence or absence of an apical or basal process with a stage of no processes, which were referred to as transient basal radial glia (tbRG) cells (Figure 1.2). All these different types of radial glia have their soma within the oSVZ, where they divide, and have been seen to undergo numerous successive rounds of proliferative divisions (Betizeau et al. 2013), that is, they are likely self-renewing and hence fulfilling one of the neural stem cell criterion. Indeed, the self-renewal of basal radial glia was also highlighted by the demonstration of a limited period of seeding cells into the oSVZ that then proliferate and expand independently from the VZ (Martínez-Martínez et al. 2016). This also allows an expansion of the SVZ independently and beyond the limited expansion of the VZ, a key process for brain folding.

And what about the cell types they generate, that is, their progeny? Are basal radial glia multipotent? Notably, the oSVZ forms at later stages and hence basal radial glial cells also appear later. For example, in the human cortex apical radial glial cells appear around gestational week 7 (GW7) and basal radial glia start appearing around gestational week 17 (GW17) (Nowakowski et al. 2017).

At this time, neurogenesis is still well under way, especially as upper layer neurons have become more numerous and are hence generated at later stages during the protracted neurogenesis. Indeed, the first observation of the oSVZ has been correlated to the generation of upper layer neurons in the primate visual cortex (Smart et al. 2002) corroborating earlier thymidine-labeling studies indicating that the proliferation of cells within the oSVZ coincides with a major wave of cortical neurogenesis (Rakic 1974). These indirect suggestions of the neurogenic nature of progenitors present in the oSVZ were then proven by the direct visualization of neurons arising from the basal neuroepithelium in mouse (Haubensak et al. 2004) and primate cortical slices (Hansen et al. 2010). Thus, basal radial glial cells generate neurons and their expansion in phylogeny is correlated to the expansion of the upper cortex layers, such as in the visual cortex. However, basal radial glia contribute both to the generation of neurons as well as glial cells. In the ferret cortex, early DiI-labelling studies have shown basal radial glial cells transiting to astroglial cells (Voigt 1989). Recent viral vector labeling showed that oSVZ cells generate predominantly future white matter astrocytes, while the VZ radial glia gives rise to migratory astrocyte progenitors that enter the cortical plate generating gray matter astrocytes (Allen et al. 2022). It is, however, still unknown if a single basal radial glial cell would generate first neurons and then astrocytes as shown for the apical radial glial cells (Gao et al. 2014), and hence would be multipotent.

As mentioned above, basal radial glial cells contribute to generate enlarged neuron numbers of the upper cortex layers by increasing the number of stem cells actively generating progeny at a given time allowing an increase in the neocortex size. In addition, basal radial glial cells have been implicated in regulating cortex folding and are particularly frequent in brains with a high gyrification index (see Chapter 5). One of their key roles in folding is to provide a fanning out radial glia scaffold for migrating neurons in a folded cortex (Borrell and Reillo 2012). In lower numbers, however, basal radial glial cells have also been observed in species with a smooth cortex, a lissencephalic cortex, such as the rodents' (Shitamukai et al. 2011), where they represent less than 5 percent of the progenitors that reside outside the VZ (Martínez-Cerdeño et al. 2012; Shitamukai et al. 2011). Moreover, a large oSVZ containing abundant basal radial glial cells is also found in the marmoset, a lissencephalic primate (Kelava et al. 2012). These observations imply that basal radial glial cells are regulated in number and contribute to, but may not be sufficient for, the formation of a large cortex with high gyrification.

A key aspect of gyrification is the uncoupling of the oSVZ from the inner proliferation zones, the iSVZ and VZ. This is crucial, as only the outer part amplifies and folds, while the apical surface remains smooth. This process of separation can be followed by tracing from the outer and inner brain surfaces using the lipophilic dye DiI. By applying DiI to the surface of the developing human brain at the beginning of neurogenesis, radial glial cells spanning the whole apical-basal thickness are labeled, just as in the mouse (Malatesta et al. 2003; Nowakowski et al. 2016). At later stages, however, basal radial glial cells without apical anchoring are observed starting from mid-neurogenic period. At this time, the application of DiI on the ventricular surface of the developing human brain labeled the truncated radial glia (Nowakowski et al. 2016) described earlier. Thus, at around mid-neurogenesis in the human cortex, the radial glia scaffold is interrupted from a physically continuous to a physically discontinuous structure. This change correlates with the change of proliferative activity from the ventricular to subventricular regions in the developing human brain at mid-neurogenesis (Nowakowski et al. 2016), and allows a separate and disproportional expansion of the outer layers and hence folding of the basal brain surface with a smooth apical surface. Thus, radial glia heterogeneity contributes to enlarging and folding brains. Generally, radial glia diversity increases in species with larger and increasingly folded cortices.

1.5 Radial Glial Cells in Phylogeny

We started out by stating how difficult it is to define neural stem cells and glial cells. One reason being that the definition of glial cells comprises all non-neuronal cells. With the more operational definition discussed in this chapter in mind, how early in phylogeny do radial glial cells appear? So far, radial glial cells have been found in other deuterostomes phyla, such as Hemichordata and Echinodermata, and evidence for their presence in protostomes such as in Annelida and Priapulida is starting to emerge (Helm et al. 2017) (Figure 1.3). These observations would suggest an early origin of radial glia in ontogeny as well as phylogeny. Radially arranged cells transversing the entire epidermis from the basal lamina to the apical surface are found in the nervous system of the annelid *O. fusiformis* (Helm et al. 2017). These cells are positive for SCO-spondin – an extracellular glycoprotein shown to be expressed and secreted by the radial glia of deuterostomes (Gobron et al. 2000; Mashanov et al. 2010). They also possess intermediate filaments and are located next to neuronal cells consistent with a support function. Moreover, they have endfeet terminating at the basal lamina and microvilli and cilia present at the apical site. Likewise, radially aligned SCO-spondin expressing cells that span the thickness of the intraepidermal nerve cordon and the adjacent epidermis were found in the priapulid *P. caudatus* (Helm et al. 2017). The function and nature of these radial-glia-like cells remain to be determined. In Echinodermata radial glia have been more studied. The two major components of the nervous system – a nerve ring around the mouth and radial nerve cords that run along each body axis of the animal (Figure 1.3) – have a neuroepithelial organization. This is formed by glial cells spanning the entire height of the neuroepithelium with a clear apico-basal polarity, their cell bodies in the apical region, the presence of a cilium on the apical surface and a long basal process stretching to the basal surface (Mashanov and Zueva 2019) (Figure 1.3A). Moreover, these cells also contain intermediate filaments and express

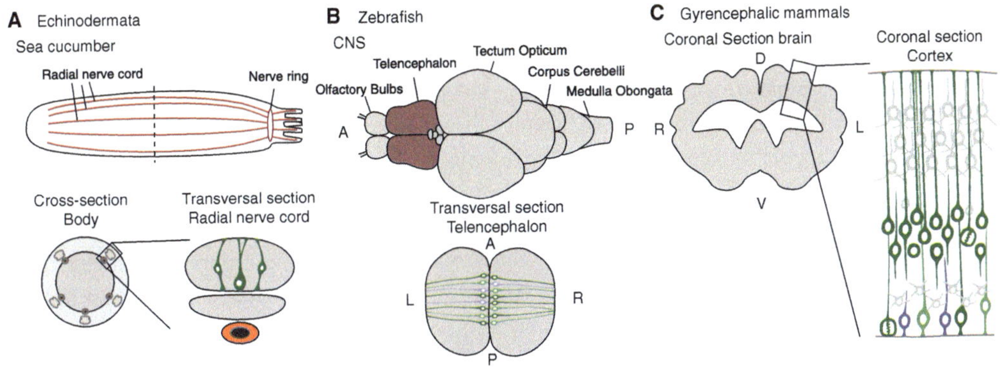

Figure 1.3 Radial glia throughout out the animal kingdom. (A) Diagram representing the general anatomy of the echinoderm nervous system. A sea cucumber is shown as an example. Each body axis is supplied with a radial nerve cord. Around the mouth, the radial nerve cords are joined together by the nerve ring. A cross-section diagram of the sea cucumber body shows their radial distribution. Within the radial nerve cord, radial glial cells illustrated in green can be found (Adapted from Mashanov and Zueva 2019). (B) Schematic representation of the adult zebrafish brain seen from dorsal. The telencephalon – the region that corresponds to the cerebral cortex – is colored dark red. A transversal section from this region is illustrated below, where radial glial cells are illustrated in different shades of green, highlighting the heterogeneity discussed in the text. (C) Schematic representation of a coronal section of a gyrencephalic developing neocortex such as in the human. Radial glial cells are illustrated in green. Note the diversity in morphology and position that these can manifest in compared to the other cases presented. CNS: central nervous system.

SCO-spondin. Interestingly, while a vast diversity of glial cells is found in chordates, radial glia is the only type of glia identified so far in Echinodermata (Mashanov and Zueva 2019). But not only are these a unique type of glia, they are also the most abundant cell type of their nervous system: in Echinodermata radial glial cells constitute between 45 and 70 percent of the total cell mass of its nervous tissue (Mashanov et al. 2010).

Importantly, like in vertebrates, these cells are responsible for both homeostatic and post-traumatic neurogenesis, and also play important roles in phagocytosis and acting as scaffolds (Mashanov and Zueva 2019). Echinodermata contain a high regenerative potential of neural tissue that has caught the attention of many researchers. Neural regeneration has been mostly studied by the complete transection of one of the five radial nerve cords present in the body of sea cucumbers as an experimental model. Within only a few weeks of the injury the connectivity of the lesioned radial nerve cord is fully restored, and its organization is indistinguishable from an undamaged region. Interestingly, it has been observed that shortly after injury, the radial glia surrounding the wound drastically change by undergoing dedifferentiation, losing their long basal process and showing high proliferative capacity in order to restore the damaged tissue. This role is reminiscent of the restorative capacity that radial glial cells have in the adult zebrafish, where they can be activated from a quiescent stage and continue to generate neurons in adult neurogenesis in the telencephalon (Alunni and Bally-Cuif 2016). In zebrafish, apically located radial glial cells appear in the telencephalon during developmental neurogenesis and remain present into adulthood, where they continue to generate new neurons in this region (Jurisch-Yaksi et al. 2020) (Figure 1.3). Apical radial glial cells thus also self-renew and generate neurons in zebrafish switching from quiescence to activation in the adult stages regulated by Notch signaling (Than-Trong et al. 2018). Live in vivo imaging of these radial glial cells in the adult dorsal telencephalon, that is, the region corresponding to the cerebral cortex, identified a novel mode of neurogenesis from these cells, namely the direct conversion to new neurons without undergoing cell division (Barbosa et al. 2015). This highlights the heterogeneity of radial glial cells at the ventricle in regard to their quiescence, self-renewal, and neurogenesis mode.

The persistence of radial glial cells into adulthood appears to be correlated to smaller brains that allow the radial processes to traverse through the entire brain thickness. Indeed, in thick brain regions, radial glial cells disappear and astrocytes emerge in adulthood covering the entire brain parenchyma and supporting synaptic and other functions of neurons supposedly better than thin processes stretching over centimeters. Indeed, even in the human brain, radial glial cells are maintained in thin epithelial-like structures (Götz 2013b). This may imply that loss of restorative neurogenesis is a byproduct of losing radial glial cells in adult brains that enlarge and need cells dispersed in the parenchyma for their support. Indeed, wherever radial glial cells are maintained into adulthood, neurogenesis continues or can be activated for repair.

Also in zebrafish, radial glial cells are heterogeneous with some in quiescent state and others activated. Radial glial cells are accompanied in the adult VZ of the zebrafish by other, non-glial stem and progenitor cells lining the ventricle (Figure 1.3B). However, so far only the earliest stem cell types, namely neuroepithelial cells and apical radial glia have been detected in the zebrafish dorsal telencephalon, thus showing a much lower degree of heterogeneity compared to the mammalian lineage. Interestingly, neuroepithelial cells were found to be particularly frequent, outnumbering the apical radial glial cells, in a species under pressure to generate neurons fast, namely the short-lived killifish (*Nothobranchius furzeri*). As these have a short lifespan they generate a mature brain in 5 weeks rather than 3 months as is the case for zebrafish (Coolen et al. 2020). Interestingly, it is a *non-glia radial neural stem cell* resembling a neuroepithelial cell, that mostly contributes to the faster neurogenesis. These cells lack S100b or GS, divide faster and express the proneural gene Neurog1 rather than Ascl1, which is expressed in the radial glial cells (Coolen et al. 2020). Thus, to speed up neurogenesis in teleosts apical progenitor heterogeneity seems to be employed. This is in contrast to the mammalian lineages where radial glia diversified and basal radial glial cells arise as principal contributors to the larger and gyrified dorsal telencephalon/ cerebral cortex development (Figure 1.3C).

Taken together, the enormous diversity of brains arising in phylogeny is generated by increasing stem and progenitor diversity during ontogeny. Within the vertebrate lineage, particularly the radial glial cells diversified into apical, subapical, truncated, and basal, radial glial cells amplify neuronal subtype generation and change the brain morphology allowing its expansion. Yet, we have explored so far only a small number of species, and still know little about the molecular characteristics corresponding (or not) to the morphological differences. Thus, exploring differences and similarities in gene expression of diverse radial glial cells and exploring them in the rich diversity of species developing very different brains, will help us understand further how ontogeny shapes the phylogeny of brains.

References

Alexandre, P. et al. (2010). Neurons derive from the more apical daughter in asymmetric divisions in the zebrafish neural tube. *Nat Neurosci* 13 (6): 673–679. doi: 10.1038/nn.2547.

Allen, D.E. et al. (2022). Fate mapping of neural stem cell niches reveals distinct origins of human cortical astrocytes. *Science* 376 (6600): 1441–1446. doi: 10.1126/science.abm5224.

Allen, N.J. and Lyons, D.A. (2018). Glia as architects of central nervous system formation and function. *Science* 362 (6411): 181–185. doi: 10.1126/science.aat0473.

Alunni, A. and Bally-Cuif, L. (2016). A comparative view of regenerative neurogenesis in vertebrates. *Dev* 143 (5): 741–753. doi: 10.1242/dev.122796.

Anthony, T.E. et al. (2004). Radial glia serve as neuronal progenitors in all regions of the central nervous system. *Neuron* 41: 881–890.

Barbosa, J.S. et al. (2015). Live imaging of adult neural stem cell behavior in the intact and injured zebrafish brain. *Science* 348 (6236): 789–793. doi: 10.1126/science.aaa2729.

Basak, O. et al. (2018). Troy+ brain stem cells cycle through quiescence and regulate their number by sensing niche occupancy. *Proc Natl Acad Sci USA* 115 (4): E610–E619. doi: 10.1073/pnas.1715911114.

Betizeau, M. et al. (2013). Precursor diversity and complexity of lineage relationships in the outer subventricular zone of the primate. *Neuron* 80 (2): 442–457. doi: 10.1016/j.neuron.2013.09.032.

Bilgic, M. et al. (2022). Single cell transcriptomics of ferrets reveal a common temporal pattern of progenitors in brain development of gyrencephalic mammals. *BioRxiv*. doi: 10.1101/2022.05.05.490846.

Borrell, V. and Reillo, I. (2012). Emerging roles of neural stem cells in cerebral cortex development and evolution. *Dev Neurobiol* 72 (7): 955–971. doi: 10.1002/dneu.22013.

Bottes, S. et al. (2021). Long-term self-renewing stem cells in the adult mouse hippocampus identified by intravital imaging. *Nat Neurosci* 24 (2): 225–233. doi: 10.1038/s41593-020-00759-4.

Camargo Ortega, G. et al. (2019). The centrosome protein AKNA regulates neurogenesis via microtubule organization. *Nature* 567 (7746): 113–117. doi: 10.1038/s41586-019-0962-4.

Coolen, M. et al. (2020). Mosaic heterochrony in neural progenitors sustains accelerated brain growth and neurogenesis in the Juvenile Killifish N. furzeri. *Curr Biol* 30 (4): 736–745.e4. doi: 10.1016/j.cub.2019.12.046.

Denoth-Lippuner, A. and Jessberger, S. (2021). Formation and integration of new neurons in the adult hippocampus. *Nat Rev Neurosci* 22 (4): 223–236. doi: 10.1038/s41583-021-00433-z.

Esgleas, M. et al. (2020). Trnp1 organizes diverse nuclear membrane-less compartments in neural stem cells. *EMBO J* 39 (16): e103373. doi: 10.15252/embj.2019103373.

Falk, S. et al. (2017). Time-specific effects of spindle positioning on embryonic progenitor pool composition and adult neural stem cell seeding. *Neuron* 93 (4): 777–791.e3. doi: 10.1016/j.neuron.2017.02.009.

Fietz, S.A. et al. (2010). OSVZ progenitors of human and ferret neocortex are epithelial-like and expand by integrin signaling. *Nat Neurosci* 13 (6): 690–699. doi: 10.1038/nn.2553.

Fujita, I. et al. (2020). Endfoot regeneration restricts radial glial state and prevents translocation into the outer subventricular zone in early mammalian brain development. *Nat Cell Biol* 22 (1): 26–37. doi: 10.1038/s41556-019-0436-9.

Fujita, S. (1963 February). The matrix cell and cytogenesis in the developing central nervous system. *J Comp Neurol* 120: 37–42. doi: 10.1002/cne.901200104.

Gaillard, A. et al. (2003). Early (E12) cortical progenitors can change their fate upon heterotopic transplantation. *Eur J Neurosci* 17 (7): 1375–1383. doi: 10.1046/j.1460-9568.2003.02576.x.

Gal, J.S. et al. (2006). Molecular and morphological heterogeneity of neural precursors in the mouse neocortical proliferative zones. *J Neurosci* 26 (3): 1045–1056. doi: 10.1523/JNEUROSCI.4499-05.2006.

Gao, P. et al. (2014). Deterministic progenitor behavior and unitary production of neurons in the neocortex. *Cell* 159 (4): 775–788. doi: 10.1016/j.cell.2014.10.027.

Gobron, S. et al. (2000). Subcommissural organ/Reissner's fiber complex. *GLIA* 32 (2): 177–191. doi: 10.1002/1098-1136(200011)32:2<177::AID-GLIA70>3.0.CO;2-V.

Götz, M. (2013a). Biology and function of glial cells. In: *Neurosciences – from Molecule to Behavior: A University Textbook* (ed. C.G. Galizia and P-M. Lledo), 163–177. Berlin Heidelberg: Springer. doi: 10.1007/978-3-642-10769-6_9.

Götz, M. (2013b). Radial glial cells. In: *Neuroglia*, 3e (ed. H. Kettenmann and B.R. Ransom), 50–61. New York: Oxford Univ. Press. doi: 10.1093/med/9780199794591.003.0005.

Götz, M. and Huttner, W.B. (2005). The cell biology of neurogenesis. *Nat Rev Mol Cell Biol* 6 (10): 777–788. doi: 10.1038/nrm1739.

Götz, M. et al. (2015). Reactive astrocytes as neural stem or progenitor cells. *GLIA* 63 (8): 1452–1468. doi: 10.1002/glia.22850.

Götz, M. et al. (1998). Pax6 controls radial glia differentiation in the cerebral cortex. *Neuron* 21: 1031–1044.

Hansen, D.V. et al. (2010). Neurogenic radial glia in the outer subventricular zone of human neocortex. *Nature* 464 (7288): 554–561. doi: 10.1038/nature08845.

Hartfuss, E. et al. (2003). Reelin signaling directly affects radial glia morphology and biochemical maturation. *Development* 130 (19): 4597–4609. doi: 10.1242/dev.00654.

Hartfuss, E. et al. (2001). Characterization of CNS precursor subtypes and radial glia. *Dev Biol* 229 (1): 15–30. doi: 10.1006/dbio.2000.9962.

Haubensak, W. et al. (2004). Neurons arise in the basal neuroepithelium of the early mammalian telencephalon. *PNAS* 101 (9): 3196–3201. doi: 10.1073/pnas.0308600100.

Haubst, N. et al. (2006). Basement membrane attachment is dispensable for radial glial cell fate and for proliferation, but affects positioning of neuronal subtypes. *Development* 133 (16): 3245–3254. doi: 10.1242/dev.02486.

Helm, C. et al. (2017). Early evolution of radial glial cells in Bilateria. *Proc Royal Soc B: Biol Sci* 284 (1859): 20170743. doi: 10.1098/rspb.2017.0743.

His, W. (1889). Die Neuroblasten und deren Entstehung im embryonalen Mark. *Abh Kgl sachs Ges Wissensch math phys Kl* 15: 311–372.

Jurisch-Yaksi, N. et al. (2020). Radial glia in the zebrafish brain. *GLIA* 68 (12): 2451–2470. doi: 10.1002/glia.23849.

Kelava, I. et al. (2012). Abundant occurrence of basal radial glia in the subventricular zone of embryonic neocortex of a lissencephalic primate, the common marmoset callithrix jacchus. *Cereb Cortex* 22 (2): 469–481. doi: 10.1093/cercor/bhr301.

Kosodo, Y. et al. (2008). Cytokinesis of neuroepithelial cells can divide their basal process before anaphase. *EMBO J* 27 (23): 3151–3163. doi: 10.1038/emboj.2008.227.

Levitt, P. and Rakic, P. (1980). Immunoperoxidase localization of glial fibrillary acidic protein in radial glial cells and astrocytes of the developing rhesus monkey brain. *J Comp Neurol* 193 (3): 815–840. doi: 10.1002/cne.901930316.

Loulier, K. et al. (2009). β1 integrin maintains integrity of the embryonic neocortical stem cell niche. *PLoS Biol* 7 (8): e1000176. doi: 10.1371/journal.pbio.1000176.

Malatesta, P. et al. (2003). Neuronal or glial progeny. *Neuron* 37: 751–764. doi: 10.1016/S0896-6273(03)00116-8.

Malatesta, P. (2000). Isolation of radial glial cells by fluorescent-activated cell sorting reveals aneuronal lineage. *Development* 127: 5253–5263.

Malik, S. et al. (2013). Neurogenesis continues in the third trimester of pregnancy and is suppressed by premature birth. *J Neurosci* 33 (2): 411–423. doi: 10.1523/JNEUROSCI.4445-12.2013.

Martínez-Cerdeño, V. et al. (2012). Comparative analysis of the subventricular zone in rat, ferret and macaque. *PLoS ONE* 7 (1): e30178. doi: 10.1371/journal.pone.0030178.

Martínez-Martínez, M.Á. et al. (2016). A restricted period for formation of outer subventricular zone defined by Cdh1 and Trnp1 levels. *Nat Commun* 7: 11812. doi: 10.1038/ncomms11812.

Mashanov, V. and Zueva, O. (2019). Radial glia in echinoderms. *Dev Neurobiol* 79 (5): 396–405. doi: 10.1002/dneu.22659.

Mashanov, V.S. et al. (2010). Organization of glial cells in the adult sea cucumber central nervous system. *GLIA* 58 (13): 1581–1593. doi: 10.1002/glia.21031.

Miyata, T. et al. (2001). Asymmetric inheritance of radial glial fibers by cortical neurons a more complete understanding of three-dimensional brain formation, however, cytogenesis by progenitor cells must be studied in the context of their in vivo. *Neuron* 31: 727–741. doi: 10.1016/S0896-6273(01)00420-2.

Noctor, S. et al. (2001). Neurons derived from radial glial cells establish radial units in neocortex. *Nature* 409: 714–420.

Nowakowski, T.J. et al. (2017). Spatiotemporal gene expression trajectories reveal developmental hierarchies of the human cortex. *Science* 358 (6368): 1318–1323. doi: 10.1126/science.aap8809.

Nowakowski, T.J. et al. (2016). Transformation of the radial glia scaffold demarcates two stages of human cerebral cortex development. *Neuron* 91 (6): 1219–1227. doi: 10.1016/j.neuron.2016.09.005.

Peters, A. and Feldman, M. (1973). The cortical plate and molecular layer of the late rat fetus*. *Zeitschrift für Anatomie und Entwicklungsgeschichte* 141 (1): 3–37.

Pilz, G.A. et al. (2013). Amplification of progenitors in the mammalian telencephalon includes a new radial glial cell type. *Nat Commun* 4: 2125. doi: 10.1038/ncomms3125.

Pinto, L. et al. (2008). Prospective isolation of functionally distinct radial glial subtypes-lineage and transcriptome analysis. *Mol Cell Neurosci* 38 (1): 15–42. doi: 10.1016/j.mcn.2008.01.012.

Rakic, P. (1971a). Guidance of neurons migrating to the fetal monkey neocortex. *Brain Res* 33 (2): 471–476.

Rakic, P. (1971b). Neuron-glia relationship during granule cell migration in developing cerebellar cortex. A Golgi and electronmicroscopic study in Macacus Rhesus. *J Comp Neurol* 141 (3): 283–312. doi: 10.1002/cne.901410303.

Rakic, P. (1974). Neurons in rhesus monkey visual cortex. *Science* 183 (4123): 425–427. doi: 10.1126/science.183.4123.425.

Reillo, I. et al. (2011). A role for intermediate radial glia in the tangential expansion of the mammalian cerebral cortex. *Cereb Cortex* 21 (7): 1674–1694. doi: 10.1093/cercor/bhq238.

Shitamukai, A. (2011). Oblique radial glial divisions in the developing mouse neocortex induce self-renewing progenitors outside the germinal zone that resemble primate outer subventricular zone progenitors. *J Neurosci* 31 (10): 3683–3695. doi: 10.1523/JNEUROSCI.4773-10.2011.

Smart, I.H.M. et al. (2002). Unique morphological features of the proliferative zones and postmitotic compartments of the neural epithelium giving rise to striate and extrastriate cortex in the monkey. *Cereb Cortex* 12 (1): 37–53.

Stahl, R. et al. (2013). Trnp1 regulates expansion and folding of the mammalian cerebral cortex by control of radial glial fate. *Cell* 153 (3): 535–549. doi: 10.1016/j.cell.2013.03.027.

Stancik, E.K. et al. (2010). Heterogeneity in ventricular zone neural precursors contributes to neuronal fate diversity in the postnatal neocortex. *J Neurosci* 30 (20): 7028–7036. doi: 10.1523/JNEUROSCI.6131-09.2010.

Than-Trong, E. et al. (2018). Neural stem cell quiescence and stemness are molecularly distinct outputs of the Notch3 signalling cascade in the vertebrate adult brain. *Development* 145 (10): dev161034. doi: 10.1242/dev.161034.

Tsunekawa, Y. et al. (2012). Cyclin D2 in the basal process of neural progenitors is linked to non-equivalent cell fates. *EMBO J* 31 (8): 1879–1892. doi: 10.1038/emboj.2012.43.

Voigt, T. (1989). Development of glial cells in the cerebral wall of ferrets. *J Comp Neurol* 289 (1): 74–88. doi: 10.1002/cne.902890106.

2

Diversity and Evolution of Human Cortical Progenitor Cell Types

Alex A. Pollen[1,2] *and Arnold R. Kriegstein*[1,2]

[1] *Eli and Edythe Broad Center for Regeneration Medicine and Stem Cell Research, University of California, San Francisco, CA, USA*
[2] *Department of Neurology, University of California, San Francisco, CA, USA*

2.1 Progenitor Cell Diversity

The developmental and evolutionary expansion of the human cortex involves diverse progenitor cell types that exhibit distinct proliferative properties, dynamic behaviors, and gene expression patterns. The neural stem and progenitor cells that produce cortical neurons and glia originate in early development from the cells that line the cerebral ventricles. Rudolf Virchow is credited with the first description in 1846 of multicellular nervous tissue support cells lining the ventricles which he referred to as neuroglia (for review see Chvátal and Verkhratsky 2018). These cells are now known as neuroepithelial cells. Wilhelm His suggested that the cell lining the ventricles could be separated into distinct progenitor cell types responsible for producing either neurons or glia; neurons were produced by neuroblasts and astroglial cells by spongioblasts, cells we now call radial glia (RG) (His 1889). Kolliker and Magini used the Golgi method to define the morphology of neuroepithelial cells including their possession of long radial fibers extending into the cortical mantle (Kölliker 1867; Magini 1888). Ramon y Cajal, agreeing with the conclusions of His, considered neuroepithelial cells distinct from neural progenitor cells that he identified as the mitotic cells dividing along the ventricular surface (Cajal 1909). However, in 1897 Schaper suggested that there was only one population of neuroblasts (Schaper 1897). When Sauer described interkinetic nuclear migration (INM) of neuroepithelial cells, it became clear that the mitotic figures lining the ventricle were neuroepithelial cells at a different phase of the cell cycle from the cells with their cell bodies away from the ventricle (Sauer 1935), but this insight did not change the concept that neurons and glia derived from distinct progenitor populations, which remained the accepted dogma for over a century.

A series of studies published in the first years of the twenty-first century demonstrated that RG, thought at the time to be glial lineage restricted cells, were actually neural progenitor cells (Malatesta et al. 2000; Miyata et al. 2001; Noctor et al. 2001). RG were shown to produce neurons in vitro (Malatesta et al. 2000) and in situ (Noctor et al. 2001). Shortly thereafter, the diversity of neural progenitor cells grew with the identification of an intermediate or basal progenitor cell type derived from the ventricular RG (vRG) coupled with the realization that these cells constitute a distinct progenitor region, the subventricular zone (Haubensak et al. 2004; Miyata et al. 2004; Noctor et al. 2004). More recently, a distinct progenitor cell type related to vRG was identified in

Neocortical Neurogenesis in Development and Evolution, First Edition. Edited by Wieland B. Huttner.

the expanded outer subventricular zone (OSVZ) of developing human cortex, the outer RG (oRG) (Hansen et al. 2010) and also described in the OSVZ of the developing ferret cortex (Fietz et al. 2012; Reillo et al. 2011) and marmoset (Kelava et al. 2012). Interestingly, the dynamic mitotic behavior of each of these progenitor cell types is distinct (Figure 2.1A). At a time when single cell genomics is providing a molecular-level definition of cell type that promises to subcluster progenitor cells into subtypes with ever more subtle defining features, it is worthwhile briefly considering

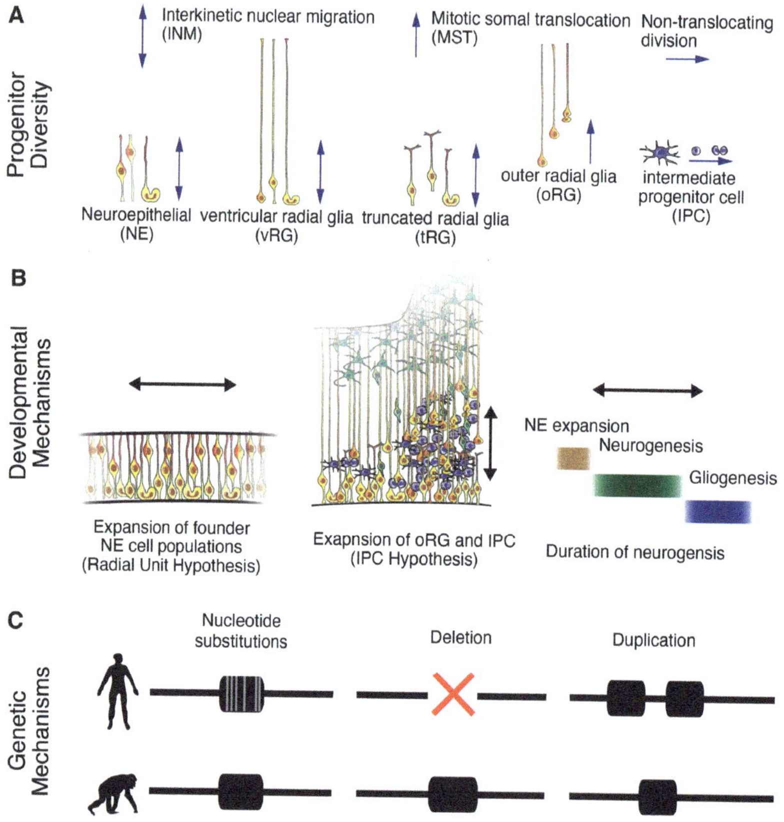

Figure 2.1 Progenitor diversity and cortical evolution. (A) Cartoons depict morphologies and cell division behaviors for major classes of cortical progenitors. Neuroepithelial (NE) cells, ventricular radial glia (vRG), and truncated radial glia (tRG) undergo interkinetic nuclear migration (INM) while intermediate progenitor cells (IPCs) do not translocate, but round up to divide, even when dividing at the ventricular surface. Outer radial glia (oRG) cells undergo mitotic somal translocation (MST). (B) Cartoons depict possible developmental mechanisms contributing to the evolutionary expansion of the cortex. Left: Increased proliferation of NE cells could expand the number of founder vRG contributing to tangential expansion of the cortex, while preserving the organization of cortical layers. Middle: Expansion of IPC and oRG populations could contribute to tangential and radial expansion of the cortex and disproportionate expansion of upper cortical layers. Right: An increased duration of neurogenesis could increase the number of neurons produced. (C) Human-specific genetic changes can modify or create functional elements through a number of mutational mechanisms, including nucleotide substitutions and structural changes, such as deletions, duplications, and inversions (not shown). Recent studies have explored accelerated rates of nucleotide substitutions in conserved noncoding sequences (left) and complete deletion of noncoding sequences (middle) as mechanisms of gene regulatory change, and coding gene duplication as a mechanism for creating entirely new genes. Future studies systematically connecting genetic changes to quantitative changes in developmental cell behavior will help to provide an integrative view of the origins of human cortical expansion.

the mitotic behaviors that help distinguish broad categories of neural progenitor cells and consider how they might contribute to distinct roles in cortical development.

2.1.1 Neuroepithelial Cells

Neuroepithelial (NE) cells constitute the founder population that will ultimately produce all the neurons and glia of the adult brain. Early in the first trimester of human development the neural plate closes to form the neural tube. At this stage the forebrain NE cells that line the lumen extend from the apical side at the ventricular surface to the basal lamina. NE cells are highly polarized along the apical–basal axis and are bound to each other at their apical end by tight junctions and adherens junctions (Aaku-Saraste et al. 1996; Stocker and Chenn 2015). NE cells undergo symmetric proliferative divisions to increase their number and expand to form the lateral telencephalic vesicles that will become the two cerebral hemispheres. As first noted by Sauer, NE cells undergo interkinetic nuclear migration (INM) as they progress through the cell cycle (Sauer 1935). DNA replication occurs during S-phase when the nuclei are located at the basal (pial) surface. The cell nuclei move to the apical surface during G2-phase and undergo mitosis during M-phase, which occurs at the ventricular surface. The nuclei then move basally and re-enter S-phase. Because NE cells are the predominant cell type within the ventricular zone, the process of INM creates a pseudostratification of the proliferative zone with nuclear position, size, and shape stratified according to cell-cycle phase. While NE cells span the apical–basal extent of the ventricular zone through interphase, time-lapse imaging of human NE cells in primary tissue and early-stage cerebral organoids demonstrates that basal fibers retract during M-phase accompanied by cell soma swelling, and that following cytokinesis the newly generated daughter cells extend new basal processes to the pia (Subramanian et al. 2017). These observations are consistent with chick and pig neural tubes described by Sauer, but it has been suggested that basal fiber splitting rather than retraction may occur in some NE cell mitoses in mouse, chicken, and zebrafish brains (Kosodo et al. 2008) however, this has not been observed in human NE cells (Subramanian et al. 2017).

At stages when the NE founder population undergoes mostly symmetric divisions to expand their numbers, NE cells present a relatively uniform appearance. However, they already demonstrate areal distinctions in terms of transcription factor expression (Bhaduri et al. 2021; La Manno et al. 2021). At slightly later stages in the second trimester, despite the lack of morphological or behavioral differences in the apical progenitors along the mediolateral or anterior-posterior axes, sharp regional boundaries can be observed when examining the expression of DNA enhancer regulatory elements (Visel et al. 2013). The discrete expression patterns of forebrain enhancers and nearby genes indicate a molecular heterogeneity of neural precursor cells within the ventricular proliferative zone and supports the concept of a protomap of cortical arealization present within this progenitor population (Rakic 1988).

2.1.2 Ventricular Radial Glia Cells

When cortical neurogenesis begins at the end of the first trimester, NE cells transform into vRG cells (Eze et al. 2021; Götz and Huttner 2005; Howard et al. 2008; Silbereis et al. 2016; Subramanian et al. 2017; Taverna et al. 2014) and express characteristics of glial cells, including the expression of specific intermediate filaments, cytoplasmic glycogen granules (Brückner and Biesold 1981; Choi and Lapham 1978; Kriegstein and Götz 2003). This transition is also accompanied by changes in the tight junctions that bind NE cells together. Occludin, a tight junction protein, is downregulated and tight junctions are lost so that unlike other epithelia, the apical junctions of vRG are composed of adherens junctions only (Aaku-Saraste et al. 1996). The junctional complexes that connect NE and vRG cells to each other are critical to maintain apicobasal polarity of the neuroepithelium and to maintain proper neural production and migration. Furthermore, mutations in junctional-related genes are causative for a range of cortical malformations (Lian and Sheen 2015; Veeraval et al. 2020).

vRG undergo INM, as NE cells do, but the mitotic behavior of RG differs from that of NE in that contact with the basal lamina is maintained throughout the cell cycle (Subramanian et al. 2017). The cortical anlage undergoes rapid radial expansion with the appearance of new stratified regions including the subventricular zone, intermediate zone, subplate, and cortical plate. The basal fibers of vRG contact the basal lamina, as do the basal fibers of NE cells, and they lengthen to maintain basal contact as the cortex expands radially. As vRG fibers lengthen, INM movements become confined to the cellular compartment spanning the ventricular zone. When the nucleus moves to the apical side and enters M-phase, cell cytoplasm streams toward the nucleus, thinning the basal process and swelling the cell soma. However, the basal processes do not retract during M-phase as they do in NE cells. Anchoring of the basal endfeet to the basal lamina is a prerequisite for establishing the RG scaffold and for the role of vRG in guiding cell migration.

NE cells and vRG are anchored by their apical endfeet to the ventricular surface where they can receive diffusible signals from the cerebrospinal fluid (CSF). CSF can signal to NE and RG cells through their primary cilia (Fuchs and Schwark 2004; Kim et al. 2010; Liu et al. 2021). For example, bone morphogenic proteins (BMPs), WNTs, FGFs, and IGF are present in the CSF with receptors expressed by RG (Dono et al. 1998; Fukumitsu et al. 2006; Lehtinen et al. 2011; Vaccarino et al. 1999). Activation or inhibition of each of these signaling pathways has been shown to influence proliferation of RG cells through a variety of downstream regulators including β-catenin, SMADs, YAP, and Notch (Draganova et al. 2015; Hatakeyama et al. 2014; Kawaguchi 2020; Li et al. 1998; Mabie et al. 1999; Zhang et al. 2010).

RG can divide symmetrically to increase their number, as do NE cells, but most often they undergo asymmetric division to self-renew and produce a daughter cell that can be a neuron, a process called direct neurogenesis, or an intermediate progenitor cell that then divides to produce neurons, a process referred to as indirect neurogenesis (Delaunay et al. 2017; Kowalczyk et al. 2009; Kriegstein et al. 2006; Uzquiano et al. 2018).

2.1.3 Intermediate Progenitor Cells

Intermediate progenitor cells (IPCs) have more limited potential than RG and most often divide terminally to produce a pair of neurons (Haubensak et al. 2004; Noctor et al. 2004). When either neurons or IPCs are first produced they migrate to the subventricular zone (SVZ) and are multipolar. However, neurons will become bipolar and begin migrating after a day or so, often after extending a process to reach the ventricle, while IPCs remain multipolar until they retract their processes and divide (Kriegstein and Noctor 2004; Noctor et al. 2004; Ohshima et al. 2007; Sakakibara et al. 2014; Tabata and Nakajima 2003). The mitotic behavior of IPCs, rounding up prior to cytokinesis, is consistent with the notion that they are dividing symmetrically to produce daughter neurons that appear to be identical and that migrate to the same cortical layer (Noctor et al. 2004). A subset of neurogenic IPCs that divide at the apical surface are known as short neural precursors (SNPs) and may be distinguished by expression of the TUBA1A gene (Gal et al. 2006). It is likely that these IPCs are among the early generated IPCs that divide at the ventricular surface prior to establishment of a distinct SVZ (Noctor et al. 2004).

Intermediate progenitor cells and those neurons that are produced directly from RG are generated through a process of delamination from the apical junction belt that resembles the process of epithelial-mesenchymal transition (Itoh et al. 2013; Singh et al. 2016). Delamination is mediated, in part, by downregulation of cadherin and related adherens junction proteins present at RG apical endfeet (Kawaguchi 2020). Proneural gene expression in RG may initiate delamination through transcriptional repression of cadherins (Itoh et al. 2013; Pacary et al. 2012; Singh and Solecki 2015). Robo signaling has also been implicated in delamination through inhibition of cadherin-based adhesions at apical processes (Borrell et al. 2012). Additionally, cytoskeleton proteins such as the centrosome related protein AKNA, have been shown to destabilize the microtubule-actin-adherens junction complex to promote delamination (Camargo Ortega et al. 2019).

2.1.4 Outer Radial Glia Cells

Outer radial glia (ORG) cells are produced by vRGs that divide with horizontal or oblique divisions resulting in basal fiber inheritance by the oRG daughter cell (Gertz et al. 2014; LaMonica et al. 2013; Martínez-Martínez et al. 2016; Shitamukai et al. 2011). In subsequent divisions, oRG cells undergo mitotic somal translocation, which contributes to migration of oRG cells away from the ventricular surface and toward the OSVZ. The ventricular daughter cell that loses its basal fiber maintains contact with the apical surface and regrows a basal fiber, but the fiber does not extend all the way to the pia and instead often bends tangentially and usually ends in a blood vessel contact (Nowakowski et al. 2016). These cells remaining at the ventricular surface are termed truncated RG (tRG) and appear to be a distinct RG subtype characterized not only by their fiber length but also by a distinct molecular signature including enriched expression of marker genes such as the heat shock protein gene, CRYAB (Nowakowski et al. 2016).

oRG cells may also be generated by delamination from ventricular RG in a process that resembles the production of intermediate progenitor cells, namely through a process where the nascent oRG cell delaminates from the adhesion belt by apical constriction or abscission (Camargo Ortega et al. 2019; Kawaguchi 2020). For example, Lzts1 is a microtubule associated protein expressed in apical RG endfeet that inhibits cadherin, induces apical contraction, and promotes delamination of RG daughter cells (Kawaue et al. 2019)(Kawaue et al. 2019). Conversely, Trnp1 is a factor associated with self-renewal of RG whose down regulation has been associated with a shift toward horizontal cleavage plane angles and an increased production of oRG cells (Stahl et al. 2013).

There are multiple regulators of apical junction integrity, and it is now clear that disruption of many of them leads to delamination and the appearance of basally located progenitor cells in mouse models, but whether these experimental manipulations reflect physiological mechanisms of oRG production is less clear. For example, BAF155 is a subunit of the chromatin remodeling BAF complex. BAF155 appears to cooperate with PAX6 to regulate the expression of genes involved in adherens junction formation and cell–cell adhesion, and reduction of BAF155 has been associated with the production of oRG-like cells in the mouse (Narayanan et al. 2018). Similarly, loss of CDC42-related proteins localized at the apical surface disrupts apical junctions and leads to delamination of progenitor cells (Cappello et al. 2006; Georgiou et al. 2008). The adaptor protein inscuteable (INSC) regulates spindle orientation during mitosis as well as cell adhesion and promotes delamination of ventricular progenitor cells in the mouse (Culurgioni et al. 2011; Gloerich et al. 2017; Konno et al. 2008; Postiglione et al. 2011). Insulinoma-associated 1 (INSM1) is a zinc-finger transcription factor expressed by vRG. Increasing expression of INSM1 in vRG leads to aberrant delamination and production of oRG-like cells in the mouse due to destabilizing apical junctions (Tavano et al. 2018).

Unlike IPCs and/or transit amplifying cells, oRGs can be considered epithelial cells as many of them contact the basal lamina and maintain contact as they divide (Hansen et al. 2010). In addition to providing a RG scaffold, oRG contact with the basal lamina via the basal fibers has been proposed to maintain the stem-like properties of oRG cells through integrin signals they receive through their basal contacts (Fietz et al. 2010). Consistent with this concept, oRG cells express receptors for integrins and a variety of extracellular matrix proteins that could regulate growth factor signaling and self-renewal (Pollen et al. 2015).

oRG cells undergo a distinct mitotic behavior that differs from interkinetic nuclear migration of NE and vRG. After centrosome duplication, and as oRG cells enter G2 phase, the nucleus translocates along the basal fiber a distance of approximately 150 microns in one hour (Hansen et al. 2010; Ostrem et al. 2014) in a process known as mitotic somal translocation (MST). MST is dependent on nonmuscle myosin II and involves activation of the Rho effector, ROCK (Ostrem et al. 2014) and differs from INM, which is driven by microtubule motors (Taverna and Huttner 2010). The consequences for brain development of this mitotic "jump" is not clear, but it appears to contribute to a developmental radial expansion of the OSVZ (Ostrem et al. 2014).

2.1.5 Systematically Defining Progenitor Cell Diversity

Classical descriptions of progenitor identity can now be supplemented using systematic single cell genomics approaches. The cell and the genome represent fundamental units in biology. Until recently, measuring properties of genome activity, such as gene expression, required mixing large numbers of cells from heterogeneous tissue samples. However, advances in microfluidics that enable sequencing nucleic acids from individual cells dissociated from tissue now support unbiased definitions of cell types based on patterns of gene expression or chromatin accessibility (Pollen et al. 2014; Quake 2022; Shapiro et al. 2013). The application of these techniques to human cortical progenitors has helped to standardize existing definitions of cell types across studies, to reveal additional markers and signaling pathways that distinguish cell types, and to generate hypotheses about lineage relationships. Single cell approaches have further revealed transcriptional heterogeneity related to cortical area, age, and germinal zone position (Bhaduri et al. 2021; Delgado et al. 2022; Nowakowski et al. 2017; Polioudakis et al. 2019; Pollen et al. 2015), and are poised to address whether we have a complete view of progenitor cell diversity in human cortical development.

While broad classes of radial glia and intermediate progenitor cells have been identified molecularly through single cell RNA sequencing, it is likely that important genomic heterogeneity remains to be discovered. The recent identification of tRG cells suggests that additional cell types and states may still await definition. Transcriptional distinctions alone are not sufficient to define novel cell subtypes and could instead represent cell states or gradients of molecular features within a cell type. Classifying a transcriptional cluster as a distinct progenitor cell type further requires integrating features of morphology, behavior, and clonal output. For example, single cell RNA sequencing approaches resolved molecular markers distinguishing oRG from vRG cells and revealed a set of oRG markers related to extracellular matrix and growth factor signaling (Pollen et al. 2015; Thomsen et al. 2016) supporting predictions that these cells themselves establish a proliferative niche in the OSVZ. The molecular distinctions of oRGs were further connected to dynamic cell behavior and clonal output by live imaging in organotypic slice culture and dissociated single cells (Pollen et al. 2015).

Integrating measures of cell identity across modalities remains challenging. Currently, measurement of properties related to cell morphology, behavior, and lineage is low throughput. In addition, high throughput single cell RNA sequencing relies on dissociating cells from tissue, which loses information about spatial position and cellular interactions. Importantly, spatial and temporal identity may be influenced by fate-determining transcriptomic and epigenomic signatures. Similarly, extrinsic signals may play a role in establishing cell identity during neural differentiation. Scalable imaging and sequence-based strategies, including spatial transcriptomics and lineage-recording strategies will further inform the extent to which molecular distinctions among human cortical progenitors are influenced by their cellular neighborhood and reflected in their function and in the daughter cell types produced (Borm et al. 2022; Delgado et al. 2022; Fang et al. 2022; Guo et al. 2020; Lein et al. 2017). Finally, the function of candidate genetic programs distinguishing cell types and states can now be tested in a human cellular and tissue context using cerebral organoids that reproduce many features of normal intrauterine brain development (Di Lullo and Kriegstein 2017; Velasco et al. 2019).

2.2 Progenitor Cell Evolution

The expansion of the cerebral cortex represents one of the most conspicuous features of human evolution. Our cortex has tripled in size since our divergence from a common ancestor with chimpanzees, and expanded over 15-fold since our divergence from the old-world monkey lineage (Herculano-Houzel 2012). These changes in size have been accompanied by changes in the composition of progenitor cells as well as the resulting daughter neurons, astrocytes, and oligodendrocytes, including an increase in the number and diversity of upper cortical layer neurons, increased diversity of astrocytes, and a protracted duration of myelination (Sousa et al. 2017). In addition, the relative size of higher order association areas and the connectivity between these areas and with dorsal thalamus has increased in humans (Buckner and Krienen 2013; Striedter 2005). Changes in cortical progenitor cell behavior are thought to underlie many of these human brain specializations. Therefore, evolutionary studies of progenitor behavior have the potential to inform our understanding of human origins. The molecular mechanisms contributing to these changes in progenitor behavior have been analyzed from a number of perspectives, including through comparative studies of development, functional studies of candidate genes, such as those underlying cortical malformations, and genome-scale analyses of human-specific mutations. Systematic studies of human-specific genetic differences have the potential to reveal which, among many plausible candidate progenitor cell behaviors and molecular pathways, contributed to expansion of the human cortex.

2.2.1 Comparative Development

Several influential models propose that cortical expansion could involve changes in the proliferation dynamics of specific progenitor populations (Figure 2.1B). The Radial Unit Hypothesis formulated by Pasko Rakic (Rakic 1978, 1988) is based on the observation that neurons migrate radially from their site of origin in the ventricular zone to their positions in the cortical plate. As successive layers of neurons are produced, a radial column of neurons originates from one or more neighboring progenitor cells of the ventricular zone. The radial units are therefore the "building blocks" of the cerebral cortex. This concept also relates to the asymmetric division mode of the neural progenitor cells, now identified as RG. Because neurogenic RG divisions are usually asymmetric, each successive daughter cell has a different birthdate, and given the correlation of birthdate with laminar position, this creates an "ontogenetic column" of related neurons that contribute to, or potentially constitute, a radial unit. Cortical areal expansion then occurs through changes in the number of radial units, driven by NE divisions, with cortical thickness and the number of neurons in each column remaining relatively unchanged.

Comparative studies suggest that additional developmental mechanisms may also contribute to evolutionary brain expansion. Analyses of cortical histology during mammalian development revealed that cortical expansion can occur independently from VZ expansion and that thickening of the SVZ may precede the formation of cortical gyri (de Juan Romero et al. 2015; Martinez-Cerdeno 2006). The intermediate progenitor hypothesis was proposed based on the observation that IPCs divide symmetrically (Kriegstein et al. 2006; Pontious et al. 2008). These symmetric IPC divisions in the SVZ amplify the neuronal output of each RG cell. In rodents most IPCs divide once to produce two neurons, but there is evidence that the IPCs produced from oRG cells in humans divide more than once (Hansen et al. 2010). In either case, because the neurons generated by IPCs are born at the same cell cycle and have the same birthdate, they are destined to migrate to the same cell layer. They will therefore increase laminar cell number and potentially promote tangential rather than radial expansion.

The extensive production of oRG cells and prolonged neurogenesis in primates further increases the number of neurons produced by vRG cells and may also contribute to the expansion of upper cortical layers. Indeed, modeling the difference in neuron output between vRG and oRGs has demonstrated the enhanced neuronal productivity of oRGs in combination with their daughter IPCs (Fietz et al. 2010; Lui et al. 2011). In primates, and especially in humans, the upper cortical layers contain a higher diversity of excitatory neuron subtypes, a feature that is primate specific (Berg et al. 2021; Dehay et al. 2015; Hutsler et al. 2005; Krienen et al. 2016; Marín-Padilla 1992). An increase in the diversity and number of upper cortical layer neurons in humans and nonhuman primates may be a consequence of the enhanced role of oRG cells in the production of upper cortical layers in these species (Nowakowski et al. 2016) in combination with the transit amplifying IPCs that they produce (Hansen et al. 2010), as these account for the majority of neural progenitors during later stages of cortical neurogenesis when upper layer neurons are generated. Thus, changes in the proportion of direct neurogenesis to indirect neurogenesis and in the number and duration of divisions of oRGs and IPCs could increase cortical size beyond that achieved by expansion of the VZ alone.

The increase in progenitor diversity in large-brain mammals has been suggested to play a role in cortical folding, which has increased in the human lineage. However, the developmental mechanisms leading to a folded cortex are complex and remain poorly understood. The presence of IPCs and oRGs coupled with their modes of division have been implicated to play a role (Borrell and Götz 2014; Lewitus et al. 2013; Lui et al. 2011; Matsumoto et al. 2020; Smart et al. 2002), as have astrocytes and their progenitor cells (Rash et al. 2019; Shinmyo et al. 2022). Although, oRG cell number does not clearly correlate with the extent of gyrification (García-Moreno et al. 2012; Kelava et al. 2012), the increased production of upper layer neurons could contribute to differential tangential growth (Nowakowski et al. 2016), a general mechanism predicted to influence folding (Bayly et al. 2014; Mota and Herculano-Houzel 2015; Tallinen et al. 2014). Additional physical forces may contribute to a folded cortical surface, including axon tension (Van Essen 2020). Cortical gyrification is likely to result from an interplay of several of these factors, but while the mechanism of cortical folding is not fully understood, neither is its function. It has been suggested that the purpose of cortical gyrification is to increase cortical area and/or to facilitate connectivity between certain regions. There is a common notion, repeated in textbooks, that cortical folding allows a larger cortex to be contained in a smaller skull. However, the most highly folded cortices are found in mammals such as elephants and whales that have the largest brains and the biggest skulls while animals with small skulls tend to be lissencephalic. This observation appears contrary to the common notion and suggests that the true reason some mammals have folded cortices is not yet known.

2.2.2 Comparative Analysis of Human and Ape Development

Understanding changes in progenitor cell behavior that emerged after humans diverged from our closest living ape relatives is challenging because developmental tissue is not accessible from these species for ethical reasons. Structural MRI studies inform the dynamics of anatomical distinctions emerging during development (Sakai et al. 2013), but cannot capture the relative contribution of distinct progenitor types. Recent studies have generated induced pluripotent stem cells (iPSCs) from chimpanzees and other nonhuman primate species that enable modeling developmental cell behavior in vitro (Gallego Romero et al. 2015; Marchetto et al. 2013; Wunderlich et al. 2014).

Studies of progenitor behavior in vitro support recent divergence in cell behaviors. Comparison of pluripotent stem cell-derived RG cultured separately and in mixed-species pools suggest that human RG have an increased proliferative capacity compared to rhesus macaque RG during deep layer neurogenesis (Otani et al. 2016). In addition, comparison of neural progenitors in day 30 organoids that may resemble NE or early RG cells revealed human-specific changes in cell cycle dynamics. Metaphase, the stage of mitosis when spindle fibers attach to chromosomes, lasts longer in human progenitors than in chimpanzee and orangutan at organoid stages corresponding to NE or early RG cells (Mora-Bermúdez et al. 2016). However, by day 52, when organoid progenitors resemble RG, the duration of metaphase shrinks in human organoids to match that of other apes. Finally, a recent study of human, chimpanzee, and gorilla NE cells proposes that a delayed maturation of human NE cells could contribute to early brain expansion (Benito-Kwiecinski et al. 2021). These studies suggest that stem cell models of human and ape neural development can localize specific stages of development in which progenitor behavior differs between species. However, each study uses a small number of individuals per species – typically one or two – making it difficult to distinguish species differences from individual variation and technical variation related to in vitro culture (Mostajo-Radji et al. 2020). Future studies can expand the number of individuals analyzed to robustly quantify species differences.

Changes in progenitor cell behavior may be manifest through changes in signaling pathway activation. Although many signaling pathways are known to influence the proliferative behavior of progenitor cell types, we still do not know which pathways changed in evolution. Comparison of gene expression changes in RG across organoids from 10 human and 8 chimpanzee individuals as well as primary samples from human and rhesus macaque revealed human-specific changes in the expression of genes involved with PI3K-AKT-mTOR signaling (Pollen et al. 2019). Notably, organoids with elevated PI3K-AKT-mTOR signaling display increased RG proliferation (Li et al. 2017) and this pathway influences cell growth, division, metabolism, and fate potential (Baser et al. 2019; Blair et al. 2018; Takei and Nawa 2014). Validation experiments in primary human and macaque demonstrated a quantitative increase in mTOR activation in human oRG cells and showed that expression of INSR and ITGB8, two genes upregulated in human organoids, was necessary for this signaling (Pollen et al. 2019). Reporters of signaling pathway activation in organoid models from many human and ape individuals could enable further quantitative determination of changes in progenitor behavior across species.

2.2.3 Candidate Molecular Pathways Influencing Cortex Size

Mechanistic studies of candidate genes have revealed many pathways that influence progenitor proliferative behavior during development and represent plausible candidate substrates for evolutionary changes. Extrinsic changes that act broadly across the cortex could have a concerted influence on cortical expansion, while local signaling or intrinsic changes in progenitors could have either concerted or region-specific influences on cortex size. The interplay of extrinsic and intrinsic factors in regulating cortex size is not well understood, but multiple plausible extrinsic factors could exert concerted evolutionary changes in progenitor behavior. For example, experimental lengthening of the gestational period can increase the duration of neurogenesis and expand upper cortical layers in mouse models (Stepien et al. 2020). Similarly, growth factors released by the choroid plexus could influence vRG behavior widely across lateral ventricles (Lehtinen et al. 2011), and circulating thyroid hormone interacts with integrin signaling to promote SVZ progenitor expansion (Stenzel et al. 2014), while the contribution of systemic factors from placenta has not yet been examined.

In addition to systemic factors, there are numerous examples of local signals and intrinsic regulation that could influence brain expansion. Studies of human patients with microcephaly have revealed that a number of genes regulating mitotic spindle formation are necessary for normal cortical development (Gilmore and Walsh 2013). Human-specific amino acid changes in several of these genes have been considered as candidate mutations influencing brain size (Hill and Walsh 2005; Vallender et al. 2008), but the impact of evolutionary changes in these widely expressed proteins is unclear. In addition, SHH, a signaling molecule and mitogen implicated in some forms of microcephaly, regulates oRG proliferation in mouse and ferret models (Matsumoto et al. 2020; Wang et al. 2016). Similarly, genes such as Insm1 and Pard3 can act in vRGs to influence oRG and IPC production by regulating the apical complex, adherens junctions, and cleavage plane along the VZ (Bultje et al. 2009; Costa et al. 2008; Tavano et al. 2018). Intrinsic changes in the regulation of cell cycle progression also influence the balance between proliferation and differentiation (Dehay and Kennedy 2007). For example, CDK and Cyclin genes that regulate G1/S transition can expand the cortex and maintain normal layering when over-expressed and are necessary for normal brain size (Nonaka-Kinoshita et al. 2013; Pilaz et al. 2009; Taverna et al. 2014). However, the necessity and sufficiency of genes for cortical expansion in development does not reveal the genes that changed in evolution or their effect size.

2.2.4 Comparative Genomics

Comparative genomics provides a path for determining causative evolutionary changes driving human progenitor cell specializations, but it has been challenging to filter causative mutations influencing brain size from the numerous neutral and small effect changes. Nucleotide substitutions account for 1.2 percent of divergence between human and chimpanzee genomes, and structural variants, including insertions, deletions, and inversions account for roughly 3 percent divergence, together representing over 100 million base pairs (Consortium, Chimpanzee Sequencing and Analysis 2005). Analyzing the consequences of individual genetic changes on progenitor behavior depends on the assumption that these mutations will have detectable effect sizes and depends on strategies for filtering for functional mutations among millions of neutral changes (Varki and Altheide 2005). Charles Darwin famously argued that nature never makes leaps, and that a large number of small effect changes together would influence traits. Although his defender Thomas Henry Huxley argued that nature does make leaps now and then, the view that evolution largely involved small effect size changes prevailed through the modern synthesis (Fisher 1930). However, evolutionary genetic studies in natural populations now suggest that mutations of medium- and large-effect size can account for substantial variation in traits under adaptive selection, supporting the premise of comparative genomics approaches, but there will be a long tail of neutral changes as well, highlighting the challenges (Albert et al. 2008; Orr 2005). Evolutionary genetics studies further suggest that mutations limiting pleiotropy by influencing tissue-specific gene regulation or by duplicating ancestral genes may act as a favored substrate for adaptive selection (Carroll 2008; King and Wilson 1975; Ohno 1970).

Based on these lessons from evolution in natural populations, several comparative genomics approaches have attempted to filter human-specific mutations for medium and large effect size candidate differences influencing progenitor cell behavior (Figure 2.1C). These approaches include identifying highly conserved regions of mammalian genomes, mainly in noncoding regulatory regions, with unexpectedly large numbers of nucleotide substitutions, termed human accelerated regions (Pollard et al. 2006; Prabhakar et al. 2006), or with unexpected deletions, termed hCONDELs (Kronenberg et al. 2018; McLean et al. 2011). In addition, coding sequences have been evaluated for an unexpectedly high ratio of human-specific amino acid substitutions compared to non-synonymous changes (Bustamante et al. 2005), for amino acid substitutions divergent from archaic humans that are near fixed in modern humans (Prüfer et al. 2014), and for duplications followed by constraint on copy number (Dennis et al. 2017). Finally, this filtering approach can further isolate changes relevant to the brain by overlapping with epigenomic features of gene regulatory enhancer or transcriptional features of tissue and progenitor cell type specificity (Camp et al. 2015; Florio et al. 2015, 2018; Pollen et al. 2019; Prescott et al. 2015)

2.2.5 Functional Studies of Candidate Genetic Changes

Comparative studies have highlighted a number of candidate regulatory mutations influencing progenitor behavior. Deletion of a ventral forebrain enhancer with conserved sequence and activity between chimpanzee and mouse near the tumor suppressor gene GADD45G represents a candidate that could release a brake on proliferation of ventral IPC populations expressing this gene (McLean et al. 2011). However, the expression domains in septum, preoptic area, and ventral diencephalon are involved with ventral forebrain neurogenesis and unlikely influence cortical inhibitory or excitatory neuron number, and the consequences of this human-specific deletion have not yet been functionally tested. Similarly, a number of forebrain enhancers with accelerated substitutions in human lineage show divergent patterns of reporter gene expression (Capra et al. 2013), and many quantitatively influence reporter gene expression in cultured cells (Girskis et al. 2021; Uebbing et al. 2021; Whalen et al. 2023), but the functional consequences are not yet known. Recently, transgenic assays in mice revealed that the human allele of an accelerated region contacting the FZD8 promoter shows greater enhancer activity than the chimpanzee allele. FZD8 mediates Wnt signaling, which is important for NE and RG proliferation, and transgenic mice with the human enhancer driving FZD8 expression also show accelerated cell cycle and shorter G1 compared to the chimpanzee enhancer (Boyd et al. 2015). Reconstruction of this mutation at the endogenous locus in mouse could further determine the effect size, and comparison of Wnt signaling between human and chimpanzee iPSC derived NE and RG cells could determine the progenitor cell types and stages where this species difference in signaling is most strongly manifest.

Comparative studies have also highlighted human-specific gene duplications likely to influence progenitor behavior. The Eichler lab identified dozens of genes duplicated in the human lineage (Dennis et al. 2017; Sudmant et al. 2010). Duplications of genome sequence can occur between chromosomes, at a distance on the same chromosome, or directly in tandem. Compared to changes in single nucleotides, such structural variation is more likely to have phenotypic consequences and be visible to selection (Abel et al. 2020). Interestingly, apes show an increased number of segmental duplications compared to other mammals (Marques-Bonet et al. 2009). These segmental duplications favor unequal crossover during recombination and act as a source for human-specific genes as well as for de novo mutations causing a range of neurodevelopmental syndromes (Dennis and Eichler 2016; Harel and Lupski 2018; Porubsky et al. 2022). Human-specific segmental duplications have generated at least 80 novel genes in the human lineage across over 30 gene families (Dennis et al. 2017; Dougherty et al. 2018; Vollger et al. 2022).

Recent studies have prioritized human-specific genes based on expression in cortical progenitor cell types and examined their influence on developmental processes. Experiments in developing mouse, ferret, and marmoset models and human and chimpanzee cerebral organoids indicate that ARHGAP11B promotes oRG proliferation and IPC number (Fischer et al. 2022; Heide and Huttner 2021). Importantly, the human specific duplication that formed ARHGAP11B was followed by a single nucleotide substitution that changed splicing, causing ARHGAP11B to localize in the mitochondrial rather than the nucleus and promote glutaminolysis (Florio et al. 2016; Namba et al. 2020). Duplication of NOTCH2 in the ancestor of African apes created truncated NOTCH2NL pseudogenes that were restored as functional genes by gene conversion and further duplicated into three NOTCH2NL paralogs specifically in humans (Fiddes et al. 2018). Interestingly, this duplication occurred in tandem with three NBPF family genes that in turn have the largest human-specific expansion of exonic regions and share specific expression domains in RG, suggesting multiple evolutionarily important events at this locus (Fiddes et al. 2019). Functional studies in developing mice, human cell lines, and organoid models indicate that the NOTCH2NL paralogs promote Notch signaling and progenitor proliferation (Fiddes et al. 2018; Florio et al. 2018; Suzuki et al. 2018). In addition, the TBC1D3 locus has undergone two large human-specific expansions, increasing the copy number of this gene, but has also undergone independent recurrent expansions in other primate lineages (Vollger et al. 2022). This gene also appears to increase RG proliferation by modulating EGF signaling and by repressing the activity of the histone lysine methyltransferase G9a (EHMT2) (Hou et al. 2021; Ju et al. 2016). Together, these studies indicate that segmental duplications, often coupled with additional mutations influencing gene function or regulation, have altered progenitor cell behavior in the human lineage.

Precise reconstruction of complex structural changes in distant animal models is challenging or impossible, making examination of the necessity of these changes in human cells important. Genome engineering in iPSCs has enabled early examples of such experiments in human organoids for NOTCH2NL and ARHGAP11B (Fiddes et al. 2018; Fischer et al. 2022). The high structural mutation rate of segmental duplications coupled with expanded medical genetics studies may further permit analyses of humans lacking human-specific genes in future studies where the effect size of these loci could be examined in a clinical context. Importantly, analysis of the genetic changes that occurred in evolution in the appropriate genetic and cellular context is crucial for weighing plausible molecular and cellular pathways that contributed to human-specific cortical progenitor behaviors.

2.2.6 Systematically Analyzing Human-specific Mutations

The combination of insights from comparative studies of development, mechanistic studies of molecular pathways influencing normal development, and functional studies of human-specific genetic changes demonstrates that an integrated understanding of the origin of human-specific progenitor cell behaviors is now a tractable goal. One of the remaining opportunities will be to transition from studies of individual candidate genes to systems-level approaches of the influence of human-specific mutations on cellular and developmental traits. Currently, it is difficult to weigh the relative influence of candidate genes on evolved progenitor traits as each locus is analyzed separately by different measures and different levels of faithful reconstruction of evolutionary genetic changes. In addition, comparative genomics prioritization strategies may highlight loci that are surprisingly divergent at the sequence level but have limited influence on cellular phenotypes when precisely reconstructed. For example, the most divergent human accelerated noncoding sequence, *HACNS1*, when precisely reconstructed in mouse models, increases the expression of Gbx2 in chondrogenic mesenchyme of developing distal limbs, but does not otherwise show detectable phenotypic changes by current metrics, despite many human-specific morphological changes in this anatomical domain (Dutrow et al. 2022). Scalable assays of many loci can help to overcome the likelihood that individual loci, even if highly divergent, will have small or no effects on phenotypes. For example, pooled reporter assays can systematically assess the impact of human-specific mutations on the capacity of *cis*-regulatory changes to influence reporter gene expression (Girskis et al. 2021; Uebbing et al. 2021; Whalen et al. 2023). However, these assays do not analyze the impact of human-specific changes at endogenous loci on cellular behavior. Future studies incorporating CRISPR screening strategies (Kampmann 2020) are now poised to analyze the functional consequences of many human mutations on progenitor cell gene expression, daughter cell fate, and behavior, but these strategies currently cannot recreate precise allelic changes and instead are best for studying the necessity of many loci in parallel.

2.3 Conclusion

Since Virchow's first description of neuroglia cells over 175 years ago, our understanding of progenitor diversity has reached a stage where we have defined many of the component cell types and can model how these populations changed in human brain evolution. Scalable molecular analyses now offer a path to furthering our resolution of these cell types and their contributions to human cortical origins. Single cell sequencing and imaging approaches have the potential to provide a complete atlas of human progenitor cell types and ultimately to link these cell types to cell behaviors and daughter cell lineages. Comparative analyses of human and chimpanzee cells using iPSC and organoid models have the potential to define cell behavior differences between humans and our closest living relatives. And genome engineering strategies implemented at scale may allow for weighing the effect size of human-specific mutations on cell behaviors. Together, the combination of classical approaches and scalable imaging, molecular, and genetic approaches will give us insights into the progenitor cell changes underlying human cortical specializations.

References

Aaku-Saraste, E. et al. (1996). Loss of occludin and functional tight junctions, but not ZO-1, during neural tube closure—remodeling of the neuroepithelium prior to neurogenesis. *Dev Biol* 180: 664–679. doi: 10.1006/dbio.1996.0336.

Abel, H.J. et al. (2020). Mapping and characterization of structural variation in 17,795 human genomes. *Nature* 583: 83–89.

Albert, A.Y.K. et al. (2008). The genetics of adaptive shape shift in stickleback. *Evolution* 62: 76–85.

Baser, A. et al. (2019). Onset of differentiation is post-transcriptionally controlled in adult neural stem cells. *Nature* 566: 100–104.

Bayly, P.V. (2014). Mechanical forces in cerebral cortical folding: a review of measurements and models. *J Mech Beh Biomed Mat* 29: 568–581.

Benito-Kwiecinski, S. et al. (2021). An early cell shape transition drives evolutionary expansion of the human forebrain. *Cell* 184: 2084–2102.e19.

Berg, J. et al. (2021). Human neocortical expansion involves glutamatergic neuron diversification. *Nature* 598: 151–158.

Bhaduri, A. et al. (2021). An atlas of cortical arealization identifies dynamic molecular signatures. *Nature* 598: 200–204.

Blair, J.D. (2018). Genetically engineered human cortical spheroid models of tuberous sclerosis. *Nat Med* 24: 1568–1578.

Borm, L.E. et al. (2022). Scalable in situ single-cell profiling by electrophoretic capture of mRNA using EEL FISH. *Nat Biotechnol* 41: 222–231. doi: 10.1038/s41587-022-01455-3.

Borrell, V. et al. (2012). Slit/Robo signaling modulates the proliferation of central nervous system progenitors. *Neuron* 76: 338–352.

Borrell, V. and Götz, M. (2014). Role of radial glial cells in cerebral cortex folding. *Curr Opin Neurobiol* 27: 39–46.

Boyd, J.L. et al. (2015). Human-chimpanzee differences in a FZD8 enhancer alter cell-cycle dynamics in the developing neocortex. *Curr Biol* 25: 772–779.

Brückner, G. and Biesold, D. (1981). Histochemistry of glycogen deposition in perinatal rat brain. *J Neurocytol* 10: 749–757.

Buckner, R.L. and Krienen, F.M. (2013). The evolution of distributed association networks in the human brain. *Trends Cogn Sci* 17: 648–665.

Bultje, R.S. et al. (2009). Mammalian Par3 regulates progenitor cell asymmetric division via Notch signaling in the developing neocortex. *Neuron* 63: 189–202.

Bustamante, C.D. et al. (2005). Natural selection on protein-coding genes in the human genome. *Nature* 437: 1153–1157.

Cajal, S.R.Y. (1909). *Histologie du système nerveux de l'homme et des vertébrés.* Paris: Maloine.

Camargo Ortega, G. et al. (2019). The centrosome protein AKNA regulates neurogenesis via microtubule organization. *Nature* 567: 113–117.

Camp, J.G. et al. (2015). Human cerebral organoids recapitulate gene expression programs of fetal neocortex development. *Proc Natl Acad Sci USA* 112: 15672–15677.

Cappello, S. et al. (2006). The Rho-GTPase cdc42 regulates neural progenitor fate at the apical surface. *Nat Neurosci* 9: 1099–1107.

Capra, J.A. et al. (2013). Many human accelerated regions are developmental enhancers. *Philos Trans Royal Soc London B: Biol Sci* 368: 20130025.

Carroll, S.B. (2008). Evo–devo and an expanding evolutionary synthesis. *Cell* 134: 25–36.

Choi, B.H. and Lapham, L.W. (1978). Radial glia in the human fetal cerebrum. *Brain Res* 148: 295–311.

Chvátal, A. and Verkhratsky, A. (2018). An early history of neuroglial research. *Neuroglia* 1: 245–257.

Consortium, Chimpanzee Sequencing and Analysis. (2005). Initial sequence of the chimpanzee genome and comparison with the human genome. *Nature* 437: 69–87.

Costa, M.R. et al. (2008). Par-complex proteins promote proliferative progenitor divisions in the developing mouse cerebral cortex. *Development* 135: 11–22.

Culurgioni, S. et al. (2011). Inscuteable and NuMA proteins bind competitively to Leu-Gly-Asn repeat-enriched protein (LGN) during asymmetric cell divisions. *Proc Natl Acad Sci USA* 108: 20998–21003.

de Juan Romero, C. et al. (2015). Discrete domains of gene expression in germinal layers distinguish the development of gyrencephaly. *EMBO J* 34: 1859–1874.

Dehay, C. and Kennedy, H. (2007). Cell-cycle control and cortical development. *Nat Rev Neurosci* 8: 438–450.

Dehay, C. et al. (2015). The outer subventricular zone and primate-specific cortical complexification. *Neuron* 85: 683–694.

Delaunay, D. et al. (2017). Division modes and physical asymmetry in cerebral cortex progenitors. *Curr Opin Neurobiol* 42: 75–83.

Delgado, R.N. et al. (2022). Individual human cortical progenitors can produce excitatory and inhibitory neurons. *Nature* 601: 397–403. doi: 10.1038/s41586-021-04230-7.

Dennis, M.Y. and Eichler, E.E. (2016). Human adaptation and evolution by segmental duplication. *Curr Opin Genet Dev* 41: 44–52.
Dennis, M.Y. et al. (2017). The evolution and population diversity of human-specific segmental duplications. *Nat Ecol Evol* 1: 69.
Di Lullo, E. and Kriegstein, A.R. (2017). The use of brain organoids to investigate neural development and disease. *Nat Rev Neurosci* 18: 573–584.
Dono, R. et al. (1998). Impaired cerebral cortex development and blood pressure regulation in FGF-2-deficient mice. *EMBO J* 17: 4213–4225.
Dougherty, M.L. et al. (2018). Transcriptional fates of human-specific segmental duplications in brain. *Genome Res* 28: 1566–1576.
Draganova, K. et al. (2015). Wnt/β-catenin signaling regulates sequential fate decisions of murine cortical precursor cells. *Stem Cells* 33: 170–182.
Dutrow, E.V. et al. (2022). Modeling uniquely human gene regulatory function via targeted humanization of the mouse genome. *Nat Commun* 13: 304.
Eze, U.C. et al. (2021). Single-cell atlas of early human brain development highlights heterogeneity of human neuroepithelial cells and early radial glia. *Nat Neurosci* 24: 584–594.
Fang, R. et al. (2022). Conservation and divergence of cortical cell organization in human and mouse revealed by MERFISH. *Science* 377: 56–62.
Fiddes, I.T. et al. (2018). Human-specific NOTCH2NL genes affect Notch signaling and cortical neurogenesis. *Cell* 173: 1356–1369.e22.
Fiddes, I.T. et al. (2019). Paired involvement of human-specific Olduvai domains and NOTCH2NL genes in human brain evolution. *Hum Genet* 138: 715–721.
Fietz, S.A. et al. (2010). OSVZ progenitors of human and ferret neocortex are epithelial-like and expand by integrin signaling. *Nat Neurosci* 13: 690–699.
Fietz, S.A. et al. (2012). Transcriptomes of germinal zones of human and mouse fetal neocortex suggest a role of extracellular matrix in progenitor self-renewal. *Proc Nat Acad Sci USA* 109: 11836–11841.
Fischer, J. et al. (2022). Human-specific ARHGAP11B ensures human-like basal progenitor levels in hominid cerebral organoids. *EMBO Rep*. 23: e54728.
Fisher, R.A. (1930). *The Genetical Theory of Natural Selection*. Oxford: Oxford University Press.
Florio, M. et al. (2015). Human-specific gene ARHGAP11B promotes basal progenitor amplification and neocortex expansion. *Science* 347: 1465–1470.
Florio, M. et al. (2018). Evolution and cell-type specificity of human-specific genes preferentially expressed in progenitors of fetal neocortex. *Elife* 7: e32332.
Florio, M. et al. (2016). A single splice site mutation in human-specific ARHGAP11B causes basal progenitor amplification. *Sci Adv* 2: e1601941–e1601941.
Fuchs, J.L. and Schwark, H.D. (2004). Neuronal primary cilia. *Cell Biol Int* 28: 111–118.
Fukumitsu, H. et al. (2006). Brain-derived neurotrophic factor participates in determination of neuronal laminar fate in the developing mouse cerebral cortex. *J Neurosci* 26: 13218–13230.
Gal, J.S. et al. (2006). Molecular and morphological heterogeneity of neural precursors in the mouse neocortical proliferative zones. *J Neurosci* 26: 1045–1056.
Gallego Romero, I. et al. (2015). A panel of induced pluripotent stem cells from chimpanzees. *Elife* 4: e07103.
García-Moreno, F. et al. (2012). Compartmentalization of cerebral cortical germinal zones in a lissencephalic primate and gyrencephalic rodent. *Cereb Cortex* 22: 482–492.
Georgiou, M. et al. (2008). Cdc42, Par6, and aPKC regulate Arp2/3-mediated endocytosis to control local adherens junction stability. *Curr Biol* 18: 1631–1638.
Gertz, C.C. et al. (2014). Diverse behaviors of outer radial glia in developing ferret and human cortex. *J Neurosci* 34: 2559–2570.

Gilmore, E.C. and Walsh, C.A. (2013). Genetic causes of microcephaly and lessons for neuronal development. *Wiley Interdiscip Rev Dev Biol* 2: 461–478.

Girskis, K.M. et al. (2021). Rewiring of human neurodevelopmental gene regulatory programs by human accelerated regions. *Neuron* 109: 3239–3251.e7.

Gloerich, M. et al. (2017). Cell division orientation is coupled to cell-cell adhesion by the E-cadherin/LGN complex. *Nat Commun* 8: 13996.

Götz, M. and Huttner, W.B. (2005). The cell biology of neurogenesis. *Nat Rev Mol Cell Biol* 6: 777–788.

Guo, S.-M. et al. (2020). Revealing architectural order with quantitative label-free imaging and deep learning. *Elife* 9: e55502. doi: 10.7554/eLife.55502.

Hansen, D.V. (2010). Neurogenic radial glia in the outer subventricular zone of human neocortex. *Nature* 464: 554–561.

Harel, T. and Lupski, J.R. (2018). Genomic disorders 20 years on–mechanisms for clinical manifestations. *Clin Genet* 93: 439–449.

Hatakeyama, J. et al. (2014). Cadherin-based adhesions in the apical endfoot are required for active Notch signaling to control neurogenesis in vertebrates. *Development* 141: 1671–1682.

Haubensak, W. (2004). Neurons arise in the basal neuroepithelium of the early mammalian telencephalon. *Proc Natl Acad Sci USA* 101: 3196–3201.

Heide, M. and Huttner, W.B. (2021). Human-specific genes, cortical progenitor cells, and microcephaly. *Cells* 10: 1209. doi: 10.3390/cells10051209.

Herculano-Houzel, S. (2012). The remarkable, yet not extraordinary, human brain as a scaled-up primate brain and its associated cost. *Proc Natl Acad Sci USA* 109 (Suppl 1): 10661–10668.

Hill, R.S. and Walsh, C.A. (2005). Molecular insights into human brain evolution. *Nature* 437: 64–67.

His, W. (1889). *Die Neuroblasten und deren Entstehung im embryonalen Mark*. Leipzig: Bei S. Hirzel.

Hou, -Q.-Q. et al. (2021). TBC1D3 promotes neural progenitor proliferation by suppressing the histone methyltransferase G9a. *Sci Adv* 7: eaba8053. doi: 10.1126/sciadv.aba8053.

Howard, B.M. et al. (2008). Radial glia cells in the developing human brain. *Neuroscientist* 14: 459–473.

Hutsler, J.J. et al. (2005). Comparative analysis of cortical layering and supragranular layer enlargement in rodent carnivore and primate species. *Brain Res* 1052: 71–81.

Itoh, Y. et al. (2013). Scratch regulates neuronal migration onset via an epithelial-mesenchymal transition-like mechanism. *Nat Neurosci* 16: 416–425.

Ju, X.-C. et al. (2016). The hominoid-specific gene TBC1D3 promotes generation of basal neural progenitors and induces cortical folding in mice. *Elife* 5: e18197. doi: 10.7554/eLife.18197.

Kampmann, M. (2020). CRISPR-based functional genomics for neurological disease. *Nat Rev Neurol* 16: 465–480.

Kawaguchi, A. (2020). Neuronal delamination and outer radial glia generation in neocortical development. *Front Cell Devel Biol* 8: 623573.

Kawaue, T. et al. (2019). Lzts1 controls both neuronal delamination and outer radial glial-like cell generation during mammalian cerebral development. *Nat Commun* 10: 2780.

Kelava, I. et al. (2012). Abundant occurrence of basal radial glia in the subventricular zone of embryonic neocortex of a lissencephalic primate, the common marmoset Callithrix jacchus. *Cereb Cortex* 22: 469–481.

Kim, S. et al. (2010). The apical complex couples cell fate and cell survival to cerebral cortical development. *Neuron* 66: 69–84.

King, M.C. and Wilson, A.C. (1975). Evolution at two levels in humans and chimpanzees. *Science* 188: 107–116.

Kölliker, A. (1867). *Handbuch der Gewebelehre des Menschen*. Leipzig: Wilhelm Engelmann.

Konno, D. et al. (2008). Neuroepithelial progenitors undergo LGN-dependent planar divisions to maintain self-renewability during mammalian neurogenesis. *Nat Cell Biol* 10: 93–101.

Kosodo, Y. et al. (2008). Cytokinesis of neuroepithelial cells can divide their basal process before anaphase. *EMBO J* 27: 3151–3163.

Kowalczyk, T. et al. (2009). Intermediate neuronal progenitors (basal progenitors) produce pyramidal–projection neurons for all layers of cerebral cortex. *Cereb Cortex* 19: 2439–2450.

Kriegstein, A., Noctor, S., and Martínez-Cerdeño, V. (2006). Patterns of neural stem and progenitor cell division may underlie evolutionary cortical expansion. *Nat Rev Neurosci* 7: 883–890.

Kriegstein, A.R. and Götz, M. (2003). Radial glia diversity. *Glia* 43: 37–43.

Kriegstein, A.R. and Noctor, S.C. (2004). Patterns of neuronal migration in the embryonic cortex. *Trends Neurosci* 27: 392–399.

Krienen, F.M. et al. (2016). Transcriptional profiles of supragranular-enriched genes associate with corticocortical network architecture in the human brain. *Proc Natl Acad Sci* 113: E469–478. doi: 10.1073/pnas.1510903113.

Kronenberg, Z.N. et al. (2018). High-resolution comparative analysis of great ape genomes. *Science* 360: eaar6343.

La Manno, G. et al. (2021). Molecular architecture of the developing mouse brain. *Nature* 596: 92–96.

LaMonica, B.E. et al. (2013). Mitotic spindle orientation predicts outer radial glial cell generation in human neocortex. *Nat Commun* 4: 1665.

Lehtinen, M.K. et al. (2011). The cerebrospinal fluid provides a proliferative niche for neural progenitor cells. *Neuron* 69: 893–905.

Lein, E. (2017). The promise of spatial transcriptomics for neuroscience in the era of molecular cell typing. *Science* 358: 64–69.

Lewitus, E. (2013). Conical expansion of the outer subventricular zone and the role of neocortical folding in evolution and development. *Front Hum Neurosci* 7: 424.

Li, W. (1998). Neuronal differentiation of precursors in the neocortical ventricular zone is triggered by BMP. *J Neurosci* 18: 8853–8862.

Li, Y. et al. (2017). Induction of expansion and folding in human cerebral organoids. *Cell Stem Cell* 20: 385–396.e3.

Lian, G. and Sheen, V.L. (2015). Cytoskeletal proteins in cortical development and disease. *Front Cell Neurosci* 9: 99.

Liu, S. et al. (2021). The essential role of primary cilia in cerebral cortical development and disorders. *Curr Top Dev Biol* 142: 99–146.

Lui, J.H. et al. (2011). Development and evolution of the human neocortex. *Cell* 146: 18–36.

Mabie, P.C. et al. (1999). Multiple roles of bone morphogenetic protein signaling in the regulation of cortical cell number and phenotype. *J Neurosci* 19: 7077–7088.

Magini, J. (1888). Nouvelles recherches histologiques sur le cerveau du foetus. *Archives Italiennes de Biologie* 10: 384–397.

Malatesta, P. et al. (2000). Isolation of radial glial cells by fluorescent-activated cell sorting reveals a neuronal lineage. *Development* 127: 5253–5263.

Marchetto, M.C.N. et al. (2013). Differential L1 regulation in pluripotent stem cells of humans and apes. *Nature* 503: 525–529.

Marín-Padilla, M. (1992). Ontogenesis of the pyramidal cell of the mammalian neocortex and developmental cytoarchitectonics: a unifying theory. *J Comp Neurol* 321: 223–240.

Marques-Bonet, T. et al. (2009). A burst of segmental duplications in the genome of the African great ape ancestor. *Nature* 457: 877–881.

Martinez-Cerdeno, V. (2006). The role of intermediate progenitor cells in the evolutionary expansion of the cerebral cortex. *Cereb Cortex* 16: i152–i161.

Martínez-Martínez, M.Á. et al. (2016). A restricted period for formation of outer subventricular zone defined by Cdh1 and Trnp1 levels. *Nat Commun* 7: 11812.

Matsumoto, N. et al. (2020). A discrete subtype of neural progenitor crucial for cortical folding in the gyrencephalic mammalian brain. *Elife* 9: e54873. doi: 10.7554/eLife.54873.

McLean, C.Y. et al. (2011). Human-specific loss of regulatory DNA and the evolution of human-specific traits. *Nature* 471: 216–219.

Miyata, T. et al. (2001). Asymmetric inheritance of radial glial fibers by cortical neurons. *Neuron* 31: 727–741.

Miyata, T. et al. (2004). Asymmetric production of surface-dividing and non-surface-dividing cortical progenitor cells. *Development* 131: 3133–3145.

Mora-Bermúdez, F. et al. (2016). Differences and similarities between human and chimpanzee neural progenitors during cerebral cortex development. *Elife* 5: e18683.

Mostajo-Radji, M.A. (2020). Reverse engineering human brain evolution using organoid models. *Brain Res* 1729: 146582.

Mota, B. and Herculano-Houzel, S. (2015). Cortical folding scales universally with surface area and thickness, not number of neurons. *Science* 349: 74–77. doi: 10.1126/science.aaa9101.

Namba, T. et al. (2020). Human-specific ARHGAP11B acts in mitochondria to expand neocortical progenitors by glutaminolysis. *Neuron* 105: 867–881.e9.

Narayanan, R. et al. (2018). Chromatin remodeling BAF155 subunit regulates the genesis of basal progenitors in developing cortex. *iScience* 4: 109–126.

Noctor, S.C. et al. (2001). Neurons derived from radial glial cells establish radial units in neocortex. *Nature* 409: 714–720.

Noctor, S.C. et al. (2004). Cortical neurons arise in symmetric and asymmetric division zones and migrate through specific phases. *Nat Neurosci* 7: 136–144.

Nonaka-Kinoshita, M. et al. (2013). Regulation of cerebral cortex size and folding by expansion of basal progenitors. *EMBO J* 32: 1817–1828.

Nowakowski, T.J. et al. (2017). Spatiotemporal gene expression trajectories reveal developmental hierarchies of the human cortex. *Science* 358: 1318–1323.

Nowakowski, T.J. et al. (2016). Transformation of the radial glia scaffold demarcates two stages of human cerebral cortex development. *Neuron* 91: 1219–1227.

Ohno, S. (1970). *Evolution by Gene Duplication*. Berlin, Heidelberg: Springer Berlin Heidelberg.

Ohshima, T. et al. (2007). Cdk5 is required for multipolar-to-bipolar transition during radial neuronal migration and proper dendrite development of pyramidal neurons in the cerebral cortex. *Development* 134: 2273–2282.

Orr, H.A. (2005). The genetic theory of adaptation: a brief history. *Nat Rev Genet* 6: 119–127.

Ostrem, B.E.L. et al. (2014). Control of outer radial glial stem cell mitosis in the human brain. *Cell Rep* 8: 656–664.

Otani, T. et al. (2016). 2D and 3D stem cell models of primate cortical development identify species-specific differences in progenitor behavior contributing to brain size. *Cell Stem Cell* 18: 467–480.

Pacary, E. et al. (2012). Crucial first steps: the transcriptional control of neuron delamination. *Neuron* 74: 209–211.

Pilaz, L.-J. et al. (2009). Forced G1-phase reduction alters mode of division, neuron number, and laminar phenotype in the cerebral cortex. *Proc Natl Acad Sci USA* 106: 21924–21929.

Polioudakis, D. et al. (2019). A single-cell transcriptomic atlas of human neocortical development during mid-gestation. *Neuron* 103: 785–801.e8.

Pollard, K.S. et al. (2006). An RNA gene expressed during cortical development evolved rapidly in humans. *Nature* 443: 167–172.
Pollen, A.A. et al. (2019). Establishing cerebral organoids as models of human-specific brain evolution. *Cell* 176: 743–756.e17.
Pollen, A.A. et al. (2015). Molecular identity of human outer radial glia during cortical development. *Cell* 163: 55–67.
Pollen, A.A. et al. (2014). Low-coverage single-cell mRNA sequencing reveals cellular heterogeneity and activated signaling pathways in developing cerebral cortex. *Nat Biotechnol* 32: 1053–1058.
Pontious, A. et al. (2008). Role of intermediate progenitor cells in cerebral cortex development. *Dev Neurosci* 30: 24–32.
Porubsky, D. et al. (2022). Recurrent inversion polymorphisms in humans associate with genetic instability and genomic disorders. *Cell* 185: 1986–2005.e26.
Postiglione, M.P. et al. (2011). Mouse inscuteable induces apical-basal spindle orientation to facilitate intermediate progenitor generation in the developing neocortex. *Neuron* 72: 269–284.
Prabhakar, S. et al. (2006). Accelerated evolution of conserved noncoding sequences in humans. *Science* 314: 786.
Prescott, S.L. et al. (2015). Enhancer divergence and cis-regulatory evolution in the human and chimp neural crest. *Cell* 163: 68–83.
Prüfer, K. et al. (2014). The complete genome sequence of a Neanderthal from the Altai Mountains. *Nature* 505: 43–49.
Quake, S.R. (2022). A decade of molecular cell atlases. *Trends Genet* 38: 805–810.
Rakic, P. (1978). Neuronal migration and contact guidance in the primate telencephalon. *Postgrad Med J* 54 (Suppl 1): 25–40.
Rakic, P. (1988). Specification of cerebral cortical areas. *Science* 241: 170–176.
Rash, B.G. et al. (2019). Gliogenesis in the outer subventricular zone promotes enlargement and gyrification of the primate cerebrum. *Proc Natl Acad Sci USA* 116: 7089–7094.
Reillo, I. et al. (2011). A role for intermediate radial glia in the tangential expansion of the mammalian cerebral cortex. *Cereb Cortex* 21: 1674–1694.
Sakai, T. et al. (2013). Developmental patterns of chimpanzee cerebral tissues provide important clues for understanding the remarkable enlargement of the human brain. *Proc Biol Sci* 280: 20122398.
Sakakibara, A. et al. (2014). Dynamics of centrosome translocation and microtubule organization in neocortical neurons during distinct modes of polarization. *Cereb Cortex* 24: 1301–1310.
Sauer, F.C. (1935). Mitosis in the neural tube. *J Comp Neurol* 62: 377–405.
Schaper, A. (1897). The earliest differentiation in the central nervous system of vertebrates. *Science* 5: 430–431.
Shapiro, E. et al. (2013). Single-cell sequencing-based technologies will revolutionize whole-organism science. *Nat Rev Genet* 14: 618–630.
Shinmyo, Y. et al. (2022). Localized astrogenesis regulates gyrification of the cerebral cortex. *Sci Adv* 8: eabi5209.
Shitamukai, A. et al. (2011). Oblique radial glial divisions in the developing mouse neocortex induce self-renewing progenitors outside the germinal zone that resemble primate outer subventricular zone progenitors. *J Neurosci* 31: 3683–3695.
Silbereis, J.C. et al. (2016). The cellular and molecular landscapes of the developing human central nervous system. *Neuron* 89: 248–268.
Singh, S. et al. (2016). Zeb1 controls neuron differentiation and germinal zone exit by a mesenchymal-epithelial-like transition. *Elife* 5: e12717. doi: 10.7554/eLife.12717.
Singh, S. and Solecki, D.J. (2015). Polarity transitions during neurogenesis and germinal zone exit in the developing central nervous system. *Front Cell Neurosci* 9: 62.

Smart, I.H.M. et al. (2002). Unique morphological features of the proliferative zones and postmitotic compartments of the neural epithelium giving rise to striate and extrastriate cortex in the monkey. *Cereb Cortex* 12: 37–53.

Sousa, A.M.M. et al. (2017). Evolution of the human nervous system function, structure, and development. *Cell* 170: 226–247.

Stahl, R. et al. (2013). Trnp1 regulates expansion and folding of the mammalian cerebral cortex by control of radial glial fate. *Cell* 153: 535–549.

Stenzel, D. et al. (2014). Integrin αvβ3 and thyroid hormones promote expansion of progenitors in embryonic neocortex. *Development* 141: 795–806.

Stepien, B.K. et al. (2020). Lengthening neurogenic period during neocortical development causes a hallmark of neocortex expansion. *Curr Biol* 30: 4227–4237.e5.

Stocker, A.M. and Chenn, A. (2015). The role of adherens junctions in the developing neocortex. *Cell Adh Mig* 9: 167–174.

Striedter, G.F. (2005). *Principles of Brain Evolution*. Sunderland, MA: Sinauer Associates.

Subramanian, L. et al. (2017). Dynamic behaviour of human neuroepithelial cells in the developing forebrain. *Nat Commun* 8: 14167.

Sudmant, P.H. et al. (2010). Diversity of human copy number variation and multicopy genes. *Science* 330: 641–646.

Suzuki, I.K. et al. (2018). Human-specific NOTCH2NL genes expand cortical neurogenesis through Delta/Notch regulation. *Cell* 173: 1370–1384.e16.

Tabata, H. and Nakajima, K. (2003). Multipolar migration: the third mode of radial neuronal migration in the developing cerebral cortex. *J Neurosci* 23: 9996–10001.

Takei, N. and Nawa, H. (2014). mTOR signaling and its roles in normal and abnormal brain development. *Front Mol Neurosci* 7: 28.

Tallinen, T. et al. (2014). Gyrification from constrained cortical expansion. *Proc Natl Acad Sci USA* 111: 12667–12672.

Tavano, S. et al. (2018). Insm1 induces neural progenitor delamination in developing neocortex via downregulation of the adherens junction belt-specific protein plekha7. *Neuron* 97: 1299–1314.e8.

Taverna, E. et al. (2014). The cell biology of neurogenesis. *Ann Rev Cell Dev Biol* 30: 465–502.

Taverna, E. and Huttner, W.B. (2010). Neural progenitor nuclei IN motion. *Neuron* 67: 906–914.

Thomsen, E.R. et al. (2016). Fixed single-cell transcriptomic characterization of human radial glial diversity. *Nat Methods* 13: 87–93.

Uebbing, S. et al. (2021). Massively parallel discovery of human-specific substitutions that alter enhancer activity. *Proc Natl Acad Sci USA* 118: e2007049118.

Uzquiano, A. et al. (2018). Cortical progenitor biology. *J Neurochem* 146: 500–525.

Vaccarino, F.M. et al. (1999). Changes in cerebral cortex size are governed by fibroblast growth factor during embryogenesis. *Nat Neurosci* 2: 848.

Vallender, E.J. et al. (2008). Genetic basis of human brain evolution. *Trends Neurosci* 31: 637–644.

Van Essen, D.C. (2020). A 2020 view of tension-based cortical morphogenesis. *Proc Natl Acad Sci USA* 117 (52): 32868–32879. doi: 10.1073/pnas.2016830117.

Varki, A. and Altheide, T.K. (2005). Comparing the human and chimpanzee genomes. *Genome Res* 15: 1746–1758.

Veeraval, L. et al. (2020). Adherens junctions: guardians of cortical development. *Front Cell Dev Biol* 8: 6.

Velasco, S. et al. (2019). Individual brain organoids reproducibly form cell diversity of the human cerebral cortex. *Nature* 570: 523–527.

Visel, A. et al. (2013). A high-resolution enhancer atlas of the developing telencephalon. *Cell* 152: 895–908. doi: 10.1016/j.cell.2012.12.041.

Vollger, M.R. et al. (2022). Segmental duplications and their variation in a complete human genome. *Science* 376: eabj6965.

Wang, L. (2016). Hedgehog signaling promotes basal progenitor expansion and the growth and folding of the neocortex. *Nat Neurosci* 19: 888–896.

Whalen, S. et al. (2023). Machine-learning dissection of human accelerated regions in primate neurodevelopment. *Neuron* 111: 857–873.e8.

Wunderlich, S. et al. (2014). Primate iPS cells as tools for evolutionary analyses. *Stem Cell Res* 12: 622–629.

Zhang, J. et al. (2010). Cortical neural precursors inhibit their own differentiation via N-cadherin maintenance of beta-catenin signaling. *Dev Cell* 18: 472–479.

3

Intermediate Progenitors in Neocortical Development and Evolution

Robert F. Hevner

Department of Pathology (Neuropathology), University of California San Diego, La Jolla, CA, USA

3.1 Definition of Intermediate Progenitors

Intermediate progenitors (IPs) are transit-amplifying cells in the developing cerebral cortex that express transcription factor Tbr2, are mitotically active, and are committed to differentiate as glutamatergic cortical neurons. They are located in the ventricular zone (VZ), the subventricular zone (SVZ), and lower intermediate zone (IZ) of developing neocortex in mammals (Englund et al. 2005; Kowalczyk et al. 2009; Miyata et al. 2004). IPs are present throughout cortical neurogenesis and generate the vast majority of glutamatergic neurons in all cortical layers, including Cajal–Retzius and subplate neurons (Kowalczyk et al. 2009; Mihalas et al. 2016).

The concept of the "transit-amplifying cell" originated from studies of epidermal keratinocyte differentiation (Watt 1988). In contrast to stem cells, transit-amplifying cells were described as "cells with a lower capacity for self-renewal and higher probability of undergoing terminal differentiation" (Jones and Watt 1993). This description aptly applies to neocortical IPs, which are also molecularly and cytologically distinct from radial glial progenitors (RGPs) – the neural stem cells of cerebral cortex during neurogenesis.

Importantly, IPs are present not only in neocortex, but also in the embryonic and postnatal hippocampus including the dentate gyrus, where they produce granule neurons (Hodge et al. 2008; Nelson et al. 2020); and in developing and postnatal subependymal zone and rostral migratory stream, where they produce some glutamatergic neurons for the olfactory bulb (Brill et al. 2009; Kahoud et al. 2014). Thus, IPs are important for neurogenesis of all pallial regions (archicortex, paleocortex, neocortex).

3.2 Historical Perspectives and the Discovery of IPs

The origins of cortical neurons have fascinated neuroscientists for more than a century, but only in the past 25 years have cortical progenitors been well characterized. In the nineteenth century, His, Cajal, and other pioneers of neuroanatomy observed that in the developing CNS, most mitotic divisions occur along the ventricular surface. They suggested that neurons are produced from rounded "germinal cells" lining the ventricles, while glial cells are derived from elongated "spongioblasts" (reviewed by Hevner 2006).

Neocortical Neurogenesis in Development and Evolution, First Edition. Edited by Wieland B. Huttner.

The first step in the discovery of IPs was the observation of abundant mitoses in the SVZ of developing cerebral cortex. In 1970, the SVZ was distinguished by consensus as an important zone of mitotic activity, especially in the cerebral hemispheres (Boulder Committee 1970). The Boulder Committee further hypothesized that cortical SVZ progenitors might produce both neurons and glia. Others hypothesized that SVZ progenitors are specialized for mainly neurogenesis (Smart 1973) or gliogenesis (Takahashi et al. 1995).

The first study to quantify abventricular mitoses (those occurring away from the ventricular surface) showed that they first appear at the onset of neurogenesis, on embryonic day (E) 10.5 in mice (Smart 1973). The SVZ became histologically distinct later (E13.5) due to progressive accumulation of abventricular progenitor cells. The same study found that most abventricular mitoses (70–80%) displayed a horizontal cleavage plane, in contrast to ventricular surface mitoses, which usually display a vertical cleavage plane (~90%). Smart (1973) concluded that "the earliest formed cells of the cortical plate probably originated from daughter cells of these peripheral mitoses." The different orientations of ventricular and abventricular mitoses were later confirmed in embryonic rat neocortex (Noctor et al. 2008).

In the period 2000 to 2010, much progress was made in definitively identifying cortical progenitor cells. Cortical projection neurons were found to arise from the pallium (cortical neuroepithelium), in contrast to interneurons (INs), which derive from subpallial progenitor zones and migrate tangentially into neocortex (Lim et al. 2018). At the onset of neurogenesis, pallial neuroepithelial cells (NECs) differentiate into RGPs, which generate neurons mainly via IPs (although NECs and RGPs may produce some early cortical neurons directly). Also, IPs were characterized as transit-amplifying cells with specific molecular and morphological properties.

Molecularly, SVZ progenitors were found to express high levels of *Svet1*, an *Unc5d* intronic RNA sequence (Sasaki et al. 2008; Tarabykin et al. 2001). Subsequently, homeobox transcription factors *Cux1* and *Cux2* were also detected at high levels in SVZ progenitors (Nieto et al. 2004; Zimmer et al. 2004). Since *Cux1* and *Cux2* are later expressed by upper layer (UL) neurons, it was hypothesized that SVZ progenitors are fated for UL neurogenesis (Nieto et al. 2004; Zimmer et al. 2004). However, other studies demonstrated that the majority of deep layer neurons are also produced from IPs (Haubensak et al. 2004; Kowalczyk et al. 2009). In 2005, transcription factor Tbr2 was identified as a specific marker of IPs (Englund et al. 2005). In 2008, the first single-cell transcriptome study of neocortical progenitors distinguished RGPs from two subtypes of Tbr2 + IPs, located in the VZ and SVZ/IZ, respectively (Kawaguchi et al. 2008).

Live-imaging microscopy of embryonic neocortex in slice cultures revealed the dynamic properties of IPs, including their origins from RGPs, and fates as PNs. In 2004, three studies showed that IPs were produced from RGPs by mitosis at the ventricular surface, and that IPs then divided in the SVZ to make neurons (Haubensak et al. 2004; Miyata et al. 2004; Noctor et al. 2004). IPs were documented at all stages of neurogenesis: early (Haubensak et al. 2004), early-middle (Miyata et al. 2004), and middle-late (Noctor et al. 2004).

3.3 Morphological Dynamics of IPs: From Apical to Basal

New IPs are initially generated by asymmetric mitosis of RGPs at the ventricular surface (Figure 3.1). For at least several hours, new IPs maintain an apical process that contacts the ventricular surface, while also extending a basal process towards the SVZ (Miyata et al. 2004). Accordingly, these new IPs typically exhibit short radial bipolar morphology in the VZ (Figure 3.1,

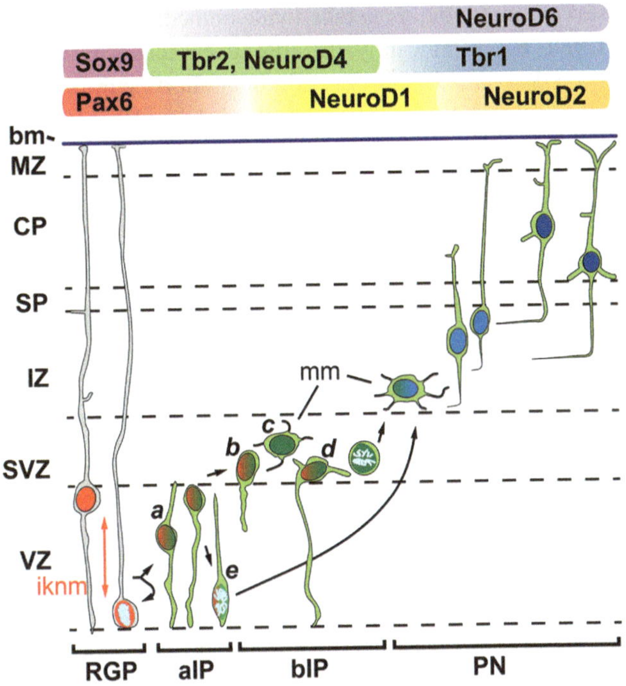

Figure 3.1 IPs are generated from RGPs and produce PNs in developing neocortex (illustrated for E14.5 mice). Stages of differentiation are indicated at the bottom; histological zones at the left; and transcription factor expression at the top. Letters indicate an aIP with short bipolar morphology (*a*), a new bIP entering the SVZ (*b*), a bIP undergoing multipolar migration (mm) in the SVZ (*c*), a bIP extending a process into the VZ (*d*), and an aIP dividing at the ventricular surface (*e*). Other abbreviations: iknm, interkinetic nuclear migration; MZ – marginal zone; CP – cortical plate; SP – subplate; IZ – intermediate zone.

cell "***a***"). The Tbr2 + IPs in the VZ have more recently been described as "apical" IPs (aIPs) (Bedogni et al. 2021). Most aIPs in embryonic mouse neocortex (60–90%, depending on the age (Kowalczyk et al. 2009)) release their apical attachment 13–23 hours after they are born (Figure 3.1, cell "***b***") (Miyata et al. 2004). These aIPs thus lose apicobasal polarity (ABP), and exit the VZ to become basal IPs (bIPs) in the SVZ.

The shift from aIP to bIP is accomplished by a form of epithelial-mesenchymal transition (EMT), in which aIPs lose ABP and acquire planar cell polarity (PCP) (Bedogni et al. 2021; Itoh et al. 2013). Upon reaching the SVZ, bIPs dynamically extend and retract short multipolar processes (Figure 3.1, cell "***c***") (Noctor et al. 2004). Such processes resemble "multipolar migration" as described for newly generated PNs (Tabata and Nakajima 2003). Indeed, *Svet1*-expressing IPs were subsequently shown to undergo multipolar migration (Sasaki et al. 2008). Also, some bIPs transiently extend a process into the VZ where they appear to contact the ventricular surface (Figure 3.1, cell "***d***") (Noctor et al. 2004). Subsequent research showed that these bIP processes often contact mitotically active RGPs, to mediate Delta-Notch signaling (Nelson et al. 2013). Eventually, bIPs divide in the VZ or SVZ to produce new projection neurons (PNs), which migrate to the inner IZ where they remain during multipolar migration, before migrating radially to reach the cortical plate.

While most aIPs migrate to the SVZ and become bIPs, a significant minority (10–30%) remain in the VZ where they retain apical surface attachment. These aIPs typically divide in the VZ at various distances from the ventricular surface, including some that divide immediately at the surface (Kowalczyk et al. 2009) (Figure 3.1, cell "*e*"). Significantly, the aIPs appear identical to other neurogenic progenitor cells that have been described in the VZ, including "short neural precursors" (SNPs) (Gal et al. 2006) and "pin-like" cells (PINs) (Ochiai et al. 2007). Like aIPs, SNPs and PINs exhibit short radial bipolar morphology and undergo neurogenic mitosis in the VZ. Since single-cell transcriptome profiling detected only RGPs and two types of IPs in embryonic mouse progenitor zones (Kawaguchi et al. 2008), SNPs and PINs are presumably identical to aIPs. The aIP terminology emphasizes that these cells have an apical attachment, and are located in relatively apical positions compared to the basal position of bIPs in the SVZ.

While bIPs lack ventricular surface attachments, they often localize adjacent to blood vessels in the SVZ (Javaherian and Kriegstein 2009; Stubbs et al. 2009). While the mechanism of this affinity is uncertain, one possibility is that IPs bind to vascular type III collagen through GPR56 (*Adgrg1*), an adhesion GPCR (G-protein coupled receptor) expressed by many IPs (Bedogni and Hevner 2021).

3.4 IP Subtypes and Transcriptomes

Transcription factor Tbr2 (NCBI Gene: *Eomes*) is expressed by aIPs and bIPs (i.e., the entire complement of IPs) throughout neurogenesis (Figure 3.2A–C) (Englund et al. 2005; Kawaguchi et al. 2008). The only other cells that express Tbr2 are Cajal–Retzius and subplate neurons, but these neurons express Tbr2 only transiently, during the preplate stage of cortical development (mouse E10.5–12.5) (Englund et al. 2005). During mid-neurogenesis (E13.5–15.5), when the SVZ becomes histologically prominent, Tbr2 + IPs accumulate in distinct histological stripes in the VZ and SVZ, representing aIPs and bIPs (Figure 3.2A, E) (Kawaguchi et al. 2008; Kowalczyk et al. 2009). During later stages of neurogenesis, Tbr2 + IPs are more widely dispersed in the VZ, SVZ, and lower IZ.

Recent molecular studies have supported the classification of IPs into aIP and bIP subtypes. During mid-corticogenesis, dozens of genes are expressed selectively by aIPs ($n = 12$), by both aIPs and bIPs ("abIP" genes; $n = 55$), or by bIPs ($n = 69$) (Figure 3.2D–E) (Bedogni and Hevner 2021). Besides *Eomes* (an abIP gene), other notable transcription factor genes expressed selectively in IPs include *Neurog2* and *Hes6* in aIPs; *Neurod4* and *Insm1* in abIPs; and *Neurod1* and *Myt1* in bIPs. Global analysis of IP-specific transcripts implicates IPs in multiple developmental functions, such as PCP and axogenesis (described in detail later).

The IP transcriptome is not homogeneous, but is modulated by spatial and temporal gradients of gene expression linked to IP maturation, laminar neurogenesis, and cortex regionalization. The differentiation of layer 4 neurons from apical progenitor mitoses on E14.5 was found to be associated with six transcriptional "waves" as cells differentiated from RGP to IP and neuron (Telley et al. 2016). Although that study focused on neurons, numerous IP-specific (or "basal progenitor"-specific) genes were also reported. At different stages of neurogenesis, maturing bIPs may express markers of layer-specific neuronal differentiation. For example, late-stage IPs express markers of upper-layer neurons (Ruan et al. 2021). These findings indicate that laminar identity is probably determined even before IPs have exited the cell cycle. This conclusion accords with previous evidence that neuronal differentiation begins in IPs, for example, as indicated by NeuN expression in mitotic IPs (Englund et al. 2005). Along the rostro-caudal axis, gradients in the expression of many genes are observed within IPs (Elsen et al. 2013).

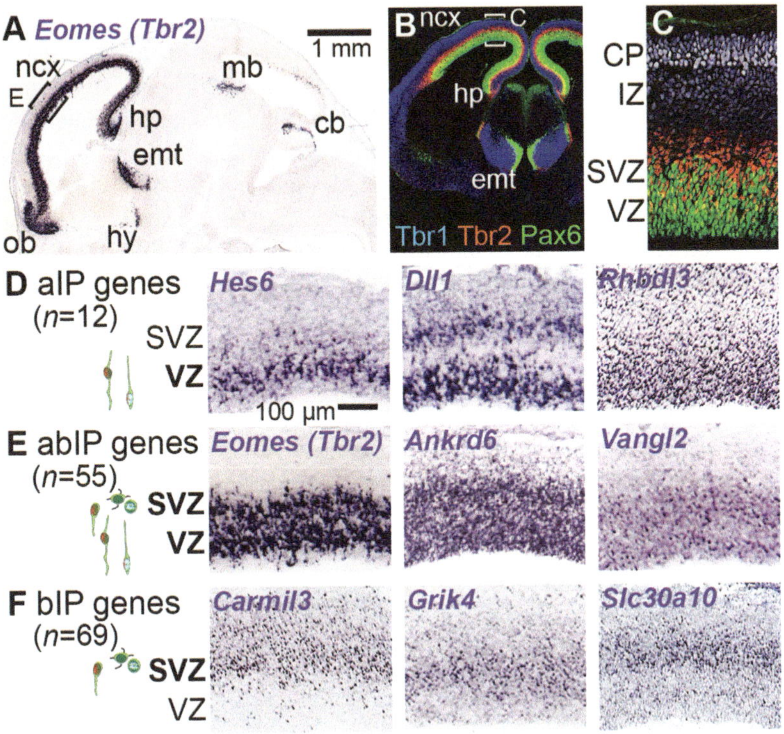

Figure 3.2 IP-selective molecular expression in E14.5 mouse neocortex. (A) *Eomes* mRNA, as detected by in situ hybridization of a sagittal brain section, is expressed in developing neocortex (ncx), olfactory bulb (ob), hippocampus (hp), eminentia thalami (emt), hypothalamus (hy), midbrain (mb), and cerebellum (cb). The bracketed area of neocortex is shown at higher magnification in (E). (B, C) Immunofluorescence detection of Pax6, Tbr2, and Tbr1 in coronal forebrain section. The bracketed area in (B) is shown at higher magnification in (C). (D) aIP-selective genes are more highly expressed in VZ than SVZ, such as *Hes6*, *Dll1*, and *Rhbdl3*. (E) abIP-selective genes display balanced expression in VZ and SVZ, including *Eomes*, *Ankrd6*, and *Vangl2*. (F) bIP-selective genes are more highly expressed in SVZ than VZ, including *Carmil3*, *Grik4*, and *Slc30a10*. The numbers of genes with each kind of selectivity are from Bedogni and Hevner (2021). In situ hybridization images (A, D, E, F) are from Genepaint (https://gp3.mpg.de).

3.5 Epigenetic Regulation and IPs

Epigenetic mechanisms regulate chromatin conformation and accessibility, to either silence or potentiate gene transcription (Hsieh and Zhao 2016; Yao et al. 2016). Many epigenetic modifications can be transmitted from parent to daughter cells across mitosis, allowing for persistent regulation of gene expression across stages of differentiation, for example from IP to PN. Moreover, conventional DNA-binding transcription factors, such as Pax6 and Tbr2, function in part by recruiting epigenetic factors to stably modify chromatin (Narayanan et al. 2018; Ninkovic et al. 2013; Sessa et al. 2017).

In developing cerebral cortex, each stage of differentiation from RGP→IP→PN is accompanied by changes in the epigenetic "landscape" of chromatin, and in the expression of specific epigenetic factors (Elsen et al. 2018). For example, abIPs specifically express Baz2a and Baz2b, components of ATP-dependent chromatin remodeling complexes in the ISWI family (Elsen et al. 2018). Indeed, all types of epigenetic mechanisms, including DNA methylation, histone covalent modifications, ATP-dependent chromatin remodeling, and noncoding RNAs such as some microRNAs, have been implicated in neocortical development (Elsen et al. 2018).

One prominent epigenetic mechanism in neocortical development involves gene silencing by histone methylation, controlled by Polycomb repressor complex 2 (PRC2) and counteracting enzymes. The PRC2 complex di- and tri-methylates histone H3 lysine 27, to deposit H3K27me3 repressive "marks" on specific regions of chromatin. PRC2-mediated gene silencing can be reversed by histone demethylase enzymes JMJD3 (*Kdm6b*) and UTX (*Kdm6a*), both of which are highly expressed in developing neocortex (Elsen et al. 2018; Lei and Jiao 2018). The transition from RGP to IP is accompanied by removal of H3K27me3 marks from the promoter regions of *Eomes* and *Neurog2*, thus releasing these genes from repression (Albert et al. 2017). Subsequently, in IPs, Tbr2 interacts with JMJD3 to guide removal of H3K27me3 marks from neuronal differentiation genes, including *Satb2* and *Tbr1* (Sessa et al. 2017). In addition, the PRC2 system regulates rostro-caudal patterning (Miró et al. 2009) and laminar neurogenesis (Telley et al. 2019).

The H3K27me3 marks placed by PRC2 can recruit another epigenetic complex, called Polycomb repressor complex 1 (PRC1), which further silences genes by depositing ubiquitin marks on histones (Tsuboi et al. 2019). Specifically, PRC1 (which can also act independently of PRC2 in some cases) mono-ubiquitylates histone H2A lysine 119 to deposit H2AK119u1 marks that drive chromatin compaction. In developing neocortex, genesis of layer 5 subcerebral projection neurons (SCPNs) is regulated by Ring1b (*Rnf2*), a ubiquitin ligase component of PRC1 that is expressed in RGPs and IPs. In mice lacking cortical Ring1b, excess layer 5 SCPNs are produced, in part because *Fezf2*, a layer 5 SCPN-specific gene, does not undergo the usual PRC1-mediated silencing (Morimoto-Suzuki et al. 2014).

Epigenetic regulation of IPs may also contribute to expansion of the neocortex, for example, in humans. Recent studies found that acetylated histone H3 lysine 9 (H3K9ac) is more abundant in human than in mouse IPs, and that this transcription-activating modification drives increased proliferation of IPs in human neocortex (Kerimoglu et al. 2021).

3.6 Regulation of IP Genesis, Amplification, and Apoptosis

The genesis, amplification, and apoptosis of IPs are controlled by a plethora of intrinsic transcriptional and epigenetic factors, as well as extrinsic signals mediated by cell-cell signaling (Bedogni and Hevner 2021).

3.6.1 IP Genesis

The initial fate choice to generate an IP is made in mitotic RGPs, which can divide *symmetrically* to produce two daughter RGPs (or less frequently, two daughter IPs), or *asymmetrically* to produce one IP and one RGP. Accordingly, molecules that drive IP genesis are expressed primarily in RGPs. Pax6, for example, is a key activator of *Eomes* transcription that is expressed mainly in RGPs, but also in new IPs (Elsen et al. 2018; Englund et al. 2005; Quinn et al. 2007). In *Pax6* null neocortex, Tbr2 levels are profoundly reduced (~2.5-fold), and abventricular mitoses are moderately decreased (Quinn et al. 2007). Another important transcriptional activator of *Eomes* is Neurogenin2, which biases RGPs towards IP genesis (Kovach et al. 2013; Ochiai et al. 2009).

Some transcription factors promote IP genesis without apparently regulating *Eomes* transcription directly. This is the case for Insm1, a transcriptional repressor that promotes the genesis and expansion of bIPs (Farkas et al. 2008). Mice with *Insm1* mutation have reduced numbers of abventricular mitoses, with equivalent reductions in Tbr2 + cells and *Eomes* mRNA levels. One key function of Insm1 is to promote IP delamination by directly repressing *Plekha7*, a component of adherens junctions at the ventricular surface (Tavano et al. 2018). Another protein that facilitates delamination is Lzts1, a leucine zipper protein that also regulates chromosome segregation (Kawaue et al. 2019). Delamination is essential for IPs to undergo EMT and thereby convert from aIPs to bIPs. Delamination is also essential for PNs generated from aIPs to exit the progenitor zones.

Given the significance of Pax6, Neurogenin2, and Insm1 in IP genesis, it is important to understand their expression patterns and interactions. Pax6 was originally proposed as a specific marker of RGPs (Götz et al. 1998). However, subsequent research showed that Pax6 is also expressed by some IPs, especially aIPs (Englund et al. 2005). Other transcription factors, such as Sox9, are more specific markers of RGPs (Kaplan et al. 2017). Neurogenin2 (*Neurog2*) expression begins in RGPs, but reaches highest levels in nascent aIPs (Bedogni and Hevner 2021; Kawaguchi et al. 2008). Transcription of *Neurog2* in neocortex is directly activated by Pax6 (Scardigli et al. 2003). The activity of Neurogenin2 protein can be blocked by Hes5, a related factor that is transcribed in RGPs in response to Notch activation (Pierfelice et al. 2011). Insm1 is expressed predominantly in aIPs and bIPs, and in IP-genic RGPs (Bedogni and Hevner 2021; Farkas et al. 2008; Kawaguchi et al. 2008).

One extrinsic factor that drives IP genesis is neutotrophin-3 (*Ntf3*), which is produced by postmitotic neurons in the cortical plate (Parthasarathy et al. 2014). In this system, neutotrophin-3 was reported to drive IP genesis from RGPs, and to drive upper layer fates.

The most potent negative regulator of IP genesis from RGPs is Delta-Notch signaling, which functions to maintain RGP stemness. Conversely, inhibition of Delta-Notch signaling rapidly induces massive differentiation of RGPs to IPs (Nelson et al. 2013; Yoon et al. 2008). Further details of Delta-Notch signaling will be given in Section 3.7 on IP functions.

The role of Tbr2 in IP genesis remains somewhat uncertain, as studies have shown different results. Complete knockout of *Eomes* in mice causes defects of trophoectoderm differentiation, resulting in failure of implantation, ultimately causing early embryonic death prior to corticogenesis (Arnold et al. 2008a). To study how Tbr2 regulates cortical development, "floxed" *Eomes* conditional knockout (cKO) mice have been produced, in which *Eomes* is inactivated only in tissues targeted by specific Cre recombinase driver genes. The first study of *Eomes* cKO cortex found that abventricular mitoses (presumptive bIPs) were significantly reduced in *Eomes*-inactivated neocortex (Sessa et al. 2008). Also, these *Eomes* cKO mice died neonatally, and exhibited complete agenesis of the corpus callosum and other forebrain commissures. However, in that study, *Foxg1*-Cre was used to recombine *Eomes*: but separately, *Foxg1*-Cre mice were found to lack IPs due to Foxg1 haploinsufficiency (Siegenthaler et al. 2008). Thus, *Eomes* cKO mice produced with *Foxg1*-Cre had underlying IP defects even before *Eomes* cKO.

Another study of *Eomes* cKO mice, recombined using *Sox1*-Cre, found that abventricular mitoses were moderately reduced. These *Eomes* cKO mice survived after birth but exhibited behavioral abnormalities, along with hypoplasia (reduced size) of the corpus callosum (Arnold et al. 2008b). While Sox1 haploinsufficiency is not currently known to affect cortical neurogenesis, *Sox1* homozygous mutations have been linked to epilepsy and defects of ventral forebrain neurogenesis (Malas et al. 2003).

A more recent study using *Nes*-Cre to recombine *Eomes* demonstrated that Tbr2 is required mainly for IP maturation, not IP genesis (Mihalas et al. 2016). In these *Eomes* cKO mice, abventricular mitoses were transiently increased (not decreased) in neocortex, and mitoses were scattered ectopically in the IZ/CP as well as VZ/SVZ. Furthermore, cells expressing Pax6 and Insm1 were increased and dispersed ectopically outside the VZ/SVZ. Since Pax6 and Insm1 are IP-genic transcription factors that are transcriptionally repressed by Tbr2 (Elsen et al. 2018), the results in these mice suggested that Tbr2 is actually required to *repress* transcriptional programs of IP genesis. The mutant mice also had a small anterior commissure, but the corpus callosum was relatively normal. Importantly, the *Nestin*-Cre transgene was inserted without disrupting the endogenous *Nes* gene, minimizing the likelihood of Cre driver effects on cortical development (Mihalas et al. 2016).

3.6.2 IP Amplification

Observations from live-slice imaging initially suggested that IPs typically divide once to generate a pair of postmitotic PNs, and do not necessarily self-amplify (Haubensak et al. 2004; Miyata et al. 2004; Noctor et al. 2004). However, alternative approaches that follow the entire developmental output of IPs, such as genetic lineage tracing, indicated that IPs may produce smaller or larger clones between 1–32 PNs (Mihalas et al. 2018; Vasistha et al. 2015; Wu et al. 2005). The most precise method of clonal analysis, called mosaic analysis with double markers (MADM), indicated that IPs produce clones of 1–12 PNs, which may occupy multiple layers of cortex (Mihalas et al. 2018). The genesis of different layer PNs from individual IPs showed that IPs are not committed to produce a single laminar fate. Surprisingly, most IPs (~2/3) produced clones consisting of only a single PN, indicating that the other daughter cell underwent apoptosis (Mihalas et al. 2018). Thus, both amplification and apoptosis may regulate neurogenesis from IPs. As mentioned above, Insm1 may promote amplification as well as genesis of IPs, although the mechanisms of this regulation are unclear (Farkas et al. 2008). Transcription factor Cux-2 is reported to restrict IP proliferation, such that Cux-2 deficient mice have increased IP proliferation and generation of upper layer neurons (Cubelos et al. 2008). Another molecule that may promote IP amplification is Boc, a Shh co-receptor that promotes symmetric progenitor divisions, and is selectively expressed by aIPs (Araújo et al. 2014; Bedogni and Hevner 2021).

3.6.3 IP Apoptosis

The factors that control apoptosis of IPs and daughter PNs are poorly understood. Studies have shown that apoptosis occurs in the embryonic VZ/SVZ, but its reported prevalence appears highly variable (Blaschke et al. 1996; Thomaidou et al. 1997). Interestingly, apoptosis of IPs and daughter cells may be triggered by microglia, which have been observed ingesting Tbr2+ cells in the embryonic VZ/SVZ (Cunningham et al. 2013). Microglia-mediated apoptosis of new neurons has also been documented in the developing and adult hippocampus (Sierra et al. 2010; Wakselman et al. 2008). Developmental apoptosis of single daughter cells, as observed in IP lineages (Mihalas and Hevner 2018), may be a "binary cell death decision" as in other systems, for example, developing *Drosophila* sensory organs where asymmetric inheritance of Numb has been linked to cell survival (Orgogozo et al. 2002). Besides modulating cell numbers, apoptosis may also function in cellular quality control, and in tissue morphogenesis (Voss and Strasser 2020). Indeed, the forces generated by apoptosis induce epithelial folding in *Drosophila* (Monier and Suzanne 2021). This raises the possibility that apoptosis might have a role in folding of the cerebral cortex, not only by modulating the number of locally generated PNs, but also by generating mechanical forces within the cortical mantle.

3.7 Developmental Functions of IPs

The discovery of IPs quickly prompted novel hypotheses about their possible roles in upper layer neurogenesis (Nieto et al. 2004; Zimmer et al. 2004), and evolutionary cerebral expansion and gyrification (Kriegstein et al. 2006). In subsequent years, IPs have emerged as key mediators of several important functions (Figure 3.3).

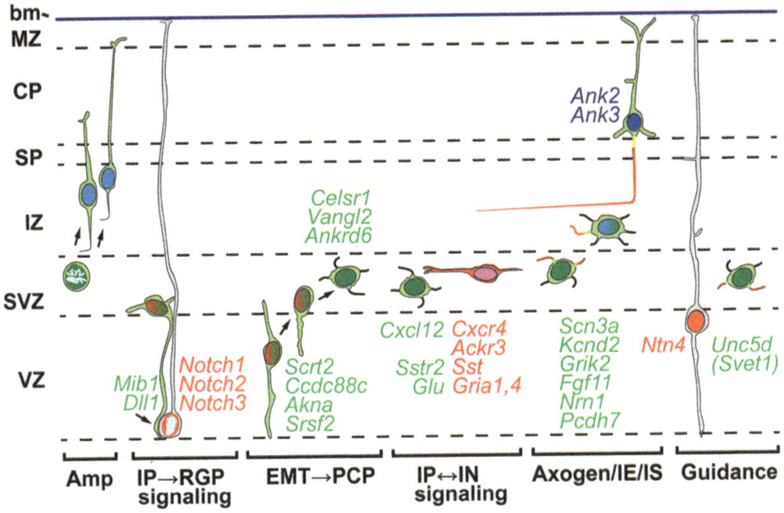

Figure 3.3 Developmental functions of IPs include amplification (Amp) of neurogenesis; IP-RGP signaling; EMT; PCP; IP-IN signaling; initiation of axogenesis (Axo), intrinsic excitability (IE), and initial segment (IS) formation; axon guidance/polarization; and rostro-caudal patterning (not shown). Some of the genes implicated in each function are shown, with IP-selective genes in green, and genes expressed by IP-interacting cell types in red. Definitive markers of initial segment formation (*Ank2*, *Ank3*) are not expressed in IPs, but are expressed in postmitotic PNs. Abbreviations: MZ – marginal zone; CP – cortical plate; SP – subplate; IZ – intermediate zone; SVZ – subventricular zone; VZ – ventricular zone.

3.7.1 Upper Layer Hypothesis

The "upper layer hypothesis" of IP commitment to upper layer neurogenesis is contradicted by multiple studies showing that IPs produce PNs for all cortical layers (Haubensak et al. 2004; Kowalczyk et al. 2009; Pontious et al. 2008). Indeed, clonal analysis has revealed that an individual IP can produce PNs for multiple cortical layers, and therefore are not committed to a specific laminar fate (Mihalas and Hevner 2018). On the other hand, one recent study appeared to indicate that most deep layer neurons are produced directly from RGPs (Cárdenas et al. 2018). However, the experiments in that study were predicated on the assumption that RGPs are the only progenitors that contact the ventricular surface. But as reviewed above, aIPs have apical processes that contact the ventricular surface, make adherens junctions, and have plasma membrane exposed to the ventricle (Gal et al. 2006; Kowalczyk et al. 2009; Miyata et al. 2004). Ventricular contacts are lost only when IPs enter the SVZ and differentiate as bIPs. The related proposal that upper layer neurons are a special feature of mammalian cortex that evolved concurrently with IPs has likewise been contradicted, by studies showing that chicken brains also contain upper layer-like neurons, albeit organized in nuclear clusters rather than layers (Suzuki et al. 2012). Also, it is not clear that IPs are restricted to mammals, as reviewed below in the section on IP evolution.

3.7.2 Radial Amplification of PNs

The idea that IPs serve to amplify neurogenesis from RGPs, dubbed the "radial amplification hypothesis" (Pontious et al. 2008), has been clouded by evidence that most IPs produce only a single PN, at least in mice (Mihalas and Hevner 2018). In this case, the neurogenic output from an RGP would be the same by IP-mediated neurogenesis as by direct neurogenesis. A more compelling case may be made that abventricular IP mitoses reduce crowding of the VZ, as suggested decades ago (Smart 1973). However, the previous observations apply to mice, while the development of larger brains (such as human) might require greater amplification of IPs (Kriegstein et al. 2006). Another potential advantage of producing multiple PNs from a single IP could also be that the impact of de novo mutations in progenitor cells may be minimized, since IPs generate smaller cohorts of PNs than do RGPs (Gao et al. 2014; Kaplan et al. 2017; Mihalas and Hevner 2018).

3.7.3 Gyrification

Larger mammalian brains, as in ferrets and humans, generally have surface gyri that could theoretically arise in part by spatially regulated amplification of IPs. Indeed, increased numbers of IPs have been observed beneath prospective gyri in the developing brains of ferrets (Toda et al. 2016). On the other hand, gyrus formation is a complex process that involves multiple mechanisms, including passive folding of the entire cerebral wall in some cases (e.g., medial temporal lobe), as well as "gyrogenesis" or "gyrus-building" by local thickening of the cerebral wall (Sun and Hevner 2014). Presumably, IPs contribute to the formation of many but not all gyri.

3.7.4 Delta-Notch Signaling

The balance between RGP self-amplification (retaining stemness) and differentiation to produce IPs is potently regulated by Delta-Notch signaling, an evolutionarily conserved mechanism of balanced cell differentiation (Pierfelice et al. 2011) (Figure 3.3). In developing cerebral cortex, RGPs express Notch receptors (Notch1–3) that detect Delta ligands (especially Delta-like-1, or Dll1) presented by IPs (Nelson et al. 2013). For Dll1 to effectively activate Notch receptors, the Dll1 must be modified by Mib1, a ubiquitin E3 ligase (Yoon et al. 2008). Both Dll1 and Mib1 are selectively expressed by IPs, making IPs the most effective drivers of active Dll1 expression and Notch signaling (Bedogni and Hevner 2021; Nelson et al. 2013). The Dll1 ligands are presented to dividing RGPs by IP processes that extend through the VZ (Nelson et al. 2013). The extension of IP processes that contact the ventricular surface was previously interpreted as a stage of IP cell migration (Noctor et al. 2004). Interference with Delta-Notch signaling, by *Mib1* inactivation or by chemical inhibition, causes rapid differentiation of RGPs to Tbr2+ IPs (Nelson et al. 2013; Yoon et al. 2008). In humans, where basal RGPs (bRGPs) in the OSVZ play a prominent role in neurogenesis, the bRGPs are likewise dependent on Delta-Notch signaling (Hansen et al. 2010), presumably from IPs.

3.7.5 Epithelial-mesenchymal Transition and Planar Cell Polarity

As aIPs migrate to the SVZ and become bIPs, they undergo a type of EMT, which results in loss of ABP and gain of PCP (Bedogni and Hevner 2021; Itoh et al. 2013). New PNs generated from aIPs likewise undergo this change in polarity. The initial state of ABP is inherited from RGPs, which have adherens junctions that not only anchor the RGP to the ventricular surface, but also divide the RGP into basolateral and apical compartments. The apical surface of the RGP is in fact very small, accounting for only ~ 1 percent of the total plasma membrane surface area, while the basolateral compartment of the RGP is much larger, as it extends from the VZ to the pial surface (Taverna et al. 2014). The adherens junctions on newly generated aIPs may subsequently be lost in the transition to bIP, or retained for those aIPs that persist in the VZ (Gal et al. 2006). In other systems, the process of EMT has been associated with specific genes, such as *Scrt2*, *Ccdc88c*, *Akna*, and *Srsf2*, which are all selectively expressed by IPs (Bedogni and Hevner 2021; Itoh et al. 2013). As EMT progresses, IPs and new PNs downregulate RGP-selective genes that support ABP, and upregulate genes that support PCP, including IP-selective *Celsr1*, *Vangl2*, and *Ankrd6* (Bedogni and Hevner 2021). Indeed, IPs express a full complement of "core" PCP genes that may orient IPs along tangential axes within the cerebral wall. Core PCP components may potentially be organized in IPs by Wnt-PCP signaling, as Wnt signaling is graded along tangential axes (Bedogni and Hevner 2021; Machon et al. 2007). One potential function of PCP in IPs and new PNs is to polarize cells for axon selection and orientation, as reviewed next.

3.7.6 IPs in Axon Development

Previous studies have shown that IPs express many molecules that are important in axogenesis, axon guidance, and axon physiology. The Wnt-PCP pathway is among these. Wnt-PCP signaling orients axon growth in *C. elegans* and zebrafish (Ackley 2014; Sun et al. 2016), and is essential for the development of cortical axon pathways (Qu et al. 2014; Wang et al. 2002). Another IP-selective molecule that may orient axon growth is netrin receptor Unc5d, which may respond to netrin-4, produced by RGPs in a high-rostral gradient (Bedogni and Hevner 2021). Axon development may also be promoted by IP expression of molecules that mediate *intrinsic excitability* and *initial segment* differentiation, including sodium channel Scn3a, potassium channel Kcnd2, and glutamate receptor Grik2 (Bedogni and Hevner 2021; Smith et al. 2018). A role for IPs in axon development may seem counterintuitive because IPs are dividing and do not have an axon. However, studies in other systems have demonstrated that axon specification and orientation can begin in progenitor cells (Adler et al. 2006; Killeen and Sybingco 2008). In chick neural crest, for example, progenitor cell polarity can be "inherited" by daughter neurons through a mechanism involving Septin7, which localizes to membrane sites designated for process outgrowth (Boubakar et al. 2017). In neocortex, Septin7 is known to be essential for callosal and corticospinal axon development (Ageta-Ishihara et al. 2013). These observations suggest that IPs may serve to "prime" daughter PNs for axon development. Consistent with this idea, bIPs extend and retract short multipolar processes (Noctor et al. 2004), apparently as a form of "multipolar migration" (Sasaki et al. 2008). In fact, "multipolar migration" is associated with little or no translational movement of the cell body (Tabata and Nakajima 2003), but more likely represents exploration of the local environment by IPs and newly generated PNs to identify appropriate existing axons with which to directionally fasciculate. This proposed mechanism is known as the "touch-and-go" model of neocortical axon growth (Namba et al. 2014).

3.7.7 Interneuron Guidance and Reciprocal Signaling

Unlike PNs, neocortical GABAergic INs are produced in the subcortical ganglionic eminences, and migrate tangentially into neocortex through streams in the marginal zone, subplate, and SVZ (Lim et al. 2018). Migration of INs through the SVZ stream is guided by IPs that secrete SDF-1 (*Cxcl12*), which attracts INs that express the cognate receptors Cxcr4 and Ackr3 (Sessa et al. 2010; Wang et al. 2011). The production of SDF-1 by IPs is dependent on Tbr2 (Sessa et al. 2010). Further interactions between IPs and INs are suggested by transcriptome profiling: IPs express the molecular machinery to package and release glutamate, while INs express glutamate receptors Gria1 and Gria4 (Bedogni and Hevner 2021). Thus, IPs may secrete glutamate to activate ion currents in INs, although the purpose of such signaling is unknown. Conversely, many migrating INs produce the neuropeptide somatostatin, while bIPs express somatostatin receptor Sstr2 (Bedogni and Hevner 2021; Kawaguchi et al. 2008). The significance of this potential signaling from INs to IPs is likewise unknown.

3.7.8 IPs in Rostro-caudal Patterning

The general layout of cortical areas (motor areas rostral, sensory areas caudal) is defined by intrinsic patterning of the cortical neuroepithelium (or pallium), and subsequent interactions with inputs such as thalamocortical projections (O'Leary et al. 2007). Signaling centers around the pallium secrete factors that induce transcription factor gradients to form a "protomap" of cortical areas in NECs and RGPs. As IPs are generated from these less differentiated precursors, transcription factors that define the protomap are downregulated, and IPs instead express other molecular gradients that define an "intermediate map" of cortical regions (Elsen et al. 2013). The intermediate map is defined and regulated in part by Tbr2, which is expressed in a high rostral–low caudal gradient. Deficiency of Tbr2 in *Eomes* cKO mice disrupts rostro-caudal patterning, such that rostral differentiation is decreased and caudal differentiation is increased (Elsen et al. 2013). The intermediate map is in turn translated to cortical PNs, which express another distinct set of molecular gradients. Among these, Tbr1 is expressed in a high rostral-low caudal gradient, and deficiency of Tbr1 also disrupts cortical patterning (Bedogni et al. 2010).

3.8 IPs, Tbr2, and Cerebral Cortex Evolution

To determine the evolutionary origins of cortical IPs, many comparative studies have examined Tbr2 expression, abventricular mitoses, and SVZ histology in the developing forebrain of diverse vertebrate species (Table 3.1). However, the evolutionary picture is not yet clear, as not all studies agree. Rigorously defined, IPs are mitotically active Tbr2 + cells, but not all previous studies have shown colocalization of Tbr2 with mitotic markers.

3.8.1 Mammals

Tbr2 + IPs appear to be present in all placental (eutherian) mammals, but the evidence is less clear for marsupial (metatherian) and monotreme (prototherian) mammals. Each group is reviewed separately next.

Table 3.1 Tbr2 and progenitor cells in neocortex (or equivalent) of diverse vertebrates.[1]

Taxon	Species	Scientific name	Tbr2 in VZ	Tbr2 in SVZ	Basal mitoses	Basal IPs	Basal RGPs
Placental mammals	Human	*Homo sapiens*	+	+	+	+	+
	Macaque	*Macaca mulatta*	+	+	+	+	+
	Marmoset	*Callithrix jacchus*	+	+	+	+	+
	Ferret	*Mustela furo*	+	+	+	+	+
	Rat	*Rattus norvegicus*	+	+	+	+	+
	Mouse	*Mus musculus*	+	+	+	+	+
Marsupial mammals	Opossum	*Monodelphis domestica*	+	+	+	± (rare)	+
	Tammar wallaby	*Macropus eugenii*	+	+	+	+	+
Monotreme mammals	Platypus	*Ornithorhynchus anatinus*	unk	unk	+	unk	unk
	Short-beaked echidna	*Tachyglossus aculeatus*	unk	unk	+	unk	unk

Table 3.1 (Continued)

Taxon	Species	Scientific name	Tbr2 in VZ	Tbr2 in SVZ	Basal mitoses	Basal IPs	Basal RGPs
Birds	Chicken	*Gallus gallus domesticus*	+	+	+	±[2]	+
	Mourning dove	*Zenaida macroura*	+	+	unk	unk	unk
Crocodilian reptiles	American alligator	*Alligator mississipiensis*	unk	unk	–	–	–
Testudine reptiles	Red-eared slider turtle	*Trachemys scripta elegans*	+	+	+	±[3]	unk
	European pond turtle	*Emys orbicularis*	unk	unk	+	unk	unk
Lepidosaur reptiles	Madagascar gecko	*Paroedura pictus*	+	–	–	–	–
	Green anole lizard	*Anolis carolinensis*	+	–	–	–	–
	African house snake	*Lamprophis fuliginosus*	unk	unk	–	–	–
Amphibians	African clawed frog	*Xenopus laevis*	+	+	+	–	unk
	Axolotl	*Ambystoma mexicanum*	unk	unk	+	unk	unk
Bony fish	Zebrafish	*Danio rerio*	+	+	+	–[4]	unk
Cartilaginous fish	Small-spotted catshark	*Scyliorhinus canicula*	+	+	+	±[5]	unk

[1] See text for references. Abbreviations: unk, unknown.
[2] Tbr2/pH3 double labeled cells seen only on induction by electroporation with dnR1/2 + Dll1 (Cárdenas et al. 2018); Tbr2/BrdU double labeling was shown at low mag only (Suzuki et al. 2012); Tbr2 with condensed chromatin was not illustrated (Martínez-Cerdeño et al. 2016).
[3] Tbr2/PCNA double IHC was used (Clinton et al. 2014; Martínez-Cerdeño et al. 2016).
[4] A single basal mitosis weakly expressed Tbr2 reporter (McIntosh et al. 2017).
[5] Tbr2 ISH/PH3 IHC (Docampo-Seara et al. 2018).

3.8.1.1 Eutheria

Tbr2 + IPs have been demonstrated with high confidence across diverse groups including rodents, carnivores, and primates including humans (Englund et al. 2005; Fietz et al. 2010; Hansen et al. 2010; Martínez-Cerdeño et al. 2012; Noctor et al. 2008; Toda et al. 2016). Humans and some other species have more complex progenitor zones than mice, but the essential properties of IPs appear to be conserved among eutherians.

3.8.1.2 Metatheria

Opossums and wallabies have basal mitoses, and show Tbr2 expression in the VZ and presumptive SVZ (Cheung et al. 2010; Nomura et al. 2016; Puzzolo and Mallamaci 2010; Sauerland et al. 2018). Wallabies were shown to have IPs by Tbr2 colocalization with mitotic markers (Sauerland et al. 2018). In contrast, mitotically active Tbr2 + IPs were described as "extremely rare" in opossums (Puzzolo and Mallamaci 2010). Rather, in opossums, most basal progenitors expressed Pax6 or Sox2, consistent with bRGPs. The discrepancy between opossums and wallabies suggests that not all marsupials have IPs.

3.8.1.3 Prototheria

Echidna and platypus exhibit numerous basal mitotic figures in the developing neocortex (Ashwell and Hardman 2012). However, no studies of Tbr2 expression in monotremes have been reported.

3.8.2 Birds

In embryonic chick and mourning dove, Tbr2 is expressed by cells in an SVZ-like distribution, and basal mitoses have been documented in the developing chick (Cheung et al. 2007; Nomura et al. 2016; Suzuki et al. 2012). One study in chicks found that Tbr2 colocalized with acute BrdU, although confocal microscopy was not done (Suzuki et al. 2012). Another study reported that some Tbr2 + cells in chicks had condensed chromatin indicating mitosis, but this result was not illustrated (Martínez-Cerdeño et al. 2016). In another study, colocalization of Tbr2 with pH3 was observed in chick pallium only after electroporation of the developing pallium with plasmids that modified Robo1/2 and Dll1 expression (dnR1/2 + Dll1) (Cárdenas et al. 2018). Yet another study in chicks found no colocalization of Tbr2 with acute BrdU or pH3, but instead found that basal mitoses expressed markers of bRGPs (Nomura et al. 2016). The latter was the only study in birds that utilized confocal microscopy. Overall, the presence or absence of IPs in birds remains uncertain, and further research is needed.

3.8.3 Reptiles

Alligators, which are more closely related to birds than to other reptiles (Cárdenas and Borrell 2020), display no basal mitoses in the developing pallium (Charvet et al. 2009). No data on Tbr2 expression in alligators is available. Turtles, in contrast, do exhibit basal mitoses, and express Tbr2 in the VZ as well as a rudimentary SVZ-like zone (Cheung et al. 2007; Clinton et al. 2014; Martínez-Cerdeño et al. 2016, 2006). However, data on whether the Tbr2+ cells in turtle pallium are mitotically active seem inconclusive. Some studies of developing turtle illustrated a few cells with colocalization of Tbr2 and PCNA, but no other markers of mitotic activity (Clinton et al. 2014; Martínez-Cerdeño et al. 2016). These studies were not definitive, because PCNA has a relatively long half-life and can be detected in postmitotic cells that recently divided (Allegranza et al. 1991). In lizards and snakes, Tbr2 expression appears limited to the VZ, and no basal mitoses are detected (Cárdenas et al. 2018; Martínez-Cerdeño et al. 2016; Nomura et al. 2013). In geckos, Tbr2+ cells showed no colocalization with acute BrdU (Nomura et al. 2013). One study stated that "mitotic Tbr2+ cells are present in the prenatal cortex of lizard" but showed no supportive evidence (Martínez-Cerdeño et al. 2016). Thus, in reptiles as in birds, more research is needed to definitively assess the presence or absence of IPs.

3.8.4 Amphibians

Basal mitotic figures have been documented in the developing frog and axolotl pallium, and Tbr2 in developing frogs is expressed in VZ and SVZ-like patterns (Moreno and González 2017; Nomura et al. 2016). However, Tbr2 did not colocalize with acute BrdU in frog pallium, and it was concluded that the Tbr2 + cells were "not mitotic" (Moreno and González 2017). Thus, IPs may not be present in amphibian pallium.

3.8.5 Fish

Remarkably, VZ and SVZ-like expression of Tbr2 has been documented in the developing pallium of a bony fish (zebrafish) and a cartilaginous fish (catshark), indicating that this transcription factor has been involved in the regulation of pallial neurogenesis at least since the origin of gnathostomes (Docampo-Seara et al. 2018; McIntosh et al. 2017; Mione et al. 2001). In zebrafish, no Tbr2 + mitotically active cells were observed by multiple methods, except a single dividing cell (among dozens of mitoses monitored) with low-level expression of a fluorescent Tbr2 reporter by live imaging (possibly representing the onset of glutamatergic neuronal differentiation coinciding with the end of RGP mitosis) (McIntosh et al. 2017). Thus, zebrafish appear to lack IPs. In catshark, some pH3 + cells appeared to express *Tbr2* mRNA, as observed by in situ hybridization (ISH), in embryonic but not juvenile or adult pallium (Docampo-Seara et al. 2018, 2020). The studies in embryonic catshark suggest that Tbr2 + IPs may have arisen in the common ancestors of all gnathostomes.

3.8.6 Conclusions on the Evolution of IPs

Further studies will be necessary to replicate and expand on previous comparative studies, but two major conclusions are currently possible. First, IPs appear to be present in all placental mammals. Second, Tbr2 has been part of the pallial neurogenic program at least since the origin of gnathostomes, possibly in IPs but also possibly in newly postmitotic neurons. In future research, more rigorous documentation of Tbr2 colocalization with markers of proliferation will be beneficial. The most rigorous studies should test several markers of proliferation (not only PCNA) for colocalization with Tbr2, and should document colocalization at high magnification in confocal planes. Until we know with high confidence when IPs arose in evolution, their relevance to mammalian-specific features such as gyrencephaly and laminar organization will remain uncertain.

3.9 IPs and Human Brain Malformations

Genetic analysis of an autosomal recessive microcephaly syndrome found that it was caused by a chromosomal translocation [t(3;10)(p24;q23)] that silenced brain expression of *EOMES* (Baala et al. 2007). In addition to severe microcephaly, affected individuals exhibited agenesis of the corpus callosum, polymicrogyria, and ventriculomegaly, and usually died in early childhood. As TBR2 is specifically expressed by IPs in developing human neocortex (Hansen et al. 2010), mutations that silence *EOMES* primarily disrupt IP development.

3.10 Future Directions

Many gaps remain in our knowledge of IPs in cortical development and evolution. Regarding development, further studies of IP roles in axogenesis are needed. The possibility that IPs are polarized by axon guidance molecules and Wnt-PCP signaling merits investigation, for example, to determine if PCP proteins are asymmetrically distributed on IPs in vivo. The possible influences of IP and daughter PN apoptosis on neurogenesis and force generation need further study, and the role of IPs in gyrus development should be examined in more species. The full range of interactions between IPs and INs, especially the potential effects of glutamate and somatostatin signaling, remain to be characterized. Regarding evolution, more species must be examined, and more attention should be paid to rigorous colocalization of Tbr2 with proliferation markers. Given the many roles of IPs in cortical development that have already been documented, it would not be surprising if novel functions are discovered as well.

References

Ackley, B.D. (2014). Wnt-signaling and planar cell polarity genes regulate axon guidance along the anteroposterior axis in C. elegans. *Dev Neurobiol* 74 (8): 781–796. doi: 10.1002/dneu.22146.

Adler, C.E. et al. (2006). UNC-6/Netrin induces neuronal asymmetry and defines the site of axon formation. *Nat Neurosci* 9 (4): 511–518. doi: 10.1038/nn1666.

Ageta-Ishihara, N. et al. (2013). Septins promote dendrite and axon development by negatively regulating microtubule stability via HDAC6-mediated deacetylation. *Nat Commun* 4: 2532. doi: 10.1038/ncomms3532.

Albert, M. et al. (2017). Epigenome profiling and editing of neocortical progenitor cells during development. *EMBO J* 36 (17): 2642–2658. doi: 10.15252/embj.201796764.

Allegranza, A. et al. (1991). Proliferating cell nuclear antigen expression in central nervous system neoplasms. *Virchows Arch A, Pathol Anat Histopathol* 419 (5): 417–423. doi: 10.1007/BF01605076.

Araújo, G.L. et al. (2014). Sonic hedgehog signaling regulates mode of cell division of early cerebral cortex progenitors and increases astrogliogenesis. *Front Cell Neurosci* 8: 77. doi: 10.3389/fncel.2014.00077.

Arnold, S.J. et al. (2008a). Pivotal roles for eomesodermin during axis formation, epithelium-to-mesenchyme transition and endoderm specification in the mouse. *Development* 135 (3): 501–511. doi: 10.1242/dev.014357.

Arnold, S.J. et al. (2008b). The T-box transcription factor Eomes/Tbr2 regulates neurogenesis in the cortical subventricular zone. *Genes Dev* 22 (18): 2479–2484. doi: 10.1101/gad.475408.

Ashwell, K.W. and Hardman, C.D. (2012). Distinct development of the cerebral cortex in platypus and echidna. *Brain, Behav Evol* 79 (1): 57–72. doi: 10.1159/000334188.

Baala, L. et al. (2007). Homozygous silencing of T-box transcription factor *EOMES* leads to microcephaly with polymicrogyria and corpus callosum agenesis. *Nat Genet* 39 (4): 454–456. doi: 10.1038/ng1993.

Bedogni, F. and Hevner, R.F. (2021). Cell-type-specific gene expression in developing mouse neocortex. *Front Mol Neurosci* 14: 686034. doi: 10.3389/fnmol.2021.686034.

Bedogni, F. et al. (2010). Tbr1 regulates regional and laminar identity of postmitotic neurons in developing neocortex. *Proc Natl Acad Sci USA* 107 (29): 13129–13134. doi: 10.1073/pnas.1002285107.

Blaschke, A.J. et al. (1996). Widespread programmed cell death in proliferative and postmitotic regions of the fetal cerebral cortex. *Development* 122 (4): 1165–1174. doi: 10.1242/dev.122.4.1165.

Boubakar, L. et al. (2017). Molecular memory of morphologies by septins during neuron generation allows early polarity inheritance. *Neuron* 95 (4): 834–851.e5. doi: 10.1016/j.neuron.2017.07.027.

Boulder Committee. (1970). Embryonic vertebrate central nervous system: revised terminology. *Anat Record* 166 (2): 257–261. doi: 10.1002/ar.1091660214.

Brill, M.S. et al. (2009). Adult generation of glutamatergic olfactory bulb interneurons. *Nat Neurosci* 12 (12): 1524–1533. doi: 10.1038/nn.2416.

Bulfone, A. et al. (1999). Expression pattern of the Tbr2 (Eomesodermin) gene during mouse and chick brain development. *Mech Dev* 84 (1–2): 133–138. doi: 10.1016/s0925-4773(99)00053-2.

Cárdenas, A. and Borrell, V. (2020). Molecular and cellular evolution of corticogenesis in amniotes. *Cell Mol Life Sci* 77 (8): 1435–1460. doi: 10.1007/s00018-019-03315-x.

Cárdenas, A. et al. (2018). Evolution of cortical neurogenesis in amniotes controlled by Robo signaling levels. *Cell* 174 (3): 590–606.e21. doi: 10.1016/j.cell.2018.06.007.

Charvet, C.J. et al. (2009). Phylogeny of the telencephalic subventricular zone in sauropsids. *Brain, Behav Evol* 73 (4): 285–294. doi: 10.1159/000230673.

Cheung, A.F. et al. (2010). The subventricular zone is the developmental milestone of a 6-layered neocortex. *Cereb Cortex* 20 (5): 1071–1081. doi: 10.1093/cercor/bhp168.

Cheung, A.F. et al. (2007). Comparative aspects of cortical neurogenesis in vertebrates. *J Anat* 211 (2): 164–176. doi: 10.1111/j.1469-7580.2007.00769.x.

Clinton, B.K. et al. (2014). Radial glia in the proliferative ventricular zone of the embryonic and adult turtle, Trachemys scripta elegans. *Neurogenesis (Austin)* 1 (1): e970905. doi: 10.4161/23262125.2014.970905.

Cubelos, B. et al. (2008). Cux-2 controls the proliferation of neuronal intermediate precursors of the cortical subventricular zone. *Cereb Cortex* 18 (8): 1758–1770. doi: 10.1093/cercor/bhm199.

Cunningham, C.L. et al. (2013 March 6). Microglia regulate the number of neural precursor cells in the developing cerebral cortex. *J Neurosci* 33 (10): 4216–4233. doi: 10.1523/JNEUROSCI.3441-12.2013.

Docampo-Seara, A. et al. (2018). Study of pallial neurogenesis in shark embryos and the evolutionary origin of the subventricular zone. *Brain Struct Funct* 223 (8): 3593–3612. doi: 10.1007/s00429-018-1705-2.

Docampo-Seara, A. et al. (2020). Characterization of neurogenic niches in the telencephalon of juvenile and adult sharks. *Brain Struct Funct* 225 (2): 817–839. doi: 10.1007/s00429-020-02038-1.

Elsen, G.E. et al. (2018). The epigenetic factor landscape of developing neocortex is regulated by transcription factors Pax6→ Tbr2→ Tbr1. *Front Neurosci* 12: 571. doi: 10.3389/fnins.2018.00571.

Elsen, G.E. et al. (2013). The protomap is propagated to cortical plate neurons through an Eomes-dependent intermediate map. *Proc Natl Acad Sci USA* 110 (10): 4081–4086. doi: 10.1073/pnas.1209076110.

Englund, C. et al. (2005). Pax6, Tbr2, and Tbr1 are expressed sequentially by radial glia, intermediate progenitor cells, and postmitotic neurons in developing neocortex. *J Neurosci* 25 (1): 247–251. doi: 10.1523/JNEUROSCI.2899-04.2005.

Farkas, L.M. et al. (2008). Insulinoma-associated 1 has a panneurogenic role and promotes the generation and expansion of basal progenitors in the developing mouse neocortex. *Neuron* 60 (1): 40–55. doi: 10.1016/j.neuron.2008.09.020.

Fietz, S.A. et al. (2010). OSVZ progenitors of human and ferret neocortex are epithelial-like and expand by integrin signaling. *Nat Neurosci* 13 (6): 690–699. doi: 10.1038/nn.2553.

Gal, J.S. et al. (2006). Molecular and morphological heterogeneity of neural precursors in the mouse neocortical proliferative zones. *J Neurosci* 26 (3): 1045–1056. doi: 10.1523/JNEUROSCI.4499-05.2006.

Gao, P. et al. (2014 November 6). Deterministic progenitor behavior and unitary production of neurons in the neocortex. *Cell* 159 (4): 775–788. doi: 10.1016/j.cell.2014.10.027.

Götz, M. et al. (1998). Pax6 controls radial glia differentiation in the cerebral cortex. *Neuron* 21 (5): 1031–1044. doi: 10.1016/s0896-6273(00)80621-2.

Hansen, D.V. et al. (2010). Neurogenic radial glia in the outer subventricular zone of human neocortex. *Nature* 464 (7288): 554–561. doi: 10.1038/nature08845.

Haubensak, W. et al. (2004). Neurons arise in the basal neuroepithelium of the early mammalian telencephalon. *Proc Natl Acad Sci USA* 101 (9): 3196–3201. doi: 10.1073/pnas.0308600100.

Hevner, R.F. (2006). From radial glia to pyramidal-projection neuron. *Mol Neurobiol* 33 (1): 33–50. doi: 10.1385/MN:33:1:033.

Hodge, R.D. et al. (2008). Intermediate progenitors in adult hippocampal neurogenesis. *J Neurosci* 28 (14): 3707–3717. doi: 10.1523/JNEUROSCI.4280-07.2008.

Hsieh, J. and Zhao, X. (2016). Genetics and epigenetics in adult neurogenesis. *Cold Spring Harb Perspect Biol* 8 (6): a018911. doi: 10.1101/cshperspect.a018911.

Itoh, Y. et al. (2013). Scratch regulates neuronal migration onset via an epithelial-mesenchymal transition-like mechanism. *Nat Neurosci* 16 (4): 416–425. doi: 10.1038/nn.3336.

Javaherian, A. and Kriegstein, A. (2009). A stem cell niche for intermediate progenitor cells of the embryonic cortex. *Cereb Cortex* 19 (Suppl 1): i70–7. doi: 10.1093/cercor/bhp029.

Jones, P.H. and Watt, F.M. (1993). Separation of human epidermal stem cells from transit amplifying cells on the basis of differences in integrin function and expression. *Cell* 73 (4): 713–724. doi: 10.1016/0092-8674(93)90251-k.

Kahoud, R.J. et al. (2014). Conditional ablation of Tbr2 results in abnormal development of the olfactory bulbs and subventricular zone-rostral migratory stream. *Dev Dyn* 243 (3): 440–450. doi: 10.1002/dvdy.24090.

Kaplan, E.S. et al. (2017). Neocortical Sox9+ radial glia generate glutamatergic neurons for all layers, but lack discernible evidence of early laminar fate restriction. *Neural Dev* 12 (1): 14. doi: 10.1186/s13064-017-0091-4.

Kawaguchi, A. et al. (2008). Single-cell gene profiling defines differential progenitor subclasses in mammalian neurogenesis. *Development* 135 (18): 3113–3124. doi: 10.1242/dev.022616.

Kawaue, T. et al. (2019). Lzts1 controls both neuronal delamination and outer radial glial-like cell generation during mammalian cerebral development. *Nat Commun* 10 (1): 2780. doi: 10.1038/s41467-019-10730-y.

Kerimoglu, C. et al. (2021). H3 acetylation selectively promotes basal progenitor proliferation and neocortex expansion. *Sci Adv* 7 (38): eabc6792. doi: 10.1126/sciadv.abc6792.

Killeen, M.T. and Sybingco, S.S. (2008). Netrin, Slit and Wnt receptors allow axons to choose the axis of migration. *Dev Biol* 323 (2): 143–151. doi: 10.1016/j.ydbio.2008.08.027.

Kovach, C. et al. (2013). Neurog2 simultaneously activates and represses alternative gene expression programs in the developing neocortex. *Cereb Cortex* 23 (8): 1884–1900. doi: 10.1093/cercor/bhs176.

Kowalczyk, T. et al. (2009). Intermediate neuronal progenitors (basal progenitors) produce pyramidal-projection neurons for all layers of cerebral cortex. *Cereb Cortex* 19 (10): 2439–2450. doi: 10.1093/cercor/bhn260.

Kriegstein, A. et al. (2006). Patterns of neural stem and progenitor cell division may underlie evolutionary cortical expansion. *Nat Rev Neurosci* 7 (11): 883–890. doi: 10.1038/nrn2008.

Lei, X. and Jiao, J. (2018). UTX affects neural stem cell proliferation and differentiation through PTEN signaling. *Stem Cell Rep* 10 (4): 1193–1207. doi: 10.1016/j.stemcr.2018.02.008.

Lim, L. et al. (2018). Development and functional diversification of cortical interneurons. *Neuron* 100 (2): 294–313. doi: 10.1016/j.neuron.2018.10.009.

Machon, O. et al. (2007). A dynamic gradient of Wnt signaling controls initiation of neurogenesis in the mammalian cortex and cellular specification in the hippocampus. *Dev Biol* 311 (1): 223–237. doi: 10.1016/j.ydbio.2007.08.038.

Malas, S. et al. (2003). Sox1-deficient mice suffer from epilepsy associated with abnormal ventral forebrain development and olfactory cortex hyperexcitability. *Neuroscience* 119 (2): 421–432. doi: 10.1016/s0306-4522(03)00158-1.

Martínez-Cerdeño, V. et al. (2012). Comparative analysis of the subventricular zone in rat, ferret and macaque. *PLoS One* 7 (1): e30178. doi: 10.1371/journal.pone.0030178.

Martínez-Cerdeño, V. et al. (2016). Evolutionary origin of Tbr2-expressing precursor cells and the subventricular zone in the developing cortex. *J Comp Neurol* 524 (3): 433–447. doi: 10.1002/cne.23879.

Martínez-Cerdeño, V. (2006). The role of intermediate progenitor cells in the evolutionary expansion of the cerebral cortex. *Cereb Cortex* 16 (Suppl 1): i152–61. doi: 10.1093/cercor/bhk017.

McIntosh, R. et al. (2017). Spatial distribution and characterization of non-apical progenitors in the zebrafish embryo central nervous system. *Open Biol* 7 (2): 160312. doi: 10.1098/rsob.160312.

Mihalas, A.B. et al. (2016). Intermediate progenitor cohorts differentially generate cortical layers and require Tbr2 for timely acquisition of neuronal subtype identity. *Cell Rep* 16 (1): 92–105. doi: 10.1016/j.celrep.2016.05.072.

Mihalas, A.B. and Hevner, R.F. (2018). Clonal analysis reveals laminar fate multipotency and daughter cell apoptosis of mouse cortical intermediate progenitors. *Development* 145 (17): dev164335. doi: 10.1242/dev.164335.

Mione, M. et al. (2001). Overlapping expression of zebrafish T-brain-1 and eomesodermin during forebrain development. *Mech Dev* 100 (1): 93–97. doi: 10.1016/s0925-4773(00)00501-3.

Miró, X. et al. (2009). Haploinsufficiency of the murine polycomb gene Suz12 results in diverse malformations of the brain and neural tube. *Dis Models Mech* 2 (7–8): 412–418. doi: 10.1242/dmm.001602.

Miyata, T. et al. (2004). Asymmetric production of surface-dividing and non-surface-dividing cortical progenitor cells. *Development* 131 (13): 3133–3145. doi: 10.1242/dev.01173.

Monier, B. and Suzanne, M. (2021). Orchestration of force generation and nuclear collapse in apoptotic cells. *Int J Mol Sci* 22 (19): 10257. doi: 10.3390/ijms221910257.

Moreno, N. and González, A. (2017). Pattern of neurogenesis and identification of neuronal progenitor subtypes during pallial development in *Xenopus laevis*. *Front Neuroanat* 11: 24. doi: 10.3389/fnana.2017.00024.

Morimoto-Suzuki, N. et al. (2014). The polycomb component Ring1B regulates the timed termination of subcerebral projection neuron production during mouse neocortical development. *Development* 141 (22): 4343–4353. doi: 10.1242/dev.112276.

Namba, T. et al. (2014). Pioneering axons regulate neuronal polarization in the developing cerebral cortex. *Neuron* 81 (4): 814–829. doi: 10.1016/j.neuron.2013.12.015.

Narayanan, R. et al. (2018). Chromatin remodeling BAF155 subunit regulates the genesis of basal progenitors in developing cortex. *iScience* 4: 109–126. doi: 10.1016/j.isci.2018.05.014.

Nelson, B.R. et al. (2013). Dynamic interactions between intermediate neurogenic progenitors and radial glia in embryonic mouse neocortex: potential role in Dll1-Notch signaling. *J Neurosci* 33 (21): 9122–9139. doi: 10.1523/JNEUROSCI.0791-13.2013.

Nelson, B.R. et al. (2020). Intermediate progenitors support migration of neural stem cells into dentate gyrus outer neurogenic niches. *Elife* 9: e53777. doi: 10.7554/eLife.53777.

Nieto, M. et al. (2004). Expression of Cux-1 and Cux-2 in the subventricular zone and upper layers II-IV of the cerebral cortex. *J Comp Neurol* 479 (2): 168–180. doi: 10.1002/cne.20322.

Ninkovic, J. et al. (2013). The BAF complex interacts with Pax6 in adult neural progenitors to establish a neurogenic cross-regulatory transcriptional network. *Cell Stem Cell* 13 (4): 403–418. doi: 10.1016/j.stem.2013.07.002.

Noctor, S.C. et al. (2004). Cortical neurons arise in symmetric and asymmetric division zones and migrate through specific phases. *Nat Neurosci* 7 (2): 136–144. doi: 10.1038/nn1172.

Noctor, S.C. et al. (2008). Distinct behaviors of neural stem and progenitor cells underlie cortical neurogenesis. *J Comp Neurol* 508 (1): 28–44. doi: 10.1002/cne.21669.

Nomura, T. et al. (2013). Changes in the regulation of cortical neurogenesis contribute to encephalization during amniote brain evolution. *Nat Commun* 4: 2206. doi: 10.1038/ncomms3206.

Nomura, T. et al. (2016). The evolution of basal progenitors in the developing non-mammalian brain. *Development* 143 (1): 66–74. doi: 10.1242/dev.127100.

O'Leary, D.D. et al. (2007). Area patterning of the mammalian cortex. *Neuron* 56 (2): 252–269. doi: 10.1016/j.neuron.2007.10.010.

Ochiai, W. et al. (2007). Transformation of pin-like ventricular zone cells into cortical neurons. *Neurosci Res* 57 (2): 326–329. doi: 10.1016/j.neures.2006.10.015.

Ochiai, W. et al. (2009). Periventricular notch activation and asymmetric Ngn2 and Tbr2 expression in pair-generated neocortical daughter cells. *Mol Cell Neurosci* 40 (2): 225–233. doi: 10.1016/j.mcn.2008.10.007.

Orgogozo, V. et al. (2002). Binary cell death decision regulated by unequal partitioning of Numb at mitosis. *Development* 129 (20): 4677–4684. doi: 10.1242/dev.129.20.4677.

Parthasarathy, S. et al. (2014). Ntf3 acts downstream of Sip1 in cortical postmitotic neurons to control progenitor cell fate through feedback signaling. *Development* 141 (17): 3324–3330. doi: 10.1242/dev.114173.

Pierfelice, T. et al. (2011). Notch in the vertebrate nervous system. *Neuron* 69 (5): 840–855. doi: 10.1016/j.neuron.2011.02.031.

Pontious, A. et al. (2008). Role of intermediate progenitor cells in cerebral cortex development. *Dev Neurosci* 30 (1–3): 24–32. doi: 10.1159/000109848.

Puzzolo, E. and Mallamaci, A. (2010). Cortico-cerebral histogenesis in the opossum Monodelphis domestica. *Neural Dev* 5: 8. doi: 10.1186/1749-8104-5-8.

Qu, Y. et al. (2014). Genetic evidence that Celsr3 and Celsr2, together with Fzd3, regulate forebrain wiring in a Vangl-independent manner. *Proc Natl Acad Sci USA* 111 (29): E2996–3004. doi: 10.1073/pnas.1402105111.

Quinn, J.C. et al. (2007). Pax6 controls cerebral cortical cell number by regulating exit from the cell cycle and specifies cortical cell identity by a cell autonomous mechanism. *Dev Biol* 302 (1): 50–65. doi: 10.1016/j.ydbio.2006.08.035.

Ruan, X. et al. (2021 March 9). Progenitor cell diversity in the developing mouse neocortex. *Proc Natl Acad Sci USA* 118 (10): e2018866118. doi: 10.1073/pnas.2018866118.

Sasaki, S. et al. (2008). The cortical subventricular zone-specific molecule Svet1 is part of the nuclear RNA coded by the putative netrin receptor gene Unc5d and is expressed in multipolar migrating cells. *Mol Cell Neurosci* 38 (4): 474–483. doi: 10.1016/j.mcn.2008.04.002.

Sauerland, C. et al. (2018). The basal radial glia occurs in marsupials and underlies the evolution of an expanded neocortex in therian mammals. *Cereb Cortex* 28 (1): 145–157. doi: 10.1093/cercor/bhw360.

Scardigli, R. et al. (2003). Direct and concentration-dependent regulation of the proneural gene Neurogenin2 by Pax6. *Development* 130 (14): 3269–3281. doi: 10.1242/dev.00539.

Sessa, A. et al. (2017). The Tbr2 molecular network controls cortical neuronal differentiation through complementary genetic and epigenetic pathways. *Cereb Cortex* 27 (6): 3378–3396. doi: 10.1093/cercor/bhw270.

Sessa, A. et al. (2010). Tbr2-positive intermediate (basal) neuronal progenitors safeguard cerebral cortex expansion by controlling amplification of pallial glutamatergic neurons and attraction of subpallial GABAergic interneurons. *Genes Dev* 24 (16): 1816–1826. doi: 10.1101/gad.575410.

Sessa, A. et al. (2008). Tbr2 directs conversion of radial glia into basal precursors and guides neuronal amplification by indirect neurogenesis in the developing neocortex. *Neuron* 60 (1): 56–69. doi: 10.1016/j.neuron.2008.09.028.

Siegenthaler, J.A. et al. (2008). Foxg1 haploinsufficiency reduces the population of cortical intermediate progenitor cells. *Cereb Cortex* 18 (8): 1865–1875. doi: 10.1093/cercor/bhm209.

Sierra, A. et al. (2010). Microglia shape adult hippocampal neurogenesis through apoptosis-coupled phagocytosis. *Cell Stem Cell* 7 (4): 483–495. doi: 10.1016/j.stem.2010.08.014.

Smart, I.H.M. (1973). Proliferative characteristics of the ependymal layer during the early development of the mouse neocortex. *J Anat* 116 (Pt 1): 67–91.

Smith, R.S. et al. (2018). Sodium channel SCN3A (NaV1.3) regulation of human cerebral cortical folding and oral motor development. *Neuron* 99 (5): 905–913.e7. doi: 10.1016/j.neuron.2018.07.052.

Stubbs, D. et al. (2009). Neurovascular congruence during cerebral cortical development. *Cereb Cortex* 19 (Suppl 1): i32–41. doi: 10.1093/cercor/bhp040.

Sun, S.D. et al. (2016). Planar cell polarity genes Frizzled3a, Vangl2, and Scribble are required for spinal commissural axon guidance. *BMC Neurosci* 17 (1): 83. doi: 10.1186/s12868-016-0318-z.

Sun, T. and Hevner, R.F. (2014). Growth and folding of the mammalian cerebral cortex: from molecules to malformations. *Nat Rev Neurosci* 15 (4): 217–232. doi: 10.1038/nrn3707.

Suzuki, I.K. et al. (2012). The temporal sequence of the mammalian neocortical neurogenetic program drives mediolateral pattern in the chick pallium. *Dev Cell* 22 (4): 863–870. doi: 10.1016/j.devcel.2012.01.004.

Tabata, H. and Nakajima, K. (2003). Multipolar migration. *J Neurosci* 23 (31): 9996–10001. doi: 10.1523/JNEUROSCI.23-31-09996.2003.

Takahashi, T. et al. (1995). Early ontogeny of the secondary proliferative population of the embryonic murine cerebral wall. *J Neurosci* 15 (9): 6058–6068. doi: 10.1523/JNEUROSCI.15-09-06058.1995.

Tarabykin, V. et al. (2001). Cortical upper layer neurons derive from the subventricular zone as indicated by Svet1 gene expression. *Development* 128 (11): 1983–1993. doi: 10.1242/dev.128.11.1983.

Tavano, S. et al. (2018). Insm1 induces neural progenitor delamination in developing neocortex via downregulation of the adherens junction belt-specific protein Plekha7. *Neuron* 97 (6): 1299–1314.e8. doi: 10.1016/j.neuron.2018.01.052.

Taverna, E. et al. (2014). The cell biology of neurogenesis. *Ann Rev Cell Dev Biol* 30: 465–502. doi: 10.1146/annurev-cellbio-101011-155801.

Telley, L. et al. (2019). Temporal patterning of apical progenitors and their daughter neurons in the developing neocortex. *Science* 364 (6440): eaav2522. doi: 10.1126/science.aav2522.

Telley, L. et al. (2016). Sequential transcriptional waves direct the differentiation of newborn neurons in the mouse neocortex. *Science* 351 (6280): 1443–1446. doi: 10.1126/science.aad8361.

Thomaidou, D. et al. (1997). Apoptosis and its relation to the cell cycle in the developing cerebral cortex. *J Neurosci* 17 (3): 1075–1085. doi: 10.1523/JNEUROSCI.17-03-01075.1997.

Toda, T. et al. (2016). An essential role of SVZ progenitors in cortical folding in gyrencephalic mammals. *Sci Rep* 6: 29578. doi: 10.1038/srep29578.

Tsuboi, M. et al. (2019 December). Diverse gene regulatory mechanisms mediated by Polycomb group proteins during neural development. *Curr Opin Neurobiol* 59: 164–173. doi: 10.1016/j.conb.2019.07.003.

Vasistha, N.A. et al. (2015). Cortical and clonal contribution of Tbr2 expressing progenitors in the developing mouse brain. *Cereb Cortex* 25 (10): 3290–3302. doi: 10.1093/cercor/bhu125.

Vitali, I. et al. (2018). Progenitor hyperpolarization regulates the sequential generation of neuronal subtypes in the developing neocortex. *Cell* 174 (5): 1264–1276.e15. doi: 10.1016/j.cell.2018.06.036.

Voss, A.K. and Strasser, A. (2020). The essentials of developmental apoptosis. *F1000Research* 9: F1000. Faculty Rev-148. doi: 10.12688/f1000research.21571.1.

Wakselman, S. et al. (2008). Developmental neuronal death in hippocampus requires the microglial CD11b integrin and DAP12 immunoreceptor. *J Neurosci* 28 (32): 8138–8143. doi: 10.1523/JNEUROSCI.1006-08.2008.

Wang, Y. et al. (2011). CXCR4 and CXCR7 have distinct functions in regulating interneuron migration. *Neuron* 69 (1): 61–76. doi: 10.1016/j.ncuron.2010.12.005.

Wang, Y. et al. (2002). Frizzled-3 is required for the development of major fiber tracts in the rostral CNS. *J Neurosci* 22 (19): 8563–8573. doi: 10.1523/JNEUROSCI.22-19-08563.2002.

Watt, F.M. (1988). Epidermal stem cells in culture. *J Cell Sci* 10 (Supplement): 85–94. doi: 10.1242/jcs.1988.supplement_10.7.

Wu, S.X. et al. (2005). Pyramidal neurons of upper cortical layers generated by NEX-positive progenitor cells in the subventricular zone. *Proc Natl Acad Sci USA* 102 (47): 17172–17177. doi: 10.1073/pnas.0508560102.

Yao, B. et al. (2016). Epigenetic mechanisms in neurogenesis. *Nat Rev Neurosci* 17 (9): 537–549. doi: 10.1038/nrn.2016.70.

Yoon, K.J. et al. (2008). Mind bomb 1-expressing intermediate progenitors generate notch signaling to maintain radial glial cells. *Neuron* 58 (4): 519–531. doi: 10.1016/j.neuron.2008.03.018.

Zimmer, C. et al. (2004). Dynamics of Cux2 expression suggests that an early pool of SVZ precursors is fated to become upper cortical layer neurons. *Cereb Cortex* 14 (12): 1408–1420. doi: 10.1093/cercor/bhh102.

4

Area V1 Development, a Model System to Link Corticogenesis to Adult Cortex Structure and Function

Colette Dehay[1,*] *and Henry Kennedy*[1,2,*]

[1] *Univ Lyon, Université Claude Bernard Lyon 1, Inserm, Stem Cell and Brain Research Institute U1208, F-69500 Bron, France*
[2] *Institute of Neuroscience, State Key Laboratory of Neuroscience, Chinese Academy of Sciences (CAS) Key Laboratory of Primate Neurobiology, CAS, Shanghai 200031, China*
[*] *Corresponding authors*

4.1 Introduction

One hallmark of the human and nonhuman primate cerebral cortical cytoarchitecture is a highly expanded supragranular (SG) compartment. This SG expansion is driven primarily by changes in gene regulation (Won et al. 2019) and is accompanied by increased cellular diversity (Berg et al. 2021; Hodge et al. 2019). SG neurons are endowed with particular features and the interareal connectivity of the SG neurons largely determines the stringent cortical hierarchy that constrains information flow through the cortex (Vezoli et al. 2021). Quantitative connectivity analyses have highlighted major differences in the nature and organization of the cortical networks between primates and rodents (Gamanut et al. 2018; Horvat et al. 2016; Markov et al. 2013; Oh et al. 2014; Zingg et al. 2014). Combined, the scaling and connectomic differences observed in these species (Herculano-Houzel et al. 2007) are thought to shape the functional properties of the neocortex and determine varying degrees of cortical complexity (Wang and Kennedy 2016). Species-specific developmental features, including quantitative and qualitative differences in developmental mechanisms, underlie the observed diversity in structure and function of the neocortex.

The cerebral cortex is parceled in distinct functional areas, the number of which is higher in primates compared to rodents. Areal diversity shows a higher degree of sophistication in human and non-human primates than in rodents, as reflected by differences in the number, density, lamination, and connectivity patterns of neurons in functionally distinct areas (DeFelipe 2011; DeFelipe et al. 2002). In all documented primates, the primary visual cortex (V1) located in the occipital lobe at the most caudal pole of the cortex, contains proportionally more neurons compared to other cortical areas (Collins et al. 2010; Powell and Hendrickson 1981; Rockel et al. 1980). Of note, V1 is clearly distinguishable from other cortical areas by its distinctive neuronal lamination and expanded SG and a sub-compartmented granular layer 4 (Figure 4.1A). In the adult, the lamination pattern seen in V1 terminates abruptly at the border with area V2. The areal boundaries of area V1 with adjacent area V2 can be detected early during mid-corticogenesis by AchE expression (Dehay et al. 1993). This precocious marked aeralization makes these two visual areas unrivalled

Neocortical Neurogenesis in Development and Evolution, First Edition. Edited by Wieland B. Huttner.

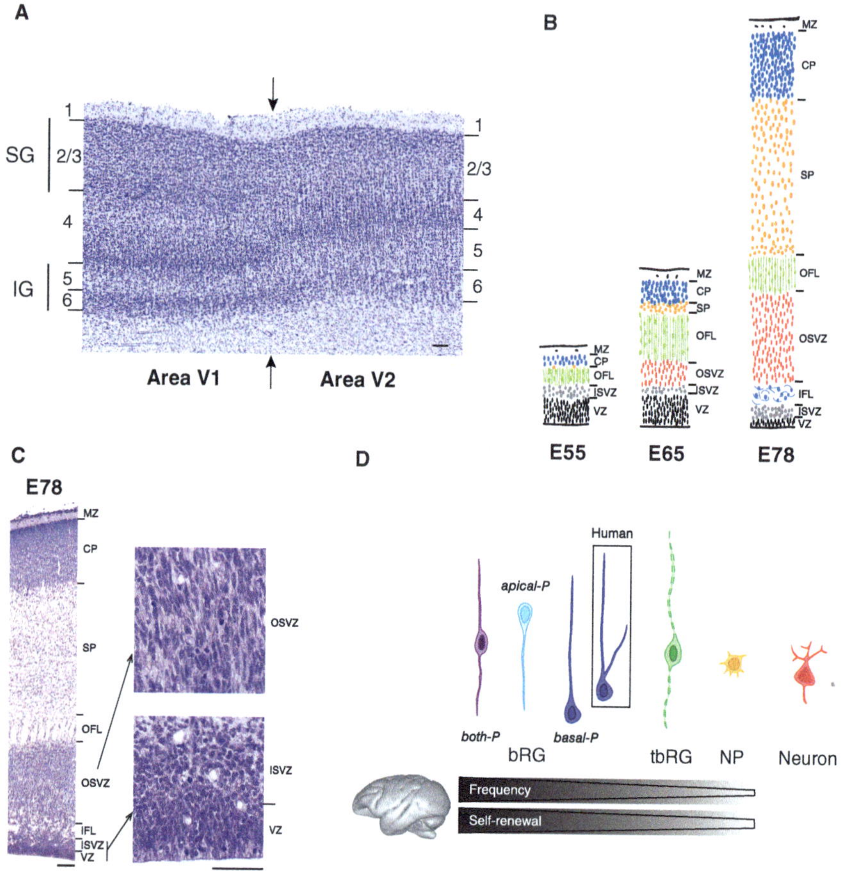

Figure 4.1 Summary of conspicuous features of the OSVZ in the presumptive Area V1 of the macaque monkey. (A) Nissl-stained section cutting through area V1 and area V2 in the adult macaque cortex. Note the conspicuous features of area V1 with enlarged SG layers and the compartmented layer 4. The border between area V1 and area V2 is clearly visible (arrow head). (B) Drawings of transects through presumptive area 17 in the macaque at key developmental stages. Note the VZ decline and OSVZ expansion at the time of SG neuron production. The OSVZ is bordered apically by IFL, basally by OFL. E65 corresponds to the production of infragranular (IG) and E78 to that of SG layers. (C) Higher-power views of the GZ in presumptive area V1. Note the conspicuous radial organization of the OSVZ (upper panel). View of the ISVZ and VZ (lower panel). Mitotic figures are seen among the irregularly orientated nuclei of the ISVZ. In the VZ, nuclei are radially arranged and mitotic figures lie towards the ventricular surface, indicating ongoing interkinetic nuclear migration typical of the VZ (adapted from Kennedy et al. 2021). (D) OSVZ progenitors include a prevalence of radially oriented progenitors bearing apical and/or basal processes. Non-polarized progenitors (NP) are scarcer. Four bRGs cell types have been identified in the macaque (Betizeau et al. 2013): bipolar bRGs bearing a basal and apical process (both-P); bRGs bearing an apical process (apical-P); bRGs bearing a basal process (basal-P); bRGs exhibiting transient apical and/or basal processes (tbRGs). In human cortex, an additional type bearing a bifurcated basal process has been observed (Kalebic et al. 2019). Self-renewal abilities are increased in bipolar bRGs. Scale bars: 10μm (A); 100μm (C). Abbreviations: Ventricular Zone (VZ); Subventricular Zone (SVZ); Inner SVZ (ISVZ); Outer SVZ (OSVZ); Inner Fibre Layer (IFL); Outer Fibre Layer (OFL); Subplate (SP); Cortical Plate (CP); Marginal Zone (MZ).

models to study the developmental mechanisms underlying cytoarchitectural areal specification in primates. We shall focus our review on findings related to the development of the macaque area V1 and explore the role of OSVZ in shaping adult cortical structure and connectivity.

The generation of a thicker area V1 in primates with high numbers of SG neurons is due to a combination of critical underlying mechanisms including a prolonged developmental period dedicated to SG neuron generation and unique properties of the cortical progenitors and organization of germinal zones (GZ). The construction and shaping of the primate interareal networks are largely determined by the finely tuned generation of SG neurons during corticogenesis as well as by the prolonged pre- and postnatal pruning of connections originating from the SG neurons.

Generation of the six-layered cortex is completed prenatally in primates. Whereas in the mouse, the neurogenic period lasts about 9–10 days (from embryonic day E10.5 to E18–19.5) (Stepien et al. 2020), it lasts 65 days in the macaque monkey and circa 110 days in human (from gestation weeks 10 to 25) (Clancy et al. 2001; Lewitus et al. 2014). There are temporal differences in the timing and rate of neuron production during neurogenesis across different regions of the neocortex (Rakic 1974; Smart and Smart 1982) with a 3 weeks lag in the caudal cortex compared to rostral areas in monkeys (Finlay and Uchiyama 2015; Rakic 1974). Of note, initiation of neurogenesis across the cortex is nearly synchronous while the time of its cessation varies (Lewitus et al. 2014). This rostro-caudal gradient of cortical neurogenesis impacts the tightly regulated spatiotemporal sequence of neuron generation across the cortex to give rise to regional and areal differences in cytoarchitecture, neuron numbers and densities as well as in relative growth rates between cortical areas (Charvet 2014). In this respect, note that area V1, which shows the highest number of SG neurons, is located at the most caudal pole of the cortex (Collins 2011; Collins et al. 2010).

4.2 The Outer Subventricular Zone: A Uniquely Specialized and Enlarged Progenitor Pool in the Visual Primate Cortex

Two decades ago, a detailed investigation of the morphological features of the developing cortex in the mouse and monkey revealed major cytoarchitectural differences (Smart et al. 2002). With respect to the GZs this study identified in the monkey the emergence and expansion of a compartment of the subventricular zone (SVZ) that shows a highly radial organization that was coined the outer subventricular zone (OSVZ) to distinguish it from a classically randomly organized subventricular zone in the monkey that was referred to as ISVZ (Figure 4.1B, C). The architecture of the monkey GZ in the occipital lobe, in presumptive area V1, includes two conspicuous fiber layers: the IFL (inner) and the OFL (outer). The OSVZ and ISVZ are separated by the IFL, largely corresponding to corticofugal axons (Saito et al. 2019), while OFL laying external to the OSVZ corresponds to ingrowing thalamocortical axons in the monkey (Borello et al. 2018; Smart et al. 2002).

The existence of the OSVZ and ISVZ as distinct pools of basally located progenitors has subsequently been amply confirmed in the human developing cortex (Fietz et al. 2010; Hansen et al. 2010; Zecevic et al. 2005). The presence of a dense, radially structured and expanded OSVZ is considered characteristic of developing primate cortex in the primate order (Kelava et al. 2012; Martinez-Cerdeno et al. 2012). Although claims of OSVZ (or OSVZ-like GZ) have been made in non-primates with large and/or convoluted cortices, including large-brained rodents (agouti) (Fietz et al. 2010; Garcia-Moreno et al. 2012; Reillo et al. 2011), they are distinct from the densely packed architecture of the primate OSVZ where there is a pronounced pseudo-stratification, reminiscent of the VZ neuroepithelium. Hence the so-called OSVZ of non-primates in fact corresponds to a sparser basal progenitor layer located between the cell-dense ISVZ and the intermediate zone (IZ) (Reillo et al. 2011).

During the course of primate corticogenesis, there is a drastic expansion of the OSVZ prior to and during the major phase of SG neuron production accompanied by a steady dwindling of the ventricular zone (VZ) (Fietz et al. 2010; Hansen et al. 2010; Lukaszewicz et al. 2005; Smart et al. 2002) that is not observed in rodents (Smart and Smart 1982). Further, contrary to rodent, birth-dating experiments in the embryonic monkey have demonstrated that the bulk of SG neurons are generated by OSVZ progenitors (Lukaszewicz et al. 2006, 2005).

4.3 Primate OSVZ Progenitors are Endowed with Extended Proliferative Abilities

The progenitors of the primate OSVZ, referred to as bRGs (basal radial glia) (Fietz et al. 2010) or oRGs (outer radial glia) (Hansen et al. 2010), are characterized by a high degree of morphological diversity (Betizeau et al. 2013; Kalebic et al. 2019; Pebworth et al. 2021) and the vast majority (>75%) exhibit radial glial morphological features (Betizeau et al. 2013; Florio and Huttner 2014; Kalebic et al. 2019; Lui et al. 2011). Remarkably, all OSVZ progenitor subtypes are able to undergo proliferative symmetric as well as neurogenic divisions (Betizeau et al. 2013). Live imaging studies in both macaque and human reveal a correlation between the morphological properties of progenitors and their proliferative behavior: bRGs with a higher number of processes exhibit increased rates of proliferation (Betizeau et al. 2013; Kalebic et al. 2019; Kalebic and Huttner 2020; Pilz et al. 2013) (Figure 4.1D), although no correlation has been observed between the transcriptomic signature and progenitor morphology (Pebworth et al. 2021).

Live imaging on embryonic macaque and human cortex shows that a salient feature of the OSVZ progenitors is the highly dynamic nature of their processes (Betizeau et al. 2013; Kalebic et al. 2019; LaMonica et al. 2013). These dynamic processes could provide the substrate to sense and integrate signals from VZ and ISVZ apical processes as well as from the basal processes of the post-mitotic neurons in the subplate and cortical plate (Nelson et al. 2013; Polleux et al. 2001; Seuntjens et al. 2009). The integration of these local, extrinsic signals from the germinal and postmitotic microenvironments likely impact on cell-cycle and/or neurogenic rates (Dehay et al. 2001; Reillo et al. 2011).

A large number of studies have identified the expression of proliferation promoting genes and miRNAs in the human and nonhuman primate OSVZ (Arcila et al. 2014; Eze et al. 2021; Fiddes et al. 2018; Florio et al. 2018; Heide et al. 2017; Johnson et al. 2015; Liu et al. 2017; Nowakowski et al. 2018; Pinson and Huttner 2021; Pollen et al. 2015, 2014; Suzuki et al. 2018). Recent fascinating breakthroughs from the Huttner's group have uncovered major mechanisms regarding the genetic underpinnings of the extensive proliferative abilities of OSVZ progenitors in humans. They showed that a human duplicated gene, ARHGAP11B, was specifically expressed in the human OSVZ progenitors (Florio et al. 2015). Using transgenesis in a lissencephalic nonhuman primate, they showed that ARHGAP11B was responsible for the expansion of the primate cortex (Heide et al. 2020). Importantly, ARHGAP11B enhances glutaminolysis (Namba et al. 2020, 2021) which in turn promotes cell-cycle progression and proliferation of BPs (Iwata and Vanderhaeghen 2020).

4.4 The Key Role of G1 Phase Regulation in the Primate OSVZ Progenitors Expansion

The developmental expansion of the OSVZ progenitor pool is linked to the temporal modulation of cell-cycle dynamics (Betizeau et al. 2013; Lukaszewicz et al. 2005) (Figure 4.2). Two cell-cycle parameters determine the rate of the progenitor pool expansion: cell-cycle duration and the mode

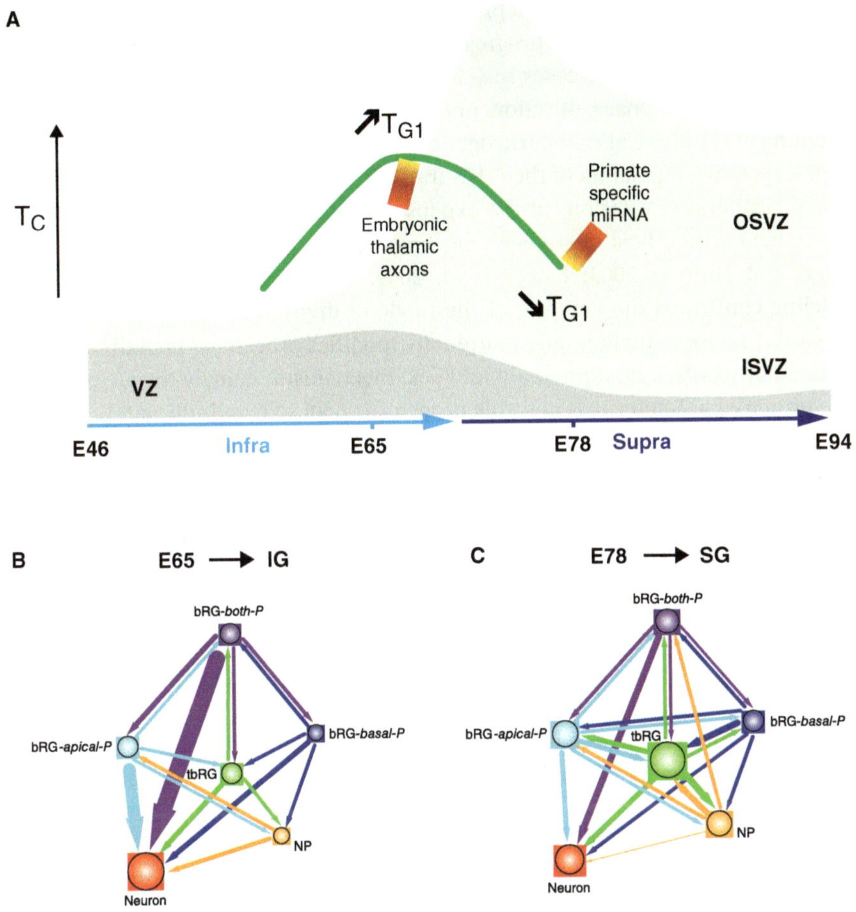

Figure 4.2 Dynamics of cortical progenitors underlying area V1 histogenesis. (A) The tempo of cell-cycle dynamics is shown for progenitors of infragranular (IG) and supragranular (SG) neurons. Cell-cycle duration (T_C) increases until mid-corticogenesis and decreases at the time of SG neuron production. T_C lengthening is associated with an increase in differentiative divisions while T_C shortening is accompanied by an increase in proliferative divisions, resulting in an amplification of the progenitor pool (shading profile) generating SG neurons. Primate-specific miRNAs targeting cell-cycle progression genes and embryonic thalamic axons impact on cell-cycle kinetics (adapted from Dehay et al. 2015) (B, C) Bidirectional and non-hierarchical lineages relationships show increased complexity during the generation of SG neurons. State transition diagrams illustrating the lineage relationships in the OSVZ of the macaque occipital cortex at E65 and E78 (Betizeau et al. 2013). Nodes represent progenitor types (states) and directed edges the transitions between progenitors. Size of nodes is proportional to the frequency of each progenitor type with respect to the total numbers of precursors, thickness of the arrows indicates transition frequency with respect to the total number of transitions. The position of the nodes with respect to the vertical axis is determined by the mean rank of occurrence of each precursor type in the lineage trees. All transitions except neurogenic are bidirectional. Note the different topology of state transition diagrams for IG and SG neurons progenitors, indicating a higher complexity for SG progenitor lineages (adapted from Betizeau et al. 2013).

of division (proliferative or differentiative). While mouse cortical progenitors cell cycle length ranges from 8–26.5 h (Arai et al. 2011; Takahashi et al. 1995), cortical progenitors of embryonic human and nonhuman primate show a longer cell cycle, ranging from 22–63 hours (Betizeau et al. 2013; Kornack and Rakic 1998) (Pollen et al. 2015; Subramanian et al. 2017).

In mouse cortical progenitors, cell-cycle variations – as observed at the population level – are mostly due to changes in G1 phase duration. During rodent corticogenesis, there is an overall lengthening of cell-cycle duration, paralleled by a progressive increase in rates of divisions leading to differentiation (Takahashi et al. 1995). This progressive lengthening of cell cycle in rodents during corticogenesis is primarily due to increases in G1 phase duration (Arai et al. 2011; Calegari et al. 2005; Gal et al. 2006). G1 phase duration and mode of division are causally related. Experimental shortening of G1 phase at mid-corticogenesis in vivo via in utero electroporation of Cyclin D and Cyclin E (positive regulators of the G1/S transition) targeted at mouse VZ progenitors increases rates of proliferative divisions at the expense of differentiation (Pilaz et al. 2009). This result is in agreement with a host of studies reporting correlative links between these two parameters (Calegari and Huttner 2003; Lange et al. 2009; Lukaszewicz et al. 2005, 2002). Mathematical modeling confirmed the key role of the mode of division in the progenitor pool amplification whereas G1 phase reduction only marginally modifies progenitor pool dimensions (Pilaz et al. 2009). In other words, a fundamental biological mechanism, namely the G1 phase of the cell-cycle is the primary parameter that controls progenitor pool size and ultimately neuron generation rates.

In the monkey, the cell-cycle duration of VZ (Kornack and Rakic 1995) and OSVZ (Lukaszewicz et al. 2005) progenitors has been measured at the population level via early in vivo studies, using injection of S phase markers. More recently, cell-cycle duration has been explored at the single-cell level using ex vivo via time-lapse video imaging on organotypic slices (Betizeau et al. 2013). Performed at key points of corticogenesis these studies showed that the cell-cycle duration of OSVZ progenitors is shorter than that of VZ progenitors. The cell-cycle duration of OSVZ progenitors lengthens between E50 and E65, prior to shortening at E78 (Figure 4.2). This reduction in cell-cycle duration at mid-corticogenesis is largely due to a shortening of the G1 phase (Betizeau et al. 2013), which is accompanied by reduced rates of cell-cycle exit and an expansion of the OSVZ progenitor pool during SG neuron production (Betizeau et al. 2013; Hansen et al. 2010; Smart et al. 2002). These results point to the time course of cell-cycle regulation, and more specifically how G1 phase duration determines the tempo of the primate OSVZ expansion (Betizeau et al. 2013) (Figure 4.2).

Remarkably, a large fraction of primate-specific miRNAs that are selectively and differentially expressed in the OSVZ progenitors, target cell-cycle genes, including genes that control the G1/S transition (Arcila et al. 2014; Dehay et al. 2015; Tomasello et al. 2022). This suggests that the G1/S transition constitutes an evolutionary target for regulation of cortical expansion, in agreement with recent advance in the genetic underpinning of cell-cycle control in primates (Girskis et al. 2021). *PPP1R17*, a repressor of protein phosphatase complexes 1 (PP1) and 2A (PP2A) (Endo 2012), which are regulators of the G1/S transition (Wlodarchak and Xing 2016), is expressed in human cortical progenitors (Noctor et al. 2004; Pollen et al. 2015; Zhong et al. 2018). *PPP1R17* expression during corticogenesis shows species-specific differences, which are being strongly expressed in primates but not detectable in ferret or mice at comparable developmental stages (Girskis et al. 2021). Importantly, *PPP1R17* expression is observed in the ISVZ and OSVZ of the prenatal cortex of macaque and human – preferentially in Tbr2 expressing progenitors – but not in the VZ. Together with the primate-specific miRNAS (Arcila et al. 2014), *PPP1R17* expression in the OSVZ progenitors point to primate-specific innovation targeting G1/S transition.

4.5 G1 Phase Regulation Underpins Cortical Cytoarchitecture

As summarized in the previous section, the shortening of G1 phase at mid-corticogenesis in OSVZ progenitors is accompanied by an upsurge in symmetric proliferative divisions, which ensures the timely amplification of the SG neurons progenitor pool in the visual cortex (Betizeau et al. 2013) (Figure 4.2).

The consequences of G1 phase modulation in cortical progenitors on neuron production and cortical structure have been explored in different species (Lange et al. 2009; Nonaka-Kinoshita et al. 2013; Pilaz et al. 2009). Experimental shortening of the G1 phase in VZ progenitors via in utero electroporation of Cyclin E and Cyclin D1 has been shown to promote symmetric proliferative divisions and an increased generation of SVZ progenitors. Under these experimental conditions, SVZ progenitors show high levels of self-renewing proliferative divisions at the expense of neurogenesis (Pilaz et al. 2009). Long-term survival studies following induced G1 phase reduction results in cytoarchitectural modifications including an expanded SG compartment (Pilaz et al. 2009). A number of studies converge to show that the shortening of the G1 phase in mouse cortex (Lange et al. 2009; Mairet-Coello et al. 2012; Nonaka-Kinoshita et al. 2013; Pilaz et al. 2009; Stahl et al. 2013; Volpe et al. 2006) selectively promotes proliferative divisions in a transiently amplified pool of SVZ progenitors. These studies show that this results in an enlarged SG compartment thereby mimicking primate corticogenesis. The control of the G1 phase duration appears therefore as a key mechanism to modulate neuron numbers in the adult via the control of OSVZ expansion.

In addition to its temporal regulation (Betizeau et al. 2013; Kornack and Rakic 1998) the cell-cycle dynamics of OSVZ progenitors are spatially controlled (Dehay et al. 1993; Lukaszewicz et al. 2005). This finely tuned spatiotemporal regulation of OSVZ proliferation has direct consequences on the histogenesis of cytoarchitecturally distinct areas, via the control of SG neuron production, as has been demonstrated in the primate occipital cortex, both empirically and computationally (Lukaszewicz et al. 2005). As mentioned earlier, in the prenatal macaque monkey it is possible to identify the GZ generating area V1 and area V2, thereby providing a unique opportunity to directly relate proliferative events to the arealization process. In the presumptive macaque monkey visual cortex, in vivo and ex vivo studies have shown that the OSVZ progenitors of area V1 have a reduced duration of cell-cycle and an augmented proliferative mode of division compared to OSVZ progenitors in area V2 (Lukaszewicz et al. 2005). Mathematical modelling indicates that these area-specific changes that are selectively detected in the OSVZ progenitors, at thc time of SG neuron production and not in the VZ during lower layer neurons production (Dehay et al. 1993; Lukaszewicz et al. 2005) are responsible for the increased SG compartment in area V1 compared to area V2 (Lukaszewicz et al. 2005).

4.6 Extrinsic Control of OSVZ Progenitors Cell-cycle by Thalamocortical Axons in Area V1

The organization of the thalamocortical connections exhibits distinctive order-specific features both during development and in the mature cortex. In the mouse, embryonic thalamocortical axons grow dorsally in the embryonic cortex at some distance from the GZ (Dehay et al. 2001; Gerstmann et al. 2015; Miller et al. 1993). By contrast, in primates the embryonic thalamocortical axons of the primary visual cortex come into close proximity with cortical progenitors. The OFL, which in macaque is present from very early stages at E46, is located immediately external to the OSVZ, stains with AChE (Borello et al. 2018; Pebworth et al. 2021; Smart et al. 2002), and can be traced back to AChE positive lateral geniculate axons in rodents (Robertson et al. 1988; Woodward and Coull 1984) and likewise in primates on horizontal slices at mid-corticogenesis (Borello et al. 2018). Given the absence of fiber pathways in the OSVZ, these observations indicate that the corticofugal axons run dorsally to the corticopetal axons in the macaque, an inversion of the normal pattern found in rodents and non-primates (Bicknese et al. 1994; Kennedy et al. 1994; Robertson et al. 1988; Woodward and Coull 1984).

This anatomical organization can be considered a major adaptation feature ensuring thalamic control of cortical expansion in primates. It results in a radial heterogeneity within the OSVZ of area V1, with its most outer part being enriched in embryonic thalamic axons (Borello et al. 2018; Smart et al. 2002). In situ observations have revealed increased rates of proliferation and symmetric proliferative divisions in the outer tier of the OSVZ (Pace et al. 2018). This finding corroborates observations made in mouse corticogenesis where it has been shown that embryonic thalamocortical axons release a diffusible mitogenic factor that promotes the G1/S transition of cortical progenitors thereby shortening the G1 phase and promoting proliferative divisions (Dehay et al. 2001). Interestingly, miRNA profiling in the primate GZ of the visual cortex revealed a molecular heterogeneity in the radial thickness of the OSVZ in area V1. The OSVZ was subdivided in three horizontal compartments, which showed distinct miRNA signatures at E78, during peak production of SG neurons, and at a time where the bulk of thalamocortical axons are observed in the OFL (Borello et al. 2018; Pace et al. 2018). Specifically, this analysis revealed that the outer tier of area V1 OSVZ exhibits a distinctive profile of differentially expressed miRNAs, over 50 percent of which are primate specific. Remarkably, a significant fraction of the target genes of these primate-specific miRNAs are cell-cycle related genes, including G1/S transition control (Arcila et al. 2014).

Together these observations raise the hypothesis that the upsurge in proliferation and shortening in cell-cycle duration specifically observed in the OSVZ SG layer progenitor pool (Betizeau et al. 2013; Lukaszewicz et al. 2005) is triggered by thalamocortical axons, possibly via primate-specific miRNAs (Figure 4.2A).

Of note, the heterochrony of mouse vs. primate corticogenesis (Kennedy and Dehay 1993) results in primate thalamocortical axons being in a position to interact with OSVZ progenitors for a much extended time window compared to the interaction of thalamic fibers with SVZ progenitors in the mouse cortex (Dehay et al. 2001; Gerstmann et al. 2015). This, together with the anatomical features of the primate thalamocortical axons early trajectory translates in an early and enhanced instructive role of the sensory periphery on corticogenesis in primates compared to non-primate species.

This early influence of thalamocortical axons on the proliferation of OSVZ progenitors in area V1 has major consequences on the adult cortical architecture. The absence of the retina at early stages of development was found to lead to a loss of neurons at postnatal stages in the lateral geniculate nucleus, thereby largely deafferenting the developing visual cortex (Rakic et al. 1986). Enucleation in the ferret during early postnatal development, at the stage of SG neuron production (Jackson et al. 1989), results in a reduced proliferation of OSVZ progenitors and a reduction of the LGN and of the visual cortex (Reillo et al. 2011). The absence of the retina in the fetal macaque led to a large reduction of striate cortex, suggesting that cortex destined to become area V1 assumed a default phenotype (referred to as default extrastriate cortex – DEC) (Rakic 1988b). The drastic depletion in thalamocortical axons in anophtalmic primates causes an alteration of cortical parcellation and abnormal gyrification in this model of congenital blindness (Dehay et al. 1989; Rakic 1988b). Subsequently, histological examination of the DEC confirmed Pasko Rakic's hypothesis and showed that it constituted a phenotypically hybrid cortex exhibiting the combined cellular and histochemical features of area V1 and area V2 (Dehay et al. 1996a, 1996b). Recent studies reveal extensive modifications of cortico-cortical connectivity in anophthalmic primates (Magrou et al. 2018, 2020).

4.7 Complex Lineages in OSVZ Progenitors and Generation of SG Neuron Diversity

Ex vivo live imaging in the macaque embryonic cortex revealed that primate SG neurons are generated through indirect neurogenesis, following numerous rounds of division and via complex, stochastic, and non-hierarchical progenitor lineages, including bidirectional transitions (Betizeau et al. 2013). These lineage relationships are temporally modulated, and show increased complexity in SG progenitors compared to infragranular neuron progenitors (Betizeau et al. 2013) (Figure 4.2B). In addition to their impact on the expansion of the progenitor pool, the local and extrinsic signals converging on the OSVZ (cf. earlier, Figure 4.2A) are predicted to be pivotal in modulating the stochastic lineages via their influence on distinct transcriptional sequences in progenitors that will in turn determine postmitotic transcriptional programs generating SG neuronal diversity (Telley et al. 2019). The spatiotemporal orchestration of these extracellular signals might therefore convey flexibility in the phenotypic fine tuning of SG neurons during the protracted primate corticogenesis (Nowakowski et al. 2016). Interestingly, single-cell transcriptomic studies have revealed an increased diversity of glutamatergic SG neuron types in human neocortex compared to the mouse (Hodge et al. 2019), correlated to an increased morphological and electrophysiological diversity (Berg et al. 2021)

The relative contribution of intrinsic developmental programs and extrinsic signals to neuron fate determination and ultimately assembly of circuits, is still incompletely understood (Borello et al. 2018; Dehay and Kennedy 2007; Jabaudon 2017). Elegant work by the Jabaudon group on the mouse cortex has highlighted the possible role of the temporal regulation of the expression of generic genes in generating cortical neuron and circuit diversity (Klingler et al. 2021). In addition to early gene expression patterns, DNA mosaicism in postmitotic neurons is considered to contribute to neuronal functional diversity (Breuss et al. 2022; Jabaudon 2017; Telley et al. 2016).

4.8 The Role of OSVZ beyond Proliferation: An Area-specific Scaffold for Radial Migration

Radial migration dynamics and their control show major differences in primates and rodents. In the rodent embryonic cortex, the radial migration scaffold is provided by the basal processes of the VZ progenitors that bear an apical (anchored to the ventricle) and a basal process (anchored to the basal membrane). While the overwhelming majority of primate bRGs extend a long basal process directed to the cortical plate (CP) (Betizeau et al. 2013; Fietz et al. 2010; Hansen et al. 2010), only a fraction (40%) exhibit an apical process, which moreover is not anchored in the ventricular border (Betizeau et al. 2013). The scaffolding cues for radial migrating neurons therefore differ between primates and rodents (Casingal et al. 2022; Cortay et al. 2020; Nowakowski et al. 2016).

A salient feature of rodent postmitotic neurons during the early stages of their radial migration is not conserved in primates. In rodents, the vast majority of early postmitotic cortical neurons initially show a prolonged pause (up to 48 hours) and start migrating from their birthplace via multipolar migration, during which they switch direction of movement before polarizing and embarking on radial trajectory (Bielas et al. 2004; Noctor et al. 2004; Tabata and Nakajima 2003). By contrast, the overwhelming majority (>80%) of primate early postmitotic neurons are bipolar and show only a restricted pause before embarking on their radial migrational path (Cortay et al.

2020). Of the VZ and OSVZ cycling progenitors in the NHP 90 percent correspond to four morphotypes showing a polarized morphology, which have a significantly higher neurogenic potential than the 10 percent of unpolarized progenitors (Betizeau et al. 2013). This observation suggests that inheritance of the bipolar morphology set the optimal conditions for effective initial steps of radial migration in NHP, by contrast with the rodent situation where a large majority of late-born pyramidal precursors are generated from unpolarized intermediate Tbr2 expressing progenitors with multipolar morphologies and highly dynamic processes (Kowalczyk et al. 2009; Kriegstein and Alvarez-Buylla 2009; Nelson et al. 2013).

Rates of neuron production and radial migration must be exquisitely orchestrated to ensure a coherent histogenetic process. The spatiotemporal variations in SG neuron production rates (Betizeau et al. 2013; Lukaszewicz et al. 2005) combined with the pronounced areal cytoarchitectonic differences observed between V1 and V2 (Lukaszewicz et al. 2005; Rockel et al. 1980) put significant constraints on the dynamics of radial migration in the primate occipital cortex. Investigation of the radial scaffold at mid-corticogenesis revealed differences in the density of radial basal processes in the SP of the primate visual cortex. In agreement with the higher numbers of bRGs in V1 OSVZ compared to V2 OSVZ (Betizeau et al. 2013; Lukaszewicz et al. 2005) a higher density of radial glia processes was observed in V1 compared to V2.

Live imaging of organotypic slices of the embryonic primate visual cortex shows that whereas V1 SG neurons show linear, strictly radial migration trajectories, V2 SG neurons show "abradial" trajectories, deviating from a radial path (Cortay et al. 2020). In addition, laminar and area-specific distinctive morphodynamic features of radially migrating IG and SG neurons have been reported. Specifically, radial migration velocity of SG neurons was observed to be significantly higher than that of IG neuron, on par with the higher production rates of SG neuron (Cortay et al. 2020). Laminar and areal differences in radial migration kinetics in the primate visual cortex are correlated with differences in morphology and membrane dynamics (Cortay et al. 2020). Whereas V1 SG neurons show straight membrane growth of the leading process associated with strict radial trajectories, V2 SG neurons show ruffling membrane growth underlying their "abradial" migration trajectories (Cortay et al. 2020), in the SP. The detailed study of the germinal zone of the primate visual cortex highlights a dual-pillar role of the OSVZ in the establishment of area-specific cytoarchitectural features: first by generating area-specific numbers of SG neurons and second in providing an area-specific scaffolding that constrains the properties of their radial migration.

The radiality of migration not only contributes to the organization of the ontogenic cortical columns (Jones and Rakic 2010; Rakic 1988b), in mouse it has also been shown to influence cortical circuitry assembly. Clonally related neurons share functional properties and preferentially interconnectivity (Gao et al. 2014; Li et al. 2012; Ohtsuki et al. 2012; Yu et al. 2009). The pronounced radial organization of V1 cortical neurons in primates (Rockland and Ichinohe 2004), which is likely to result from the strict radial migration trajectories, could therefore have functional consequences on V1 connectivity. The radial characteristics of migration observed in V1 SG migrating neurons could be linked to the high adult SG neuron density compared to other cortical areas. By contrast, the relative dispersion of postmitotic neurons, which is likely to result from the nonlinear migration trajectories in area V2, could also impact V2 functional connectivity. For instance, the communication via gap junctions between neurons generated by clonally related siblings are predicted to be less developed in V2 than in V1. Another possibility is that the functional radial units would be wider in V2, which could impact the local cortical network function and information processing. The spatial modulation of migration in order to accommodate area variation in SG neuron density could constitute an important adaptive feature as high SG neurons densities would favor the sparse coding strategy observed in these neurons that is thought to allow enhanced computational capacities (Harris and Mrsic-Flogel 2013).

4.9 Bringing into Line Understanding of the Development of Cortex with Modern Concepts of Cortical Function

So far we have reviewed the molecular and anatomical features that ensure unique properties of the OSVZ, which reaches its apogee in the primate area V1. We have argued for example, that the complex lineages of the OSVZ can underly the sophisticated circuits of SG layer neurons, prompting the conclusion that an unusual developmental process may underly an unexpectedly complex function. A number of recent considerations of the organizational features of the visual system suggest that area V1, the so-called primary visual area, can be expected to display a surprising degree of engagement in higher cognitive functions (Hochstein and Ahissar 2002; Vezoli et al. 2021). In addition there is a body of results showing that indeed area V1 is endowed with a unique potential: congenitally blind individuals exhibit an extraordinary plasticity and their area V1 routinely takes on complex linguistic functions, which is not the case following the deafferentation of any other cortical region including the auditory cortex (Amedi et al. 2004, 2003; Bedny et al. 2011). These observations suggest that area V1 deprived of its visual input is indeed an incredibly valuable piece of brain "real estate" that is immediately solicited by higher cognitive function namely language. Recent work suggests that the recruitment of the occipital cortex for high-level cognition function as observed in blind individuals relates to the intrinsic computational properties of the solicited region (Crollen et al. 2019). While it has been suggested that the nature of the "real estate" is largely determined by its location in the cortical hierarchy (Bedny 2017), recent genomic analysis shows that primate area V1 exhibits numerous genomic specificities suggesting that its computational power could be related to its unique transcriptomic cytoarchitecture (Jorstad et al. 2022).

Area V1 being a primary area sits at the base of the cortical hierarchy, and is the source of feedforward pathways ascending the cortical hierarchy which are reciprocated by feedback projections from higher order areas (Felleman and Van Essen 1991; Markov et al. 2014). Unraveling the role of the feedforward pathways has been a major part of the success story of neuroscience of the past 50 years that has shown that in the ascending pathway the converging inputs at successive levels of the hierarchy, fashion the receptive field properties of the individual cortical areas. This relatively straight forward interpretation of the feedforward pathway contrasts with the altogether more mysterious function of the yet twice as numerous feedback pathways (Bullier 2006; Markov et al. 2014). Globally, feedforward processes are envisioned to sequentially transform high-dimensional sensory representations such as an image into low-dimensional representations such as an object category located at higher hierarchical levels. Conceivably feedback pathways invert this process, thereby generating high-dimensional representations from low-dimensional variables (Hinton and Ghahramani 1997; Vezoli et al. 2021). However, it is only very recently that there has been empirical investigation on how top-down generative networks are supported by feedback connections (Bastos et al. 2012; Kosslyn 1994; Mumford 1992; Senden et al. 2019). Increasingly, evidence is coming from human imaging and nonhuman primate electrophysiology studies of spatial and temporal activation of area V1 in response to imagined objects (Emmerling et al. 2016; Hinton 2007b, 2007a; Naselaris et al. 2015; Senden et al. 2019; van Kerkoerle et al. 2017; Vezoli et al. 2021). These findings are coherent with the demonstration that imagery, imagination, and perception share the same neuronal machinery in area V1 and extensively throughout the visual cortex (Dijkstra et al. 2020, 2021, 2017).

What are the factors that trigger and guide the development of this valuable piece of brain estate? This includes the afferent specification of area V1 in terms of the ascending visual pathways as described earlier in their role in shaping first the proliferation of the early progenitors of the OSVZ and later relaying the influence of the environment on the maturation of the cortex (Wiesel 1982). This role of the sensory periphery in shaping the developmental biology of the cortex has been investigated since the 1960s, and was part of the conceptual issues of the competing theories of protomap vs. protocortex (O'Leary 1989; Dehay and Kennedy 2007; Kennedy and Dehay 1993; Magrou et al. 2018; Rakic 1988a).

In our description of the top-down generative networks provided we are referring to a large body of work that argues for a radical inversion of recent systems and cognitive neuroscience; namely that rather than the brain extracting information from the sensory epithelia it is implementing a process of active inference as originally proposed by Helmholtz in 1925 (Friston 2018; Rao and Ballard 1999; von Helmholtz 1925). This recent reinterpretation of brain function is anchored in hierarchical processing where predictive errors or surprises are proposed to be fed up the hierarchy and predictions played down the cortical hierarchy (Bastos et al. 2012; Markov and Kennedy 2013). This computational theory of brain function known as predictive coding or processing bears powerful explanatory power in terms of cognitive function, but also in computational neuroscience and brain diseases. Despite its conceptual attractivity, predictive processing is proving to be difficult to validate experimentally, although powerful breakthroughs are being reported in particular in respect to long-term priors as required for a developmental function (Hardstone et al. 2021). The reason for this difficulty is that while classical systems neuroscience looks at the response of neurons to manipulation of stimuli *exterior* to the brain (that is in the sensory environment); predictive processing requires addressing experimental manipulation of a stimulus originating from *within* the brain, and thereby examining how activity related to predictions integrates with the feedforward stream. We propose that development of the cortex will also be shaped by descending processes, which will be equally difficult to isolate. A systems-level example of this is provided by looking at the feedback to area V1, which shows that, contrary to what has been thought, there is a heterogeneity of feedback processes to different retinotopic subdivisions of area V1 (Wang et al. 2022). It turns out that the connectivity profiles of the upper and lower visual field show remarkable differences in terms of inputs from the ventral and dorsal stream in line with the well-established psychophysical properties predicted by Previc in his ecological theory of vision (Previc 1990). These findings raise numerous questions concerning visual function but also regarding the developmental mechanisms ensuring such a complex compartmentalization of the feedback pathways. The growing field of single-cell multi-omics is already revealing exciting insights into links between development and modern theories of brain function and will allow relating findings in experimental animal models to human neurobiology (Park et al. 2022). Already cell-type and gene-expression gradients are providing important insights into the hierarchical organization of cortex (Wang 2022). A particularly promising avenue of research is the recent demonstration in mouse of targetable prediction error units (O'Toole et al. 2022). This study was able to distinguish molecularly distinct positive and negative prediction error neurons in layers 2/3. We anticipate that the complex lineages of the SG neurons in primates (Betizeau et al. 2013) will lead to an expanded diversity of such cells. The determination of the developmental process that established them and the exploitation of their molecular signatures would constitute a major advance in understanding the primate brain.

Acknowledgments

We apologize to all colleagues whose important work could not be cited due to space limitations. This study is supported by a grant LABEX CORTEX-I ANR-11-LABX-0042 (H.K., C.D.) and LABEX DEVweCAN ANR-10-LABX-0061 (C.D.) Université de Lyon ANR-11-IDEX-0007; INSERM IRP CORTICAL_CONNECTOME (H.K., C.D.); ANR ThaCoPrim ANR21-CE16-0041 (C.D.)

References

Amedi, A. et al. (2004). Transcranial magnetic stimulation of the occipital pole interferes with verbal processing in blind subjects. *Nat Neurosci* 7 (11): 1266–1270.

Amedi, A. et al. (2003). Early "visual" cortex activation correlates with superior verbal memory performance in the blind. *Nat Neurosci* 6 (7): 758–766.

Arai, Y. et al. (2011). Neural stem and progenitor cells shorten S-phase on commitment to neuron production. *Nat Commun* 2: 154.

Arcila, M.L. et al. (2014). Novel primate miRNAs co-evolved with ancient target genes in germinal zone-specific expression patterns. *Neuron* 81 (6): 1255–1262.

Bastos, A.M. et al. (2012). Canonical microcircuits for predictive coding. *Neuron* 76 (4): 695–711.

Bedny, M. (2017). Evidence from blindness for a cognitively pluripotent cortex. *Trends Cogn Sci* 21 (9): 637–648. doi: 10.1016/j.tics.2017.06.003.

Bedny, M. et al. (2011). Language processing in the occipital cortex of congenitally blind adults. *Proc Natl Acad Sci USA* 108 (11): 4429–4434.

Berg, J. et al. (2021). Human neocortical expansion involves glutamatergic neuron diversification. *Nature* 598 (7879): 151–158.

Betizeau, M. et al. (2013). Precursor diversity and complexity of lineage relationships in the outer subventricular zone (OSVZ) of the primate. *Neuron* 80: 442–457.

Bicknese, A.R. et al. (1994). Thalamocortical axons extend along a chondroitin sulfate proteoglycan-enriched pathway coincident with the neocortical subplate and distinct from the efferent path. *J Neurosci* 14 (6): 3500–3510.

Bielas, S. et al. (2004). Cortical neuronal migration mutants suggest separate but intersecting pathways. *Ann Rev Cell Devel Biol* 20: 593–618.

Borello, U. et al. (2018). The logistics of afferent cortical specification in mice and men. *Semin Cell Dev Biol* 76: 112–119.

Breuss, M.W. et al. (2022). Somatic mosaicism reveals clonal distributions of neocortical development. *Nature* 604 (7907): 689–696.

Bullier, J. (2006). What is fed back? In: *23 Problems in Systems Neuroscience* (ed. J.L. van Hemmen and T.J. Sejnowski), 103–132. New York: Oxford University Press.

Calegari, F. et al. (2005). Selective lengthening of the cell cycle in the neurogenic subpopulation of neural progenitor cells during mouse brain development. *J Neurosci* 25 (28): 6533–6538.

Calegari, F. and Huttner, W.B. (2003). An inhibition of cyclin-dependent kinases that lengthens, but does not arrest, neuroepithelial cell cycle induces premature neurogenesis. *J Cell Sci* 116 (Pt 24): 4947–4955.

Casingal, C.R. et al. (2022). Coordinating cerebral cortical construction and connectivity. *Neuron* 110 (7): 1100–1115.

Charvet, C.J. (2014). Distinct developmental growth patterns account for the disproportionate expansion of the rostral and caudal isocortex in evolution. *Front Hum Neurosci* 8: 190.

Clancy, B. et al. (2001). Translating developmental time across mammalian species. *Neuroscience* 105 (1): 7–17.

Collins, C.E. (2011). Variability in neuron densities across the cortical sheet in primates. *Brain, Behav Evol* 78 (1): 37–50.

Collins, C.E. et al. (2010). Neuron densities vary across and within cortical areas in primates. *Proc Natl Acad Sci USA* 107 (36): 15927–15932.

Cortay, V. et al. (2020). Radial migration dynamics is modulated in a laminar and area-specific manner during primate corticogenesis. *Front Cell Dev Biol* 8: 588814.

Crollen, V. et al. (2019). Recruitment of the occipital cortex by arithmetic processing follows computational bias in the congenitally blind. *Neuroimage* 186: 549–556.

DeFelipe, J. (2011). The evolution of the brain, the human nature of cortical circuits, and intellectual creativity. *Front Neuroanat* 5: 29.

DeFelipe, J. et al. (2002). Neocortical circuits. *J Neurocytol* 31 (3–5): 387–416.

Dehay, C. et al. (1993). Modulation of the cell cycle contributes to the parcellation of the primate visual cortex. *Nature* 366: 464–466.

Dehay, C. et al. (1996a). Contribution of thalamic input to the specification of cytoarchitectonic cortical fields in the primate. *J Comp Neurol* 367 (1): 70–89.

Dehay, C. et al. (1996b). Phenotypic characterisation of respecified visual cortex subsequent to prenatal enucleation in the monkey. *J Comp Neurol* 376 (3): 386–402.

Dehay, C. et al. (1989). Maturation and connectivity of the visual cortex in monkey is altered by prenatal removal of retinal input. *Nature* 337: 265–267.

Dehay, C. and Kennedy, H. (2007). Cell-cycle control and cortical development. *Nat Rev Neurosci* 8 (6): 438–450.

Dehay, C. (2015). The outer subventricular zone and primate-specific cortical complexification. *Neuron* 85 (4): 683–694.

Dehay, C. et al. (2001). Cell-cycle kinetics of neocortical precursors are influenced by embryonic thalamic axons. *J Neurosci* 21: 201–214.

Dijkstra, N. et al. (2020). Neural dynamics of perceptual inference and its reversal during imagery. *Elife* 9: e53588.

Dijkstra, N. et al. (2021). No evidence for neural overlap between unconsciously processed and imagined stimuli. *eNeuro* 8 (5): ENEURO.0228-0221.2021.

Dijkstra, N. et al. (2017). Distinct top-down and bottom-up brain connectivity during visual perception and imagery. *Sci Rep* 7 (1): 5677.

Emmerling, T.C. et al. (2016). Decoding the direction of imagined visual motion using 7T ultra-high field fMRI. *Neuroimage* 125: 61–73.

Endo, S. (2012). G-substrate: the cerebellum and beyond. *Prog Mol Biol Transl Sci* 106: 381–416.

Eze, U.C. et al. (2021). Single-cell atlas of early human brain development highlights heterogeneity of human neuroepithelial cells and early radial glia. *Nat Neurosci* 24 (4): 584–594.

Felleman, D.J. and Van Essen, D.C. (1991). Distributed hierarchical processing in the primate cerebral cortex. *Cereb Cortex* 1 (1): 1–47.

Fiddes, I.T. et al. (2018). Human-specific NOTCH2NL genes affect notch signaling and cortical neurogenesis. *Cell* 173 (6): 1356–1369 e1322.

Fietz, S.A. et al. (2010). OSVZ progenitors of human and ferret neocortex are epithelial-like and expand by integrin signaling. *Nat Neurosci* 13 (6): 690–699.

Finlay, B.L. and Uchiyama, R. (2015). Developmental mechanisms channeling cortical evolution. *Trends Neurosci* 38 (2): 69–76.

Florio, M. et al. (2015). Human-specific gene ARHGAP11B promotes basal progenitor amplification and neocortex expansion. *Science* 347 (6229): 1465–1470.

Florio, M. et al. (2018). Evolution and cell-type specificity of human-specific genes preferentially expressed in progenitors of fetal neocortex. *Elife* 7: e32332.

Florio, M. and Huttner, W.B. (2014). Neural progenitors, neurogenesis and the evolution of the neocortex. *Development* 141 (11): 2182–2194.

Friston, K. (2018). Does predictive coding have a future? *Nat Neurosci* 21 (8): 1019–1021.

Gal, J.S. et al. (2006). Molecular and morphological heterogeneity of neural precursors in the mouse neocortical proliferative zones. *J Neurosci* 26 (3): 1045–1056.

Gamanut, R. et al. (2018). The mouse cortical connectome, characterized by an ultra-dense cortical graph, maintains specificity by distinct connectivity profiles. *Neuron* 97 (3): 698–715 e610.

Gao, P. et al. (2014). Deterministic progenitor behavior and unitary production of neurons in the neocortex. *Cell* 159 (4): 775–788.

Garcia-Moreno, F. et al. (2012). Compartmentalization of cerebral cortical germinal zones in a lissencephalic primate and gyrencephalic rodent. *Cereb Cortex* 22 (2): 482–492.

Gerstmann, K. et al. (2015). Thalamic afferents influence cortical progenitors via ephrin A5-EphA4 interactions. *Development* 142 (1): 140–150.

Girskis, K.M. et al. (2021). Rewiring of human neurodevelopmental gene regulatory programs by human accelerated regions. *Neuron* 109 (20): 3239–3251 e3237.

Hansen, D.V. et al. (2010). Neurogenic radial glia in the outer subventricular zone of human neocortex. *Nature* 464 (7288): 554–561.

Hardstone, R. et al. (2021). Long-term priors influence visual perception through recruitment of long-range feedback. *Nat Commun* 12 (1): 6288.

Harris, K.D. and Mrsic-Flogel, T.D. (2013). Cortical connectivity and sensory coding. *Nature* 503 (7474): 51–58.

Heide, M. et al. (2020). Human-specific ARHGAP11B increases size and folding of primate neocortex in the fetal marmoset. *Science* 369 (6503): 546–550. doi: 10.1126/science.abb2401. eabb2401.

Heide, M. et al. (2017). Novel gene function and regulation in neocortex expansion. *Curr Opin Cell Biol* 49: 22–30.

Herculano-Houzel, S. et al. (2007). Cellular scaling rules for primate brains. *Proc Natl Acad Sci USA* 104 (9): 3562–3567.

Hinton, G.E. (2007a). Learning multiple layers of representation. *Trends Cogn Sci* 11 (10): 428–434.

Hinton, G.E. (2007b). To recognize shapes, first learn to generate images. *Prog Brain Res* 165: 535–547.

Hinton, G.E. and Ghahramani, Z. (1997). Generative models for discovering sparse distributed representations. *Phil Trans Royal Soc London. Series B, Biol Sci* 352 (1358): 1177–1190.

Hochstein, S. and Ahissar, M. (2002). View from the top. *Neuron* 36 (5): 791–804.

Hodge, R.D. et al. (2019). Conserved cell types with divergent features in human versus mouse cortex. *Nature* 573 (7772): 61–68.

Horvat, S. et al. (2016). Spatial embedding and wiring cost constrain the functional layout of the cortical network of rodents and primates. *PLoS Biol* 14 (7): e1002512.

Iwata, R. and Vanderhaeghen, P. (2020). Tempus fugit. *Science* 369 (6510): 1431–1432.

Jabaudon, D. (2017). Fate and freedom in developing neocortical circuits. *Nat Commun* 8: 16042.

Jackson, C.A. (1989). Visual cortex development in the ferret. I. Genesis and migration of visual cortical neurons. *J Neurosci* 9 (4): 1242–1253.

Johnson, M.B. et al. (2015). Single-cell analysis reveals transcriptional heterogeneity of neural progenitors in human cortex. *Nat Neurosci* 18 (5): 637–646.

Jones, E.G. and Rakic, P. (2010). Radial columns in cortical architecture: it is the composition that counts. *Cereb Cortex* 20 (10): 2261–2264.

Jorstad, N. L. et al. (2022 November). Transcriptomic cytoarchitecture reveals principles of human neocortex organization. *BioRxiv*: 515349. doi: 10.1101/2022.11.06.515349.

Kalebic, N. et al. (2019). Neocortical expansion due to increased proliferation of basal progenitors is linked to changes in their morphology. *Cell Stem Cell* 24 (4): 535–550 e539.

Kalebic, N. and Huttner, W.B. (2020). Basal progenitor morphology and neocortex evolution. *Trends Neurosci* 43 (11): 843–853.

Kelava, I. et al. (2012). Abundant occurrence of basal radial glia in the subventricular zone of embryonic neocortex of a lissencephalic primate, the common marmoset callithrix jacchus. *Cereb Cortex* 22: 469–481.

Kennedy, H. and Dehay, C. (1993). Cortical specification of mice and men. *Cereb Cortex* 3 (3): 27–35.

Kennedy, H. et al. (1994). Topography of developing thalamic and cortical pathways in the visual system of the cat. *J Comp Neurol* 348 (2): 298–319.

Kennedy, H. et al. (2021). Determinants of primate neurogenesis and the deployment of top-down generative networks in the cortical hierarchy. *Curr Opin Neurobiol* 66: 69–76.

Klingler, E. et al. (2021). Temporal controls over inter-areal cortical projection neuron fate diversity. *Nature* 599 (7885): 453–457.

Kornack, D.R. and Rakic, P. (1995). Radial and horizontal deployment of clonally related cells in the primate neocortex. *Neuron* 15: 311–321.

Kornack, D.R. and Rakic, P. (1998). Changes in cell-cycle kinetics during the development and evolution of primate neocortex. *Proc Natl Acad Sci USA* 95: 1242–1246.

Kosslyn, S.M. (1994). *Image and Brain*. Cambridge, MA: MIT Press.

Kowalczyk, T. et al. (2009). Intermediate neuronal progenitors (basal progenitors) produce pyramidal-projection neurons for all layers of cerebral cortex. *Cereb Cortex* 19 (10): 2439–2450.

Kriegstein, A. and Alvarez-Buylla, A. (2009). The glial nature of embryonic and adult neural stem cells. *Ann Rev Neurosci* 32: 149–184.

LaMonica, B.E. et al. (2013). Mitotic spindle orientation predicts outer radial glial cell generation in human neocortex. *Nat Commun* 4: 1665.

Lange, C. et al. (2009). Cdk4/cyclinD1 overexpression in neural stem cells shortens G1, delays neurogenesis, and promotes the generation and expansion of basal progenitors. *Cell Stem Cell* 5 (3): 320–331.

Lewitus, E. et al. (2014). An adaptive threshold in mammalian neocortical evolution. *PLoS Biol* 12 (11): e1002000.

Li, Y. et al. (2012). Clonally related visual cortical neurons show similar stimulus feature selectivity. *Nature* 486 (7401): 118–121.

Liu, J. et al. (2017). The primate-specific gene TMEM14B marks outer radial glia cells and promotes cortical expansion and folding. *Cell Stem Cell* 21 (5): 635–649 e638.

Lui, J.H. et al. (2011). Development and evolution of the human neocortex. *Cell* 146 (1): 18–36.

Lukaszewicz, A. et al. (2006). The concerted modulation of proliferation and migration contributes to the specification of the cytoarchitecture and dimensions of cortical areas. *Cereb Cortex* 16 (Suppl 1): i26–34.

Lukaszewicz, A. et al. (2002). Contrasting effects of basic fibroblast growth factor and neurotrophin 3 on cell cycle kinetics of mouse cortical stem cells. *J Neurosci* 22 (15): 6610–6622.

Lukaszewicz, A. et al. (2005). G1 phase regulation, area-specific cell cycle control, and cytoarchitectonics in the primate cortex. *Neuron* 47 (3): 353–364.

Magrou, L. et al. (2018). How areal specification shapes the local and interareal circuits in a macaque model of congenital blindness. *Cereb Cortex* 28 (8): 3017–3034.

Magrou, L. et al. (2020). Unique features of subcortical circuits in a macaque model of congenital blindness. *Cereb Cortex* 30 (3): 1407–1421.

Mairet-Coello, G. et al. (2012). p57(KIP2) regulates radial glia and intermediate precursor cell cycle dynamics and lower layer neurogenesis in developing cerebral cortex. *Development* 139 (3): 475–487.

Markov, N.T. et al. (2013). Cortical high-density counter-stream architectures. *Science* 342 (6158): 1238406.

Markov, N.T. and Kennedy, H. (2013). The importance of being hierarchical. *Curr Opin Neurobiol* 23 (2): 187–194.

Markov, N.T. et al. (2014). The anatomy of hierarchy. *J Comp Neurol* 522 (1): 225–259.

Martinez-Cerdeno, V. et al. (2012). Comparative analysis of the subventricular zone in rat, ferret and macaque. *PLoS One* 7 (1): e30178.

Miller, B. et al. (1993). The early development of thalamocortical and corticothalamic projections. *J Comp Neurol* 335 (1): 16–41.

Mumford, D. (1992). On the computational architecture of the neocortex. II. The role of cortico-cortical loops. *Biol Cybern* 66 (3): 241–251.

Namba, T. et al. (2020). Human-specific ARHGAP11B acts in mitochondria to expand neocortical progenitors by glutaminolysis. *Neuron* 105 (5): 867–881 e869.

Namba, T. et al. (2021). Metabolic regulation of neocortical expansion in development and evolution. *Neuron* 109 (3): 408–419.

Naselaris, T. et al. (2015). A voxel-wise encoding model for early visual areas decodes mental images of remembered scenes. *Neuroimage* 105: 215–228.

Nelson, B.R. et al. (2013). Dynamic interactions between intermediate neurogenic progenitors and radial glia in embryonic mouse neocortex. *J Neurosci* 33 (21): 9122–9139.

Noctor, S.C. et al. (2004). Cortical neurons arise in symmetric and asymmetric division zones and migrate through specific phases. *Nat Neurosci* 7 (2): 136–144.

Nonaka-Kinoshita, M. et al. (2013). Regulation of cerebral cortex size and folding by expansion of basal progenitors. *EMBO J* 32 (13): 1817–1828.

Nowakowski, T.J. et al. (2016). Transformation of the radial glia scaffold demarcates two stages of human cerebral cortex development. *Neuron* 91 (6): 1219–1227.

Nowakowski, T.J. et al. (2018). Regulation of cell-type-specific transcriptomes by microRNA networks during human brain development. *Nat Neurosci* 21 (12): 1784–1792.

O'Leary, D.D.M. (1989). Do cortical areas emerge from a protocortex? *Trends Neurosci* 12: 400–406.

O'Toole, S.M. et al. (2022). Prediction error neurons in mouse cortex are molecularly targetable cell types. *BioRxiv*. doi: 10.1101/2022.07.20.500837.

Oh, S.W. et al. (2014). A mesoscale connectome of the mouse brain. *Nature* 508 (7495): 207–214.

Ohtsuki, G. et al. (2012). Similarity of visual selectivity among clonally related neurons in visual cortex. *Neuron* 75 (1): 65–72.

Pace, C. et al. (2018). Role of thalamocortical axons in areal specification of the primate visual cortex. Cortical Evolution. Las Palmas, Spain.

Park, S.H.E. et al. (2022). Corticogenesis across species at single-cell resolution. *Dev Neurobiol* 82 (6): 517–532. Epub ahead of print 2022/ 08/07. doi: 10.1002/dneu.22896.

Pebworth, M.P. et al. (2021). Human intermediate progenitor diversity during cortical development. *Proc Natl Acad Sci USA* 118: 26.

Pilaz, L.J. et al. (2009). Forced G1-phase reduction alters mode of division, neuron number, and laminar phenotype in the cerebral cortex. *Proc Natl Acad Sci USA* 106: 21924–21929.

Pilz, G.A. et al. (2013). Amplification of progenitors in the mammalian telencephalon includes a new radial glial cell type. *Nat Commun* 4: 2125.

Pinson, A. and Huttner, W.B. (2021). Neocortex expansion in development and evolution-from genes to progenitor cell biology. *Curr Opin Cell Biol* 73: 9–18.

Pollen, A.A. et al. (2015). Molecular identity of human outer radial glia during cortical development. *Cell* 163 (1): 55–67.

Pollen, A.A. et al. (2014). Low-coverage single-cell mRNA sequencing reveals cellular heterogeneity and activated signaling pathways in developing cerebral cortex. *Nat Biotechnol* 32 (10): 1053–1058.

Polleux, F. et al. (2001). Pre- and post-mitotic events contribute to the progressive acquisition of area-specific connectional fate in the neocortex. *Cereb Cortex* 11 (11): 1027–1039.

Powell, T.P.S. and Hendrickson, A.E. (1981). Similarity in number of neurons through the depth of the cortex in the binocular and monocular parts of area 17 of the monkey. *Brain Res* 216: 409–413.

Previc, F.H. (1990). Functional specialization in the lower and upper visual fields in humans. *Behav Brain Sci* 13: 519–575.

Rakic, P. (1974). Neurons in rhesus monkey visual cortex. *Science* 183: 425–427.

Rakic, P. (1988a). Intrinsic and extrinsic determinants of neocortical parcellation: a radial unit model. In: *Neurobiology of Neocortex* (eds. P. Rakic and W. Singer), 5–27. New York: Wiley-Interscience.

Rakic, P. (1988b). Specification of cerebral cortical areas. *Science* 241: 170–176.

Rakic, P. et al. (1986). Concurrent overproduction of synapses in diverse regions of the primate cerebral cortex. *Science* 232: 232–235.

Rao, R.P. and Ballard, D.H. (1999). Predictive coding in the visual cortex. *Nat Neurosci* 2 (1): 79–87.

Reillo, I. et al. (2011). A role for intermediate radial glia in the tangential expansion of the mammalian cerebral cortex. *Cereb Cortex* 21 (7): 1674–1694.

Robertson, R.T. et al. (1988). Investigations of the origins of transient acetylcholinesterase activity in developing rat visual cortex. *Dev Brain Res* 41: 1–23.

Rockel, A.J. et al. (1980). The basic uniformity in structure of the neocortex. *Brain* 103: 221–244.

Rockland, K.S. and Ichinohe, N. (2004). Some thoughts on cortical minicolumns. *Exp Brain Res* 158 (3): 265–277.

Saito, K. et al. (2019). Characterization of the inner and outer fiber layers in the developing cerebral cortex of gyrencephalic ferrets. *Cereb Cortex* 29 (10): 4303–4311.

Senden, M. et al. (2019). Reconstructing imagined letters from early visual cortex reveals tight topographic correspondence between visual mental imagery and perception. *Brain Struct Funct* 224 (3): 1167–1183.

Seuntjens, E. et al. (2009). Sip1 regulates sequential fate decisions by feedback signaling from postmitotic neurons to progenitors. *Nat Neurosci* 12 (11): 1373–1380.

Smart, I.H. et al. (2002). Unique morphological features of the proliferative zones and postmitotic compartments of the neural epithelium giving rise to striate and extrastriate cortex in the monkey. *Cereb Cortex* 12 (1): 37–53.

Smart, I.H.M. and Smart, M. (1982). Growth patterns in the lateral wall of the mouse telencephalon. *J Anat* 134: 273–298.

Stahl, R. et al. (2013). Trnp1 regulates expansion and folding of the mammalian cerebral cortex by control of radial glial fate. *Cell* 153 (3): 535–549.

Stepien, B.K. et al. (2020). Lengthening neurogenic period during neocortical development causes a hallmark of neocortex expansion. *Curr Biol* 30 (21): 4227–4237 e4225.

Subramanian, L. et al. (2017). Dynamic behaviour of human neuroepithelial cells in the developing forebrain. *Nat Commun* 8: 14167.

Suzuki, I.K. et al. (2018). Human-specific NOTCH2NL genes expand cortical neurogenesis through Delta/Notch regulation. *Cell* 173 (6): 1370–1384 e1316.

Tabata, H. and Nakajima, K. (2003). Multipolar migration. *J Neurosci* 23 (31): 9996–10001.

Takahashi, T. et al. (1995). The cell cycle of the pseudostratified ventricular epithelium of the embryonic murine cerebral wall. *J Neurosci* 15 (9): 6046–6057.

Telley, L. et al. (2019). Temporal patterning of apical progenitors and their daughter neurons in the developing neocortex. *Science* 364: 6440.

Telley, L. et al. (2016). Sequential transcriptional waves direct the differentiation of newborn neurons in the mouse neocortex. *Science* 351 (6280): 1443–1446.

Tomasello, U. et al. (2022). miR-137 and miR-122, two outer subventricular zone non-coding RNAs, regulate basal progenitor expansion and neuronal differentiation. *Cell Rep* 38 (7): 110381.

van Kerkoerle, T. et al. (2017). Layer-specificity in the effects of attention and working memory on activity in primary visual cortex. *Nat Commun* 8: 13804.

Vezoli, J. et al. (2021). Cortical hierarchy, dual counterstream architecture and the importance of top-down generative networks. *Neuroimage* 225: 117479.

Volpe, M. et al. (2006). trnp. *DNA and Cell Biology* 25 (6): 331–339.

von Helmholtz, H. (1925). *Helmholtz's Treatise on Physiological Optics*. Rochester, NY: Optical Society of America.

Wang, M. et al. (2022). Retinotopic organization of feedback projections in primate early visual cortex. *BioRxiv*. doi: 10.1101/2022.04.27.489651.

Wang, X.J. (2022). Theory of the multiregional neocortex. *Ann Rev Neurosci* 45: 533–560.

Wang, X.J. and Kennedy, H. (2016). Brain structure and dynamics across scales. *Curr Opin Neurobiol* 37: 92–98.

Wiesel, T.N. (1982). Postnatal development of the visual cortex and the influence of environment. *Nature* 299: 583–591.

Wlodarchak, N. and Xing, Y. (2016). PP2A as a master regulator of the cell cycle. *Cri Rev Biochem Mol Biol* 51 (3): 162–184.

Won, H. et al. (2019). Human evolved regulatory elements modulate genes involved in cortical expansion and neurodevelopmental disease susceptibility. *Nat Commun* 10 (1): 2396.

Woodward, W.R. and Coull, B.M. (1984). Localization and organization of geniculocortical and corticofugal fiber tracts within the subcortical white matter. *Neuroscience* 12 (4): 1089–1099.

Yu, Y.C. et al. (2009). Specific synapses develop preferentially among sister excitatory neurons in the neocortex. *Nature* 458 (7237): 501–504.

Zecevic, N. et al. (2005). Contributions of cortical subventricular zone to the development of the human cerebral cortex. *J Comp Neurol* 491 (2): 109–122.

Zhong, S. et al. (2018). A single-cell RNA-seq survey of the developmental landscape of the human prefrontal cortex. *Nature* 555 (7697): 524–528.

Zingg, B. et al. (2014). Neural networks of the mouse neocortex. *Cell* 156 (5): 1096–1111.

5

Neocortical Neurogenesis in Amniote Evolution

Virginia Fernández and Víctor Borrell

Institute of Neuroscience, CSIC - UMH, San Juan de Alicante, Spain

5.1 Introduction

The size, cytoarchitecture, and cell composition of the brain vary dramatically across amniotes, the group of vertebrates that includes sauropsids (reptiles and birds), synapsids (mammals), and all their extinct relatives. In general terms, brain size scales with body size following a linear allometric power law, with a scaling coefficient relatively stable across vertebrates, estimated between 2/3 and 3/4. Birds and mammals are of particular interest in this context because they independently evolved brains relatively larger than other vertebrate classes (Jerison 1975). In contrast, reptiles have small brains relative to body size and also reduced densities of neurons compared to the rest of amniotes, resulting in average total neuron count nearly 20 times lower than birds and mammals of comparable body size. Thus, evolution in amniotes involved major events that profoundly altered their brain size compared to the body (Smaers et al. 2021).

The evolutionary expansion of the brain affected most profoundly the dorsal pallium, the embryonic territory that gives rise to the neocortex (NCx) in mammals. The NCx is the seat of higher cognitive functions, and is organized in six main layers of neuronal and glial cells. Neurons may connect locally with other cortical neurons, or project their axons to other brain regions outside the NCx. Neurons in different cortical layers are also interconnected, forming functional columns. These general organizational features are robustly conserved across mammals (Dugas-Ford and Ragsdale 2015). In a subset of mammals (gyrencephalic) the neocortex went through an additional evolutionary innovation, the formation of folds, which allowed a further increase in neocortical surface area while limiting the increase in cranial volume, in contrast with the smooth cortex of lissencephalic mammals. The emergence of folds, or *gyri*, also brought together cortical regions that are distant in smooth cortices, thus also having an impact on cortical connectivity and function (Borrell and Calegari 2014; Borrell and Götz 2014; Reillo and Borrell 2012). The neocortex was a mammalian innovation, but other amniotes develop homologues and analogues to the mammalian cerebral cortex, such as the hyperpallium in birds and the three-layered dorsal cortex in reptiles (Fujita et al. 2019). All these brain structures are characterized by the expression of common key genes during embryonic development that define brain regional identity, and at the cellular level there is also significant analogy in neuron types and their connectivity (Puelles 2001) (Figure 5.1).

Neocortical Neurogenesis in Development and Evolution, First Edition. Edited by Wieland B. Huttner.

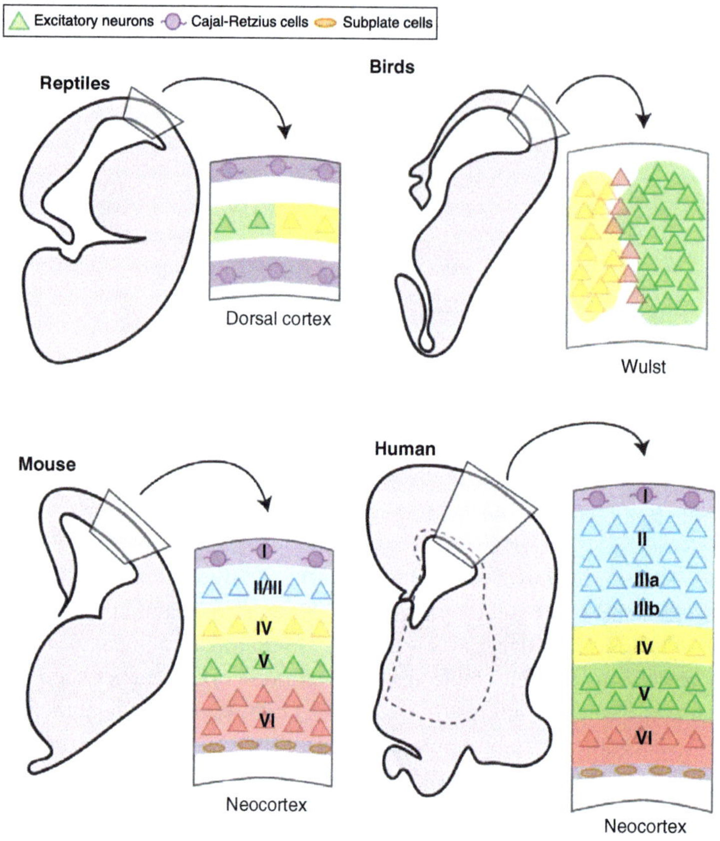

Figure 5.1 Cell distribution in the pallium of amniotes. Outline of brain sections at embryonic stages of (from left to right) reptile, bird, mouse, and human. Schemes show and the distribution of excitatory neurons (red, green, yellow, and blue), cells secreting reelin (purple) and subplate cells (orange). Only reptiles have a layer of pyramidal neurons in the dorsal cortex. Birds have a nuclear distribution of neurons in the Wulst. Mammals have a six-layered cortex with different size of each layer depending on the species. Note that humans have a dramatic enlargement of layers II/III.

The size and shape of brain structures, such as the cerebral cortex and its homologs, are determined by the final number of neuronal and glial cells, and their density. Accordingly, the size of the cerebral cortex is determined by the proliferation of progenitor cells, the differentiation of neurons and glia, and programmed cell death during development. At early stages of embryonic development, the rostral domain of the neural tube expands dramatically, giving rise to the two telencephalic vesicles. Then, the dorsal half of these vesicles is molecularly specified as the cortical primordium, to develop into the cerebral cortex. The early cortical primordium is formed by a single layer of neural progenitors, known as neuroepithelial cells (NECs). The behavior of NECs before the onset of neurogenesis is highly conserved across amniotes. At the onset of neurogenesis, NECs transform into a more committed type of progenitor cell named apical radial glia cell (aRGC), which will then go on to produce progenitor cells, neurons, and glia. Neurogenesis involves activating specific cell proliferation programs that generate the full repertoire of neuronal types and, ultimately, of cortical phenotypes (García-Moreno and Molnár 2020). In general terms, a progenitor cell may produce neurons directly, via a neurogenic division, or indirectly via an extra step generating an intermediate progenitor. Indirect neurogenesis takes more time but allows the expansion of the progenitor pool before the production of neurons, and this process increases exponentially the final number of neurons. In this chapter, we focus on the cellular and genetic mechanisms of cortical progenitor cell proliferation and their regulation across amniotes. We especially highlight mechanisms involved in neurogenesis, and the main differences across amniote phylogeny that lead to the formation of homologue structures but with different tissue architectures.

5.2 Cerebral Cortex Development in Mouse

The mouse has been traditionally used as the primary animal model to understand the development of the mammalian cerebral cortex, and to infer mechanisms of human cortical development and the underlying human neurodevelopmental disorders (Rakic 2009). In placental mammals (including human and mouse), the vast majority of neurons is generated during embryonic development (Polleux and Anton 2005). In mouse, cortical neurogenesis begins at embryonic day 11 (E11), reaches its maximum circa E15 and finishes shortly prior to birth (Bayer and Altman 1991; Polleux and Anton 2005).

5.2.1 Progenitors in Ventricular Zone: NECs and aRGCs

All excitatory neurons of the cerebral cortex derive from the lineage of apical progenitor cells that are located in the apical side of the cortical primordium where they form the primary germinal layer, the ventricular zone (VZ). Multiple types of apical progenitor cells exist in the VZ. Prior to neurogenesis these are all NECs, and during neurogenesis the predominant type by far is apical aRGCs, with a very minor presence of other progenitor cell types. For a comprehensive description of cortical progenitor cell types across amniotes, we refer the reader to Chapter 1.

5.2.1.1 NECs

At early stages of brain development, prior to the onset of neurogenesis, the cortical primordium is composed uniquely by a monolayer of neural stem cells named neuroepithelial cells (NECs) (Bayer and Altman 1991). NECs have apico-basal polarity and are attached to each other by their apical domain via adherens, tight, and gap junctions, which also allow molecular and electrical communication (Paridaen and Huttner 2014). NECs are typically expansive, undergoing symmetric proliferative divisions that exponentially increase their number (Miyata et al. 2010) (Figure 5.2). The duration of this preneurogenic period determines the number of NEC cell cycles and, hence, the abundance of the starting pool of progenitors at the onset of neurogenesis. NECs undergo mitosis at the apical surface, and during the rest of the cell cycle their nucleus moves along the apico-basal axis, in a process called interkinetic nuclear migration (INM). INM is characterized by the movement of the cell nucleus towards the basal side of the neuroepithelium during the G1 phase, which then remains in the basal side during DNA synthesis (S phase), followed by the movement toward the apical side during G2, to finally undergo mitosis again at the apical surface (Taverna and Huttner 2010). INM of NECs is not synchronized, so at any moment there are NEC nuclei along the entire thickness of the VZ, conferring its typical pseudostratified appearance (Figure 5.2). The size of the NEC pool at the onset of neurogenesis has critical consequences on cortical size. Experimental manipulations of the developing mouse neocortex that expand NECs, either by promoting cell cycle re-entry or decreasing apoptosis, lead to an increase in surface area and folding of the neuroepithelium (Chenn and Walsh 2002; Kingsbury et al. 2003; Siegenthaler et al. 2009).

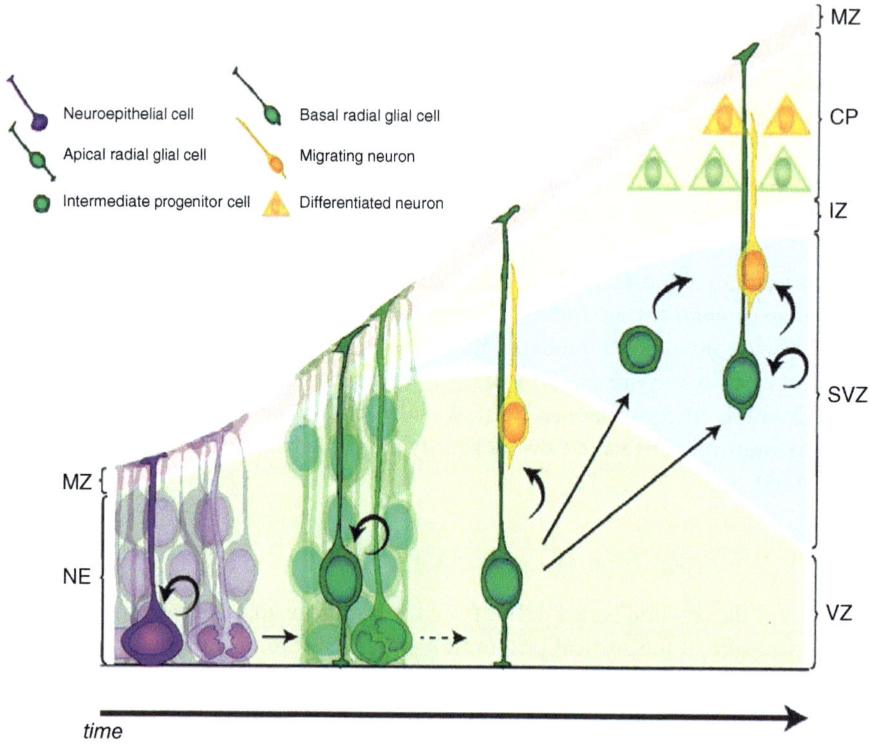

Figure 5.2 Stem cells in the developing cerebral cortex. Schema of the main types of progenitor cells and their lineage in the developing cerebral cortex. Prior to neurogenesis, NECs self-amplify undergoing symmetric divisions, to then generate aRGCs. aRGCs self-amplify to increase the pool of progenitors and at the onset of neurogenesis, they divide asymmetrically to generate neurons, directly or indirectly through secondary progenitors (IPCs or bRGCs). NE, neuroepithelium; MZ, marginal zone; VZ, ventricular zone; CP, cortical plate; IZ, intermediate zone; SVZ, subventricular zone.

The onset of neurogenesis is bookmarked by a change in cell properties of NECs, which lose tight junctions and acquire features typical of glial cells, including expression of the paired-box transcription factor Pax6, Brain lipid binding protein (Blbp), Vimentin, Slc1a3 (Glast), and S100b. These changes characterize the conversion of NECs into aRGCs. This transition in cell identity is critically regulated by Notch signaling, and expression of its downstream transcription factors Hes1 and Hes5 (Gaiano et al. 2000), as well as by Fgf10-mediated signaling, which promotes the generation of aRGCs and maintenance of their identity (Kang et al. 2009; Sahara and O'Leary 2009).

5.2.1.2 aRGCs

Apical RGCs are the primary type of neural progenitor cell in the cerebral cortex, giving rise to all cortical excitatory neurons and glia generated locally (Malatesta et al. 2003; Miyata et al. 2001; Noctor et al. 2001). Thus, aRGCs are more fate restricted than NECs while maintaining some of their typical characteristics, such as apico-basal polarity (contacting the basal lamina and the apical surface) and cell-cell attachment via their apico-lateral domain, in this case via adherens junctions (Figure 5.1). Similar to NECs, aRGCs also undergo INM, going through mitosis also in the apical, ventricular surface (Taverna et al. 2014). The apico-basal polarity of aRGCs, and the exposure of their apical cell membrane to the lumen of the telencephalic ventricle, are key in determining their biology, cellular lineage, and fate (Götz and Huttner 2005; Kriegstein and Götz 2003). For example, mutations altering apico-basal polarity cause changes in the plane of cell division, INM, proliferation and, eventually, in neurogenesis (Cappello et al. 2006; Sottocornola et al. 2010).

At the onset of neurogenesis, aRGCs undergo mostly self-amplifying divisions, producing two aRGCs. As neurogenesis proceeds, they gradually switch to asymmetric divisions, generating one aRGC plus a different type of cell. This other cell may be a secondary type of progenitor, or a neuron, both of which move away from the ventricular surface to the most basal (outer) part of the cortical primordium. In contrast, the cell body of aRGCs remains in INM at the apical domain of the cortical primordium, now conforming the clearly distinguishable VZ (Angevine et al. 1970). The progressive accumulation of newborn neurons above the VZ increases the thickness of the cortical primordium, which is coupled with the elongation of the basal process of aRGCs (radial fiber) that remains attached to the basal lamina.

Self-amplifying aRGCs divide with a vertical mitotic cleavage plane (perpendicular to the apical surface), resulting in an equal distribution of apical membrane and cellular components, thus producing two daughter cells of the same type (aRGCs). Following the same principle, cell divisions with an oblique mitotic plane produce an asymmetric distribution of cellular components, where the cell that inherits the apical membrane retains aRGC identity, and the other daughter cell becomes an intermediate progenitor or a postmitotic neuron (Huttner and Kosodo 2005). aRGCs dividing with a horizontal cleavage plane (parallel to the ventricular surface) produce a particular type of secondary progenitor: basal RGC (bRGC; see later). Typically, the daughter cell that inherits the basal process becomes a bRGC, and the cell inheriting the apical membrane remains an aRGC (LaMonica et al. 2013). The orientation of the mitotic cleavage plane in the mammalian cerebral cortex is regulated by multiple molecular factors, including Lgn, Insc, and Lis1 (Postiglione et al. 2011; Shitamukai et al. 2011; Yingling et al. 2008). In addition, the occurrence of symmetric or asymmetric cell divisions is regulated by proteins related to apical adherent junctions, such as Notch signaling, Par3, Par6, and Prominin-1 (CD133) (Bultje et al. 2009; Costa et al. 2008; Götz and Huttner 2005; Hatakeyama et al. 2004; Imayoshi et al. 2010; Kriegstein and Alvarez-Buylla 2009). Proliferative divisions are also regulated by a subset of genes controlling cell cycle re-entry like *Cdk4*, *Fgf*, and *CyclinD1* (Lange et al. 2009). Other important signaling pathways regulating cortical progenitor proliferation are the Wnt, Bmp, MAPK, Notch, retinoic acid, and Trnp1 pathways (see Fernández et al. 2016 for more details).

In the mouse cerebral cortex, the average duration of the cell cycle in aRGCs increases as neurogenesis proceeds (Govindan and Jabaudon 2017). Interestingly, increased duration of mitosis in aRGCs increases asymmetric divisions, thus decreasing self-amplification (Arai et al. 2011). The proliferation of aRCGs can also be modulated by microRNAs. During early brain development, a decrease in the expression *let-7* leads to the over-expression of *Irs2*, which promotes aRGC self-amplification at the expense of neuronal differentiation (Fernández et al. 2020). Another example of miRNAs regulating cortical progenitor proliferation and lineage is the case of *miR-3607*. Its ectopic expression in mouse neocortex increases Wnt/β-cat signaling, causing the amplification of RGCs and expansion of the VZ (Chinnappa et al. 2022).

5.2.2 Progenitors in the Subventricular Zone: IPCs and bRGCs

Neuron production in the neocortex stems from aRGCs. These progenitor cells are located only in the VZ, so the size of this population is limited to the maximum number of dividing cells that fit the apical VZ surface. However, aRGCs can generate secondary types of progenitor cells that locate basally and generate a secondary basal germinal zone, the subventricular zone (SVZ). The emergence of this second mitotic compartment expands the neurogenic potential of VZ progenitors, leading to the generation of greater numbers of neurons within the same restricted area (Cheung et al. 2010; Fish et al. 2008; García-Moreno and Molnár 2020; Noctor et al. 2004; Smart et al. 2002).

Basal progenitors are common in the developing brain of all amniotes. However, only mammals seem to have developed a *bona fide* SVZ in the cerebral cortex. In sauropsids, areas analog to the cerebral cortex contain sparse basal progenitors without forming a well-defined SVZ. Only the ventral pallium of reptiles and the dorsal ventricular ridge (DVR) of selected avian species form a genuine SVZ, but not so their cortex homolog. In mammals, the size and cellular complexity of the SVZ is very variable, especially between lissencephalic (e.g., mouse) and gyrencephalic (e.g., human) species. Thus, understanding how aRGCs produce basal progenitors may explain the differences in brain size observed across the amniote clade.

5.2.2.1 IPCs

As pointed out earlier, the asymmetric division of aRGCs can generate one neuron and a secondary progenitor, which will be located in the SVZ (Figure 5.2). In mouse, the SVZ is populated mainly (but not exclusively) by intermediate progenitor cells (IPCs). IPCs are multipolar progenitor cells that reside and divide in the SVZ, and contrary to aRGCs do not undergo INM and express the t-box transcription factor Tbr2 (Englund et al. 2005). In mouse, the vast majority of IPCs divide once to produce two excitatory neurons (usually do not self-amplify). Because each IPC self-consumes at mitosis, they are much less abundant than aRGCs (Kowalczyk et al. 2009). As neurogenesis progresses, there is a lower requirement for aRGC self-renewal and a greater need for neuron production, so there is a gradual predominance of asymmetric aRGC divisions producing IPCs and, hence, neurons (Kowalczyk et al. 2009; Noctor et al. 2004). In mice, Tbr2 is required for IPC specification and proliferation, as its loss causes a dramatic reduction of IPCs and their differentiated progenies. Upon Tbr2 loss, aRGCs switch from progenitor (indirect) to neurogenic (direct) asymmetric divisions, thus reducing the generation of IPCs. This shift from indirect to direct neurogenesis leads to an initial imbalance toward neuron production (neurons are generated instead of progenitors), but this early consumption of progenitors soon leads to a compromised neuron production, and cortical thickness is reduced (Sessa et al. 2008). In fact, around 80 percent of cortical excitatory neurons go through a stage of Tbr2 expression, suggesting that Tbr2 is necessary for excitatory neuron differentiation and subtype specification (Lv et al. 2019).

A hypothesis to explain the generation of IPCs in amniote evolution explores the effect of heterochrony in cell division dynamics, where a delayed cell cycle exit might underlie the formation of the SVZ (Charvet and Striedter 2011; García-Moreno and Molnár 2020). This hypothesis suggests that newborn neural-committed cells (neuroblasts) derived from aRGCs fail to exit from the cell cycle, but still move towards basal positions (as postmitotic neurons do). Radial migration of these immature neuroblasts might be arrested in the SVZ and remain cycling for some time, increasing the neurogenic output. In the mammalian cortex, such delay in cell cycle exit may happen on Tbr2-expressing neuroblasts (Arnold et al. 2008; Englund et al. 2005; Sessa et al. 2008; Vasistha et al. 2015).

5.2.2.2 bRGCs

The SVZ is also populated by bRGCs (Figure 5.2) (Fietz et al. 2010; Reillo et al. 2011), also known as oRGs (Hansen et al. 2010). These secondary progenitors exhibit many similarities with aRGCs, including a basal process extended radially across the cortical thickness and contacting its basal lamina, and the expression of Pax6, Sox2, Vimentin, and Nestin (Shitamukai et al. 2011; Wang et al. 2011). In human, nonhuman primates, and carnivores, bRGCs frequently also express Tbr2 and Hopx, are very abundant, and highly amplificative (Martínez-Martínez et al. 2016; Pilz et al. 2013; Reillo et al. 2011). In the mouse neocortex, the abundance of bRGCs is minimal compared to gyrencephalic species, and they are exclusively neurogenic, without self-amplification or self-renewal (Wang et al. 2011). bRGCs divide in the SVZ and do not perform INM, as opposed to aRGCs. A unique feature of primate bRGCs is that immediately prior to mitotic division their soma moves basally along the basal process, in a movement called mitotic somal translocation (MST) (Betizeau et al. 2013; Hansen et al. 2010).

bRGCs are produced by aRGCs after asymmetric divisions, with the mitotic cleavage plane either oblique or parallel to the ventricular surface. The daughter cell that receives the basal process becomes a bRGC, and the other cell may become a newborn neuron, an IPC, or even an aRGC that remains anchored to the ventricular surface and regrows a new basal process (LaMonica et al. 2013; Shitamukai et al. 2011). Experiments in the mouse neocortex have been able to force aRGC mitoses to occur with the cleavage plane parallel to the ventricular surface. This produces one daughter progenitor cell apically anchored, and another one delaminated, but without affecting the rate of neuron production (Konno et al. 2007). The production of bRGCs from aRGCs is strongly increased by the downregulation of Trnp1 (nuclear protein), even in the murine neocortex where bRGCs are otherwise very scarce (Stahl et al. 2013). Conversely, the over-expression of Trnp1 leads to the expansion of aRGCs at the expense of IPCs, causing the tangential growth of the cortical VZ surface.

5.2.3 Neuronal Radial Migration

Corticogenesis begins with the formation of a layer of pioneer neurons, named preplate. The preplate is composed by a combination of neurons generated locally, and Cajal–Retzius (CR) cells, which are neurons born at the borders of the dorsal pallium that migrate tangentially to cover the entire cortex. The first cohort of neurons born destined to form the future gray matter migrate radially and intercalate within the preplate, splitting it into the marginal zone (MZ), containing CR cells, and subplate, containing the locally generated pioneer neurons. The subplate is also present in sauropsids (Kostovic and Rakic 1990), and it provides a stable platform for the transient accumulation of afferent connections while the cortex is being constructed (Allendoerfer and Shatz 2003; Kanold and Luhmann 2010). CR cells are the major source of Reelin in the mammalian neocortex, which is essential for the inside-out organization of neocortical layers.

Newborn neurons originated in the cortical germinal zones are intimately associated with the radial fibers of RGCs, and use them as guide and substrate to migrate radially from their place of birth to the vicinity of the cortical surface, where they finish migration and begin to differentiate (Figure 5.2). In the mammalian neocortex, late-born neurons migrate over the layer of early-born neurons to reach a more superficial position above them, thus establishing a gradient of inside-first to outside-last (inside-out) distribution of neurons (Pasko 1974). This process is repeated with every new cohort of newborn neurons, until its characteristic six neuronal layers are formed. The cell–cell interaction between migrating neurons and the scaffold of RGC radial fibers is subject to precise molecular regulation, and its disruption leads to severe defects of neuronal positioning and layer formation in the cortex (Anton et al. 1997; Anton et al. 1999; Elias et al. 2007; Pasko 1974; Rakic 1978; Sidman and Rakic 1973). Due to this dependence of radially migrating neurons on radial fibers, the trajectory of these fibers determines the migratory route and final location of new neurons along the cortical surface (Rakic 1995). Thus, neurons born from a given RGC are usually located at close proximity in the mature cerebral cortex (Gao et al. 2014; Gupta et al. 2003; O'Leary and Borngasser 2006; Soriano et al. 1995). In reptiles, Reelin expressing cells are located in the apical and the basal parts of the cortex (Figure 5.1), and the radial migration of neurons establishes an outside-in gradient of neuron distribution (García-Moreno et al. 2018).

5.3 Sauropsids

The sauropsid lineage is composed of reptiles and birds, subclassified into lepidosaurs (including snakes, lizards, and tuatara) and archosaurs (birds, crocodilians, and turtles). Understanding cortical development in sauropsids is key to understanding the evolution of the mammalian cerebral cortex. Importantly, the structural organization of the brain in birds is extraordinarily different from mammals, and yet some species from these two clades share a similar level of cognitive performance, demonstrating evolutionary convergence of features important for cognition. As mentioned previously, the brain-to-body size ratio in birds and mammals is larger than in other vertebrate classes, such as reptiles, and this feature evolved in an independent manner (Jerison 1975; Smaers et al. 2021). Interestingly, whereas differences in duration of the neurogenic period may affect the final number of neurons produced (Montiel et al. 2016), convergent characteristics between mammalian and avian brains occurred independently from the duration of their neurogenic period, which in all sauropsids is much shorter than in mammals.

5.3.1 Homologies and Organization of the Pallium

In reptiles and birds, the brain structure homolog to the "6-layered" mammalian neocortex is the dorsal cortex (reptiles) and the hyperpallium or "Wulst" (birds), which contain elements of neuronal circuitry equivalent to the mammalian cerebral cortex, but with a different arrangement (Karten 2013). The dorsal cortex of reptiles is a relatively simple structure composed of three distinct layers: two cell-sparse plexiform layers (inner and outer) and a cell-dense neuronal layer in between (Figure 5.1). A similarly simple organization is also found in evolutionarily ancestral regions of the mammalian brain, such as the hippocampus and the piriform cortex (Cárdenas et al. 2018). Single-cell transcriptomic analyses comparing the brain of mammals and reptiles reveal the molecular conservation of several of these brain structures, including the hippocampal region, the avian DVR with the mammalian ventral pallium, and the anterior dorsal cortex of reptiles with the mammalian neocortex (Tosches et al. 2018). Birds have a large dorsal pallium, which unlike reptiles and mammals it is not organized in layers but in nuclei (Figure 5.1) (Dugas-Ford et al. 2012; Karten 2013). The avian homolog to the reptilian dorsal cortex and the mammalian neocortex is called "Wulst" or hyperpallium (Reiner et al. 2004). The Wulst processes mainly visual and somatosensory inputs, and it is especially developed in birds with high visual capacities such as raptors (Franchini 2021; Puelles 2001, 2017). In addition to the dorsal pallium, reptiles and birds develop the DVR, a big telencephalic structure that processes the main sensory inputs and is analog to the mammalian lateral neocortex. It must be noted that the evolutionary origin of the mammalian neocortex, and its homology with birds and reptiles, still remains the focus of a long-standing debate (Butler et al. 2011; Montiel et al. 2016; Puelles 2017; Striedter 2005).

5.3.1.1 Conservation and Divergence of Progenitor Cell Types

aRGCs are the most conserved type of cortical progenitor cell across amniotes. The main and distinctive morphological and molecular features of aRGCs are highly conserved, including apical mitosis, basal process extended towards the basal lamina, apical adherent junctions, and Pax6 expression (De Juan Romero and Borrell 2015). Although expression of Pax6 is a highly conserved characteristic of aRGCs across amniotes, the downstream effects of this expression vary slightly between species. In the chick pallium, high levels of Pax6 promote aRGC differentiation independently from developmental stage, whereas in mouse high Pax6 may promote either aRGC proliferation or neuronal differentiation, depending on developmental stage (Nomura et al. 2018). Different species also have a different abundance of aRGCs at the onset of cortical neurogenesis, depending on the initial expansion of NECs, as mentioned earlier. Intriguingly, aRGCs in birds and reptiles display a curved basal process (Nomura et al. 2014), potentially a common feature among nonmammalian amniotes and distinctive from mammals, where this process is radially straight.

Signals mediated by cell–cell interaction such as Notch receptors control the cellular dynamics during cortical development. Notch signaling is an evolutionary conserved pathway critical in fate determination of neural progenitor cells, where differential levels of Notch signaling between cortical progenitors directly impact the rate of neurogenesis in different amniote species (Nomura et al. 2013, 2014). Interestingly, Notch has a species-specific thermal sensitivity in the developing amniote brain, where hypothermia increases canonical Notch activity and reduces neurogenesis in chick neural progenitors (Nomura et al. 2022).

In the majority of reptiles, the proliferative and neurogenic activities of aRGCs in the dorsal cortex are very limited, such that they undergo only direct neurogenesis, without producing basal progenitors (Figure 5.3), and the final number of cortical neurons is relatively small (Cárdenas et al. 2018; Martínez-Cerdeño et al. 2006, 2016). In birds, aRGCs in the Wulst or hyperpallium combine direct with indirect neurogenesis (Figure 5.3) (Cárdenas et al. 2018; Martínez-Cerdeño et al. 2016; Nomura et al. 2013). Remarkably, direct neurogenesis predominates in the medial region of the dorsal pallium, whereas indirect neurogenesis predominates in the lateral region, as observed in chick embryos (Cárdenas et al. 2018). Avian indirect neurogenesis produces two different types of basal progenitors that exhibit morphological and molecular characteristics reminiscent of those in mammals: multipolar cells similar to IPCs, and morphologically polarized cells that resemble bRGCs (Nomura et al. 2016).

5.3.1.2 Absence of a Bona Fide SVZ

The SVZ as a distinct secondary germinal layer is only present in the mammalian neocortex (García-Moreno et al. 2018; Nomura et al. 2016), but some researchers have postulated that it is present in both leading domains of the amniote pallium: the mammalian dorsal pallium (i.e. neocortex) (García-Moreno et al. 2012; Smart et al. 2002), and DVR of selected avian species, while not in the Wulst (Charvet and Striedter 2011; Striedter and Charvet 2009). Basal progenitors do also exist in other parts of the embryonic brain, but there these progenitors are not clustered as a distinct, segregated, and organized compartment of cycling neural progenitors, located at a distance from the ventricular surface, which raises the question of how the SVZ emerged during evolution.

Regarding the molecular control of pallial progenitors in sauropsids, we found a conserved mechanism across amniote taxa that controls the shift from direct to indirect neurogenesis. Functional experiments in mouse, chick, and snake embryos, and in human cerebral organoids, demonstrate that the combination of high Slit/Robo and low Dll1 signaling is both necessary and sufficient to drive direct neurogenesis. The experimental decrease in *Robo* levels and increase in

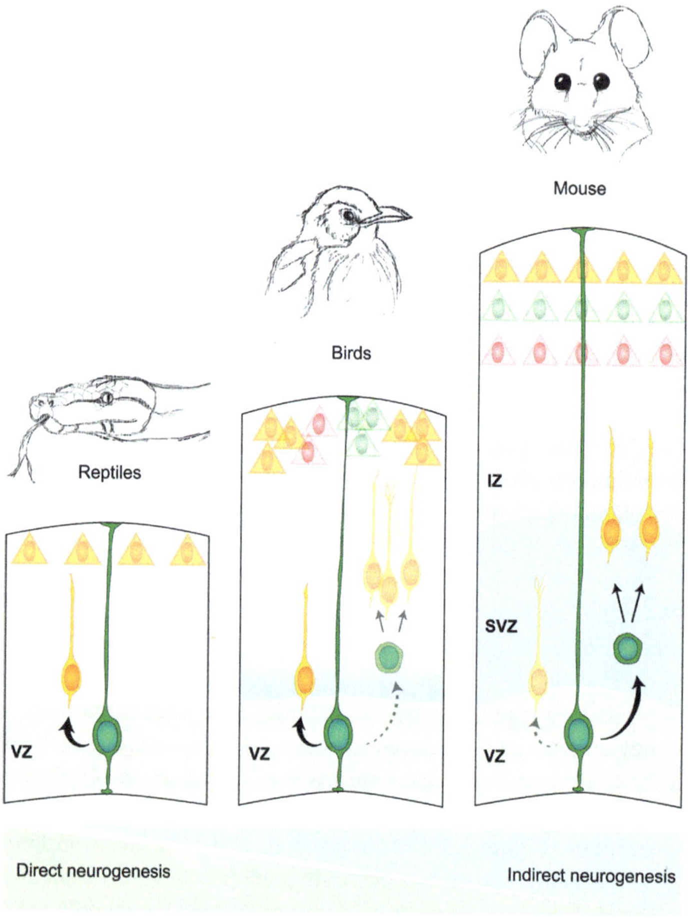

Figure 5.3 Different types of neurogenesis and neuron number in the pallium of amniotes. Drawings of representative reptile, bird, and rodent and schemas of their embryonic pallium showing the germinal layers, types of neural progenitor cells, and preferential mode of neurogenesis. Reptiles have ventricular zone (VZ) and apical radial glial cells (aRGCS). Thus, neurons are produced by direct neurogenesis. Birds have a non-bona fide subventricular zone (SVZ), populated by intermediate progenitor cells (IPCs, blurred blue), and a low proportion of neurons are generated though indirect neurogenesis. In mouse, indirect neurogenesis become much more predominant. New-born neurons migrate through the intermediate zone (IZ, gray) to reach their final position in the neuronal layer or cortical plate. Arrow thickness represents the relative frequency of each mode of neurogenesis.

Dll1 levels in aRGCs of snakes and birds promotes indirect neurogenesis via the generation of IPCs (Cárdenas et al. 2018). Basal progenitors in the chick dorsal pallium are molecularly heterogeneous, some expressing Pax6 (marker of RGCs) and some expressing Tbr2 (marker of mouse IPCs) (Cárdenas et al. 2018). This evidence has been challenged by Nomura and colleagues, who reported that basal cells in the chick pallium express Tbr2 but don't undergo mitosis, and hence they are not IPCs but neuroblasts committed to the neuronal glutamatergic lineage. Altogether, these results suggest that the proliferative activity in Tbr2 expressing cells is not completely conserved across amniotes (Nomura et al. 2016). In addition to IPCs, cells resembling the mammalian bRGCs have been also found in avian embryos (Fietz et al. 2010; Hansen et al. 2010; Nomura et al. 2016). In chick, bRGC-like cells express characteristic markers such as Pax6 and Sox2, their cell body is located basally to the VZ, and they extend apically and basally directed radial processes (Nomura et al. 2016). These observations suggest that basal radial glia-like cells may have emerged in ancestral amniotes, and then have undergone secondary loss in many of the nonmammalian lineages (e.g., reptiles).

5.3.1.3 Generation and Spatial Distribution of Neurons

The generation of different neuronal subtypes in the pallium depends on the temporal and spatial specification of progenitor cells. In mammals, apical progenitors produce different subtypes of neurons in a temporal-dependent manner (Suzuki et al. 2012). Studies in chick suggest that this temporal sequence of cortical neuron generation was already present in the stem amniote (Suzuki et al. 2012). However, this temporal code has not been preferentially selected in avian evolution, where the pallial germinal zone generates different types of excitatory neurons in a spatial-dependent manner (Nomura et al. 2008; Suzuki et al. 2012). In chick, dorsal pallial progenitors located in the medial domain generate neurons that express molecular markers typical of mammalian deep cortical layers, whereas progenitors in the lateral domain generate neurons that express markers of upper-layer neurons. Recent studies show that some progenitor cells in the pallium of chick and gecko are multipotent, such that they can generate different types of neurons in a spatial-independent manner (Nomura et al. 2018). Unfortunately, it is still not known if in the reptilian pallium neurons are generated following preferentially a spatial or a temporal-dependent strategy. It is also not clear if areas in the sauropsid dorsal pallium containing neurons that express markers of neocortical upper or lower layers can be defined as homologous to the corresponding mammalian neocortical layers (Montiel et al. 2016).

In birds, the hyperpallium follows a developing program without the tangential ingression of neurons from other pallial territories, contrary to what is observed in mice. These typically correspond to subplate and CR cells, so the molecular clues provided in mammals by these transient neuron populations may be altogether missing in birds (García-Moreno et al. 2018). Considering that in mammals these two layers of cells regulate the radial migration and proper positioning of neurons within the six-layered neocortex, their absence may be a key reason for the organization of neurons in the avian pallium not in layers, but in nuclei.

5.4 Higher Mammals: Increase in Cortical Size and Complexity

During mammalian evolution, neocortical size and complexity increased disproportionately compared to other brain structures. Cortical size differs dramatically between mammalian species (Teffer and Semendeferi 2012), mainly related to changes in its surface area rather than thickness. The size of the neocortex is critical for normal brain function, and microcephaly (small brain) or macrocephaly (large brain) are linked to severe cognitive deficits in humans (Sun and Hevner 2014). Neocortical thickness increases parallel to brain size across mammals, such that the human neocortex is three times thicker than in mouse (Hofman 1988; Zhang and Sejnowski 2000). The evolutionary expansion of cortical thickness in mammals was disproportionately greater in upper neuronal layers (2/3) compared to lower layers (Marín-Padilla 1992; Molnár et al. 2006) (Figure 5.1). Given the inside-out gradient of neurogenesis in the neocortex, this specific enlargement of upper layers has been linked to the production of neurons at late stages of neurogenesis, possibly linked to the dramatic expansion of the SVZ and its cellular composition. For example, at early stages of development aRGCs generate secondary progenitors at the expense of producing few neurons, but at late stages of neurogenesis most progenitors self-consume generating a vast amount of neurons, destined to upper layers and hence expanding them (Nowakowski et al. 2016; Pollen et al. 2015; Smart et al. 2002). The length of gestation also has a direct influence on the length of the neurogenic period (Stepien et al. 2020). In mouse, cortical neurogenesis lasts 9–10 days from a total of 19 gestational days, while in human it lasts circa 110 days out of 280 gestational days (Lewitus et al. 2014; Stepien et al. 2021). In the human lineage, neocortical expansion is not proportional across all areas and layers, with the rostral cortex (including the frontal and prefrontal areas) substantially more enlarged than caudal areas (Brodmann 1912; Deacon 1997; Donahue et al. 2018; McBride et al. 1999; Passingham and Smaers 2014; Rilling 2006; Schoenemann et al. 2005; Semendeferi and Damasio 2000; Semendeferi et al. 2002; Smaers et al. 2017). Depending on the species, the mammalian neocortex may be lissencephalic (smooth, or without folds, as in mice), or gyrencephalic (folded, as in carnivores and primates). Gyrification is typical of large cortices, such as those of large rodents (i.e., capybara) and primates (humans), whereas species with a small cortex (e.g., mouse, marmoset) are lissencephalic (Zilles et al. 2013).

5.4.1 Progenitor Cell Behavior and Regulation

5.4.1.1 NECs

In gyrencephalic species, the period of NECs expansion is longer than in lissencephalic rodents. This delay in the beginning of neurogenesis promotes an increase in the NEC pool, contributing to the expansion of the neocortex (Rakic 1995 2009). This seems to be regulated by the Wnt and Notch signaling pathways. Transcriptomic comparison of NECs and aRGCs in ferret has shown that expression of Wnt signaling genes such as *Lef1*, *Zic1*, and *Axin2* are specifically enriched in NECs, while expression of Notch signaling genes are enriched in aRGCs. Moreover, cell adhesion proteins such as fibronectins, integrins, and cadherins are upregulated during the early NEC-to-aRGC transition, suggesting that cell–cell interactions are another key factor controlling this process (Govindan and Jabaudon 2017). In apes, this NEC-to-aRGC transition requires a specific change in cell shape. At early stages of development, NECs have a thick apical process, and just prior to the onset of neurogenesis this apical process thins out, with the corresponding volume reduction. This subtle change in morphology is regulated by the transcription factor Zeb2, and is key for the onset of neurogenesis. Studies in cerebral organoids demonstrate that the NEC-to-aRGC transition is delayed in humans compared to other great apes, which is associated with differences in INM and cell-cycle length, and ultimately leads to the formation of larger brain organoids (Benito-Kwiecinski et al. 2021).

5.4.1.2 aRGCs and the Generation of bRGCs

In gyrencephalic species, the initial high self-amplification of VZ progenitors, and the greater abundance of founder NECs at earlier stages, directly translates into a much greater abundance of aRGCs than in species with a smooth cortex, giving rise to a larger VZ. In addition to the classical type of aRGCs found in all amniotes, the neocortex of gyrencephalic species displays apical RGCs in two additional morphological types not found in lissencephalic species: subapical progenitors (SAPs) and truncated Radial Glia (tRGC) (these are further elaborated in the chapter by Merino and Götz). SAPs have the general morphology of aRGCs but undergo mitosis in the basal domain of the VZ, in contrast to the typical divisions of aRGCs at the apical surface. SAPs are considered highly productive neurogenic progenitors because they undergo self-amplifying divisions before producing two neurons by symmetric terminal division. SAPs are quite abundant in gyrencephalic species but extremely scarce in lissencephalic ones (Pilz et al. 2013). tRGCs were initially discovered in human embryos at late stages of cortical development, and characterized by the loss of contact of the basal process with the cortical basal lamina, which in fact retracts to the vicinity of VZ/ISVZ, hence having a "truncated" basal process (Nowakowski et al. 2016). These progenitor cells evolve from the prototypical aRGCs since circa gestational week (GW) 17, and characteristically express CRYAB and NR4A1 (Nowakowski et al. 2016).

At the molecular level, a key gene that regulates the behavior and lineage of aRGCs, with relevance in gyrencephalic species, is Trnp1 (Stahl et al. 2013), a DNA-associated protein highly expressed in self-amplifying aRGCs (Pinto et al. 2008). Expression levels of *Trnp1* in aRGCs change during development, from the highest levels at early developmental stages, to then gradually decrease as neurogenesis progresses. Over-expression of *Trnp1* in aRGCs induces their symmetric amplificative division (producing two aRGCs), with the consequent decrease in the generation of secondary progenitors and neurons. Conversely, downregulation of *Trnp1* increases the production of secondary progenitors (both IPCs and bRGCs) and neurons (Stahl et al. 2013). Analysis of *Trnp1* expression in the developing cortex of ferret and human showed that this is specifically low in cortical regions fated to generate folds, and high in prospective fissures, highlighting its key role in cortical folding (de Juan Romero et al. 2015; Stahl et al. 2013).

Several genes are exclusively expressed in human aRGCs, many of which regulate their cellular progeny, including the abundance of secondary progenitor cells. One of these genes is platelet-derived growth factor D (PDGFD), a protein-coding gene expressed in human pallial aRGCs. Pharmacological inhibition of the PDGFD-PDGFRβ signaling cascade in human embryonic brain slices disrupts the normal cell cycle progression of aRGCs, whereas the ectopic expression of PDGFD or its receptor PDGFRβ in the developing mouse cortex promotes the generation of bRGCs, otherwise scarce (Lui et al. 2014). In 2015, Florio and colleagues identified the Rho GTPase-Activating Protein 11B (ARHGAP11B) as a human-specific gene specifically expressed in aRGCs that promotes the production of basal progenitors, and drives folding of the mouse cortex when ectopically expressed (Florio et al. 2015). ARHGAP11B emerged during the recent human lineage after separation from the chimpanzee, as a partial duplication of ARHGAP11A (Antonacci et al. 2014) (see Chapter 8). Ectopic expression of ARHGAP11B in the embryonic mouse neocortex promotes the massive production of secondary progenitors from aRGCs, many of which are bRGCs, hence diving the generation of cortical folds. Subsequent studies identified three additional human-specific genes, evolved from Notch2 (NOTCH2NL A through C), that were generated by multiple rounds of gene duplication and conversion. NOTCH2NL is highly enriched in human cortical progenitors and its ectopic expression in mouse embryos promotes cortical progenitor amplification and delays their differentiation, while its downregulation induces neuronal differentiation (Fiddes et al. 2018; Suzuki et al. 2018). Human duplications in NOTCH2NL are associated with abnormally large brains (i.e., megalencephaly; Fiddes et al. 2018).

Genes specific to great apes have also been identified, such as TBC1D3, which emerged after several gene duplications during evolution and are related to brain development and bRGC production. Ectopic expression of TBC1D3 in mouse cortical aRGCs induces the generation of bRGCs and subsequent cortical folding (Ju et al. 2016). In line with this finding, Liu and colleagues (2017) identified TMEM14B as a primate-specific marker for bRGCs. Genetic manipulations to express this gene in the VZ of the mouse neocortex promoted secondary progenitor production, together with the expansion of the SVZ and, in some cases, the generation of cortical folds (Liu et al. 2017; Uzquiano et al. 2018). The biological relevance of all these studies is the discovery of genes with key roles in human brain evolution, which suffice to generate cortical expansion and folding in an evolutionary distant context, such as the small and smooth mouse neocortex. This opens the gate to a deeper understanding of the evolution of human brain development (Wong et al. 2015).

5.4.1.3 Outer Subventricular Zone Formation and Expansion

Basal progenitors are much more proliferative and abundant in gyrencephalic than in lissencephalic mammals, which form an enlarged and thick SVZ (Figure 5.2). In contrast to small rodents, with a smooth cortex, bRGCs are very abundant in gyrencephalic species, where these self-amplify dramatically increasing the production of neurons and promoting cortex folding (Fietz et al. 2010; Pilz et al. 2013; Reillo et al. 2011). Compared with the developing mouse cortex, where the SVZ contains a relatively low number of progenitors, in gyrencephalic species the SVZ is the predominant germinal layer, containing a much greater number of progenitor cells. In primates, not only the number but also the diversity of basal progenitor cell types in the SVZ is much greater than in other species. Multiple morphotypes have been described in the embryonic neocortex of macaque monkeys, including bRGCs with only a basal process, only an apical process, with both processes, or even with the transient extension and retraction of these processes (Betizeau et al. 2013). More detailed analyses in ferret, a small carnivore, identified additional morphotypes of bRGC: with two basal processes (bRGC-2-basal-P), and with two basal and one apical process (bRGC-apical-2-basal-P) (Kalebic et al. 2019). These extra processes in bRGCs are thought to improve their capacity for proliferation, and thus contribute to increase the pool of SVZ progenitors (Kalebic et al. 2019). As a result of this great expansion of cortical basal progenitors in gyrencephalic species, the SVZ is subdivided in two different compartments: inner and outer (ISVZ and OSVZ) (Smart et al. 2002; Dehay and Kennedy 2007; Reillo et al. 2011). The ISVZ is immediately basal to the VZ and contains a high density of progenitor cells, whereas the OSVZ is located basal to the ISVZ and has decreased cell density. The OSVZ is by far the thickest germinal compartment of the developing cortex in gyrencephalic species, and thought to contribute most significantly to cortical expansion and folding. Within the OSVZ, bRGCs are extremely abundant, highly proliferative, diverse, and with very plastic lineage dynamics. Altogether, this contributes to a dramatic increase in neurogenesis and cortical expansion (Betizeau et al. 2013; Fietz et al. 2010; Hansen et al. 2010; LaMonica et al. 2013; Lukaszewicz et al. 2005; Reillo et al. 2011; Smart et al. 2002). ISVZ and OSVZ are separated by a distinct fiber-rich layer called the inner fiber layer, and an outer fiber layer is located basal to the OSVZ. Both fiber layers are particularly prominent in primates (Smart et al. 2002).

The cellular composition of ISVZ and OSVZ is very similar, both containing bRGCs and IPCs. This is in agreement with the closely related gene expression profiles of ISVZ and OSVZ in the human and ferret developing neocortex (Fietz et al. 2010; Miller et al. 2014). IPCs located in the SVZ may be generated from the VZ or from bRGCs located in the SVZ. Downregulation of the transcription factor Eomes/Tbr2 reduces the abundance of IPCs and bRGCs in the gyrencephalic ferret, specifically suppressing the generation of upper layer neurons and preventing cortex folding (Toda et al. 2016). This is in agreement with the role of Tbr2 in mouse neocortex development (Sessa et al. 2008), suggesting that the effect of Tbr2 on the generation of IPCs is conserved across mammals (Cárdenas and Borrell 2020). bRGCs are also generated by aRGCs (in the VZ) or by bRGCs already in the SVZ that undergo self-amplification. Studies in ferret by Martínez-Martínez and colleagues identified a brief time window during embryonic development when aRGCs generate a massive number of bRGCs by self-consumption, which then become the founder progenitor cells of the OSVZ. After this brief period, the OSVZ becomes a germinal layer independent from the lineage of aRGCs in VZ, expanding exclusively by progenitor cell self-renewal. The time window for bRGC seeding of the OSVZ is defined by the transient and coincident downregulation of *Cdh1* and *Trnp1* in the VZ; the subsequent upregulation of these two genes blocks the production of OSVZ bRGCs, and bookmarks the beginning of its independent lineage (Martínez-Martínez et al. 2016).

Some of the mechanisms regulating bRGC behavior and lineage are conserved with aRGCs, but the morphological and spatial characteristics of bRGCs make them a unique cell type. Contrary to early notions (Hansen et al. 2010), bRGCs in gyrencephalic species are highly proliferative, re-entering cell cycle several times and, thus, expanding their population (Betizeau et al. 2013). In contrast to IPCs, which divide with random cleavage planes, the majority of bRGCs divide with a horizontal cleavage plane. After cell division, the basal daughter inherits the basal process and maintains bRGC identity, whereas the apical daughter cell becomes a neuron or an IPC (Hansen et al. 2010). Extracellular matrix components together with other signals in direct contact with the basal process or cell body of bRGCs create a microenvironment in the OSVZ that controls their proliferation (Fietz et al. 2010; Pollen et al. 2015).

Similar to aRGCs, the Notch signaling pathway plays important roles in the regulation of OSVZ progenitors, especially controlling bRGC behavior. Inhibition of Notch signaling in human bRGCs induces their neuronal differentiation (Hansen et al. 2010). Similarly, Sonic hedgehog (SHH) signaling levels regulate the generation of bRGCs (Wang et al. 2016). SHH is strongly expressed in human fetal neocortex when compared with mouse. Its ectopic expression in mouse neocortex causes the expansion of bRGCs and IPCs, and the formation of neocortical folds. Conversely, the blockade of SHH signaling in human cerebral organoids decreases specifically the abundance of bRGCs. SHH signaling may actually increase the proliferation of a specific subtype of bRGC, characterized by the expression of Hopx. Suppression of SHH signaling in the developing ferret cortex reduces Hopx-expressing bRGCs and the generation of upper-layer neurons, together with a decrease in cortical folding. Given that SHH signaling is more active in the neocortex of gyrencephalic than of lissencephalic species, it seems that this pathway is of significant importance in cortex folding (Del-Valle-Anton and Borrell 2022; Matsumoto et al. 2020).

In addition to protein-coding genes, different miRNAs also play key roles as regulators of bRGC proliferation. Tomasello and colleagues (2022) showed that *miR-137* promotes bRGC self-amplification together with the generation of upper layer neurons, while expression of *miR-122* decreases neuronal differentiation. These findings indicate that cortical expansion is also regulated by the cell type-specific expression of miRNAs during development (Tomasello et al. 2022).

5.4.1.4 Radial Migration of Neurons and Tangential Expansion

The radial unit hypothesis postulated by Pasko Rakic more than three decades ago advanced our understanding of how the developing neocortex is organized. This hypothesis postulates that progenitor cells residing in the ventricular surface (aRGCs, or proliferative units) form a protomap of the future mature cerebral cortex. aRGCs give rise to neurons that will use the basal fibers of the former as substrate and guide for their radial migration from the neurogenic layers to the cortical surface. Thus, the protomap made by ventricular progenitors is radially projected onto the cytoarchitectonic cortical areas formed by postmitotic neurons (Rakic 1988). Following this seminal idea, subsequent models have been developed to explain human brain development, especially regarding the existence and importance of the OSVZ and bRGCs, which contribute to the tangential dispersion of migrating neurons and lead to cortical folding (Kriegstein et al. 2006; Nowakowski et al. 2016; Reillo et al. 2011). The currently accepted model of the development of cortical folds postulates that folding depends on the presence of extra basal fibers provided by bRGCs. These basal processes from bRGCs intercalate within the existing scaffold of basal fibers from aRGCs, modifying the parallel disposition of these fibers toward a fanned array, which causes the tangential dispersion of radially migrating neurons (Figure 5.4). The extra bRGC basal processes guide neurons in laterally dispersive trajectories, while maintaining their radial glia-dependent locomotive migration (Gertz and Kriegstein 2015). A further modification of this model, proposed by Nowakowski and colleagues, adds a new level of complexity in human cortical development, where tRGCs at the VZ do not extend their basal process beyond the ISVZ, thus setting a gap in the radial fiber scaffold between VZ and OSVZ. The model proposes that the absence in OSVZ of radial fibers from aRGCs allows space for the expansion of bRGCs, and neurons generated in the OSVZ

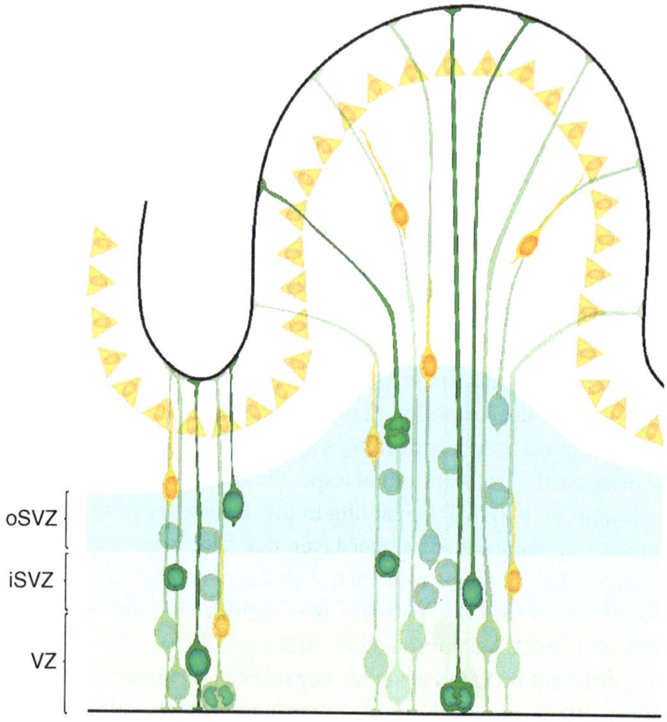

Figure 5.4 Cell mechanism of tangential expansion that generates cortical folding. Differential arrangement of the radial fiber scaffold in the cerebral cortex in a sulcus (left) or in a gyrus (right). In sulci, the radial glia scaffold is parallel and there is no net lateral dispersion of pyramidal neurons (yellow). In gyri, the radial fiber scaffold acquires a fan-like organization due to the intercalation of radial fibers from bRGCs. As a result, radially migrating neurons follow divergent trajectories and end far from their birth place; this increases cortical surface area and ultimately promotes folding. VZ, ventricular zone; iSVZ, inner subventricular zone; oSVZ, outer subventricular zone.

after this period will only migrate following the basal fibers of bRGCs (Nowakowski et al. 2016). Although the picture is far from complete, this model may explain the dramatic increase in surface area between upper layers (II–IV) and lower layers (V and VI) of the human neocortex, which is believed key for cortex folding (Nowakowski et al. 2016).

As presented in this chapter, multiple cellular and molecular mechanisms changed during evolution generating a wide range of cortical phenotypes, with specific cytoarchitectonic, hodological, and cellular characteristics. In each species, the behavior of progenitor cells, starting with NECs and aRGCs, and following with IPCs and bRGCs, determines the main strategy of embryonic neurogenesis (e.g., direct vs. indirect neurogenesis), with a dramatic impact on the final size and shape of their brain. Within mammals, the progeny of secondary progenitor cells (e.g., amplification of progenitors vs. neurogenesis) determines the size and thickness of the SVZ. This may eventually split in two subcompartments rich in highly proliferative progenitor cells (ISVZ and OSVZ), and thus contribute to the folding of the cerebral cortex, a central process in mammalian brain development and evolution.

References

Allendoerfer, K.L. and Shatz, C.J. (2003). The subplate, a transient neocortical structure. *Ann Rev Neurosci* 17: 185–218. doi: 10.1146/annurev.ne.17.030194.001153.

Angevine, J.B. et al. (1970). Embryonic vertebrate central nervous system. *Anat Record* 166 (2): 257–261. doi: 10.1002/AR.1091660214.

Anton, E.S. (1997). Role of GGF/neuregulin signaling in interactions between migrating neurons and radial glia in the developing cerebral cortex. *Development* 124 (18): 3501–3510. doi: 10.1242/DEV.124.18.3501.

Anton, E.S. et al. (1999). Distinct functions of alpha3 and alpha(v) integrin receptors in neuronal migration and laminar organization of the cerebral cortex. *Neuron* 22 (2): 277–289. doi: 10.1016/S0896-6273(00)81089-2.

Antonacci, F. et al. (2014). Palindromic GOLGA8 core duplicons promote chromosome 15q13.3 microdeletion and evolutionary instability. *Nat Genet* 46 (12): 1293–1302. doi: 10.1038/NG.3120.

Arai, Y. et al. (2011). Neural stem and progenitor cells shorten S-phase on commitment to neuron production. *Nat Commun* 2 (1): 1–12. doi: 10.1038/ncomms1155.

Arnold, S.J. et al. (2008). The T-box transcription factor Eomes/Tbr2 regulates neurogenesis in the cortical subventricular zone. *Genes Dev* 22 (18): 2479. doi: 10.1101/GAD.475408.

Bayer, S.A. and Altman, J. (1991). *Neocortical Development*. New York: Raven Press.

Benito-Kwiecinski, S. et al. (2021). An early cell shape transition drives evolutionary expansion of the human forebrain. *Cell* 184 (8): 2084–2102.e19. doi: 10.1016/J.CELL.2021.02.050.

Betizeau, M. et al. (2013). Precursor diversity and complexity of lineage relationships in the outer subventricular zone of the primate. *Neuron* 80 (2): 442–457. doi: 10.1016/j.neuron.2013.09.032.

Borrell, V. and Calegari, F. (2014). Mechanisms of brain evolution. *Neurosci Res* 86: 14–24. doi: 10.1016/J.NEURES.2014.04.004.

Borrell, V. and Götz, M. (2014). Role of radial glial cells in cerebral cortex folding. *Curr Opin Neurobiol* 27: 39–46. doi: 10.1016/j.conb.2014.02.007.

Brodmann, K. (1912). *Neue Ergebnisse über die vergleichende histologische Lokalisation der Grosshirnrinde mit besonderer Berücksichtigung des Stirnhirns*. https://scholar.google.com/scholar_lookup?journal=Anat.+Anzeiger.&title=Neue+ergebnisse+über+die+vergleichende+histologische+lokalisation+der+grosshirnrinde+mit+besonderer+berücksichtigung+des+stirnhirns.&author=K.+Brodmann&volume=41&publication_year=1912 (accessed 2 June 2022).

Bultje, R.S. et al. (2009). Mammalian Par3 regulates progenitor cell asymmetric division via Notch signaling in the developing neocortex. *Neuron* 63 (2): 189–202. doi: 10.1016/J.NEURON.2009.07.004.

Butler, A.B. et al. (2011). Evolution of the amniote pallium and the origins of mammalian neocortex. *Ann New York Acad Sci* 1225 (1): 14–27. doi: 10.1111/J.1749-6632.2011.06006.X.

Cappello, S. et al. (2006). The Rho-GTPase cdc42 regulates neural progenitor fate at the apical surface. *Nat Neurosci* 9 (9): 1099–1107. doi: 10.1038/nn1744.

Cárdenas, A. et al. (2018). Evolution of cortical neurogenesis in amniotes controlled by robo signaling levels. *Cell* 174 (3): 590–606.e21. doi: 10.1016/J.CELL.2018.06.007.

Cárdenas, A. and Borrell, V. (2020). Molecular and cellular evolution of corticogenesis in amniotes. *Cell Mol Life Sci: CMLS* 77 (8): 1435–1460. doi: 10.1007/s00018-019-03315-x.

Charvet, C.J. and Striedter, G.F. (2011). Causes and consequences of expanded subventricular zones. *Eur J Neurosci* 34 (6): 988–993. doi: 10.1111/J.1460-9568.2011.07818.X.

Chenn, A. and Walsh, C.A. (2002). Regulation of cerebral cortical size by control of cell cycle exit in neural precursors. *Science* 297 (5580): 365–369. doi: 10.1126/SCIENCE.1074192/SUPPL_FILE/1074192S1_THUMB.GIF.

Cheung, A.F.P. et al. (2010). The subventricular zone is the developmental milestone of a 6-layered neocortex. *Cereb Cortex* 20 (5): 1071–1081. doi: 10.1093/CERCOR/BHP168.

Chinnappa, K. et al. (2022). Secondary loss of miR-3607 reduced cortical progenitor amplification during rodent evolution. *Sci Adv* 8 (2): eabj4010. doi: 10.1126/SCIADV.ABJ4010.

Costa, M.R. et al. (2008). Par-complex proteins promote proliferative progenitor divisions in the developing mouse cerebral cortex. *Development* 135 (1): 11–22. doi: 10.1242/DEV.009951.

Deacon, T.W. (1997). What makes the human brain different? *Ann Rev Anthropol* 26 (1): 337–357. doi: 10.1146/annurev.anthro.26.1.337.

Dehay, C. and Kennedy, H. (2007). Cell-cycle control and cortical development. *Nat Rev Neurosci* 8 (6): 438–450. doi: 10.1038/nrn2097.

Del-Valle-Anton, L. and Borrell, V. (2022). Folding brains. *Physiol Rev* 102 (2): 511–550. doi: 10.1152/PHYSREV.00016.2021.

Donahue, C.J. et al. (2018). Quantitative assessment of prefrontal cortex in humans relative to nonhuman primates. *Proc Natl Acad Sci USA* 115 (22): E5183–E5192. doi: 10.1073/PNAS.1721653115.

Dugas-Ford, J. and Ragsdale, C.W. (2015). Levels of homology and the problem of neocortex. Annu Rev Neurosci 38: 351–368. doi: 10.1146/annurev-neuro-071714-033911.

Dugas-Ford, J. et al. (2012). Cell-type homologies and the origins of the neocortex. *Proc Natl Acad Sci USA* 109 (42): 16974–16979. doi: 10.1073/PNAS.1204773109/-/DCSUPPLEMENTAL.

de Juan Romero, C. et al. (2015). Discrete domains of gene expression in germinal layers distinguish the development of gyrencephaly. *EMBO J* 34 (14): 1859–1874. doi: 10.15252/EMBJ.201591176.

De Juan Romero, C. and Borrell, V. (2015). Coevolution of radial glial cells and the cerebral cortex. *Glia* 63 (8): 1303. doi: 10.1002/GLIA.22827.

Elias, L.A.B.B. et al. (2007). Gap junction adhesion is necessary for radial migration in the neocortex. *Nature* 448 (7156): 901–907. doi: 10.1038/NATURE06063.

Englund, C. et al. (2005). Pax6, Tbr2, and Tbr1 are expressed sequentially by radial glia, intermediate progenitor cells, and postmitotic neurons in developing neocortex. *J Neurosci* 25 (1): 247–251. doi: 10.1523/JNEUROSCI.2899-04.2005.

Fernández, V. et al. (2020). Repression of Irs2 by let-7 miRNAs is essential for homeostasis of the telencephalic neuroepithelium. *EMBO J* 39 (21): e105479. doi: 10.15252/embj.2020105479.

Fernández, V. et al. (2016). Cerebral cortex expansion and folding: what have we learned? *EMBO J* 35 (10): 1021–1044. doi: 10.15252/embj.201593701.

Fiddes, I.T. et al. (2018). Human-specific NOTCH2NL genes affect Notch signaling and cortical neurogenesis. *Cell* 173 (6): 1356–1369.e22. doi: 10.1016/J.CELL.2018.03.051.

Fietz, S.A. et al. (2010). OSVZ progenitors of human and ferret neocortex are epithelial-like and expand by integrin signaling. Nat Neurosci 13 (6): 690–699.

Fish, J.L. et al. (2008). Making bigger brains – the evolution of neural-progenitor-cell division. *J Cell Sci* 121 (17): 2783–2793. doi: 10.1242/JCS.023465.

Florio, M. et al. (2015). Human-specific gene ARHGAP11B promotes basal progenitor amplification and neocortex expansion. *Science* 347 (6229): 1465–1470.

Franchini, L.F. (2021). Genetic mechanisms underlying cortical evolution in mammals. *Front Cell Dev Biol* 9: 591017. doi: 10.3389/FCELL.2021.591017.

Fujita, T. et al. (2019). The chick pallium displays divergent expression patterns of chick orthologues of mammalian neocortical deep layer-specific genes. *Sci Rep* 9 (1): 1–13. doi: 10.1038/s41598-019-56960-4.

Gaiano, N. et al. (2000). Radial glial identity is promoted by Notch1 signaling in the murine forebrain. *Neuron* 26 (2): 395–404. doi: 10.1016/S0896-6273(00)81172-1.

Gao, P. et al. (2014). Deterministic progenitor behavior and unitary production of neurons in the neocortex. *Cell* 159 (4): 775–788. doi: 10.1016/J.CELL.2014.10.027.

García-Moreno, F. et al. (2012). Compartmentalization of cerebral cortical germinal zones in a lissencephalic primate and gyrencephalic rodent. *Cereb Cortex* 22 (2): 482–492. doi: 10.1093/CERCOR/BHR312.

García-Moreno, F. et al. (2018). Absence of tangentially migrating glutamatergic neurons in the developing avian brain. *Cell Rep* 22 (1): 96–109. doi: 10.1016/J.CELREP.2017.12.032.

García-Moreno, F. and Molnár, Z. (2020). Variations of telencephalic development that paved the way for neocortical evolution. *Prog Neurobiol* 194: 101865. doi: 10.1016/J.PNEUROBIO.2020.101865.

Gertz, C.C. and Kriegstein, A.R. (2015). Neuronal migration dynamics in the developing ferret cortex. *J Neurosci* 35 (42): 14307–14315. doi: 10.1523/JNEUROSCI.2198-15.2015.

Götz, M. and Huttner, W.B. (2005). The cell biology of neurogenesis. *Nat Rev Mol Cell Biol* 6 (10): 777–788. doi: 10.1038/nrm1739.

Govindan, S. and Jabaudon, D. (2017). Coupling progenitor and neuronal diversity in the developing neocortex. *FEBS Lett* 591 (24): 3960–3977. doi: 10.1002/1873-3468.12846.

Gupta, A. et al. (2003). Layering defect in p35 deficiency is linked to improper neuronal-glial interaction in radial migration. *Nat Neurosci* 6 (12): 1284–1291. doi: 10.1038/NN1151.

Hansen, D.V. et al. (2010). Neurogenic radial glia in the outer subventricular zone of human neocortex. *Nature* 464 (7288): 554–561.

Hatakeyama, J. et al. (2004). Hes genes regulate size, shape and histogenesis of the nervous system by control of the timing of neural stem cell differentiation. *Development* 131 (22): 5539–5550.

Hofman, M.A. (1988). Size and shape of the cerebral cortex in mammals. II. The cortical volume. *Brain, Behav Evol* 32 (1): 17–26. doi: 10.1159/000116529.

Huttner, W.B. and Kosodo, Y. (2005). Symmetric versus asymmetric cell division during neurogenesis in the developing vertebrate central nervous system. *Curr Opin Cell Biol* 17 (6): 648–657. doi: 10.1016/J.CEB.2005.10.005.

Imayoshi, I. et al. (2010). Essential roles of Notch signaling in maintenance of neural stem cells in developing and adult brains. *J Neurosci* 30 (9): 3489–3498. doi: 10.1523/JNEUROSCI.4987-09.2010.

Jerison, H.J. (1975). Review: evolution of the brain and intelligence on JSTOR. *Evolution of the Brain and Intelligence*. https://www.jstor.org/stable/2741455 (accessed 2 June 2022).

Ju, X.C. et al. (2016 August 9). The hominoid-specific gene TBC1D3 promotes generation of basal neural progenitors and induces cortical folding in mice. *Elife* 5: e18197.

Kalebic, N. et al. (2019). Neocortical expansion due to increased proliferation of basal progenitors is linked to changes in their morphology. *Cell Stem Cell* 24 (4): 535–550.e9. doi: 10.1016/J.STEM.2019.02.017.

Kang, W. et al. (2009). The transition from radial glial to intermediate progenitor cell is inhibited by FGF signaling during corticogenesis. *J Neurosci* 29 (46): 14571–14580. doi: 10.1523/JNEUROSCI.3844-09.2009.

Kanold, P.O. and Luhmann, H.J. (2010). The subplate and early cortical circuits. *Ann Rev Neurosci* 33: 23–48. doi: 10.1146/ANNUREV-NEURO-060909-153244.

Karten, H.J. (2013). Neocortical evolution: neuronal circuits arise independently of lamination. *Curr Biol* 23 (1): R12–5. doi: 10.1016/J.CUB.2012.11.013.

Kingsbury, M.A. et al. (2003). Non-proliferative effects of lysophosphatidic acid enhance cortical growth and folding. *Nat Neurosci* 6 (12): 1292–1299. doi: 10.1038/NN1157.

Konno, D. et al. (2007). Neuroepithelial progenitors undergo LGN-dependent planar divisions to maintain self-renewability during mammalian neurogenesis. *Nat Cell Biol* 10 (1): 93–101. doi: 10.1038/ncb1673.

Kostovic, I. and Rakic, P. (1990). Developmental history of the transient subplate zone in the visual and somatosensory cortex of the macaque monkey and human brain. *J Comp Neurol* 297 (3): 441–470. doi: 10.1002/CNE.902970309.

Kowalczyk, T. et al. (2009). Intermediate neuronal progenitors (basal progenitors) produce pyramidal-projection neurons for all layers of cerebral cortex. *Cereb Cortex* 19 (10): 2439–2450. doi: 10.1093/cercor/bhn260.

Kriegstein, A. and Alvarez-Buylla, A. (2009). The glial nature of embryonic and adult neural stem cells. *Ann Rev Neurosci* 32: 149–184. doi: 10.1146/annurev.neuro.051508.135600.

Kriegstein, A., Noctor, S., and Martínez-Cerdeño, V. (2006). Patterns of neural stem and progenitor cell division may underlie evolutionary cortical expansion. *Nat Rev Neurosci* 7 (11): 883–890. doi: 10.1038/NRN2008.

Kriegstein, A.R. and Götz, M. (2003). Radial glia diversity. *Glia* 43 (1): 37–43. doi: 10.1002/GLIA.10250.

LaMonica, B.E. et al. (2013). Mitotic spindle orientation predicts outer radial glial cell generation in human neocortex. Nat Commun 4 (1): 1665.

Lange, C. et al. (2009). Cdk4/cyclinD1 overexpression in neural stem cells shortens G1, delays neurogenesis, and promotes the generation and expansion of basal progenitors. *Cell Stem Cell* 5 (3): 320–331. doi: 10.1016/J.STEM.2009.05.026.

Lewitus, E. et al. (2014). An adaptive threshold in mammalian neocortical evolution. *PLoS Biol* 12 (11): e1002000. doi: 10.1371/JOURNAL.PBIO.1002000.

Liu, J. et al. (2017). The primate-specific gene TMEM14B marks outer radial glia cells and promotes cortical expansion and folding. *Cell Stem Cell* 21 (5): 635–649.e8.

Lui, J.H. et al. (2014). Radial glia require PDGFD-PDGFRβ signalling in human but not mouse neocortex. *Nature* 515 (7526): 264–268. doi: 10.1038/NATURE13973.

Lukaszewicz, A. et al. (2005). G1 phase regulation, area-specific cell cycle control, and cytoarchitectonics in the primate cortex. *Neuron* 47 (3): 353–364. doi: 10.1016/j.neuron.2005.06.032.

Lv, X. et al. (2019). TBR2 coordinates neurogenesis expansion and precise microcircuit organization via Protocadherin 19 in the mammalian cortex. *Nat Commun* 10 (1): 1–15. doi: 10.1038/s41467-019-11854-x.

Malatesta, P. et al. (2003). Neuronal or glial progeny. *Neuron* 37 (5): 751–764. doi: 10.1016/S0896-6273(03)00116-8.

Marín-Padilla, M. (1992). Ontogenesis of the pyramidal cell of the mammalian neocortex and developmental cytoarchitectonics. *J Comp Neurol* 321 (2): 223–240. doi: 10.1002/CNE.903210205.

Martínez-Cerdeño, V. et al. (2016). Evolutionary origin of Tbr2-expressing precursor cells and the subventricular zone in the developing cortex. *J Comp Neurol* 524 (3): 433–447. doi: 10.1002/CNE.23879.

Martínez-Cerdeño, V. et al. (2006). The role of intermediate progenitor cells in the evolutionary expansion of the cerebral cortex. *Cereb Cortex* 16 (Suppl 1): i152–61. doi: 10.1093/CERCOR/BHK017.

Martínez-Martínez, M.Á. et al. (2016). A restricted period for formation of outer subventricular zone defined by Cdh1 and Trnp1 levels. *Nat Commun* 7 (1): 1–15. doi: 10.1038/ncomms11812.

Matsumoto, N. et al. (2020). A discrete subtype of neural progenitor crucial for cortical folding in the gyrencephalic mammalian brain. *Elife* 9: e54873. doi: 10.7554/ELIFE.54873.

McBride, T. et al. (1999). A comparative volumetric analysis of the prefrontal cortex in human and baboon MRI. *Brain, Behav Evol* 54 (3): 159–166. doi: 10.1159/000006620.

Miller, J.A. et al. (2014). Transcriptional landscape of the prenatal human brain. *Nature* 508 (7495): 199–206. doi: 10.1038/NATURE13185.

Miyata, T. et al. (2001). Asymmetric inheritance of radial glial fibers by cortical neurons. *Neuron* 31 (5): 727–741. doi: 10.1016/S0896-6273(01)00420-2.

Miyata, T. et al. (2010). Mechanisms that regulate the number of neurons during mouse neocortical development. *Curr Opin Neurobiol* 20 (1): 22–28. doi: 10.1016/J.CONB.2010.01.001.

Molnár, Z. et al. (2006). Comparative aspects of cerebral cortical development. *Eur J Neurosci* 23 (4): 921–934. doi: 10.1111/J.1460-9568.2006.04611.X.

Montiel, J.F. et al. (2016). From sauropsids to mammals and back. *J Comp Neurol* 524 (3): 630–645. doi: 10.1002/CNE.23871.

Noctor, S.C. et al. (2001). Neurons derived from radial glial cells establish radial units in neocortex. *Nature* 409 (6821): 714–720. doi: 10.1038/35055553.

Noctor, S.C. et al. (2004). Cortical neurons arise in symmetric and asymmetric division zones and migrate through specific phases. *Nat Neurosci* 7 (2): 136–144. doi: 10.1038/NN1172.

Nomura, T. et al. (2008). Patterns of neurogenesis and amplitude of Reelin expression are essential for making a mammalian-type cortex. *PloS one* 3 (1): e1454. doi: 10.1371/JOURNAL.PONE.0001454.

Nomura, T. et al. (2013). Changes in the regulation of cortical neurogenesis contribute to encephalization during amniote brain evolution. *Nat Commun* 4: 2206.

Nomura, T. et al. (2014). Reconstruction of ancestral brains. *Neurosci Res* 86: 25–36. doi: 10.1016/J.NEURES.2014.03.004.

Nomura, T. et al. (2016). The evolution of basal progenitors in the developing non-mammalian brain. *Development* 143 (1): 66–74. doi: 10.1242/DEV.127100.

Nomura, T. et al. (2018). Species-specific mechanisms of neuron subtype specification reveal evolutionary plasticity of amniote brain development. *Cell Rep* 22 (12): 3142–3151. doi: 10.1016/J.CELREP.2018.02.086.

Nomura, T. et al. (2022). Temperature sensitivity of Notch signaling underlies species-specific developmental plasticity and robustness in amniote brains. *Nat Commun* 13 (1): 1–14. doi: 10.1038/s41467-021-27707-5.

Nowakowski, T.J. et al. (2016). Transformation of the radial glia scaffold demarcates two stages of human cerebral cortex development. *Neuron* 91 (6): 1219–1227. doi: 10.1016/J.NEURON.2016.09.005.

O'Leary, D.D.M. and Borngasser, D. (2006). Cortical ventricular zone progenitors and their progeny maintain spatial relationships and radial patterning during preplate development indicating an early protomap. *Cereb Cortex* 16 (Suppl 1): i46–56. doi: 10.1093/CERCOR/BHK019.

Paridaen, J.T. and Huttner, W.B. (2014). Neurogenesis during development of the vertebrate central nervous system. *EMBO Rep* 15 (4): 351–364.

Pasko, R. (1974). Neurons in rhesus monkey visual cortex. *Science* 183 (4123): 425–427. doi: 10.1126/science.183.4123.425.

Passingham, R.E. and Smaers, J.B. (2014). Is the prefrontal cortex especially enlarged in the human brain allometric relations and remapping factors. *Brain, Behav Evol* 84 (2): 156–166. doi: 10.1159/000365183.

Pilz, G.-A.-A. et al. (2013). Amplification of progenitors in the mammalian telencephalon includes a new radial glial cell type. *Nat Commun* 4: 2125. doi: 10.1038/ncomms3125.

Pinto, L. et al. (2008). Prospective isolation of functionally distinct radial glial subtypes–lineage and transcriptome analysis. *Mol Cell Neurosci* 38 (1): 15–42. doi: 10.1016/J.MCN.2008.01.012.

Pollen, A.A. et al. (2015). Molecular identity of human outer radial glia during cortical development. *Cell* 163 (1): 55–67. doi: 10.1016/J.CELL.2015.09.004.

Polleux, F. and Anton, E.S. (2005). Neuronal migration in the developing brain BT. In: *Developmental Neurobiology* (ed. M.S. Rao and M. Jacobson†), 223–239. Boston, MA: Springer US. doi: 10.1007/0-387-28117-7_8.

Postiglione, M.P. et al. (2011). Mouse inscuteable induces apical-basal spindle orientation to facilitate intermediate progenitor generation in the developing neocortex. *Neuron* 72 (2): 269–284. doi: 10.1016/J.NEURON.2011.09.022.

Puelles, L. (2001). Thoughts on the development, structure and evolution of the mammalian and avian telencephalic pallium. *Phil Trans Royal Soc London. Series B, Biol Sci* 356 (1414): 1583–1598. doi: 10.1098/RSTB.2001.0973.

Puelles, L. (2017). Comments on the updated tetrapartite pallium model in the mouse and chick, featuring a homologous claustro-insular complex. *Brain, Behav Evol* 90 (2): 171–189. doi: 10.1159/000479782.

Rakic, P. (1978). Neuronal migration and contact guidance in the primate telencephalon. *Postgrad Med J* 54 (Suppl 1): 25–40.

Rakic, P. (1988). Specification of cerebral cortical areas. *Science* 241 (4862): 170–176. doi: 10.1126/SCIENCE.3291116.

Rakic, P. (1995). A small step for the cell, a giant leap for mankind. 18 (9): 383–388. doi: 10.1016/0166-2236(95)93934-P.

Rakic, P. (2009). Evolution of the neocortex: a perspective from developmental biology. *Nat Rev Neurosci* 10 (10): 724–735. doi: 10.1038/nrn2719.

Reillo, I. et al. (2011). A role for intermediate radial glia in the tangential expansion of the mammalian cerebral cortex. *Cereb Cortex* 21 (7): 1674–1694. doi: 10.1093/CERCOR/BHQ238.

Reillo, I. and Borrell, V. (2012). Germinal zones in the developing cerebral cortex of ferret: ontogeny, cell cycle kinetics, and diversity of progenitors. *Cereb Cortex* 22 (9): 2039–2054. doi: 10.1093/CERCOR/BHR284.

Reiner, A. et al. (2004). Revised nomenclature for avian telencephalon and some related brainstem nuclei. *J Comp Neurol* 473 (3): 377. doi: 10.1002/CNE.20118.

Rilling, J.K. (2006). Human and nonhuman primate brains. *Evol Anthropol: Issues, News, Rev* 15 (2): 65–77. doi: 10.1002/EVAN.20095.

Sahara, S. and O'Leary, D.D.M. (2009). Fgf10 regulates transition period of cortical stem cell differentiation to radial glia controlling generation of neurons and basal progenitors. *Neuron* 63 (1): 48–62.

Schoenemann, P.T. et al. (2005). Prefrontal white matter volume is disproportionately larger in humans than in other primates. *Nat Neurosci* 8 (2): 242–252. doi: 10.1038/NN1394.

Semendeferi, K. et al. (2002). Humans and great apes share a large frontal cortex. *Nat Neurosci* 5 (3): 272–276. doi: 10.1038/NN814.

Semendeferi, K. and Damasio, H. (2000). The brain and its main anatomical subdivisions in living hominoids using magnetic resonance imaging. *J Hum Evol* 38 (2): 317–332. doi: 10.1006/JHEV.1999.0381.

Sessa, A. et al. (2008). Tbr2 directs conversion of radial glia into basal precursors and guides neuronal amplification by indirect neurogenesis in the developing neocortex. *Neuron* 60 (1): 56. doi: 10.1016/J.NEURON.2008.09.028.

Shitamukai, A. et al. (2011). Oblique radial glial divisions in the developing mouse neocortex induce self-renewing progenitors outside the germinal zone that resemble primate outer subventricular zone progenitors. *J Neurosci* 31 (10): 3683–3695. doi: 10.1523/JNEUROSCI.4773-10.2011.

Sidman, R.L. and Rakic, P. (1973). Neuronal migration, with special reference to developing human brain: a review. *Brain Res* 62 (1): 1–35. doi: 10.1016/0006-8993(73)90617-3.

Siegenthaler, J.A. et al. (2009). Retinoic acid from the meninges regulates cortical neuron generation. *Cell* 139 (3): 597–609. doi: 10.1016/J.CELL.2009.10.004/ATTACHMENT/B04259B6-AFFD-4E5F-B20C-B9B883DD28D1/MMC1.PDF.

Smaers, J.B. et al. (2017). Exceptional evolutionary expansion of prefrontal cortex in great apes and humans. *Curr Biol* 27 (10): 1549. doi: 10.1016/J.CUB.2017.05.015.

Smaers, J.B. et al. (2021). The evolution of mammalian brain size. *Sci Adv* 7 (18): 9. doi: 10.1126/SCIADV.ABE2101.

Smart, I.H.M.M. et al. (2002). Unique morphological features of the proliferative zones and postmitotic compartments of the neural epithelium giving rise to striate and extrastriate cortex in the monkey. *Cereb Cortex* 12 (1): 37–53. doi: 10.1093/CERCOR/12.1.37.

Soriano, E. et al. (1995). Molecular heterogeneity of progenitors and radial migration in the developing cerebral cortex revealed by transgene expression. *Proc Natl Acad Sci USA* 92 (25): 11676–11680. doi: 10.1073/PNAS.92.25.11676.

Sottocornola, R. et al. (2010). ASPP2 binds Par-3 and controls the polarity and proliferation of neural progenitors during CNS development. *Dev Cell* 19 (1): 126–137. doi: 10.1016/J.DEVCEL.2010.06.003.

Stahl, R. et al. (2013). Trnp1 regulates expansion and folding of the mammalian cerebral cortex by control of radial glial fate. *Cell* 153 (3): 535–549.

Stepien, B.K. et al. (2020). Lengthening neurogenic period during neocortical development causes a hallmark of neocortex expansion. *Curr Biol* 30 (21): 4227–4237.e5. doi: 10.1016/J.CUB.2020.08.046.

Stepien, B.K. et al. (2021). Length of the neurogenic period—a key determinant for the generation of upper-layer neurons during neocortex development and evolution. *Front Cell Dev Biol* 9: 1218. doi: 10.3389/FCELL.2021.676911/BIBTEX.

Striedter, G.F. (2005). *Principles of Brain Evolution.* https://psycnet.apa.org/record/2004-21314-000 (Accessed 2 June 2022).

Striedter, G.F. and Charvet, C.J. (2009). Telencephalon enlargement by the convergent evolution of expanded subventricular zones. *Biol Lett* 5 (1): 134–137. doi: 10.1098/rsbl.2008.0439.

Sun, T. and Hevner, R.F. (2014). Growth and folding of the mammalian cerebral cortex: from molecules to malformations. *Nat Rev Neurosci* 15 (4): 217. doi: 10.1038/NRN3707.

Suzuki, I.K. et al. (2012). The temporal sequence of the mammalian neocortical neurogenetic program drives mediolateral pattern in the chick pallium. *Dev Cell* 22 (4): 863–870. doi: 10.1016/J.DEVCEL.2012.01.004.

Suzuki, I.K. et al. (2018). Human-specific NOTCH2NL genes expand cortical neurogenesis through Delta/Notch regulation. *Cell* 173 (6): 1370–1384.e16. doi: 10.1016/J.CELL.2018.03.067.

Taverna, E. et al. (2014). The cell biology of neurogenesis. *Ann Rev Cell Dev Biol* 30: 465–502. doi: 10.1146/ANNUREV-CELLBIO-101011-155801.

Taverna, E. and Huttner, W.B. (2010). Neural progenitor nuclei IN motion. *Neuron* 67 (6): 906–914. doi: 10.1016/J.NEURON.2010.08.027.

Teffer, K. and Semendeferi, K. (2012). Human prefrontal cortex. *Prog Brain Res* 195: 191–218. doi: 10.1016/B978-0-444-53860-4.00009-RX.

Toda, T. et al. (2016). An essential role of SVZ progenitors in cortical folding in gyrencephalic mammals. *Sci Rep* 6 (1): 1–12. doi: 10.1038/srep29578.

Tomasello, U. et al. (2022). miR-137 and miR-122, two outer subventricular zone non-coding RNAs, regulate basal progenitor expansion and neuronal differentiation. *Cell Rep* 38 (7): 110381. doi: 10.1016/J.CELREP.2022.110381.

Tosches, M.A. et al. (2018). Evolution of pallium, hippocampus, and cortical cell types revealed by single-cell transcriptomics in reptiles. *Science* 360 (6391): 881–888. doi: 10.1126/SCIENCE.AAR4237.

Uzquiano, A. et al. (2018). Cortical progenitor biology. *J Neurochem* 146 (5): 500–525. doi: 10.1111/JNC.14338.

Vasistha, N.A. et al. (2015). Cortical and clonal contribution of Tbr2 expressing progenitors in the developing mouse brain. *Cereb Cortex* 25 (10): 3290–3302. doi: 10.1093/CERCOR/BHU125.

Wang, L. et al. (2016). Hedgehog signaling promotes basal progenitor expansion and the growth and folding of the neocortex. *Nat Neurosci* 19 (7): 888–896. doi: 10.1038/NN.4307.

Wang, X. et al. (2011). A new subtype of progenitor cell in the mouse embryonic neocortex. *Nat Neurosci* 14 (5): 555–561. doi: 10.1038/nn.2807.

Wong, F.K. et al. (2015). Sustained Pax6 expression generates primate-like basal radial glia in developing mouse neocortex. *PLoS Biol* 13 (8): e1002217. doi: 10.1371/JOURNAL.PBIO.1002217.

Yingling, J. et al. (2008). Neuroepithelial stem cell proliferation requires LIS1 for precise spindle orientation and symmetric division. *Cell* 132 (3): 474–486. doi: 10.1016/J.CELL.2008.01.026.

Zhang, K. and Sejnowski, T.J. (2000). A universal scaling law between gray matter and white matter of cerebral cortex. *Proc Natl Acad Sci USA* 97 (10): 5621–5626. doi: 10.1073/PNAS.090504197.

Zilles, K. et al. (2013). Development of cortical folding during evolution and ontogeny. *Trends Neurosci* 36 (5): 275–284. doi: 10.1016/J.TINS.2013.01.006.

6

Dynamic Transcriptional Control of Neural Stem Cells

Ryoichiro Kageyama[1,2,3,4,5,*] *and Hiromi Shimojo*[1,6]

[1] *Institute for Frontier Life and Medical Sciences, Kyoto University, Shogoin-Kawahara, Sakyo-ku, Kyoto, Japan*
[2] *Kyoto University Graduate School of Medicine, Kyoto, Japan*
[3] *Kyoto University Graduate School of Biostudies, Kyoto, Japan*
[4] *Institute for Integrated Cell-Material Sciences, Kyoto University, Kyoto, Japan*
[5] *RIKEN Center for Brain Science, Wako Japan*
[6] *Graduate School of Frontier Biosciences, Osaka University, Suita, Osaka, Japan*
* *Corresponding author*

6.1 Introduction

In the developing nervous system, neuroepithelial cells proliferate actively, elongate gradually, and become radial glial cells that retain their cell bodies in the ventricular zone (VZ) and extend their processes, called radial fibers, to the external surface of the neural tube. Neuroepithelial cells undergo symmetric cell division, in which each cell produces two neuroepithelial cells, whereas radial glial cells undergo asymmetric cell division, in which each cell produces two distinct cell types, one radial glial cell and one intermediate progenitor (INP). INPs migrate from the VZ into the outer layer, which is called the subventricular zone (SVZ), where they divide further and differentiate into mature neurons. Radial glial cells give rise to deep layer neurons first and then superficial layer neurons. After producing neurons, radial glial cells finally differentiate into glial cells (oligodendrocytes and astrocytes). Neuroepithelial cells and radial glial cells are collectively called neural stem cells (NSCs).

In this chapter, we discuss the significance of the expression dynamics of basic helix-loop-helix (bHLH) transcription factors in the regulation of the proliferation and differentiation of NSCs.

6.2 Regulation of NSC Proliferation and Differentiation by bHLH Transcription Factors

The proliferation and differentiation of NSCs are controlled by bHLH transcription factors, including proneural factors such as achaete-scute family transcription factor 1 (Ascl1) and neurogenin2 (Neurog2) and Notch-signaling effectors such as Hes family transcription factor 1 (Hes1) and Hes5 (Bertrand et al. 2002; Imayoshi and Kageyama 2014; Ross et al. 2003). Ascl1 and Neurog2 upregulate the expression of genes involved in neuronal differentiation, while Hes1 and Hes5 repress *Ascl1* and *Neurog2* expression, inhibit neuronal differentiation, and maintain NSCs. However, Hes1 and Hes5 can also promote astrocyte differentiation at later stages (Ohtsuka et al. 2001),

Neocortical Neurogenesis in Development and Evolution, First Edition. Edited by Wieland B. Huttner.

suggesting that they have dual functions, that is, maintaining NSCs and promoting astrocyte differentiation (Figure 6.1). Furthermore, chromatin immunoprecipitation-chip analysis showed that Ascl1 binds directly not only to the promoters of genes involved in cell cycle exit, neurotransmitter biosynthesis, and neurite outgrowth, which are important in neuronal differentiation, but also to the promoters of genes involved in cell cycle progression, including those essential for the G1/S transition and entry into mitosis (Castro et al. 2011). Furthermore, when Ascl1 is acutely inactivated, NSCs in the VZ exit the cell cycle prematurely (Castro et al. 2011). These results suggest that Ascl1 also has dual functions: promoting NSC proliferation and neuronal differentiation (Figure 6.1). Another bHLH factor, oligodendrocyte transcription factor 2 (Olig2), promotes the differentiation of NSCs to oligodendrocyte precursor cells (Lu et al. 2002; Takebayashi et al. 2002; Zhou and Anderson 2002). Interestingly, at early developmental stages, Olig2 inhibits the differentiation of NSCs and promotes their proliferation. This proliferative activity of Olig2 is regulated by the phosphorylation of a triple serine motif at its N-terminal region, which is non-phosphorylated in differentiating oligodendrocyte precursor cells (Sun et al. 2011). When phosphorylated at these positions, the proliferative function of Olig2 becomes dominant over its differentiation functions. Thus, Olig2 also has dual functions, that is, NSC proliferation and oligodendrocyte differentiation (Figure 6.1). These results indicate that the bHLH factors Ascl1, Olig2, and Hes1 exhibit opposing dual functions: the promotion of NSC proliferation and the specification of neurons, oligodendrocytes, and astrocytes, respectively.

The next question is how these bHLH factors coordinate their opposing functions. Time-lapse imaging analyses showed that *Ascl1*, *Olig2*, and *Hes1* are expressed in an oscillatory manner by NSCs, but are upregulated in a sustained manner by differentiating neurons, oligodendrocytes, and astrocytes, respectively (Figure 6.1). These observations suggest that the expression dynamics are very important for the opposing functions of these bHLH genes. To address this notion, an

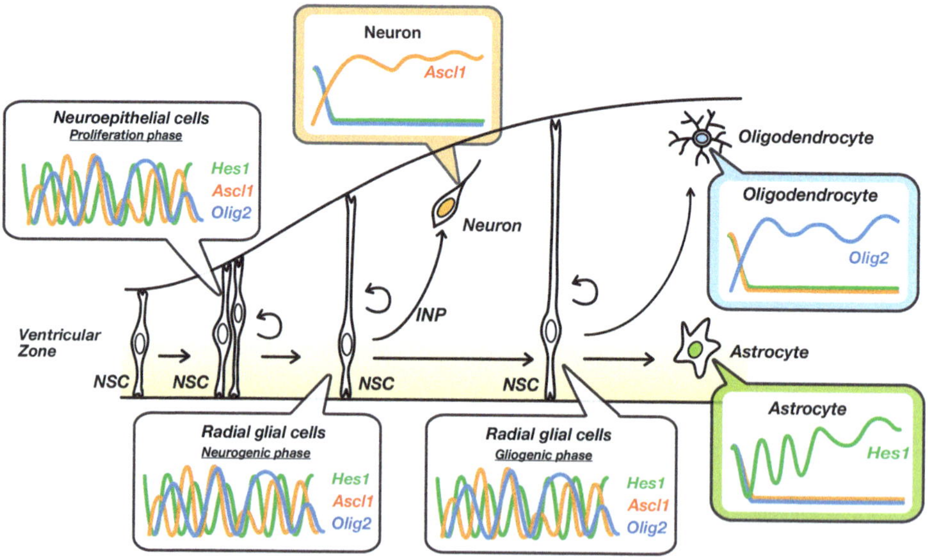

Figure 6.1 Expression dynamics of basic helix-loop-helix (bHLH) factors in proliferating neural stem cells (NSCs) and differentiating cells. NSCs proliferate actively while giving rise to neurons, oligodendrocytes, and astrocytes. The bHLH factors Ascl1, Olig2, and Hes1 are expressed in an oscillatory manner in proliferating NSCs, but are upregulated in differentiating neurons, oligodendrocytes, and astrocytes, respectively. INP, intermediate progenitor.

optogenetic approach using GAVPO has been employed to control the expression dynamics of Ascl1. GAVPO is a light-activatable protein consisting of the light-inducible dimerizing protein Vivid (VVD), a Gal4 DNA-binding domain, and a p65 transcriptional activation domain (Figure 6.2A) (Wang et al. 2012). Blue-light illumination activates VVD, forming a dimer, and the dimeric form of the Gal4 DNA-binding domain binds to the upstream activator sequence (UAS) sequences. Then, the p65 transcriptional activation domain upregulates gene expression under the control of the UAS sequences (Figure 6.2A). Under dark conditions, GAVPO becomes a monomer, and the monomeric form of the Gal4 DNA-binding domain cannot interact with the UAS, thereby repressing gene expression (Figure 6.2A). Blue-light illumination with 3-hour intervals induces oscillatory expression with 3-hour periodicity, while blue-light illumination with 30-minute intervals induces sustained expression (Imayoshi et al. 2013; Isomura et al. 2017). The significance of gene expression dynamics was examined by introducing this Ascl1-inducible system into *Ascl1*-null NSCs. Light-induced sustained Ascl1 expression enhances neuronal differentiation, whereas light-induced oscillatory Ascl1 expression activates NSC proliferation (Figure 6.2B). Thus, oscillatory versus sustained expression dynamics of Ascl1 regulate the choice between NSC proliferation and neuronal differentiation (Imayoshi et al. 2013). These data suggest that the expression dynamics of bHLH factors are important for them to exert their opposing functions in a coordinated manner.

How does the expression of these bHLH factors oscillate in NSCs? Hes1, a transcriptional repressor, can repress not only proneural genes, such as *Ascl1* and *Neurog2*, but also *Hes1* itself by binding directly to its own promoter (negative feedback) (Figure 6.3A). However, when the Hes1

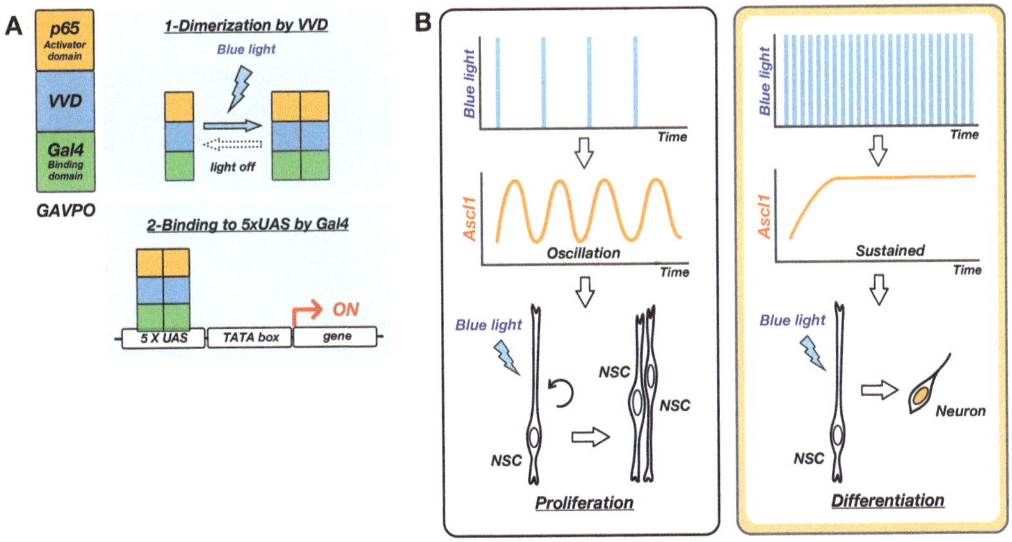

Figure 6.2 Optogenetic control of gene expression dynamics. (A) GAVPO consists of the light-inducible dimerizing protein Vivid (VVD), a Gal4 DNA-binding domain, and a p65 transcriptional activation domain. Blue-light illumination activates VVD, forming a dimer, and the dimeric form of the Gal4 DNA-binding domain binds to the upstream activator sequence (UAS) sequence. Then, the p65 transcriptional activation domain upregulates the gene expression under the control of the UAS sequences. Under dark conditions, GAVPO becomes a monomer, which cannot interact with the UAS, thereby repressing gene expression. (B) By changing the blue-light illumination pattern, the GAVPO system can induce oscillatory or sustained expression of Ascl1. Ascl1 oscillations activate NSC proliferation, whereas sustained Ascl1 expression enhances neuronal differentiation.

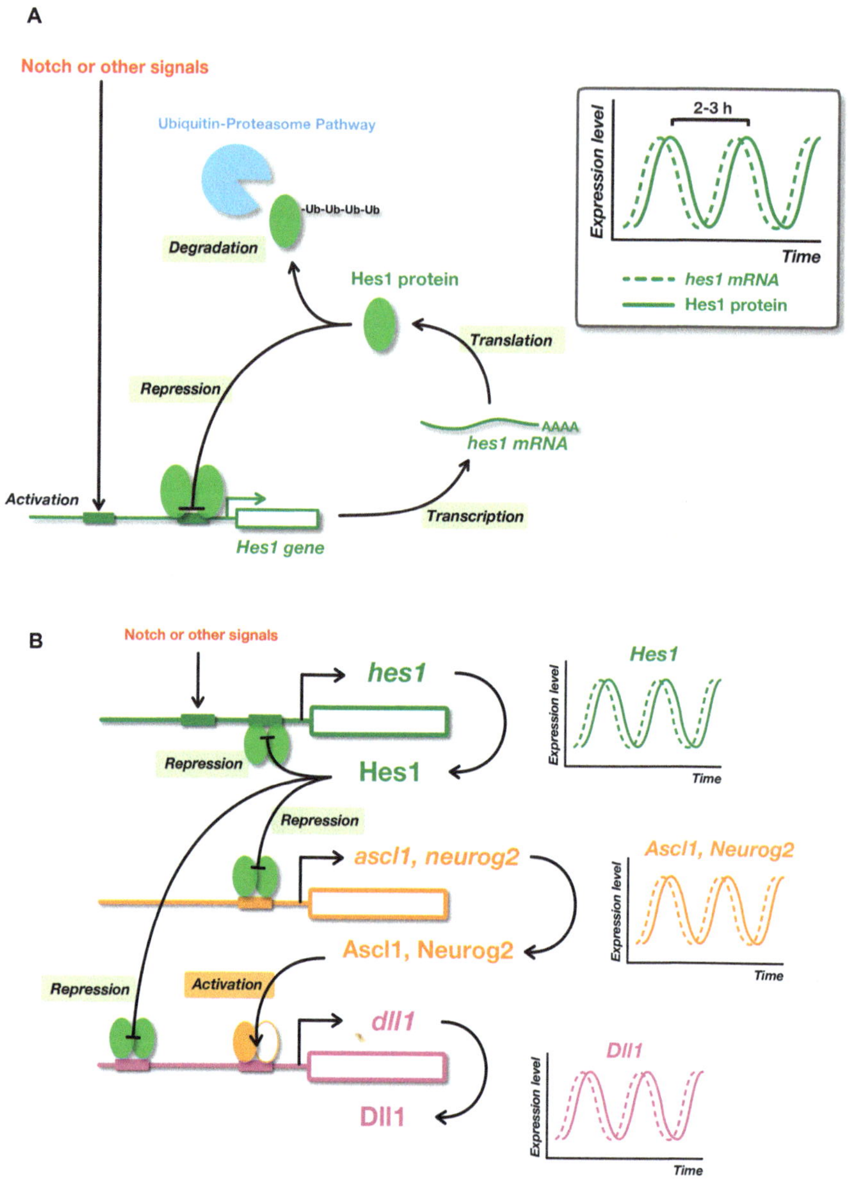

Figure 6.3 Oscillatory expression in NSCs. (A) When Hes1 expression is induced, it represses its own expression by binding directly to its own promoter (negative feedback). As a result, both *Hes1* mRNA and Hes1 protein disappear rapidly, because they are extremely unstable, which allows the next round of expression. In this way, Hes1 expression oscillates autonomously with a period of 2–3 hours in mouse NSCs. (B) Hes1 drives the oscillatory expression of proneural genes, and Hes1 and proneural gene oscillations drive Dll1 oscillations.

promoter is repressed by negative feedback, both *Hes1* mRNA and Hes1 protein disappear rapidly, because they are extremely unstable, which allows the next round of expression. In this way, Hes1 expression oscillates autonomously with a period of 2–3 hours in mouse NSCs (Figure 6.3A) (Hirata et al. 2002; Shimojo et al. 2008). Hes1 oscillations then periodically repress Ascl1, Neurog2, and Olig2 expression, which also oscillates in NSCs (Figure 6.3B) (Imayoshi et al. 2013; Shimojo et al. 2008). Thus, oscillatory expression of multiple bHLH factors is the underlying mechanism for multipotency of NSCs.

6.3 Dynamic Control of Notch Signaling in NSCs

Among the bHLH genes, *Hes1* and its related genes are essential for the maintenance of NSCs. *Hes1*-null mice frequently show anencephaly in the 129 background because NSCs are depleted, but have almost normal brains in other backgrounds such as C57BL/6 and mixed backgrounds, suggesting that *Hes1*-related genes compensate for *Hes1* in brain development (Ishibashi et al. 1995). Indeed, in *Hes1;Hes5* double- knockout mice, the expression of proneural genes is upregulated, leading to severe premature neuronal differentiation, rapid depletion of NSCs, and disorganized structures of the developing nervous system in the latter backgrounds (Hatakeyama et al. 2004; Ohtsuka et al. 1999). In *Hes1;Hes3;Hes5* triple-knockout mice, even more severe and wider defects of premature neurogenesis and NSC depletion occur, although NSCs are maintained and proliferate almost normally in the developing telencephalon (Hatakeyama et al. 2004). In the *Hes1;Hes3;Hes5*;Hes-related family bHLH transcription factor with YRPW motif 1 (*Hey1*) knockout mice, virtually all NSCs are exhausted even in the developing telencephalon, indicating that these Hes/Hey factors cooperatively regulate NSC maintenance in the developing nervous system (Sueda et al. 2019).

The expression of these Hes/Hey factors is controlled by Notch signaling. The proneural factors Ascl1 and Neurog2 induce the expression of Notch ligands such as Delta-like 1 (Dll1), which activate Notch signaling in neighboring cells (Figure 6.4A). Upon activation of Notch signaling, Notch proteins are cleaved, releasing the Notch intracellular domain (NICD), an active form of Notch signaling, which then enters the nucleus and forms a complex with the DNA-binding protein, named recombination signal binding protein for immunoglobulin kappa J region (RBPj), and the coactivator Mastermind-like (Maml) (Kopan and Ilagan 2009). The NICD-RBPj-Maml complex is a transcriptional activator that induces Hes1 and Hes5 expression (Figure 6.4A). These findings indicate that Ascl1- or Neurog2-expressing differentiating neurons and INPs activate Notch signaling in their neighboring cells, which are inhibited from neuronal differentiation, a process called lateral inhibition. When *Hes1* and *Hes5* are knocked out, lateral inhibition does not work properly: *Ascl1* and *Neurog2* are upregulated and accelerate neuronal differentiation, depleting NSCs prematurely. Similarly, in *RBPj*-null mice, all NSCs are prematurely exhausted, as in *Hes1;Hes3;Hes5* and *Hes1;Hes3;Hes5;Hey1* knockout mice (Hatakeyama et al. 2004; Imayoshi et al. 2010; Sueda et al. 2019). Thus, Notch signaling is essential for the maintenance of NSCs, particularly during asymmetric cell division, in which each NSC (radial glial cell) produces one NSC (radial glial cell) and one INP. When Notch signaling is impaired, both daughter cells become INPs and undergo neuronal differentiation, depleting NSCs.

The above observations suggest that INPs and neurons regulate the maintenance of NSCs by expressing Dll1; however, this raises the question of how NSCs are maintained at early stages before INPs and neurons are generated. Accumulating evidence suggests that Notch signaling regulation is not as simple as a one-way pathway from differentiating INPs and neurons to neighboring NSCs. Actually, Ascl1, Neurog2, and Dll1 are expressed by NSCs in a salt-and-pepper pattern (i.e., a mixture of positive and negative cells) in the early stages of neural development, particularly before INPs and neurons are born (Kageyama et al. 2008; Shimojo et al. 2008). These findings indicate that Ascl1, Neurog2, and Dll1 are also expressed by NSCs, raising the possibility that NSCs mutually activate Notch signaling. Time-lapse imaging analysis showed that all these factors are expressed in an oscillatory manner with a 2–3-hour periodicity in mouse NSCs. Dll1 oscillation is driven by periodic activation by Ascl1 and Neurog2 and repression by Hes1 (Figure 6.3). When Hes1 expression is high, Ascl1, Neurog2, and Dll1 expression is low, while

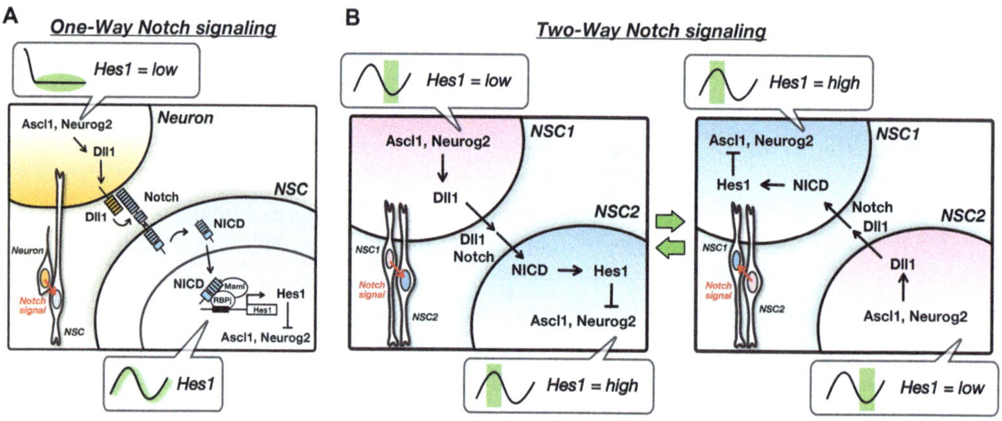

Figure 6.4 Notch signaling in lateral inhibition. (A) One-way Notch signaling. Ascl1 and Neurog2 induce Dll1 expression, which activates Notch signaling in neighboring cells. Upon activation of Notch signaling, Notch proteins are cleaved, releasing NICD, which then enters the nucleus and forms a complex with the DNA-binding protein RBPj and the co-activator Maml. The NICD-RBPj-Maml complex is a transcriptional activator that induces Hes1 expression. (B) Two-way Notch signaling. When Hes1 expression is low in a certain NSC (NSC1), Ascl1 and Neurog2 expression is upregulated, inducing Dll1 expression, and high Dll1 expression activates Notch signaling in its neighboring NSC (NSC2), which expresses high levels of Hes1. However, Hes1 expression is downregulated at 1–1.5 hour later in the latter cell (NSC2), resulting in high Ascl1, Neurog2, and Dll1 expression, which activates Notch signaling in the former cell (NSC1). Thus, depending on these oscillations, NSCs can mutually activate Notch signaling, inhibiting the neuronal differentiation of each other, and maintaining a group of cells in an undifferentiated state.

when Hes1 expression is low, Ascl1, Neurog2, and Dll1 expression is high, showing an inverse correlation between Hes1 and the other factors. On the basis of this observation, the current view of Notch signaling is as follows. When Hes1 expression is low in certain NSCs, Ascl1 and Neurog2 expression is upregulated, inducing Dll1 expression, and high Dll1 levels activate Notch signaling in neighboring NSCs, which express high levels of Hes1 (Figure 6.4B). However, because of oscillatory expression, Hes1 levels are downregulated at 1–1.5 hours later in the latter cells, resulting in high Ascl1, Neurog2, and Dll1 expression, which activates Notch signaling in the former cells (Figure 6.4B). Thus, depending on these oscillations, NSCs can mutually activate Notch signaling, inhibiting the neuronal differentiation of each other, and maintaining a group of cells in an undifferentiated state (Kageyama et al. 2008; Shimojo et al. 2008). This two-way regulation is important particularly at the early stages of neural development before INPs and neurons are generated. As development proceeds, this two-way regulation disappears and Dll1 signals are produced only by differentiating INPs and neurons.

6.4 Regulation of Boundary Cell or Astrocyte Formation by Sustained Hes1 Expression

The developing nervous system is partitioned into many compartments by boundaries, such as the zona limitans intrathalamica (Zli), isthmus, and the roof and floor plates. The Zli is the boundary between the thalamus and prethalamus, whereas the isthmus is the boundary between the midbrain and hindbrain. The roof and floor plates separate the right and left halves of the neural tube. Boundaries are formed by specialized neuroepithelial or radial glial cells, which have unique features, including slow proliferation, delayed or no neurogenesis, and organizer activity that regulates the specificity of neighboring compartments. For example, the Zli and isthmus function as organizing centers by secreting sonic hedgehog (Shh) and fibroblast growth factor 8, respectively, and regulate the regional specification of neighboring compartments (Kiecker and Lumsden 2005). The roof and floor plates secrete Wnt and Shh, respectively, and regulate dorso-ventral specification of the neural tube. Cells migrate within each compartment but do not usually cross boundaries; thus, each compartment forms a unit that consists of a distinct set of cell types (Kiecker and Lumsden 2005).

The mechanism by which compartment and boundary cells are formed remains to be determined, but it is known that the *Hes1* expression dynamics are different between compartment and boundary cells (Baek et al. 2006). Notably, boundary cells express Hes1 at high levels in a sustained manner and do not express proneural genes, suggesting that sustained Hes1 expression contributes to the non-proliferative and non-neurogenic properties of boundary cells. The inactivation of *Hes1* and *Hes1*-related genes leads to the ectopic expression of proneural genes and downregulation of signaling molecules in the boundary regions, whereas sustained Hes1 expression represses proneural gene expression and inhibits NSC proliferation (Baek et al. 2006; Hirata et al. 2001). High Hes1 expression also inhibits cell-cycle progression in various cell types such as fibroblasts and progenitor cells, suggesting that the requirement for Hes1 oscillations in cell proliferation is not specific to NSCs (Noda et al. 2011; Sang et al. 2008; Yu et al. 2006). Similarly, adult NSCs are mostly quiescent (non-proliferative) and express high levels of Hes1, continuously repressing *Ascl1* expression (Sueda et al. 2019). When Ascl1 oscillations are induced, such quiescent NSCs are activated to start proliferating and to make new neurons (Sueda et al. 2019). Thus, high and sustained Hes1 expression and the resultant suppression of proneural genes are important for the non-proliferative and non-neurogenic properties of boundary cells. The next question is how sustained Hes1 expression differentially controls astrocyte differentiation and boundary cell formation.

High and sustained Hes1 expression induces astrocyte differentiation at the later stages of neural development, but not at the early stages. The exact mechanism by which NSCs respond differently to high and sustained Hes1 expression depending on stage remains to be clarified. In compound proneural gene mutant mice (*Neurog2;Ascl1* and *Ascl1;Math3* double-knockout mice), neuronal differentiation is inhibited, leading to NSC maintenance at the early stages, and astrocyte formation is prematurely induced only at the later stages (Nieto et al. 2001; Tomita et al. 2000), suggesting that the intrinsic properties of NSCs may change as development proceeds. It has been shown that the competency of astrocyte differentiation is controlled by epigenetic modifications (Namihira and Nakashima 2013). As the promoter sequences of astrocytic genes, including glial fibrillary acidic protein (*Gfap*) and S100 calcium binding protein B (*S100β*), are highly methylated in early-stage NSCs, the response of astrocytic genes is inhibited (Takizawa et al. 2001). As development proceeds, the DNA sequences of astrocytic genes become demethylated, making NSCs responsive to astrocyte-inducing signals. In addition to DNA methylation, histone methylation is also involved in astrocyte formation. The H3K9 methyltransferase ESET and high mobility group A (HMGA) proteins repress accelerated astrocyte production (Kishi et al. 2012; Tan et al. 2012), whereas Polycomb promotes a neurogenic to astrogenic fate transition (Hirabayashi et al. 2009). Thus, the timing of astrocyte formation during brain development is controlled by epigenetic modifications such as DNA and histone methylation.

6.5 Regulation of NSC Proliferation by Oscillatory Hes1 Expression

The significance of oscillatory expression in neural development in vivo has been analyzed by dampening Hes1 oscillations. Two approaches have been taken to dampen Hes1 oscillations, based on mathematical modeling (Figure 6.5). As stated above, Hes1 oscillations are controlled by negative feedback, but delayed negative feedback (with a delay, τ_1, in Figure 6.5A) is very important for oscillatory expression: accelerated negative feedback (shorter τ_1) dampens oscillations, leading to steady expression (Takashima et al. 2011). Hes1 oscillations drive Dll1 oscillations by periodic repression, and then Dll1 oscillations activate Notch signaling periodically and induce Hes1 expression in neighboring NSCs (Figure 6.5A). This regulation can be simplified as a double-negative feedback loop, where Hes1 represses its own expression with a delay τ_1 within the same cell, while repressing Hes1 expression with a delay τ_2 in a neighboring cell (Figure 6.5A). According to mathematical modeling (Figure 6.5B), the delay in this negative feedback (τ_2 in Figure 6.5A) is also very important for oscillatory dynamics. With various τ_2 values, neighboring cells exhibit in-phase oscillations, similar to Hes7 oscillations in the presomitic mesoderm (Bessho et al. 2001), or out-of-phase oscillations, as observed in NSCs (Figure 6.5C). However, when τ_2 is shortened or elongated,

A

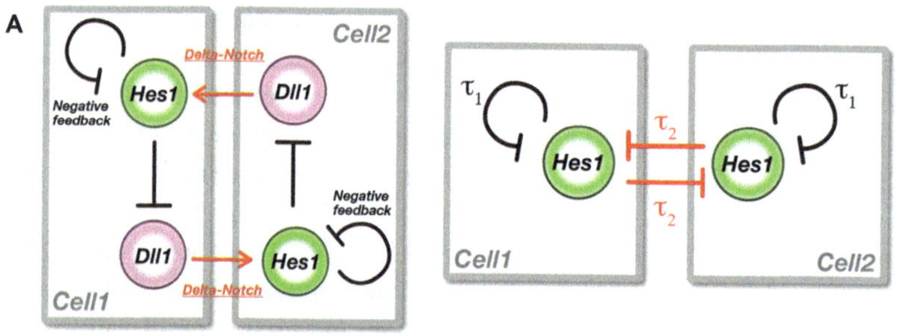

B

$$\frac{d}{dt}X_1(t) = v\frac{K_1^m}{K_1^m + X_1(t-\tau_1)^m}\frac{K_2^n}{K_2^n + X_2(t-\tau_2)^n} - rX_1(t)$$

$$\frac{d}{dt}X_2(t) = v\frac{K_1^m}{K_1^m + X_2(t-\tau_1)^m}\frac{K_2^n}{K_2^n + X_1(t-\tau_2)^n} - rX_2(t)$$

C

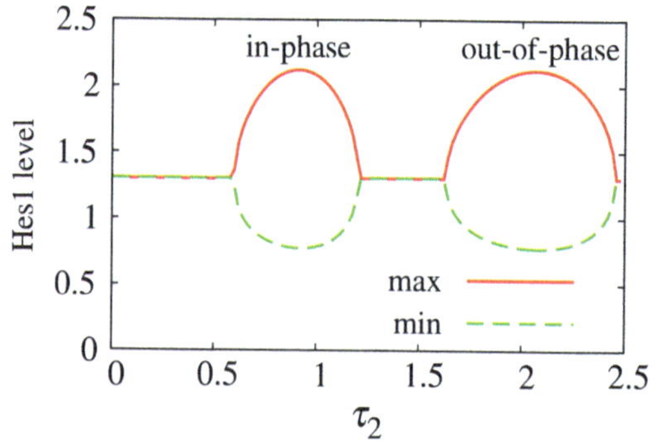

Figure 6.5 Mathematical modeling of oscillatory dynamics. (A) Mathematical modeling of double-negative feedback loops. (Left) Hes1 forms a negative feedback loop. Hes1 represses Dll1 expression in the same cell, while Dll1 induces Hes1 expression in a neighboring cell. (Right) The regulation shown (left) can be simplified as a double-negative feedback loop. Hes1 represses its own expression with a delay τ_1 within the same cell, while repressing Hes1 expression with a delay τ_2 in a neighboring cell. (B) Differential equations for Hes1 oscillations. $X_1(t)$ and $X_2(t)$ represent Hes1 levels in two neighboring cells. (C) In-phase and out-of-phase oscillations and amplitude/oscillation death depending on τ_2 values. The red and green lines represent the highest and lowest levels of Hes1 expression, respectively. The distance between these two lines indicates the amplitude of oscillation.

in-phase and out-of-phase oscillations are both dampened, and in the most extreme cases, expression becomes steady, a condition known as amplitude/oscillation death (Figure 6.5C) (Ramana Reddy et al. 1998).

The first approach to dampen Hes1 oscillations is to shorten the τ_1 value for Hes1 protein expression, that is, accelerate negative feedback. To accelerate negative feedback, the time delay required for Hes1 protein expression was shortened. Intronic delay, which includes the transcription of introns and the removal of intronic sequences by splicing, constitutes a major part of the time delay required for Hes1 protein expression. As the *Hes1* gene does not have intronic enhancer or silencer sequences, all introns can be removed from the *Hes1* locus (*Hes1*-intron[–]) without a significant effect on its average expression levels. In such mutant mice, Hes1 oscillations in NSCs are dampened, and NSC proliferation decreases slightly. The phenotype is rather mild, probably because Hes1 oscillations are not abolished completely, that is, Hes1 expression still oscillates in the mutant mice, although its amplitude is smaller. Another reason is that the functions of *Hes1* can be compensated for by *Hes1*-related genes, such as *Hes3* and *Hes5*. Indeed, although *Hes3;Hes5* null mice are almost normal, the introduction of the *Hes1*-intron(–) mutation significantly inhibits NSC proliferation and accelerates neurogenesis, leading to microcephaly (Ochi et al. 2020).

The other approach to dampen oscillations is to shorten or elongate the τ_2 value, or change the time delay required for Dll1-Notch signaling transmission between cells. To this end, the *Dll1* gene was shortened by deleting all introns (type 1 mutant) or elongated by inserting an extra sequence (type 2 mutant) (Figure 6.6A) (Shimojo et al. 2016). The shortened and elongated *Dll1* genes exhibit

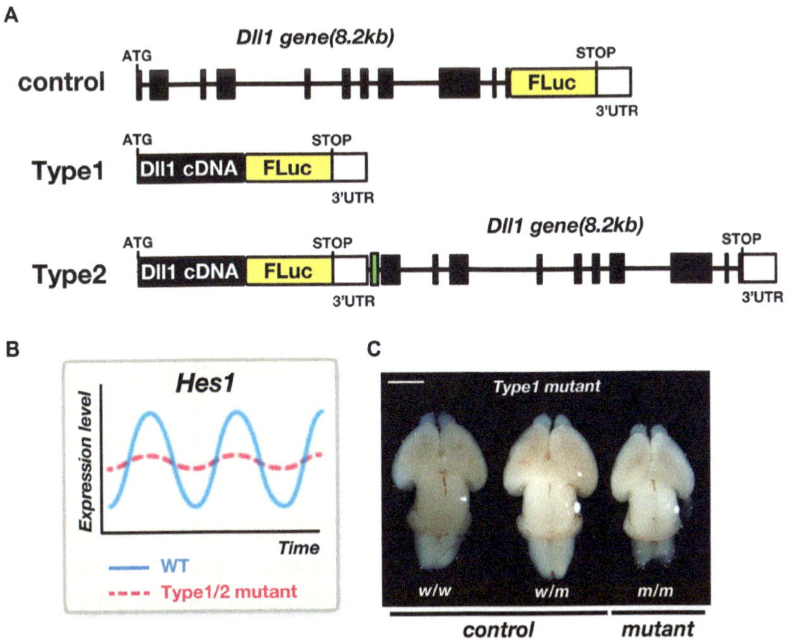

Figure 6.6 The phenotypes of Dll1 type 1 and type 2 mutant mice. (A) Structures of control, shortened (type1), and elongated (type 2) *Dll1* genes. Dll1 expression from the shortened (type 1) and elongated (type 2) *Dll1* genes is accelerated (shorter τ_2) and delayed (longer τ_2), respectively. (B) Hes1 oscillations are dampened in both *Dll1* type 1 and type 2 mutant NSCs (red broken line). WT, wild-type. (C) Compared to control mice, NSC proliferation is impaired in both Dll1 type 1 and type 2 mutant mice, which show microcephaly.

accelerated and delayed Dll1 expression, respectively. As a result, the time delay in Dll1-Notch signaling transmission is shortened and elongated in type 1 and type 2 Dll1 mutants, respectively. Furthermore, Dll1 expression levels are not affected much by deleting all introns, because the *Dll1* gene has no intronic enhancer or silencer sequences. Notably, both types of *Dll1* mutant mice exhibit dampened Hes1 oscillations in NSCs (Figure 6.6B) and dampened Hes7 oscillations in the presomitic mesoderm (Shimojo et al. 2016). Dampened Hes1 oscillations inhibit the proliferation of NSCs, accelerate neuronal differentiation, and lead to microcephaly (Figure 6.6C) while dampened Hes7 oscillations lead to severe fusion of somites and their derivatives, such as vertebrae and ribs (Shimojo et al. 2016). These studies clearly indicate that oscillatory expression in NSCs is important for normal brain morphogenesis in vivo.

The oscillations observed in the developing nervous system are anti-phase or out-of-phase between neighboring NSCs, unlike the in-phase oscillations of Hes7 in the presomitic mesoderm. However, the significance of anti-phase or out-of-phase oscillations in NSCs is not known. NSCs are required to produce diverse cell types during neural development, and anti-phase or out-of-phase oscillations may be useful for the generation of the diverse responses of NSCs. For example, Hes1-low cells could respond to certain signals, but Hes1-high cells could not. Further analysis is required to test this hypothesis.

6.6 Conclusions

Hes1 oscillations drive the oscillatory expression of proneural genes such as *Ascl1*, leading to an active state, whereas high and sustained Hes1 expression suppresses proneural gene expression, leading to quiescence, as in boundary cells. In other developmental contexts, high and sustained Hes1 expression is associated with astrocyte differentiation. Therefore, Hes1 expression dynamics are a key regulatory mechanism for generating various types of cells in the developing nervous system. Similarly, in the adult brain, Hes1 oscillations activate NSCs to initiate neurogenesis, while high and sustained Hes1 expression makes NSCs quiescent (Sueda et al. 2019). However, the mechanisms by which oscillatory and sustained Hes1 expression is controlled and how such different expression dynamics differentially control cell cycle progression remain to be determined. It was recently shown that a combination of over-expressing PLAG1-like zinc finger 2 (Plagl2) and knocking-down dual specificity tyrosine phosphorylation-regulated kinase 1a (Dyrk1a) can efficiently induce Ascl1 oscillations and thereby activate quiescent NSCs (Kaise et al. 2022). Further understanding of the significance of gene expression dynamics will be useful for the manipulation of NSCs and the development of regenerative medicine.

Acknowledgments

This work was supported by Grant-in-Aid for Scientific Research on Innovative Areas (16H06480 to Ryoichiro Kageyama) and Specially Promoted Research (21H04976 to Ryoichiro Kageyama) from Ministry of Education, Culture, Sports, Science, and Technology (MEXT), Japan, and AMED-CREST (JP21gm1110002 to Ryoichiro Kageyama) from Japan Agency for Medical Research and Development.

References

Baek, J.H. et al. (2006). Persistent and high levels of Hes1 expression regulate boundary formation in the developing central nervous system. *Development* 133: 2467–2476.

Bertrand, N. et al. (2002). Proneural genes and the specification of neural cell types. *Nat Rev Neurosci* 3: 517–530.

Bessho, Y. et al. (2001). Dynamic expression and essential functions of *Hes7* in somite segmentation. *Genes Dev* 15: 2642–2647.

Castro, D.S. et al. (2011). A novel function of the proneural factor Ascl1 in progenitor proliferation identified by genome-wide characterization of its targets. *Genes Dev* 25: 930–945.

Hatakeyama, J. et al. (2004). *Hes* genes regulate size, shape and histogenesis of the nervous system by control of the timing of neural stem cell differentiation. *Development* 131: 5539–5550.

Hirabayashi, Y. et al. (2009). Polycomb limits the neurogenic competence of neural precursor cells to promote astrogenic fate transition. *Neuron* 63: 600–613.

Hirata, H. et al. (2001). *Hes1* and *Hes3* regulate maintenance of the isthmic organizer and development of the mid/hindbrain. *EMBO J* 20: 4454–4466.

Hirata, H. et al. (2002). Oscillatory expression of the bHLH factor Hes1 regulated by a negative feedback loop. *Science* 298: 840–843.

Imayoshi, I. et al. (2013). Oscillatory control of factors determining multipotency and fate in mouse neural progenitors. *Science* 342: 1203–1208.

Imayoshi, I. and Kageyama, R. (2014). bHLH factors in self-renewal, multipotency, and fate choice of neural progenitor cells. *Neuron* 82: 9–23.

Imayoshi, I. et al. (2010). Essential roles of Notch signaling in maintenance of neural stem cells in developing and adult brains. *J Neurosci* 3: 3489–3498.

Ishibashi, M. et al. (1995). Targeted disruption of mammalian *hairy* and *Enhancer of split* homolog-1 (*HES-1*) leads to up-regulation of neural helix-loop-helix factors, premature neurogenesis and severe neural tube defects. *Genes Dev* 9: 3136–3148.

Isomura, A. et al. (2017). Optogenetic perturbation and bioluminescence imaging to analyze cell-to-cell transfer of oscillatory information. *Genes Dev* 31: 524–535.

Kageyama, R. et al. (2008). Dynamic Notch signaling in neural progenitor cells and a revised view of lateral inhibition. *Nat Neurosci* 11: 1247–1251.

Kaise, T. et al. (2022). Functional rejuvenation of aged neural stem cells by Plagl2 and anti-Dyrk1a activity. *Genes Dev* 36: 23–37.

Kiecker, C. and Lumsden, A. (2005). Compartments and their boundaries in vertebrate brain development. *Nat Rev Neurosci* 6: 553–564.

Kishi, Y. et al. (2012). HMGA regulates the global chromatin state and neurogenic potential in neocortical precursor cells. *Nat Neurosci* 15: 1127–1133.

Kopan, R. and Ilagan, M.X. (2009). The canonical Notch signaling pathway. *Cell* 137: 216–233.

Lu, Q.R. et al. (2002). Common developmental requirement for Olig function indicates a motor neuron/oligodendrocyte connection. *Cell* 109: 75–86.

Namihira, M. and Nakashima, K. (2013). Mechanisms of astrocytogenesis in the mammalian brain. *Curr Opin Neurobiol* 23: 921–927.

Nieto, M. et al. (2001). Neural bHLH genes control the neuronal versus glial fate decision in cortical progenitors. *Neuron* 29: 401–413.

Noda, N. et al. (2011). Hes1 is required for contact inhibition of cell proliferation in 3T3-L1 preadipocytes. *Genes Cells* 16: 704–713.

Ochi, S. et al. (2020). Oscillatory expression of Hes1 regulates cell proliferation and neuronal differentiation in the embryonic brain. *Development* 147: dev182204.

Ohtsuka, T. et al. (1999). *Hes1* and *Hes5* as Notch effectors in mammalian neuronal differentiation. *EMBO J* 18: 2196–2207.

Ohtsuka, T. et al. (2001). Roles of Notch signaling in expansion of neural stem cells of the developing brain. *J Biol Chem* 276: 30467–30474.

Ramana Reddy, D.V. et al. (1998). Experimental evidence of time delay induced death in coupled limit cycle oscillators. *Phys Rev Lett* 80: 5109–5112.

Ross, S.E. et al. (2003). Basic helix-loop-helix factors in cortical development. *Neuron* 39: 13–25.

Sang, L. et al. (2008). Control of the reversibility of cellular quiescence by the transcriptional repressor HES1. *Science* 321: 1095–1100.

Shimojo, H. et al. (2016). Oscillatory control of Delta-like1 in cell interactions regulates dynamic gene expression and tissue morphogenesis. *Genes Dev* 30: 102–116.

Shimojo, H. et al. (2008). Oscillations in Notch signaling regulate maintenance of neural progenitors. *Neuron* 58: 52–64.

Sueda, R. et al. (2019). High Hes1 expression and resultant Ascl1 suppression regulate quiescent versus active neural stem cells in the adult mouse brain. *Genes Dev* 33: 511–523.

Sun, Y. et al. (2011). Phosphorylation state of Olig2 regulates proliferation of neural progenitors. *Neuron* 69: 906–917.

Takashima, Y. et al. (2011). Intronic delay is essential for oscillatory expression in the segmentation clock. *Proc Natl Acad Sci USA* 108: 3300–3305.

Takebayashi, H. et al. (2002). The basic helix-loop-helix factor olig2 is essential for the development of motoneuron and oligodendrocyte lineages. *Curr Biol* 12: 1157–1163.

Takizawa, T. et al. (2001). DNA methylation is a critical cell-intrinsic determinant of astrocyte differentiation in the fetal brain. *Dev Cell* 1: 749–758.

Tan, S.-L. et al. (2012). Essential roles of the histone methyltransferase ESET in the epigenetic control of neural progenitor cells during development. *Development* 139: 3806–3816.

Tomita, K. et al. (2000). Mammalian *achaete-scute* and *atonal* homologs regulate neuronal versus glial fate determination in the central nervous system. *EMBO J* 19: 5460–5472.

Wang, X. et al. (2012). Spatiotemporal control of gene expression by a light-switchable transgene system. *Nat Methods* 9: 266–269.

Yu, X. et al. (2006). HES1 inhibits cycling of hematopoietic progenitor cells via DNA binding. *Stem Cells* 24: 876–888.

Zhou, Q. and Anderson, D.J. (2002). The bHLH transcription factors OLIG2 and OLIG1 couple neuronal and glial subtype specification. *Cell* 109: 61–73.

7

Mechanical and Physical Interactions Involving Neocortical Progenitor Cells

Takaki Miyata

Nagoya University Graduate School of Medicine 65 Tsurumai, Showa, Nagoya, 466–8550 Aichi, Japan

7.1 Introduction

In recent decades, the mechanisms underlying neocortical neurogenesis by neural progenitor cells (NPCs) whose nuclei/somata functionally constitute the ventricular zone (VZ) (Chenn 1995; Davis and Temple 1994; Malatesta et al. 2000; Miyata et al. 2001; Noctor et al. 2001; Smart 1973; Takahashi et al. 1993) (corresponding to the apical radial glia: Taverna et al. 2014) have been elucidated in detail by investigations from a molecular or chemical viewpoint. By contrast, however, questions from a physical or mechanical viewpoint, such as what mechanical forces these NPCs are generating, receiving, and using within the growing cerebral wall (Sauer 1935; Smart 1965), have been almost entirely unexplored until recently. It is also unknown how the three-dimensional (3D) morphology of the VZ-forming NPCs and the behaviors of these cells, including division at the apical surface (Figure 7.1) and the cell-cycle-dependent movement of the nucleus/soma, called interkinetic nuclear migration (IKNM) (Sauer 1935; Schaper 1897; reviewed in Kosodo 2012; Lee and Norden 2013; Miyata 2008; Miyata et al. 2015; Reiner et al. 2012; Spear and Erickson 2012a; Taverna and Huttner 2010) (Figure 7.1), are associated with or influenced by mechanical factors.

This chapter summarizes recent findings on the physical aspects of VZ-forming NPCs in the developing neocortex, mainly focusing on the mouse as a traditional but still mysterious model system. The first part will show that the ventricular/apical surface of the cerebral wall is contractile and in tension due to actomyosin function in NPCs' apical endfeet (Figure 7.2A, B) and that normal subapical crowding generated by the apical contractility enables an elasticity-mediated passive boosting phase in basalward IKNM, thereby supporting the collective productivity of NPCs (Figure 7.2C, D). The VZ avoids subapical overcrowding to ensure normal neurogenesis/histogenesis through sequential rather than simultaneous departure of sibling daughter cell nuclei/somata from the apical surface (Figure 7.1 and 7.2D). Overcrowding experimentally induced by artificial retraction of the basal fiber or over-proliferation seems to be "sensed" by NPCs at/near the apical surface, making them detach from the apical surface (Figure 7.2E).

The second part of the chapter summarizes how NPCs and differentiating neurons interact physically, thereby collaboratively playing roles in the spreading/expansion of the neocortical neuronal zone in the ventral direction (Figure 7.3) and the safe maintenance of the VZ and cytogenesis there (Figure 7.2F). The second part will also provide new results, obtained from microsurgical experiments (Figure 7.4), showing that NPCs are under apicobasal tension because

Neocortical Neurogenesis in Development and Evolution, First Edition. Edited by Wieland B. Huttner.

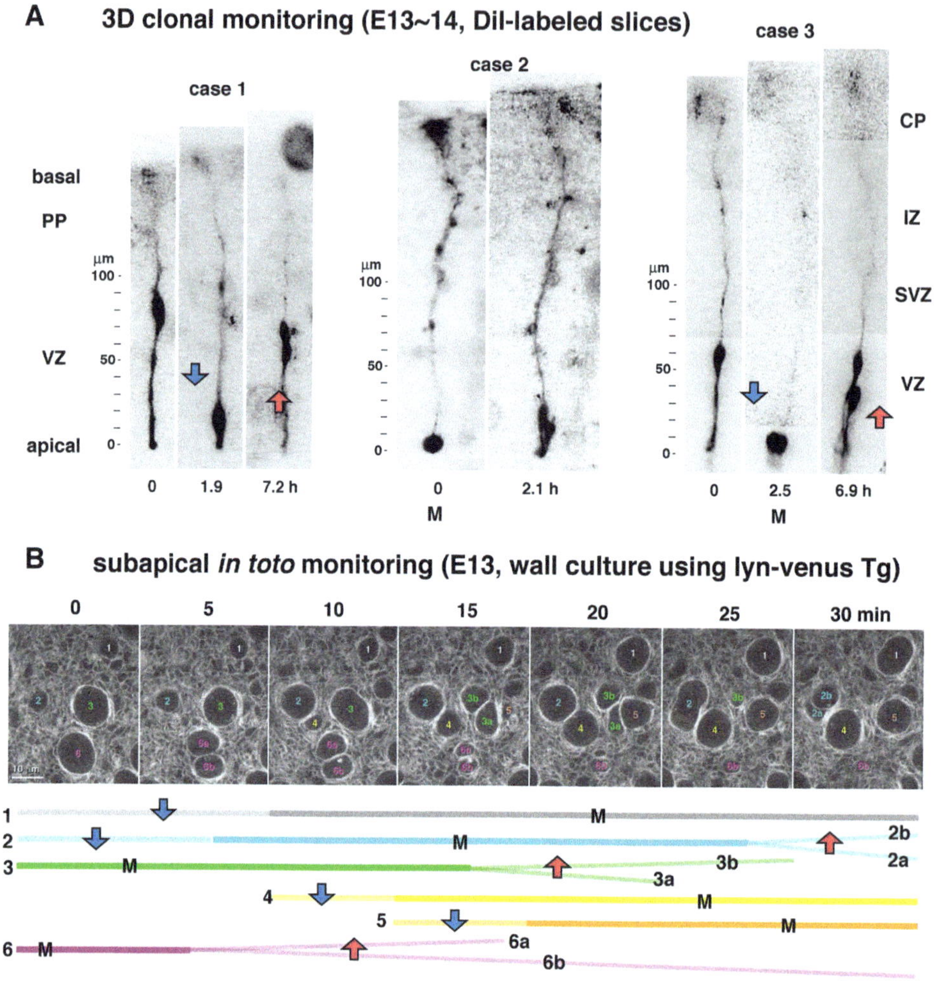

Figure 7.1 Clonal and in toto live imaging of VZ-forming NPCs. (A) Time-lapse monitoring of apicobasally spanning neural progenitor cells (NPCs) labeled sparsely with DiI from the basal surface of E13 ~ E14 mouse cerebral pallial walls. They correspond to the apical radial glial cells, divide at the apical surface, keep the basal process/fiber during M phase, with their nuclear/somal movements toward the apical surface (thick blue arrow) before mitosis and with the nuclear/somal movements of their daughter cells away from the apical surface (thick red arrow). The apicobasal length of NPCs, that is, the thickness of cultured slices, increased during observation. Each basal process/fiber is inherited by one of the two daughter cells, and fiber inheritance contributes to the sequential departure of daughter cell nuclei/somata from the subapical area, with a fiber-inheriting daughter cell's nucleus/soma leaving basally more quickly than its sibling cell's nucleus/soma. (B) In toto live (horizontal sectional) monitoring at the level of 5 μm from the apical surface in a cerebral wall prepared from an E13 Lyn-Venus transgenic mouse, which shows the plasma membrane of all cells (Okamoto et al. 2013; Shinoda et al. 2018). Six NPC somata (numbered) are schematically tracked below, forming lineage trees with mitosis (M) and daughter cells (a and b) and somal movements (apicalward, blue; basalward, red).

they are stretched passively by the progressive addition and dense intramural packing of neurons and that tangential contractility of the apical surface assists in a proper 3D packing of the progressively increasing neurons and are thereby underlying an orthogonal thickening of the wall. The third part will show, with a spatially wider view in the embryonic head before osteogenesis, that the cerebral wall, including NPCs, is under mechanical confinement by the surrounding

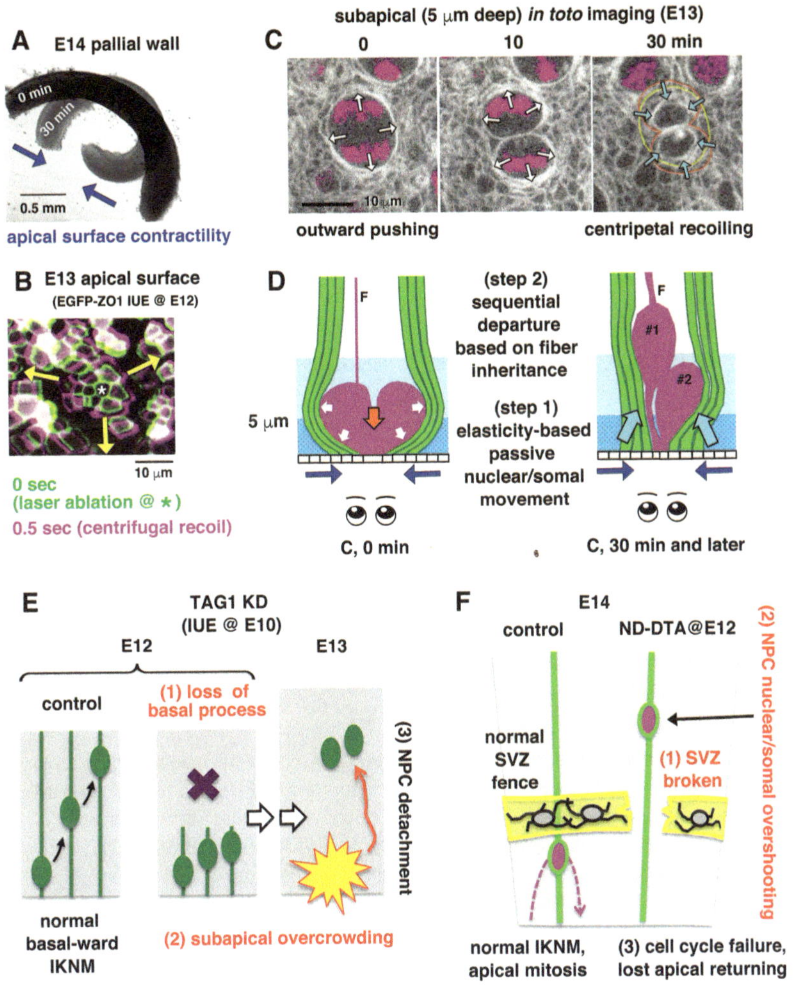

Figure 7.2 Contractility of the apical surface underlies the mechanical behaviors of ventricular-zone NPCs. (A) Time lapse of an E14 mouse cerebral wall slice in culture medium; the slice spontaneously bent/curled toward the inner/apical side in 30 minutes. Although this is a slice prepared horizontally (along the anterior–posterior axis), very similar bending/curling occurs in coronal slices prepared along the dorso-ventral axis. (B) Live laser ablation to the apical surface en face observed with GFP-ZO1. Upon ablation of an NPC apex (asterisk), the surrounding areas recoiled centrifugally (arrow). (C) Horizontal in toto observation (nuclei/chromosome, H2B-mCherry [magenta]; membrane, Lyn-Venus [white]; at 5 μm from the apical surface) of an M-phase NPC (0 minutes) and its daughter cells (10 minutes and 30 minutes) together with the surrounding space filled densely with neighboring NPCs' apical processes, suggesting outward pushing by the M-phase cell and subsequent centripetal recoiling of the surrounding tissue (Shinoda et al. 2018). (D) Schematic illustrations cross-sectionally depicting a dividing NPC (left) and its daughter cells (right) during step 1 (elasticity-based passive nuclear/somal departure, by 30 minutes) and step 2 (sequential nuclear/somal displacement [#1 → #2] based on the asymmetric inheritance of the basal fiber, F, by #1) under physiological subapical crowding/compression due to apical contraction. (E) Subapical overcrowding of NPCs (E12) due to the retraction of their basal processes, which was induced by knockdown of TAG-1 (E10) (Okamoto et al. 2013). Overcrowded NPCs detached themselves from the apical surface (E13) and underwent abnormal heterotopic divisions (~E15), suggesting that NPCs may sense excessive mechanical stimuli at/near the apical surface. (F) When cells comprising the SVZ were acutely ablated via IUE with a vector expressing diphtheria toxin A under the NeuroD promoter (ND-DTA), NPCs' nuclei/somata went too far during basalward IKNM, and they failed to proceed with the cell cycle and did not come back to divide at the apical surface, indicating that SVZ plays a mechanical role in safegaurding NPCs' IKNM range and apical mitosis (Watanabe et al. 2018).

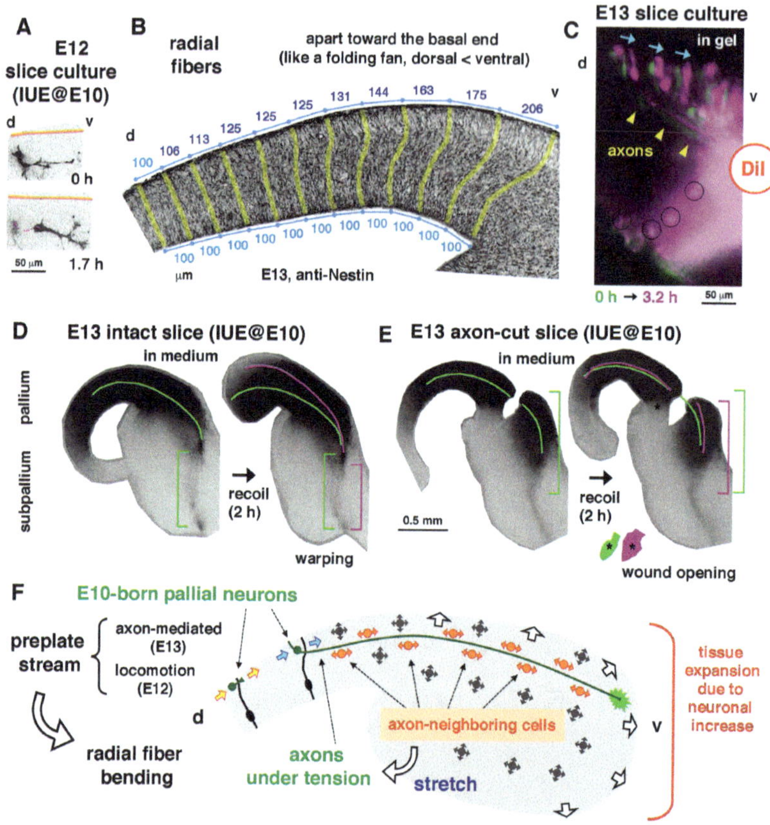

Figure 7.3 Dorsal-to-ventral streaming of the preplate underlies the bending of radial fibers. (A) A single preplate (PP) neuron in an E12 slice, which was prepared following in utero electroporation (IUE) with a plasmid vector for sparse expression of GFP at E10. The GFP-labeled E10-born neurons migrated ventrally. This tangential locomotion-like migration is the first physical contributor to the bending of radial fibers. (B) Anti-Nestin immunohistochemistry at E13, showing a dorsal (d)-to-ventral (v) gradient of the bending of radial fibers (RFs). In the ventral region close to the pallio-striatal angle, the basal terminal of each radial fiber (yellow highlighted every 100 μm at the apical surface) is observed much more ventrally than at the apical terminal, separating two basal terminals much wider (up to 206 μm) than in the dorsal-most region (100 μm, as always at the apical surface) and bending the distal RFs ventrally. (C) Time-lapse observation of PP-like neurons labeled retrogradely with DiI through their axons, showing that somata of the axon-bearing PP-like neurons (7 ~ 8 cells identifiable) all moved ventrally at the same pace (blue arrow), while cells in the ventricular zone (three, circled) did not move ventrally at all. (D) An E13 cerebral wall slice that had been labeled heavily with GFP via IUE at E10 to visualize PP (future subplate) neurons and their corticofugal axons (intrapallial part traced in green or magenta). It spontaneously warped outward, with simultaneous curling at the dorsal-most part. Shortening of the axon route is clearly visible at the subpallial region. (E) Another E13 cerebral wall slice in which PP neurons and axons (intrapallial part traced in green or magenta) had been visualized, but an incision was made to cut the axon route. This slice did not warp; the wound merely opened. (F) Schematic illustration depicting the mechanical mechanisms underlying the dorsal-to-ventral bending of RFs. Initially (from E11 to E12), PP neurons migrating ventrally in a locomotion-like manner (yellow arrow) may directly push the distal part of RFs and may also shift the endfeet of RFs by remodeling/expanding the basal surface (because PP neurons themselves can comprise the basal surface). Then, at E13, approximately 40 percent of the PP neurons have extended axons to the subpallial regions. Along the route of these PP axons in vivo, new neurons continuously increasing their number may be under mutual compression, thereby passively stretching the PP axons. When a slice is surgically made and kept freely in culture medium, such compressed (thus stretcher) neurons may locally recoil laterally (to displace toward the cut edge and beyond, as exemplified in Figure 7.4B, C), thereby allowing the prestretched axons that were in tension to elastically recoil to shorten themselves, thus warping the entire wall. When the slice is embedded/held in collagen gel, its warping is blocked, and as the whole tissue grows with the terminals of PP-derived axons going further and new neurons (non-PP pallial-derived neurons and subpallial neurons) added, the PP-derived axons may be stretched. Consequently, a traction force may be given to PP neurons' somata (blue arrow), resulting in the ventral streaming of PP neurons' somata, as shown in C. This axonal traction for PP streaming is the second (E13) driving force underlying the ventral bending of RFs and explains why RF bending occurs deeply (at the level between the subplate and upper intermediate zone). (Addendum to Saito et al. 2019).

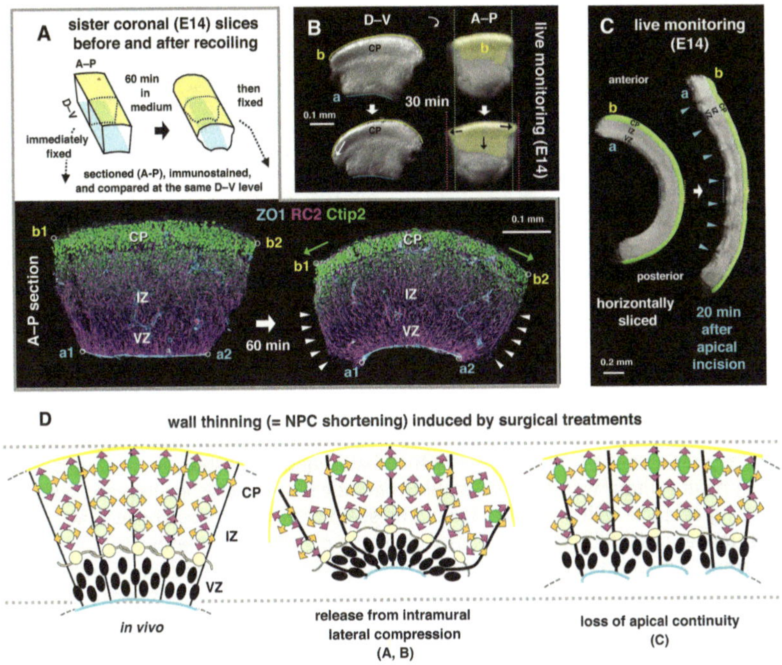

Figure 7.4 Passive stretching of NPCs/radial fibers by compressively packed neurons with assistance from the contractile apical surface. (A) *Type I* surgery (1, making coronal slices). Top illustration, coronal slices prepared along the D–V axis were then cryosectioned perpendicularly (along the A–P axis, at the same D–V level). Bottom photomicrographs, cryosection-based immunohistochemical comparison between slices before (left, fixed soon after live slicing) and after outward recoiling of the intramurally packed neurons (right, fixed 60 minutes later). The basal surface of the 60-minute-old wall had expanded, with a wider and thinner CP consisting of Ctip2$^+$ neurons. At the section edges (the anterior or posterior borders), bulging of the intermediate zone (IZ) coincided with outward bending of RC2$^+$ radial fibers (arrowhead). Ratio of the length of the section edges (e.g., traced from a1 to b1, curved) to the length of a straight line drawn between a1 and b1 (% curve/straight) was calculated to quantitatively evaluate the degree of bulging (bulging index, BI). BI was significantly greater ($p < 0.005$, Wilcoxon rank sum exact test) in cryosections made from the 60-minute-old coronal slices after recoiling (1.03 ± 0.03 [n = 6]) than in those from slices before recoiling (1.20 ± 0.09 [n = 6]). (B) *Type I* surgery (2, making cubes). Continuous observation of an E14 cerebral wall cube for 30 minutes. a, apical. b, basal. Consistent with Figure 7.1A, the width of the apical surface decreased (p = 0.0013 [paired t test], to 85.7 ± 7.3% of the original [n = 9]), while the width of the basal surface increased (p = 0.0003 [paired t test], to 112.5 ± 6.1% of the original [n = 9]). The width of the CP also increased (p = 0.003 [paired t test], to 113.2 ± 8.0% of the original [n = 9]). The widening of the basal surface was comparable between the D–V plane (to 111.1 ± 6.0%) and the A–P plane (to 112.2 ± 4.8%) (p = 0.69 [paired t test, n = 8]). The widening of the CP was also comparable between the D–V plane (to 113.6 ± 8.5%) and the A–P plane (to 111.0 ± 2.7%) (p = 0.43 [paired t test, n = 8]). The thickness of the entire wall decreased (p = 0.009 [paired t test], to 85.1 ± 7.0% of the original [n = 9]). The thickness of the CP also decreased ($p = 5.74 \times 10^{-6}$ [paired t test], to 72.2 ± 6.0% of the original [n = 9]). (C) *Type II* surgery (apical incisions). Live observation of an E14 horizontal cerebral wall slice (prepared continuously along the anterior-posterior axis) before and after (20 minutes) incising onto the apical surface (blue arrowhead). After incision, which reduced the apical concavity, the lateral length of the slice measured at the level of SVZ significantly increased (p = 0.008 [Wilcoxon signed rank test with continuity correction], to 109.7 ± 4.9% of the original length [n = 8]), whereas the wall thickness significantly decreased (p = 0.0002 [paired t test], to 84.8 ± 5.2% of the original thickness [n = 8]). Experiments where incisions were made in the basal surface did not show thinning or lengthening of the wall (n = 3/3); only curling to the apical side was observed, as in the control (unincised) slices. a, apical. b, basal. (D) Schematic illustrations summarizing the results of wall thinning when it was relieved from intramural lateral compression (A, B) or when its apically continuous contractility was broken (C), showing that NPCs/radial fibers are passively stretched by the dense packing of neurons under geometrical and mechanical assistance by the contractile apical surface.

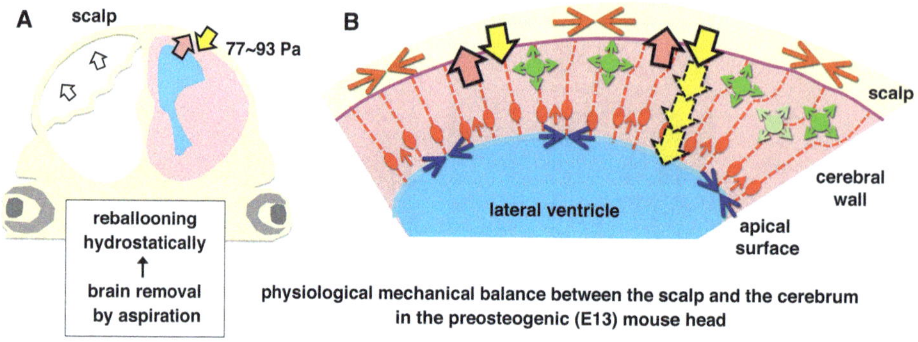

Figure 7.5 Mechanical relationship between the cerebral hemispheric wall and the scalp in the preosteogenic mouse head. (A) Measurement of pressure at which mechanical confrontation between the embryonic brain and the elastic scalp (consisting of the epidermal and mesenchymal layers) is established. An E13 head was emptied by aspirating out the brain and was then ballooned hydrostatically; the pressure needed to restore the original head contour was 77 ~ 93 Pa. (B) Schematic illustration showing mechanical forces existing in the developing cerebral wall and the surrounding scalp of an E13 mouse head. Since confinement by the scalp influences brain morphogenesis as well as the distribution of embryonic cerebrospinal fluid (yellow arrows with dashed lines), NPCs that comprise the wall and face the ventricle may also be under mechanical influences from both the basal surface and the apical surface. (Addendum to Tsujikawa et al. 2022).

embryonic scalp, which is elastic and contractile (Figure 7.5). This chapter will provide a basis for future elucidation of mechanochemical coupling (Hannezo and Heisenberg 2019) in neocortical neurogenesis.

7.2 Mechanical Forces Generated, Used, and Managed by Neocortical VZ Cells

7.2.1 The Ventricular Zone is Dynamically Composed of Bidirectionally Moving Nuclei/somata of NPCs

When cerebral wall slices prepared from embryonic day 12 (E12) ~ E14 mice are cultured in collagen gel, they thicken through extensive cell production by NPCs. An intra-VZ event by which force generation by NPCs is most clearly recognizable is IKNM (Figure 7.1A). Pulling forces (via dynein during G2 phase or via kinesin during G1 phase) or squeezing forces (via actomyosin during G2 and G1 phases) act intracellularly on the nucleus to move it toward (G2 phase) or away from (G1 phase) the apical surface (Norden et al. 2009; Schenk et al. 2009; Spear and Erickson 2012b; Tsai et al. 2005, 2010).

Execution of IKNM by neighboring different NPCs in a chronologically non-synchronized (thus spatially staggered) manner collectively generates a pseudostratified VZ structure. 3D in toto (all-cell) observation of NPCs and their daughter cells has provided us with a platform to quantitatively monitor all nuclear/somal trafficking in the VZ (Okamoto et al. 2013; Shinoda et al. 2018). Tangential observation under visualization of all cell membranes shows that in a space near the apical surface (= subapical space) filled densely with NPCs' apical processes, somata of NPCs entering M phase emerge frequently and almost diffusely to round up and divide, suggesting a physiological level of crowding (Figure 7.1B).

7.2.2 The Apical Surface is Actively Contractile

Although mesoscopic inspections give the impression that a 3D dome-like cerebral pallial wall structure is static, its apical concavity is established actively (in an energy-consuming manner) by a force-generation mechanism. Surgical tests demonstrated that the apical surface containing the dynamically dividing cells (Figure 7.1B) was contractile and in tension (Figure 7.2A). Slicing relieves a wall from a 3D mechanical balance that exists in vivo (represented by pulling forces from multiple directions along the apical surface), enabling them to freely bend or curl in the culture medium along one axis over a long distance to increase the apical concavity (Okamoto et al. 2013). This bending/curling is blocked when actomyosin is pharmacologically inhibited (Nagasaka et al. 2016; Shinoda et al. 2018). Laser ablation under en face high-power observation reveals that cut edges immediately recoil, reflecting the contractility of NPCs' apices (Figure 7.2B) (Okamoto et al. 2013; Shinoda et al. 2018).

7.2.3 Normal Subapical Crowding Induces Elasticity-mediated Passive Nucleokinesis

The contractile/narrowing property of the apical surface makes the subapical space compressive, providing a tissue-level elasticity. The elastic modulus measured by atomic force microscopy (AFM) on/near the apical surface of the pallial walls is much greater (1400 Pa) (Nagasaka et al. 2016) than that in more basal VZ regions (~100 Pa) (Iwashita et al. 2014) and is reduced (to 800 ~ 900 Pa) by inhibition of actomyosin (Nagasaka et al. 2016). The soma of each NPC at M phase pushes outwardly/centrifugally the subapical space, leading to a consequent centripetal recoil of the subapical space, which passively supports an initial (~30 minutes) step of basal nucleokinesis by the NPC's daughter cells (Shinoda et al. 2018) (Figure 7.2C, D). The velocity of nucleokinesis is greater during this elasticity-mediated boosting step (initial 30 minutes) than in the next 30 minutes during live monitoring, and the absence of this crowding-based boosting mechanism collapses the overall IKNM and the integrity of a mathematically simulated "virtual VZ" (Shinoda et al. 2018).

7.2.4 Overcrowding, Likely Sensed Periapically by NPCs, Disrupts VZ Integrity

Nevertheless, if NPCs are too crowded at or near the apical surface beyond a useful level of crowding, such overcrowding leads to abnormal detachment of NPCs from the apical surface (Figure 7.2E). Overcrowding-induced delamination occurs when NPCs are acutely retracted from the basal surface and shortened (via artificial removal of TAG-1) (Okamoto et al. 2013). Since apices of the shortened TAG1-lacking NPCs expanded and bulged toward the lumen, it is possible that these morphological abnormalities at or near the apical surface are tightly associated with mechanisms (molecularly yet unknown) that allow NPCs to "sense" overcrowding. This delamination might be a form of endogenous "first aid" on a mechanical emergency when quick re-optimization of pressure (decompression) is needed for NPCs while preserving the total number of divisions, at least tentatively, using ectopic mitoses, although the overall tissue integrity is subsequently disrupted. Intra-VZ over-proliferation (via overactivation of Wnt3a or Yap signaling) also leads to NPC delamination and ectopic mitosis (Cappello et al. 2013; Chenn and Walsh 2002; Lavado et al. 2018; Liu et al. 2018; Saito et al. 2018).

To streamline basalward IKNM within the subapical space that is fragile to overcrowding, nuclei/somata of two daughter cells generated apically from a single parent NPC move sequentially via asymmetric inheritance of the parent cell's basal fiber by one daughter cell (Miyata et al. 2001) (Figures 7.1A and 7.2D). A fiber-inheriting daughter cell's nucleus/soma departs the subapical space earlier than the nucleus/soma of its sibling cell that has not inherited the fiber, avoiding "bottleneck" problems (Okamoto et al. 2013). Mathematical simulation to reproduce a VZ virtually (Shinoda et al. 2018) confirmed an essential role of this "staggered commuting."

7.2.5 Curvature and Stiffness of the Apical Surface in Region Specificity and Evolution

The loss of cdc42 (Cappello et al. 2006) or N-cadherin (Kadowaki et al. 2007) in the pallial region locally converts the apical surface from a normal concave shape to a convex contour similar to that of the ganglionic eminences (GEs). The normal apically convex shape of the GEs becomes evident from E11 ~ E12, which subsequently leads to inward growth of the striatum into the lateral ventricle, while the pallial wall maintains the concavity, apparently promoting space efficiency (i.e., avoiding mechanical competition between the neighboring pallial and striatal regions) in the fetal cranium. Comparisons using AFM showed that the pallial apical surface is stiffer (1300 ~ 1500 Pa) than the GE apical surface (650 ~ 800 Pa) at E12 ~ E14 (Nagasaka and Miyata 2021). Factors underlying this difference are that NPCs' apices are denser and F-actin is denser along the pallial apical surface than along the GE apical surface. Laser ablation on the apical surface combined with inhibition of actomyosin showed that recoiling observed along the convex apical surface of the GE includes an actomyosin-independent (thus passively stretched) element more than in the concave pallial apical surface.

Comparisons of IKNM behaviors and VZ densification in the developing pallium between mice and ferrets (Okamoto et al. 2014) suggest that IKNM patterns can be modulated in a species-specific manner, and physical situations in the VZ may be one of the possible contributing factors to IKNM, as also suggested in Drosophila wing disc epithelia (Hecht et al. 2022; Kirkland et al. 2020). A comparative AFM analysis showed that the pallial apical surface is stiffer (1700 Pa) in E28 ~ E30 ferrets than in E13 mice (1400 Pa) (Nagasaka et al. 2016). Interestingly, a recent study compared neocortical organoids derived from human, gorilla, and chimpanzee cells to show that the concavity of the organoid apical surface (human < ape) underlies the human–ape difference in cerebral expansion (Benito-Kwiecinski et al. 2021).

7.3 Mechanical Influences of Differentiating Neurons on Progenitor Cells

7.3.1 The SVZ Mechanically Fences IKNM and the VZ and Safeguards Apical Cytogenesis

Force originating from the apical surface (highlighted earlier) seems to propagate throughout the VZ, passively assisting in the overall basal IKNM (Kosodo et al. 2011; Norden et al. 2009; Shinoda et al. 2018). Under such a net apical-to-basal force, NPC nuclei/somata are mechanically barriered by the subventricular zone (SVZ), consisting of a dense array of multipolar differentiating cells (i.e., neurons and intermediate progenitors) (Watanabe et al. 2018) (Figure 7.2F). While the IKNM trajectory should normally be within 100 μm (within the VZ), acute drilling of the SVZ (through cell ablation by diphtheria toxin A via in utero electroporation [IUE]) results in the overshooting of NPC nuclei/somata to 200 μm (beyond the SVZ to the intermediate zone) (Watanabe et al. 2018). The overshot nuclei/somata cannot return to the apical surface and even to the VZ, which is consistent with their cell cycle arrest during S phase (detected using Fucci imaging) in the overshot nuclei because completion of S phase is required for apicalward IKNM (Kosodo et al. 2011). This might also be explained by potential insufficiency of dynein-related molecules that normally work near the apical surface (Hu et al. 2013). This result indicates that the SVZ is an essential physical barrier to safeguard VZ structure and cytogenesis at the apical surface.

7.3.2 The Earliest-born Neurons' Dorsal-to-ventral Streaming Deflects RFs, Setting up Ventrally Spread Corticogenesis

The radial fibers (RFs) of NPCs are arced, at their distal/basal part, in the lateral/ventral direction (Figure 7.1A) (Gadisseux et al. 1989). This fiber arcing emerges at E11 in the lateral pallial wall region and then widely spreads (most extensively ventrally and mildly dorsally) (Figure 7.3). Live imaging and neuron-ablation experiments have revealed that RFs are bent depending on a mechanical force externally provided from neurons that are generated earliest (around E10) and subsequently stream ventrally forming a transient layer called the preplate (PP) until E13 (Saito et al. 2019). It is likely that a pushing force applied to the distal RFs from the soma of the PP neurons is driven initially (E11 ~ E12) by the locomotion mode of migration (with an intermittent fast phase based on cell-autonomous traction along the leading process and a slower adhesion-mediated passive-like phase) (Figure 7.3A) and then (E13) by streaming of PP neurons using long-range tension along the axons extended corticofugally (Figure 7.3C–F). Artificial reduction of PP neurons by E11 results in a weaker RF deflection and insufficient ventral spreading of layers to be formed by later-born neurons during the mid-embryonic period, with dorsally shrunken (ventrally narrower) neocortical maps postnatally (Saito et al. 2019). This result indicates a mechanical priming role of the early PP stream for the ventral expansion of the neocortex through a route modification to the RF system, which is responsible for the guidance of neocortical neurons along RFs (Rakic 1972). It would be interesting to study whether the mechanical force potentially received by NPCs at their RFs from the PP stream (dorsal < ventral) might modulate NPCs' cytogenetic and/or morphogenetic properties along the dorsoventral axis.

7.3.3 Compressively Packed Neurons Stretch Axons along the Dorso-ventral Axis

Tension along the corticofugal axons extended from PP neurons (which massively include neurons eventually constituting the subplate) can be assessed in a spontaneous warping response (i.e., outward/basalward bending) of coronal slices (Saito et al. 2019). In contrast to the aforementioned curling of the wall to the apical side, which is dependent on actomyosin, this outward warping, which coincides (or coexists in a sequence) with the apical curling (Figure 7.3D), is not blocked by actomyosin inhibitors. In vivo, the PP-derived axons running in an outer zone of the pallial and subpallial walls are thought to be passively stretched by non-PP neurons that are packed along the PP axons and compressed under a 3D mechanical balance established within the embryonic cerebral hemisphere (Figure 7.3F). Once hemispheres are sliced (0.2 ~ 0.3 mm thick) and resultant slices are kept (~2 hours) in culture medium, a pressure relief (i.e., tissue-level elastic recoil) occurs involving such neurons that had previously been compressively packed in vivo. Dislocation or spreading of these axon-neighboring neurons bilaterally toward/to the cut edges of each slice and beyond (shown in Figure 7.4) simultaneously allows the pre-stretched PP axons to orthogonally recoil/shorten along the dorso-ventral axis, which outwardly warps the pallial wall (Figure 7.3D). When the axons are also cut, the wall does not warp; the wound merely opens (Figure 7.3E). However, during long-term observation of slices embedded in collagen gel (not allowed to freely curl or warp), a massive supply of new neurons may arise along the axons whose terminals are also growing further, passively stretching the axons and generating a pulling force from them to the somata of PP neurons in the pallial wall (Figure 7.3F), thereby reproducing the dorsal-to-ventral PP stream as evidenced in vivo via pulse-chase experiments based on IUE (Saito et al. 2019).

7.3.4 Compressively Packed Neurons also Apicobasally Stretch RFs

A microsurgical test that cut single fluorescently labeled RFs in slice culture by a pulled glass capillary (internally fluorescently labeled) showed that the cut edges immediately recoiled (i.e., separated from each other), and the RFs were thus in tension along the apicobasal axis (Miyata and Ogawa 2007). Accordingly, whether the mechanical influence of compressively packed neurons on long fiber structures (i.e., stretching), as recognized in the PP-derived axons along the dorsoventral axis, also applies orthogonally along the apicobasal axis of the wall to NPCs and RFs was tested, as follows. Quantitative analysis of the thickness of the E14 mouse pallial wall (= apicobasal length of NPCs), as well as the width of it, was performed immediately after surgical treatments and 20 ~ 60 min later.

When tangential continuity of the wall was suddenly reduced (*type I* surgery) to a degree to obtain/leave coronal slices (0.2 ~ 0.3 mm thick) (Figure 7.4A) or to leave only a cube-like structure (Figure 7.4B), such slices or cubes observed in culture medium spontaneously changed their overall shapes in 30 ~ 60 min. In addition to the occurrence of the naturally expected narrowing of the apical surface, remarkably observed (statistically significant) changes were the tangential expansion of the outer/basal surface, the expansion/bulging of the neuronal zones consisting of the cortical plate (CP) and the intermediate zone (IZ), the thinning of the CP, and the thinning of the entire wall (Figure 7.4A–D). These results indicate that pressure-relieving recoil of the intramural neurons lateral to and beyond the slice edges upon surgery always resulted in thinning of the neuronal layers and shortening of NPCs along the apicobasal axis. It is therefore suggested that in vivo neurons, packed in a manner compressed centripetally parallel to the wall surfaces (along the circumferential plane including the anterior-posterior and dorso-ventral axes), use their counteractingly expansive property to orthogonally (thus apicobasally) stratify themselves to thicken the CP and to stretch NPCs/RFs (i.e., to thicken the wall).

It would be interesting to study to what extent the total RF/NPC extension this passive stretch mechanism accounts for. Related questions would be whether or how a possible feedback mechanism is driven for the active RF growth by this passive stretch, as known for axons as "stretch growth" (Falconieri et al. 2022; Fan et al. 2017; Pfister et al. 2004) and whether the passive stretch of RFs is associated with Ca^{2+} activity along RFs (Rash et al. 2016) or mRNA transport and local translation at the basal endfeet (Pilaz et al. 2016; Tsunekawa et al. 2012). It is also curious whether this passive RF stretch works as a mechanical "ruler" for chemically controlling NPCs' neurogenesis or underlies the physical folding of the CP in gyrencephalic species (Llinares-Benadero and Borrell 2019; Long et al. 2018; Nowakowski et al. 2016), perhaps through functional and/or morphological segregation into gyrus-forming RFs and sulcus-forming RFs, as implicated in epithelial folding (Wang 2021).

7.3.5 Apical Surface Contractility Underlies Wall Thickening via Circumferential Compression of Intramural Components and Inward Pulling

Interestingly, the orthogonal coupling or convertibility of the intramural mechanical force (i.e., compression and thus elastically expansive property of the packed neurons) from along the tangential axis to along the apicobasal axis is supported by the apical surface via its spatially continuous contractility, which was revealed by another surgical test (*type II* surgery) (Figure 7.4C). When slices prepared long (>1 mm) along the anterior–posterior axis were subjected to shallow incisions (0.2 ~ 0.3 mm apart) onto the apical surface, the apical concavity naturally decreased, making the VZ thinner and tangentially wider, and the lateral length of the slice measured at the level of SVZ increased, whereas the wall thickness decreased (Figure 7.4C, D) in 20 minutes.

Without continuity of the apical surface, circumferential compression of neurons and VZ cells weakened, consequently reducing the apicobasal stratification of these cells. Additionally, due to NPCs' apicobasal spanning, tangential contractility along the apical surface by itself generates an inward pulling force along NPCs/RFs, partly contributing to (or at least playing a permissive role in) the thickening of the wall via neuronal packing and stratification. Consistent with the latter model, the observed thinning of the embryonic mouse cerebral wall as well as shortening of NPCs/RFs induced by apical incisions (Figure 7.4C) is reminiscent of the thinning of the wall of human organoids exposed to actomyosin inhibitors (oblate-shaped, not incised) (Karzbrun et al. 2018) and the shortening of NPCs/RFs in the embryonic mouse cerebral wall when the β1 integrin signal was blocked at the apical surface with intraventricular antibody injection (Loulier et al. 2009).

7.4 Mechanical Influences on NPCs from the Components that Sandwich the Cerebral Wall

Lessons from the intra-VZ as well as the intramural mechanical interactions involving NPCs, as noted earlier, also motivate us to wonder whether or how the components existing inside and outside the cerebral wall might interact mechanically with NPCs. Internally, the ventricle that the apical surface (i.e., endfeet of NPCs) directly faces is filled with embryonic cerebrospinal fluid (eCSF). Withdrawal of eCSF via intubation results in failed brain growth (Desmond and Jacobson 1977; Pexieder and Jelinek 1970) (in chick embryos), while excessive intraluminal pressure induced by β-D-xyloside (Alonso et al. 1998, 1999) or by a gravity-fed drip (Desmond et al. 2005) leads to an enlargement of the brain (in chick and rat embryos) and increases mitotic indices (in chick embryos), suggesting hydraulic pressure provided by eCSF on NPC functions (Garcia et al. 2019).

Externally, the preosteogenic (~E13) mesenchymal and overlying epidermal layers (together referred to as scalp layers) are elastic and contractile, inwardly pushing (at a pressure of approximately 77 ~ 93 Pa) the outwardly growing mouse brains, thereby modulating brain morphogenesis (contributing to bending of the brainstem and centripetal packing of the bilateral cerebral hemispheres) and eCSF homeostasis (Tsujikawa et al. 2022) (Figure 7.5). While tangential tension generated in the scalp by outward brain enlargement facilitates the proliferation of scalp cells (Tsujikawa et al. 2022), the possibility of inverse mechanical influences from the scalp on neurogenesis by NPCs, either directly via constriction or indirectly via pressurization of eCSF, needs to be studied. Whether mechanically interdependent development also applies to between the cerebrum and the meninges (DeSisto et al. 2020; Kume et al. 1998) is also be an important question.

7.5 Discussion and Perspectives

Based on the qualitative understanding of physical situations in the developing neocortex as introduced in this chapter, interdisciplinary scopes, as follow, can be shared for future elucidation of mechanochemical coupling in neurogenesis by NPCs.

7.5.1 Sensing and Actuation

From the viewpoint of mechanics or mechanical engineering, the developing neocortex that should execute a mission of dynamic morphogenesis coupled with extensive cell production can be taken as a system equipped with sophisticated sensors and actuators. Regarding sensing, mechanical forces existing in, across, and on the cerebral wall have been summarized and updated in this chapter. However, it is not yet known how these physical stimuli are received by which types of cells, in which intramural locations, in which molecular devices (e.g., cytoskeletons and cell-surface mechanoreceptors) (Canales Coutiño and Major 2021; Inman and Smutny 2021), or how such stimulus reception might further be intracellularly transduced for downstream events (Hannezo and Heisenberg 2019). Since the involvement of stretch-mediated Ca^{2+} influx has been shown to participate in the growth and differentiation of multiple epithelial/stem cell systems (Gudipaty et al. 2017; He et al. 2018; Pathak et al. 2014), it would be interesting to discover whether Ca^{2+} waves in the neocortical VZ, which are suggested to involve $P2Y_1$ ATP receptors and FGF and Notch signaling and influence proliferation/neurogenesis (Rash et al. 2016; Weissman et al. 2004), can also be triggered mechanically.

Regarding actuation, this chapter suggests the following three types of morphogenetic actuators in the developing cerebral wall. First, as a conventional type, cellular movements exhibited actively in an energy-consuming manner, represented by mitosis, IKNM, and neuronal migration, can be recognized. Contractility of the apical surface is also categorized into this type. Second, cell-number increase (tissue volume increase) is another important actuation underlying tissue-level morphogenesis. Third, passive mechanisms (such as by using elasticity) occurring based on physical environments, including the former two actuators and the specific cellular and tissue morphologies or geometries (such as fiber or surface), are another important, although relatively unexplored, actuator for corticogenesis. Given the benefit of passive actuation for minimizing energy expenditure (Cavagna et al. 1977; Roberts 2016; Tucker 1970), it would be interesting to study the relationships between the metabolic strategies taken by NPCs (Namba et al. 2021) and the composition and the choice of actuation modes during development and evolution.

The apical surface, where the apicobasally spanning NPCs are assembled tangentially at their apical endfeet, is unique as a key actuator, not only generating tangential tension but also contributing to mechanical events along the orthogonal axis (i.e., wall thickening, RF tension) (Figure 7.4). Given this mechanical crosstalk at the apical surface and that NPCs seem to sense overcrowding there (Figure 7.2), it can be speculated that the apical surface (or nearby) would be an important place for a cerebral wall to install sensor devices, which could assist the apical surface in acting as a mechanical organizer. If mechanosensors truly exist there, they could be useful for the wall to monitor mechanical fluctuations occurring circumferentially and radially (i.e., sensitive to a wide variety of stimuli from those internally along the wall to others across the wall), which would be beneficial in making appropriate feedback-based actuations.

A related question would be whether NPCs mutually adjust their IKNM behaviors based on mechanical stimuli (e.g., pushing or sheer stress) from the neighbors; in Drosophila wing disc epithelia it is suggested that crowding slows down IKNM (Hecht et al. 2022). If this was the case, asking whether the possible mechanically induced acceleration or deceleration of the nucleus in each NPC involves fine-tuning of cell cycle progression in the VZ would also be fruitful.

7.5.2 Prestress and Self-tightening

In architecture or building science, an understanding of 3D structures, such as bridges, towers, and domes, for design and construction is based on the assessment of forces as well as mechanical properties related to materials. Previous studies targeting brain formation that focused on cell assembly or stratification, traditionally, did not sufficiently dissect forces and inter-material (cell–cell) mechanical relationships in such a way. This chapter has depicted a new overview on the intramural (tissue-level) “prestresses” (though still qualitative) in the mid-embryonic mouse cerebral wall. Prestress has originally been used to describe the tension along the intracellular filamentous cytoskeletal structures as a basis for the concept of “tensegrity” (tensional integrity) (Ingber 1993; Stamenović et al. 1996; Wang et al. 1993, 2002) and has also recently been discussed at the tissue level (Ingber et al. 2014; van Kelle et al. 2019). Usually, a “compression element” makes a nearby structure possess a prestress (to be a “tension element”), and these two different elements are mechanically counterbalanced. As shown here, after surgical treatments irreversible tissue displacements have revealed hidden prestresses along the apical surface, the circumferential axons, and the NPCs/RFs, which had individually been balanced with compressive packing of cells, raising the question of whether the developing cerebral hemispheric wall has tensegrity architecture.

Interestingly, mechanical similarities are seen between the wall of the embryonic cerebral hemisphere and the walls of wooden casks and hollow trees, regarding how tensile and compressive structures/elements are situated circumferentially along the dome-like wall. In a cask, longitudinal wooden staves (to be circumferentially compressed) are held by steel hoops (to be under tension) from the outside and/or inside using radial bolts across the staves, which is similar to a strategy for ensuring mechanical stability to what is observed in the tree trunk hollowed by central decay (Mattheck et al. 2015). The cerebral wall is packed with compressed neurons and circumferentially “hooped” by the contractile apical surface inside and the stretched axons outside, with orthogonally supportive RFs (Nakagawa et al. 2019), giving an impression of a similar action of self-tightening for mechanical stability.

7.5.3 Measurement and Simulation

Intratissue stresses generated by pushing or pulling between cells do not usually immediately dissipate because cells are crowded under physiological conditions. Instead, these stresses may be stored transiently or cumulatively. Such stresses may play important roles in vivo (Hannezo and Heisenberg 2019; Wang 2021). Development/morphogenesis of the neocortex would be described better if histories of forces/stresses were added to those of cells and molecules. Although surgical tests have been useful in revealing tension/prestresses and compressions, measurements based on observation on oil droplets introduced into tissues (Campàs et al. 2014; Mongera et al. 2018) or on Brillouin microscopy (Elsayad et al. 2019) will enable less-invasive mechanical assessment in situ. Combining other available methodologies to measure the stiffness of cells and tissues (by AFM) (Franze 2011) and to apply pulling or pushing forces to cells and tissues (by aspirators or chambers for stretching and compressing) (Campàs 2016; Franze 2013) would facilitate functional analysis.

Simulations performed physically (Miyata and Ogawa 2007; Saito et al. 2019; Shinoda et al. 2018) have been helpful in identifying the roles of elasticity related to NPCs. Mathematically, particle-based models (Kosodo et al. 2011; Shinoda et al. 2018) have been used to reproduce IKNM and a virtual VZ. The finite-element method (Filas et al. 2012; Garcia et al. 2017, 2019; Karzbrun et al. 2018) and the vertex model (Eiraku et al. 2011; Okamoto et al. 2013) are useful for inferring which mechanical force would result in which morphogenetic outcome during brain development. Awareness of the mechanical phenomena involving the neocortical NPCs, as summarized in this chapter, and the concomitant quantitative measurement of forces in, along, or across the developing cerebral wall, in combination with appropriate simulations, will facilitate the understanding of physiological and pathological mechanical events and their coupling with chemical and genetic regulation during neocortical formation.

Acknowledgment

The author would like to thank MEXT Grant-in-Aid for Scientific Research on Innovative Areas "Cross-talk between moving cells and microenvironment as a basis of emerging order" (22111006) for its support and also JSPS Grant-in-Aid for Scientific Research (16H02457, 19K22683, 21H00363, and 21H02656). The author thanks Dr Masaharu Ogawa for inspiring developmental neuroscience and Drs Masatsugu Toyota, Shinichiro Sawa, Ken'ichi Kawaguchi, and Taku Demura for interdisciplinary discussions. The author also thanks previous and current T.M. team members for providing images, statistical or technical assistance, and helpful discussions.

References

Alonso, M.I. et al. (1998). Disruption of proteoglycans in neural tube fluid by β-D-xyloside alters brain enlargement in chick embryos. *Anat Rec* 252 (4): 499–508. doi: 10.1002/(SICI)1097-0185(199812)252:4<499:AID-AR1>3.0.CO;2-1.

Alonso, M.I. et al. (1999). Involvement of sulfated proteoglycans in embryonic brain expansion at earliest stages of development in rat embryos. *Cells, Tissues, Organs* 165 (1): 1–9. doi: 10.1159/000016667.

Benito-Kwiecinski, S. et al. (2021). An early cell shape transition drives evolutionary expansion of the human forebrain. *Cell* 184 (8): 2084–2102.e19. doi: 10.1016/j.cell.2021.02.050.

Campàs, O. (2016). A toolbox to explore the mechanics of living embryonic tissues. *Semin Cell Dev Biol* 55: 119–130. doi: 10.1016/j.semcdb.2016.03.011.

Campàs, O. et al. (2014). Quantifying cell-generated mechanical forces within living embryonic tissues. *Nat Methods* 11 (2): 183–189. doi: 10.1038/nmeth.2761.

Canales Coutiño, B. and Major, R. (2021). Mechanosensitive ion channels in cell migration. *Cells Dev* 166: 203683. doi: 10.1016/j.cdev.2021.203683.

Cappello, S. et al. (2006). The rho-GTPase cdc42 regulates neural progenitor fate at the apical surface. *Nat Neurosci* 9 (9): 1099–1107. doi: 10.1038/nn1744.

Cappello, S. et al. (2013). Mutations in genes encoding the cadherin receptor-ligand pair DCHS1 and FAT4 disrupt cerebral cortical development. *Nat Genet* 45 (11): 1300–1308. doi: 10.1038/ng.2765.

Cavagna, G.A. et al. (1977). Mechanical work in terrestrial locomotion: two basic mechanisms for minimizing energy expenditure. *Am J Physiol-Regul, Integr Comp Physiol* 233 (5): R243–R261. doi: 10.1152/ajpregu.1977.233.5.R243.

Chenn, A. and McConnell, S.K. (1995). Cleavage orientation and the asymmetric inheritance of Notch1 immunoreactivity in mammalian neurogenesis. *Cell* 82 (4): 631–641. doi: 10.1016/0092-8674(95)90035-7.

Chenn, A. and Walsh, C.A. (2002). Regulation of cerebral cortical size by control of cell cycle exit in neural precursors. *Science* 297 (5580): 365–369. doi: 10.1126/science.1074192.

Davis, A.A. and Temple, S. (1994). A self-renewing multipotential stem cell in embryonic rat cerebral cortex. *Nature* 372 (6503): 263–266. doi: 10.1038/372263a0.

DeSisto, J. et al. (2020). Single-cell transcriptomic analyses of the developing meninges reveal meningeal fibroblast diversity and function. *Dev Cell* 54 (1): 43–59.e4. doi: 10.1016/j.devcel.2020.06.009.

Desmond, M.E. and Jacobson, A.G. (1977). Embryonic brain enlargement requires cerebrospinal fluid pressure. *Dev Biol* 57 (1): 188–198. doi: 10.1016/0012-1606(77)90364-5.

Desmond, M.E. et al. (2005). Internal luminal pressure during early chick embryonic brain growth. *Anat Rec. Part A, Disc Mol, Cell, Evol Biol* 285 (2): 737–747. doi: 10.1002/ar.a.20211.

Eiraku, M. et al. (2011). Self-organizing optic-cup morphogenesis in three-dimensional culture. *Nature* 472 (7341): 51–56. doi: 10.1038/nature09941.

Elsayad, K. et al. (2019). Probing mechanical properties in biology using Brillouin microscopy. *Trends Cell Biol* 29 (8): 608–611. doi: 10.1016/j.tcb.2019.04.002.

Falconieri, A. et al. (2022). Magnetically-actuated microposts stimulate axon growth. *Biophys J* 121 (3): 374–382. doi: 10.1016/j.bpj.2021.12.041.

Fan, A. et al. (2017). Coupled circumferential and axial tension driven by actin and myosin influences in vivo axon diameter. *Sci Rep* 7 (1): 14188. doi: 10.1038/s41598-017-13830-1.

Filas, B.A. et al. (2012). Regional differences in actomyosin contraction shape the primary vesicles in the embryonic chicken brain. *Phys Biol* 9 (6): 066007. doi: 10.1088/1478-3975/9/6/066007. 16.PMID: 23160445.

Franze, K. (2011). Atomic force microscopy and its contribution to understanding the development of the nervous system. *Curr Opin Genet Dev* 21: 530–537. doi: 10.1016/j.gde.2011.07.001.

Franze, K. (2013). The mechanical control of nervous system development. *Development* 140: 3069–3077. doi: 10.1242/dev.079145.

Gadisseux, J.F. et al. (1989). Dynamic structure of the radial glial fiber system of the developing murine cerebral wall. an immunocytochemical analysis. *Brain Res Dev Brain Res* 50 (1): 55–67. doi: 10.1016/0165-3806(89)90126-0.

Garcia, K.E. et al. (2017). Contraction and stress-dependent growth shape the forebrain of the early chicken embryo. *J Mech Behav Biomed Mater* 65: 383–397. doi: 10.1016/j.jmbbm.2016.08.010.

Garcia, K.E. et al. (2019). Molecular and mechanical signals determine morphogenesis of the cerebral hemispheres in the chicken embryo. *Development* 146 (20): dev174318. doi: 10.1242/dev.174318.

Gudipaty, S.A. et al. (2017). Mechanical stretch triggers rapid epithelial cell division through Piezo1. *Nature* 543 (7643): 118–121. doi: 10.1038/nature21407.

Hannezo, E. and Heisenberg, C.P. (2019). Mechanochemical feedback loops in development and disease. *Cell* 178 (1): 12–25. doi: 10.1016/j.cell.2019.05.052.

He, L. et al. (2018). Mechanical regulation of stem-cell differentiation by the stretch-activated Piezo channel. *Nature* 555 (7694): 103–106. doi: 10.1038/nature25744.

Hecht, S. et al. (2022). Mechanical constraints to cell-cycle progression in a pseudostratified epithelium. *Curr Biol* 22: S0960-9822(22)00395-5. doi: 10.1016/j.cub.2022.03.004.

Hu, D.J.-K. et al. (2013). Dynein recruitment to nuclear pores activates apical nuclear migration and mitotic entry in brain progenitor cells. *Cell* 154 (6): 1300–1313. doi: 10.1016/j.cell.2013.08.024.

Ingber, D.E. (1993). Cellular tensegrity: defining new rules of biological design that govern the cytoskeleton. *J Cell Sci* 104 (Pt 3): 613–627. doi: 10.1242/jcs.104.3.613.

Ingber, D.E. et al. (2014). Tensegrity, cellular biophysics, and the mechanics of living systems. *Rep Prog Phys* 77 (4): 046603. doi: 10.1088/0034-4885/77/4/046603.

Inman, A. and Smutny, M. (2021). Feeling the force. *Sem Cell Dev Biol* 120: 53–65. doi: 10.1016/j.semcdb.2021.06.006.

Iwashita, M. et al. (2014). Systematic profiling of spatiotemporal tissue and cellular stiffness in the developing brain. *Development* 141 (19): 3793–3798. doi: 10.1242/dev.109637.

Kadowaki, M. et al. (2007). N-cadherin mediates cortical organization in the mouse brain. *Dev Biol* 304 (1): 22–33. doi: 10.1016/j.ydbio.2006.12.014.

Karzbrun, E. et al. (2018). Human brain organoids on a chip reveal the physics of folding. *Nat Phys* 4 (5): 515–522. doi: 10.1038/s41567-018-0046-7.

Kirkland, N.J. et al. (2020). Tissue mechanics regulate mitotic nuclear dynamics during epithelial development. *Curr Biol* 30 (13): 2419–2432.e4. doi: 10.1016/j.cub.2020.04.041.

Kosodo, Y. (2012). Interkinetic nuclear migration: beyond a hallmark of neurogenesis. *Cell Mol Life Sci* 69 (16): 2727–2738. doi: 10.1007/s00018-012-0952-2.

Kosodo, Y. et al. (2011). Regulation of interkinetic nuclear migration by cell cycle-coupled active and passive mechanisms in the developing brain. *EMBO J* 30 (9): 1690–1704. doi: 10.1038/emboj.2011.81.

Kume, T. et al. (1998). The forkhead/winged helix gene Mf1 is disrupted in the pleiotropic mouse mutation congenital hydrocephalus. *Cell* 93 (6): 985–996. doi: 10.1016/s0092-8674(00)81204-0.

Lavado, A. et al. (2018). The Hippo pathway prevents YAP/TAZ-driven hypertranscription and controls neural progenitor number. *Dev Cell* 47 (5): 576–591.e8. doi: 10.1016/j.devcel.2018.09.021.

Lee, H.O. and Norden, C. (2013). Mechanisms controlling arrangements and movements of nuclei in pseudostratified epithelia. *Trends Cell Biol* 23 (3): 141–150. doi: 10.1016/j.tcb.2012.11.001.

Liu, W.A. et al. (2018). PARD3 dysfunction in conjunction with dynamic HIPPO signaling drives cortical enlargement with massive heterotopia. *Genes Dev* 32 (11–12): 763–780. doi: 10.1101/gad.313171.118.

Llinares-Benadero, C. and Borrell, V. (2019). Deconstructing cortical folding: genetic, cellular and mechanical determinants. *Nat Rev Neurosci* 20 (3): 161–176. doi: 10.1038/s41583-018-0112-2.

Long, K.R. et al. (2018). Extracellular matrix components HAPLN1, lumican, and collagen I cause hyaluronic acid-dependent folding of the developing human neocortex. *Neuron* 99 (4): 702–719.e6. doi: 10.1016/j.neuron.2018.07.013.

Loulier, K. et al. (2009). Beta1 integrin maintains integrity of the embryonic neocortical stem cell niche. *PLoS Biol* 7 (8): e1000176. doi: 10.1371/journal.pbio.1000176.

Malatesta, P. et al. (2000). Isolation of radial glial cells by fluorescent-activated cell sorting reveals a neuronal lineage. *Development* 127 (24): 5253–5263. doi: 10.1242/dev.127.24.5253.

Mattheck, C. et al. (2015). *The Body Language of Trees. Encyclopedia of Visual Tree Assessment.* Karlsruhe, Germany: Karlsruhe Institute for Technology.

Miyata, T. (2008). Development of three-dimensional architecture of the neuroepithelium. *Dev, Growth Differ* 50 (Suppl 1): S105–S112. doi: 10.1111/j.1440-169X.2007.00980.x.

Miyata, T. et al. (2001). Asymmetric inheritance of radial glial fibers by cortical neurons. *Neuron* 31 (5): 727–741. doi: 10.1016/s0896-6273(01)00420-2.

Miyata, T. and Ogawa, M. (2007). Twisting of neocortical progenitor cells underlies a spring-like mechanism for daughter-cell migration. *Curr Biol* 17 (2): 146–151. doi: 10.1016/j.cub.2006.11.023.

Miyata, T. et al. (2015). Interkinetic nuclear migration generates and opposes ventricular-zone crowding: insight into tissue mechanics. *Front Cell Neurosci* 8: 473. doi: 10.3389/fncel.2014.00473.

Mongera, A. et al. (2018). A fluid-to-solid jamming transition underlies vertebrate body axis elongation. *Nature* 561 (7723): 401–405. doi: 10.1038/s41586-018-0479-2.

Nagasaka, A. and Miyata, T. (2021). Comparison of the mechanical properties between the convex and concave inner/apical surfaces of the developing cerebrum. *Front Cell Dev Biol* 9: 702068. doi: 10.3389/fcell.2021.702068.

Nagasaka, A. et al. (2016). Differences in the mechanical properties of the developing cerebral cortical proliferative zone between mice and ferrets at both the tissue and single-cell levels. *Front Cell Dev Biol* 4: 139. doi: 10.3389/fcell.2016.00139.

Nakagawa, N. et al. (2019). Memo1-mediated tiling of radial glial cells facilitates cerebral cortical development. *Neuron* 103 (5): 836–852.e5. doi: 10.1016/j.neuron.2019.05.049.

Namba, T. et al. (2021). Metabolic regulation of neocortical expansion in development and evolution. *Neuron* 109: 408–419. doi: 10.1016/j.neuron.2020.11.014.

Noctor, S.C. et al. (2001). Neurons derived from radial glial cells establish radial units in neocortex. *Nature* 409 (6821): 714–720. doi: 10.1038/35055553.

Norden, C. et al. (2009). Actomyosin is the main driver of interkinetic nuclear migration in the retina. *Cell* 138 (6): 1195–1208. doi: 10.1016/j.cell.2009.06.032.

Nowakowski, T.J. et al. (2016). Transformation of the radial glia scaffold demarcates two stages of human cerebral cortex development. *Neuron* 91 (6): 1219–1227. doi: 10.1016/j.neuron.2016.09.005.

Okamoto, M. et al. (2013). TAG-1–assisted progenitor elongation streamlines nuclear migration to optimize subapical crowding. *Nat Neurosci* 16 (11): 1556–1566. doi: 10.1038/nn.3525.

Okamoto, M. et al. (2014). Ferret–mouse differences in interkinetic nuclear migration and cellular densification in the neocortical ventricular zone. *J Neurosci Res* 86: 88–95. doi: 10.1016/j.neures.2014.10.006.

Pathak, M.M. et al. (2014). Stretch-activated ion channel Piezo1 directs lineage choice in human neural stem cells. *Proc Natl Acad Sci USA* 111 (45): 16148–16153. doi: 10.1073/pnas.1409802111.

Pexieder, T. and Jelinek, R. (1970). Pressure of the CSF and the morphogenesis of CNS. II. Pressure necessary for normal development of brain vesicle. *Folia Morphol (Praha)* 18 (2): 181–192.

Pfister, B.J. et al. (2004). Extreme stretch growth of integrated axons. *J Neurosci* 24 (36): 7978–7983. doi: 10.1523/JNEUROSCI.1974-04.2004.

Pilaz, L.-J. et al. (2016). Dynamic mRNA transport and local translation in radial glial progenitors of the developing brain. *Curr Biol* 26 (24): 3383–3392. doi: 10.1016/j.cub.2016.10.040.

Rakic, P. (1972). Mode of cell migration to the superficial layers of fetal monkey cortex. *J Comp Neurol* 145 (1): 61–83. doi: 10.1002/cne.901450105.

Rash, B.G. et al. (2016). Biderectional radial Ca^{2+} activity regulates neurogenesis and migration during early cortical column formation. *Sci Adv* 2 (2): e1501733. doi: 10.1126/sciadv.1501733.

Reiner, O., Sapir, T., and Gerlitz, G. (2012). Interkinetic nuclear movement in the ventricular zone of the cortex. *J Mol Neurosci* 46 (3): 516–526. doi: 10.1007/s12031-011-9633-0.

Roberts, T.J. (2016). Contribution of elastic tissues to the mechanics and energetics of muscle function during movement. *J Exp Biol* 219 (Pt 2): 266–275. doi: 10.1242/jeb.124446.

Saito, K. et al. (2018). Neural progenitor cells undergoing Yap/Tead-mediated enhanced self-renewal form heterotopias more easily in the diencephalon than in the telencephalon. *Neurochem Int* 43 (1): 180–189. doi: 10.1007/s11064-017-2390-x.

Saito, K. et al. (2019). Dorsal-to-ventral cortical expansion is physically primed by ventral streaming of early embryonic preplate neurons. *Cell Rep* 29 (6): 1555–1567. doi: 10.1016/j.celrep.2019.09.075.

Sauer, F.C. (1935). Mitosis in the neural tube. *J Comp Neurol* 62: 377–405.

Schaper, A. (1897). The earliest differentiation in the central nervous system of vertebrates. *Science* 5: 430–431.

Schenk, J. et al. (2009). Myosin II is required for interkinetic nuclear migration of neural progenitors. *Proc Natl Acad Sci USA* 106 (38): 16487–16492. doi: 10.1073/pnas.0908928106.

Shinoda, T. et al. (2018). Elasticity-based boosting of neuroepithelial nucleokinesis via indirect energy transfer from mother to daughter. *PLOS Biol* 16 (4): e2004426. doi: 10.1371/journal.pbio.2004426.

Smart, I.H.M. (1965). The operation of ependymal "choke" in neurogenesis. *J Anat* 99: 941–943.

Smart, I.H.M. (1973). Proliferative characteristics of the ependymal layer during the early development of the mouse neocortex. *J Anat* 116 (pt 1): 67–91. PMID: 4777782. PMCID: PMC1271551.

Spear, P. and Erickson, C. (2012a). Interkinetic nuclear migration: a mysterious process in search of a function. *Dev, Growth Differ* 54 (3): 306–316. doi: 10.1111/j.1440-169X.2012.01342.x.

Spear, P.C. and Erickson, C.A. (2012b). Apical movement during nuclear migration is a two-step process. *Dev Biol* 370 (1): 33–41. doi: 10.1016/j.ydbio.2012.06.031.

Stamenović, D. et al. (1996). A microstructural approach to cytoskeletal mechanics based on tensegrity. *J Theor Biol* 181 (2): 125–136. doi: 10.1006/jtbi.1996.0120.

Takahashi, T. et al. (1993). Cell cycle parameters and patterns of nuclear movement in the neocortical proliferative zone of the fetal mouse. *J Neurosci* 13 (2): 820–833. doi: 10.1523/JNEUROSCI.13-02-00820.1993.

Taverna, E. et al. (2014). The cell biology of neurogenesis. *Ann Rev Cell Dev Biol* 30: 465–502. doi: 10.1146/annurev-cellbio-101011-155801.

Taverna, E. and Huttner, W.B. (2010). Neural progenitor nuclei in motion. *Neuron* 67 (6): 906–914. doi: 10.1016/j.neuron.2010.08.027.

Tsai, J.-W. et al. (2005). LIS1 RNA interference blocks neural stem cell division, morphogenesis, and motility at multiple stages. *J Cell Biol* 170 (6): 935–945. doi: 10.1083/jcb.200505166.

Tsai, J.W. et al. (2010). Kinesin 3 and cytoplasmic dynein mediate interkinetic nuclear migration in neural stem cells. *Nat Neurosci* 13 (12): 1463–1471. doi: 10.1038/nn.2665.

Tsujikawa, K. et al. (2022). Developmentally interdependent stretcher–compressor relationship between the embryonic brain and the surrounding scalp in the preosteogenic head. *Dev Dyn* 251 (7): 1107–1122. doi: 10.1002/dvdy.451.

Tsunekawa, Y. et al. (2012). Cyclin D2 in the basal process of neural progenitors is linked to non-equivalent cell fates. *EMBO J* 31 (8): 1879–1892. doi: 10.1038/emboj.2012.43.

Tucker, V.A. (1970). Energetic cost of locomotion in animals. *Comp Biochem Physiol* 34 (4): 841–846. doi: 10.1016/0010-406x(70)91006-6.

van Kelle, M.A.J. et al. (2019). Increased cell traction-induced prestress in dynamically cultured microtissues. *Front Bioeng Biotechnol* 7: 41. doi: 10.3389/fbioe.2019.00041.

Wang, N. et al. (1993). Mechanotransduction across the cell surface and through the cytoskeleton. *Science* 260 (5111): 1124–1127. doi: 10.1126/science.7684161.

Wang, N. et al. (2002). Cell prestress. I. stiffness and prestress are closely associated in adherent contractile cells. *Am J Physiol-Cell Physiol* 282 (3): C606–C616. doi: 10.1152/ajpcell.00269.2001.

Wang, Y.-C. (2021). The origin and the mechanism of mechanical polarity during epithelial folding. *Semin Cell Dev Biol* 120: 94–107. doi: 10.1016/j.semcdb.2021.05.027.

Watanabe, Y. et al. (2018). Differentiating cells mechanically limit the interkinetic nuclear migration of progenitor cells to secure apical cytogenesis. *Development* 145 (14): dev162883. doi: 10.1242/dev.162883.

Weissman, T.A. et al. (2004). Calcium waves propagate through radial glial cells and modulate proliferation in the developing neocortex. *Neuron* 43 (5): 647–661. doi: 10.1016/j.neuron.2004.08.015.

8

The Role of Human-specific Genes and Amino Acid Substitutions for Neocortex Expansion and Modern Human vs. Neanderthal Differences in Neocortical Neurogenesis

Lei Xing, Anneline Pinson*, Felipe Mora-Bermúdez*, and Wieland B. Huttner*

Max Planck Institute of Molecular Cell Biology and Genetics, Dresden, Germany
** Joint first authors*

8.1 Introduction

The neocortex is the largest and evolutionarily the youngest part of the cerebral cortex. As a hallmark of mammalian brain evolution, the expansion of the neocortex during the development of humans as compared to that of other primates is considered to be the structural basis of the enhanced cognitive abilities of humans. The primary cause of the expansion of the neocortex in human is the increased production of neurons, especially of the late-born upper-layer neurons, which are generated by cortical neural stem and progenitor cells (cNSPCs) during cortical development (Rakic 2009).

This increased production of cortical neurons can be achieved in principle in two ways. First, by an increase in the length of the neurogenic period, that is, the period during which cortical neurons are generated from cNSPCs. Evidence in support of this has come from both mathematical modeling (Lewitus et al. 2014) and experimental (Stepien et al. 2020) studies. Second, by an increase in the pool size of the relevant class of cNSPCs and in their proliferative capacity (Dehay et al. 2015; Fernandez et al. 2016; Florio and Huttner 2014; Lui et al. 2011; Miller et al. 2019; Rakic 2009). Here, we will focus on this latter way of increasing the production of cortical neurons.

After describing the key features of the principal two classes of cNSPCs and the various cNSPC types therein, we will focus on two themes. First, we will summarize the role of human-specific genes, notably *ARHGAP11B*, in the evolutionary expansion of the human neocortex. Second, we will discuss recent evidence demonstrating that human-specific amino acid substitutions in proteins with crucial roles in cNSPC function imply key differences in cortical neurogenesis between modern humans and Neanderthals.

8.2 Cortical Neural Stem and Progenitor Cells

cNSPCs reside in the developing neocortical wall, which exhibits apical-basal polarity, with the apical side facing the cerebral ventricles and the basal side corresponding to the pial surface (Götz and Huttner 2005; Huttner and Brand 1997). Based on the location of mitosis, cNSPCs can be categorized into two different principal classes: apical progenitors (APs) and basal progenitors (BPs) (Götz and Huttner 2005; Taverna et al. 2014).

Neocortical Neurogenesis in Development and Evolution, First Edition. Edited by Wieland B. Huttner.

8.2.1 Apical Progenitors

APs can be classified into three main types, neuroepithelial cells (NECs), apical (or ventricular) radial glia (aRG) and apical intermediate progenitors (aIPs). At the early stage of cortical development, before the onset of neurogenesis, NECs in the neural tube function as the primary cNSPCs and undergo symmetric proliferative divisions to self-amplify and expand their pool size (Fish et al. 2006; Noctor et al. 2007). At the onset of neurogenesis, NECs transform into aRG, which switch to asymmetric self-renewing differentiative divisions, with most of them generating BPs (indirect neurogenesis) rather than neurons (direct neurogenesis). Like NECs, aRG reside in the ventricular zone (VZ) of the developing neocortex and undergo mitosis at the surface of the cerebral ventricles (Huttner and Kosodo 2005; Kosodo et al. 2004). Similar to NECs, aRG exhibit apical and basal polarity and have contact with both the apical (ventricular) surface and the pial surface, via their apical and basal processes, respectively (Götz and Huttner 2005; Hartfuss et al. 2001; Kriegstein and Götz 2003). aIPs, previously known as short neural precursors, maintain the contact with the ventricular surface, like aRG, but lose their basal process-mediated contact with the pial surface, in contrast to aRG (Gal et al. 2006; Tyler and Haydar 2013).

Despite their variety, these three types of APs share some common features. (i) The apical endfoot of all APs is integrated into the apical junction belt and provides apical plasma membrane, which has direct contact with the cerebrospinal fluid (CSF) in the cerebral ventricles. This allows APs to receive pro-proliferative signals from the CSF, notably through their primary cilium (Lehtinen and Walsh 2011; Lehtinen et al. 2011; Paridaen et al. 2015). (ii) When APs progress through the cell cycle, they exhibit a characteristic movement of their nuclei called interkinetic nuclear migration (INM) (Lee and Norden 2013; Taverna et al. 2014). After mitosis at the ventricular surface, the nuclei of APs move basally during the G1 phase of the cell cycle to the basal side of the VZ, where they undergo S phase (Sauer 1935; Sauer and Walker 1959; Taverna and Huttner 2010). This is followed by the migration of the nuclei apically during the G2 phase of the cell cycle for the next round of mitosis at the ventricular surface. INM allows APs to cleverly utilize the limited space of ventricular surface for mitosis, as the nuclei of interphase APs move away to increase the space for apical mitoses, and hence allows for an increase in the number of AP mitoses per unit time. This in turn allows for an increased generation of APs and their progeny.

8.2.2 Basal Progenitors – Advantages for Neocortex Expansion

BPs can be classified into two main types, basal (or outer) radial glia (bRG) and basal intermediate progenitors (bIPs) (Götz and Huttner 2005; Kriegstein and Götz 2003). bRG exhibit basal polarity and characteristically exhibit a basal process that may reach the pial surface. bRG may in addition exhibit an apically directed process, which however does not reach the ventricular surface (Fietz et al. 2010; Hansen et al. 2010; Reillo et al. 2011). bIPs lack apical-basal cell polarity and typically exhibit multiple short processes (Haubensak et al. 2004; Miyata et al. 2004; Noctor et al. 2004). Both types of BPs have delaminated from the apical surface and have translocated their cell bodies to a basal location for mitosis, typically in the subventricular zone (SVZ).

During mammalian evolution, BPs play a pivotal role in contributing to neocortex expansion due to the following advantages they have over APs.

i) The emergence of BPs provided a different yet more efficient pathway for neuron generation, referred to as indirect neurogenesis. The opposite to indirect neurogenesis, referred to as direct neurogenesis, is typically seen in the developing spinal cord, when a NEC undergoes asymmetric cell division to give rise to a NEC and a neuron, which results in one neuron per NEC mitosis (Kosodo et al. 2008; Rousso et al. 2012). Such direct neurogenesis, either from a NEC or an aRG, occurs rarely in the developing neocortex (Fietz et al. 2010; Hansen et al. 2010; Haubensak et al. 2004; Kriegstein et al. 2006; Miyata et al. 2004; Noctor et al. 2004; Reillo et al. 2011). To generate the large numbers of neurons that populate the neocortex, especially the expanded neocortex in human, direct neurogenesis is not sufficient. This limitation is overcome by indirect neurogenesis, when an aRG undergoes asymmetric cell division to give rise to one aRG and one BP. The latter can self-amplify and thereafter, or without self-amplification, divide to give rise to one or two neurons per each BP mitosis (Florio and Huttner 2014). This way of indirect neurogenesis can significantly increase the number of neurons derived from one AP mitosis, and typically takes place in the developing primate neocortex, including human (Florio and Huttner 2014; Lui et al. 2011).

ii) By being able to undergo mitosis basally, BPs can massively increase the number of mitoses, in contrast to APs whose mitosis is limited to the apical domain at the ventricular surface of the VZ. Although in some species such as mouse, the cell cycle of BPs can be longer than that of APs, the use of the entire thickness of the SVZ for basal mitoses allows much more BP mitoses to occur simultaneously, which generates a large number of neurons in a more time-efficient way (Arai et al. 2011; Dehay et al. 2015; Smart et al. 2002). Thus, more neurons can be generated from BPs than from APs.

iii) Residing in the SVZ and lacking contact with the ventricles, BPs are away from, and no longer directly exposed to, potential pro-proliferation signals in the CSF. However, this localization allows the mitotic BPs to have better access to pro-proliferation signals in the fetal blood stream, as the SVZ is highly vascularized with the so-called honeycomb vessels, whereas the VZ (Komabayashi-Suzuki et al. 2019), especially the region close to the apical surface, is considered avascular. Many growth factors (Lui et al. 2014; Matsumoto et al. 2017), neurotransmitters (Xing and Huttner 2020; Xing et al. 2020), and morphogens (Ferent et al. 2020) derived from the fetal blood stream as well as locally produced extracellular matrix (Fietz et al. 2012; Stenzel et al. 2014) have been identified to be specific in stimulating the proliferation of BPs but not APs.

In addition to these three major advantages that BPs have, the abundance and proliferative capacity of BPs are considered to be key factors underlying the evolutionary expansion of the human neocortex (Borrell 2019; Kalebic and Huttner 2020; Sauerland et al. 2018; Xing et al. 2021b). In species with a small and lissencephalic neocortex, such as the mouse, BPs, both bRG (accounting for less than 10% of the total BPs) and bIPs (accounting for over 90% of the total BPs), are in lower abundance and possess lower proliferative capacities (Shitamukai et al. 2011; Wang et al. 2011) than in species with a large and gyrencephalic neocortex, such as human. BPs in the former species tend to undergo consumptive division to give rise to two neurons. In contrast, human BPs (which comprise about half bRG and half bIPs) exist not only in higher abundance compared to mouse, but possess higher proliferative capacities to undergo proliferative division and give rise to more progenitors (Fietz et al. 2010; Hansen et al. 2010). This in turn contributes to the thickening of the human SVZ, which is split into two distinct zones, a thinner inner SVZ (iSVZ) and a thicker outer SVZ (oSVZ), to host the increased abundance of BPs in the developing neocortex (Dehay et al. 2015; Smart et al. 2002). Thus, intrinsic and extrinsic factors that promote and maintain the proliferative capacities of BPs are key regulators for the evolutionary expansion of the human neocortex.

8.3 Human-specific Genes Preferentially Expressed in cNSPCs – ARHGAP11B

During human evolution, the emergence of human-specific genes may have contributed to the higher proliferative capacities of human BPs, which ultimately led to the drastically increased neocortex size and neuron number. Thus, the human-specific genes that are expressed preferentially in the cNSPCs, especially BPs, are the prime candidates for exerting specific roles in the evolutionary expansion of the human neocortex. Transcriptomic analyses of the fetal human and the embryonic mouse neocortex have revealed a list of human-specific genes that are preferentially expressed in cNSPCs compared to neurons (Fietz et al. 2012; Florio et al. 2015, 2018; Johnson et al. 2015; Miller et al. 2014; Pollen et al. 2015). One human-specific gene, *ARHGAP11B*, has been reported to exert key functions in neocortex development and hence has been implicated in the evolution of the human neocortex (Fischer et al. 2022; Florio et al. 2015; Heide et al. 2020; Kalebic et al. 2018; Namba et al. 2020; Xing et al. 2021a) it will be our focus in this section. Another human-specific gene, *NOTCH2NL*, will be briefly addressed later.

8.3.1 *ARHGAP11B* – Molecular Features and Expression in cNSPCs

ARHGAP11B arose by a partial duplication of the ubiquitous gene *ARHGAP11A* around 5 million years ago, after the human lineage and the chimpanzee lineage had segregated from one another (Antonacci et al. 2014; Dougherty et al. 2018; Meyer et al. 2012; Riley et al. 2002; Sudmant et al. 2010). Subsequent to the partial gene duplication, a single C– > G base substitution in exon 5 of the *ARHGAP11B* gene generated a new GU-purine splice-donor site (Florio et al. 2015, 2016). Upon mRNA splicing, using this new splice donor site results in the loss of 55 nucleotides of exon 5 and in a reading frame shift. Human *ARHGAP11A* encodes a Rho guanosine triphosphatase-activating protein (RhoGAP), located in the cell nucleus, with its GAP domain ranging from amino acid residues 46 to 246 (Kagawa et al. 2013; Namba et al. 2020; Zanin et al. 2013). The reading frame shift caused by the C– > G base substitution in *ARHGAP11B* happens at amino acid residue 221, which leaves ARHGAP11B a truncated GAP domain (residues 46–220), with no RhoGAP activity in vivo, and a human-specific 47 amino acid C-terminal sequence (amino acids 221 to 267) that is crucial for its function (Florio et al. 2015, 2016). Interestingly, the crucial C– > G base substitution is also found in the genome of Neanderthals, whose brains were at least as large as those of modern humans but more elongated along the rostral-caudal axis, and in the genome of Denisovans (Florio et al. 2016). Thus, the C– > G base substitution, which is thought to have happened after the partial gene duplication event (Antonacci et al. 2014; Florio et al. 2016; Riley et al. 2002), most likely occurred before the segregation between the modern human versus the Neanderthal/Denisovan lineages, that is, before ≈ 500,000 years ago.

In fetal human neocortical tissue, ARHGAP11B mRNA and protein are predominantly found in the germinal zones, including VZ, iSVZ, and oSVZ, and accordingly in cNSPCs, including aRG, bRG, and bIPs, but not in the CP and in neurons (Fietz et al. 2012; Florio et al. 2015, 2018; Namba et al. 2020). Taken together, *ARHGAP11B* is a cNSPC-enriched human-specific gene that may exert a novel molecular function in cNSPCs.

8.3.2 *ARHGAP11B* – Basal Progenitor Amplification

To explore the function of *ARHGAP11B* in corticogenesis, *ARHGAP11B* was ectopically over-expressed in the developing mouse and ferret neocortex by in utero electroporation (Florio et al. 2015; Kalebic et al. 2018). *ARHGAP11B* over-expression induced features associated with neocortical expansion, including the increase in the abundance and proliferation of BPs (Florio et al. 2015; Kalebic et al. 2018). Specifically, in the developing neocortex of the mouse, which is a lissencephalic species, *ARHGAP11B* over-expression increased the abundance of mitotic BPs by three-fold and the abundance of total BPs by 50 percent, accompanied by the thickening of the SVZ (Florio et al. 2015) (see Figure 8.1A).

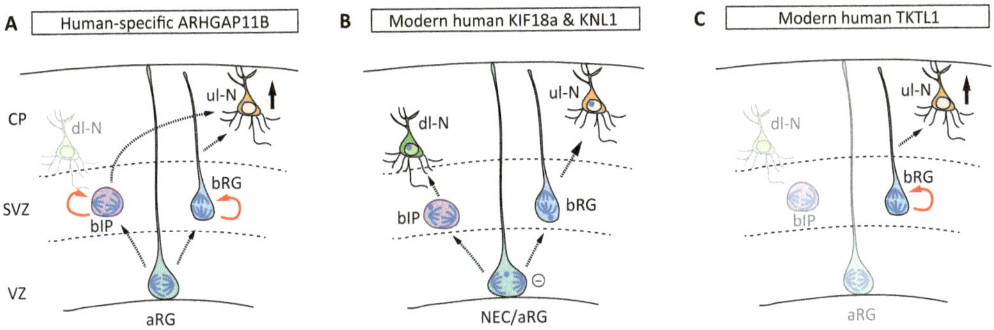

Figure 8.1 Effects of human-specific *ARHGAP11B* (A) and human-specific amino acid substitutions in either KIF18a and KNL1 (B) or TKTL1 (C) on cNSPCs and cortical neurogenesis. Illustration showing the major cNSPC types and cortical neurogenesis in a highly simplified manner: NEC, neuroepithelial cell; aRG, apical radial glia (both turquoise); bIP, basal intermediate progenitor (purple); bRG, basal radial glia (blue); dl-N, deep-layer neuron (green); ul-N, upper-layer neuron (orange). Chromosomes of mitotic NECs, aRG, bIPs, and bRG are shown in dark blue. aRG in the ventricular zone (VZ) give rise to both bIPs and bRG, which migrate to the subventricular zone (SVZ); both bIPs and bRG can generate deep-layer neurons as well as upper-layer neurons, which migrate to the cortical plate (CP). Other cortical zones such as the intermediate zone are not shown for clarity.

(A) The protein encoded by human-specific *ARHGAP11B* increases the generation of bIPs and bRG from aRG (dashed arrows) and promotes the proliferation of bIPs and bRG (red arrows), which eventually results in an increase (solid arrow) in upper-layer neurons (dashed arrows).

(B) The three modern human-specific amino acid substitutions in KIF18a (R- > K) and KNL1 (H- > R, G- > S) reduce (minus sign) the chromosome segregation errors that occur upon NEC/aRG mitosis (dark blue dot, lagging chromosome); these errors, which are less with modern human KIF18a and KNL1 than ancestral KIF18a and KNL1, may be inherited by the entire NEC/aRG progeny (dashed arrows).

(C) The single modern human-specific amino acid substitution in TKTL1 (K- > R) promotes the proliferation specifically of bRG (red arrow), which eventually results in an increase (solid arrow) in upper-layer neurons (dashed arrow).

(A, C) Cell types not affected by *ARHGAP11B* (A) or modern human TKTL1 (C) are shown dimmed.

To further dissect the effects of *ARHGAP11B* in increasing BP abundance, *ARHGAP11B* mRNA was microinjected into the aRG in organotypic slices of the developing mouse neocortex. Analysis on the daughter cell pairs born from targeted aRG revealed that there was an aRG division mode switch upon *ARHGAP11B* expression, from symmetric-proliferative and asymmetric-differentiative to symmetric-differentiative divisions yielding two BPs, thereby increasing the generation of BPs (Florio et al. 2015). Moreover, both the clone size of the aRG progeny upon *ARHGAP11B* mRNA microinjection and the proportion of cycling cells in the SVZ upon *ARHGAP11B* electroporation were increased (Florio et al. 2015). Therefore, *ARHGAP11B* increased BP abundance by promoting the self-amplification of BPs.

In the developing neocortex of the ferret, which is a gyrencephalic species, *ARHGAP11B* overexpression by in utero electroporation increased the number of mitotic bRG by almost four-fold and the abundance of total BPs by almost three-fold, in particular the proliferative bRG type (Kalebic et al. 2018). The effect of *ARHGAP11B* in BP amplification in the developing ferret neocortex is substantially greater and significantly different from the observations in embryonic mouse neocortex. This is due to the difference in the proliferative capacities of BPs between mouse and ferret (Fietz et al. 2010; Hansen et al. 2010). Mouse BPs, even the low-abundance bRG, have been shown to undergo mostly neurogenic cell divisions with limited proliferative capacity (Shitamukai et al. 2011; Wang et al. 2011). In contrast, ferret bRG and some bIPs are known to be highly proliferative and give rise to more BPs (Fietz et al. 2010). The greater increase in bRG in the developing ferret neocortex is thought to result from the promotion of the proliferative division of ferret bRG induced by *ARHGAP11B* over-expression (Kalebic et al. 2018).

It is important to note that in these two studies with mouse and ferret, *ARHGAP11B* expression was induced by using a strong constitutive promoter, which results in unphysiologically high levels of expression (Florio et al. 2015; Kalebic et al. 2018). This raised the question if a physiological level of *ARHGAP11B* would increase BP levels in the developing neocortex. To this end, a stable transgenic mouse line was generated to express *AHRGAP11B* at a physiological level by converting one allele of the mouse *Arhgap11a* gene into a mutant *ARHGAP11B* gene using the CRISPR/Cas9 genome editing technology (Xing et al. 2021a). The physiological expression of *ARHGAP11B*, which was driven by the endogenous mouse *Arhgap11a* promoter, increased mitotic BPs by 50 percent, including both mitotic bRG and mitotic bIPs, and total abundance of BPs by 40 percent in the *ARHGAP11B*-transgenic mice (Xing et al. 2021a). Of note, the increased level of BPs in these transgenic mice was due to the promotion of BP proliferation when *ARHGAP11B* was expressed physiologically in BPs, not due to the increased generation of BPs from APs when *ARHGAP11B* was over-expressed in APs by in utero electroporation (Florio et al. 2015; Xing et al. 2021a).

In line with this, physiologically relevant expression of *ARHGAP11B*, which was driven by the human *ARHGAP11B* promoter, was shown to be sufficient to increase the levels of mitotic bRG and mitotic bIPs by almost three-fold and two-fold, respectively, in the developing neocortex of the common marmoset, which is a lissencephalic nonhuman primate (Heide et al. 2020). The increase in total mitotic BPs was more significant in the oSVZ, the thickness of which was also increased, than in the iSVZ, similar to the findings in the *ARHGAP11B*-over-expressing developing ferret neocortex (Heide et al. 2020; Kalebic et al. 2018). Considering the different proliferative capacities between BPs in rodent, carnivore, and primate, this suggests that *ARHGAP11B* has a greater potential and ability to promote the proliferation of BPs possessing higher proliferative capacities. Another nonhuman primate model system used to test the function of *ARHGAP11B* was chimpanzee cerebral organoids. When over-expressed in chimpanzee cerebral organoids, *ARHGAP11B* increased the abundance of BPs, including bRG, similar to findings reported in other in vivo animal model systems (Fischer et al. 2022). Taken together, the human-specific *ARHGAP11B* gene increases the abundance of BPs and promotes the proliferation of BPs, which may have contributed to the evolutionary expansion of the human neocortex.

8.3.3 *ARHGAP11B* – Neocortex Expansion

As a consequence of the increased BP proliferation and abundance in the developing neocortex, *ARHGAP11B* expression also led to increased cortical neuron numbers, expanded the neocortex, and induced cortical folding (Florio et al. 2015; Heide et al. 2020; Kalebic et al. 2018; Xing et al. 2021a). Within the six-layered neocortex, layers II–IV are the evolutionarily youngest and mammalian-characteristic layers (Molnar et al. 2006). Particularly, the increase in the number of the last-born neurons for layers II and III is considered as one of the fundamental characteristics of the evolutionary expansion of the mammalian neocortex. When *ARHGAP11B* was over-expressed in the developing mouse neocortex by in utero electroporation, the number of upper-layer neurons was increased by 50 percent (Xing et al. 2021a). In developing ferret neocortex, the upper-layer neuron increase induced by *ARHGAP11B* over-expression was much greater, by 5.6-fold (Kalebic et al. 2018). The number of callosal projection neurons, which play a key role in the high-level associative connectivity, was also increased upon *ARHGAP11B* over-expression in the developing ferret neocortex (Kalebic et al. 2018). Similarly, in the *ARHGAP11B*-transgenic mice and *ARHGAP11B*-expressing marmoset fetuses, the increases in upper-layer neurons and callosal projection neurons were also observed (Heide et al. 2020; Xing et al. 2021a). Specifically, *ARHGAP11B*-transgenic mice have shown a 20 percent increase in callosal projection neurons during development, whereas the *ARHGAP11B*-expressing marmoset fetuses have shown 40 percent and 50 percent increases in callosal projection neurons and upper-layer neurons, respectively (Heide et al. 2020; Xing et al. 2021a).

The increases in upper-layer neurons and callosal projection neurons induced by *ARHGAP11B* led to neocortex expansion in developing mouse, ferret, and marmoset neocortex (Heide et al. 2020; Kalebic et al. 2018; Xing et al. 2021a). In the *ARHGAP11B*-over-expressing ferret neocortex, the thickness of the targeted gyrus, and the lateral area were increased, which reflect neocortex expansion in both radial and tangential dimensions (Kalebic et al. 2018). The *ARHGAP11B*-transgenic mice also showed neocortex expansion in the radial and tangential direction, which was indicated by the overall enlarged neocortex size, especially the neocortex width, as well as the increases in neocortical thickness and perimeter (Xing et al. 2021a). Interestingly, in the fetal marmoset neocortex, *ARHGAP11B* did not induce neocortex expansion in the tangential (medial-lateral) direction, rather in the radial and longitudinal (rostral-caudal) directions, potentially due to the differences in *ARHGAP11B* expression patterns and experimental settings in the marmoset fetuses vs. mouse and ferret embryos (Heide et al. 2020). Remarkably, the *ARHGAP11B*-expressing marmoset fetuses not only showed larger neocortex size, but exhibited surface folds (Heide et al. 2020). The gyrification index (GI) in the *ARHGAP11B*-expressing marmoset fetuses was increased to 1.08, compared to the normally smooth surface with a GI of 1.0 (Heide et al. 2020). Cortical folding was also evident in half of the cases, when *ARHGAP11B* was over-expressed in the developing mouse neocortex by in utero electroporation (Florio et al. 2015).

8.3.4 *ARHGAP11B* – Enhanced Cognitive Abilities

Importantly, in contrast to the previous transient expression of *ARHGAP11B* in embryonic mouse, embryonic ferret, and fetal marmoset neocortex, the *ARHGAP11B*-transgenic mouse line that expresses *ARHGAP11B* physiologically in the neocortex allowed us to extend our studies from developmental stages to the adult stage (Xing et al. 2021a). Key aspects of the neocortex expansion observed in the *ARHGAP11B*-transgenic mouse embryos were found to persist into adulthood, including the increases in CP thickness, especially the thickness of layers II and III, and in upper-layer neuron number (Xing et al. 2021a). As these features have been assumed to be associated with the emergence of higher cognitive abilities in humans, it was therefore intriguing to explore whether these transgenic mice carrying human-specific gene *ARHGAP11B* show any altered behaviors associated with higher cognitive abilities. Behavioral tests using IntelliCage revealed that the *ARHGAP11B*-transgenic mice show enhanced memory flexibility (Xing et al. 2021a). The initial formation of memory is dependent on the hippocampus; however, the neocortex is believed to be the site of long-term memory storage (Clark 2018; Mercer et al. 2008; Vann and Albasser 2011). In the behavioral study of the *ARHGAP11B*-transgenic mice, hippocampus-dependent learning and memory were not different between wild-type and *ARHGAP11B*-transgenic mice when using the Barnes maze test; however, the hippocampus-independent memory flexibility was increased in the latter mice when using the IntelliCage test (Xing et al. 2021a). More specifically, no difference was observed in the *ARHGAP11B*-transgenic mice for the initial place learning during the acquisition step at the beginning of the test, which is consistent with the findings from the Barnes maze test on the hippocampus-dependent memory formation. However, during the reversal steps, the overall error rate was significantly lower for both male and female *ARHGAP11B*-transgenic mice compared to wild-type mice (Xing et al. 2021a). This is in line with findings on the neocortex expansion and upper-layer neuron number increase.

8.3.5 *ARHGAP11B* – Mechanism of Action

How does the human-specific gene *ARHGAP11B* promote BP proliferation and induce neocortex expansion and folding? To study the molecular mechanisms underlying ARHGAP11B function, its subcellular localization needs to be examined first. When mouse fibroblast cells (NIH 3T3) were transfected with a plasmid encoding either human *ARHGAP11A* or *ARHGAP11B*, immunofluorescence analysis revealed that ARHGAP11A is localized in the cell nucleus (Namba et al. 2020), as previously reported (Zanin et al. 2013). However, ARHGAP11B was not found in the cell nucleus, but in mitochondria (Namba et al. 2020). This subcellular localization is due to the presence of a mitochondrial targeting sequence in the N-terminal domain of ARHGAP11B, which is sufficient and required to direct the ARHGAP11B protein into the mitochondrial matrix (Namba et al. 2020). Although ARHGAP11A has the identical mitochondrial targeting sequence, the two nuclear localization signals also contained in the larger ARHGAP11A protein, which are absent in the shorter ARHGAP11B protein, are thought to direct ARHGAP11A to the cell nucleus instead of mitochondria. Another reason that ARHGAP11A is localized in the nucleus is that the C-terminal domain of ARHGAP11A is sterically close to its N-terminal domain, which likely masks the mitochondrial targeting sequence and inhibits its ability to direct ARHGAP11A to mitochondria (Namba et al. 2020).

The mitochondrial localization of ARHGAP11B was not only documented in the transfected NIH 3T3 cells, but also in fetal human cNSPCs (Namba et al. 2020). In these *ARHGAP11B*-expressing human cNSPCs, ARHGAP11B physically interacts with adenine nucleotide translocase, which resides in the inner mitochondrial membrane, and inhibits its function in regulating the opening of the mitochondrial permeability transition pore (mPTP). Thus, via its human-specific C-terminal sequence, ARHGAP11B delays the onset of mPTP opening. Since mPTP opening leads to the release of calcium from mitochondria, the inhibition of mPTP opening induced by ARHGAP11B increases mitochondrial calcium concentration, and eventually results in an enhancement of glutaminolysis (Namba et al. 2020). Glutaminolysis, the metabolic pathway that converts glutamine to glutamate and then to alpha-ketoglutarate, has been described as a hallmark of proliferative cells such as cancer cells (Yang et al. 2017). Taken together, at the mechanistic level, the human-specific gene *ARHGAP11B* increases BP proliferation by regulating cell metabolism, that is, enhancing glutaminolysis, and thereby ultimately has contributed to the evolutionary expansion of the human neocortex (Namba et al. 2020).

8.4 Human-specific Amino Acid Substitutions in cNSPC-active Proteins – Differences in Cortical Neurogenesis between Modern Humans and Neanderthals

8.4.1 Chromosome Segregation upon Apical Progenitor Mitosis

8.4.1.1 Mitotic Differences among Hominid Neural Stem and Progenitor Cells

The generation of around 16 billion neocortical neurons, as well as the macroglial cells that support them, is a momentous task for the developing human fetus. For this, cell division is logically a foundational process, as the cNSPCs must divide profusely to eventually generate all these specialized cells. Decades of research have established a tight link between cNSPC division and other aspects of their cell and developmental biology (Bystron et al. 2008; Mora-Bermúdez et al. 2020; Sauer 1935; Smart et al. 2002; Taverna et al. 2014).

8.4.1.2 Spindle Orientation of Apical Progenitors

It is widely thought that the division of cNSPCs not only serves to multiply them, but can also participate in determining their identity and fate. This is achieved by, for example, cell divisions generating different degrees of daughter cell structural symmetry. For APs before and during early neurogenesis, a classical indicator of the probable level of symmetry of a division is the cleavage plane angle with respect to the apical, ventricular surface. Angles perpendicular to the apical surface favor symmetric, proliferative divisions, by facilitating the inheritance of the epithelial components to both daughter cells. Oblique and horizontal angles tend to instead favor asymmetric divisions, with the daughter cells each inheriting only some of the epithelial components, which can favor a neurogenic cell fate (Di Pietro et al. 2016; Homem et al. 2015; Mora-Bermudez and Huttner 2015; Nano and Basto 2017; Smart 1972a, 1972b).

When comparing brain development in species with typically very different brain sizes, like rodents and primates, a higher proportion of symmetric proliferative divisions and asymmetric self-renewing divisions, compared to asymmetric neurogenic and symmetric neurogenic divisions, can help grow the pool of cNSPCs, thereby eventually increasing the final neuronal output. This can be achieved by prolonging the duration of developmental phases where those proliferative and self-renewing divisions are numerous, for example before and during early neurogenesis. This is thought to be a major mechanism for the increase in size and neuron content in apes, including humans (Herculano-Houzel 2012; Lewitus et al. 2014; Mora-Bermudez et al. 2022b; Rakic 1995).

8.4.1.3 Metaphase Prolongation of Apical Progenitors

With regards to differences among hominids, a study that focused on comparing the cNSPC divisions of humans and other great apes identified a difference, albeit an unexpected one (Mora-Bermudez et al. 2016). AP spindle and cleavage plane dynamics were compared in cerebral organoids of humans and chimpanzees, as a candidate mechanism to explain brain size differences among these species. Ultimately however, no such differences were found. Instead, a temporal difference was noticed. In APs at early neurogenic stages (organoids at ≈ 30 days of growth), human metaphase was shown to be around 50 percent longer than in chimpanzees (Mora-Bermudez et al. 2016).

Metaphase duration of APs was also measured in other species to probe if the difference constituted a specific prolongation in humans, or a specific shortening in chimpanzees. When compared to that of orangutans, the human metaphase was also around 50 percent longer, and when compared to that of mice, the difference was even greater, with the human metaphase being more than twice as long (Mora-Bermudez et al. 2016). A shorter metaphase is therefore likely the ancestral state, and a prolongation is likely the derived characteristic, and especially so in humans. This raises the possibility that a metaphase prolongation of APs may be an evolutionary advantage that has been selected for.

Metaphase is the last of the mitotic phases where chromosomes can prepare for segregation, and it may be intuitive to think that a larger karyotype would require more preparation time. However, there is no evidence that metaphase duration is correlated with the number of chromosomes per species. Chimpanzees and orangutans both have 48 chromosomes, 2 *more* than humans, yet they have *shorter* AP metaphases. Furthermore, mice have 42 chromosomes, just 4 less than humans, yet their APs metaphase lasts for less than half that of humans (Mora-Bermudez et al. 2016).

Another interesting aspect is that metaphase prolongation did not persist during development, as it was no longer seen when comparing organoid APs in a more advanced neurogenic stage (≈50 days of growth) (Mora-Bermudez et al. 2016). This could mean that it is a developmentally regulated feature of early cNSPCs. Further work was consistent with this view, finding no difference in the human vs. chimpanzee induced pluripotent stem cells (iPSCs) used to grow the organoids. Also, no difference was seen when comparing human and chimpanzee B-lymphocytes (Mora-Bermudez et al. 2016), another highly proliferative type of cell but not of the neural lineage. These observations suggest that metaphase prolongation could be a specific feature of early and highly proliferative APs, such as NECs and early aRG (Mora-Bermudez et al. 2016).

Previous to these observations, the only known specific role for metaphase in neurogenesis was in establishing the position and orientation of the mitotic spindle for symmetric vs. asymmetric AP divisions, as briefly summarized earlier. Since no spindle and cleavage plane orientation differences were seen concurrently with the metaphase prolongation in human vs. chimpanzee APs, this suggested an independent and unknown role for metaphase prolongation in neocortex development, with potential evolutionary consequences.

8.4.1.4 Mitotic Differences between Modern and Archaic Human Apical Progenitors

In addition to differences between present-day humans and other primates, it has also become possible to investigate potential physiological differences to the extinct relatives of modern humans, such as Neanderthals and Denisovans. This is primarily thanks to the whole-genome sequencing of an increasing number of individuals from those species (Hajdinjak et al. 2021; Mafessoni et al. 2020; Prüfer et al. 2014). These genomes also provided clues to investigate human metaphase prolongation. Around 31,000 base pair substitutions between modern and archaic humans have been found, of which around one hundred are in the sequence of proteins (Kuhlwilm and Boeckx 2019; Prüfer et al. 2014). Of those hundred, six changes in three proteins stand out as possibly playing a role in the cNSPC divisions of the developing brain. KIF18a (or Kinesin 8) with one amino acid difference, KNL1 (or CASC5) with two differences, and SPAG5 (or Astrin) with three differences, have a high expression in the germinal layers of the neocortex and have been shown in cell biological studies to participate in chromosome segregation and kinetochore function during mitosis (see e.g., Cheeseman et al. 2008; Hafner et al. 2014; Manning et al. 2010; Stumpff et al. 2012; Thein et al. 2007; Zhang et al. 2017). Also remarkable is the fact that rodents, monkeys, and many other organisms have the same six amino acids in those positions as Neanderthals, whereas the particular combination found in modern humans seems to be specific. These observations suggested the possibility that the six amino acid differences in KIF18a, KNL1, and SPAG5 could be involved in metaphase prolongation.

Evidence for this was obtained in a study that examined differences in neocortical development between modern and archaic humans and involved the use of native brain tissue. The above-mentioned six Neanderthal-like amino acids naturally present in mice were changed to the modern human variants. Live brain tissue imaging showed an AP metaphase prolongation in these gene-edited mice, and further screening of individual and combinations of amino acids variants showed that, in the mouse background, only the three amino acid substitutions in KIF18a and KNL1, but not those three in SPAG5, caused an AP metaphase prolongation. Further evidence was obtained in human cerebral organoids grown from gene-edited embryonic stem cells (ESCs), where the three modern human amino acids in KIF18a and KNL1 were changed to the ancestral, Neanderthal-like variants. The APs in the organoids grown from these ESCs showed a shorter metaphase, confirming, in a human background, that the three modern human amino acids in KIF18a and KNL1 cause an AP metaphase prolongation (see Figure 8.1B) (Mora-Bermudez et al. 2022a).

8.4.1.5 Mechanism Underlying Metaphase Prolongation

Insight into the biochemical mechanism underlying the metaphase prolongation came when the number of spindle assembly checkpoint (SAC)-positive kinetochores was shown to increase in the gene-edited mouse APs with the modern human variants of KIF18a and KNL1. Conversely, this number decreased in the human cerebral organoid APs with the ancestral variants. This suggests that a more active SAC causes a prolongation of metaphase, as SAC activation in just one kinetochore has been shown to be capable of delaying anaphase onset until all chromosomes are bi-oriented and all kinetochores have amphitelic attachments to the spindle poles (Musacchio and Salmon 2007; Rieder et al. 1994). Consistent with these results, the numbers of SAC-positive AP kinetochores were higher in native human developing neocortex tissue, as well as in human iPSC-derived cerebral organoids, when compared to those in chimpanzee organoids, which have the same amino acid variants in KIF18a and KNL1 as Neanderthals (Mora-Bermudez et al. 2022a).

8.4.1.6 Metaphase Prolongation and Increased Chromosome Segregation Accuracy

Ensuring chromosome segregation accuracy to generate daughter cells with the correct number and type of chromosomes is the main function of the SAC (Foley and Kapoor 2013; Musacchio 2015). Therefore, SAC activity being higher when the modern human variants of KIF18a and KNL1 were present suggested a function in chromosome segregation. Counting lagging chromosomes in anaphase and telophase showed that the number of these segregation errors was around twice as high in APs with the ancestral variants of KIF18a and KNL1, such as mouse, chimpanzee and "Neanderthalized" human APs, compared to APs with the derived variants, such a "modern-humanized" and modern human APs (Mora-Bermudez et al. 2022a).

In addition to spindle orientation, metaphase prolongation is therefore a second metaphase-specific process employed by APs during neurogenesis, especially in humans. Whereas spindle orientation is used to control neuronal output by modulating division symmetry, metaphase prolongation seems to reduce the incidence of chromosome segregation mistakes in the progeny of cNSPCs of modern humans compared to that of other hominids and animals. This is particularly relevant in light of the fact that the size of the progeny of cNSPCs of modern humans is the largest among primates. Genomics data suggests that other single amino-acid differences between modern and archaic humans may also be somehow involved in mitosis or tubulin regulation, perhaps in the brain or other tissues (Peyregne et al. 2022).

In general terms, the proportion of mitotic APs making chromosome segregation mistakes, including those with the ancestral variants of KIF18a and KNL1, is rather low (around 2% or less). This makes intuitive sense when considering that organisms will generally benefit when their tissues can develop from cells with as few chromosomal errors as possible. In the case of the brain, and specifically of the neocortex, the neurons therein have an extremely high connectivity, with thousands of connections per single neuron. In such dense interconnected networks, even a low number of mistakes may have consequences throughout brain areas. This idea is further supported by the fact that the increased chromosome segregation errors in non-modern-human species are found mostly at the telophase of early APs, when the chances of rescuing these errors are rapidly decreasing as the cell is already reforming the daughter nuclei and undergoing cytokinesis and abscission (Mora-Bermudez et al. 2022a). It therefore seems plausible that many of these mistakes will be passed on to the whole AP progeny. Such mistakes may then be present in entire radial units (Rakic 1988, 2000), and it is conceivable that the presence of such suboptimal cortical columns, interspersed throughout the neocortex even if only in a low percentage, may sensibly affect the cognitive processes that are the hallmark of the neocortex. Experiments that compare the cognitive performance of whole organisms, for example with mice that have either the ancestral or the derived set of amino acids in KIF18a and KNL1, will be key to further exploration of this topic.

8.4.2 Neuron Production by Basal Radial Glia

8.4.2.1 NOVA1

The first role of a single modern human-specific amino acid substitution in a protein implicated in brain development was reported by Muotri and colleagues (Trujillo et al. 2021). The splicing regulator neuro-oncological ventral antigen 1 (NOVA1) contains an isoleucine-to-valine amino acid change in modern humans compared to Neanderthals. Cortical organoids expressing archaic NOVA1 variant were reported to exhibit a slower development and changes in synaptic gene expression compared to cortical organoids expressing modern human NOVA1 (Trujillo et al. 2021). Of note, heterozygous deletions of target DNA have been reported for the iPSCs used to generate these cortical organoids (Maricic et al. 2021). Thus, it cannot be excluded that the phenotype observed upon editing of NOVA1 is in fact due to these deletions. However, further analyses by Sanger sequencing of NOVA1 PCR products obtained from the genomic DNA of the various clones used identified a deletion in only one of these clones (Herai et al. 2021).

8.4.2.2 Transketolase-like 1

Endocast analyses have revealed that the endocranial volume of modern humans and Neanderthals was similar (Gunz et al. 2019). This suggests that modern humans and Neanderthals had similar brain and neocortex size. However, a similar brain size does not automatically imply a similar number of neurons. Moreover, while Neanderthals and modern humans had similar brain size, their brain morphology was different. The modern human brain has a globular shape, whereas the Neanderthal brain was more elongated (Gunz et al. 2019). An additional difference between the modern human and the Neanderthal brain, pertaining to the number of neocortical neurons, has recently been reported (Pinson et al. 2022). Specifically, the protein transketolase-like 1 (TKTL1) was shown to be important for modern human frontal neocortex development and could potentially explain some of the differences that appeared during hominin neocortex evolution (Pinson et al. 2022). Thus, besides the aforementioned KIF18a, KNL1, SPAG5, and NOVA1, TKTL1 is another protein carrying an amino acid substitution (lysine-to-arginine) that distinguishes modern humans from extinct archaic humans, Neanderthals, and Denisovans (Prüfer et al. 2014).

8.4.2.2.1 Basal Radial Glia Abundance

In fetal human neocortical tissue, *TKTL1* mRNA is preferentially expressed in cNSPCs (Fietz et al. 2012; Florio et al. 2015; Johnson et al. 2015; Pinson et al. 2022; Pollen et al. 2015). Its expression increases with cortical development and is higher in the frontal lobe than the occipital lobe (Miller et al. 2014; Pinson et al. 2022). Ectopic expression of modern human TKTL1 (hTKTL1) in embryonic mouse neocortex, a model organism with a smooth (lissencephalic) neocortex, increases bRG abundance without affecting the abundance of APs and bIPs (see Figure 8.1C). Thus, bRG, which typically represent only 5–10 percent of all mitotic BPs in embryonic mouse neocortex (Kelava et al. 2012; Wang et al. 2011), account for 33 percent of all mitotic BPs in hTKTL1-electroporated mouse neocortex (Pinson et al. 2022). The ability of TKTL1 to increase bRG abundance relies on the modern human-specific amino acid substitution, as ectopic expression of archaic human TKTL1 (aTKTL1) has no effect on cNSPC abundance.

The physiological relevance of hTKTL1 in the control of bRG abundance was demonstrated by the finding that CRISPR/Cas9-mediated knockout of *hTKTL1* in human neocortical tissue ex vivo reduces bRG abundance. Moreover, aTKTL1-expressing cerebral organoids generated from CRISPR/Cas9-edited human embryonic stem cells had less bRG than hTKTL1-expressing organoids (Pinson et al. 2022). Of note, a role of hTKTL1 in bRG proliferation is consistent with previous reports that hTKTL1 is associated with tumor cell proliferation (Diaz-Moralli et al. 2016;

Peltonen et al. 2020; Sun et al. 2010; Yuan et al. 2010). This in turn is in line with the notion that cancer cells are recapitulating developmental programs and with recent observations that these cells may even use pathways that led to the evolutionary expansion of the neocortex. Some ependymoma cells were reported to have a gene expression pattern similar to radial glia cells (Taylor et al. 2005). Moreover, the radial glia gene FABP-7 has been shown to be expressed in some glioblastoma cells (De Rosa et al. 2012; Mita et al. 2007). Further evidence along these lines comes from the finding that some invasive glioblastoma cells are similar to bRG (Bhaduri et al. 2020; Wang et al. 2020). These cells, like bRG, undergo mitotic somal translocation (Bhaduri et al. 2020). Furthermore, the expression of the human-specific gene *NOTCH2NL*, involved in cNSPC proliferation (Fiddes et al. 2018; Florio et al. 2018; Suzuki et al. 2018), contributes to the increased proliferation of H3.3G34R-mutant glioma cells (Funato et al. 2021).

8.4.2.2.2 Basal Radial Glia Morphology – Basal Process and Proliferative Capacity

In a gyrencephalic (folded neocortex) species, the ferret, hTKTL1 expression in the developing neocortex by in utero electroporation increases not only bRG abundance but also the number of bRG processes (Pinson et al. 2022). bRG are polarized cells that were initially reported as bearing a single basal process (bRG-b) (Fietz et al. 2010; Hansen et al. 2010; Reillo et al. 2011). However, additional morphotypes have been identified in the developing macaque neocortex (apically directed process-bearing bRG (bRG-a), apically directed and basal process-bearing bRG (bRG-ab) and bRG that alternate between stages (transient bRG)) (Betizeau et al. 2013). Recently, two additional morphotypes were characterized in embryonic ferret and fetal human neocortices, but not in embryonic mouse neocortex: bRG with a bifurcated basal process (bRG-b_{bf}) and bRG with an apically directed and a bifurcated basal process (bRG-ab_{bf}) (Kalebic et al. 2019). The first hint that bRG processes are linked to cell proliferation came from the report that bRG-ab have higher self-renewing capacity than bRG-b and bRG-a (Betizeau et al. 2013). More recently, a study of the morpho-regulatory protein PALMDELPHIN has uncovered a causal relationship between bRG processes and cell proliferation. Indeed, when expressed in embryonic mouse and ferret neocortex, the human membrane-bound PALMDELPHIN protein drives BP process growth and, as a result, induces cell proliferation. Conversely, *PALMDELPHIN* knockout in fetal human neocortical tissue reduces the number of BP processes and cell proliferation (Kalebic et al. 2019; Kalebic and Huttner 2020). The relevance of bRG with more than one process in neocortical evolution is reflected by the higher proportion of these morphotypes in human and macaque neocortices than in ferret and mouse neocortices (Betizeau et al. 2013; Kalebic et al. 2019; Kalebic and Huttner 2020). These data highlight that bRG cell biology, and more specifically morphological aspects related to their number of processes, are a key regulator of primate neocortical development and evolution.

8.4.2.2.3 Neuron Production

Neurons are generated by two types of BPs, bRG and bIPs. Reflecting the cell polarity of bRG, and more specifically the presence of a process, their neuron-generating divisions are asymmetric self-renewing divisions generating a bRG and a neuron. Compared to the neuron-generating symmetric consumptive divisions of the nonpolar bIPs, the self-renewing division of bRG are more efficient to produce neurons over time (Fietz et al. 2010). In line with this model, hTKTL1 expression in embryonic mouse and ferret neocortices increases late-born upper-layer neuron production without affecting early-born deep-layer neuron production (Pinson et al. 2022). This is particularly relevant as upper-layer neuron enrichment is considered to be an essential aspect of neocortex expansion and evolution in primates and humans. Furthermore, aTKTL1-expressing cerebral organoids generated from CRISPR/Cas9-edited human embryonic stem cells had less neurons than the hTKTL1-expressing organoids (Pinson et al. 2022).

8.4.2.2.4 Metabolic Pathways

During recent years, metabolism has emerged as an essential aspect of human neocortical development (Namba et al. 2021). As aforementioned, the human-specific gene *ARHGAP11B*, the protein of which is located in mitochondria, increases BP proliferation by promoting glutaminolysis (Namba et al. 2020). In addition, a single amino acid substitution between Neanderthals and modern humans in the enzyme adenylosuccinate lyase (ADSL) has been associated with differences in purine synthesis in the adult brain. Specifically, postnatal mice that are humanized for ADSL have a reduction in purine synthesis in their brain compared to wild-type mice. In contrast, Neanderthalized human cells have a greater level of purine biosynthesis than wild-type cells. These results were corroborated by the finding that purine metabolism is lower in the prefrontal cortex, primary visual cortex, and cerebellum of adult modern humans than of chimpanzee and macaque (Stepanova et al. 2021).

TKTL1 belongs to the transketolase family. The founding member of this family, TKT, is a thiamine-dependent enzyme that catalyzes two different two-substrates reactions in the non-oxidative part of the pentose phosphate pathway (PPP) (Coy et al. 2005; Patra and Hay 2014). PPP, also known as the phosphogluconate pathway or the hexose monophosphate shunt, is a metabolic pathway that is essential to: (i) maintain carbon homeostasis; (ii) produce NADPH, the electron donor that provides reducing power for anabolic reactions and is key to maintaining the redox balance; (iii) provide precursors for nucleic acid and amino acid synthesis; and (iv) feed glycolysis. PPP is important for cell proliferation and has been associated with cancer cell proliferation (Jiang et al. 2014; Patra and Hay 2014). Notably, PPP enzyme expression is increased in rapidly dividing glioblastoma cells (Kathagen-Buhmann et al. 2016). Whether TKTL1 is enzymatically active has been subject to debate (Deshpande et al. 2019; Diaz-Moralli et al. 2016; Schneider et al. 2012), but a reported action of TKTL1 is the cleavage of xylulose 5-phosphate, a metabolite in the PPP, into glyceraldehyde 3-phosphate and acetate (Coy et al. 2005; Diaz-Moralli et al. 2016).

Pharmacological inhibition of the PPP in hTKTL1-electroporated embryonic mouse neocortex suppresses the hTKTL1-induced increase in bRG abundance, thus confirming that TKTL1 acts through the PPP (Pinson et al. 2022). Glyceraldehyde 3-phosphate and acetate can both be metabolized to acetyl-CoA, a precursor for fatty acid synthesis. Accordingly, the acetyl-CoA concentration is elevated in hTKTL1-expressing mouse bRG compared to control mouse bRG and aTKTL1-expressing mouse bRG. Pharmacological inhibition of fatty acid synthesis abolishes the hTKTL1-induced increase in bRG abundance, suggesting that elevated fatty acid synthesis is involved in hTKTL1 action in bRG (Pinson et al. 2022). Of note, fatty acid synthesis likely increases bRG proliferation by providing membrane lipids used for process growth.

Fatty acid synthesis is an important regulator of cell proliferation. Conditional deletion or pharmacological inhibition of the multiprotein enzyme fatty acid synthase (FASN) in the embryonic mouse telencephalon induces microcephaly, highlighting the importance of de novo lipogenesis in mouse brain development (Gonzalez-Bohorquez et al. 2022). Likewise, pharmacological inhibition or CRISPR/Cas9-mediated genetic ablation of FASN in human forebrain organoids disturbs AP cell polarity, reduces bRG proliferation, and reduces neuron production (Gonzalez-Bohorquez et al. 2022). Furthermore, a FASN point mutation has been linked to intellectual disabilities in humans and to learning and memory deficits in mice (Bowers et al. 2020; Najmabadi et al. 2011). Fatty acid catabolism, known as β-oxidation, is also essential for the developing brain. Thus, a reduction in fatty acid β-oxidation induces a switch in the mode of cNSPC division from asymmetric self-renewing divisions to symmetric differentiative divisions (Xie et al. 2016). Palmitoylation, the post-translational modification that covalently adds fatty acids to proteins, is essential to maintain the full level of BPs in fetal human neocortex, but not in embryonic mouse neocortex (Kalebic et al. 2019). Taking together, these studies highlight that changes in metabolic pathways are responsible, at least partially, for the increased cNSPC proliferation that occurred during human evolution.

8.5 Concluding Remarks

Human-specific genes and modern-human specific amino acid substitutions in proteins with functional relevance for cNSPCs have played an important role in the evolution of the human neocortex. Technical advances in gene editing and the establishment of cerebral organoid culture over the past decade have provided new avenues to study not only the development of the brain in species whose fetal tissue is difficult to obtain, but also the consequences of genetic changes for brain development. Deciphering the links between gene expression and the cell biological features of cNSPCs has allowed the identification of important genes essential for the amplification of the cNSPC pool, and more specifically of BPs, that occurred during the evolution of the human neocortex. It also appears that minimizing the number of chromosome segregation mistakes in this larger number of cNSPCs may have been an additional advantage in the evolution of the modern human brain.

References

Antonacci, F. et al. (2014). Palindromic *GOLGA8* core duplicons promote chromosome 15q13.3 microdeletion and evolutionary instability. *Nat Genet* 46: 1293–1302.

Arai, Y. et al. (2011). Neural stem and progenitor cells shorten S-phase on commitment to neuron production. *Nat Commun* 2: 154.

Betizeau, M. et al. (2013). Precursor diversity and complexity of lineage relationships in the outer subventricular zone of the primate. *Neuron* 80: 442–457.

Bhaduri, A. et al. (2020). Outer radial glia-like cancer stem cells contribute to heterogeneity of glioblastoma. *Cell Stem Cell* 26: 48–63 e46.

Borrell, V. (2019). Recent advances in understanding neocortical development. *F1000Res* 8.

Bowers, M. et al. (2020). FASN-dependent lipid metabolism links neurogenic stem/progenitor cell activity to learning and memory deficits. *Cell Stem Cell* 27: 98–109 e111.

Bystron, I. et al. (2008). Development of the human cerebral cortex. *Nat Rev Neurosci* 9: 110–122.

Cheeseman, I.M. et al. (2008). KNL1 and the CENP-H/I/K complex coordinately direct kinetochore assembly in vertebrates. *Mol Biol Cell* 19: 587–594.

Clark, R.E. (2018). A history and overview of the behavioral neuroscience of learning and memory. *Curr Topics Behav Neurosci* 37: 1–11. doi: 10.1007/7854_2017_37.rost.

Coy, J.F. et al. (2005). Mutations in the transketolase-like gene TKTL1: clinical implications for neurodegenerative diseases, diabetes and cancer. *Clin Lab* 51: 257–273.

De Rosa, A. et al. (2012). A radial glia gene marker, fatty acid binding protein 7 (FABP7), is involved in proliferation and invasion of glioblastoma cells. *PLoS One* 7: e52113.

Dehay, C. et al. (2015). The outer subventricular zone and primate-specific cortical complexification. *Neuron* 85: 683–694.

Deshpande, G.P. et al. (2019). The human transketolase-like proteins TKTL1 and TKTL2 are bona fide transketolases. *BMC Struct Biol* 19: 2.

Di Pietro, F. et al. (2016). Regulation of mitotic spindle orientation. *EMBO Rep* 17: 1106–1130.

Diaz-Moralli, S. et al. (2016). A key role for transketolase-like 1 in tumor metabolic reprogramming. *Oncotarget* 7: 51875–51897.

Dougherty, M.L. et al. (2018). Transcriptional fates of human-specific segmental duplications in brain. *Genome Res* 28: 1566–1576.

Ferent, J. et al. (2020). Extracellular control of radial glia proliferation and scaffolding during cortical development and pathology. *Front Cell Dev Biol* 8: 578341.

Fernandez, V. et al. (2016). Cerebral cortex expansion and folding. *EMBO J* 35: 1021–1044.

Fiddes, I.T. et al. (2018). Human-specific *NOTCH2NL* genes affect notch signaling and cortical neurogenesis. *Cell* 173: 1356–1369 e1322.

Fietz, S.A. et al. (2010). OSVZ progenitors of human and ferret neocortex are epithelial-like and expand by integrin signaling. *Nature Neuroscience* 13: 690–699.

Fietz, S.A. et al. (2012). Transcriptomes of germinal zones of human and mouse fetal neocortex suggest a role of extracellular matrix in progenitor self-renewal. *Proc Natl Acad Sci USA* 109: 11836–11841.

Fischer, J. et al. (2022). Human-specific *ARHGAP11B* ensures human-like basal progenitor levels in hominid cerebral organoids. *EMBO Rep* e54728.

Fish, J.L. et al. (2006). Aspm specifically maintains symmetric proliferative divisions of neuroepithelial cells. *Proc Natl Acad Sci USA* 103: 10438–10443.

Florio, M. et al. (2015). Human-specific gene *ARHGAP11B* promotes basal progenitor amplification and neocortex expansion. *Science* 347: 1465–1470.

Florio, M. et al. (2018). Evolution and cell-type specificity of human-specific genes preferentially expressed in progenitors of fetal neocortex. *Elife* 7: e32332.

Florio, M. and Huttner, W.B. (2014). Neural progenitors, neurogenesis and the evolution of the neocortex. *Development* 141: 2182–2194.

Florio, M. et al. (2016). A single splice site mutation in human-specific *ARHGAP11B* causes basal progenitor amplification. *Sci Adv* 2: e1601941.

Foley, E.A. and Kapoor, T.M. (2013). Microtubule attachment and spindle assembly checkpoint signalling at the kinetochore. *Nat Rev Mol Cell Biol* 14: 25–37.

Funato, K. et al. (2021). Dissecting the impact of regional identity and the oncogenic role of human-specific *NOTCH2NL* in an hESC model of H3.3G34R-mutant glioma. *Cell Stem Cell* 28: 894–905 e897.

Gal, J.S. et al. (2006). Molecular and morphological heterogeneity of neural precursors in the mouse neocortical proliferative zones. *J Neurosci* 26: 1045–1056.

Gonzalez-Bohorquez, D. et al. (2022). FASN-dependent de novo lipogenesis is required for brain development. *Proc Natl Acad Sci USA* 119: e2112040119.

Götz, M. and Huttner, W.B. (2005). The cell biology of neurogenesis. *Nat Rev Mol Cell Biol* 6: 777–788.

Gunz, P. et al. (2019). Neandertal introgression sheds light on modern human endocranial globularity. *Curr Biol* 29: 120–127.e125.

Hafner, J. et al. (2014). Pre-anaphase chromosome oscillations are regulated by the antagonistic activities of Cdk1 and PP1 on Kif18A. *Nat Commun* 5: 4397.

Hajdinjak, M. et al. (2021). Initial Upper Palaeolithic humans in Europe had recent Neanderthal ancestry. *Nature* 592: 253–257.

Hansen, D.V. et al. (2010). Neurogenic radial glia in the outer subventricular zone of human neocortex. *Nature* 464: 554–561.

Hartfuss, E. et al. (2001). Characterization of CNS precursor subtypes and radial glia. *Dev Biol* 229: 15–30.

Haubensak, W. et al. (2004). Neurons arise in the basal neuroepithelium of the early mammalian telencephalon. *Proc Natl Acad Sci USA* 101: 3196–3201.

Heide, M. et al. (2020). Human-specific *ARHGAP11B* increases size and folding of primate neocortex in the fetal marmoset. *Science* 369: 546–550.

Herai, R.H. et al. (2021). Response to comment on "Reintroduction of the archaic variant of *NOVA1* in cortical organoids alters neurodevelopment". *Science* 374: eabi9881.

Herculano-Houzel, S. (2012). The remarkable, yet not extraordinary, human brain as a scaled-up primate brain and its associated cost. *Proc Natl Acad Sci USA* 109 (1): 10661–10668.

Homem, C.C. et al. (2015). Proliferation control in neural stem and progenitor cells. *Nat Rev Neurosci* 16: 647–659.

Huttner, W.B. and Brand, M. (1997). Asymmetric division and polarity of neuroepithelial cells. *Curr Opin Neurobiol* 7: 29–39.

Huttner, W.B. and Kosodo, Y. (2005). Symmetric versus asymmetric cell division during neurogenesis in the developing vertebrate central nervous system. *Curr Opin Cell Biol* 17: 648–657.

Jiang, P. et al. (2014). Regulation of the pentose phosphate pathway in cancer. *Protein & Cell* 5: 592–602.

Johnson, M.B. et al. (2015). Single-cell analysis reveals transcriptional heterogeneity of neural progenitors in human cortex. *Nat Neurosci* 18: 637–646.

Kagawa, Y. et al. (2013). Cell cycle-dependent Rho GTPase activity dynamically regulates cancer cell motility and invasion in vivo. *PLoS One* 8: e83629.

Kalebic, N. et al. (2018). Human-specific *ARHGAP11B* induces hallmarks of neocortical expansion in developing ferret neocortex. *Elife* 7: e41241.

Kalebic, N. et al. (2019). Neocortical expansion due to increased proliferation of basal progenitors is linked to changes in their morphology. *Cell Stem Cell* 24: 535–550 e539.

Kalebic, N. and Huttner, W.B. (2020). Basal progenitor morphology and neocortex evolution. *Trends Neurosci* 43: 843–853.

Kathagen-Buhmann, A. et al. (2016). Glycolysis and the pentose phosphate pathway are differentially associated with the dichotomous regulation of glioblastoma cell migration versus proliferation. *Neuro Oncol* 18: 1219–1229.

Kelava, I. et al. (2012). Abundant occurrence of basal radial glia in the subventricular zone of embryonic neocortex of a lissencephalic primate, the common marmoset Callithrix jacchus. *Cereb Cortex* 22: 469–481.

Komabayashi-Suzuki, M. et al. (2019). Spatiotemporally dependent vascularization is differently utilized among neural progenitor subtypes during neocortical development. *Cell Rep* 29: 1113–1129 e1115.

Kosodo, Y. et al. (2004). Asymmetric distribution of the apical plasma membrane during neurogenic divisions of mammalian neuroepithelial cells. *EMBO J* 23: 2314–2324.

Kosodo, Y. et al. (2008). Cytokinesis of neuroepithelial cells can divide their basal process before anaphase. *EMBO J* 27: 3151–3163.

Kriegstein, A. et al. (2006). Patterns of neural stem and progenitor cell division may underlie evolutionary cortical expansion. *Nat Rev Neurosci* 7: 883–890.

Kriegstein, A.R. and Götz, M. (2003). Radial glia diversity. *Glia* 43: 37–43.

Kuhlwilm, M. and Boeckx, C. (2019). A catalog of single nucleotide changes distinguishing modern humans from archaic hominins. *Sci Rep* 9: 8463.

Lee, H.O. and Norden, C. (2013). Mechanisms controlling arrangements and movements of nuclei in pseudostratified epithelia. *Trends Cell Biol* 23: 141–150.

Lehtinen, M.K. and Walsh, C.A. (2011). Neurogenesis at the brain-cerebrospinal fluid interface. *Ann Rev Cell Dev Biol* 27: 653–679.

Lehtinen, M.K. et al. (2011). The cerebrospinal fluid provides a proliferative niche for neural progenitor cells. *Neuron* 69: 893–905.

Lewitus, E. et al. (2014). An adaptive threshold in mammalian neocortical evolution. *PLoS Biol* 12: e1002000.

Lui, J.H. et al. (2011). Development and evolution of the human neocortex. *Cell* 146: 18–36.

Lui, J.H. et al. (2014). Radial glia require PDGFD-PDGFRbeta signalling in human but not mouse neocortex. *Nature* 515: 264–268.

Mafessoni, F. et al. (2020). A high-coverage Neandertal genome from Chagyrskaya Cave. *Proc Natl Acad Sci USA* 117: 15132–15136.

Manning, A.L. et al. (2010). CLASP1, astrin and Kif2b form a molecular switch that regulates kinetochore-microtubule dynamics to promote mitotic progression and fidelity. *EMBO J* 29: 3531–3543.

Maricic, T. et al. (2021). Comment on "Reintroduction of the archaic variant of *NOVA1* in cortical organoids alters neurodevelopment". *Science* 374: eabi6060.

Matsumoto, N. et al. (2017). Gyrification of the cerebral cortex requires FGF signaling in the mammalian brain. *Elife* 6: e29285.

Mercer, T.R. et al. (2008). Noncoding RNAs in long-term memory formation. *Neuroscientist* 14: 434–445.

Meyer, M. et al. (2012). A high-coverage genome sequence from an archaic Denisovan individual. *Science* 338: 222–226.

Miller, D.J. et al. (2019). Shared and derived features of cellular diversity in the human cerebral cortex. *Curr Opin Neurobiol* 56: 117–124.

Miller, J.A. et al. (2014). Transcriptional landscape of the prenatal human brain. *Nature* 508: 199–206.

Mita, R. et al. (2007). B-FABP-expressing radial glial cells: the malignant glioma cell of origin? *Neoplasia* 9: 734–744.

Miyata, T. et al. (2004). Asymmetric production of surface-dividing and non-surface-dividing cortical progenitor cells. *Development* 131: 3133–3145.

Molnar, Z. et al. (2006). Comparative aspects of cerebral cortical development. *Eur J Neurosci* 23: 921–934.

Mora-Bermudez, F. et al. (2016). Differences and similarities between human and chimpanzee neural progenitors during cerebral cortex development. *Elife* 5: e18683.

Mora-Bermudez, F. and Huttner, W.B. (2015). Novel insights into mammalian embryonic neural stem cell division: focus on microtubules. *Mol Biol Cell* 26: 4302–4306.

Mora-Bermudez, F. et al. (2022a). Longer metaphase and fewer chromosome segregation errors in modern human than Neanderthal brain development. *Sci Adv* 8: eabn7702.

Mora-Bermudez, F. et al. (2022b). From stem and progenitor cells to neurons in the developing neocortex. *FEBS J* 289: 1524–1535.

Mora-Bermúdez, F. et al. (2020). Neural stem cells in cerebral cortex development. In: *Neuroscience in the 21st Century: From Basic to Clinical* (ed. D.W. Pfaff, N.D. Volkow, and J. Rubenstein), 1–32. New York: Springer New York.

Musacchio, A. (2015). The molecular biology of spindle assembly checkpoint signaling dynamics. *Curr Biol* 25: R1002–1018.

Musacchio, A. and Salmon, E.D. (2007). The spindle-assembly checkpoint in space and time. *Nat Rev Mol Cell Biol* 8: 379–393.

Najmabadi, H. et al. (2011). Deep sequencing reveals 50 novel genes for recessive cognitive disorders. *Nature* 478: 57–63.

Namba, T. et al. (2020). Human-specific *ARHGAP11B* acts in mitochondria to expand neocortical progenitors by glutaminolysis. *Neuron* 105: 867–881 e869.

Namba, T. et al. (2021). Metabolic regulation of neocortical expansion in development and evolution. *Neuron* 109: 408–419.

Nano, M. and Basto, R. (2017). Consequences of centrosome dysfunction during brain development. *Adv Exp Med Biol* 1002: 19–45.

Noctor, S.C. et al. (2004). Cortical neurons arise in symmetric and asymmetric division zones and migrate through specific phases. *Nat Neurosci* 7: 136–144.

Noctor, S.C. et al. (2007). Neural stem and progenitor cells in cortical development. *Novartis Found Symp* 288: 59–73. discussion 73–58, 96–58.

Paridaen, J.T. et al. (2015). Analysis of primary cilia in the developing mouse brain. *Methods Cell Biol* 127: 93–129.

Patra, K.C. and Hay, N. (2014). The pentose phosphate pathway and cancer. *Trends Biochem Sci* 39: 347–354.

Peltonen, R. et al. (2020). High TKTL1 expression as a sign of poor prognosis in colorectal cancer with synchronous rather than metachronous liver metastases. *Cancer Biol Ther* 21: 826–831.

Peyregne, S. et al. (2022). The evolutionary history of human spindle genes includes back-and-forth gene flow with Neandertals. *Elife* 11: e75464.

Pinson, A. et al. (2022). Human TKTL1 implies greater neurogenesis in frontal neocortex of modern humans than Neanderthals. *Science* 377: eabl6422.

Pollen, A.A. et al. (2015). Molecular identity of human outer radial glia during cortical development. *Cell* 163: 55–67.

Prüfer, K. et al. (2014). The complete genome sequence of a Neanderthal from the Altai Mountains. *Nature* 505: 43–49.

Rakic, P. (1988). Specification of cerebral cortical areas. *Science* 241: 170–176.

Rakic, P. (1995). A small step for the cell, a giant leap for mankind. *Trends Neurosci* 18: 383–388.

Rakic, P. (2000). Radial unit hypothesis of neocortical expansion. *Novartis Found Symp* 228: 30–42. Discussion 42–52.

Rakic, P. (2009). Evolution of the neocortex: a perspective from developmental biology. *Nat Rev Neurosci* 10: 724–735.

Reillo, I. et al. (2011). A role for intermediate radial glia in the tangential expansion of the mammalian cerebral cortex. *Cereb Cortex* 21: 1674–1694.

Rieder, C.L. et al. (1994). Anaphase onset in vertebrate somatic cells is controlled by a checkpoint that monitors sister kinetochore attachment to the spindle. *J Cell Biol* 127: 1301–1310.

Riley, B. et al. (2002). A 3-Mb map of a large Segmental duplication overlapping the alpha7-nicotinic acetylcholine receptor gene (CHRNA7) at human 15q13-q14. *Genomics* 79: 197–209.

Rousso, D.L. et al. (2012). Foxp-mediated suppression of N-cadherin regulates neuroepithelial character and progenitor maintenance in the CNS. *Neuron* 74: 314–330.

Sauer, F.C. (1935). Mitosis in the neural tube. *J Comp Neurol* 62: 377–405.

Sauer, M.E. and Walker, B.E. (1959). Radioautographic study of interkinetic nuclear migration in the neural tube. *Proc Soc Exp Biol Med* 101: 557–560.

Sauerland, C. et al. (2018). The basal radial glia occurs in marsupials and underlies the evolution of an expanded neocortex in therian mammals. *Cereb Cortex* 28: 145–157.

Schneider, S. et al. (2012). A delta38 deletion variant of human transketolase as a model of transketolase-like protein 1 exhibits no enzymatic activity. *PLoS One* 7: e48321.

Shitamukai, A. et al. (2011). Oblique radial glial divisions in the developing mouse neocortex induce self-renewing progenitors outside the germinal zone that resemble primate outer subventricular zone progenitors. *J Neurosci* 31: 3683–3695.

Smart, I.H. et al. (2002). Unique morphological features of the proliferative zones and postmitotic compartments of the neural epithelium giving rise to striate and extrastriate cortex in the monkey. *Cereb Cortex* 12: 37–53.

Smart, I.H.M. (1972a). Proliferative characteristics of the ependymal layer during the early development of the spinal cord in the mouse. *J Anat* 111: 365–380.

Smart, I.H.M. (1972b). Proliferative characteristics of the ependymal layer during the early development of the mouse diencephalon, as revealed by recording the number, location, and plane of cleavage of mitotic figures. *J Anat* 113: 109–129.

Stenzel, D. et al. (2014). Integrin alphavbeta3 and thyroid hormones promote expansion of progenitors in embryonic neocortex. *Development* 141: 795–806.

Stepanova, V. et al. (2021). Reduced purine biosynthesis in humans after their divergence from Neandertals. *Elife* 10: e58741.

Stepien, B.K. et al. (2020). Lengthening neurogenic period during neocortical development causes a hallmark of neocortex expansion. *Curr Biol* 30: 4227–4237 e4225.

Stumpff, J. et al. (2012). Kif18A and chromokinesins confine centromere movements via microtubule growth suppression and spatial control of kinetochore tension. *Dev Cell* 22: 1017–1029.

Sudmant, P.H. et al. (2010). Diversity of human copy number variation and multicopy genes. *Science* 330: 641–646.

Sun, W. et al. (2010). TKTL1 is activated by promoter hypomethylation and contributes to head and neck squamous cell carcinoma carcinogenesis through increased aerobic glycolysis and HIF1alpha stabilization. *Clin Cancer Res* 16: 857–866.

Suzuki, I.K. et al. (2018). Human-specific *NOTCH2NL* genes expand cortical neurogenesis through Delta/Notch regulation. *Cell* 173: 1370–1384 e1316.

Taverna, E. et al. (2014). The cell biology of neurogenesis. *Ann Rev Cell Dev Biol* 30: 465–502.

Taverna, E. and Huttner, W.B. (2010). Neural progenitor nuclei IN motion. *Neuron* 67: 906–914.

Taylor, M.D. et al. (2005). Radial glia cells are candidate stem cells of ependymoma. *Cancer Cell* 8: 323–335.

Thein, K.H. et al. (2007). Astrin is required for the maintenance of sister chromatid cohesion and centrosome integrity. *J Cell Biol* 178: 345–354.

Trujillo, C.A. et al. (2021). Reintroduction of the archaic variant of *NOVA1* in cortical organoids alters neurodevelopment. *Science* 371: eaax2537.

Tyler, W.A. and Haydar, T.F. (2013). Multiplex genetic fate mapping reveals a novel route of neocortical neurogenesis, which is altered in the Ts65Dn mouse model of Down syndrome. *J Neurosci* 33: 5106–5119.

Vann, S.D. and Albasser, M.M. (2011). Hippocampus and neocortex: recognition and spatial memory. *Curr Opin Neurobiol* 21: 440–445.

Wang, R. et al. (2020). Adult human glioblastomas harbor radial glia-like cells. *Stem Cell Rep* 15: 275–277.

Wang, X. et al. (2011). A new subtype of progenitor cell in the mouse embryonic neocortex. *Nat Neurosci* 14: 555–561.

Xie, Z. et al. (2016). Inborn errors of long-chain fatty acid beta-oxidation link neural stem cell self-renewal to autism. *Cell Reports* 14: 991–999.

Xing, L. and Huttner, W.B. (2020). Neurotransmitters as modulators of neura progenitor cell proliferation during mammalian neocortex development. *Front Cell Dev Biol* 8: 391.

Xing, L. et al. (2020). Serotonin receptor 2A activation promotes evolutionarily relevant basal progenitor proliferation in the developing neocortex. *Neuron* 108: 1113–1129 e1116.

Xing, L. et al. (2021a). Expression of human-specific *ARHGAP11B* in mice leads to neocortex expansion and increased memory flexibility. *EMBO J* 40: e107093.

Xing, L. et al. (2021b). How neural stem cells contribute to neocortex development. *Biochem Soc Trans* 49 (5): 1997–2006.

Yang, L. et al. (2017). Glutaminolysis: a hallmark of cancer metabolism. *Ann Rev Biomed Eng* 19: 163–194.

Yuan, W. et al. (2010). Silencing of TKTL1 by siRNA inhibits proliferation of human gastric cancer cells in vitro and in vivo. *Cancer Biol Ther* 9: 710–716.

Zanin, E. et al. (2013). A conserved RhoGAP limits M phase contractility and coordinates with microtubule asters to confine RhoA during cytokinesis. *Dev Cell* 26: 496–510.

Zhang, G. et al. (2017). Bub1 positions Mad1 close to KNL1 MELT repeats to promote checkpoint signalling. *Nat Commun* 8: 15822.

Part 2

Progenitor Lineages

9

Temporal Scaling: A Link between Conserved Neurogenic Processes and Differential Size in Mammalian Cortical Development

Quan Wu, Merve Bilgic, and Fumio Matsuzaki

RIKEN Center for Biosystems Dynamics Research, 2-2-3 Minatojima-Minamimachi, Chuo-ku, Kobe 650-0047, Japan

9.1 Conserved Fundamental Processes of the Cortical Development

The size and complexity of mammalian brains are highly variable depending on species, from small smooth brains to large folded brains (Cárdenas and Borrell 2020). The size difference reaches the order of 10^3 when compared mice and elephants. Even across such a huge diversity of scale, basic processes are conserved across mammalian cortical neurogenesis; neuroepithelia initially expand by the proliferation of neuroepithelial cells via symmetric divisions (Götz and Huttner 2005). Those cells become multipotent neural stem cells (NSC), known as radial glial cells (RGCs; Miyata et al. 2001; Noctor et al. 2001; Tamamaki et al. 2001). RGCs subsequently undergo a transition into asymmetric division mode to generate neurons or differentiated progenitors (termed intermediate progenitor cells (IPCs; Haubensak et al. 2004; Miyata et al. 2004; Noctor et al. 2004). In mice, RGCs directly generate postmitotic immature neurons during early neurogenesis. This direct neurogenesis shift to indirect neurogenesis is where RGCs successively produce mitotic active IPC, which mostly divide once to generate a pair of neurons. Interestingly, doubling of neurons by indirect neurogenesis from a RGC division is a widely used strategy from insects (ganglion mother cells) to vertebrates (IPC), while the cell lineage of RGCs is diversified in gyrencephalic mammals for further amplification of a NSC clone size as described later.

RGC progressively generate neurons in the deep layers (DL), then upper layers (UL), and finally generate glial cells (Rowitch and Kriegstein 2010). During this process, RGC division occurs at the ventricular zone (VZ), and IPC divide into neurons in the subventricular zone (SVZ). Neurons accumulate in the six-layered cortical plate from the deep layers to upper layers in an inside-out manner (Figure 9.1). A consensus is that a fundamental gene network is conserved across mammalian species to control these common processes.

9.2 The Formation of the Variety in Neural Stem Cells Promoting the Expansion of Brain Size in Evolution

9.2.1 Formation of New Germinal Zone during Corticogenesis

In the past decade, there has been rapid progress in understanding the development of brains with expanded cortical sizes and high complexity such as those of primates including humans

Neocortical Neurogenesis in Development and Evolution, First Edition. Edited by Wieland B. Huttner.

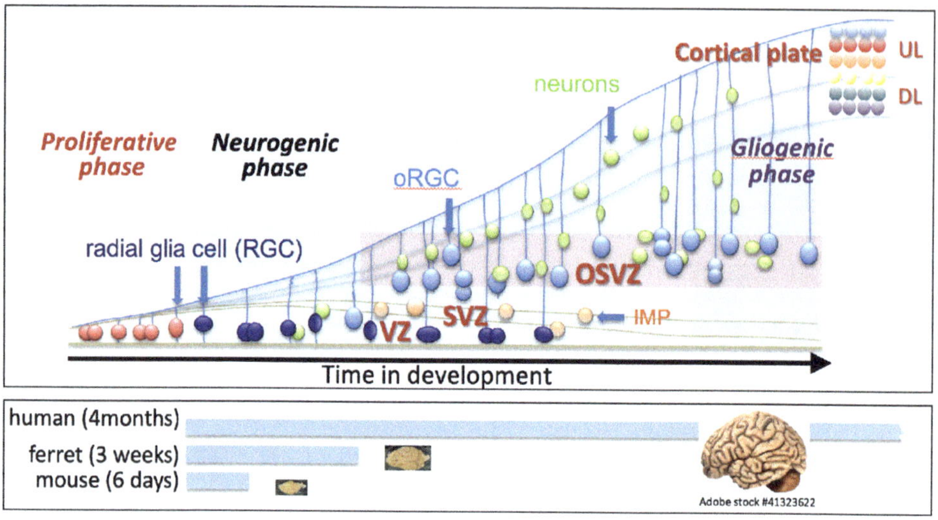

Figure 9.1 Mammalian cortical development.

and also of ferrets belonging to *Carnivora*, a gyrencephalic mammalian species. In the majority of gyrencephalic species, if not all, the SVZ expands during cortical development to form a new germinal zone termed the outer subventricular zone (OSVZ) (Smart et al. 2002). The expanded cortical size of those species has been largely attributed to the emergence of the OSVZ. This germinal zone contains outer RGC (oRGC) that are also termed basal RGC (bRGC), which lacks the apical attachment (Fietz et al. 2010; Hansen et al. 2010; Reillo et al. 2011). Whereas a similar type of RGC lacking the apical endfoot emerges even in lissencephalic species such as mice (Konno et al. 2008; Shitamukai et al. 2011; Wang et al. 2011), they do not necessarily form a germinal zone or contribute to an increase in the neuronal population. In contrast, the OSVZ grows significantly in most gyrencephalic species, presumably by an enhanced proliferative division of oRGCs and their progeny, leading to the amplification of neuronal and glial populations in the cortex (Rash et al. 2019).

9.2.2 Evolutional Implication of the OSVZ and Gyrification

The cerebral cortices develop the OSVZ in many phylogenic trajectories, in parallel, during mammalian evolution. Considering this and the presence of oRG-like cells in lissencephalic species, the ancestor of mammals likely possessed the potential to form oRG-like cells rather than convergence. Additional evolutional changes in gene expression of oRGCs and other cells must have been required to impact the nature of oRGCs themselves and the environments surrounding those cells that were acting as stem cell niche in mammalian species, which led to a drastic expansion of brain size and complexity (Fietz et al. 2012; Long and Huttner 2022). We also note that gyrencephaly has also evolved in many phylogenic branches from Echidna of monotremes to primates, suggesting that the ancestoral mammals also possessed the potential for gyrification. Generally, the larger the cortical size, the more folded the cortex. Several studies suggest that gyrification occurs when the two layers with different tensions (or extensibility) are tightly apposed, just like the white matter and gray matter of the cerebral cortex (Greiner et al. 2021) or the superficial neural layers and deep neural layers (Tallinen et al. 2014). Because neurons born in the OSVZ contribute to the expansion of the superficial neuronal layers, the development of the OSVZ might enhance the difference in the neuron number between the superficial layers and deep layers. This may lead to differential tensions of these two parts of the cortical layer, resulting in the formation of the deeper gyri.

9.3 Variety of Progenitor Cells in the VZ

9.3.1 Truncated RGC is a Progenitor Subtype across Species

A new subtype of neural progenitor cells in the VZ, instead of in the OSVZ, has been reported in humans and rhesus macaques (DeAzevedo et al. 2003; Nowakowski et al. 2016, 2016; Sidman and Rakic 1973). Those cells, due to the absence of a long basal process, are termed truncated RG (tRG). We found that the same cell type is present from the late neurogenic to early gliogenic stage in ferrets by a series of single cell transcriptomes of ferret progenitor cells (Bilgic et al. 2022). Our pseudo-time trajectory and histochemical analyses indicate that the descendants of tRG are fated to either ependymal cells or astroglia cells and suggest that this is the case for humans. Preliminary results in the investigation of the mechanisms that underlie the formation of tRG suggest that apical RGC generate their sibling cells maintaining the apical endfoot, and undergo asymmetric divisions, which produce a daughter that apically attaches, leading to be a tRG that expresses Cryab, a marker of tRG (Nowakowski et al. 2016). In mice, we do not observe tRG in the dorsal cortex. Indeed, the ependymal layer is not formed in this region, the ventricular surface of this area is fused with that of the ventral side, resulting in the disappearance of a ventricle in the adult stage, which is distinct from gyrencephalic species.

9.3.2 A Novel IPC Subtype Undergoing Interkinetic Nuclear Migration

In ferret neurogenesis, the RGC sibling cells remaining at the apical surface, as described earlier, are frequently observed throughout neurogenesis (Tsunekawa et al. pers. comm.). These cells have a short basal process that progressively extends but does not reach the cortical layer, which is in contrast to the apical RGC. Those RGC siblings surprisingly express Hes1/Hes5, major transcription factors downstream of Notch signaling for self-renewal, and consistently undergo interkinetic nuclear migration during cell cycling just like the sister RGCs. We, therefore, tentatively named this type of progenitors short RGC (sRGC). However, their mitotic activity is limited and those cells give rise to neurons directly or migrating IPC after one or two cell cycles (none or very few sRGC go through three cell cycles) and also produce tRG at the later neurogenic stage by asymmetric division, as described earlier. In mice, although short neural precursors (SNP) were identified (Gal et al. 2006), they are different from those identified as sRGC in ferrets. As far as has been examined, SNP are committed IPC that are still attached to the apical surface, and neither express Hes1/Hes5 nor undergo an interkinetic nuclear migration. Therefore, sRGC are not SNP but a subtype of intermediate progenitors with a partial stem cell property.

9.3.3 Enormous Heterogeneity of Cell Lineages of RGC in the Presence sRGC

In the mid-neurogenesis of ferret cortex, the population of short RGC is not small (approximately up to 30% in ferrets), and in time-lapse imaging of ferret cortical slices in culture they appear to emerge randomly in a RGC lineage, causing the RGC lineages high diversity (Tsunekawa et al. pers. comm.), in contrast to the stereotyped division pattern of lissencephalic rodent RGC.

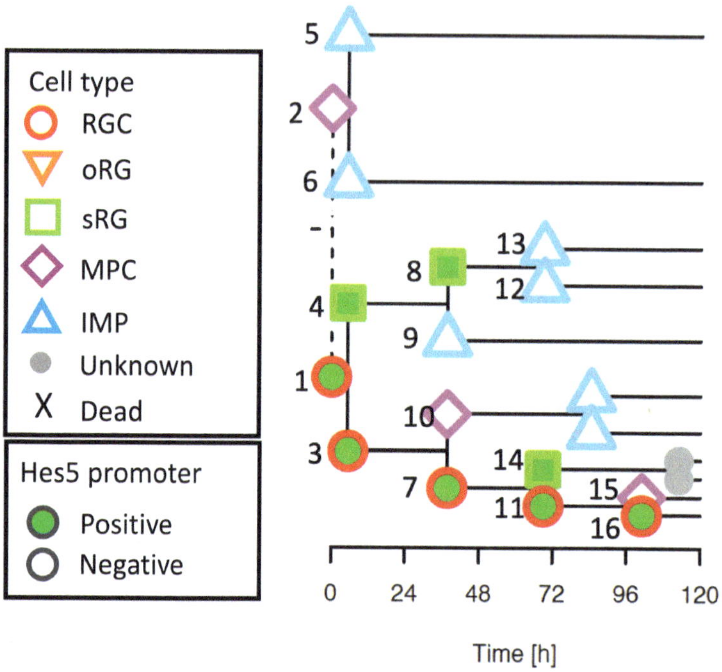

Figure 9.2 An example of division pattern of ferret aRGC. Cell division patterns were obtained by time-lapse imaging of slice-cultured ferret developing neocortex. Notch activity was monitored by its Hes5 reporter. MPC is the multipolar progenitor cell.

Because the presence of this type of IPC in the VZ contributes to an increase in neurons, this might be identifiable as a peculiar characteristic of mammalian species with an expanded cortex. This hypothesis needs to be tested in other mammalian species with a large brain such as humans.

9.4 Temporal Scaling of Brain Development

9.4.1 Time Course of Cortical Development Scales

As described above, processes that form the cerebral cortex organization of the six neuronal layers are conserved across mammalian species, whereas mammals have evolved mechanisms expanding neuronal populations (via an increase in both RGC population and in individual clone sizes), leading to an explosive expansion of the cortical size. These dual aspects of mammalian cerebral cortices must be coordinated during corticogenesis to form neuronal circuits that perform highly complex tasks as in human beings. One important mechanism of this coordination would be an extension of the developmental period of the cerebral cortex. Indeed, it has been shown that an extension in the neurogenic period leads to an increase in RGC clone size (Stepien et al. 2020). However, the temporal extension of corticogenesis is not just an extension of the period but needs to be coordinated with the gene regulatory network (GRN) that controls the temporal pattern of RGC and sequential birth of diverse neurons. This requires scaling mechanisms for gene expression and temporal sequences of birth and the differentiation of diverse progenitor cells (see Figure 9.3).

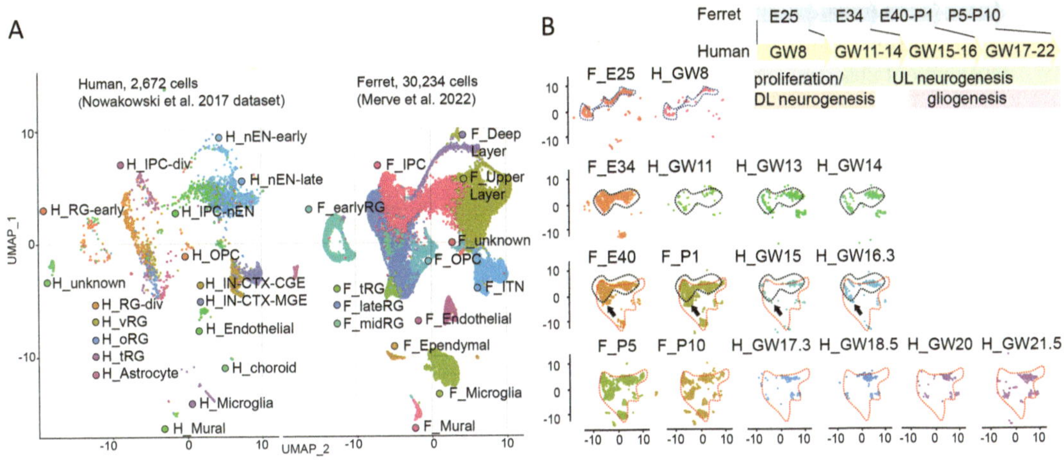

Figure 9.3 Comparison of temporal pattern of progenitor populations. (A) A developmental set of single cell transcriptomes of ferrets and humans (Nowakowski et al. 2017) merged by mutual nearest neighbors followed by canonical correlation analysis. (B) Cell clusters are resolved into individual dates to show that the temporal pattern of progenitor clusters is parallel between species, namely, a scaling mechanism operates. The upper right panel shows corresponding stages of humans and ferrets. H: human; F: ferret. E25 = embryonic day 25. P5 = postnatal day 5. GW13 = gestation week 13. Arrows in [F_E40, and P1 and H_GW15, and 16.3] indicate tRG clusters. After Bilgic et al. (2022).

9.4.2 Mechanisms Underlying Scaling in Developmental Time

The brain is a remarkable example of developmental time scaling associated with a variety of sizes. The developmental time period for cortical neurogenesis varies from species to species, ranging from 1 week in mice, to 3 weeks in ferrets, and 16 weeks in humans. What underlies such extraordinary changes in developmental time scale? A general mechanism that might be involved in developmental time scale is the synthesis and turnover rate of RNAs and proteins. Protein turnover was recently proposed to be associated with differential developmental timing in somitogenesis and motor neuron development (Matsuda et al. 2020; Rayon et al. 2020). However, the protein turnover rate is 2–2.5-fold faster in mouse than in human cells. Thus, it is unlikely that the synthesis and turnover rates of RNA and proteins could alone account for the temporal scaling between human and mouse corticogenesis (approximately more than 10-fold difference), although they could contribute significantly.

9.4.3 Evolution of Gene Regulatory Network and Species-specific Genes

Based on the most orthodox way of considering brain evolution, evolution largely depends on the changes in the regulatory mechanisms of gene expression (Davidson and Erwin 2006). At the genomic level, the emergence of species-specific genes is a typical change that may impact the developmental time scale (Ivakhnitskaia et al. 2016). Recently, many studies have been performed to investigate species-specific changes in the GRN underlying neurogenesis, based on species-specific genes or mutations (Florio et al. 2015; Lui et al. 2014; Namba et al. 2020; Suzuki et al. 2018). PDGFD (platelet-derived growth factor D) is specifically expressed in human RGC although it is not a human specific gene (Florio et al. 2015). NOTCH2NL is a truncated form that was generated in gene duplication and promotes stem cell renewal by an elevated Notch activity via the sis-inhibition of Delta activity (Suzuki et al. 2018). ARHGAP11B is preferentially expressed in non-VZ progenitors and promotes

TCA cycle in mitochondria metabolism (Namba et al. 2020). While these human-specific genes certainly contribute to the expansion of the human cortex, they do not explain the graded scaling of development observed across many species.

9.4.4 Contribution of Epigenetic Control of Gene Regulatory Network

Chromatin remodeling perhaps plays a critical role in temporal scaling because it particularly undergoes dynamic and global changes during cortical neurogenesis (Sanosaka et al. 2017). Transition of NSC from the neurogenic to gliogenic state is regulated by Histone H3 lysine 27 trimethylation (H3K27me3), a repressive histone methylation (Hirabayashi et al. 2009), and DNA methylation (Namihira et al. 2009). Indeed, loci susceptible to H3K27me3 shift, largely over the genome from early to late neurogenesis (Bilgic et al. 2022; Wu et al. 2022), raise their possible indispensable role in temporal scaling of cortical neurogenesis.

9.4.5 Impacts of Metabolism and Mitochondria

Differences in metabolism among species have long been considered to underlie changes in lifespan and growth (Glazier 2015; West et al. 2001), although metabolism's relationship with developmental time scaling remains unclear. Metabolism and mitochondria have recently been found to drive cell-fate decisions in adult stem cells and during embryogenesis including neurogenesis (Iwata et al. 2020; Knobloch et al. 2017; Namba et al. 2020; Pernas and Scorrano 2016; Shyh-Chang et al. 2013). Several groups revealed that mitochondria dynamics directly influence the balance between self-renewal and differentiation of RGC, partly via changes in the oxidative phosphorylation activity (Iwata et al. 2020; Khacho et al. 2016; Namba et al. 2020). Intriguingly, it was recently identified that differences in the rates of mitochondria dynamics and metabolism between mouse vs. human cortical neurons influenced the speed of their maturation (Iwata et al. 2023). This raises the hypothesis that species-specific differences in the mitochondrial metabolism in cortical progenitors influence the temporal scaling of neurogenesis. Metabolism could also control chromatin remodeling; key mitochondrial metabolites operate as rate-limiting substrates or regulators of histone modifications (Ly et al. 2020; Reid et al. 2017), although possible mechanisms remain to be explored.

9.5 Conclusion

Time scale is highly variable depending on species in many biological contexts including developmental duration, heart beats, and lifespan. Whereas the time of biological processes has been long known to scale allometrically (nonlinearly) with the size of organisms and metabolic quantities (West et al. 1997), there is no clear "mechanistic" explanation about how time scales in a biological event. Cortical development is a striking example from 1 week in mice to 15 weeks in humans. Scaling temporal progression is a powerful mechanism that coordinates conserved GRN of corticogenesis and a striking diversity in the cortical size. Here we propose three mechanisms of different layers: epigenetic remodeling, mitochondrial metabolism, and synthesis and turnover of RNA/protein, are major contributors to temporal scaling.

References

Bilgic, M. et al. (2022). Single cell transcriptomics of ferrets reveal a common temporal pattern of progenitors in brain development of gyrencephalic mammals. *BioRxiv*. doi: 10.1101/2022.05.05.490846.

Cárdenas, A. and Borrell, V. (2020). Molecular and cellular evolution of corticogenesis in amniotes. *Cell Mol Life Sci* 77: 1435–1460.

Davidson, E.H. and Erwin, D.H. (2006). Gene regulatory networks and the evolution of animal body plans. *Science* 311: 796–797.

DeAzevedo, L.C. et al. (2003). Cortical radial glial cells in human fetuses. *J Neurobiol* 55: 288–298.

Fietz, S.A. et al. (2010). OSVZ progenitors of human and ferret neocortex are epithelial-like and expand by integrin signaling. *Nat Neurosci* 13: 690–699.

Fietz, S.A. et al. (2012). Transcriptomes of germinal zones of human and mouse fetal neocortex suggest a role of extracellular matrix in progenitor self-renewal. *Proc Natl Acad Sci USA* 109: 11836–11841.

Florio, M. et al. (2015). Human-specific gene ARHGAP11B promotes basal progenitor amplification and neocortex expansion. *Science* 347: 1465–1470.

Gal, J.S. et al. (2006). Molecular and morphological heterogeneity of neural precursors in the mouse neocortical proliferative zones. *J Neurosci* 26: 1045–1056.

Glazier, D.S. (2015). Is metabolic rate a universal "pacemaker" for biological processes? *Biol Rev* 90: 377–407.

Götz, M. and Huttner, W.B. (2005). The cell biology of neurogenesis. *Nat Rev Mol Cell Biol* 6: 777–788.

Greiner, A. et al. (2021). Physical aspects of cortical folding. *Soft Matter* 17: 1210–1222.

Hansen, D.V. et al. (2010). Neurogenic radial glia in the outer subventricular zone of human neocortex. *Nature* 464 (7288): 554–561.

Haubensak, W. et al. (2004). Neurons arise in the basal neuroepithelium of the early mammalian telencephalon: a major site of neurogenesis. *Proc Natl Acad Sci USA* 101 (9): 3196–3201.

Hirabayashi, Y. et al. (2009). Polycomb limits the neurogenic competence of neural precursor cells to promote astrogenic fate transition. *Neuron* 63: 600–613.

Ivakhnitskaia, E. et al. (2016). Timing mechanisms in neuronal pathfinding, synaptic reorganization, and neuronal regeneration. *Dev, Growth Diff* 58: 88–93.

Iwata, R. et al. (2023). Mitochondria metabolism sets the species-specific tempo of neuronal development. *Science* 379 (6632): eabn4705. doi: 10.1126/science.abn4705.

Iwata, R. et al. (2020). Mitochondrial dynamics in postmitotic cells regulate neurogenesis. *Science* 369: 858–862.

Khacho, M. et al. (2016). Mitochondrial dynamics impacts stem cell identity and fate decisions by regulating a nuclear transcriptional program. *Cell Stem Cell* 19: 232–247.

Knobloch, M. et al. (2017). A fatty acid oxidation-dependent metabolic shift regulates adult neural stem cell activity. *Cell Reports* 20: 2144–2155.

Konno, D. et al. (2008). Neuroepithelial progenitors undergo LGN-dependent planar divisions to maintain self-renewability during mammalian neurogenesis. *Nat Cell Biol* 10: 93–101.

Long, K.R. and Huttner, W.B. (2022). The role of the extracellular matrix in neural progenitor cell proliferation and cortical folding during human neocortex development. *Front Cell Neurosci* 15: 804649.

Lui, J.H. et al. (2014). Radial glia require PDGFD-PDGFRβ signalling in human but not mouse neocortex. *Nature* 515: 264–268.

Ly, C.H. et al. (2020). A metabolic roadmap for somatic stem cell fate. *Cell Metab* 31: 1052–1067.

Matsuda, M. et al. (2020). Recapitulating the human segmentation clock with pluripotent stem cells. *Nature* 580: 124–129.

Miyata, T. et al. (2001). Asymmetric inheritance of radial glial fibers by cortical neurons. *Neuron* 31: 727–741.

Miyata, T. et al. (2004). Asymmetric production of surface-dividing and non-surface-dividing cortical progenitor cells. *Development* 131: 3133–3145.

Namba, T. et al. (2020). Human-specific ARHGAP11B acts in mitochondria to expand neocortical progenitors by glutaminolysis. *Neuron* 105: 867–881.e9.

Namihira, M. et al. (2009). Committed neuronal precursors confer astrocytic potential on residual neural precursor cells. *Dev Cell* 16: 245–255.

Noctor, S.C. et al. (2001). Neurons derived from radial glial cells establish radial units in neocortex. *Nature* 409: 714–720.

Noctor, S.C. et al. (2004). Cortical neurons arise in symmetric and asymmetric division zones and migrate through specific phases. *Nature Neuroscience* 7: 136–144.

Nowakowski, T.J. et al. (2017). Spatiotemporal gene expression trajectories reveal developmental hierarchies of the human cortex. *Science* 358: 1318–1323.

Nowakowski, T.J. et al. (2016). Transformation of the radial glia scaffold demarcates two stages of human cerebral cortex development. *Neuron* 91: 1219–1227.

Pernas, L. and Scorrano, L. (2016). Mito-morphosis. *Ann Rev Physiol* 78: 505–531.

Rash, B.G. et al. (2019). Gliogenesis in the outer subventricular zone promotes enlargement and gyrification of the primate cerebrum. *Proc Natl Acad Sci USA* 116: 7089–7094.

Rayon, T. et al. (2020). Species-specific pace of development is associated with differences in protein stability. *Science* 369: eaba7667.

Reid, M.A. et al. (2017). The impact of cellular metabolism on chromatin dynamics and epigenetics. *Nat Cell Biol* 19: 1298.

Reillo, I. et al. (2011). A role for intermediate radial glia in the tangential expansion of the mammalian cerebral cortex. *Cereb Cortex* 21: 1674–1694.

Rowitch, D.H. and Kriegstein, A.R. (2010). Developmental genetics of vertebrate glial-cell specification. *Nature* 468: 214–222.

Sanosaka, T. et al. (2017). DNA methylome analysis identifies transcription factor-based epigenomic signatures of multilineage competence in neural stem/progenitor cells. *Cell Rep* 20: 2992–3003.

Shitamukai, A. et al. (2011). Oblique radial glial divisions in the developing mouse neocortex induce self-renewing progenitors outside the germinal zone that resemble primate outer subventricular zone progenitors. *J Neurosci* 31: 3683–3695.

Shyh-Chang, N. et al. (2013). Stem cell metabolism in tissue development and aging. *Development* 140: 2535–2547.

Sidman, R.L. and Rakic, P. (1973). Neuronal migration, with special reference to developing human brain: a review. *Brain Res* 62: 1–35.

Smart, I.H.M. et al. (2002). Unique morphological features of the proliferative zones and postmitotic compartments of the neural epithelium giving rise to striate and extrastriate cortex in the Monkey. *Cereb Cortex* 12: 37–53.

Stepien, B.K. et al. (2020). Lengthening neurogenic period during neocortical development causes a hallmark of neocortex expansion. *Curr Biol* 30: 4227–4237.e5.

Suzuki, I.K. et al. (2018). Human-specific NOTCH2NL genes expand cortical neurogenesis through Delta/Notch regulation. *Cell* 173: 1370–1384.e16.

Tallinen, T. et al. (2014). Gyrification from constrained cortical expansion. *Proc Natl Acad Sci USA* 111: 12667–12672.

Tamamaki, N. et al. (2001). Radial glia is a progenitor of neocortical neurons in the developing cerebral cortex. *Neurosci Res* 41: 51–60.

Wang, X. et al. (2011). A new subtype of progenitor cell in the mouse embryonic neocortex. *Nat Neurosci* 14: 555–562.

West, G.B. et al. (1997). A general model for the origin of allometric scaling laws in biology. *Science* 276: 122–126.

West, G.B. et al. (2001). A general model for ontogenetic growth. *Nature* 413 (6856): 628–631.

Wu, Q. et al. (2022). Selective translation of epigenetic modifiers affects the temporal pattern and differentiation of neural stem cells. *Nat Commun* 13 (1): 1–18.

10

Interplay of Cell-autonomous Gene Function and Tissue-wide Mechanisms Regulating Radial Glial Progenitor Lineage Progression

Ana Villalba[1,], Nicole Amberg[1,*], and Simon Hippenmeyer[1,#]*

[1] *Institute of Science and Technology Austria, Am Campus 1, Klosterneuburg 3400, Austria*
* *Both authors equally contributed*
# *Corresponding author*

10.1 Introduction

10.1.1 Cortical Development

The mammalian brain stands as, by far, the most complex biological structure. In particular, the cerebral cortex has evolved into a critical structure for cognitive and behavioral brain functions. To give rise to a correctly sized cerebral cortex, coordinated production of a vast number of cell types and molecular scaffolds with a fine cooperative regulation is necessary. In a precise temporal manner, cortical progenitor cells will generate all excitatory projection neurons and glial cell types of the neocortex. The underlying developmental stages are known as neurogenesis and gliogenesis, respectively (Figure 10.1A–C).

Cortical development starts from a limited number of neuroepithelial stem cells (NECs), which self-amplify and subsequently transit to apical radial glial progenitor cells (aRGPs) (Taverna et al. 2014). aRGPs are highly polarized progenitor cells located in the ventricular zone (VZ), with a short apical process attached to the ventricular surface and a long basal process that extends until the basal lamina (Sidman and Rakic 1973). At the initiation of neurogenesis, most aRGPs divide in a self-amplifying mode while a modest number directly produce a small proportion of neurons (Florio and Huttner 2014; Haubensak et al. 2004). As development proceeds, the asymmetric division rate increases, with aRGPs directly giving rise to either new-born neurons in a defined sequential manner or secondary progenitors such as intermediate progenitors (IPs) or basal radial glial progenitor cells (bRGPs) (Malatesta et al. 2003; Miyata et al. 2004). Secondary progenitors migrate radially, populate the subventricular zone (SVZ) and provide an additional amplification step to increase the final neuronal output (Miyata et al. 2004; Noctor et al. 2004, 2008). Newly generated neurons migrate radially along the basal processes and form the cortical plate (CP) (Ayala et al. 2007; Evsyukova et al. 2013; Valiente and Marin 2010). Within the CP, neurons organize in an inside-out manner, meaning that later generated neurons will pass through previously formed and already mature neurons in the CP to settle down in upper layers (Noctor et al. 2004; Rakic 1974). Radial glial progenitor (RGP) lineage (i.e., the whole progeny of a single progenitor cell) progression seems highly determined and thus predictable. Recent clonal RGP lineage tracing experiments have revealed that murine aRGPs produce a unitary output of about eight to nine neurons

Neocortical Neurogenesis in Development and Evolution, First Edition. Edited by Wieland B. Huttner.

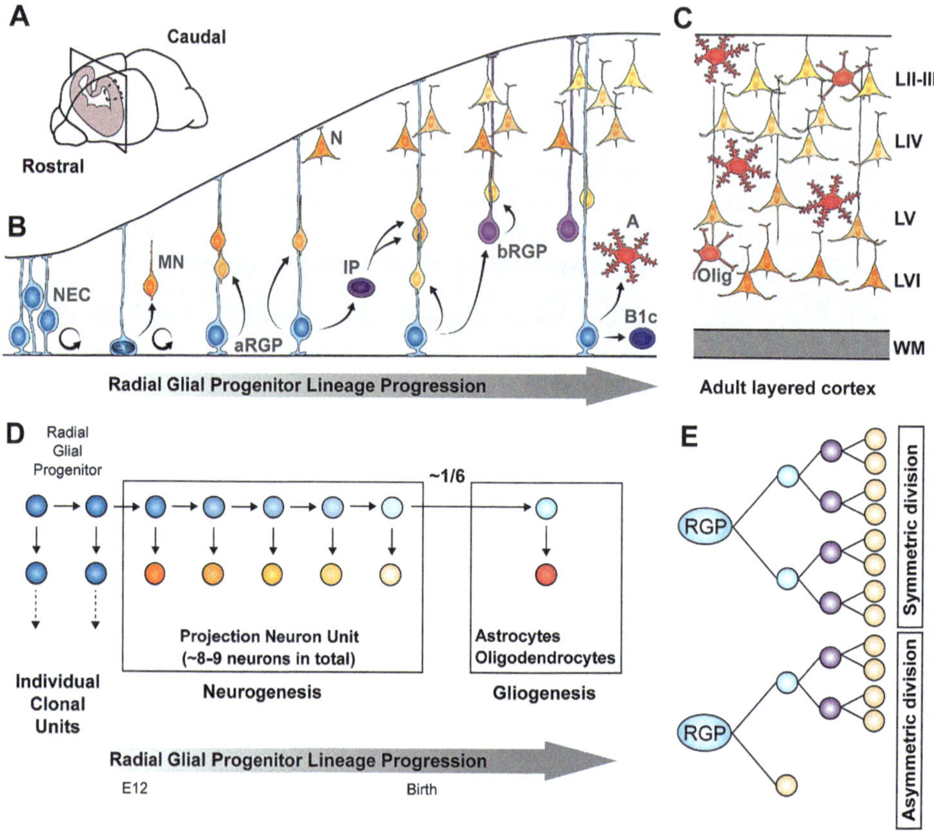

Figure 10.1 The quantitative framework of cortical development. (A) Schematic illustration of the mammalian embryonic forebrain with a coronal section of the telencephalon. (B) Schematic summary of mammalian cortical development through apical radial glial progenitor cell (aRGP) lineage progression from cortical primordium to gliogenesis and early adult neural stem cell production. (C) Illustration of adult layered cortex. (D) Deterministic RGP behavior during cortical development gives rise to an eight to nine neuronal unitary output and one out of six generates glia. (E) Schematic illustration of RGPs division patterns: symmetric division and asymmetric division. Light blue cell, neural stem cell (NEC) and apical radial glial progenitor (aRGP); dark blue cell, type B1 progenitor cell (B1c); purple cells, secondary progenitors, dark purple, intermediate progenitor (IP); light purple, basal radial glial progenitor (bRGP); orange cells, migrating (MN) and mature neurons (N); dark pink, glial cells, astrocytes (A) or oligodendrocytes (Olig); orange gradient indicates different neuronal cell types.

before one out of six aRGPs switch to glia production (Beattie and Hippenmeyer 2017; Gao et al. 2014) (Figure 10.1D). Although RGP lineage progression appears to be highly sequential and predictable in murine cerebral cortex, some stochastic factors might control neuronal output too and cannot be ruled out (Llorca et al. 2019).

Cortical stem and progenitor cells divide either symmetrically or asymmetrically. In the first case, the progeny will possess the same identity, while asymmetric divisions give rise to two distinct types of cells (Figures 10.1E and 10.3A). Each division can either self-renew the progenitor cell or consume it, independently of the division mode. In self-renewing divisions, at least one of the daughter cells will maintain progenitor cell identity. In consumptive divisions, both daughter cells are distinctly different to the mother stem cell. Consequently, four possible combinations of cell division may occur: asymmetric self-renewing, asymmetric consumptive, symmetric proliferative, or symmetric consumptive (Fernandez et al. 2016; Gotz and Huttner 2005; Llinares-Benadero and Borrell 2019; Taverna et al. 2014).

Deviations from the standard cell division modes during development generate profound abnormalities in the mature neocortex, such as microcephaly or megalencephaly (Sun and Hevner 2014). In addition, along evolution, slight changes in the principles of lineage progression may imply evolutionary cellular and tissue-wide differences between species (Cardenas et al. 2018; Florio et al. 2015). Thus, with regards to the neocortex and neurogenesis, an exquisite orchestration of multiple molecular pathways and signals need to be tightly regulated in order to regulate correct lineage progression and cortex formation. Although the above inaugural quantitative framework has been established at single cell level in mice, the precise cellular and molecular mechanisms underlying faithful and orderly aRGP lineage progression are still not well understood and are still under investigation. The proliferative behavior of individual aRGPs is subject to multiple parameters and layers of regulation, determining fate decisions and thus their final cellular output. Developmental instructions comprise not only intrinsic signaling pathways to orchestrate their individual proliferative activity but also extracellular signals that may affect global tissue behavior (Figure 10.2). To address experimentally how aRGP lineage progression is regulated one may directly study an isolated progenitor in culture systems. However, such an experimental design would lack all the extracellular and systemic signals to which the progenitor cells are exposed in an intact tissue. Thus, in vivo approaches and animal models confer a complete system that allow the assessment of aRGPs in their natural environment. However, the presence of extracellular and systemic signals also involves a higher level of complexity for the interpretation of experimental results.

10.1.2 Cell-autonomous Gene Function vs. Tissue-wide Regulation of RGP Lineage Progression

As the source for all cortical excitatory projection neurons, aRGPs are the prime target of regulatory signals that may come from a variety of sources (close or distant from the targeted cells). Extrinsic factors comprise diverse components and range from highly systemic to rather locally restricted signals (Figure 10.2).

The brain is equipped with an intricate vasculature system that supplies the developing brain tissue with oxygen; systemic signals (such as environmental components, signaling molecules, hormonal and nutritional supplies) and immune cells. The endothelial blood brain barrier (BBB) constrains the access of a wide range of metabolically important molecules to the brain. Angiogenesis and neurogenesis take place simultaneously to ensure proper coverage of oxygen and other molecules for the developing brain (Figure 10.2B) (Vogenstahl et al. 2022). As such, the vascular system provides an entangled connection between systemic and local cues by establishing the supply of further blood-derived factors as the brain grows (Kadry et al. 2020; Rash et al. 2018). Indeed, as an example, maternal hyperglycemia can interfere with aRGPs behavior by altering intracellular calcium signaling, impairing mitochondrial transport and thus, leading to disruption of the basal processes extended from aRGPs (Rash et al. 2018). The BBB is directly connected to cerebrospinal fluid homeostasis (CSF) due to the choroid plexus barrier, and thus, also takes a central part in the regulation of neurogenesis via CSF-derived factors (Bueno and Garcia-Fernàndez 2016; Kadry et al. 2020). The CSF is a protein-rich fluid that fills the brain cavities and ventricles. Thus, CSF-derived factors are in intimate contact with cells lining the ventricular surface and exert an important function in regulating aRGP behavior (Figure 10.2B). Some components present in the CSF are well known regulators of neurogenesis such as sonic hedgehog, insulin-like growth

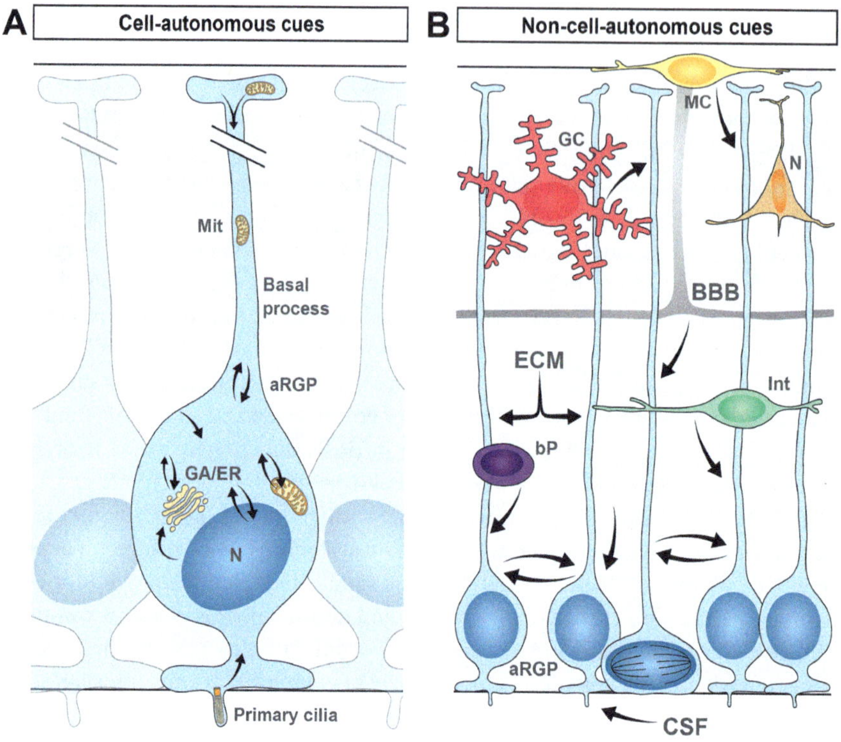

Figure 10.2 Comparative extrinsic and intrinsic cues affecting aRGPs during cortical development. (A) Cell-autonomous cues. Within individual progenitor cells, different pathways cell-autonomously regulate aRGP self-amplification, cell cycle length, division mode, and fate involving cellular compartments as basal process signaling to the process and to the soma, plasma-membrane signaling to cytoplasm, Golgi and endoplasmic reticulum signaling from the nucleus to/from cytoplasm, mitochondrial communication to/from cytoplasm, nuclear signaling to/from cytoplasm and signals coming from the primary cilium. (B) Non-cell-autonomous cues. Tissue-wide effects may come from wide and different distal sources (as BBB or CSF) and/or close direct interactions (ECM or cell–cell contacts). Light blue cell, apical radial glial progenitor (aRGP); yellow cell, meningeal cell (MC); dark pink, glial cells (GC); orange cell, migrating and mature neurons (N); turquoise cell, interneuron (Int); purple cell, secondary or basal progenitor (bP); gray vasculature; mitochondria (Mit); Golgi apparatus or endoplasmic reticulum (GA/ER); blood brain barrier (BBB); extracellular matrix (ECM); cerebrospinal fluid (CSF). Black arrows indicate source/target and directionality of the signaling.

factor, fibroblast growth factor-2, Wnt signaling, slit proteins and retinoic acid (Borrell et al. 2012; Bueno and Garcia-Fernàndez 2016; Huang et al. 2010; Johansson et al. 2013; Lehtinen and Walsh 2011; Lehtinen et al. 2011; Martín et al. 2006; Raballo et al. 2000). Both, the vascular system and CSF allow signaling molecules to reach distal targets in a systemic manner by widely affecting the entire tissue. They can however also act locally with a region-specific distribution and thereby establish regional signaling gradients (Cavanagh et al. 1983; Zappaterra et al. 2007).

Diffusible factors derived from the BBB and the CSF, as well as directly released from neural cells present in the developing cortex, disseminate through a macromolecular network, the extracellular matrix (ECM), until they reach their final target. Thus, the ECM can act as a mesh that helps to generate a signaling gradient from the source to the targets by generating microenvironments that differently affect progenitor cell behavior. In addition, ECM molecules can influence progenitor cell proliferation, differentiation and migration by direct contact (Figure 10.2B) (Long and Huttner 2019). It is of note, that the ECM has been highly related with evolutionary cortical expansion (Fietz et al. 2012; Florio et al. 2015; Pollen et al. 2015).

aRGP proliferative behavior can be shaped by signals from neighboring cells in a directed manner as well. Cell–cell interactions represent a rather local type of extrinsic cue within growing tissues. The interactions may be direct via physical cell-cell contact (e.g., cell adhesion molecules, Notch signaling, or Gap junctions) or indirect via soluble signaling molecules, such as growth factors or morphogens (Ferent et al. 2020). Extrinsic cues influencing RGP lineage progression (Figure 10.2B) may be generated by other apical progenitors (Rash et al. 2016; Vitali et al. 2018; Weissman et al. 2004) but also from secondary progenitors (Nelson et al. 2013), neurons (Dehay et al. 1996; LoTurco et al. 1995; Seuntjens et al. 2009), Cajal–Retzius cells (Lakomá et al. 2011) and meningeal cells (Siegenthaler et al. 2009). Further invasion by other cellular lineages, such as interneurons (Silva et al. 2018), microglia (Ueno and Yamashita 2014), and vascular cells (Nie et al. 2010; Segarra et al. 2018) contributes to an increasingly complex cellular landscape within the developing cortex.

Within the neocortex, individual aRGPs in vivo are embedded within the neocortical ventricular stem cell niche and thus operate in a complex cellular environment. Individual aRGPs are exposed to all of the above listed extrinsic signals at the same time and need to consequently integrate them for faithful execution of proper developmental programs. Beyond all the extrinsic cues, multiple intrinsic signals also affect aRGP behavior and fate, and thus, cortical neurogenesis (Figure 10.2A). Several intracellular pathways regulate aRGP self-amplification, cell cycle length, division mode, and fate, leading to a precise control of lineage progression (Betizeau et al. 2013; Pilz et al. 2013; Taverna et al. 2014; Turrero Garcia et al. 2016). Among others, certain transcription factors (as Hes1, Pax6, Foxg1, Sox9, and Trnp1) and diverse signaling cascades (as Notch, Shh, or Wnt pathways) have been extensively related to aRGP intrinsic behavior regulation (Villalba et al. 2021). In conclusion, cells are exposed to a variety of cues, which may be equated as non-cell-autonomous (extrinsic) and cell-autonomous (intrinsic) contributors to cortical neurogenesis (Figure 10.2). Upon precise dissection of cell-autonomous gene function or non-cell-autonomous mechanisms, we will gain a detailed understanding of the cellular and molecular mechanisms controlling cortical development.

To study tissue development and more precisely, a gene function, two main experimental approaches exist: gain-of-function (i.e., over-expression) or loss-of-function (i.e., knockdown and knockout) of the gene. The latter allows the observation of an effect (phenotype) based on gene deletion and permits the inference of gene function. However, the gene may exert a cell-autonomous or tissue-wide function, for example, secreted molecules being either absent or over-expressed. Cell-autonomous gene function is defined as a genetic condition in which a phenotype is detected within an individual cell harboring a genetic alteration of a particular gene of interest.

Genetic mosaic tissues can arise naturally from a somatic mutation, (i.e., a spontaneous mutation in a non-germ cell and inherited by its cellular progeny). Alternatively, cell-autonomous phenotypes can be studied obtaining a sparse knockout (KO) scenario whereby the mutant cells are surrounded by genotypically different cells (i.e., mosaic tissue). By this approach, even essential genes can be manipulated without inducing lethality enabling their study. Generating genetic sparse KO (mosaics tissues) as experimental paradigms also has the advantage of direct comparisons between mutant and non-mutant cells within the same tissue (Contreras et al. 2021). Conversely, a tissue-wide effect corresponds to a trait in which genotypically mutant cells promote other cells to present a mutant phenotype regardless of their genotype. As previously described, a phenotype might be triggered by diverse sources as BBB, CSF, ECM, and other cell types in different manners. The observed phenotype in an individual cell in conditional (cKO) or full knockout (KO) most often reflect a combination of both cell-autonomous gene function and environment-derived cues that may remedy or exacerbate any observed phenotype. It is thus important in genetic loss-of-function paradigms to qualitatively and quantitatively determine the relative contributions of the intrinsic and extrinsic components to the overall loss-of-function phenotype.

Currently, most studies utilize experimental paradigms with global and/or whole tissue-wide loss of gene function, where the analysis of RGP lineage progression lacks single cell resolution. Consequently, whether global tissue-wide mechanisms shape the cell-autonomous requirement or function of key regulators in individual aRGPs is mostly unclear. To overcome this limitation, progenitor cells need to be sparsely labeled and genetically modified in a stable and permanent manner. In the most optimal case, the entire progeny of the stem cell will maintain the label after several rounds of division and the reporter construct integrates into the genome, that is, expression of a fluorescent protein. To this end, numerous genetic approaches have been developed to pursue high-resolution lineage tracing in vivo (Buckingham and Meilhac 2011; Dumas et al. 2022; Kretzschmar and Watt 2012; Woodworth et al. 2017) like Brainbow (Loulier et al. 2014), CloNe (García-Moreno et al. 2014), or Star Track (Garcia-Marques and López-Mascaraque 2013). On top of labeling an individual cell, the study of a gene function also requires genetic manipulation, such as gene KO, on the single cell level. The visualization and manipulation of genetically defined cells at single cell resolution enables detangling the precise progenitor division pattern and mapping the whole lineage of cells produced by an individual progenitor (Figures 10.1D and 10.3A). Combining lineage tracing with genetic manipulation of individual cells provides also a powerful insight into cell-autonomous phenotypes. By contrasting sparse gene deletion with tissue-wide KO paradigms, scientists can assess the cell-autonomous and non-cell-autonomous mechanisms underlying faithful RGP lineage progression. The genetic tool Mosaic Analysis with Double Markers (MADM) is a unique genetic technique used in mice allowing for fluorescent labelling with concomitant genetic manipulation at the single cell level without the requirement of additional surgical manipulation of the embryos (Figure 10.3) (Contreras et al. 2021; Zong et al. 2005).

10.1.3 The MADM Principle

MADM relies on Cre/loxP-dependent interchromosomal recombination to generate differentially labeled wild-type (WT) and mutant cells in an otherwise heterozygous background in mice. For MADM, two reciprocally chimeric marker genes are targeted separately to identical loci on homologous chromosomes. The chimeric marker genes (GT and TG alleles) consist of partial coding sequences for green fluorescent protein (GFP[G]) and tandem dimer Tomato (tdT[T],) separated by an intron containing a LoxP site. Following Cre recombinase-mediated interchromosomal recombination during mitosis, functional green and red fluorescent proteins are reconstituted. Depending on the cell division mode, distinct color-labelled cells are generated: recombination in G2 of the cell cycle followed by X segregation (G2-X events) results in one red and one green labelled daughter cell. Interchromosomal recombination followed by G2-Z events, or during G1 or G0 results in one double-labelled yellow cell and one unlabeled cell (Contreras et al. 2021; Hippenmeyer et al. 2010; Zong et al. 2005). The particular Cre-driver promoter will provide a specific lineage labeling. Combination of tamoxifen-inducible CreER will generate individual clones at precise spatiotemporal resolution and thus allow assessment of the function of genes of interest in regulating RGP division patterns and unitary output. This strategy provides a unique temporally controlled experimental design giving insights about exact clone birth date and cell division patterns (i.e., symmetric or asymmetric division) (Beattie and Hippenmeyer 2017; Gao et al. 2014; Hippenmeyer et al. 2010). The division pattern can be deducted from the size of the red and green subclones. A comparable subclone size is indicative of symmetric RGP divisions, while one large and one small subclone with the small clone harboring less than three cells is indicative of asymmetric division pattern (Figure 10.3A).

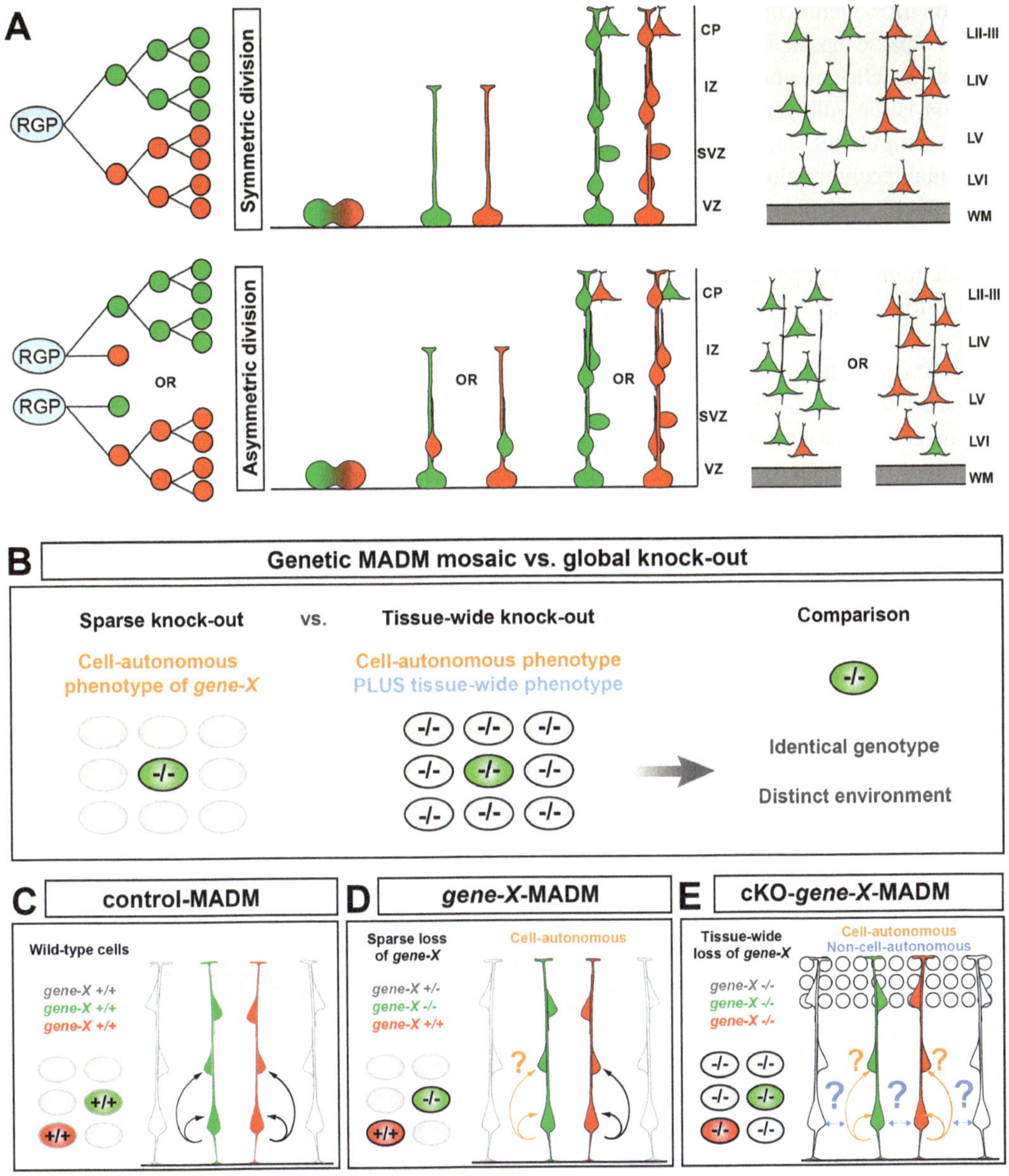

Figure 10.3 The MADM experimental platform enables to study cell-autonomous and non-cell-autonomous gene function. (A) MADM clone in symmetrically proliferative and asymmetrically neurogenic dividing RGPs. The quantification of the output of the red and green subclone allows to distinguish between the two distinct RGP division modes. (B) MADM experimental dissection of cell-autonomous and non-cell-autonomous phenotypes regulating aRGP lineage progression. The assay relies on a comparable analysis of MADM paradigms with labeled sparse cells surrounded by genotypically distinct cells to determine the cell-autonomous and non-cell-autonomous role of a particular gene in development. (C) Control MADM situation in which labeled cells remain in a WT environment and, thus, all cells present the same genotype. (D) Sparse genetic loss of *gene-X* in an otherwise heterozygous background. Green cells present a complete loss of the *gene-X* while red cells are WT for the same gene. Due to the sparse clonal condition, it is possible to analyze cell-autonomous phenotypes by comparing green to red cells (mutant cells vs. WT cells). (E) Tissue-wide genetic loss of the *gene-X*. All cells show a functional disruption of the gene independent of their labeling. The phenotype will represent a mixture of cell-autonomous and tissue-wide mechanisms. The non-cell-autonomous component of the phenotype can be assessed by direct comparison of the green cells from the sparse KO platform to the green cells from the global cKO paradigm.

Upon introduction of an engineered gene of interest (here called *gene-X*) distally to the TG allele, genetic sparse mosaic KO animals can be generated in which red cells will be WT, green cells will be *gene-X*-deficient, and yellow and unlabeled cells will be heterozygous for *gene-X*. Importantly, MADM is the only genetic manipulation system that provides 100 percent correlation between gene manipulation and dual color marker labeling (Figure 10.3A). Since the required interchromosomal recombination is a rare event, the resulting labelling is sparse and offers a great opportunity to achieve detailed high-resolution imaging of single clones and single cells. Not only that, MADM also conserves intact information about cellular localization within the tissue, providing spatial information parallel to the genetic manipulation (in contrast to DNA barcodes-based techniques for example). Thus, MADM constitutes an ideal system for qualitative and quantitative analysis.

MADM provides several unique advantages for studying gene function. Upon introduction of targeted gene mutations distal to the MADM cassettes, genetic sparse KO comprising WT and mutant cells can be generated within a heterozygous environment. Thus, sparse mutant clones are generated in an otherwise normal genetic background given the gene is not dosage-sensitive (Laukoter et al. 2020a). The MADM system allows contrasting of the sparse gene elimination with a whole tissue ablation paradigm to genetically dissect the interplay of *gene-X* cell-autonomous and global tissue requirement (i.e., non-cell-autonomous phenotypes). The sparse gene deletion in a mosaic animal gives MADM the unique power to assess cell-autonomous gene function, while comparison with a whole-tissue deletion paradigm can unravel potential non-cell-autonomous gene effects (Figure 10.3B) (Amberg et al. 2022; Beattie et al. 2017; Contreras et al. 2021; Hansen et al. 2022).

In order to use the MADM system as a platform to assess cell-autonomous and non-cell-autonomous gene function, the first step is the establishment of an experimental paradigm that allows comparison of MADM-labelled WT cells in a normal brain (Figure 10.3C), *gene-X* mutant cells in a heterozygous brain (Figure 10.3D), and *gene-X* mutant cells in a global tissue KO brain (Figure 10.3E). Importantly, the genotype of the *gene-X* mutant cells in the genetic sparse KO is identical to the green *gene-X* mutant cells in the global tissue KO model. However, a different cellular and genetic environment surrounding the mutant cells distinguishes both conditions. In the case of the genetic sparse KO, individual *gene-X* mutant RGPs and their progeny are encompassed by a local microenvironment consisting of heterozygous and WT cells. If individual mutant RGPs exhibit a phenotype, *gene-X* has a cell-autonomous function in RGP lineage progression. In the global tissue KO mice, mutant cells are surrounded by a *gene-X* mutant environment (Figure 10.3B–E). It is thus possible that a phenotype of mutant cells in an all-mutant environment may get exacerbated due to systemic and/or community effects. Therefore, the phenotype of sparse *gene-X* mutant cells might differ from the phenotype of global tissue KO cells. Such a difference will elucidate cell-autonomous and non-cell-autonomous phenotypes of *gene-X* in RGPs.

Studies making use of MADM will identify the importance of the local stem cell niche environment and thus non-cell-autonomous contributions in concert with cell-autonomous gene function in RGP proliferation and lineage progression. More generally, single cell phenotypes in *gene-X* global tissue KO animals will reflect a combination of both, cell-autonomous gene function and environment-derived cues, which may remedy or exacerbate any observed phenotype. Thus, the main assay for discrimination between cell-autonomous and non-cell-autonomous effects consists of subtractive phenotypic analysis at single cell resolution by comparing sparse and global-tissue KO of genes of interest (Figure 10.3C–E). Taken together, MADM provides an unambiguous quantitative readout of gene function at the single-cell level and thus, presents an optimal technology to determine gene function during neural stem cell lineage progression.

In this chapter, we will highlight several cellular processes where the application of MADM technology has been able to uncover, precisely, cell-type and stage-specific functions of particular genes in cortical stem cell lineage progression.

10.2 Cellular Features Orchestrating aRGP Lineage Progression

Given the multitude of cellular mechanisms that can be affected upon a genetic alteration, we have grouped the selected cellular features that are highlighted in this chapter by their major cellular function in the developing cortex.

10.2.1 Cell Polarity in RGP Lineage Progression

aRGPs show high polarization allowing them to be exposed to different microenvironments (as CSF, meninges, or ECM). The morphological polarization of aRGPs is concomitant to a polarized organization of their intracellular components. Intracellular proteins, membrane elements, mRNA, and organelles are distributed in an asymmetric manner within the cell and normally localized close to subcellular sites where their dedicated biological function is required. Through using localized component distribution, cells are able to respond locally within the individual cell. For instance, Pilaz et al. 2016 reported that basal processes showed local protein translation as a local response independent of the somatic one (Pilaz et al. 2016). Therefore, faithful aRGP lineage progression (of e.g., neurogenesis) requires a precise regulation and maintenance of the asymmetrical cellular morphology and thus, the asymmetric distribution of intracellular components (Arai et al. 2017; Taverna et al. 2014; Villalba et al. 2021).

10.2.1.1 Distinct and Sequential Roles of *Lgl1* along Cortical Development

One of the first identified key regulators for intracellular polarity, from Drosophila to mammals, is the Lethal giant larvae 1 (*Lgl1*) genc (Bcattie et al. 2017; Betschinger et al. 2003; Jossin et al. 2017; Klezovitch et al. 2004; Vasioukhin and Vasioukhin 2006). Early studies in Drosophila showed that the LGL1 signaling protein is involved in apico-basal polarity, epithelial tissue organization, and tumor-like growth control (Bilder and Bilder 2001; Bilder et al. 2000; Humbert et al. 2003) by counteracting the protein complexes responsible for maintenance of the apical membrane domain (Yamanaka et al. 2003). In vivo results in mammals parallel previous observations in invertebrates and demonstrated that *Lgl1* loss-of-function in neural progenitors causes a disruption of cell polarity. *Lgl1*-cKO studies showed that LGL1 directly binds and promotes the internalization of N-cadherin by aPKC mediated phosphorylation, restricting the apical junctional complexed to the basolateral-apical boundary (Jossin et al. 2017). Such alterations compromised the VZ integrity resulting in a severe and progressive disorganization, apoptosis and an aberrant proliferation of aRGPs forming rosettes (Beattie et al. 2017; Jossin et al. 2017; Klezovitch et al. 2004). As a consequence, *Lgl1*-cKO mice or dense in utero electroporation of a short hairpin (sh) RNA against *Lgl1* (sh-*Lgl1*) generate a massive disorganization of the cerebral cortex composed of an ectopic second layer of gray matter, resembling a subcortical band heterotopia mainly formed by late born neurons (Beattie et al. 2017; Jossin et al. 2017). Global KO loss of *Lgl1* results in neonatal death (Beattie et al. 2017; Jossin et al. 2017; Klezovitch et al. 2004).

In order to detangle the mechanisms by which *Lgl1* regulates cell polarity maintenance and proliferation in a cell-autonomous manner, Beattie et al. 2017 (Beattie et al. 2017), established distinct MADM paradigms with sparse and whole-tissue *Lgl1* deletion. In the sparse deletion paradigm, the MADM system allows the generation of individual *Lgl1*$^{-/-}$ mutant cells within a "normal" cellular environment. If the aberrant aRGP proliferation and cortical heterotopia as observed in *Lgl1* whole-tissue KO mice (Beattie et al. 2017; Jossin et al. 2017; Klezovitch et al. 2004) arise as a cell-autonomous *Lgl1* function, one would expect increased aRGP proliferation and thus higher numbers of green *Lgl1*$^{-/-}$ mutant neurons as compared to red WT neurons. Contrary to expectations, the green *Lgl1* mutant / red WT ratio of cortical projection neurons was equal to one, demonstrating that *Lgl1* is not cell-autonomously required for aRGP-mediated neurogenesis.

At later stages of RGP lineage progression, sparse *Lgl1* ablation led to increment the early proliferative postnatal astrocyte progenitors and thus, astrocyte generation. Although it is out of the scope for this review, it should be noted that *Lgl1* is also cell-autonomously essential for adult NSC lineage progression in the postnatal V-SVZ niche though the maintenance of type B1 cells morphology and integrity (Beattie et al. 2017).

Thus, MADM experiments were able to dissect sequential functions of *Lgl1*: a non-cell-autonomous one along neurogenesis, where a community effect induces tissue disorganization, proliferation alterations, and apoptosis; and a cell-autonomous function later in development where *Lgl1* regulates gliogenesis, postnatal neurogenesis, and V-SVZ niche integrity (Figure 10.4B) (Beattie et al. 2017; Ortiz-Álvarez et al. 2019).

10.2.2 Cell Division Regulation during Neocortical Development

Precise control of the mitotic process is an essential feature of multicellular organisms to regulate tissue integrity. Cell cycle regulation may occur via mitotic checkpoints, which orchestrate cell cycle progression and are thus important for the maintenance of the stem cell pool (Barnum and O'Connell 2014). Furthermore, mitotic spindle orientation and plane of cleavage in mammals is an important determinant of cell fate (LaMonica et al. 2013; Lancaster and Knoblich 2012; Taverna et al. 2014). It has been suggested that the spindle orientation dictates the division mode of aRGPs, or in other words, whether a cell division yields aRGP expansion or the generation of new neurons although the relationship between mitotic cleavage and the cell fate remains unclear (Konno et al. 2008; Lancaster and Knoblich 2012; Noctor et al. 2008).

10.2.2.1 The Cellular Landscape Influences *Sp2* Gene Function to Regulate Lower- or Upper-layer Neuron Formation

The zinc finger protein Specificity protein (*Sp*)2 belongs to the glutamine-rich Sp family of transcription factors. In contrast to the other *Sp* family members, *Sp2* shows weak DNA binding and little if any transcriptional activity in various mammalian cell lines (Moorefield et al. 2004). In the nervous system, *Sp2* has been shown to be an essential regulator of cell cycle progression. Global tissue KO of *Sp2* using *Emx1*-Cre results in strongly reduced cortical thickness during embryonic development (Liang et al. 2013). In cKO mice, the cortical plate is extremely thin at E14.5, while the VZ displays a significant expansion by containing a high number of mitotic cells (as identified by staining for the M phase marker Phospho-Histone 3 (PH3)). The high amount of PH3 positive aRGPs was caused by M phase arrest, which led to a reduced production of aRGPs and neurons over developmental time.

The cell-autonomous function of *Sp2* in cell cycle progression was identified by deletion of *Sp2* using MADM, which clearly established that individual *Sp2*$^{-/-}$ aRGPs are M phase arrested (Liang et al. 2013). Later studies using MADM could determine that loss of *Sp2* in neurogenic progenitors results in prolonged mitosis due to extension of early mitotic stages (Johnson and Ghashghaei 2020). The disruption of mitotic progression is correlated with depletion of the populations of upper layer neurons in the cortex. In contrast, early cortical neural stem cells proliferate and

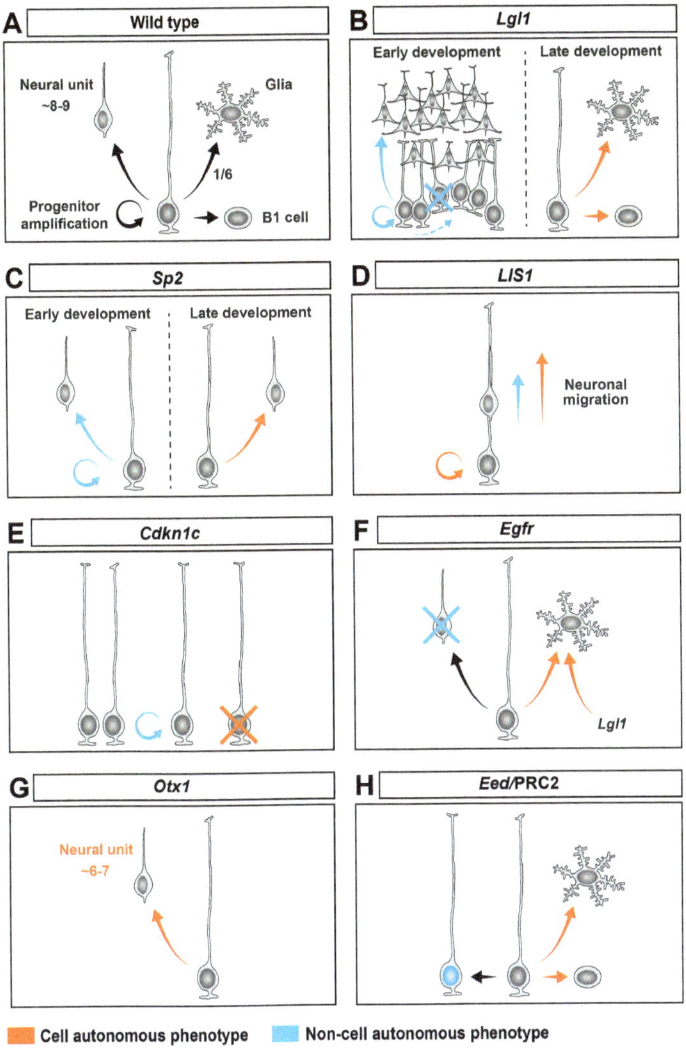

Figure 10.4 Cell-autonomous gene functions and tissue-wide effects at sequential stages during RGP lineage progression. (A) WT aRGP lineage progression. aRGPs self-amplify, give rise to a unit of eight to nine neurons, with one out of six aRGPs progress to generate glia and others to produce V-SVZ type B1 adult progenitors. (B) During neurogenesis, tissue-wide loss of *Lgl1* induces proliferation disruption, apoptosis, and tissue disorganization with rosettes formation, and double cortex in a non-cell-autonomous manner. Later, *Lgl1* cell-autonomously regulates gliogenesis, postnatal neurogenesis, and V-SVZ niche integrity. (C) The imprinted *Cdkn1c* locus promotes growth in a non-cell-autonomous manner but also executes an essential cell-autonomous anti-apoptotic function. (D) *Sp2* non-cell-autonomously regulates cell cycle progression along early embryonic development while regulates neurogenesis in a stage-specific manner (first tissue-wide dependent and later cell-autonomously dependent). (E) *Lis1* regulates neural progenitor proliferation and dosage-dependent migration in a cell-autonomous manner. However, *Lis1* also exerts a non-cell-autonomous function in neuronal migration on the global tissue level. (F) *Egfr* is required for gliogenesis and astrocyte survival in a cell-autonomous manner but prevents neuronal cell death through a tissue wide-effect. (G) *Otx1* cell-autonomously controls unitary neuron output size. (H) *Eed*/PRC2 cell-autonomously controls astrocyte progenitor proliferation and astrocyte maturation as well as adult neurogenesis but regulates the correct temporal patterning of neurogenesis in a non-cell-autonomous manner. Circled arrows indicate progenitor amplification, horizontal straight arrows point to transition, vertical straight arrows denote migration, bended arrows show cell production, dashed arrow indicate tissue disruption, crosses imply cell loss, orange color stands for cell-autonomous phenotype and blue indicates non-cell-autonomous.

expand normally in the absence of *Sp2* (Johnson and Ghashghaei 2020). Altogether, the findings from these studies implicate *Sp2*-dependent mechanisms as novel regulators of cell cycle progression a regulation of neurogenesis in the embryonic brain in a stage-specific manner (Figure 10.4C).

10.2.2.2 *Lis1* Cell-autonomously Regulates aRGP Proliferation during Symmetrical Division State

Lissencephaly-1 (*Lis1*) is a central component of a protein complex coupling the nucleus and the centrosome (Morris and Morris 2000). As such, *Lis1* was found to be essential for the precise control of mitotic spindle orientation in both neuroepithelial stem cells and aRGPs, and thus, in cell division regulation (Schwamborn and Knoblich 2008; Yingling et al. 2008). Conditional tissue-wide KO of *Lis1* in NECs, where cleavage is uniformly vertical and symmetrical, provokes rapid apoptosis of those cells. However, the asymmetrically dividing aRGPs, are less affected. Thus, the control of symmetric cell division, which is essential to expand the pool of neuroepithelial stem cells, is mediated through spindle orientation determined in a *Lis1*-dependent manner (Yingling et al. 2008). Using sparse deletion of *Lis1* from individual aRGPs in a MADM context, it was shown that the essential role of *Lis1* for neural progenitor proliferation is cell-autonomous dependent as the production of *Lis1* mutant cells was reduced compared to the WT cells (Hippenmeyer et al. 2010).

In mice, the comparison between WT ($Lis1^{+/+}$), null heterozygotes ($Lis1^{ko/+}$), compound heterozygote ($Lis1^{ko/hc}$), and conditional null ($Lis1^{ko/hc}$;Cre) showed that LIS1 cell-autonomously regulates neuronal radial migration efficiency in a dosage-sensitive manner (Hippenmeyer 2014; Hippenmeyer et al. 2010; Wynshaw-Boris 2007). Additionally, MADM usage allowed showing a community effect in non-radial migration and cell-to-cell communication (Figure 10.4D) (Hippenmeyer et al. 2010). As migration is out of the scope of this chapter, for more insights into neural migration and the interplay of cell-autonomous versus non-cell-autonomous effects discussions refer to the suggested publications: Hansen et al. 2022; Hansen and Hippenmeyer 2020 and Hippenmeyer 2014.

Importantly, such non-cell-autonomous functions could explain the clinical symptoms of human Lissencephaly, whereby cells with a 50 percent reduction in LIS1 protein levels exhibit inappropriate community effects or fail to signal to each other. This may in turn exacerbate the already-impaired, intrinsic migratory capacity of $Lis1^{+/-}$ neurons. We will however not go into further details at this point and refer to Chapter 18.

10.2.2.3 The Cell-autonomous Neuron Survival Regulation by *Cdkn1c* is Masked by a Cellular Community Effect on Growth

The regulation of the cell cycle progression can be also achieved by modulating the activity of the cell cycle drivers as *Cdkn1c* does. *Cdkn1c* acts as a growth/tumor suppressor by inhibiting the activity of cyclin-dependent kinases, which are the main orchestrators of the cell cycle progression (Hochegger et al. 2008). *Cdkn1c* is a paternal imprinted gene that encodes for the cyclin-dependent kinase inhibitor $p57^{KIP2}$. Imprinting refers to an epigenetic phenomenon that results in the mono-allelic expression inactivation (completely or partially) of a gene in a parent-of-origin-specific manner (Laukoter et al. 2020a; Laukoter et al. 2020b; Pauler et al. 2021). In other words, certain genes are expressed only from the allele inherited from the father, while others are only expressed when inherited from the mother. As the parental inheritance needs to be considered during all experimental steps, genes showing imprinted expression are difficult to study. Also, as their standard role is dependent of a unique dose (parental or maternal), these genes are highly dose sensitive. Two expressed alleles or the suppression of the expressed one leads to an abnormal gene dosage promoting altered phenotypes. Thus, the imprinted cell-autonomous gene dosage effect has been poorly understood, mainly due to the lack of assays allowing single-cell resolution of phenotypic analysis. The MADM technology provides an unprecedented advantage to assess the function of imprinted genes at the individual cell level (Pauler et al. 2021). Besides the sparse generation of labelled cells, MADM interchromosomal recombination flips the maternal origin allele with the paternal origin allele, resolving into the coupling of each fluorescent protein to one of the maternal or paternal alleles. G2-X event segregates the two recombinant chromosomes into different daughter cells. Thus, depending on the parental mating, the labeled cell will inherit two copies of the maternal or the parental alleles and consequently, double-dose or a complete suppression of the gene expression (uniparental chromosome disomy, UPD). G2-Z events generating yellow cells result in no alteration of the imprinted pattern and thus represent a control cell within the same tissue. Thereby, the MADM technique allows for the precise analysis of imprinted and dosage-sensitive genes such as *Cdkn1c* and to dissect their cell-autonomous or tissue-wide function (Laukoter et al. 2020a; Pauler et al. 2021).

Cdkn1c loss of function in the whole animal results in a growth gain. Besides the whole-body increase compared to a WT mouse, *Cdkn1c*$^{-/-}$ mice also develop macrocephaly and cortical hyperplasia (Mairet-Coello et al. 2012). Based on the *Cdkn1c*$^{-/-}$ phenotype, it was expected that *Cdkn1c* cell-autonomous role would be related to growth and proliferation. Contrary to expectations, MADM sparse *Cdkn1c* mutant cells (paternal UPD) showed an equal growth/proliferation potential than maternal UPD aRGPs independently of genomic imprinting. Thus, *Cdkn1c* does not cell-autonomously regulate aRGP proliferative behavior and/or maturation (Laukoter et al. 2020a; Pauler et al. 2021). Therefore, macrocephaly in *Cdkn1c* full knockout likely reflects global organism overgrowth rather than an individual cell consequence of genetic *Cdkn1c* deletion. Stainings for the cell death marker Caspase activated 3 showed a reduction in cell survival upon MADM sparse and global ablation of *Cdkn1c* regardless of the imprinting status. Thus *Cdkn1c* cell-autonomously controls cell death in a highly dosage-dependent manner by promoting cellular survival of differentiating and maturing cortical projection neurons and (to lesser extent) proliferating aRGPs (Laukoter et al. 2020a; Pauler et al. 2021).

The cell-autonomous growth phenotype after *Cdkn1c* ablation parallels the downregulation of genes related to neurogenesis and upregulation of genes involved in cell death. However, the general growth promoted by global *Cdkn1c* ablation (Mairet-Coello et al. 2012) is dominant over the imprinting status of the genomic *Cdkn1c* locus, precluding to detangle a cell-autonomous role in a global mutant (Figure 10.4E) (Laukoter et al. 2020a; Pauler et al. 2021). This paradoxical example in which loss of a gene can either promote growth in a tissue wide manner but also favors cell death within an individual cell, highlights the benefits of using a technology as MADM.

10.2.3 Cell Survival Regulation during RGP Lineage Progression

During development, the cerebral cortex is not only sculpted by neuron production, but also by neuronal cell death (Wong and Marín 2019). Excess neurons are removed by apoptosis to ensure correct and precise synaptic network connection and cortical size. However, most neural cells are entitled to survive long periods. Unbalanced cell survival regulation thus results in severe neurodevelopmental alterations such as autism spectrum disorders, macrocephaly, or polymicrogyria (Butler et al. 2005; Buxbaum et al. 2007; Eriksson et al. 2001; Wong et al. 2018).

10.2.3.1 *Egfr* is Cell-autonomously Required for Astrocyte Production, but Orchestrates Neuronal Survival in a Non-cell-autonomous Manner through Glia-neuron Interactions

Egfr (epidermal growth factor receptor) is a member of the structurally related tyrosine kinase family of ErbB receptors. Its activation by direct binding of Epidermal Growth Factor (EGF) among different growth factors leads to dimerization and activation of the intrinsic tyrosine kinase via autophosphorylation of key tyrosine residues. These phosphorylated sites act as binding residues for downstream signaling cascades activation (Sibilia et al. 1998). In the neocortex, EGFR expression increases during late-embryonic and early-postnatal development concomitant with the onset of gliogenesis (Burrows et al. 1997; Kornblum et al. 1998; Seroogy et al. 1995). Over-expression of EGFR by retroviral infections in aRGPs shifts the lineage towards late developmental traits such as astrocyte production (Burrows et al. 1997). Moreover, migrating cells over-expressing EGFR are found distributed away from proliferative zones, biased toward the deepest CP layer and the marginal zone, which are typical locations of fetal astroglial cells (Burrows et al. 1997).

In contrast, *Egfr* ablation induces a high degree of neurodegeneration right after birth (Sibilia et al. 1998; Wagner et al. 2006). *Egfr*$^{-/-}$ mice showed an increase in nuclear condensation and Akt-caspase-dependent apoptosis in the cerebral cortex and olfactory bulbs concomitant with a reduction in cell density affecting both neurons and glial cells (Sibilia et al. 1998; Wagner et al. 2006). *Egfr* deletion in gliogenic clones using the MADM technique revealed that *Egfr* is cell-autonomously required for gliogenesis in the mouse cerebral cortex, but not for neurogenesis (Beattie et al. 2017; Zhang et al. 2020). Thus, it is suggested that the massive neural degeneration observed in *Egfr*$^{-/-}$ mice arises in a non-cell-autonomous manner reflected by a local lack of trophic support by glial cells (Beattie et al. 2017; Kornblum et al. 1998; Sibilia et al. 1998; Wagner et al. 2006). Upon sparse mosaic deletion, where individual *Egfr*$^{+/+}$ progenitors have double the dosage of *Egfr* relative to the surrounding heterozygous *Egfr*$^{+/-}$ cells, *Egfr*$^{+/+}$ astrocytes are overabundant in the cortex (Beattie et al. 2017; Zhang et al. 2020). These results suggest a dosage-sensitive requirement of *Egfr* for cortical astrocyte production. It has been demonstrated that functional *Egfr* is involved in the excessive astrocyte production induced by *Lgl1* ablation in a synergistic manner, as double ablation of *Lgl1* and *Egfr* led to an almost complete absence on astrocyte production (Beattie et al. 2017). To sum up, *Egfr* is cell-autonomously required for gliogenesis and glial survival, but affects neuronal survival in a non-cell-autonomous manner on the global tissue level (Figure 10.4F) (Beattie et al. 2017; Zhang et al. 2020).

10.2.4 Transcriptional Regulation Guiding Faithful Cortical Development

Executing correct and robust transcriptional programs is crucial for the developmental progression and thus, RGP lineage progression. Understanding the orchestration of cortical development necessarily requires a tight transcriptional regulation as a basic process for cellular behavior and fate specification. Correct unfolding of temporally dynamic gene expression programs involves a wide variety of components, such as sequence-specific transcription factors, chromatin modifiers, and co-regulators. An enhanced knowledge of this topic will be developed by others authors within this book.

10.2.4.1 *Otx1* Regulates Neurogenesis Cell-autonomously in a Layer-independent Manner

One key transcriptional regulator during cortical development is the transcription factor *Otx1* (Orthodenticle Homeobox 1). In mice, *Otx1* is highly expressed in E12.5 – E13.5 aRGPs, at that moment generating the deep layer 5 and 6 cortical projection neurons (Telagirdon gene browser (Frantz et al. 1994; Telley et al. 2019)). Due to this unique expression pattern, OTX1 has been postulated to control the production of deep-layer neurons specifically.

The function of *Otx1* in cortical development has been studied at the single progenitor as well as on the global community level. *Otx1* null mice present a reduced number of neurons in the cortex and thus display microcephaly (Acampora et al. 1996). However, results from global tissue KO studies are not able to determine whether the microcephaly emerges from a cell-autonomous function of *Otx1* in the developing neocortex.

To gain more insight into the *Otx1* related molecular regulation of aRGP behavior and unitary neuronal production, Gao et al. 2014 examined the function of OTX1 using MADM clonal analysis. The MADM system allowed the sparse generation of individual green WT and red *Otx1*$^{-/-}$ progenitors, which could be assessed for their neurogenic capacity by comparing the size of the neuron populations in individual clones with respect to their color (i.e., genotype) (Figure 10.3A). Interestingly, the red majority neuron number (originating from an *Otx1*$^{-/-}$ self-renewing aRGP) was significantly reduced when compared to the green majority neuron number (originating from a WT self-renewing aRGP) in individual clones, suggesting a decreased neurogenic capacity in *Otx1*$^{-/-}$ aRGPs. As anticipated from the previous full KO study (Frantz et al. 1994), the total size of "*Otx1*$^{-/-}$ units" was substantially decreased from eight to nine neurons being generated from a WT progenitor to a total of approximately six to seven neurons produced from an *Otx1*$^{-/-}$ progenitor (Gao et al. 2014). This decrease in unitary neuronal output by aRGPs largely accounted for the microcephaly and ~20–30 percent reduced neocortical thickness observed in *Otx1*$^{-/-}$ animals (Acampora et al. 1996; Gao et al. 2014).

Given that *Otx1* is predominantly expressed in aRGPs when deep-layer neurons are produced, (Gao et al. 2014) tested whether the reduction of neuronal production in *Otx1*$^{-/-}$ clones is selective for deep-layer neurons. Surprisingly, the reduction applied to both superficial-layer and deep-layer neurons.

Together, these results strongly suggest that OTX1 plays an important cell-autonomous role in controlling the size of the unitary neuron output by individual aRGPs through the production of both the deep and superficial layer neurons, despite its expression in aRGPs being downregulated during superficial-layer neuron genesis (Figure 10.4G). The study by Gao et al. (Gao et al. 2014) thus provides a clear example that the early expression of a transcription factor in aRGPs influences late neuronal production, which could for example, be achieved by controlling the late expression of other critical factors required for the production of superficial-layer neurons. Importantly, these data suggest that the seemingly "correlated" expression of certain transcription factors in aRGPs and postmitotic neurons does not necessarily reflect an exclusive lineage bias towards a specific cellular fate acquisition (Gao et al. 2014).

10.2.4.2 *Eed*/PRC2 is not Cell-autonomously Required during Neurogenesis but at the Later Stage during Astrocyte Production

Eed (embryonic ectoderm development) constitutes one of the three core components of the epigenetic regulator Polycomb Repressive Complex 2 (PRC2). Single-cell RNAsequencing (scRNAseq) experiments in mice have unraveled spatiotemporally defined expression patterns of PRC2, showing high expression in E12.5 aRGPs and low expression in later aRGPs and in projection neurons (Telley et al. 2019). Tissue-wide deletion of *Eed* using *Emx1*-Cre results in alterations in temporal patterning of aRGPs. aRGP display proliferation defects from E14.5 onwards and switch too early to the generation of later-born neurons. Thus, *Eed* cKO suffers from a diminished generation of late-born upper layer neurons and dramatic microcephaly (Telley et al. 2019).

By carrying out MADM-based clonal analysis to probe cell-autonomous PRC2 function at true single aRGP cell level, Amberg et al. (2022) could not detect a significant difference in the numbers of *Eed*$^{-/-}$ mutant when compared to *Eed*$^{+/+}$ control neurons. The total unit size was ~eight to nine neurons for each genotype. Due to its cell-intrinsic mode of action, PRC2 activity is generally thought to be a cell-autonomous one. However, upon analyzing the functional requirement of PRC2 at individual aRGP cell level in a MADM-based approach Amberg et al. (2022) could show that PRC2 is not cell-autonomously required in the control of neurogenesis but rather plays a critical role at the global tissue-wide level.

Although *Eed*$^{-/-}$ cells in sparse and global tissue KO paradigms have identical genotypes they exist in distinct genetic and cellular environments (predominantly "normal" environment in sparse or *Eed*$^{-/-}$ in global KO). Given the dramatic phenotypic difference in individual MADM-labeled *Eed*$^{-/-}$ mutant cells depending on their genetic and cellular environment, the authors used RNAseq to assess molecular correlates hinting at global tissue-wide deregulation of gene expression due to PRC2 loss of function. Their results imply that PRC2-dependent transcriptional control, regulating aRGP lineage progression and cell survival, strongly depends on the genetic tissue-wide landscape and cellular environment.

Eed$^{-/-}$ mutant cells from sparse KO showed more similar transcriptome to WT but significantly distinct gene expression when compared to *Eed*$^{-/-}$ cells from global KO cortices. Thus, variable global gene expression in mutant *Eed*$^{-/-}$ cells appears to correlate with their genetic/cellular environment. Only global tissue-wide KO, but not sparse deletion, of *Eed* translated to reduced proliferative potential in aRGPs and increased apoptosis.

However, upon later stages of neurogenesis aRGPs obtain gliogenic potential and the authors tested the requirement of PRC2 in aRGP lineage progression towards gliogenesis at the individual progenitor level. Their data show that the neurogenic-to-gliogenic switch in aRGPs was not compromised upon loss of PRC2 activity, but that PRC2 cell-autonomously controls proliferation in astrocyte progenitors and astrocyte maturation (Figure 10.4H) (Amberg et al. 2022).

10.3 Concluding Remarks

The regulation of cerebral cortex development, and thus faithful RGP lineage progression, is a highly complex process subject to tight genetic regulation of cell-intrinsic mechanisms and systemic effects. With the development of more advanced experimental paradigms, we are starting to unravel and to understand these regulatory mechanisms in greater detail. Classical genetic approaches include the generation of whole tissue mutants and the study of the resulting phenotype. However, an individual cell is a non-isolated unit in close contact to other cell types and structures. Alterations in the normal cellular behavior are very likely to affect its environment by sending aberrant types of signals, exhibiting reduced contact or even modifying the extracellular matrix. On the whole-tissue level, the sum of these alterations may promote aggravated phenotypes. Consequently, whole-tissue phenotypes can result in misleading conclusions about precise gene function.

For a fine comprehension of gene function, it is therefore essential to distinguish between cell-autonomous and non-cell-autonomous phenotypes. As both phenotypes are taking place at the same time in a whole-tissue mutant, such accurate discernment requires particular and specific tools enabling to detangle both mechanisms (Figure 10.2). The genetic tool MADM stands out nowadays as an ideal technique to dissect cell-autonomous gene function and non-cell-autonomous tissue-wide and/or community effects (Figure 10.3B-E). The MADM technique allows for the generation of sparse mutant clones in an otherwise "normal" cellular background, and to contrast the sparse with a whole-tissue deletion paradigm dissecting intrinsic and extrinsic mechanisms (Figure 10.3B). The selection of tissue- or cell-type-specific Cre-drivers allows precise targeting of particular genetic lineages of interest. Tamoxifen-inducible CreER strains provide an accurate spatiotemporally controlled experimental design (Beattie and Hippenmeyer 2017; Beattie et al. 2020; Gao et al. 2014; Zong et al. 2005).

In this chapter, we have highlighted several cases were the distinction between cell-autonomous and non-cell-autonomous phenotypes was crucial to gain a deeper understanding of gene function at precise steps of RGP lineage progression. These cases emphasize how the experimental techniques and paradigms used will impact the conclusions reached (Figure 10.4). Without the proper discrimination of cell-autonomous and non-cell-autonomous gene function, one might overlook particular phenotypes, such as distinct and even apparently opposite phenotypes. Such is the case for the loss of *Cdkn1c*, which despite its tissue-wide role in proliferation and growth also controls cell survival in a cell-autonomous manner (Laukoter et al. 2020a). Thus, in a whole-tissue mutant displaying overgrowth, the systemic growth phenotype masks the apoptosis induction. Alternatively, a gene can exhibit distinct sequential functions along development as shown for the *Lgl1* gene or the *Sp2* gene. Sparse *Lgl1* deletion does not impact embryonic neurogenesis or aRGP amplification, but it is cell-autonomously involved in gliogenesis and adult type B1 progenitor maintenance during late developmental processes (Beattie et al. 2017). However, the complete tissue-wide ablation of *Lgl1* revealed a severe neurogenesis phenotype with subcortical band heterotopia formation, alteration in aRGP proliferation and tissue integrity disruption. For *Sp2*, non-cell-autonomous effects drive early proliferation and neurogenesis, while late in development neurons are generated in a cell-autonomous manner (Johnson and Ghashghaei 2020; Liang et al. 2013). In some instances, the community effect is a direct consequence of the individual cell-autonomous phenotype, as the neural cell death caused by the absence of supporting glia in *Egfr* mutants (Beattie et al. 2017; Zhang et al. 2020). In other cases, the mutant cellular landscape exacerbates the cell-autonomous phenotype (like the altered cell adhesion in *Lgl1* mutants (Beattie et al. 2017; Jossin et al. 2017)). Certain molecular characteristics might suggest correlations that cannot be causally linked with the phenotype, as shown for *Otx1*. Due to high *Otx1* expression at early neurogenic stages (Telley et al. 2019), one might postulate that it controls deep-layer neurons generation and *Otx1*$^{-/-}$ microcephaly results as a lack of deep-layer neurons (Frantz et al. 1994; Telley et al. 2019). However, clonal analysis could uncover that *Otx1* has an essential cell-autonomous role throughout neurogenesis and thus controls neuron production in a layer-independent manner (Gao et al. 2014). PRC2 was assumed to regulate neurogenesis in a cell-autonomous manner based on its cell-intrinsic mode of action as epigenetic regulator. Yet, MADM experiments employing clonal analysis could demonstrate that PRC2 is not cell-autonomously required during neurogenesis but at later stages of RGP lineage progression in astrocyte production (Amberg et al. 2022). All these studies highlight the tremendous importance of the interplay between cell-autonomous and systemic mechanisms for faithful cortical development.

Since alterations in neurogenesis based on gene mutations can lead to neurodevelopmental disorders, a precise understanding of the correct developmental processes is crucial for a detailed understanding of disease origins. Occasionally, the mutations found in a patient are not present in the germ line but comprise a somatic cell mosaicism. Postzygotic mutations may take place at any point during cortical development leading to severe neurological disorders or cancer (Bizzotto and Walsh 2022; D'Gama and Walsh 2018; Frank 2014; Jamuar et al. 2014). Somatic mutations imply that mutant cells will be surrounded by non-mutant cells and the phenotype of the disease in humans might be a result of both, cell-autonomous and tissue-wide effects. Thus, the need of approaches that distinguish cell-autonomous and tissue-wide phenotypes become clearly essential in these cases. Future discoveries might help the understanding of somatic-mutation-related diseases and the contribution of the cellular environment and/or the cell-autonomous effects. Indeed, there are already known examples of human diseases that imply an interplay between cell intrinsic and extrinsic effects. In the mentioned case of *LIS1*, somatic mutations affecting only a portion of migrating neurons can result in emergence of a "double cortex," as opposed to the severe complete lissencephaly upon whole mutant tissue (Poduri et al. 2013; Sicca et al. 2003). Thus, the cell-autonomous disruption of progenitor proliferation and neuronal migration does not completely explain the observed phenotype in human patients, highlighting the importance of a comprehensive understanding of all the different cues orchestrating progenitor behavior. Similarly, instead of a complete lissencephaly, males with somatic mutations in *DCX* (located in X-chromosome) can exhibit a "double cortex" in a similar way as happens with chromosome X-inactivation mosaics in females, as only some neurons carry the mutation (Gleeson et al. 2000; Poduri et al. 2013). Another example are focal malformations of cortical development, produced by postzygotic somatic mutations that activate the phosphatidylinositol-4,5-bisphosphate-3-kinase (PI3K)–protein kinase B (AKT)–mammalian target of rapamycin (mTOR) pathway. Mutant progenitor cells induce alterations in migration of non-mutant cells by a tissue-wide-mediated dyslamination. The ectopically produced neurons localize to the white matter and contribute to epilepsy (Baek et al. 2015). The mechanisms of the disease remain still poorly understood, as the precise effects exerted by the mutant cells on the whole tissue are not fully uncovered yet. However, the quantity or density of mutant cells is suggested to correlate with disease severity (Baek et al. 2015). Thus, a deeper understanding of the interplay between cell-autonomous and systemic mechanisms will have profound implications for our understanding of human disease that derive from postzygotic mutation and their possible therapies.

Acknowledgments

We thank all lab members for discussion. Nicole Amberg received funding from the FWF Firnberg-Programm (T 1031). The work was supported by ISTA institutional funds and by the European Research Council (ERC) under the European Union's Horizon 2020 research and innovation program (grant agreement 725780 LinPro) to S.H.

References

Acampora, D. et al. (1996). Epilepsy and brain abnormalities in mice lacking the Otx1 gene. *Nat Genet* 14: 218–222. doi: 10.1038/ng1096-218.

Amberg, N. et al. (2022 November 4). Tissue-wide genetic and cellular landscape shapes the execution of sequential PRC2 functions in neural stem cell lineage progression. *Sci Adv* 8 (44): eabq1263. doi: 10.1126/sciadv.abq1263. Epub 2022 Nov 2. PMID: 36322669; PMCID: PMC9629739.

Arai, Y. et al. (2017). Neural progenitor cell polarity and cortical development. *Front Cell Neurosci* 11 (384): 1–11. doi: 10.3389/fncel.2017.00384.

Ayala, R. et al. (2007). Trekking across the brain. *Cell* 128 (1): 29–43. doi: 10.1016/j.cell.2006.12.021.

Baek, S.T. et al. (2015). An AKT3-FOXG1-reelin network underlies defective migration in human focal malformations of cortical development. *Nat Med* 21: 1445–1454. doi: 10.1038/nm.3982.

Barnum, K.J. and O'Connell, M.J. (2014). Cell cycle regulation by checkpoints. *Methods Mol Biol* 1170 (2): 29–40. doi: 10.1007/978-1-4939-0888-2_2.

Beattie, R. and Hippenmeyer, S. (2017). Mechanisms of radial glia progenitor cell lineage progression. *FEBS Lett* 591 (24): 3993–4008. doi: 10.1002/1873-3468.12906.

Beattie, R. et al. (2017). Mosaic analysis with double markers reveals distinct sequential functions of Lgl1 in neural stem cells. *Neuron* 94 (3): 517–533.e3. doi: 10.1016/j.neuron.2017.04.012.

Beattie, R. et al. (2020). Lineage tracing and clonal analysis in developing cerebral cortex using mosaic analysis with double markers (MADM). *J Vis Exp: JoVE* E61147 (159): 1–14. doi: 10.3791/61147.

Betizeau, M. et al. (2013). Precursor diversity and complexity of lineage relationships in the outer subventricular zone of the primate. *Neuron* 80 (2): 442–457. doi: 10.1016/j.neuron.2013.09.032.

Betschinger, J. et al. (2003). The Par complex directs asymmetric cell division by phosphorylating the cytoskeletal protein Lgl. *Nature* 422: 326–330. doi: 10.1038/nature01486.

Bilder, D. and Bilder, D. (2001). Cell polarity. *Curr Biol* 11 (4): R132–R135. doi: 10.1016/s0960-9822(01)00060-4.

Bilder, D. et al. (2000). Cooperative regulation of cell polarity and growth by Drosophila tumor suppressors. *Science* 289 (5476): 113–116. doi: 10.1126/science.289.5476.113.

Bizzotto, S. and Walsh, C.A. (2022). Genetic mosaicism in the human brain. *Nat Rev Neurosci* 23: 275–286. doi: 10.1038/s41583-022-00572-x.

Borrell, V. et al. (2012). Slit/Robo signaling modulates the proliferation of central nervous system progenitors. *Neuron* 76 (2): 338–352. doi: 10.1016/j.neuron.2012.08.003S0896-6273(12)00706-4[pii].

Buckingham, M. and Meilhac, S.M. (2011). Tracing cells for tracking cell lineage and clonal behavior. *Dev Cell* 21 (3): 394–409. doi: 10.1016/j.devcel.2011.07.019.

Bueno, D. and Garcia-Fernàndez, J. (2016). Evolutionary development of embryonic cerebrospinal fluid composition and regulation. *Fluids Barriers CNS* 13 (5): 1–12. doi: 10.1186/s12987-016-0029-y.

Burrows, R.C. et al. (1997). Response diversity and the timing of progenitor cell maturation are regulated by developmental changes in EGFR expression in the cortex. *Neuron* 19 (2): 251–267. doi: 10.1016/s0896-6273(00)80937-x.

Butler, M.G. et al. (2005). Subset of individuals with autism spectrum disorders and extreme macrocephaly associated with germline PTEN tumour suppressor gene mutations. *J Med Genet* 42 (4): 318–321. doi: 10.1136/jmg.2004.024646.

Buxbaum, J.D. et al. (2007). Mutation screening of the PTEN gene in patients with autism spectrum disorders and macrocephaly. *Am J Med Genet* 144B (4): 484–491. doi: 10.1002/ajmg.b.30493.

Cardenas, A. et al. (2018). Evolution of cortical neurogenesis in amniotes controlled by robo signaling levels. *Cell* 174 (3): 590–606 e21. doi: 10.1016/j.cell.2018.06.007.

Cavanagh, M.E. et al. (1983). Comparison of proteins in CSF of lateral and IVth ventricles during early development of fetal sheep. *Dev Brain Res* 11 (2): 159–167. doi: 10.1016/0165-3806(83)90213-4.

Contreras, X. et al. (2021). A genome-wide library of MADM mice for single-cell genetic mosaic analysis. *Cell Rep* 35 (12): 1–18. doi: 10.1016/j.celrep.2021.109274.

D'Gama, A.M. and Walsh, C.A. (2018). Somatic mosaicism and neurodevelopmental disease. *Nat Neurosci* 21: 1504–1514. doi: 10.1038/s41593-018-0257-3.

Dehay, C. et al. (1996). Contribution of thalamic input to the specification of cytoarchitectonic cortical fields in the primate. *J Comp Neurol* 367 (1): 70–89. doi: 10.1002/(sici)1096-9861(19960325)367:1<70:aid-cne6>3.0.co;2-g.

Dumas, L. et al. (2022). Multicolor strategies for investigating clonal expansion and tissue plasticity. *Cell Mol Life Sci* 79 (141): 1–37. doi: 10.1007/s00018-021-04077-1.

Eriksson, S.H. et al. (2001). Persistent reelin-expressing Cajal-Retzius cells in polymicrogyria. *Brain* 124 (7): 1350–1361. doi: 10.1093/brain/124.7.1350.

Evsyukova, I. et al. (2013). Integrative mechanisms of oriented neuronal migration in the developing brain. *Ann Rev Cell Dev Biol* 29: 299–353. doi: 10.1146/annurev-cellbio-101512-122400.

Ferent, J. et al. (2020). Extracellular control of radial glia proliferation and scaffolding during cortical development and pathology. *Front Cell Dev Biol* 8 (578341): 1–35. doi: 10.3389/fcell.2020.578341.

Fernandez, V. et al. (2016). Cerebral cortex expansion and folding: what have we learned? *EMBO J* 35 (10): 1021–1044. doi: 10.15252/embj.201593701.

Fietz, S.A. et al. (2012). Transcriptomes of germinal zones of human and mouse fetal neocortex suggest a role of extracellular matrix in progenitor self-renewal. *Proc Natl Acad Sci USA* 109 (29): 11836–11841. doi: 10.1073/pnas.1209647109.

Florio, M. et al. (2015). Human-specific gene ARHGAP11B promotes basal progenitor amplification and neocortex expansion. *Science* 347 (6229): 1465–1470. doi: 10.1126/science.aaa1975.

Florio, M. and Huttner, W.B. (2014). Neural progenitors, neurogenesis and the evolution of the neocortex. *Development* 141 (11): 2182–2194. doi: 10.1242/dev.090571.

Frank, S.A. (2014). Somatic mosaicism and disease. *Curr Biol* 24 (12): R577–R581. doi: 10.1016/j.cub.2014.05.021.

Frantz, G.D. et al. (1994). Otx1 and Otx2 define layers and regions in developing cerebral cortex and cerebellum. *J Neurosci* 14 (10): 5725–5740. https://www.ncbi.nlm.nih.gov/pubmed/7931541.

Gao, P. et al. (2014). Deterministic progenitor behavior and unitary production of neurons in the neocortex. *Cell* 159 (4): 775–788. doi: 10.1016/j.cell.2014.10.027.

García-Marques, J. and López-Mascaraque, L. (2013). Clonal identity determines astrocyte cortical heterogeneity. *Cereb Cortex* 23 (6): 1463–1472. doi: 10.1093/cercor/bhs134.

García-Moreno, F. et al. (2014). CLoNe is a new method to target single progenitors and study their progeny in mouse and chick. *Development* 141 (7): 1589–1598. doi: 10.1242/dev.105254.

Gleeson, J.G. et al. (2000). Somatic and germline mosaic mutations in the doublecortin gene are associated with variable phenotypes. *Am J Hum Genet* 67 (3): 574–581. doi: 10.1086/303043.

Gotz, M. and Huttner, W.B. (2005). The cell biology of neurogenesis. *Nat Rev Mol Cell Biol* 6 (10): 777–788. doi: 10.1038/nrm1739.

Hansen, A.H. and Hippenmeyer, S. (2020). Non-cell-autonomous mechanisms in radial projection neuron migration in the developing cerebral cortex. In: *Frontiers in Cell and Developmental Biology*, 8 (574382): 1–13. https://www.frontiersin.org/article/10.3389/fcell.2020.574382.

Hansen, A.H. et al. (2022). Tissue-wide effects override cell-intrinsic gene function in radial neuron migration. *Oxford Open Neurosci* 1 (1): 1–25. doi: 10.1093/oons/kvac009.

Haubensak, W. et al. (2004). Neurons arise in the basal neuroepithelium of the early mammalian telencephalon. *Proc Natl Acad Sci USA* 101 (9): 3196–3201. doi: 10.1073/pnas.0308600100.

Hippenmeyer, S. (2014). Molecular pathways controlling the sequential steps of cortical projection neuron migration BT. In: *Cellular and Molecular Control of Neuronal Migration* (ed. L. Nguyen and S. Hippenmeyer), 1–24. Netherlands: Springer. doi: 10.1007/978-94-007-7687-6_1.

Hippenmeyer, S. et al. (2010). Genetic mosaic dissection of Lis1 and Ndel1 in neuronal migration. *Neuron* 68 (4): 695–709. doi: 10.1016/j.neuron.2010.09.027.

Hochegger, H. et al. (2008). Cyclin-dependent kinases and cell-cycle transitions: does one fit all? *Nat Rev Mol Cell Biol* 9: 910–916. doi: 10.1038/nrm2510.

Huang, X. et al. (2010). Transventricular delivery of Sonic hedgehog is essential to cerebellar ventricular zone development. *Proc Natl Acad Sci USA* 107 (18): 8422–8427. doi: 10.1073/pnas.0911838107.

Humbert, P.O. et al. (2003). Dlg, Scribble and Lgl in cell polarity, cell proliferation and cancer. *BioEssays* 25 (6): 542–553. doi: 10.1002/bies.10286.

Jamuar, S.S. et al. (2014). Somatic mutations in cerebral cortical malformations. *New Engl J Med* 371 (8): 733–743. doi: 10.1056/nejmoa1314432.

Johansson, P.A. et al. (2013). The transcription factor Otx2 regulates choroid plexus development and function. *Development* 140 (5): 1055–1066. doi: 10.1242/dev.090860.

Johnson, C.A. and Ghashghaei, H.T. (2020). Sp2 regulates late neurogenic but not early expansive divisions of neural stem cells underlying population growth in the mouse cortex. *Development* 147 (4): 1–13. doi: 10.1242/dev.186056.

Jossin, Y. et al. (2017). Llgl1 connects cell polarity with cell-cell adhesion in embryonic neural stem cells. *Dev Cell* 41 (5): 481–495.E5. doi: 10.1016/j.devcel.2017.05.002.

Kadry, H. et al. (2020). A blood–brain barrier overview on structure, function, impairment, and biomarkers of integrity. *Fluids Barriers CNS* 17 (69): 1–24. doi: 10.1186/s12987-020-00230-3.

Klezovitch, O. et al. (2004). Loss of cell polarity causes severe brain dysplasia in Lgl1 knockout mice. *Genes Dev* 18: 559–571. doi: 10.1101/gad.1178004.

Konno, D. et al. (2008). Neuroepithelial progenitors undergo LGN-dependent planar divisions to maintain self-renewability during mammalian neurogenesis. *Nat Cell Biol* 10 (1): 93–101. doi: 10.1038/ncb1673.

Kornblum, H.I. et al. (1998). Abnormal astrocyte development and neuronal death in mice lacking the epidermal growth factor receptor. *J Neurosci Res* 53 (6): 697–717. doi: 10.1002/(sici)1097-4547(19980915)53:6<697::aid-jnr8>3.0.co;2-0.

Kretzschmar, K. and Watt, F.M. (2012). Lineage tracing. *Cell* 148 (1–2): 33–45. doi: 10.1016/j.cell.2012.01.002.

Lakomá, J. et al. (2011). Reelin sets the pace of neocortical neurogenesis. *Development* 138 (23): 5223–5234. doi: 10.1242/dev.063776.

LaMonica, B.E. et al. (2013). Mitotic spindle orientation predicts outer radial glial cell generation in human neocortex. *Nat Commun* 4 (1665): 1–11. doi: 10.1038/ncomms2647.

Lancaster, M.A. and Knoblich, J.A. (2012). Spindle orientation in mammalian cerebral cortical development. *Curr Opin Neurobiol* 22 (5): 737–746. doi: 10.1016/j.conb.2012.04.003.

Laukoter, S. et al. (2020a). Imprinted Cdkn1c genomic locus cell-autonomously promotes cell survival in cerebral cortex development. *Nat Commun* 11 (1): 1–14. doi: 10.1038/s41467-019-14077-2.

Laukoter, S. et al. (2020b). Cell-type specificity of genomic imprinting in cerebral cortex. *Neuron* 107 (6): 1160–1179. doi: 10.1016/j.neuron.2020.06.031.

Lehtinen, M.K. and Walsh, C.A. (2011). Neurogenesis at the brain-cerebrospinal fluid interface. *Ann Rev Cell Dev Biol* 27: 653–679. doi: 10.1146/annurev-cellbio-092910-154026.

Lehtinen, M.K. et al. (2011). The cerebrospinal fluid provides a proliferative niche for neural progenitor cells. *Neuron* 69 (5): 893–905. doi: 10.1016/j.neuron.2011.01.023.

Liang, H. et al. (2013). Neural development is dependent on the function of specificity protein 2 in cell cycle progression. *Development* 140 (3): 552–561. doi: 10.1242/dev.085621.

Llinares-Benadero, C. and Borrell, V. (2019). Deconstructing cortical folding: genetic, cellular and mechanical determinants. *Nat Rev Neurosci* 20 (3): 161–176. doi: 10.1038/s41583-018-0112-2.

Llorca, A. et al. (2019). A stochastic framework of neurogenesis underlies the assembly of neocortical cytoarchitecture. *Elife* 8: e51381. doi: 10.7554/elife.51381.

Long, K.R. and Huttner, W.B. (2019). How the extracellular matrix shapes neural development. *Open Biol* 9 (1): 180216. doi: 10.1098/rsob.180216.

LoTurco, J.J. et al. (1995). GABA and glutamate depolarize cortical progenitor cells and inhibit DNA synthesis. *Neuron* 15 (6): 1287–1298. doi: 10.1016/0896-6273(95)90008-x.

Loulier, K. et al. (2014). Multiplex cell and lineage tracking with combinatorial labels. *Neuron* 81 (3): 505–520. doi: 10.1016/j.neuron.2013.12.016.

Mairet-Coello, G. et al. (2012). P57KIP2 regulates radial glia and intermediate precursor cell cycle dynamics and lower layer neurogenesis in developing cerebral cortex. *Development* 139 (3): 475–487. doi: 10.1242/dev.067314.

Malatesta, P. et al. (2003). Neuronal or glial progeny. *Neuron* 37 (5): 751–764. doi: 10.1016/s0896-6273(03)00116-8.

Martín, C. et al. (2006). FGF2 plays a key role in embryonic cerebrospinal fluid trophic properties over chick embryo neuroepithelial stem cells. *Dev Biol* 297 (2): 402–416. doi: 10.1016/j.ydbio.2006.05.010.

Miyata, T. et al. (2004). Asymmetric production of surface-dividing and non-surface-dividing cortical progenitor cells. *Development* 131 (13): 3133–3145. doi: 10.1242/dev.01173.

Moorefield, K.S. et al. (2004). Sp2 DNA binding activity and trans-activation are negatively regulated in mammalian cells*. *J Biol Chem* 279 (14): 13911–13924. doi: 10.1074/jbc.m313589200.

Morris, N.R. and Morris, N.R. (2000). Nuclear migration. From fungi to the mammalian brain. *J Cell Biol* 148 (6): 1097–1102. doi: 10.1083/jcb.148.6.1097.

Nelson, B.R. et al. (2013). Dynamic interactions between intermediate neurogenic progenitors and radial glia in embryonic mouse neocortex. *J Neurosci* 33 (21): 9122–9139. doi: 10.1523/jneurosci.0791-13.2013.

Nie, K. et al. (2010). Proliferation but not migration is associated with blood vessels during development of the rostral migratory stream. *Dev Neurosci* 32 (3): 163–172. doi: 10.1159/000301135.

Noctor, S.C. et al. (2004). Cortical neurons arise in symmetric and asymmetric division zones and migrate through specific phases. *Nat Neurosci* 7: 136–144. doi: 10.1038/nn1172.

Noctor, S.C. et al. (2008). Distinct behaviors of neural stem and progenitor cells underlie cortical neurogenesis. *J Comp Neurol* 508 (1): 28–44. doi: 10.1002/cne.21669.

Ortiz-Álvarez, G. et al. (2019). Adult neural stem cells and multiciliated ependymal cells share a common lineage regulated by the geminin family members. *Neuron* 102 (1): 159–172.e7. doi: 10.1016/j.neuron.2019.01.051.

Pauler, F.M. et al. (2021). Inducible uniparental chromosome disomy to probe genomic imprinting at single-cell level in brain and beyond. *Neurochem Int* 145 (104986): 1–17. doi: 10.1016/j.neuint.2021.104986.

Pilaz, L.-J. et al. (2016). Dynamic mRNA transport and local translation in radial glial progenitors of the developing brain. *Curr Biol* 26 (24): 3383–3392. doi: 10.1016/j.cub.2016.10.040.

Pilz, G.-A. et al. (2013). Amplification of progenitors in the mammalian telencephalon includes a new radial glial cell type. *Nat Commun* 4 (2125): 1–11. doi: 10.1038/ncomms3125.

Poduri, A. et al. (2013). Somatic mutation, genomic variation, and neurological disease. *Science* 341 (6141): 43–51. doi: 10.1126/science.1237758.

Pollen, A.A. et al. (2015). Molecular identity of human outer radial glia during cortical development. *Cell* 163 (1): 55–67. doi: 10.1016/j.cell.2015.09.004.

Raballo, R. et al. (2000). Basic fibroblast growth factor (Fgf2) is necessary for cell proliferation and neurogenesis in the developing cerebral cortex. *J Neurosci* 20 (13): 5012–5023. doi: 10.1523/jneurosci.20-13-05012.2000.

Rakic, P. (1974). Neurons in rhesus monkey visual cortex. *Science* 183 (4123): 425–427. doi: 10.1126/science.183.4123.425.

Rash, B.G. et al. (2016). Bidirectional radial Ca(2+) activity regulates neurogenesis and migration during early cortical column formation. *Sci Adv* 2 (2): 1–10. doi: 10.1126/sciadv.1501733.

Rash, B.G. et al. (2018). Metabolic regulation and glucose sensitivity of cortical radial glial cells. *Proc Natl Acad Sci USA* 115 (40): 10142–10147. doi: 10.1073/pnas.1808066115.

Schwamborn, J.C. and Knoblich, J.A. (2008). LIS1 and spindle orientation in neuroepithelial cells. *Cell Stem Cell* 2 (3): 193–194. doi: 10.1016/j.stem.2008.02.010.

Segarra, M. et al. (2018). Endothelial Dab1 signaling orchestrates neuro-glia-vessel communication in the central nervous system. *Science* 361 (6404): 1–15. doi: 10.1126/science.aao2861.

Seroogy, K.B. et al. (1995). Proliferative zones of postnatal rat brain express epidermal growth factor receptor mRNA. *Brain Res* 670 (1): 157–164. doi: 10.1016/0006-8993(94)01300-7.

Seuntjens, E. et al. (2009). Sip1 regulates sequential fate decisions by feedback signaling from postmitotic neurons to progenitors. *Nat Neurosci* 12: 1373–1380. doi: 10.1038/nn.2409.

Sibilia, M. et al. (1998). A strain-independent postnatal neurodegeneration in mice lacking the EGF receptor. *EMBO J* 17 (3): 719–731. doi: 10.1093/emboj/17.3.719.

Sicca, F. et al. (2003). Mosaic mutations of the LIS1 gene cause subcortical band heterotopia. *Neurology* 61 (8): 1042–1046. doi: 10.1212/wnl.61.8.1042.

Sidman, R.L. and Rakic, P. (1973). Neuronal migration, with special reference to developing human brain: a review. *Brain Res* 62 (1): 1–35. doi: 10.1016/0006-8993(73)90617-3.

Siegenthaler, J.A. et al. (2009). Retinoic acid from the meninges regulates cortical neuron generation. *Cell* 139 (3): 597–609. doi: 10.1016/j.cell.2009.10.004.

Silva, C.G.Da. et al. (2018). Cell-intrinsic control of interneuron migration drives cortical morphogenesis. *Cell* 172 (5): 1063–1078.e19. doi: 10.1016/j.cell.2018.01.031.

Sun, T. and Hevner, R.F. (2014). Growth and folding of the mammalian cerebral cortex: from molecules to malformations. *Nat Rev Neurosci* 15 (4): 217–232. doi: 10.1038/nrn3707.

Taverna, E. et al. (2014). The cell biology of neurogenesis: toward an understanding of the development and evolution of the neocortex. *Ann Rev Cell Dev Biol* 30: 465–502. doi: 10.1146/annurev-cellbio-101011-155801.

Telley, L. et al. (2019). Temporal patterning of apical progenitors and their daughter neurons in the developing neocortex. *Science* 364 (6440): 1–7. doi: 10.1126/science.aav2522.

Turrero Garcia, M. et al. (2016). S-phase duration is the main target of cell cycle regulation in neural progenitors of developing ferret neocortex. *J Comp Neurol* 524 (3): 456–470. doi: 10.1002/cne.23801.

Ueno, M. and Yamashita, T. (2014). Bidirectional tuning of microglia in the developing brain: from neurogenesis to neural circuit formation. *Curr Opin Neurobiol* 27: 8–15. doi: 10.1016/j.conb.2014.02.004.

Valiente, M. and Marin, O. (2010). Neuronal migration mechanisms in development and disease. *Curr Opin Neurobiol* 20 (1): 68–78. doi: 10.1016/j.conb.2009.12.003S0959-4388(09)00179-2[pii].

Vasioukhin, V. and Vasioukhin, V. (2006). Lethal giant puzzle of Lgl. *Dev Neurosci* 28 (1–2): 13–24. doi: 10.1159/000090749.

Villalba, A. et al. (2021). Chapter One – The regulation of cortical neurogenesis. In: *Current Topics in Developmental Biology* (ed. G.J. Bashaw), vol. 142, 1–66. Academic Press. doi: 10.1016/bs.ctdb.2020.10.003.

Vitali, I. et al. (2018). Progenitor hyperpolarization regulates the sequential generation of neuronal subtypes in the developing neocortex. *Cell* 174 (5): 1264–1276.e15. doi: 10.1016/j.cell.2018.06.036.

Vogenstahl, J. et al. (2022). Vascular regulation of developmental neurogenesis. *Front Cell Dev Biol* 10: 890852. doi: 10.3389/fcell.2022.890852.

Wagner, B. et al. (2006). Neuronal survival depends on EGFR signaling in cortical but not midbrain astrocytes. *EMBO J* 25 (4): 752–762. doi: 10.1038/sj.emboj.7600988.

Weissman, T.A. et al. (2004). Calcium waves propagate through radial glial cells and modulate proliferation in the developing neocortex. *Neuron* 43 (5): 647–661. doi: 10.1016/j.neuron.2004.08.015.

Wong, F.K. et al. (2018). Pyramidal cell regulation of interneuron survival sculpts cortical networks. *Nature* 557 (7707): 668–673. doi: 10.1038/s41586-018-0139-6.

Wong, F.K. and Marín, O. (2019). Developmental cell death in the cerebral cortex. *Ann Rev Cell Dev Biol* 35: 523–542. doi: 10.1146/annurev-cellbio-100818-125204.

Woodworth, M.B. et al. (2017). Building a lineage from single cells: genetic techniques for cell lineage tracking. *Nat Rev Genet* 18: 230–244. doi: 10.1038/nrg.2016.159.

Wynshaw-Boris, A. (2007). Lissencephaly and LIS1. *Clin Genet* 72 (4): 296–304. doi: 10.1111/j.1399-0004.2007.00888.x.

Yamanaka, T. et al. (2003). Mammalian Lgl forms a protein complex with PAR-6 and aPKC independently of PAR-3 to regulate epithelial cell polarity. *Curr Biol* 13 (9): 734–743. doi: 10.1016/s0960-9822(03)00244-6.

Yingling, J. et al. (2008). Neuroepithelial stem cell proliferation requires LIS1 for precise spindle orientation and symmetric division. *Cell* 132 (3): 474–486. doi: 10.1016/j.cell.2008.01.026.

Zappaterra, M.D. et al. (2007). A comparative proteomic analysis of human and rat embryonic cerebrospinal fluid. *J Proteome Res* 6 (9): 3537–3548. doi: 10.1021/pr070247w.

Zhang, X. et al. (2020). Clonal analysis of gliogenesis in the cerebral cortex reveals stochastic expansion of glia and cell autonomous responses to Egfr dosage. *Cells* 9 (12): 2662. doi: 10.3390/cells9122662.

Zong, H. et al. (2005). Mosaic analysis with double markers in mice. *Cell* 121 (3): 479–492. doi: 10.1016/j.cell.2005.02.012.

Part 3

Generation of Neuron Types

11

Generation of Projection Neuron Diversity in the Neocortex

From Embryos to Organoids

Ana Uzquiano[1,2] *and Paola Arlotta*[1,2,*]

[1] *Department of Stem Cell & Regenerative Biology Harvard University, Cambridge, MA, USA*
[2] *Stanley Center for Psychiatric Research Broad Institute of MIT and Harvard, Cambridge, MA, USA*
* *Corresponding author*

11.1 Introduction

The neocortex is the youngest part of the mammalian brain and has undergone a vast expansion throughout evolution that is particularly noticeable in humans. As a result of this evolutionary expansion, the neocortex contains an unparalleled diversity of cell types generated through a series of orchestrated events critical for proper cortical circuit assembly and function. The extraordinary complexity of the neocortex requires extensive investigation to decipher how this structure develops across mammalian species, especially in humans. Abnormal cortical development often translates to severe neurodevelopmental and neuropsychiatric diseases with biological substrates that remain poorly understood, driving an additional motivation to unveil the rules dictating cerebral cortex assembly.

The basic structure and function of neocortical organization has been known for many years. Over the past decade, the emergence of single-cell genomics, a fast-evolving field, has provided a first glimpse into remaining questions such as different transcriptional cell types and states present across several species, including humans. Additionally, profiling of individual cells during long periods of cortical development is resulting in unprecedented maps of mammalian corticogenesis, that are in turn leveraged to decipher the molecular strategies that build cortical cellular diversity. Still, many questions remain open. For example, what are the codes that dictate the timing and fate of the progeny produced by the different cortical progenitors? How does this process differ across species with different cortical complexity? Is there a previously unidentified degree of transcriptional divergence in between species with different cortical size that could be further related to cellular physiology? And finally, which are the human-specific features related to these processes, that could eventually result in the highly evolved human neocortex?

Here, we cover key concepts in the cellular diversity of the cerebral cortex with a special focus on the developmental rules underlying the generation and diversification of cortical excitatory projection neurons. We then review the emergence and establishment of brain organoids as models to study human features of cortical development and the unprecedented opportunity these model systems offer to investigate how cellular specification is achieved in human cortical cells.

Neocortical Neurogenesis in Development and Evolution, First Edition. Edited by Wieland B. Huttner.

11.2 Basic Principles of Cellular Organization and Composition of the Cerebral Cortex

Since the nineteenth century, neuroscientists have been aware that regions with specialized function could be identified in the cerebral cortex. Indeed, on the tangential axis, the neocortex is parcellated into functional areas with defined boundaries, different cytoarchitectonic features, and different patterns of afferent-efferent connectivity. There are four primary areas: the somatosensory cortex (which processes sensory modalities), the auditory cortex (which processes sound), the visual cortex (which processes the sense of sight), and the motor cortex (which outputs information to control motor behavior) (Rash and Grove 2006). Additionally, there is a specialized region in the human brain, the prefrontal cortex, that has expanded in size and complexity to act as an important processing center for high-function cognitive abilities (e.g., memory, planning, decision-making). For review on cortical areas and ongoing efforts to investigate areal development, we refer the readers to Nano et al. (2021).

On its radial dimension, the neocortex is characterized by the organization of neurons into six horizontal layers, historically defined as supragranular (layer I/II–III), granular (layer IV), and infragranular (layers V and VI) (Figure 11.1). Layers contain different classes of neurons and vary in thickness and tissue architecture depending on their areal identity (reviewed in Greig et al. (2013)). The afferent-efferent connections established by cortical neurons are highly interconnected with the cortical layer in which they reside. For instance, projection neurons in superficial layers mainly project to intracortical targets, while projection neurons in deep layers connect with subcortical and subcerebral regions. The two primary neuronal populations of the cortex existing in these six-layers are excitatory projection neurons (PN) produced by the progenitors of the dorsal telencephalon (see later) and GABAergic interneurons that largely arise from ventral regions, namely the ganglionic eminences (GE), and migrate extensively to reach the developing cortex (for a review on interneuron diversity and development, see Lim et al. 2018). PN make up the vast majority of cortical neurons, around 70–80 percent, while interneurons constitute the remaining 20–30 percent. Of note, the interneuron percentage is higher in primates and thus humans than in rodents (Clowry 2015). The cerebral cortex is also populated by glial cells, namely astrocytes, oligodendrocytes, and microglia, which have multiple functions across cortical development to ensure correct cortical circuit assembly, plasticity, and function (Farhy-Tselnicker and Allen 2018; Mount and Monje 2017; Thion et al. 2018).

11.3 Diversity of Excitatory Projection Neurons

PN are excitatory glutamatergic neurons that connect the cerebral cortex to the entirety of its distal intracortical, subcortical, and subcerebral targets. As proposed by Ramon y Cajal in the early twentieth century, the nomenclature we still use to distinguish PN is based on their connectivity: PN are broadly classified as intracortical (i.e., projecting to other regions of the cortex) or corticofugal (CFuPN; i.e., projecting to non-cortical targets) neurons (Figure 11.1). Intracortical PN are mostly localized in the upper layers II/III of the cortex although they can be found in all cortical layers. They are further subdivided into commissural or associate PN. Commissural PN project their axons to the opposite hemisphere, mainly though the corpus callosum (CC), hence constituting the callosal projection neuron (CPN) population, or alternatively through the anterior commissure. On the other hand, associative PN project their axons to a different layer or cortical column in the same hemisphere. CFuPN are mainly located in the deep layers of the cortex and can be

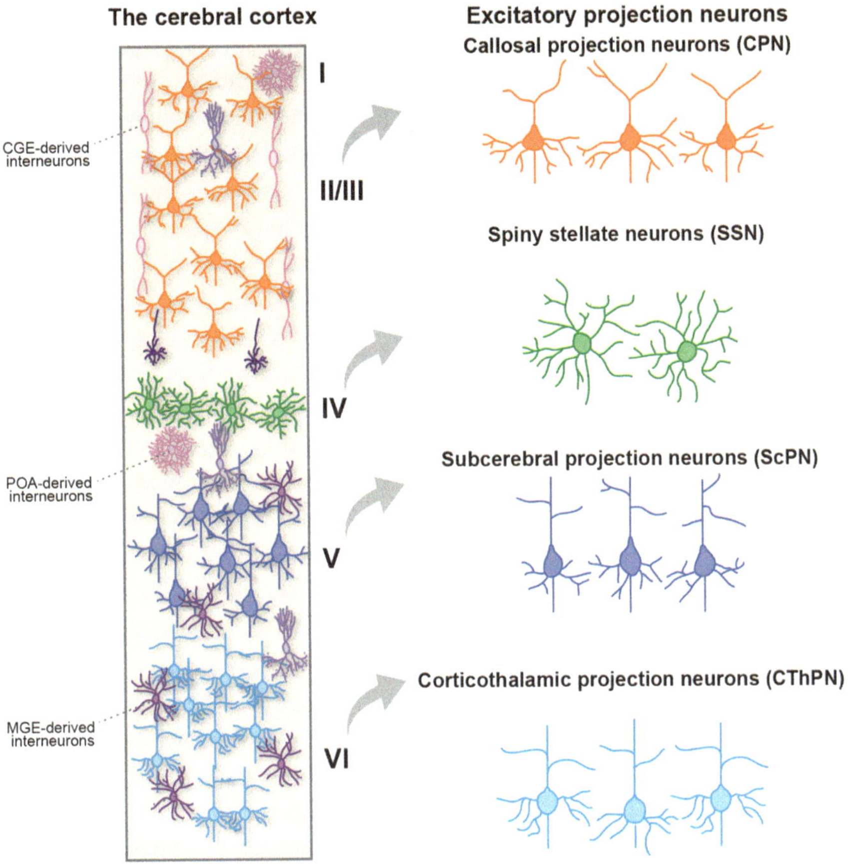

Figure 11.1 Distribution of excitatory projection neurons and inhibitory interneurons in the six-layer mammalian cortex. On the right: specific projection neurons populating each cortical layer. CGE: caudal ganglionic eminence; POA: preoptic area; MGE: medial ganglionic eminence.

further classified in corticothalamic PN (CThPN) and subcerebral PN (ScPN) (Figure 11.1). CThPN are located in layer VI and project to several nucleus of the thalamus to modulate sensory information while ScPN are located in layer Vb and project to different targets below the brain, including the pons and other nuclei of the brainstem (corticopontine PN), the superior colliculus (corticotectal PN), and the spinal cord (corticospinal motor neurons; CSMN) (Molyneaux et al. 2007; Lodato and Arlotta 2015).

The molecular profiling of defined PN began with approaches such as retrograde labelling of different neuronal types (Arlotta et al. 2005; Catapano et al. 2008; LaVail 1978; Molyneaux et al. 2009), genetic labelling (Josh Huang and Zeng 2013), and nuclear immunostaining with antibodies allowing fluorescence-activated cell sorting (FACS) of distinctly labelled neuronal types (Molyneaux et al. 2015). These techniques allowed the first molecular characterization of cortical neuron subtypes in the rodent cortex. Refined versions of these approaches are still proving useful. For example, this technique has allowed the molecular characterization of PN in the human cortex (Zuccaro et al. 2021) and to decipher the molecular divergence and similarities between different subtypes of intracortical PN (Klingler et al. 2019). The combination of these initial approaches with more advanced technology, such as single-cell RNA sequencing (scRNA-seq), has led to the development of MAP-seq (multiplexed analysis of projections by sequencing) (Kebschull et al. 2016).

By using MAP-seq, a technique that combines retrograde labeling, afferent individual cell barcoding, and scRNA-seq, Klingler and colleagues (2021) discovered a temporal molecular shift in the development of motor cortex PN and somatosensory PN in the primary somatosensory cortex. This indicated that these cell types that target different cortical regions share transcriptional programs through their development rather than displaying distinct molecular trajectories (Klingler et al. 2021).

These initial studies uncovered the first set of PN subtype-specific signature genes that are still actively used to identify the different PN populations outlined above (Molyneaux et al. 2015), and whose function in PN development is still studied to date. In this initial work researchers performed deep characterization of CThPN, allowing molecular distinction of the different subtypes and identifying genes specific for each of these PN subtypes (Arlotta et al. 2005). For instance, Tle4 identifies CThPN but not CSMN, while CSMN are characterized by the expression of markers such as Ldb2 or Fezf2 but CThPN are not (Arlotta et al. 2005; Lodato et al. 2014; Molyneaux et al. 2015). In these initial studies, CPN were also extensively characterized, revealing molecular identifiers of this population such as Cux2, Inhba, Btg1, Lp1, Cited2, and PlexinD1 (Molyneaux et al. 2009). Of note, CPN localized in superficial and deep layers expressed few genes that molecularly distinguish them (Molyneaux et al. 2009). Recent work has investigated whether transcriptional diversity of intracortically projecting neurons could be associated with their projection target or is instead driven by laminar location. Assessment of the transcriptional profile of upper layer CPN, deep layer CPN, and spiny stellate neurons (SSN) – located in layer IV and projecting locally within cortical columns (Lefort et al. 2009; Staiger et al. 2004) – revealed a projection-based organization of transcriptional programs, with deep layer CPN showing a closer transcriptional profile to upper layer CPN than SSN (Klingler et al. 2019).

The evolutionary expansion of CPN in human and nonhuman primates, and the association of this cell type with human cognitive abilities, makes it an interesting and imperative subject of study. Several groups have assessed the differences of CPN across species at the electrophysiological (Deitcher et al. 2017; Gidon et al. 2020; Kalmbach et al. 2018) and molecular levels (Fame et al. 2017; Berg et al. 2021). It has been described that, for instance, while the expression of some genes identifying discrete populations of CPN in the mouse cortex is consistent in macaques, other genes show a divergent pattern of expression, indicating variable levels of conservation across these species (Fame et al. 2017). A step further, Berg and colleagues (2021) described an increase in transcriptional subtypes of CPN in humans when compared to mouse, indicating an increased diversification of this neuronal population in the human cerebral cortex (Berg et al. 2021). Additionally, the molecular signatures of human CPN, when compared to the mouse, have been shown to differ the most between species and across all PN, further highlighting the divergence of the CPN population in the human versus mouse cortex (Zuccaro et al. 2021).

The fast-evolving field of single-cell genomics is simultaneously challenging and shaping the classic classification of cortical PN. Zeisel and colleagues (2015) performed the first unbiased sampling of the mouse somatosensory cortex identifying diverse neuronal cell types fitting with previously molecularly defined cortical neuron subtypes (Zeisel et al. 2015). This initial work was followed by single-cell profiling of the mouse primary visual cortex (Tasic et al. 2018) and the anterior lateral cortex (Tasic et al. 2018) upon microdissection of cortical layers and FACS-purification of specific neuronal populations. These studies led to the annotation of more than 50 PN in both regions, including previously defined subtypes, novel transcriptional subtypes, as well as area-specific subtypes (Tasic et al. 2018). These initial works were followed by further profiling at single-cell resolution in other areas of the mouse cortex, such as the motor cortex, not only in the transcriptome but also in the epigenome space (Bakken et al. 2021; Yao et al. 2021). In addition to this research, which mainly focused on the mouse cerebral cortex, seminal work emerging in the past few years has profiled the cerebral cortex of other species at single-cell resolution, including humans (Bakken et al. 2021; Berg et al. 2021; Hodge et al. 2019; Yuan et al. 2020). This recent research is allowing an in-depth investigation of the cellular composition in the human cerebral cortex and is beginning to reveal shared and divergent molecular features of cortical cell types across different species (Hodge et al. 2019; Luo et al. 2017). Additionally, this work is revealing increased diversification of specific PN populations in the human cerebral cortex when compared to mouse, as stressed above for CPN (Berg et al. 2021).

PN subtypes with different transcriptional identities may also differ in physiological properties, ultimately dictating neuronal function and neural network assembly. The development of techniques such as Patch-seq (Cadwell et al. 2016) allow us to characterize the electrophysiological and transcriptional profiles of individual cells. Although this technology was first applied in the mouse neocortex (Cadwell et al. 2016), the investigation of the physiological and transcriptional properties of individual PN in the human cortex is now also possible (Bakken et al. 2021; Berg et al. 2021; Kalmbach et al. 2021). These studies are beginning to reveal convergent and divergent features of human PN in both the transcriptome and physiological space when compared to mouse PN (Berg et al. 2021; Kalmbach et al. 2021). Understanding these species-specific differences to uncover uniquely human properties will lead to the identification of human-specific traits of neural networks that may underlie human computational capacity.

11.4 Developmental Origin of Projection Neurons: Progenitor Strategies

All excitatory PN of the neocortex are generated from neural progenitors of the dorsal telencephalon within the anterior part of the neural tube. In mice, neurogenesis spans from embryonic day (E) 11 to E19, whereas in humans, neurogenesis is a protracted process spanning approximately from gestational week (GW) 5 to GW20 (Silbereis et al. 2016). Pioneer birth-dating studies confirmed by other approaches showed that PN generation follows a precise temporal sequence with PN of the deep layers generated first, followed by production of upper layer neurons. Therefore, PN populate the cortex in an inside-out pattern of migration. Interestingly, recent work showed that neurons produced at earlier stages of corticogenesis display a more heterogeneous pattern in terms of location as compared to neurons produced at later stages (Magrinelli et al. 2022).

Before the onset of neurogenesis, neural progenitors populating the early dorsal telencephalon are neuroepithelial cells (NE). NE display a characteristic apico-basal polarity with an apical process reaching the ventricle and a basal process attached to the basement membrane; thus, these cells span the entire neuroepithelium. NE divide in a symmetric proliferative manner to expand their population. At the onset of neurogenesis, NE transit from a purely proliferative to a neurogenic state, giving rise to the aRG population. aRG derive from NE at the onset of neurogenesis and although they are broadly transcriptionally similar to NE, aRG express astroglial markers and upregulate the expression of certain transcription factors (TF) such as Pax6. aRG retain a neuroepithelial character as well as an apico-basal polarity with their basal process acting as a crucial guide for migration of newborn neurons. Their soma is restricted to the proliferative ventricular zone (VZ), in the vicinity of the ventricle, and they contact the cerebrospinal fluid via their apical process. aRG can undergo symmetrical proliferative divisions but can also divide asymmetrically to produce other progenitor types (i.e., basal progenitors) that will go on to produce neurons (indirect neurogenesis), or alternatively, generate neurons directly (direct neurogenesis). In mice, this process of direct neurogenesis generates only 10–20 percent of the total PN population (Kowalczyk et al. 2009), with the vast majority of PN generated by intermediate progenitors (IP) instead (Kowalczyk et al. 2009; Vasistha et al. 2015). IP are multipolar, transit-amplifying progenitors, that divide in a basally located germinal zone: the subventricular zone. In species with complex and gyrified cortices, the subventricular zone (SVZ) is split into the inner and outer SVZ, with IP residing mostly in the inner region. In the mouse, IP are mainly neurogenic, and divide symmetrically to produce two neurons. In species with more complex brains, such as humans, IP can self-renew several times before performing a terminal division resulting in two neurons. Furthermore, in species with a gyrified neocortex, such as humans and nonhuman primates, there is another highly abundant type of basal progenitor localized in the SVZ, termed outer or basal radial glia (oRG/bRG). oRG are highly polarized progenitors that can display different morphologies with or without apical and/or basal processes (Betizeau et al. 2013; Coquand et al. 2022). As opposed to aRG, their apical process never reaches the ventricular surface while, like aRG, their basal process is important for neuronal migration and contributes to the tangential dispersion of neurons. oRG have a high proliferative capacity and self-renew several times before producing postmitotic progeny. They predominantly contribute to the final neuronal output by generating CPN of the upper cortical layers (see Figure 11.2; for a review on cortical progenitors, see Taverna et al. (2014); Vaid and Huttner (2022)).

The existence of such a wide variety of cortical progenitors and PN pose a series of questions that remain a subject of debate: Are progenitors progressively and predictably restricted in their potential neuronal outcomes? Are there progenitors pre-committed to generate distinct PN types?

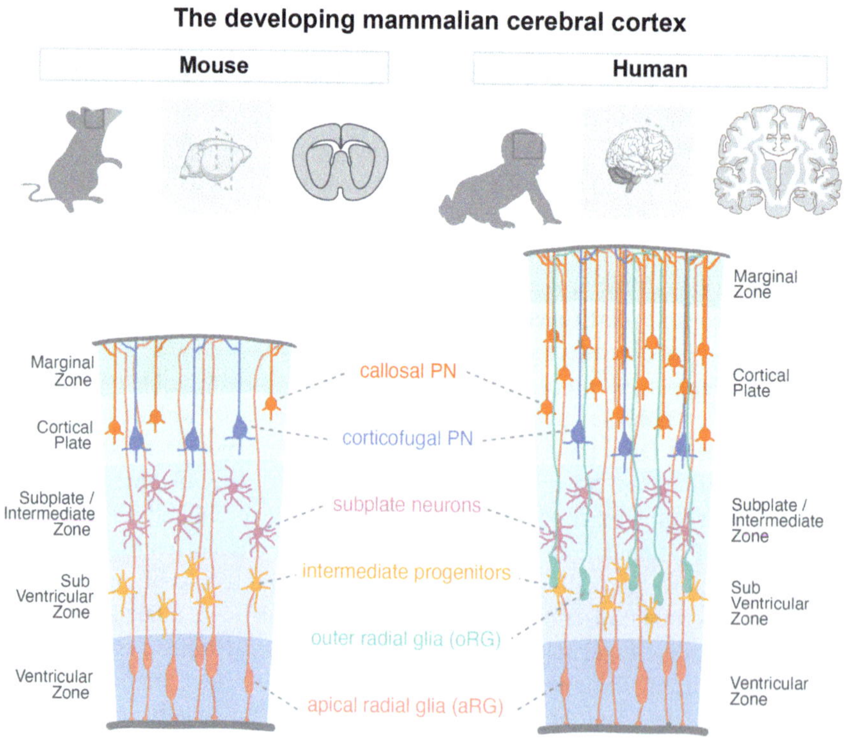

Figure 11.2 The developing mammalian cortex. Schematic representation of the mouse and human developing cerebral cortex. This displays the human expansion of specific populations such as outer radial glia progenitor cells and callosal projection neurons of the upper cortical layers. PN: projection neuron.

Pioneer experiments in the 1990s began to address these questions by interrogating the fate potential of cortical progenitors in heterochronic transplantation paradigms. These experiments leveraged the use of [^{3}H] thymidine to label cycling progenitors in the ferret germinal zones. They found that early cortical progenitors are multipotent whereas late progenitors cannot produce earlier PN even when transplanted into a younger environment (Frantz and McConnell 1996). This work demonstrated a temporal and progressive restriction of progenitor fate potential, which was then confirmed by initial lineage tracing and retroviral infection experiments in the mouse neocortex. Here, individually labelled early progenitors of the VZ produced neurons of all cortical layers (Luskin et al. 1988; Walsh and Cepko 1993). More recently, studies using mouse transgenic lines also support these initial findings (Cadwell et al. 2020; Gao et al. 2014). Work leveraging mosaic analysis with double markers (MADM) further confirmed this temporal competence restriction and provided a quantitative evaluation of the neuronal output produced by individual aRG once they enter a neurogenic state (Gao et al. 2014). *In vitro* studies also support this model, showing that early progenitors in culture give rise to PN in the same temporal order as *in vivo* (Shen et al. 2006). Similar results were gathered when patterning embryonic stem cells (ES) and induced pluripotent stem cells (iPS) to a cortical progenitor fate across multiple species, including mouse, human, and nonhuman primates (Gaspard et al. 2008; Otani et al. 2016; Shi et al. 2012). Importantly, and as further discussed later, this temporal sequence of PN production is also maintained in cortical organoids (Eiraku et al. 2008; Kadoshima et al. 2013; Uzquiano et al. 2022). In humans, the temporal production of deep and upper layer PN has also been confirmed through approaches such as retrospective lineage tracing, which assesses the presence of somatic mutations across multiple cortical PN (Huang et al. 2020). Therefore, mounting evidence supports that cortical progenitors undergo changes in fate potential over time, most likely mediated by several factors including changes in the length of cell cycle (reviewed in Uzquiano et al. (2018)) or in their physiological properties (Vitali et al. 2018).

Recent work by Oberst and colleagues (2019) has challenged the longstanding hypothesis that neurogenic fate progression implies cortical progenitor fate restriction (Oberst et al. 2019). In this work, late mouse cortical progenitors were transplanted into a younger environment. Heterochronic transplantation of late aRG into a younger VZ resulted in the production of deep layer PN, and therefore a change in the neurogenic potential of the late progenitor that would have produced upper layer PN. In contrast, heterochronic transplantation of late IP into a younger environment did not alter its neurogenic potential: these progenitors continued producing upper layer PN. These results contrast the pioneer work performed in ferrets (Frantz and McConnell 1996). However, as the authors of this new study note, they isolated cortical progenitors of different identities separately while the initial study isolated all cycling progenitors (presumably both aRG and abundant IP). These results indicate that mouse aRG are plastic throughout long periods of corticogenesis, whereas other progenitor types are not (i.e., IP). Whether this scenario also occurs in other species still needs to be confirmed. Additionally, these results raise questions about the neurogenic potential and plasticity of other progenitor cell types, such as oRG.

Further fate-mapping and lineage tracing studies were performed to probe the fate potential of cortical progenitors and determine if some progenitors could be fate-committed to produce distinct types of PN. Over the past decade multiple studies have assessed this longstanding question and the results are mixed to this day. Franco and colleagues (2012) showed that aRG expressing the TF Cux2 (marker of CPN and selected interneurons of layer II/III) mainly produce upper layer neurons. To this end, the authors used a knock-in mouse (Cux2-CreERT2) to fate-map Cux2-positive early aRG and their progeny. This approach showed that Cux2-positive aRG are present in the VZ as early as E10.5, and while deep layer CFuPN are generated, these Cux2-positive aRG mainly divide to then produce upper layer PN at later stages of corticogenesis. In addition, when forced to differentiate in an early environment, Cux2-positive aRG still produced upper layer neurons, suggesting that they are intrinsically pre-fated independently of temporal restrictions (Franco et al. 2012). These results indicate that certain progenitor subpopulations are pre-fated and could thus contribute to generating PN diversity. Supporting the presence of pre-fated progenitors, Llorca and colleagues (2019) performed lineage tracing experiments in the mouse neocortex combining genetic fate-mapping, retroviral labeling, and MADM (Llorca et al. 2019). After extensive assessment of clonal neuron positioning, they found that a small number of clones were composed only by cells populating the upper layers of the cortex (Llorca et al. 2019). In agreement with this result, recent work assessing clonal relationships in the mouse telencephalon using lentiviral barcoding coupled with single-cell transcriptomics also suggests the existence of cortical clones exclusively composed by upper layer PN (Ratz et al. 2022). However, careful interpretation of this data is critical due to inherent technical difficulties of the experiments performed which may include cell loss or barcode dropout.

Despite these results, several studies have contradicted the model in which PN diversity may be achieved due to the presence of pre-fated progenitor cells. For instance, work from Guo et al. (2013) used the same Cux2-ERT2 reporter line used by Franco and colleagues (2012) to fate-map progenitors and failed to obtain the same results, instead demonstrating the presence of multipotent progenitors capable of generating all different types of PN. In parallel, they used a Fezf2-CreERT2 bacterial artificial chromosome (BAC) line and reported similar results when performing fate-mapping of progenitors from this line (Guo et al. 2013). Using lineage-tracing with MADM, Gao and colleagues (2014) reported that clones derived from early aRG span all cortical layers (Gao et al. 2014). In agreement with the absence of pre-fated progenitors at early stages of cortical development, extensive single-cell transcriptomics studies have not found heterogeneity in the transcriptome of early aRG and rather support a model in which PN diversification occurs post-mitotically (Di Bella et al. 2021; Telley et al. 2019). These studies are further reinforced by recent work in which clonal relationships of the mouse cortex were assessed at single-cell resolution and clones composed exclusively of specific PN were not reported (Bandler et al. 2022).

It is worth noting that the disagreement among studies may be a result of both models coexisting simultaneously: it is plausible that the VZ may be composed of different progenitors with different fate potentials.

The work discussed above focuses mainly on the temporal restriction and potential fate commitment of aRG. However, further studies have assessed the contribution of basal progenitors to PN output and diversity. The neuronal subtype produced by IP has been a controversial topic: while some studies performed in mice support that IP mainly generate upper layer neurons (Tarabykin et al. 2001; Zimmer et al. 2004) opposing work indicates that they produce PN of all cortical layers (Vasistha et al. 2015). Mihalas and colleagues (2016) showed that while IP have the potential to generate neurons of all layers, the birth-date of these progenitors could influence the neuronal progeny produced. The authors showed that early generated IP mainly produce deep layer PN but production of upper layers PN could be derived from both early and late born IP (Mihalas et al. 2016). Interestingly, IP may not only contribute to the preferential generation of a PN subtype: production of neurons from an IP lineage may also contribute to the establishment of certain morphological and physiological neuronal properties. Neurons derived from IP differ from those produced directly from aRG in their apical dendrite morphology as well as in their action potential patterns (Tyler et al. 2015; Guillamon-Vivancos et al. 2019). This work suggests that lineage origin may be important not only to determine PN identity, but also to instruct the acquisition of other properties that then configure neuronal function.

Assessing the neuronal fates of PN clones derived from oRG is still a challenging task due to the low number of these progenitors in the cerebral cortex of the mouse (Figure 11.2) and the species-specific features they display in terms of proliferative behavior and molecular profile (Betizeau et al. 2013; Coquand et al. 2022; Fietz et al. 2010; Gertz et al. 2014; Hansen et al. 2010; Reillo and Borrell 2012; Shitamukai et al. 2011; Vaid et al. 2018; Wang et al. 2011). Although oRG have been described to generate both deep and upper PN (Pollen et al. 2015), they have primarily been reported to mainly produce CPN of the upper layers in the cortex of humans and nonhuman primates (Betizeau et al. 2013; Lukaszewicz et al. 2005; Nowakowski et al. 2016; Ostrem et al. 2017). Related to this, CPN have been recently described to display a higher transcriptional heterogeneity in the human adult cortex when compared to the mouse (Berg et al. 2021). Therefore, it would be important to decipher the potential contribution of the different cortical progenitor types leading to this divergence and to understand if oRG, abundant in the human but not mouse developing cortex, could underlie this species-specific feature pertaining to CPN transcriptional diversity.

The work discussed above mainly focuses on studies using the mouse as a model system to reveal principles of mammalian corticogenesis and PN production and diversification; however, assessing these principles in other species, specifically human and nonhuman primates, is still challenging due to ethical limitations and scarce access to fetal tissue. Delgado et al. (2022), performed prospective lineage tracing in the human fetal cortex by infecting VZ progenitors of GW15 and GW18 fetal specimens with a lentiviral barcoding library followed by single-cell transcriptomics of the progeny six weeks after infection. These experiments led to the characterization of clonal composition in the human fetal cortex. Interestingly, a few clones contained both excitatory PN and inhibitory interneurons with a CGE-like transcriptional identity, suggesting that interneurons could be produced by dorsal progenitors in humans (Delgado et al. 2022). Further understanding how human progenitors progress throughout corticogenesis, the progeny they produce, and the relationships established in the human cortex, is crucial in understanding how the human cerebral cortex produces the diversity of PN populations and how the size of these populations is determined. As discussed later, human brain organoids have emerged as model systems to study human cortical development, providing an outstanding opportunity to address these questions.

11.5 The Molecular Logic Underlying Projection Neuron Diversification: Postmitotic Mechanisms

The molecular programs that unfold as cortical progenitors progress through neurogenesis are key in determining neuronal fate commitment and lineage determination. However, these progenitor mechanisms coexist with regulatory events restricted to early postmitotic stages that also contribute to the establishment and refinement of PN subtype identities.

Transcriptional characterization of PN subtypes has led to the identification of neuron subtype-specific TF which are expressed in early postmitotic neurons (Heavner et al. 2020; Molyneaux et al. 2015). In this chapter we mainly focus on the role of TF in postmitotic PN identity establishment, however, it is worth noting that other factors such as microRNAs (Diaz et al. 2020) or epigenetic states including chromatin accessibility and DNA methylation (Noack et al. 2022) also contribute to PN identity acquisition.

In early postmitotic neurons, TF that are expressed postmitotically regulate each other to refine PN subtype identity (Greig et al. 2013; Lodato and Arlotta 2015; Srinivasan et al. 2012). First, focusing on CPN specification, several TF have been described to promote CPN identity by repressing CFuPN fates. Satb2, a chromatin remodeling protein restricted to postmitotic CPN

(Alcamo et al. 2008; Britanova et al. 2008) and its interacting-protein Ski (Baranek et al. 2012), repress the ScPN marker Bcl11b, also known to control axon fasciculation and extension (Arlotta et al. 2005). Absence of Satb2 or Ski results in ectopic expression of Bcl11b in CPN that do not extend projections through the CC and instead project to ipsilateral subcortical targets (Alcamo et al. 2008; Baranek et al. 2012). Recently, the TF Myt1 and Myt1l have also been reported to regulate Bcl11b and Satb2 expression in early CFuPN: Myt1 represses Bcl11b expression, and concomitantly, both Myt1 and Myt1l enhance expression of Satb2, therefore promoting a CPN fate (Heavner et al. 2020). Additionally, and further reinforcing the importance of Satb2 in CPN specification, the absence of Satb2 causes the lack of expression of several subtype-specific markers of CPN (Alcamo et al. 2008; Britanova et al. 2008). The TF Lhx2, an additional marker of CPN (Bulchand et al. 2003; Molyneaux et al. 2015), has also been shown to regulate the expression of the TF Fezf2 and Sox11, which are determinants of ScPN identity (Arlotta et al. 2005; Molyneaux et al. 2005). To regulate the expression of these TF, Lhx2 interacts with the chromatin remodeling complex NuRD (Muralidharan et al. 2017). Loss of Lhx2 in the mouse developing cortex leads to an increase in Fezf2 and Sox11 expression, both in the VZ and cortical plate, due to an increase in active epigenetic histone marks at the loci of these genes (Muralidharan et al. 2017).

Tbr1 is another TF that progressively refines PN subtype identity. Tbr1 is expressed in subplate neurons, CThPN and CPN. In the absence of Tbr1, the subplate is no longer distinguishable and CThPN express aberrantly high levels of Fezf2 and Bcl11b (Arlotta et al. 2005; Molyneaux et al. 2015). This results in the abnormal development of Tbr1-depleted CThPN that fail to project to the thalamus and project instead to subcerebral targets (Han et al. 2011; McKenna et al. 2011). Fog2, an additional TF important for CFuPN fate acquisition and diversification, has also been reported to regulate the diversification and function of CThPN, in part by regulating the expression level of Bcl11b. Fog2 loss of function leads to an aberrant upregulation of Bcl11b in CThPN and the acquisition of a mixed CThPN/ScPN molecular identity, which additionally display abnormal axonal extension (Galazo et al. 2016). Another TF important for refining the identity of PN populating deep layers of the cortex is Sox5. This TF is required to ensure that both subplate and CFuPN are generated in the correct temporal sequence. When Sox5 is absent, subplate neurons acquire molecular features of a precocious ScPN fate. Loss of Sox5 also impacts the specification of CThPN, which are incorrectly differentiated (Lai et al. 2008). Ctip1 is also an important TF that regulates the postmitotic development of PN that populate the deep layers of the cortex, ensuring that each subtype is produced in the right proportion in a given functional area (Woodworth et al. 2016). The TF Bhlhb5 and Lmo4 are expressed exclusively in postmitotic neurons and are important for CSMN specification in the caudal motor cortex and the rostral motor cortex, respectively. Absence of these TF lead to aberrant axonal projections from these two cortical regions to their corresponding targets (Cederquist et al. 2013; Joshi et al. 2008).

Recent work leveraging the use of single-cell transcriptomics is providing further insight into the global regulatory mechanisms that govern neuronal differentiation and diversification. In these studies scRNA-seq or assay for transposase-accessible chromatin (ATAC) sequencing are combined with computational algorithms that infer the developmental trajectory of different cortical lineages and in turn provide an unprecedented array of candidate genes and TF involved in PN differentiation and commitment (Di Bella et al. 2021; Nowakowski et al. 2017; Telley et al. 2019; Trevino et al. 2021; Ziffra et al. 2021). In the most complete up-to-date mouse developing cortex atlas, a total of ~98,000 cells from the putative somatosensory cortex were profiled at single-cell resolution both in the transcriptome and epigenome space and throughout early embryonic stages (E10.5) to postnatal day 4. By applying URD, an algorithm that generates branch trajectory trees based on transcriptional similarity (Farrell et al. 2018), the authors reveal sets of TF that could act as molecular codes to discriminate between branches of the trajectory tree, which broadly correspond to different cortical lineages. Therefore, this provides the molecular codes that potentially regulate the acquisition of different PN subtype fates. In addition, this analysis also provides the molecular cascade of genes expressed throughout the differentiation of each PN lineage. These genes likely act postmitotically to further refine PN subtype identity (Di Bella et al. 2021). Therefore, this work provides a comprehensive collection of all the molecular states of each cortical lineage across time, exposing the mechanistic principles by which the mammalian cerebral cortex generates its cellular diversity, and providing a resource to decode the effectors regulating PN specification. Approaches based on scalable genetic assays, such as Perturb-seq (Dixit et al. 2016), grant functional insight and validation of this vast array of newly identified molecular candidates mediating PN diversification in the mouse cerebral cortex.

This work, spanning decades of research, revealed fundamental principles and key genes regulating PN differentiation and diversification by using the mouse as a model system. Recently, the profiling of individual human fetal cells at single-cell resolution is allowing the identification of the molecular rules governing such processes in the human cerebral cortex (Nowakowski et al. 2017; Trevino et al. 2021; Ziffra et al. 2021). For instance, Nowakowski and colleagues (2017) performed scRNA-seq of human fetal cells (GW17–18) and described a common neuronal differentiation program that is conserved across different cortical areas and even shared across dorsal and ventral lineages. Aiming to understand the regulatory logic of neurogenesis in humans, Ziffra and colleagues (2021) performed scATAC-seq of the fetal cortex (GW17–20) to identify the trajectories of chromatin accessibility underlying differentiation and maturation of PN and revealed a hierarchy of TF involved in neurogenesis. These studies allowed an unprecedented insight into the regulatory logic underlying neuronal generation and specification in the human cerebral cortex. However, certain limitations need to be overcome to exploit these resources to their full potential. For instance, in most studies excitatory PN are not classified into subtypes thus hampering the identification of gene candidates refining PN subtype identity. Deciphering the factors that govern diversification of human PN subtypes becomes crucial given the different features that PN subtypes display across species, not only in terms of molecular profile and transcriptional heterogeneity, but also in terms of physiology. Additionally, the issue of scarce fetal tissue available for experimental use is exacerbated for late stages of fetal development when processes such as cellular diversification occur. This leads to the inability to profile human fetal cells across a longitudinal time course spanning all major events of cortical development. Therefore, this hinders the investigation of late events in cortical development and of protracted processes such as PN subtype identity acquisition and refinement. As discussed below, human cortical organoids, cultured across long periods *in vitro*, offer an unprecedented opportunity to study these late events of human cortical development.

11.6 The Emergence of Human Brain Organoids as Model Systems to Investigate Human-specific Features of Cortical Development

Our brain differs from that of even our closest primate relatives. However, as it can be appreciated in the previous sections of this chapter, much of our current knowledge pertaining to cortical development and function comes from studies in model organism lacking the enormous morphological and genetic complexity characteristic of humans (e.g., rodents). The cellular and molecular mechanisms underlying human cortical development are still largely unknown.

Human cortical development is a protracted process that occurs largely *in utero* and is thus experimentally inaccessible. Following an extensive period of apical progenitor proliferation, neurogenesis extends for over 3 months. As discussed earlier, work using human fetal tissue has proven critical to our knowledge of human cortical development. However, these studies rely on fetal tissue availability, and only provide a snapshot of a specific time point in cortical development. Therefore, tractable experimental models are needed to dissect the cellular and molecular mechanisms underlying human cortical development and evolution. These models are also crucial to dissect the biological substrates underlying severe neuropsychiatric and neurodevelopmental disorders.

In the past decade, brain organoids have emerged as powerful models to investigate human brain development and diseases. Brain organoids are 3D *in vitro* cultures derived from ES or iPS, which spontaneously develop some of the cellular diversity and architectural features characteristic of the endogenous brain through a process of self-organization. Pioneering work showed that, depending on the culture protocol, brain organoids can intrinsically generate multiple regions of the developing brain (self-patterned/whole brain organoids) (Lancaster et al. 2013), or can be directed toward a particular brain region after treatment with small molecules that promote a specific cell fate (Figure 11.3) (patterned/region-specific brain organoids) (Eiraku et al. 2008; Kadoshima et al. 2013).

Whole brain organoids are largely produced through self-organization and minimal patterning, leveraging the bias of the early ectoderm to generate cells of the dorsal forebrain (Espuny-Camacho et al. 2013). Therefore, these models provide a unique platform to investigate the intrinsic capacity of neural stem cells to generate different brain cell types and self-assemble into distinct brain regions within the same organoid (Benito-Kwiecinski and Lancaster 2020), which are not randomly localized and are separated by boundaries mimicking borders found *in vivo* (Renner et al. 2017). After seminal work by Lancaster and colleagues (2013) to establish this organoid model, whole brain organoid protocols were further improved to allow for extensive periods of *in vitro* culture and enhanced neuronal maturation, which resulted in the presence of neuronal activity patterns (Quadrato et al. 2017). Although whole brain organoids could be considered less artificial

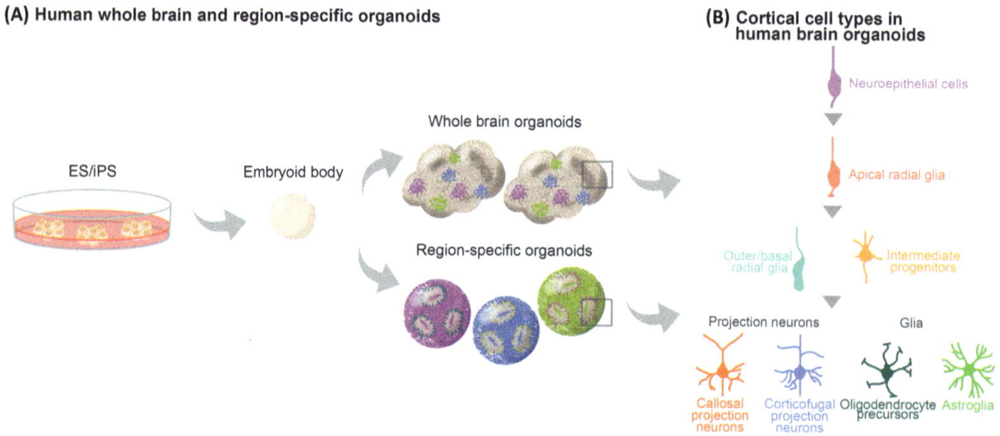

Figure 11.3 Human brain organoids have emerged as models to study human-specific events of cortical development. (A) Brain organoids are generated from embryonic stem cells (ES) or induced pluripotent stem cells (iPS). Depending on the protocol, organoids can be self-patterned, resulting in whole brain organoids, or patterned using small molecules, leading to the generation of region-specific organoids. (B) Cortical cell types present in human brain organoids.

than patterned organoids and more reflective of endogenous principles of brain development (Velasco et al. 2020), one big limitation of this type of organoid model is the high variability of cell types produced and overall morphology found across individual organoids and experimental batches (Del Dosso et al. 2020; Velasco et al. 2020). This lack of reproducibility limits the use of this type of organoids for the investigation of developmental and disease-associated processes and has led to a wider use of patterned protocols that show an improved cellular and morphological reproducibility.

Patterned brain organoids generate select brain regions through application of extrinsic factors that direct cells to acquire a specific regional identity. These protocols have an initial step of inhibition of the SMAD pathway (Chambers et al. 2009), known to promote the generation of epidermis over neural ectoderm. This SMAD (suppressor of mothers against decapentaplegic) inhibition can be dual or partial and can be achieved by applying small molecules to inhibit the TFGβ or/and BMP pathways. Wnt inhibition is also often employed to represses mesodermal identities and promote generation of anterior neuroectoderm (ten Berge et al. 2008). Initial work on these patterned protocols mainly focused on the generation of cerebral cortex organoids (cortical organoids) (Eiraku et al. 2008; Kadoshima et al. 2013; Mariani et al. 2015; Paşca et al. 2015), and these approaches used to generate cerebral cortex organoids have been continuously improved to enhance reproducibility and scalability (Amiri et al. 2018; Sloan et al. 2018; Velasco et al. 2019). Although we mostly focus on the promise of cortical organoids to decipher human-specific features of brain development it is worth noting that protocols for the generation of many other brain regions have also been developed, improved, and characterized, including thalamus (Xiang et al. 2019), hypothalamus (Qian et al. 2016), midbrain (Fiorenzano et al. 2021; Jo et al. 2016; Monzel et al. 2017; Qian et al. 2016), cerebellum (Muguruma et al. 2015), and choroid plexus (Pellegrini et al. 2020). As discussed later, this also offers an opportunity to connect organoids from multiple brain regions, whose interaction is required to ensure proper development of the brain, including the cerebral cortex.

11.7 Cortical Cell Type Diversity and Cellular Specification in Human Brain Organoids: An Opportunity to Decipher How Human Neurons are Made

Many studies have shown that the human brain and cortical organoids can produce a large diversity of the cell types that compose the human endogenous developing cortex (Figure 11.3) (Bhaduri et al. 2020; Kadoshima et al. 2013; Lancaster et al. 2013; Pollen et al. 2019; Quadrato et al. 2017; Trujillo et al. 2019; Uzquiano et al. 2022; Velasco et al. 2019; Yoon et al. 2019). Certain cortical organoid models have been shown to generate this large compendium of cortical cell types in a reproducible fashion (Velasco et al. 2019; Yoon et al. 2019), from early stages of organoid development up to long periods of *in vitro* culture (Uzquiano et al. 2022). Additionally, the temporal sequence in which these cortical cells are produced mimics the cellular transitions of the endogenous developing cortex. Organoids are first populated by NE that then transition into aRG (Benito-Kwiecinski et al. 2021; Eze et al. 2021), including human-specific aRG states found in the endogenous human brain but not in mouse (Eze et al. 2021). IP and oRG are also present in human brain organoids validating these models as an unprecedented opportunity to investigate human-specific mechanisms controlling oRG production, behavior, and progeny (Andrews et al. 2020; Coquand et al. 2022; Kyrousi et al. 2021). As basal progenitors are produced, PN are also generated following the same temporal sequence as in the endogenous cerebral cortex: CFuPN emerge first, followed by CPN. Production of CPN is concomitant to the emergence of oRG (Uzquiano et al. 2022), and consistent with the production of CPN from oRG (Betizeau et al. 2013; Lukaszewicz et al. 2005; Nowakowski et al. 2016). Finally, following neurogenesis, gliogenesis begins and results in the generation of astrocytes and oligodendrocyte precursor cells (OPC) (Pollen et al. 2019; Trujillo et al. 2019; Uzquiano et al. 2022; Velasco et al. 2019; Yoon et al. 2019). As previously mentioned, this agrees with previous work indicating the intrinsic capacity of cortical neural progenitors to generate their cell progeny in a controlled temporal sequence, even when cell type production occurs *in vitro*.

At late stages of cortical organoid development an interneuron population is also produced (Giandomenico et al. 2019; Trujillo et al. 2019; Uzquiano et al. 2022; Velasco et al. 2019), but these cells do not appear to have a GE origin and/or identity (Uzquiano et al. 2022; Velasco et al. 2019). Their developmental timing and gene expression profile suggests that they could be either cortically derived interneurons destined to the olfactory bulb (Fuentealba et al. 2015; Kohwi et al. 2007; Young et al. 2007), or interestingly, a recently identified interneuron population emerging from human cortical progenitors of the dorsal telencephalon (Delgado et al. 2022), although further work is needed to understand the developmental origin of this interneuron population present in organoids.

As described earlier, human brain organoids generate a large diversity of differentiated cell types of the human cerebral cortex, including PN, astroglia, and interneurons. Therefore, these models provide a platform for understanding the regulatory logic underlying cell type diversification in the human cerebral cortex. However, to leverage human brain organoids to decipher molecular programs of cell identity acquisition, it is necessary to understand how the cell types generated in these models resemble their fetal endogenous counterparts. For this, extensive comparisons of organoid and fetal cells have been performed (Velasco et al. 2019), (Bhaduri et al. 2020; Cheroni et al. 2022; Gordon et al. 2021; Trevino et al. 2020; Uzquiano et al. 2022). Of particular value are the studies that have compared organoids and fetal tissue at single-cell resolution, allowing comparisons of cell type identity of organoid cell types with their endogenous fetal counterparts (Bhaduri et al. 2020; Uzquiano et al. 2022; Velasco et al. 2019). This work performed across different organoid models and by different labs has shown close correspondence between organoid and fetal cells (Bhaduri et al. 2020; Gordon et al. 2021; Trevino et al. 2020; Uzquiano et al. 2022; Velasco et al. 2019). Notably, although it is possible that certain cells produced in organoids acquire abnormal metabolic signatures, upon transplantation into the mouse brain or under specific culture protocols, identity acquisition of most cell types is not impaired by metabolic abnormalities (Bhaduri et al. 2020; Uzquiano et al. 2022; Vértesy et al. 2022). A specific population of neurons with a strong metabolic signature that localize to the organoid core has been recently reported (Uzquiano et al. 2022; Vértesy et al. 2022); these cells express pan-neuronal markers but lack PN subtype-specific genes (Uzquiano et al. 2022). These metabolically challenged neurons represent an "unspecified" or "undifferentiated" PN state, which is likely to emerge due to the hypoxic environment created in the organoid core as the organoid size increases. Additionally, the absence of other features of the endogenous fetal brain known to contribute to the acquisition of cell identity (e.g., thalamocortical inputs) (Antón-Bolaños et al. 2018; Pouchelon et al. 2014) may also contribute to the emergence of this "unspecified" state of PN.

The high degree of fidelity of cortical cell type identity in organoids with their fetal endogenous counterparts empowers human brain organoids as a model to investigate the molecular mechanisms underlying cellular diversification. Additionally, recent work has shown that organoids can reproduce long developmental trajectories of cerebral cortex development (Uzquiano et al. 2022), further suggesting that these models may be used for investigation of the developmental events associated with the acquisition of cell type identity. Indeed, cortical organoids have already been used to define the molecular cascades associated with distinct human cortical lineages, leading to the identification of human-specific candidate genes associated with PN diversification (Uzquiano et al. 2022). To establish this finding the authors applied the URD algorithm (Farrell et al. 2018) to the compendium of cortical cells present in cortical organoids across 6 months of *in vitro* development, generating a branched-trajectory tree composed of human organoid cortical cells. After revealing sets of TF that potentially act as molecular codes to discriminate between different branches of the trajectory tree and the molecular cascades associated with each lineage (namely CFuPN, CPN, astroglia, and OPC), the authors compared this human cortical organoid tree with an equivalent tree of the mouse developing cortex (Di Bella et al. 2021). This comparison revealed genes associated with a given cortical lineage in humans but not in mice (e.g., HS6ST3, associated with CPN lineage in human cortical organoid tree, but not expressed in the mouse developing cortex). They also uncovered TF important for the neurogenesis-gliogenesis switch in the human cortex that do not have a mouse ortholog (e.g., ZNF26, ZNF37A) (Uzquiano et al. 2022). Therefore, work in human cortical organoids is beginning to expose the molecular programs underlying the generation and specification of human cortical cells. Organoids are experimentally tractable model systems amenable to techniques such as genetic modification and high-throughput assays. Multiplexed gene-perturbation approaches using CRISPR-Cas9 technology, which allow study of mutation in multiple genes in parallel, have recently been successfully implemented in brain organoids (Esk et al. 2020; Fleck et al. 2021). These techniques are now required to accelerate the functional validation of the newly emerging human-specific molecular candidates mediating fate commitment.

Algorithms such as URD use pseudotime to arrange cells based on transcriptional similarity to model and reconstruct dynamic processes of development across time. However, by applying these approaches, information about the developmental history of individual cells may be missing. For example, this includes information about cell division rates, reversibility of states, or differences between clones (Wagner and Klein 2020). *Bona fide* lineage analysis is required for this, in which empirical developmental relationships between progenitor cells and their progeny are traced and revealed. Human brain organoids can be leveraged to prospectively trace lineage relationships of the human brain, as shown by a recent study in which a barcode-based lineage tracing approach was implemented in whole brain organoids (He et al. 2022). Therefore, the tractability of brain organoids and their protracted development provide an opportunity to reveal lineage relationships of the human cerebral cortex and understand how different human progenitors behave in terms of cell division rates and postmitotic progeny produced. This may uncover the neurogenic potential of different human progenitors, as well as the assessment of clone composition in the human cerebral cortex. To this end, careful experimental planning is needed given the potential variability in the results depending on the organoid protocol used (e.g., whole brain organoids vs. cortical organoids) and the initial progenitor cell being traced (e.g., initial iPS vs. an already committed cortical progenitor).

Notably, organoids can be generated from nonhuman primates, allowing the study of human specific brain biology elements that are not shared with even our closest relatives (Benito-Kwiecinski et al. 2021; Kanton et al. 2019; Pollen et al. 2019). Several studies have now leveraged brain organoids from different primates to investigate human-specific features of cortical progenitor biology (Benito-Kwiecinski et al. 2021; Mora-Bermúdez et al. 2016). We envision the use of these organoids to investigate how lineage relationships, cortical clones, and more generally events of neuronal diversification, differ in the human cerebral cortex when compared to other primates.

It is worth noting that although cortical organoids generate a large diversity of the cell types that populate the human cerebral cortex, certain additional features of the endogenous brain are currently missing in these models and must be incorporated to realize their potential more fully. For instance, certain cell types known to play important roles in several steps of corticogenesis are not present in current cortical organoid models. These include oligodendrocytes, microglia, and GE-derived interneurons. Recent studies have begun to develop modified organoid protocols to promote differentiation and maturation of oligodendrocytes (Kim et al. 2019; Madhavan et al. 2018; Marton et al. 2019) and integrate microglia (Cakir et al. 2019; Popova et al. 2021). Toward the goal of modelling interaction between cortical excitatory neurons and GE-interneurons, (Bagley et al. 2017) and Birey et al. (2017) pioneered the establishment of ventral telencephalon organoids, that generate interneurons of medial and lateral GE identities. These ventral organoids were successfully fused to cortical organoids to generate "assembloids" that contain GE-interneuron populations that migrate from the ventral compartment into the dorsal compartment and form functional synapses with glutamatergic PN (Bagley et al. 2017; Birey et al. 2022). Other assembloid systems have also been developed to model interactions between distant brain regions (Andersen et al. 2020; Miura et al. 2020; Xiang et al. 2019). These strategies pave the way for the modelling of interactions between the cortex and other brain regions known to be critical in driving and modulating sensory input. Establishment of multi-organoid models incorporating, for instance, retinal, thalamic, and cortical organoids may help us model the impact of extra-cortical input on human PN specification, maturation, and function.

11.8 Concluding Remarks

Over the past decades, the development of the mammalian cerebral cortex development has been the subject of many studies. Given the unparalleled neuronal diversity present in the cerebral cortex, many questions have arisen related to the molecular logic underlying neuronal diversification. This area of research has further intensified due to the emergence of single-cell profiling approaches, which are revealing neuronal subtypes and states previously inaccessible, and are providing novel insights into the molecular effectors shaping neuronal diversity. The advent of this single-cell technology is also leading to interspecies comparisons, allowing investigation of human-specific events of cortical cell type emergence and specification. This is proving possible thanks to the emergence of human brain organoids as powerful tractable models through which to study human-specific features of cortical development, offering an unprecedented opportunity to decipher how human neurons are made. All combined, the parallel advances occurring over the past years are revolutionizing our knowledge of how PN diversity is achieved in the mammalian cerebral cortex, and are offering previously inaccessible opportunities to unearth processes of cell identity acquisition and diversification that are specific of the human brain.

Acknowledgments

We thank Lila Lyons for editing the manuscript and Bruna Paulsen for help creating the illustrations. Work in the Arlotta lab related to the topics of this chapter is supported by grants from the Stanley Center for Psychiatric Research, the Broad Institute of MIT and Harvard, the National Institutes of Health (R01MH112940, P50MH094271, U01MH115727, and RF1MH123977 to P.A.).

Conflict of Interest Statement

Paola Arlotta is a SAB member at Herophilus, Rumi Therapeutics, and Foresite Labs, and is a co-founder of Vesalius.

References

Alcamo, E.A. et al. (2008). Satb2 regulates callosal projection neuron identity in the developing cerebral cortex. *Neuron* 57 (3): 364–377.
Amiri, A. et al. (2018). Transcriptome and epigenome landscape of human cortical development modeled in organoids. *Science* 362 (6420): eaat6720.
Andersen, J. et al. (2020). Generation of functional human 3D cortico-motor assembloids. *Cell* 183 (7): 1913–1929.e1926.
Andrews, M.G. et al. (2020). mTOR signaling regulates the morphology and migration of outer radial glia in developing human cortex. *Elife* 9: e58737.
Antón-Bolaños, N. et al. (2018). Developmental interactions between thalamus and cortex. *Curr Opin Neurobiol* 52: 33–41.
Arlotta, P. et al. (2005). Neuronal subtype-specific genes that control corticospinal motor neuron development in vivo. *Neuron* 45 (2): 207–221.
Bagley, J.A. et al. (2017). Fused cerebral organoids model interactions between brain regions. *Nat Methods* 14 (7): 743–751.
Bakken, T.E. et al. (2021). Comparative cellular analysis of motor cortex in human, marmoset and mouse. *Nature* 598 (7879): 111–119.
Bandler, R.C. et al. (2022). Single-cell delineation of lineage and genetic identity in the mouse brain. *Nature* 601 (7893): 404–409.
Baranek, C. et al. (2012). Protooncogene Ski cooperates with the chromatin-remodeling factor Satb2 in specifying callosal neurons. *Proc Natl Acad Sci* 109 (9): 3546–3551.
Benito-Kwiecinski, S. et al. (2021 April 15). An early cell shape transition drives evolutionary expansion of the human forebrain. *Cell* 184 (8): 2084–2102.e2019.
Benito-Kwiecinski, S. and Lancaster, M.A. (2020). Brain organoids. *Cold Spring Harbor Perspectives in Biology* 12 (8): a035709.
Berg, J. et al. (2021). Human neocortical expansion involves glutamatergic neuron diversification. *Nature* 598 (7879): 151–158.
Betizeau, M. et al. (2013). Precursor diversity and complexity of lineage relationships in the outer subventricular zone of the primate. *Neuron* 80 (2): 442–457.
Bhaduri, A. et al. (2020). Cell stress in cortical organoids impairs molecular subtype specification. *Nature* 578 (7793): 142–148.
Birey, F. et al. (2017). Assembly of functionally integrated human forebrain spheroids. *Nature* 545 (7652): 54–59.
Birey, F. et al. (2022). Dissecting the molecular basis of human interneuron migration in forebrain assembloids from Timothy syndrome. *Cell Stem Cell* 29 (2): 248–264.e247.
Britanova, O. et al. (2008). Satb2 is a postmitotic determinant for upper-layer neuron specification in the neocortex. *Neuron* 57 (3): 378–392.
Bulchand, S. et al. (2003). Dynamic spatiotemporal expression of LIM genes and cofactors in the embryonic and postnatal cerebral cortex. *Dev Dyn* 226 (3): 460–469.
Cadwell, C.R. et al. (2016). Electrophysiological, transcriptomic and morphologic profiling of single neurons using Patch-seq. *Nat Biotechnol* 34 (2): 199–203.
Cadwell, C.R. et al. (2020). Cell type composition and circuit organization of clonally related excitatory neurons in the juvenile mouse neocortex. *Elife* 9: e52951.
Cakir, B. et al. (2019). Engineering of human brain organoids with a functional vascular-like system. *Nat Methods* 16 (11): 1169–1175.
Catapano, L.A. et al. (2008). Neuroanatomical tracing of neuronal projections with Fluoro-Gold. *Methods Mol Biol* 438: 353–359.

Cederquist, G.Y. et al. (2013). Lmo4 establishes rostral motor cortex projection neuron subtype diversity. *J Neurosci* 33 (15): 6321–6332.

Chambers, S.M. et al. (2009). Highly efficient neural conversion of human ES and iPS cells by dual inhibition of SMAD signaling. *Nat Biotechnol* 27 (3): 275–280.

Cheroni, C. et al. (2022). Benchmarking brain organoid recapitulation of fetal corticogenesis. *BioRxiv*. doi: 10.1101/2022.04.22.488753.

Clowry, G.J. (2015). An enhanced role and expanded developmental origins for gamma-aminobutyric acidergic interneurons in the human cerebral cortex. *J Anat* 227 (4): 384–393.

Coquand, L. et al. (2022). A cell fate decision map reveals abundant direct neurogenesis in the human developing neocortex. *BioRxiv*. doi: 10.1101/2022.02.01.478661.

Deitcher, Y. et al. (2017). Comprehensive morpho-electrotonic analysis shows 2 distinct classes of L2 and L3 pyramidal neurons in human temporal cortex. *Cereb Cortex* 27 (11): 5398–5414.

Del Dosso, A. et al. (2020). Upgrading the physiological relevance of human brain organoids. *Neuron* 107 (6): 1014–1028.

Delgado, R.N. et al. (2022). Individual human cortical progenitors can produce excitatory and inhibitory neurons. *Nature* 601 (7893): 397–403.

Di Bella, D.J. et al. (2021). Molecular logic of cellular diversification in the mouse cerebral cortex. *Nature* 595 (7868): 554–559.

Diaz, J.L. et al. (2020). An evolutionarily acquired microRNA shapes development of mammalian cortical projections. *Proc Natl Acad Sci* 117 (46): 29113–29122.

Dixit, A. et al. (2016). Perturb-Seq. *Cell* 167 (7): 1853–1866.

Eiraku, M. et al. (2008). Self-organized formation of polarized cortical tissues from ESCs and its active manipulation by extrinsic signals. *Cell Stem Cell* 3 (5): 519–532.

Esk, C. et al. (2020). A human tissue screen identifies a regulator of ER secretion as a brain-size determinant. *Science* 370 (6519): 935–941.

Espuny-Camacho, I. et al. (2013). Pyramidal neurons derived from human pluripotent stem cells integrate efficiently into mouse brain circuits in vivo. *Neuron* 77 (3): 440–456.

Eze, U.C. et al. (2021). Single-cell atlas of early human brain development highlights heterogeneity of human neuroepithelial cells and early radial glia. *Nat Neurosci* 24 (4): 584–594.

Fame, R.M. et al. (2017). Subtype-specific genes that characterize subpopulations of callosal projection neurons in mouse identify molecularly homologous populations in macaque cortex. *Cereb Cortex* 27 (3): 1817–1830.

Farhy-Tselnicker, I. and Allen, N.J. (2018). Astrocytes, neurons, synapses: a tripartite view on cortical circuit development. *Neural Dev* 13 (1): 7.

Farrell, J.A. et al. (2018). Single-cell reconstruction of developmental trajectories during zebrafish embryogenesis. *Science* 360 (6392): eaar3131.

Fietz, S.A. et al. (2010). OSVZ progenitors of human and ferret neocortex are epithelial-like and expand by integrin signaling. *Nat Neurosci* 13 (6): 690–699.

Fiorenzano, A. et al. (2021). Single-cell transcriptomics captures features of human midbrain development and dopamine neuron diversity in brain organoids. *Nat Commun* 12 (1): 7302.

Fleck, J.S. et al. (2021). Inferring and perturbing cell fate regulomes in human cerebral organoids. *BioRxiv*. doi: 10.1101/2021.08.24.457460.

Franco, S.J. et al. (2012). Fate-restricted neural progenitors in the mammalian cerebral cortex. *Science* 337 (6095): 746–749.

Frantz, G.D. and McConnell, S.K. (1996). Restriction of late cerebral cortical progenitors to an upper-layer fate. *Neuron* 17 (1): 55–61.

Fuentealba, L.C. et al. (2015). Embryonic origin of postnatal neural stem cells. *Cell* 161 (7): 1644–1655.

Galazo, M.J. et al. (2016). Corticothalamic projection neuron development beyond subtype specification. *Neuron* 91 (1): 90–106.

Gao, P. et al. (2014). Deterministic progenitor behavior and unitary production of neurons in the neocortex. *Cell* 159 (4): 775–788.

Gaspard, N. et al. (2008). An intrinsic mechanism of corticogenesis from embryonic stem cells. *Nature* 455 (7211): 351–357.

Gertz, C.C. et al. (2014). Diverse behaviors of outer radial glia in developing ferret and human cortex. *J Neurosci* 34 (7): 2559–2570.

Giandomenico, S.L. et al. (2019). Cerebral organoids at the air-liquid interface generate diverse nerve tracts with functional output. *Nat Neurosci* 22 (4): 669–679.

Gidon, A. et al. (2020). Dendritic action potentials and computation in human layer 2/3 cortical neurons. *Science* 367 (6473): 83–87.

Gordon, A. et al. (2021). Long-term maturation of human cortical organoids matches key early postnatal transitions. *Nat Neurosci* 24 (3): 331–342.

Greig, L.C. et al. (2013). Molecular logic of neocortical projection neuron specification, development and diversity. *Nat Rev Neurosci* 14 (11): 755–769.

Guillamon-Vivancos, T. et al. (2019). Distinct neocortical progenitor lineages fine-tune neuronal diversity in a layer-specific manner. *Cereb Cortex* 29 (3): 1121–1138.

Guo, C. et al. (2013). Fezf2 expression identifies a multipotent progenitor for neocortical projection neurons, astrocytes, and oligodendrocytes. *Neuron* 80 (5): 1167–1174.

Han, W. et al. (2011). TBR1 directly represses Fezf2 to control the laminar origin and development of the corticospinal tract. *Proc Natl Acad Sci* 108 (7): 3041–3046.

Hansen, D.V. et al. (2010). Neurogenic radial glia in the outer subventricular zone of human neocortex. *Nature* 464 (7288): 554–561.

He, Z. et al. (2022). Lineage recording in human cerebral organoids. *Nat Methods* 19 (1): 90–99.

Heavner, W.E. et al. (2020). Transcription factor expression defines subclasses of developing projection neurons highly similar to single-cell RNA-seq subtypes. *Proc Natl Acad Sci* 117 (40): 25074–25084.

Hodge, R.D. et al. (2019). Conserved cell types with divergent features in human versus mouse cortex. *Nature* 573 (7772): 61–68.

Huang, A.Y. et al. (2020). Parallel RNA and DNA analysis after deep sequencing (PRDD-seq) reveals cell type-specific lineage patterns in human brain. *Proc Natl Acad Sci* 117 (25): 13886–13895.

Jo, J. et al. (2016). Midbrain-like organoids from human pluripotent stem cells contain functional dopaminergic and neuromelanin-producing neurons. *Cell Stem Cell* 19 (2): 248–257.

Josh Huang, Z. and Zeng, H. (2013). Genetic approaches to neural circuits in the mouse. *Ann Rev Neurosci* 36: 183–215.

Joshi, P.S. et al. (2008). Bhlhb5 regulates the postmitotic acquisition of area identities in layers II-V of the developing neocortex. *Neuron* 60 (2): 258–272.

Kadoshima, T. et al. (2013). Self-organization of axial polarity, inside-out layer pattern, and species-specific progenitor dynamics in human ES cell-derived neocortex. *Proc Natl Acad Sci* 110 (50): 20284–20289.

Kalmbach, B.E. et al. (2018). h-channels contribute to divergent intrinsic membrane properties of supragranular pyramidal neurons in human versus mouse cerebral cortex. *Neuron* 100 (5): 1194–1208.e1195.

Kalmbach, B.E. et al. (2021). Signature morpho-electric, transcriptomic, and dendritic properties of human layer 5 neocortical pyramidal neurons. *Neuron* 109 (18): 2914–2927. e2915.

Kanton, S. et al. (2019). Organoid single-cell genomic atlas uncovers human-specific features of brain development. *Nature* 574 (7778): 418–422.

Kebschull, J.M. et al. (2016). High-throughput mapping of single-neuron projections by sequencing of barcoded RNA. *Neuron* 91 (5): 975–987.

Kim, H. et al. (2019). Pluripotent stem cell-derived cerebral organoids reveal human oligodendrogenesis with dorsal and ventral origins. *Stem Cell Rep* 12 (5): 890–905.

Klingler, E. et al. (2019). A translaminar genetic logic for the circuit identity of intracortically projecting neurons. *Curr Biol* 29 (2): 332–339.e335.

Klingler, E. et al. (2021). Temporal controls over inter-areal cortical projection neuron fate diversity. *Nature* 599 (7885): 453–457.

Kohwi, M. et al. (2007). A subpopulation of olfactory bulb GABAergic interneurons is derived from Emx1-and Dlx5/6-expressing progenitors. *J Neurosci* 27 (26): 6878–6891.

Kowalczyk, T. et al. (2009). Intermediate neuronal progenitors (basal progenitors) produce pyramidal–projection neurons for all layers of cerebral cortex. *Cereb Cortex* 19 (10): 2439–2450.

Kyrousi, C. et al. (2021). Extracellular LGALS3BP regulates neural progenitor position and relates to human cortical complexity. *Nat Commun* 12 (1): 6298.

Lai, T. et al. (2008). SOX5 controls the sequential generation of distinct corticofugal neuron subtypes. *Neuron* 57 (2): 232–247.

Lancaster, M.A. et al. (2013). Cerebral organoids model human brain development and microcephaly. *Nature* 501 (7467): 373–379.

LaVail, J.H. (1978). A review of the retrograde transport technique. *Neuroanat Res Tech* 2: 355–384.

Lefort, S. et al. (2009). The excitatory neuronal network of the C2 barrel column in mouse primary somatosensory cortex. *Neuron* 61 (2): 301–316.

Lim, L. et al. (2018). Development and functional diversification of cortical interneurons. *Neuron* 100 (2): 294–313.

Llorca, A. et al. (2019). A stochastic framework of neurogenesis underlies the assembly of neocortical cytoarchitecture. *Elife* 8: e51381.

Lodato, S. and Arlotta, P. (2015). Generating neuronal diversity in the mammalian cerebral cortex. *Ann Rev Cell Dev Biol* 31: 699–720.

Lodato, S. et al. (2014). Gene co-regulation by Fezf2 selects neurotransmitter identity and connectivity of corticospinal neurons. *Nat Neurosci* 17 (8): 1046–1054.

Lukaszewicz, A. et al. (2005). G1 phase regulation, area-specific cell cycle control, and cytoarchitectonics in the primate cortex. *Neuron* 47 (3): 353–364.

Luo, C. et al. (2017). Single-cell methylomes identify neuronal subtypes and regulatory elements in mammalian cortex. *Science* 357 (6351): 600–604.

Luskin, M.B. et al. (1988). Cell lineage in the cerebral cortex of the mouse studied in vivo and in vitro with a recombinant retrovirus. *Neuron* 1 (8): 635–647.

Madhavan, M. et al. (2018). Induction of myelinating oligodendrocytes in human cortical spheroids. *Nat Methods* 15 (9): 700–706.

Magrinelli, E. et al. (2022). Heterogeneous fates of simultaneously-born neurons in the cortical ventricular zone. *Sci Rep* 12 (1): 1–11.

Mariani, J. et al. (2015). FOXG1-dependent dysregulation of GABA/glutamate neuron differentiation in autism spectrum disorders. *Cell* 162 (2): 375–390.

Marton, R.M. et al. (2019). Differentiation and maturation of oligodendrocytes in human three-dimensional neural cultures. *Nat Neurosci* 22 (3): 484–491.

McKenna, W.L. et al. (2011). Tbr1 and Fezf2 regulate alternate corticofugal neuronal identities during neocortical development. *J Neurosci* 31 (2): 549–564.

Mihalas, A.B. et al. (2016). Intermediate progenitor cohorts differentially generate cortical layers and require Tbr2 for timely acquisition of neuronal subtype identity. *Cell Rep* 16 (1): 92–105.

Miura, Y. et al. (2020). Generation of human striatal organoids and cortico-striatal assembloids from human pluripotent stem cells. *Nat Biotechnol* 38 (12): 1421–1430.

Molyneaux, B.J. et al. (2009). Novel subtype-specific genes identify distinct subpopulations of callosal projection neurons. *J Neurosci* 29 (39): 12343–12354.

Molyneaux, B.J. et al. (2005). Fezl is required for the birth and specification of corticospinal motor neurons. *Neuron* 47 (6): 817–831.

Molyneaux, B.J. et al. (2007). Neuronal subtype specification in the cerebral cortex. *Nat Rev Neurosci* 8 (6): 427–437.

Molyneaux, B.J. et al. (2015). DeCoN. *Neuron* 85 (2): 275–288.

Monzel, A.S. et al. (2017). Derivation of human midbrain-specific organoids from neuroepithelial stem cells. *Stem Cell Rep* 8 (5): 1144–1154.

Mora-Bermúdez, F. et al. (2016). Differences and similarities between human and chimpanzee neural progenitors during cerebral cortex development. *Elife* 5: e18683.

Mount, C.W. and Monje, M. (2017 August 16). Wrapped to adapt. *Neuron* 95 (4): 743–756.

Muguruma, K. et al. (2015). Self-organization of polarized cerebellar tissue in 3D culture of human pluripotent stem cells. *Cell Rep* 10 (4): 537–550.

Muralidharan, B. et al. (2017). LHX2 interacts with the NuRD complex and regulates cortical neuron subtype determinants Fezf2 and Sox11. *J Neurosci* 37 (1): 194–203.

Nano, P.R. et al. (2021). Cortical cartography: mapping arealization using single-cell omics technology. *Front Neural Circuits* 15: 788560.

Noack, F. et al. (2022). Multimodal profiling of the transcriptional regulatory landscape of the developing mouse cortex identifies Neurog2 as a key epigenome remodeler. *Nat Neurosci* 25 (2): 154–167.

Nowakowski, T.J. et al. (2017). Spatiotemporal gene expression trajectories reveal developmental hierarchies of the human cortex. *Science* 358 (6368): 1318–1323.

Nowakowski, T.J. et al. (2016). Transformation of the radial glia scaffold demarcates two stages of human cerebral cortex development. *Neuron* 91 (6): 1219–1227.

Oberst, P. et al. (2019). Temporal plasticity of apical progenitors in the developing mouse neocortex. *Nature* 573 (7774): 370–374.

Ostrem, B. et al. (2017). oRGs and mitotic somal translocation—a role in development and disease. *Curr Opin Neurobiol* 42: 61–67.

Otani, T. et al. (2016). 2D and 3D stem cell models of primate cortical development identify species-specific differences in progenitor behavior contributing to brain size. *Cell Stem Cell* 18 (4): 467–480.

Paşca, A.M. et al. (2015). Functional cortical neurons and astrocytes from human pluripotent stem cells in 3D culture. *Nat Methods* 12 (7): 671–678.

Pellegrini, L. et al. (2020). SARS-CoV-2 infects the brain choroid plexus and disrupts the blood-CSF barrier in human brain organoids. *Cell Stem Cell* 27 (6): 951–961.e955.

Pollen, A.A. et al. (2019). Establishing cerebral organoids as models of human-specific brain evolution. *Cell* 176 (4): 743–756.e717.

Pollen, A.A. et al. (2015). Molecular identity of human outer radial glia during cortical development. *Cell* 163 (1): 55–67.

Popova, G. et al. (2021). Human microglia states are conserved across experimental models and regulate neural stem cell responses in chimeric organoids. *Cell Stem Cell* 28 (12): 2153–2166.e2156.

Pouchelon, G. et al. (2014). Modality-specific thalamocortical inputs instruct the identity of postsynaptic L4 neurons. *Nature* 511 (7510): 471–474.

Qian, X. et al. (2016). Brain-region-specific organoids using mini-bioreactors for modeling ZIKV exposure. *Cell* 165 (5): 1238–1254.

Quadrato, G. et al. (2017). Cell diversity and network dynamics in photosensitive human brain organoids. *Nature* 545 (7652): 48–53.

Rash, B.G. and Grove, E.A. (2006). Area and layer patterning in the developing cerebral cortex. *Curr Opin Neurobiol* 16 (1): 25–34.

Ratz, M. et al. (2022). Clonal relations in the mouse brain revealed by single-cell and spatial transcriptomics. *Nat Neurosci* 25 (3): 285–294.

Reillo, I. and Borrell, V. (2012). Germinal zones in the developing cerebral cortex of ferret: ontogeny, cell cycle kinetics, and diversity of progenitors. *Cereb Cortex* 22 (9): 2039–2054.

Renner, M. et al. (2017). Self-organized developmental patterning and differentiation in cerebral organoids. *EMBO J* 36 (10): 1316–1329.

Shen, Q. et al. (2006). The timing of cortical neurogenesis is encoded within lineages of individual progenitor cells. *Nat Neurosci* 9 (6): 743–751.

Shi, Y. et al. (2012). Human cerebral cortex development from pluripotent stem cells to functional excitatory synapses. *Nat Neurosci* 15 (3): 477–486.

Shitamukai, A. et al. (2011). Oblique radial glial divisions in the developing mouse neocortex induce self-renewing progenitors outside the germinal zone that resemble primate outer subventricular zone progenitors. *J Neurosci* 31 (10): 3683–3695.

Silbereis, J.C. et al. (2016). The cellular and molecular landscapes of the developing human central nervous system. *Neuron* 89 (2): 248–268.

Sloan, S.A. et al. (2018). Generation and assembly of human brain region–specific three-dimensional cultures. *Nat Protoc* 13 (9): 2062–2085.

Srinivasan, K. et al. (2012). A network of genetic repression and derepression specifies projection fates in the developing neocortex. *Proc Natl Acad Sci* 109 (47): 19071–19078.

Staiger, J.F. et al. (2004). Functional diversity of layer IV spiny neurons in rat somatosensory cortex. *Cereb Cortex* 14 (6): 690–701.

Tarabykin, V. et al. (2001). Cortical upper layer neurons derive from the subventricular zone as indicated by Svet1 gene expression. *Development* 128 (11): 1983–1993.

Tasic, B. et al. (2018). Shared and distinct transcriptomic cell types across neocortical areas. *Nature* 563 (7729): 72–78.

Taverna, E. et al. (2014). The cell biology of neurogenesis: toward an understanding of the development and evolution of the neocortex. *Ann Rev Cell Dev Biol* 30 (1): 465–502.

Telley, L. et al. (2019). Temporal patterning of apical progenitors and their daughter neurons in the developing neocortex. *Science* 364 (6440): eaav2522.

ten Berge, D. et al. (2008). Wnt signaling mediates self-organization and axis formation in embryoid bodies. *Cell Stem Cell* 3 (5): 508–518.

Thion, M.S. et al. (2018). Microglia and early brain development. *Science* 362 (6411): 185–189.

Trevino, A.E. et al. (2021). Chromatin and gene-regulatory dynamics of the developing human cerebral cortex at single-cell resolution. *Cell* 184 (19): 5053–5069. e5023.

Trevino, A.E. et al. (2020). Chromatin accessibility dynamics in a model of human forebrain development. *Science* 367 (6476): eaay1645.

Trujillo, C.A. et al. (2019). Complex oscillatory waves emerging from cortical organoids model early human brain network development. *Cell Stem Cell* 25 (4): 558–569.e557.

Tyler, W.A. et al. (2015). Neural precursor lineages specify distinct neocortical pyramidal neuron types. *J Neurosci* 35 (15): 6142–6152.

Uzquiano, A. et al. (2018). Cortical progenitor biology. *J Neurochem* 146 (5): 500–525.

Uzquiano, A. et al. (2022). Proper acquisition of cell class identity in organoids allows definition of fate specification programs of the cerebral cortex. *Cell* 185 (20): 3770–3788.

Vaid, S. et al. (2018). A novel population of Hopx-dependent basal radial glial cells in the developing mouse neocortex. *Development* 145 (20): dev169276.

Vaid, S. and Huttner, W.B. (2022). Progenitor-based cell biological aspects of neocortex development and evolution. *Front Cell Dev Biol* 10: 892922.

Vasistha, N.A. et al. (2015). Cortical and clonal contribution of Tbr2 expressing progenitors in the developing mouse brain. *Cereb Cortex* 25 (10): 3290–3302.

Velasco, S. et al. (2019). Individual brain organoids reproducibly form cell diversity of the human cerebral cortex. *Nature* 570 (7762): 523–527.

Velasco, S. et al. (2020). 3D brain organoids: studying brain development and disease outside the embryo. *Ann Rev Neurosci* 43: 375–389.

Vértesy, Á. et al. (2022). Cellular stress in brain organoids is limited to a distinct and bioinformatically removable subpopulation. *BioRxiv*. doi: 10.1101/2022.03.11.483643,2022.2003.2011.483643.

Vitali, I. et al. (2018). Progenitor hyperpolarization regulates the sequential generation of neuronal subtypes in the developing neocortex. *Cell* 174 (5): 1264–1276. e1215.

Wagner, D.E. and Klein, A.M. (2020). Lineage tracing meets single-cell omics: opportunities and challenges. *Nat Rev Genet* 21 (7): 410–427.

Walsh, C. and Cepko, C.L. (1993). Clonal dispersion in proliferative layers of developing cerebral cortex. *Nature* 362 (6421): 632–635.

Wang, X. et al. (2011). A new subtype of progenitor cell in the mouse embryonic neocortex. *Nat Neurosci* 14 (5): 555–561.

Woodworth, M.B. et al. (2016). Ctip1 regulates the balance between specification of distinct projection neuron subtypes in deep cortical layers. *Cell Rep* 15 (5): 999–1012.

Xiang, Y. et al. (2019). hESC-derived thalamic organoids form reciprocal projections when fused with cortical organoids. *Cell Stem Cell* 24 (3): 487–497.e487.

Yao, Z. et al. (2021). A transcriptomic and epigenomic cell atlas of the mouse primary motor cortex. *Nature* 598 (7879): 103–110.

Yoon, S.J. et al. (2019). Reliability of human cortical organoid generation. *Nat Methods* 16 (1): 75–78.

Young, K.M. et al. (2007). Subventricular zone stem cells are heterogeneous with respect to their embryonic origins and neurogenic fates in the adult olfactory bulb. *J Neurosci* 27 (31): 8286–8296.

Yuan, X. et al. (2020). Versatile live-cell activity analysis platform for characterization of neuronal dynamics at single-cell and network level. *Nat Commun* 11 (1): 1–14.

Zeisel, A. et al. (2015). Cell types in the mouse cortex and hippocampus revealed by single-cell RNA-seq. *Science* 347 (6226): 1138–1142.

Ziffra, R.S. et al. (2021). Single-cell epigenomics reveals mechanisms of human cortical development. *Nature* 598 (7879): 205–213.

Zimmer, C. et al. (2004). Dynamics of Cux2 expression suggests that an early pool of SVZ precursors is fated to become upper cortical layer neurons. *Cereb Cortex* 14 (12): 1408–1420.

Zuccaro, E. et al. (2021). Human-specific enrichment of schizophrenia risk-genes in callosal neurons of the developing neocortex. *BioRxiv*. doi: 10.1101/2021.09.10.459747.

12

Development of Cortical Neuron Heterogeneity and Impact of Neurodevelopmental Disorders

Zhen Li, William A. Tyler, and Tarik F. Haydar

Center for Neuroscience Research, Children's National Hospital, 20010, Washington DC, USA

12.1 Identity of Precursors within the Neocortical Germinal Zones

Solving the riddle of how the complex brain emerges from a rudimentary cellular structure during early embryonic development has included disputes regarding the identity of the brain precursor population and the degree to which intrinsic programs operating in the precursor cells may predispose later features of brain development. Beginning at the end of the nineteenth century, Wilhelm His' examination of the germinal epithelium led him to postulate that two different cell types may exist within the ventricular zone (VZ) and that these cells separately generate either neurons or glia (His 1889). This concept contrasted with Schaper's contemporaneous assertion that a uniform population of VZ cells generates offspring with indifferent fates (Schaper 1897). Over the next half century, studies supporting various mechanisms of neuron and glial cell production were argued from electron micrographic and immunohistochemical studies, again alternating between the existence of fate-restricted precursor groups to temporally induced changes within what was then argued to be a very simple and uniform epithelium (Angevine 1961; Fujita 1963; Levitt et al. 1981; Levitt and Rakic 1980; Sidman et al. 1959). From the 1970s to the 1990s, the use of ^{3}H-TdR and BrdU to label cells in S phase of the cell cycle contributed to the concept that the VZ was a very well-ordered yet homogeneous population of precursors (Caviness and Takahashi 1995; Takahashi et al. 1999, 1994). During this period, the concept of inside-out temporal commitment of neurons to each of the six layers of the cortex was established using these new tools (Rakic 1975, 1985, 1988). This latter realization, coupled with the layer-specific neuronal variation and the emerging roadmap of afferent and efferent fibers from different cortical lamina, prompted renewed focus on the degree to which precursor cell variation may play a role in cortical circuit development. Recently, genetic fate mapping, time-lapse microscopy, single-cell transcriptomics, and chromatin-accessibility studies in a variety of mammalian species have provided a new look at the composition of the proliferative zones during neocortical neurogenesis, prompting new theories on how the complexities of the cortex develop.

Radial glial cells (RGCs) are at the heart of the recent developments, as they are now recognized to be the resident stem cells in the neocortex during neurogenesis. Traditional methods have identified these elongated cells in different forms, including full-span apical variants (aRGCs) with foot processes at the ventricular and pial surfaces, basal variants (bRGCs) that are only connected

Neocortical Neurogenesis in Development and Evolution, First Edition. Edited by Wieland B. Huttner.

to the pial surface with cell soma located in the subventricular and intermediate zones (SVZ, IZ) and found predominantly in the gyrencephalic brain, as well as several other bipolar and unipolar morphotypes (Betizeau et al. 2013; Li et al. 2020b; Pilz et al. 2013; Pinto and Gotz 2007; Pinto et al. 2008).

Beginning in the early 2000s, a flurry of studies demonstrated that aRGCs generate neuron daughter cells directly (Hartfuss et al. 2001; Malatesta et al. 2000; Miyata et al. 2001; Noctor et al. 2001; Tamamaki et al. 2001) in addition to their well-known structural role in the telencephalic wall by providing a substrate for neuronal migration (Rakic 1971, 1972). This finding quickly ushered in a renewed interest in the theory of precursor homogeneity, that cortical development depends chiefly upon a uniform population of RGCs that is successively tuned over the course of neurogenesis to generate cells for each cortical layer (Noctor et al. 2002). Subsequent data continues to support the notion that RGCs are the engine that drives cortical neurogenesis. Thus, the mechanisms by which these cells produce all the requisite neurons for the cortical layers, and whether the fine-tuning of their cell output (including the intermediate precursors they create) influences cortical function, remain active areas of study.

12.2 Intermediate Precursor Cells

To understand mechanistically how RGCs generate neurons, it is essential to fully characterize the daughter cell types they produce during neurogenesis. It is now clear that many of these cell types, termed intermediate progenitors, retain proliferative capacity, generate neurons, and are found in distinct germinal compartments (Englund et al. 2005; Haubensak et al. 2004; Miyata et al. 2004; Noctor et al. 2004). Examination of the fate and output potential of these intermediate precursor cell types is therefore also necessary when integrating the mechanisms of proper cortical growth and lineage diversification. Joining the aRGC within the apical compartment of the neocortical wall are apical intermediate progenitor cells (aIPCs, also termed short neural progenitors), which are bipolar radial cells that undergo interkinetic nuclear migration like aRGCs but lack the long, basal process connected to the pia that are found in aRGCs (Ellender et al. 2019; Gal et al. 2006; Pilz et al. 2013; Tyler and Haydar 2013). Serial EM reconstructions demonstrate that aIPCs conspicuously lack an ascending process during mitosis and time-lapse imaging and fate mapping indicates that this cell type does not self-renew. There are also several different morphologically separable basal precursor cell types, all of which express the transcription factor EOMES (aka Tbr2), though they are reported to have different levels of mitotic capacity and fate potential. The basal intermediate progenitors (bIPCs) are multipolar dividing cells that reside in the rodent SVZ and the inner SVZ of gyrencephalic species. bIPCs appear early in mammalian neocortical neurogenesis and remain proliferatively active throughout the neurogenesis period, generating neurons for each cortical layer (Arnold et al. 2008; Englund et al. 2005; Kowalczyk et al. 2009; Sessa et al. 2008; Vasistha et al. 2015). They undergo neuron-generating mitoses in situ, primarily dividing away from the ventricular margin unlike the aRGCs and aIPCs. bIPCs are also thought to have more limited proliferative capacity compared to RGCs, most often undergoing exhaustive symmetric division to generate two daughter neurons.

A second basal precursor cell type, bRGCs, share many properties with aRGCs including gene expression and enhanced proliferative capacity. These cells, which have their soma in the outer SVZ of gyrencephalic brains, are tethered only to the pial surface and, like bIPCs, undergo mitosis in situ (Hansen et al. 2010; Shitamukai et al. 2011; Wang et al. 2011). bRGCs have been reported to express aRGC transcription factors such as SOX2 as well as several other bRGC-specific genes such as TMEM14B, PTPRZ1 and ARHGAP11B (Florio et al. 2015; Kalebic et al. 2018; Liu et al. 2017; Pollen et al. 2015). They are numerous in the gyrencephalic cortex and were previously thought to be absent from lissencephalic brains such as those in rodents. These observations led to the hypothesis that neurogenesis via bRGCs underlies the evolution and development of larger-brained species, but a true measure of their contribution to neuronal output has not yet been established, primarily due to a paucity of tools to specifically label and fate map bRGCs, and an appropriate model with which to do so. It is now clear that bRGCs exist in different quantities in all mammalian species, including those with a lissencephalic cortex (Li et al. 2020b; Wang et al. 2011), and also are a major dorsal source of oligodendrocytes (Huang et al. 2020). Recently, it has become clear that bRGCs themselves are a heterogenous population of cells, both within and across species (Kalebic et al. 2019; Kalebic and Huttner 2020; Li et al. 2020b). Several studies have identified bRGC-like cells with distinct morphologies and cell cycle kinetics, further exemplifying the need to parse out and characterize the contributions of each of these subpopulations transcriptomically.

bRGCs in the mouse appear to express a combination of canonical aRGC and bIPC transcripts. For example, mouse bRGCs express Tbr2 mRNA and/or protein in addition to SOX2, while a potentially human-specific population of bRGCs only expresses SOX2. Despite advances in single-cell RNA-sequencing, there remains a gap between the morphologically distinguishable stem and progenitor subtypes and the number of resolvable transcriptional profiles. It is unclear whether this is a current limitation of the technology or whether the transcriptome alone can define separate cell classes.

12.3 RNA Sequencing for Determination of Cell Type

Since its inception (Ramskold et al. 2012; Shapiro et al. 2013; Tang et al. 2009), single-cell RNA sequencing (scRNAseq) has rapidly become a crucial method that many studies have relied on to classify cell types, including neural stem and progenitor cells in the brain (Darmanis et al. 2015; Di Bella et al. 2021; Li et al. 2020b; Loo et al. 2019; Mayer et al. 2018; Mi et al. 2018; Pollen et al. 2014; Saunders et al. 2018; Tasic et al. 2018; Zeisel et al. 2015). RNA sequencing studies in developing mouse and human neocortex have demonstrated that multiple groups of cortical progenitors can be identified based on transcriptome profiling. Thus far, all of the in vivo major cell classes (aRGC, bRGC, bIPC) have been identified transcriptomically, and post hoc bioinformatics techniques, including both supervised and unsupervised clustering, have suggested that several precursor groups contain subtypes. The technique provides genomic information at the highest cellular resolution currently possible at extraordinarily large scale and through put (Osumi-Sutherland et al. 2021). Heretofore unresolvable problems now appear to be in reach, including those related to cellular heterogeneity and time-dependent transcriptome changes during development, especially when single cell expression analysis is combined with advanced bioinformatics approaches such as pseudotime (Tritschler et al. 2019).

As powerful as this new technology is, it comes with significant technical challenges. The most obvious is a phenomenon known as dropout, which is when a gene expressed by a cell fails to be detected due to several underlying technical limitations (Kharchenko et al. 2014; Stegle et al. 2015). Dropout especially affects genes expressed at low levels. After messenger RNA (mRNA) is released from a single cell through the process of cell lysis, the mRNA molecule undergoes capture, reverse transcription, and amplification through multiple rounds of PCR (polymerase chain reaction) reactions to finally generate a "read" that is recorded in the sequencing library (a collection of double-stranded DNA molecules or fragments representing the transcriptome) during sequencing.

Each of the events in the process, the capture (typically through poly-dT binding of the poly-A tails of mRNA transcripts), the reverse transcription, and the amplification are random events. Thus, whether a mRNA molecule will eventually be included in the final sequencing library is uncertain. Because of these technical uncertainties, genes with high expression (more mRNA transcripts) have a higher chance of being represented in the final library, whereas genes with low expression are less likely to be recorded. In addition, the specific sequences of the mRNA transcripts can also contribute to dropout, as some sequences are harder to capture, reverse transcribe, or amplify (Kharchenko et al. 2014). These technical challenges can play a large role later in the analysis pipeline and is one reason why it is necessary to collect many thousands of cells for each experiment. The overwhelming cell numbers increase the likelihood of detecting the transcriptomic nature of the population of interest, but still the genes expressed at low rates per cell are less reliably represented in the sequencing dataset. Importantly, small differences in gene expression can play large roles in a cell's function, as in the case of various signaling molecules and transcription factors. The complication of dropout is therefore important to consider when determining distinctions between cell types.

Another challenge present in scRNAseq experiments is the flexibility and ambiguity of the bioinformatics used to interpret it (Armand et al. 2021). In addition to an often-incomplete representation of the total transcriptome from each cell due to dropout, the computational resources currently available are limiting as well, presenting problems handling the size and complexity of scRNAseq data. This is compounded by the inability of the human mind to process high dimensional data. To compensate for this, the high dimensionality of the scRNAseq dataset must first undergo dimension reduction (DR) to be interpretable. In practice, the specific parameters chosen for the DR can have a huge impact on the downstream analyses and the conclusions drawn. As an example, many popular DR techniques rely first on constructing a neighborhood graph, which in turn requires a predetermined neighborhood size, often denoted as "k." By choosing different values of k, the neighborhood size changes, which in turn changes the topology of the DR graph – sometimes subtly while other times substantially. Moreover, many of the downstream analyses including clustering, pseudotime, and correlational network analysis depend upon the topology of DR graph (Figure 12.1). By changing k and subsequently the DR graph, one may come to different interpretations as a result.

To make matters worse, there is currently no way to objectively determine an optimal k value since such an attempt would have to accommodate the vastly different characteristics (quality and source of original tissue, number of cells, sequencing depth etc.) of individual datasets. This lack of objectivity is not only associated with DR. In fact, almost all the steps of scRNAseq analysis require similar supervision and subjective input, which is why we still do not have standardized

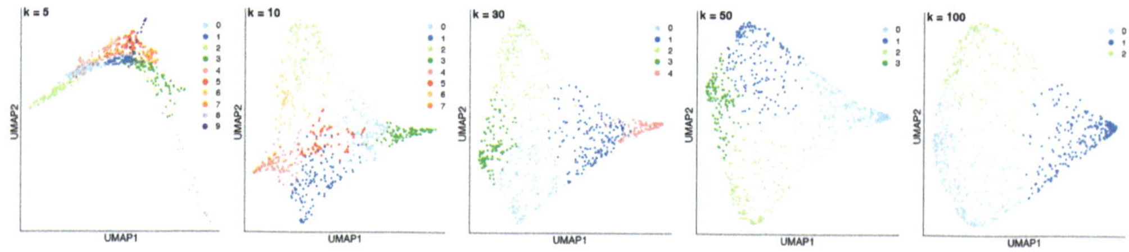

Figure 12.1 UMAPs based on similarity nearest-neighbor (SNN) graphs computed with different neighborhood size (k). Different k values were used to generate the SNN graph, followed by UMAP and clustering with default parameters in the Seurat single-cell RNA sequencing analysis pipeline. Colors represent clusters.

and automatic scRNAseq data analysis solutions. ScRNAseq studies still require researchers to be fully equipped with both biological knowledge and a sophisticated understanding of data analytics to generate reliable findings. While advanced bioinformatics techniques such as artificial intelligence may alleviate some of the issues around subjectivity and ambiguity, at the moment it means that when analyzing scRNAseq datasets, one should remain critical of the generated results and interpretation. It also means that validation of gene expression in the tissue of interest is essential and should be an integrated part of any scRNAseq study.

Studies of neural precursor cell diversity have highlighted the shortcomings of scRNAseq. For example, while studies have shown that RGCs are a diverse group of cells with different gene expression profiles related to cell surface proteins and signaling molecules, this diversity is not apparent in all scRNAseq datasets (Li et al. 2020b). On the contrary, neural precursor cells, especially RGCs, usually form an entity of their own on the DR graph and no apparent boundaries have yet been found to reliably demarcate subgroups of RGCs. In fact, the only transcriptome variability that can be discerned repeatedly in many studies is associated with cell cycle, which has led to the conclusion that RGCs are homogeneous and differ only by their mitotic states (Nowakowski et al. 2017; Telley et al. 2016). It is likely that technical dropout and low transcriptome coverage, as previously mentioned, contributes to this lack of resolution, and that the diversity of RGCs may be masked by the overwhelming unity of their stemness. In other words, one may have to look beyond the part of transcriptome that reflects the stem cell identity of RGCs to differentiate between them.

Indeed, studies have shown that once the transcriptome variability associated with cell cycle is removed, aRGC transcriptional diversity can be revealed (Li et al. 2020a; Mi et al. 2018; Yuzwa et al. 2017). At least two populations of aRGCs can be identified during the middle of mouse neurogenesis, one of which expresses *Tbr2/EOMES* transcript as elucidated by single cell sequencing, *Tbr2* promoter expression via IUE, and by in situ hybridization (Li et al. 2020a). Interestingly, these cells in the VZ do not express TBR2 protein, even though the transcript is present. This phenomenon invokes a mechanism called transcriptional priming (Laslo et al. 2006; Miyai et al. 2018; Nowakowski et al. 2013; Zahr et al. 2018), whereby a cell produces mRNA that is blocked from further translation, perhaps by 5′ capping, association with inhibiting RNA binding proteins, or miRNA. This inhibited mRNA may then be activated by unknown mechanisms in a developmentally appropriate fashion, for example during production of an IPC from an aRGC mother cell. Although the consequences of this emerged diversity in aRGCs remain to be defined functionally, the coexistence of multiple groups of aRGCs during mammalian neurogenesis may be a critical feature of cortical growth and complexity.

As datasets generated by scRNAseq studies have ever increasing cell numbers, each striving to encompass as many cell types of the brain as possible across ages and anatomical regions, the issues surrounding low coverage, technical dropout, and subjectivity also become increasingly apparent (Regev et al. 2017). When it comes to neural progenitor diversity, the reverse approach – focusing only on the progenitor niche with greater cell numbers and transcriptome coverage – may still prove to be beneficial, as the true differentiating factors between progenitors of different lineages may indeed lie within subtle transcriptome differences that can only be detected with deep coverage.

Another fundamental limitation of current scRNAseq technology is the lack of fine temporal resolution. While pseudotime analysis has been used to overcome the lack of "real-time" transcriptome data, it is far from perfect and is prone to misrepresentation of cell–cell relationships. Pseudotime is best suited for analyzing transitions in gene expression that are continuous and linear, as in the case of neuronal differentiation or during progressive cell state changes within a single cell type. When forced to describe relationships between different cell types that do not share a lineal connection, pseudotime will often impute connectivity between these cell types nonetheless, leading to arbitrary conclusions of differentiation pathways. In the end, the identity of a neural stem or progenitor cell is only meaningful in the context of what daughter cell it produces (Zeng 2022). Therefore, it is likely that the genetic fate mapping approach will remain a powerful tool to aid single cell genomics studies in discerning the true nature of neural precursor diversity (Baron and van Oudenaarden 2019; Ma et al. 2018; Vinsland and Linnarsson 2022; Woodworth et al. 2017).

12.4 Role of Neural Precursor Heterogeneity in Neocortical Development

One of the exciting new research aims for the field is to confirm that subtypes of aRGC, bIPC, and bRGC exist within the brain, to determine their individual roles in cortical development, and whether these types are found in all or only some mammalian species. Notwithstanding these continuing efforts, the constituency of the neocortical proliferative zones is more complex than imagined even 50 years ago and can therefore be thought of as a proliferative community, a lineally related and comingled population of neuron-generating cells in which individual precursor types retain important distinctions in gene expression and fate potential. Thus, it is important to discuss the ramifications of this proliferative cell diversity to the formation of the neocortical wall, beginning first with data prompting new theories for the generation of interlaminar diversity followed by recent reports highlighting the mechanisms generating neuronal diversity within an individual cortical layer.

12.4.1 Interlaminar Heterogeneity

The requirements of cortical neurogenesis include strong spatial and temporal constraints, with differences over time along the rostro-caudal and latero-medial axes within the neocortex. Thus, highly controlled techniques that can record the neuron production occurring in a particular location at a particular time are required. The existence of a diverse proliferative community greatly complicates this effort since each type of precursor may play specific roles during neurogenesis, and these roles may evolve in a spatiotemporal fashion during development. Many studies have used conditional fate mapping in transgenic animals, employing cell specific promoters (e.g., *EMX2, GLAST, EOMES*), to explore mechanisms of cortical development. While this approach can yield general results of the contribution of different cell types, it is limited in its ability to address questions that require a sharp temporal control to define the relationship between expression from an active locus and a cell's lineage. In addition, since there is considerable transcriptional overlap between multiple cell types within the neocortical wall (e.g., both aRGCs and bRGCs express SOX2, GLAST, and HOPX; bIPCs and bRGCs and some aRGCs express EOMES), transgene-based conditional fate mapping often cannot reveal the cell type-specific dependency of layer formation. Inducible models provide one solution to this problem, although interpretation of the results of these experiments may be confounded by the sensitivity and extent of recombination following tamoxifen administration. For example, this approach may bias recombination to only the highest expressing cells. It is also difficult to use this approach for a sharply delimited recombination within a lineage (for example only allowing lineage recombination for a single day of development). Another approach to temporal labeling is the FlashTag technique, in which fluorescently labeled esters are injected into the telencephalic ventricle to label mitotic progenitors present at that specific timepoint. Recent data indicate that FlashTag can be used to sharply label only the aRGCs directly generating neurons on a particular day (Telley et al. 2019, 2016). A third approach, in utero electroporation (IUE)-based fate mapping, enables spatially discrete, time-limited mapping of particular cell types and cell classes. Because the episomal plasmid delivered via IUE is diluted from precursors during subsequent cell division, IUE confers the ability to sharply label a cell lineage for a short period of development to mark temporal cohorts of neurons.

A high degree of developmental plasticity must be present in the neural precursor community to explain its ability to produce such variation in neuronal progeny over time. Indeed, recent studies using FlashTag coupled with RNA sequencing and electrophysiology indicate that apical precursors acquire demonstrable changes in gene expression and fate potential as neurogenesis proceeds. In the mouse neocortex, aRGCs express a core set of proliferation-related genes as they generate both IPCs and the neurons destined for the deeper cortical layers 5 and 6. Later in neurogenesis, aRGCs express additional gene sets including genes for ion transporters and cell-cell contact proteins as they again produce temporally appropriate IPCs as well as the neurons destined for the upper cortical layers. Thus, current evidence largely confirms historical findings that suggest the aRGC population ages over the course of neurogenesis by diversifying its gene expression profile (Desai and McConnell 2000; Guo et al. 2013), perhaps allowing for acquisition of signals operating in the local environment (i.e., feedback from the developing cortical plate); these changes to the aRGC population underlie the capacity of the germinal zones to form the architectonically and cellularly distinct cortical layers over time.

12.4.2 Intralaminar Heterogeneity: Mapping the Output of Cortical Progenitor Cell Types

A critical unresolved issue in the field is understanding the functional consequences of precursor heterogeneity. The prevailing theory to date has suggested that the fate of neurons for each layer is tuned in parental aRGCs across the neurogenic interval, and that bIPCs/bRGCs evolved merely to expand neuronal output. However, emerging data from gene expression and fate mapping approaches have indicated important distinctions between neural precursor groups, suggesting that lineage-specific output may enable more than just increasing neuron numbers. To first begin asking whether precursor cell types contribute uniquely to formation of an individual cortical layer, we developed a series of novel fate mapping strategies employing Cre expression plasmids active in either apical precursors (using *Tα1*, *Sox2*, *Fabp7*, or *Slc1a3* gene promoters) or by Tbr2-expressing precursor cells (using *Tbr2* promoter), thus broadly and simultaneously separating both direct and indirect streams of neurogenesis (Tyler and Haydar 2013; Tyler et al. 2015) (Figure 12.2). Beginning at E14.5 during the generation of layers 2 and 3 in the future somatosensory cortex, we showed that each neurogenic stream produces cortical excitatory neurons intermingled in layers 2/3 after migration and differentiation. Using patch clamp electrophysiology and morphological reconstructions, we showed that the neurons from each lineage possess significantly different basic membrane properties and dendrite morphology, *even though they reside within the same neocortical layer and were thus generated in the same temporal cohort*. Specifically, neurons born from the Tbr2-expressing precursors were highly excitable, firing more action potentials from equivalent current injections than neurons born from non-Tbr2-expressing precursors. In addition, neurons from the non- Tbr2-expressing lineage possessed apical dendrites that were significantly more elaborate than their neighbors generated from the Tbr2-expressing lineage. These studies showed that two major neurogenic production schemes, direct neurogenesis from aRGCs and indirect neurogenesis via IPCs, generate neurons in cortical layer 2/3 with explicit differences in their key mature properties and lay the foundation for interrogating how these routes ultimately shape the formation and function of neocortical circuitry.

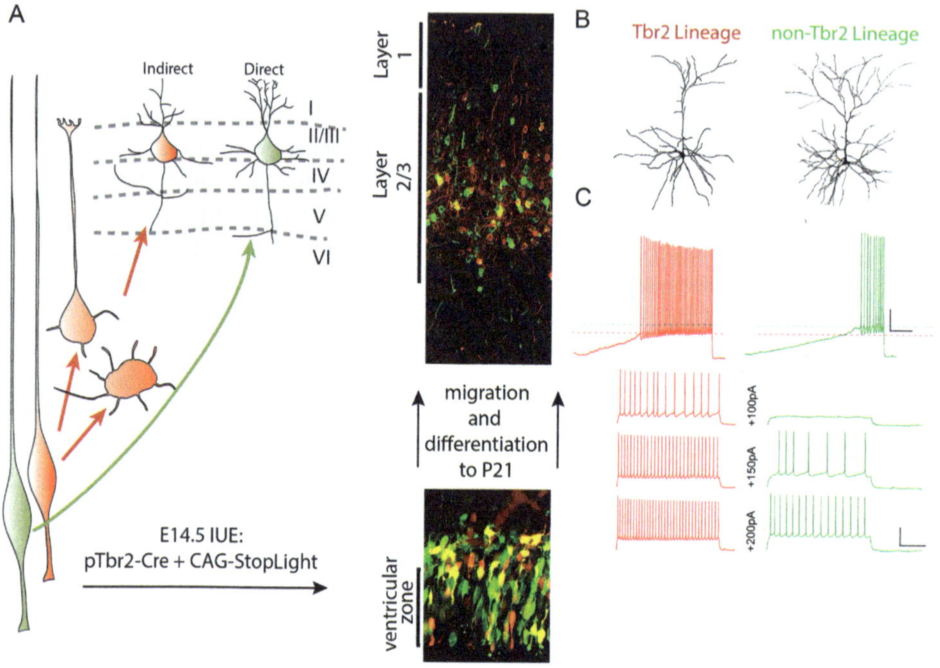

Figure 12.2 Tbr2 (EOMES) fate mapping identifies lineage-based neuronal parameters. (A) In utero electroporation (IUE) with Tbr2 promoter-Cre plasmid drives recombination of the CAG-StopLight plasmid to identify Tbr2-lineage precursors (red) and non-Tbr2-lineage precursors (green) in the ventricular zone. Tbr2-lineage precursors generate *red neurons* indirectly through IPCs whereas non-Tbr2-lineage precursors simultaneously generate *green neurons* directly from aRGCs. Inset micrographs illustrate precursors fate mapped at E15.5 in the mouse ventricular zone (24 hours post IUE). The neurons generated by these precursors migrate radially and are intermingled in cortical layer 2/3 in the postnatal cortical plate (P21 shown). (B) Tbr2-lineage layer 2/3 pyramidal neurons have simpler apical dendrite morphology and (C) higher excitability compared to non-Tbr2-lineage pyramidal neurons. Adapted from (Tyler et al. 2015).

To determine whether this lineage-based mechanism for yielding interlaminar neuronal diversity operates during the formation of other cortical layers and therefore represents a general theme of cortical development, we repeated the experiments in the cortical wall on E13.5, during the period when cortical layer 4 is formed (Guillamon-Vivancos et al. 2019). In contrast to layers 2/3 for which only pyramidal neurons are produced, layer 4 contains both pyramidal neuron and spiny stellate excitatory neurons. Although the cellular constituency of these two layers is quite different, significant differences were again found between Tbr2-expressing and non-Tbr2-expressing lineages. Similar to the findings in layer 2/3, both pyramidal and stellate neurons from the Tbr2-lineage were more excitable than their non-Tbr2 lineage neighbors. Similarly, key morphological differences emerged between cells of each lineage, highlighted by increased polarization of Tbr2 lineage stellate cells and variations in spine distribution in layer 4 pyramidal cells between lineages. These results in layer 4 therefore compliment the layer 2/3 findings with respect to lineage-specified neuronal properties, but they also indicate that each lineage can produce neurons with layer-specific properties, that is, the programs from both aRGCs and bIPCs are tuned to generate diversity between layers.

Evidence of excitatory neuron diversity has also been recently demonstrated from aIPCs during layers 2/3 and 4 generation within the somatosensory cortex (Ellender et al. 2019).

Specifically, cortical precursors were fate mapped using a tubulin alpha-1 (Tα1) promoter-driven Cre and a dual color FLEX reporter plasmid, which yielded GFP expression in aIPCs and TdTomato expression in all other transfected progenitor types. Neurons emerging from these precursor populations on E14.5 were intermingled in layers 2/3 and a minor population was also found in layer 4. Examination of cell morphology and membrane properties did not identify differences by lineage. However, in multi-patch studies within layer 2/3, aIPC-derived neurons were found to preferentially synapse with neurons derived from other progenitors instead of other aIPC-derived neurons. In addition, aIPC-derived neurons in layer 2/3 were more likely to synapse with pyramidal neurons in layer 5a whereas the neurons generated from other progenitors favored layer 5b neurons.

12.4.3 Precursor Effects on Gyrencephaly

In addition to playing a role in the complexity of cortical layers, precursor heterogeneity may also be involved in the development of the cortical convolutions evident in gyrencephalic species. The topographical map of the cortex is a complex and highly specific anatomical feature of large-brained mammals. Many theories for the mechanisms underlying gyrencephaly have been proposed, including physical forces generated by axons, local sites of extreme neuropil growth, and specialized sites of hyper- or hypo-proliferation to give rise to gyri and sulci, respectively (Borrell 2018; Reillo et al. 2017). Regarding the latter, several studies in ferret brain development have demonstrated regional differences in neural precursor proliferation prior to gyrus formation, and comparisons of microarray gene expression to neighboring regions indicate specific differences in gene expression (de Juan Romero et al. 2015). The most parsimonious explanation for the observed fidelity of cortical topography between individuals of the same species is a coordinated plan by which extrinsic influences act on neural precursor populations to perform a developmental plan that differs from that occurring in neighboring regions. Thus, the extrinsic signals (e.g., cortical afferents) must either specifically target only selected regions, or the precursors within specific regions must be tuned to react differently to a broad signal in the environment. These precursors, which may include percentages of aRGC, bIPC, and bRGC subtypes specific to that location, must also be present prior to the arrival of the extrinsic cues and therefore must be pre-positioned by an as yet unappreciated mechanism.

Taken together, the labeling strategies described here that enable temporal resolution of neuronal production demonstrate that cortical precursor diversity is an operational feature of the developing system, that it directly contributes cellular complexity to the cortical layers by providing a variegated population of parent cells that can also be fine-tuned during the formation of each cortical layer. The neuronal diversity now attributed to precursor of origin extends to cell morphology, electrophysiological behavior, and post-synaptic partnerships. Future work is needed to determine how this neuronal diversity is operationalized over the course of neurogenesis (i.e., which parameters arise from which lineages) and the extent to which environmental impacts and activity-based interactions further refine circuits in each area of the cortex. In addition, future work should include investigation of long-range intra- and subcortical projections to determine how neurons from different lineages connect to different parts of the brain.

These findings have prompted several new and important questions: How do aRGC balance the generation of intermediate progenitors with their own neuronal output and is this balance regionally controlled to generate cortical areas with specific lamina profiles and circuitry? If cortical neurogenesis depends on a complex interplay between the influences of multiple precursor groups and extrinsic cues, how does this system react to challenges during early brain development?

12.5 Consequences of Altering Neurogenesis

Both congenital and environmental stressors can lead to perturbations of cortical neurogenesis. In this section we discuss several developmental disorders that impact cortical growth and function from the perspective of the cellular diversity findings presented above.

12.5.1 Trisomy 21

In Down syndrome (DS), approximately 220 protein coding genes and more than 300 non-protein coding genes are triplicated by trisomy of chromosome 21 (Gupta et al. 2016). Since many of these genes are known to be expressed within the nervous system, such as Amyloid Precursor Protein, Superoxide Dismutase-1, DYRK1A, and several ion channel subunits, it is unsurprising that developmental abnormalities have been found in the DS nervous system. The DS cerebral cortex is microencephalic and distinct architectonic abnormalities have been found in multiple cortical regions, including alterations in cortical lamina and synapse formation in frontal cortex and the medial temporal gyrus (Golden and Hyman 1994; Stagni et al. 2018; Utagawa et al. 2022). In addition to decreases in gray matter, the development and maintenance of myelinated tracts are also affected in DS. More than just a consequence of fewer neurons and therefore fewer axons to myelinate, recent transcriptomics, animal model, and induced pluripotent stem cell studies have demonstrated that the oligodendrocyte lineage exhibits an intrinsic differentiation delay (Aziz et al. 2019; Klein and Haydar 2022; Klein et al. 2021; Lu et al. 2012; Olmos-Serrano et al. 2016). Thus, trisomy 21 is a complex genetic disorder that affects many cell types and developmental processes during brain development and the combination of these changes impacts cortical growth and processing.

Since the trisomy in DS occurs most frequently at or near fertilization, development is affected not only by a protracted period of altered gene expression but also because each cell must carry an extra chromosome, a significant burden for proliferative cells. Indeed, BrdU labeling studies on postmortem tissue have now shown impairments in neural precursor proliferation in the developing hippocampus (Contestabile et al. 2007) and cerebellum (Guidi et al. 2011). It is therefore probable that the developmental abnormalities in the DS cerebral cortex are also caused by precursor deficits, but because it is not possible to obtain adequate numbers of human specimen for controlled studies at early prenatal periods, clear answers to whether neocortical precursor cells are affected in DS have been provided mainly from mouse models.

Thus far, BrdU labeling studies in the Ts16, Ts65Dn, Ts1Cje, and Ts2Cje mouse models of DS have demonstrated reduced precursor cell numbers and slower cell cycle kinetics in the VZ compared to littermate controls, leading to slower radial expansion of the neocortical wall during neurogenesis (Chakrabarti et al. 2007; Haydar et al. 1996; Ishihara et al. 2010). In Ts65Dn, Ts1Cje, and Ts2Cje models, BrdU pulse/chase studies indicate a lower level of neuron production during this period. Interestingly, although the Ts65Dn neocortical wall is delayed in its expansion, cortical width appears to grow rapidly just before birth due to increased proliferation in the SVZ, indicating significant plasticity in the germinal zones which works to offset earlier delays by increasing neuronal production late in the neurogenesis period. Nevertheless, evidence of altered neuronal specification, differentiation, and synapse formation in the mouse and human telencephalon indicate that the delayed arrival of neurons into the cortical lamina is not sufficient for proper growth, perhaps due to the ensuing mismatch between the developmental state of the new neurons and the critical time windows that operate during early cortical differentiation.

Since much of the data from human samples and from the mouse models have used only nucleotide analog methods to measure cell proliferation, there is scant information regarding whether neural precursor subtypes are affected in DS. In an IUE study on Ts65Dn animals (Tyler and Haydar 2013), fate mapping cortical precursors using a Tubulin-alpha-1 promoter (Tα1-Cre) plasmid, previously identified as aIPCs, found significant reductions in this precursor cell type within the VZ. This finding, coupled with the increased proliferation of SVZ cells (likely to be bIPCs) later in neurogenesis (Chakrabarti et al. 2007), indicates that trisomy 21 is accompanied by alterations in specific subsets of cells that generate excitatory neurons for the cerebral cortex. The recent development of the TcMAC21 mouse and TcHSA21 rat models of DS, which contain a full copy of human chromosome 21 and therefore represent the most genetically sound models of the human condition (Kazuki et al. 2020, 2022), portend well for the field of DS neuroscience. It will be exciting to combine careful measurements of cortical growth and connectivity with fate mapping-based approaches to query the roles of specific neural precursor types during development. In addition, several labs have embarked on cortical development studies in DS using two- and three-dimensional cultures of human iPSCs, which may provide an unparalleled glimpse of the impact on neural precursor subtypes during DS cortical formation.

12.5.2 Prenatal Viral Infection

Several disorders that result in cortical malformation and altered function are caused by environmental insults during prenatal development. In recent years, much focus has been paid to the effects of prenatal infection on cortical growth and the evidence suggests that maternal immune activation and direct infection of the fetal brain can lead to developmental abnormalities. For example, human fetuses exposed to Influenza A virus (IAV) infection during the second and third trimester appear to be predisposed to neuropsychiatric disorders such as schizophrenia (Mednick et al. 1988). Studies in mouse (Fatemi et al. 2002, 2009) and nonhuman primate (Short et al. 2010) indicate that many strains of IAV, including H1N1, can lead to reductions in cortical gray matter, macrocephaly, and changes in white matter development and connectivity. The association between IAV infection and schizophrenia are particularly intriguing given the protracted period of seemingly normal development before symptoms occur in adolescence and early adulthood. The results suggest that either genetic or environmental (i.e., prenatal infection) insults can lead to alterations in cortical circuitry during prenatal and early postnatal development, particularly in the frontal cortex. Changes to this circuitry, which initially seem to be inconsequential or are compensated for during the first decades of life, can then be unmasked by a second hit (such as psychological trauma) during adolescence (Selemon and Zecevic 2015). If neural precursor subtypes contribute specific features of the cortical circuitry by producing the heterogeneous neurons comprising those circuits, vulnerability of precursor subtypes to prenatal infection or maternal immune activation must be considered possible features of the etiology of psychiatric disorders related to prenatal viral infection.

Some cortical precursor types appear to be particularly vulnerable to viral infection. In mouse model and organoid studies of prenatal Zika virus (ZIKV) infection (Chang et al. 2020; Noguchi et al. 2020; Onorati et al. 2016; Schultz et al. 2021; Shelton et al. 2021; Shi et al. 2018), it was shown that ZIKV preferentially and lethally infects aRGCs before transferring to other cell types in the neocortical wall either via cell-free particles or via cell division. This infection program can lead to severe consequences including microcephaly and profound intellectual disability. However, many babies born after prenatal exposure to ZIKV do not exhibit microcephaly or intellectual disability.

While this may be due to differences in timing of infection (i.e., which trimester was affected), neural precursor diversity may play a role in limiting the devastating impacts of prenatal ZIKV infection. For example, not all aRGCs become infected, even after a large interventricular inoculation, and other intermediate precursor cell types are not killed by ZIKV despite the fact that many cell types within the neocortical wall remain infected. These data indicate that in addition to yielding a diverse population of neurons for the cortex, the neural precursor variety described may also provide a protective function in the brain. Different precursor types exhibit varying degrees of vulnerability to viral infection and this may enable the system to compensate, albeit partially, for the loss of some aRGCs during cortical neurogenesis.

12.6 Conclusion

Modern techniques to visualize cell morphology, behavior, and gene expression in the developing brain have generated newfound appreciation for the complex populations of neural precursor cells found in the prenatal neocortex. In addition, species comparisons have demonstrated that additional cell types and compartments within the neocortical wall have appeared during mammalian evolution, presumably related to differences in brain size and complexity. Emerging evidence suggests that cortical precursor heterogeneity is likely a major contributing factor to the neuronal diversity within and between cortical layers. It appears that the developmental programs operating in the VZ and SVZ are controlled in a regional manner, enabling large architectonic distinctions in cortical lamination even between neighboring areas, for example between the neighboring primary and secondary visual areas of the cortex (Tyler 2019). Therefore, in addition to the developmental changes that yield cellular differences between layers, the germinal zones likely behave differently depending on whether they underlie a future gyrus or sulcus.

Thus far, advances in understanding how precursor variety leads to specific features of cortical shape and function have relied on advanced genomics, imaging, and electrophysiological techniques. Each of these approaches has significant drawbacks, so recognizing the impact of these limitations on the acquisition and evaluation of the data they produce is critical. For instance, the fidelity of sequencing approaches can only be assured by validating the presence of those same features in the living brain. Understanding how specific properties of local VZ and SVZ cells yield the cortical features for the area that they produce require precise spatiotemporal labeling each of the cell types in a manner that can be tracked as development ensues.

The complex developmental interplay between extrinsic influences and the multiple types of neocortical precursor cells requires an exquisite level of control that somehow emerges from the biological system of the developing brain. Paradoxically, while the multitude of different types of precursor cells constitute a system that can potentially adapt or compensate for developmental anomalies, transient interference in even one precursor type, perhaps even for a short period of time in a small area of the developing neocortical wall, can have long-lasting effects on cortical function. Upsetting the intricate role that each precursor types plays in forming subsets of neurons with specific properties may lead to subtle alterations in circuitry, resulting in intellectual deficits later in life. It is therefore clear that future work on neurodevelopmental disabilities must include an analysis of precursor diversity as a component of the etiology of the disorder. The combination of advanced techniques, species comparisons, and testing of neurodevelopmental models mentioned above sets the stage for discovering in the near future how the complex precursor populations cooperate to form the cerebral cortex.

References

Angevine, J.B. and Sidman, R.L. (1961). Autoradiographic study of cell migration during histogenesis of the cerebral cortex in the mouse. *Nature* 192: 766–768.

Armand, E.J. et al. (2021). Single-cell sequencing of brain cell transcriptomes and epigenomes. *Neuron* 109: 11–26. doi: 10.1016/j.neuron.2020.12.010.

Arnold, S.J. et al. (2008). The T-box transcription factor Eomes/Tbr2 regulates neurogenesis in the cortical subventricular zone. *Genes Dev* 22: 2479–2484. doi: 10.1101/gad.475408.

Aziz, N.M. et al. (2019). Spatiotemporal development of spinal neuronal and glial populations in the Ts65Dn mouse model of Down syndrome. *J Neurodev Disorders* 11: 35. doi: 10.1186/s11689-019-9294-9.

Baron, C.S. and van Oudenaarden, A. (2019). Unravelling cellular relationships during development and regeneration using genetic lineage tracing. *Nat Rev Mol Cell Biol* 20: 753–765. doi: 10.1038/s41580-019-0186-3.

Betizeau, M. et al. (2013). Precursor diversity and complexity of lineage relationships in the outer subventricular zone of the primate. *Neuron* 80: 442–457. doi: 10.1016/j.neuron.2013.09.032.

Borrell, V. (2018). How cells fold the cerebral cortex. *J Neurosci* 38: 776–783. doi: 10.1523/JNEUROSCI.1106-17.2017.

Caviness, V.S., Jr. and Takahashi, T. (1995). Proliferative events in the cerebral ventricular zone. *Brain Dev* 17: 159–163.

Chakrabarti, L. et al. (2007). Defects in embryonic neurogenesis and initial synapse formation in the forebrain of the Ts65Dn mouse model of Down syndrome. *J Neurosci* 27: 11483–11495.

Chang, Y. et al. (2020). Different gene networks are disturbed by Zika virus infection in a mouse microcephaly model. *Genom, Proteom Bioinform* 18: 737–748. doi: 10.1016/j.gpb.2019.06.004.

Contestabile, A. et al. (2007). Cell cycle alteration and decreased cell proliferation in the hippocampal dentate gyrus and in the neocortical germinal matrix of fetuses with Down syndrome and in Ts65Dn mice. *Hippocampus* 17: 665–678. doi: 10.1002/hipo.20308.

Darmanis, S. et al. (2015). A survey of human brain transcriptome diversity at the single cell level. *Proc Natl Acad Sci USA* 112: 7285–7290. doi: 10.1073/pnas.1507125112.

de Juan Romero, C. et al. (2015). Discrete domains of gene expression in germinal layers distinguish the development of gyrencephaly. *EMBO J* 34: 1859–1874. doi: 10.15252/embj.201591176.

Desai, A.R. and McConnell, S.K. (2000). Progressive restriction in fate potential by neural progenitors during cerebral cortical development. *Development* 127: 2863–2872. doi: 10.1242/dev.127.13.2863.

Di Bella, D.J. et al. (2021). Molecular logic of cellular diversification in the mouse cerebral cortex. *Nature* 595: 554–559. doi: 10.1038/s41586-021-03670-5.

Ellender, T.J. et al. (2019). Embryonic progenitor pools generate diversity in fine-scale excitatory cortical subnetworks. *Nat Commun* 10: 5224. doi: 10.1038/s41467-019-13206-1.

Englund, C. et al. (2005). Pax6, Tbr2, and Tbr1 are expressed sequentially by radial glia, intermediate progenitor cells, and postmitotic neurons in developing neocortex. *J Neurosci* 25: 247–251.

Fatemi, S.H. et al. (2002). Human influenza viral infection in utero alters glial fibrillary acidic protein immunoreactivity in the developing brains of neonatal mice. *Mol Psychiatry* 7: 633–640. doi: 10.1038/sj.mp.4001046.

Fatemi, S.H. et al. (2009). Abnormal expression of myelination genes and alterations in white matter fractional anisotropy following prenatal viral influenza infection at E16 in mice. *Schizophrenia Res* 112: 46–53. doi: 10.1016/j.schres.2009.04.014.

Florio, M. et al. (2015). Human-specific gene ARHGAP11B promotes basal progenitor amplification and neocortex expansion. *Science* 347: 1465–1470. doi: 10.1126/science.aaa1975.

Fujita, S. (1963). The matrix cell and cytogenesis in the developing central nervous system. *J Comp Neurol* 120: 37–42.

Gal, J.S. et al. (2006). Molecular and morphological heterogeneity of neural precursors in the mouse neocortical proliferative zones. *J Neurosci* 26: 1045–1056.
Golden, J. and Hyman, B. (1994). Development of the superior temporal neocortex is anomalous in trisomy 21. *J Neuropathol Exp Neurol* 53: 513–520.
Guidi, S. et al. (2011). Widespread proliferation impairment and hypocellularity in the cerebellum of fetuses with down syndrome. *Brain Pathol* 21: 361–373. doi: 10.1111/j.1750-3639.2010.00459.x.
Guillamon-Vivancos, T. et al. (2019). Distinct neocortical progenitor lineages fine-tune neuronal diversity in a layer-specific manner. *Cereb Cortex* 29: 1121–1138. doi: 10.1093/cercor/bhy019.
Guo, C. et al. (2013). Fezf2 expression identifies a multipotent progenitor for neocortical projection neurons, astrocytes, and oligodendrocytes. *Neuron* 80: 1167–1174. doi: 10.1016/j.neuron.2013.09.037.
Gupta, M. et al. (2016). Mouse models of Down syndrome: gene content and consequences. *Mamm Genome* 27: 538–555. doi: 10.1007/s00335-016-9661-8.
Hansen, D.V. et al. (2010). Neurogenic radial glia in the outer subventricular zone of human neocortex. *Nature* 464: 554–561. nature08845 [pii]. doi: 10.1038/nature08845.
Hartfuss, E. et al. (2001). Characterization of CNS precursor subtypes and radial glia. *Dev Biol* 229: 15–30.
Haubensak, W. et al. (2004). Neurons arise in the basal neuroepithelium of the early mammalian telencephalon. *Proc Natl Acad Sci USA* 101: 3196–3201.
Haydar, T.F. et al. (1996). Consequences of trisomy 16 for mouse brain development. *J Neurosci* 16: 6175–6182.
His, W. (1889). *Die Entwicklung des Menschlichen Gehirns wahrend der ersten Monate*. Leipzig: Hirzel.
Huang, W. et al. (2020). Origins and proliferative states of human oligodendrocyte precursor cells. *Cell* 182: 594–608 e511. doi: 10.1016/j.cell.2020.06.027.
Ishihara, K. et al. (2010). Enlarged brain ventricles and impaired neurogenesis in the Ts1Cje and Ts2Cje mouse models of Down syndrome. *Cereb Cortex* 20: 1131–1143. doi: 10.1093/cercor/bhp176.
Kalebic, N. et al. (2018). Human-specific ARHGAP11B induces hallmarks of neocortical expansion in developing ferret neocortex. *Elife* 7: e41241. doi: 10.7554/eLife.41241.
Kalebic, N. et al. (2019). Neocortical expansion due to increased proliferation of basal progenitors is linked to changes in their morphology. *Cell Stem Cell* 24: 535–550 e539. doi: 10.1016/j.stem.2019.02.017.
Kalebic, N. and Huttner, W.B. (2020). Basal progenitor morphology and neocortex evolution. *Trends Neurosci* 43: 843–853. doi: 10.1016/j.tins.2020.07.009.
Kazuki, Y. et al. (2020). A non-mosaic transchromosomic mouse model of Down syndrome carrying the long arm of human chromosome 21. *Elife* 9: e56223. doi: 10.7554/eLife.56223.
Kazuki, Y. et al. (2022). A transchromosomic rat model with human chromosome 21 shows robust Down syndrome features. *Am J Hum Genet* 109: 328–344. doi: 10.1016/j.ajhg.2021.12.015.
Kharchenko, P.V. et al. (2014). Bayesian approach to single-cell differential expression analysis. *Nat Methods* 11: 740–742. doi: 10.1038/nmeth.2967.
Klein, J.A. and Haydar, T.F. (2022). Neurodevelopment in Down syndrome. *Front Cell Neurosci* 16: 941855. doi: 10.3389/fncel.2022.941855.
Klein, J.A. et al. (2021). Sonic hedgehog pathway modulation normalizes expression of Olig2 in rostrally patterned NPCs with trisomy 21. *Front Cell Neurosci* 15: 794675. doi: 10.3389/fncel.2021.794675.
Kowalczyk, T. et al. (2009). Intermediate neuronal progenitors (basal progenitors) produce pyramidal-projection neurons for all layers of cerebral cortex. *Cereb Cortex* 19: 2439–2450. doi: 10.1093/cercor/bhn260.
Laslo, P. et al. (2006). Multilineage transcriptional priming and determination of alternate hematopoietic cell fates. *Cell* 126: 755–766. doi: 10.1016/j.cell.2006.06.052.
Levitt, P. et al. (1981). Coexistence of neuronal and glial precursor cells in the cerebral ventricular zone of the fetal monkey. *J Neurosci* 1: 27–39.

Levitt, P. and Rakic, P. (1980). Immunoperoxidase localization of glial fibrillary acidic protein in radial glial cells and astrocytes of the developing rhesus monkey brain. *J Comp Neurol* 193: 815–840.

Li, Z. et al. (2020a). Lessons from single cell sequencing in CNS cell specification and function. *Curr Opin Genet Dev* 65: 138–143. doi: 10.1016/j.gde.2020.05.043.

Li, Z. et al. (2020b). Transcriptional priming as a conserved mechanism of lineage diversification in the developing mouse and human neocortex. *Sci Adv* 6: eabd2068. doi: 10.1126/sciadv.abd2068.

Liu, J. et al. (2017). The primate-specific gene TMEM14B marks outer radial glia cells and promotes cortical expansion and folding. *Cell Stem Cell* 21: 635–649 e638. doi: 10.1016/j.stem.2017.08.013.

Loo, L. et al. (2019). Single-cell transcriptomic analysis of mouse neocortical development. *Nat Commun* 10: 134. doi: 10.1038/s41467-018-08079-9.

Lu, J. et al. (2012). OLIG2 over-expression impairs proliferation of human Down syndrome neural progenitors. *Hum Mol Genet* 21: 2330–2340. doi: 10.1093/hmg/dds052.

Ma, J. et al. (2018). Neural lineage tracing in the mammalian brain. *Curr Opin Neurobiol* 50: 7–16. doi: 10.1016/j.conb.2017.10.013.

Malatesta, P. et al. (2000). Isolation of radial glial cells by fluorescent-activated cell sorting reveals a neuronal lineage. *Development* 127: 5253–5263.

Mayer, C. et al. (2018). Developmental diversification of cortical inhibitory interneurons. *Nature* 555: 457–462. doi: 10.1038/nature25999.

Mednick, S.A. et al. (1988). Adult schizophrenia following prenatal exposure to an influenza epidemic. *Arch Gen Psychiatry* 45: 189–192. doi: 10.1001/archpsyc.1988.01800260109013.

Mi, D. et al. (2018). Early emergence of cortical interneuron diversity in the mouse embryo. *Science* 360: 81–85. doi: 10.1126/science.aar6821.

Miyai, T. et al. (2018). Three-step transcriptional priming that drives the commitment of multipotent progenitors toward B cells. *Genes Dev* 32: 112–126. doi: 10.1101/gad.309575.117.

Miyata, T. et al. (2001). Asymmetric inheritance of radial glial fibers by cortical neurons. *Neuron* 31: 727–741.

Miyata, T. et al. (2004). Asymmetric production of surface-dividing and non-surface-dividing cortical progenitor cells. *Development* 131: 3133–3145.

Noctor, S.C. et al. (2001). Neurons derived from radial glial cells establish radial units in neocortex. *Nature* 409: 714–720.

Noctor, S.C. et al. (2002). Dividing precursor cells of the embryonic cortical ventricular zone have morphological and molecular characteristics of radial glia. *J Neurosci* 22: 3161–3173.

Noctor, S.C. et al. (2004). Cortical neurons arise in symmetric and asymmetric division zones and migrate through specific phases. *Nat Neurosci* 7: 136–144.

Noguchi, K.K. et al. (2020). Zika virus infection in the developing mouse produces dramatically different neuropathology dependent on viral strain. *J Neurosci* 40: 1145–1161. doi: 10.1523/JNEUROSCI.1376-19.2019.

Nowakowski, T.J. et al. (2017). Spatiotemporal gene expression trajectories reveal developmental hierarchies of the human cortex. *Science* 358: 1318–1323. doi: 10.1126/science.aap8809.

Nowakowski, T.J. et al. (2013). MicroRNA-92b regulates the development of intermediate cortical progenitors in embryonic mouse brain. *Proc Natl Acad Sci USA* 110: 7056–7061. doi: 10.1073/pnas.1219385110.

Olmos-Serrano, J.L. et al. (2016). Down syndrome developmental brain transcriptome reveals defective oligodendrocyte differentiation and myelination. *Neuron* 89: 1208–1222. doi: 10.1016/j.neuron.2016.01.042.

Onorati, M. et al. (2016). Zika virus disrupts phospho-TBK1 localization and mitosis in human neuroepithelial stem cells and radial glia. *Cell Rep* 16: 2576–2592. doi: 10.1016/j.celrep.2016.08.038.

Osumi-Sutherland, D. et al. (2021). Cell type ontologies of the Human Cell Atlas. *Nat Cell Biol* 23: 1129–1135. doi: 10.1038/s41556-021-00787-7.

Pilz, G.A. et al. (2013). Amplification of progenitors in the mammalian telencephalon includes a new radial glial cell type. *Nat Commun* 4: 2125. doi: 10.1038/ncomms3125.

Pinto, L. and Gotz, M. (2007). Radial glial cell heterogeneity – the source of diverse progeny in the CNS. *Prog Neurobiol* 83: 2–23.

Pinto, L. et al. (2008). Prospective isolation of functionally distinct radial glial subtypes – lineage and transcriptome analysis. *Mol Cell Neurosci* 38: 15–42.

Pollen, A.A. et al. (2015). Molecular identity of human outer radial glia during cortical development. *Cell* 163: 55–67. doi: 10.1016/j.cell.2015.09.004.

Pollen, A.A. et al. (2014). Low-coverage single-cell mRNA sequencing reveals cellular heterogeneity and activated signaling pathways in developing cerebral cortex. *Nat Biotechnol* 32: 1053–1058. doi: 10.1038/nbt.2967.

Rakic, P. (1971). Guidance of neurons migrating to the fetal monkey neocortex. *Brain Res* 33: 471–476.

Rakic, P. (1972). Mode of cell migration to the superficial layers of fetal monkey neocortex. *J Comp Neurol* 145: 61–83.

Rakic, P. (1975). Timing of major ontogenetic events in the visual cortex of the rhesus monkey. *UCLA Forum Med Sci* 18: 3–40.

Rakic, P. (1985). DNA synthesis and cell division in the adult primate brain. *Ann New York Acad Sci* 457: 193–211.

Rakic, P. (1988). Specification of cerebral cortical areas. *Science* 241: 170–176.

Ramskold, D. et al. (2012). Full-length mRNA-Seq from single-cell levels of RNA and individual circulating tumor cells. *Nat Biotechnol* 30: 777–782. doi: 10.1038/nbt.2282.

Regev, A. et al. (2017). The human cell atlas. *Elife* 6: 10.7554/eLife.27041.

Reillo, I. et al. (2017). A complex code of extrinsic influences on cortical progenitor cells of higher mammals. *Cereb Cortex* 27: 4586–4606. doi: 10.1093/cercor/bhx171.

Saunders, A. et al. (2018). Molecular diversity and specializations among the cells of the adult mouse brain. *Cell* 174: 1015–1030 e1016. doi: 10.1016/j.cell.2018.07.028.

Schaper, A. (1897). The earliest differentiation in the central nervous system of vertebrates. *Science* 5: 430–431.

Schultz, V. et al. (2021). Oligodendrocytes are susceptible to Zika virus infection in a mouse model of perinatal exposure. *Glia* 69: 2023–2036. doi: 10.1002/glia.24010.

Selemon, L.D. and Zecevic, N. (2015). Schizophrenia. *Transl Psychiatry* 5: e623. doi: 10.1038/tp.2015.115.

Sessa, A. et al. (2008). Tbr2 directs conversion of radial glia into basal precursors and guides neuronal amplification by indirect neurogenesis in the developing neocortex. *Neuron* 60: 56–69. doi: 10.1016/j.neuron.2008.09.028.

Shapiro, E. et al. (2013). Single-cell sequencing-based technologies will revolutionize whole-organism science. *Nat Rev Genet* 14: 618–630. doi: 10.1038/nrg3542.

Shelton, S.M. et al. (2021). Forebrain neural precursor cells are differentially vulnerable to Zika virus infection. *eNeuro* 8: ENEURO.0108-21.2021. doi: 10.1523/ENEURO.0108-21.2021.

Shi, Y. et al. (2018). Vertical transmission of the Zika virus causes neurological disorders in mouse offspring. *Sci Rep* 8: 3541. doi: 10.1038/s41598-018-21894-w.

Shitamukai, A. et al. (2011). Oblique radial glial divisions in the developing mouse neocortex induce self-renewing progenitors outside the germinal zone that resemble primate outer subventricular zone progenitors. *J Neurosci* 31: 3683–3695. 31/ 10/3683[pii]. doi: 10.1523/JNEUROSCI.4773-10.2011.

Short, S.J. et al. (2010). Maternal influenza infection during pregnancy impacts postnatal brain development in the rhesus monkey. *Biol Psychiatry* 67: 965–973. doi: 10.1016/j.biopsych.2009.11.026.

Sidman, R. et al. (1959). Cell proliferation and migration in the primitive ependymal zone. *Exp Neurol* 1: 322–333.

Stagni, F. et al. (2018). Neurogenesis impairment. *Free Rad Biol Med* 114: 15–32. doi: 10.1016/j.freeradbiomed.2017.07.026.

Stegle, O. et al. (2015). Computational and analytical challenges in single-cell transcriptomics. *Nat Rev Genet* 16: 133–145. doi: 10.1038/nrg3833.

Takahashi, T. et al. (1999). Sequence of neuron origin and neocortical laminar fate. *J Neurosci* 19: 10357–10371.

Takahashi, T. et al. (1994). Mode of cell proliferation in the developing mouse neocortex. *Proc Natl Acad Sci USA* 91: 375–379.

Tamamaki, N. et al. (2001). Radial glia is a progenitor of neocortical neurons in the developing cerebral cortex. *Neurosci Res* 41: 51–60.

Tang, F. et al. (2009). mRNA-Seq whole-transcriptome analysis of a single cell. *Nat Methods* 6: 377–382. doi: 10.1038/nmeth.1315.

Tasic, B. et al. (2018). Shared and distinct transcriptomic cell types across neocortical areas. *Nature* 563: 72–78. doi: 10.1038/s41586-018-0654-5.

Telley, L. et al. (2019). Temporal patterning of apical progenitors and their daughter neurons in the developing neocortex. *Science* 364: eaav2522. doi: 10.1126/science.aav2522.

Telley, L. et al. (2016). Sequential transcriptional waves direct the differentiation of newborn neurons in the mouse neocortex. *Science* 351: 1443–1446. doi: 10.1126/science.aad8361.

Tritschler, S. et al. (2019). Concepts and limitations for learning developmental trajectories from single cell genomics. *Development* 146: dev170506. doi: 10.1242/dev.170506.

Tyler, W.A. and Haydar, T.F. (2013). Multiplex genetic fate mapping reveals a novel route of neocortical neurogenesis, which is altered in the Ts65Dn mouse model of Down syndrome. *J Neurosci* 33: 5106–5119. 33/ 12/5106[pii]. doi: 10.1523/JNEUROSCI.5380-12.2013.

Tyler, W.A. and Haydar, T.F. (2019). Cortical specification and neuronal migration. In: *The Neocortex* (ed. W. Singer, T.J. Sejnowski, and P. Rakic), 11–29. Cambridge, MA: MIT Press.

Tyler, W.A. et al. (2015). Neural precursor lineages specify distinct neocortical pyramidal neuron types. *J Neurosci* 35: 6142–6152. doi: 10.1523/JNEUROSCI.0335-15.2015.

Utagawa, E.C. et al. (2022). Neurogenesis and neuronal differentiation in the postnatal frontal cortex in Down syndrome. *Acta Neuropathol Commun* 10: 86. doi: 10.1186/s40478-022-01385-w.

Vasistha, N.A. et al. (2015). Cortical and clonal contribution of Tbr2 expressing progenitors in the developing mouse brain. *Cereb Cortex* 25: 3290–3302. doi: 10.1093/cercor/bhu125.

Vinsland, E. and Linnarsson, S. (2022). Single-cell RNA-sequencing of mammalian brain development. *Development* 149: dev200180. doi: 10.1242/dev.200180.

Wang, X. et al. (2011). A new subtype of progenitor cell in the mouse embryonic neocortex. *Nat Neurosci* 14: 555–561. nn.2807 [pii]. doi: 10.1038/nn.2807.

Woodworth, M.B. et al. (2017). Building a lineage from single cells: genetic techniques for cell lineage tracking. *Nat Rev Genet* 18: 230–244. doi: 10.1038/nrg.2016.159.

Yuzwa, S.A. et al. (2017). Developmental emergence of adult neural stem cells as revealed by single-cell transcriptional profiling. *Cell Rep* 21: 3970–3986. doi: 10.1016/j.celrep.2017.12.017.

Zahr, S.K. et al. (2018). A translational repression complex in developing mammalian neural stem cells that regulates neuronal specification. *Neuron* 97: 520–537 e526. doi: 10.1016/j.neuron.2017.12.045.

Zeisel, A. et al. (2015). Brain structure. Cell types in the mouse cortex and hippocampus revealed by single-cell RNA-seq. *Science* 347: 1138–1142. doi: 10.1126/science.aaa1934.

Zeng, H. (2022). What is a cell type and how to define it? *Cell* 185: 2739–2755. doi: 10.1016/j.cell.2022.06.031.

13

Developmental and Evolutionary Origins of Cortical Projection Neuron Identity and Connectivity

Navjot Kaur[1], Rothem Kovner[1], Kevin T. Gobeske[1], and Nenad Sestan[1,2,]*

[1] *Department of Neuroscience, Yale School of Medicine, New Haven, CT 06510, USA*
[2] *Departments of Comparative Medicine Genetics, Neurosurgery and Psychiatry, Wu Tsai Institute, Kavli Institute of Neuroscience, Program of Cellular Neuroscience, Neurodegeneration and Repair, and Yale Child Study Center, Yale School of Medicine, New Haven, CT 06510, USA*
* *Correspopnding author*

13.1 Laminar Organization of the Cerebral Cortex

The cerebral cortex is the outer extent of the dorsal pallium responsible for processing sensory information, controlling motor actions, and performing advanced cognitive processes. The prototypical six-layered neocortex is unique to mammals and is surrounded by two simpler three-layered allocortical structures at its edges, the piriform cortex and the hippocampus. The cerebral cortex is organized into distinct areas, each with a unique set of functions and connections (Kaas 2019; Rakic 1988; Sur and Rubenstein 2005). The laminar and areal organizations are largely established by glutamatergic excitatory projection neurons (Kwan et al. 2012b; Leone et al. 2008; Molyneaux et al. 2007). Depending on their laminar and areal location, these neurons extend long-range axons to various regions of the cortex or the nervous system forming connections between different neural circuits and allowing for specialized processing of information. The pattern and strength of these connections determine the boundaries between different areas, creating the characteristic architecture of the cortex. In this way, excitatory projection neurons act as the building blocks for cortical organization and together with GABAergic inhibitory neurons (DeFelipe et al. 2013) play a crucial role in determining the functional properties of the cortex.

The six layers (L1–L6) of neocortical excitatory neurons are distinguished by their birth order, constituent cell type, cell density, dendritic properties, axonal projection, input and output synapses, and synaptic physiology (Kumamoto and Hanashima 2014; Kwan et al. 2012b; Leone et al. 2008; Molyneaux et al. 2007; Oberlaender et al. 2012) . Most of the deep layer (L5 and L6) projection neurons form synaptic connections with neurons outside the telencephalon (also known as extratelencephalic or subcerebral neurons; ET neurons). The upper layer (L2––L4) projection neurons form synaptic connections exclusively within the telencephalon or cerebrum via intra- or interhemispheric long-range axonal projections (also known as intratelencephalic or cortico-cortical; IT neurons) (Figure 13.1).

Layer 6 (L6) projection neurons can be subtyped into three major classes based on properties of their dendritic trees and axonal projections: corticothalamic (CT) neurons, inferior temporal (IT) neurons, and claustrum-projecting neurons (Thomson 2010) (Figure 13.1). The CT neurons that emanate from deep layer 6 (L6b) are reminiscent of the subplate neurons that are instrumental in establishing the thalamocortical circuitry during development (Hoerder-Suabedissen and Molnar 2015; Kostovic et al. 2019; Kostovic and Rakic 1980; McConnell et al. 1994). Claustrum-projecting projection neurons resemble typical IT projecting neurons, having a long apical dendrite innervating L1 and a long axon remaining within the deep layers (Thomson 2010).

Neocortical Neurogenesis in Development and Evolution, First Edition. Edited by Wieland B. Huttner.

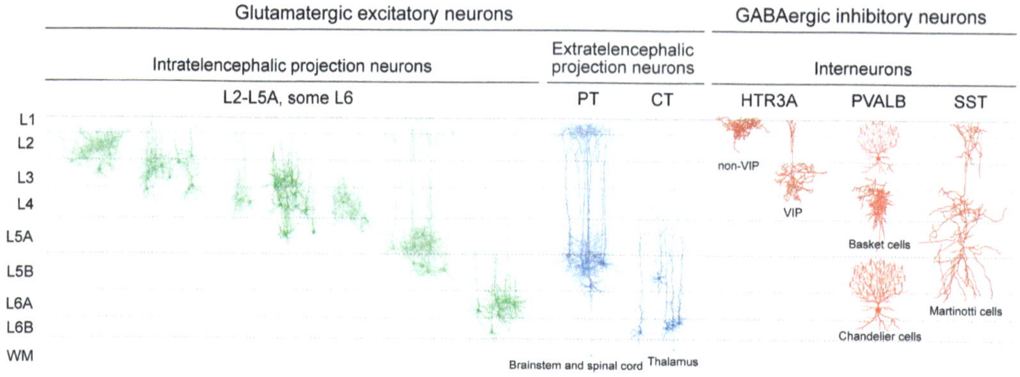

Figure 13.1 Major neuronal subtypes within the adult cerebral cortex: the neurons within the cortex are subclassified into glutamatergic excitatory neurons and GABAergic inhibitory neurons. The excitatory neurons in L2 to L5a form IT connections whereas neurons in the L5b and L6 form IT or ET axonal projections. Different subtypes of GABAergic inhibitory neurons are distributed across multiple layers. PT, pyramidal tract; CT, corticothalamic tract Adapted from Oberlaender et al. (2012).

Excitatory projection neurons in L5 include two major classes of ET and IT neurons (Kumamoto and Hanashima 2014; Molyneaux et al. 2009). ET neurons are predominantly within L5b and are thick tufted, intrinsically bursting pyramidal neurons with very large soma. IT neurons are predominantly within L5a and are thin tufted, regularly spiking neurons with small soma (Oswald et al. 2013). L5b ET neurons project to multiple regions outside the telencephalon, including the diencephalon, brainstem, and spinal cord (Figure 13.1) (Kumamoto and Hanashima 2014; Kwan et al. 2012b; Molyneaux et al. 2007; Oswald et al. 2013). Specialized magnocellular L5b ET neurons in the primary motor cortex, known as Betz cells, project long converging axons that comprise the corticospinal tract, which is the longest such structure in the human body (Rivara et al. 2003). In L5a, IT neurons project intrahemispherically to striatum, or callosally to the contralateral cortex (Molyneaux et al. 2009; Oswald et al. 2013). Additionally, in great apes, humans, elephants, and whales, specialized L5 Von Economo neurons and fork cells in anterior cingulate and fronto-insular regions have long spindle shapes allowing rapid connection of distant brain regions and are proposed to have a role in socialization, empathy, intuition, and complex decision making (Nimchinsky et al. 1999; Seeley et al. 2012).

Within L4, medium spiny excitatory neurons differ from the excitatory neurons in other layers because they do not extend long axons to other brain regions. Rather, they project to nearby neurons in adjacent layers and integrate sensory information being received from thalamic inputs (Scala et al. 2019). Upper layer IT projection neurons form cortico-cortical projections extending intrahemispherically or to the contralateral hemisphere via large axon tracts comprising the corpus callosum or the anterior commissure (Britanova et al. 2008; Leone et al. 2008; Lindwall et al. 2007). During development, considerably more upper layer neurons are produced in primates than in other species due to protracted neurogenesis (see later), leading to increased cortico-cortical connectivity (Lui et al. 2011; Miller et al. 2019).

Across all cortical layers, GABAergic inhibitory interneurons form local, modulatory synaptic connections with glutamatergic neurons. GABAergic interneurons are broadly classified into three categories. Nearly 40 percent of GABAergic neurons express parvalbumin (PVALB), 30 percent express somatostatin (SST), and 30 percent express the serotonin receptor (5HT3aR) (Figure 13.1.) (Rudy et al. 2011). Other cell types that are abundant in the cortex and essential for its function include astrocytes, oligodendrocytes, and microglia. These provide diverse and complex functions that are detailed in other chapters.

13.2 Developmental Origins of Cortical Projection Neurons

Neurogenesis leading to the formation of the cerebral cortex begins with the differentiation of the neuroepithelial cells to neurogenic radial glial cells (RGCs) around post-conception week (PCW) PCW in humans (Figure 13.2) (Silbereis et al. 2016). RGCs span the developing cortical wall, serving dual roles as both the stem cells that produce excitatory neurons and as guides for new-born neurons to reach the forming cortical plate (Breunig et al. 2011; Kriegstein and Alvarez-Buylla 2009; Kwan et al. 2012b; Rasin et al. 2007; Taverna et al. 2014). The key guiding structure of RGCs is the basal process, which traverses almost the entire thickness of the developing cortical wall (Rakic 1971) (Figure 13.2). During the transition of neuroepithelial cells to the RGCs, the microtubule cytoskeleton, intermediate filament proteins, and membrane components play an essential role in the development and maintenance of the RGCs scaffold essential for proper lamination

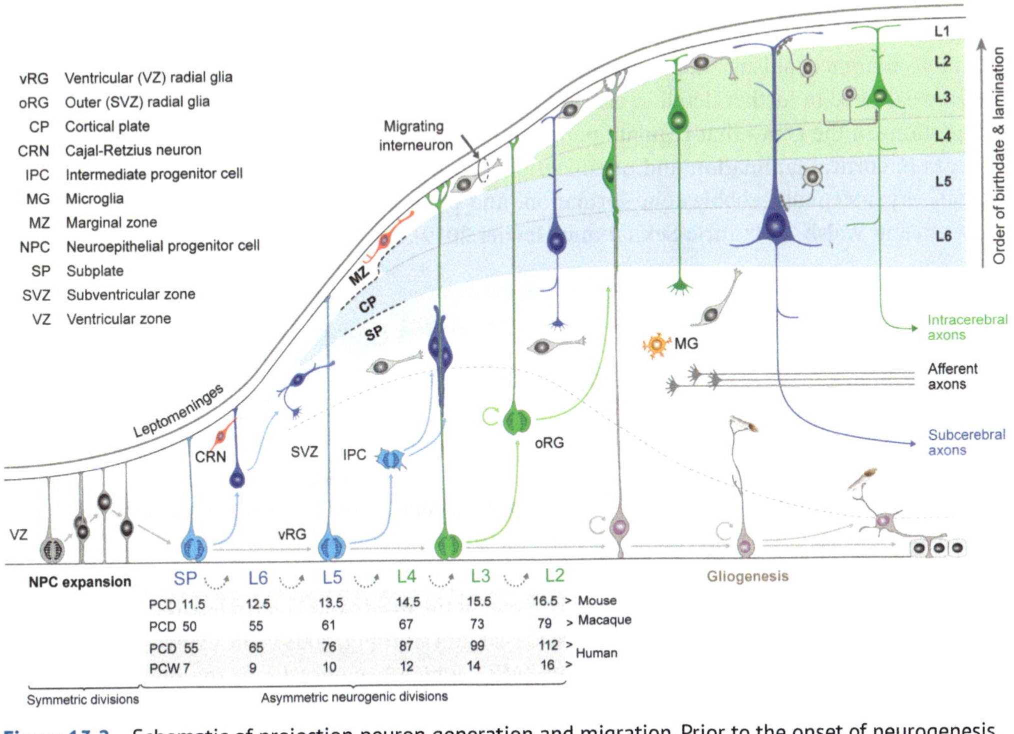

Figure 13.2 Schematic of projection neuron generation and migration. Prior to the onset of neurogenesis, neural progenitors (NPs) in the ventricular zone (VZ; blue) of the developing neocortex divide symmetrically to expand the progenitor pool, undergoing interkinetic nuclear migration (IKNM) as they progress through the cell cycle. NPs assume radial glial morphology and begin dividing asymmetrically to generate neurons, which migrate from the germinal zones guided by radial glia cells (RGC) to reach the mantle layers. The first projection neurons settle within the preplate (PP) to form the nascent cortical plate (CP), which will subsequently become layers (L) 2 to 6 of the neocortex. Some daughter cells of NPs become intermediate progenitor cells (IPCs), migrating away from the VZ and undergoing symmetric neurogenic divisions in the subventricular zone (SVZ). Outer RGCS (oRGCs) are generated from the RGCs during late mid-fetal period where the apical endfoot detaches from the VZ surface. This mode of neurogenesis contributes significantly to upper-layer neurons. At the end of neurogenesis at ~E17.5, the radial scaffold is dismantled, and NPs become gliogeneic, generating cortical and subependymal zone (SEZ) astrocytes (Ast) and giving rise to a layer of ependymal cells (EL). The tangential migration and laminar positioning of interneurons are not illustrated. BV, blood vessel; CR, Cajal–Retzius neuron; DL Pyr, deep-layer pyramidal neuron; IZ, intermediate zone; UL Pyr, upper-layer pyramidal neuron; WM, white matter. Adapted from Kwan et al. (2012b).

organization of immature excitatory neurons (Breunig et al. 2011; Kriegstein and Alvarez-Buylla 2009; Kwan et al. 2012b; Rasin et al. 2007; Taverna et al. 2014). RGC divisions also form another class of neural progenitors, the intermediate progenitor cells (IPCs) (Breunig et al. 2011; Kriegstein and Alvarez-Buylla 2009). This allows RGCs to maintain symmetric and asymmetric divisions that increase the pool of progenitor cells and generate all the pyramidal neurons within the cortex, respectively. The newly born excitatory neurons mainly attach to the radial processes of RGCs as they also begin to migrate outward to form the cortical plate (Rakic, 1971). During this process, different subtypes of excitatory projection neurons are generated through sequential divisions of neural stem/progenitor cells in the ventricular zone (VZ) and subventricular zone (SVZ) in an inside-out manner, followed by subsequent generation of astrocytes and oligodendrocytes (Figure 13.2).

In contrast to the formation and migration of glutamatergic excitatory neurons, the generation of cortical GABAergic inhibitory neurons occurs through different mechanisms and locations. GABAergic neurons primarily arise from neural progenitor cells found in the ventral forebrain neurogenic zones within the medial, lateral, and caudal ganglionic eminences. These neurons migrate tangentially towards the cortical plate (Hu et al. 2017; Marin et al. 2002; Mi et al. 2018). The molecular mechanisms that regulate the formation and migration of cortical GABAergic neurons are explored in further detail in other chapters.

Mutations in the genes that regulate neurogenesis or neuronal migration can lead to dramatic changes in cortical lamination and organization that may be expressed as microcephaly, lissencephaly, hydrocephaly, cobblestone formation, and periventricular or cortical band heterotopia (Gleeson and Walsh 2000; Juric-Sekhar and Hevner 2019).

13.3 Molecular Mechanisms Governing the Laminar Identity of Cortical Projection Neurons

The disrupted phenotypes of cortical layer formation seen in mutant mouse lines have provided the initial opportunity to understand the molecular mechanisms governing the process of neuronal migration and formation of each layer. The spontaneously occurring Reeler mouse mutant provided the initial entry point into the molecular mechanisms that govern the migration of neurons and laminar organization of the cortex, without affecting the specification of neurons themselves. In Reeler mice, there is a complete inversion of the inside-out layering pattern, due to a loss of function mutation in the *reelin* (*Reln*) gene (Tissir and Goffinet, 2003). The expression of *Reln* by the Cajal–Retzius cells in the marginal zone (MZ), which becomes L1 in the mature cortex, is essential to provide a signal for migrating nascent excitatory neurons to stop within the forming cortical plate and form an inside-out laminar organization of the cortex (Tissir and Goffinet, 2003). In absence of *Reln*, the subplate neurons reach the upper most layer just below the MZ. As a result, subplate neurons extend to upper layers just below the MZ and thalamocortical projections pierce the cortical plate obliquely to reach the subplate neurons within the upper layers before turning sharply inwards to invade the L4 neurons.

More recent studies have identified the essential role of transcription factors (TFs) and their interaction with the cis- and trans-regulatory elements in the specification of glutamatergic neurons within each layer of the cerebral cortex (Kwan et al. 2012b; Leone et al. 2008; Molyneaux et al. 2007; Shibata et al. 2015). A TF critical for specification of laminar identity and one of the best understood in the context of developmental and evolutionary regulation is FEZF2 (also known as FEZL or ZFP312). Related studies show that *Fezf2* is selectively enriched in L5 and L6 pyramidal neurons (Gray et al. 2004; Hirata et al. 2004; Inoue et al. 2004) and required for their proper specification of deep L5/6 projection neurons and the formation of their long-range pathway, such as the corticospinal tract (Chen et al. 2005a, 2005b; Molyneaux et al. 2005), a major pathway controlling skilled voluntary movements. Notably, *Fezf2* regulates corticospinal tract formation in a cell autonomous fashion (Chen et al. 2005b; Kaur et al. 2020; Shim et al. 2012) and post-mitotically (Tsyporin et al. 2021). Upstream regulation of *Fezf2* within L5 is controlled by the TFs SOX4 and SOX11, which bind to a neocortex-specific enhancer of *Fezf2* (Shim et al. 2012). Yet in nascent L6 neurons, expression of *Fezf2* is downregulated by SOX5 and TBR1 (Fazel Darbandi et al. 2018; Han et al. 2011; Kwan et al. 2008; Lai et al. 2008; McKenna et al. 2011; Shim et al. 2012), which inhibit the same enhancer. Mechanistically, *Tbr1* and *Sox5*, which are expressed by the subplate and L6 neurons in early cortical development (Hevner et al. 2001; Kwan et al. 2008), bind the cis-regulatory enhancer element of *Fezf2*, and suppress its expression. This *Tbr1* and *Sox5* dependent suppression of *Fezf2* expression is crucial for specification of L5b corticospinal neurons (Han et al. 2011; Kwan et al. 2008). Therefore, these regulatory interactions maintain high expression of *Fezf2* in L5 corticospinal neurons and lower expression in L6 neurons. This regulatory process is tightly controlled, as the forced increase of *Fezf2* expression in nascent L6 neurons (Kwan et al. 2008) can respecify them into corticospinal neurons normally found only in L5; and ectopic expression in upper layer callosal projection neurons can specify the acquisition of molecular characteristics and axonal projections typical of deep layer ET neurons (Chen et al. 2005a; Rouaux and Arlotta 2013). These studies revealed that the identity and connectivity of nascent cortical projection neurons are plastic, and that they can be molecularly reprogrammed – at least in their earlier stages.

In addition to TFs, critical enhancer elements have also been identified. By identifying key enhancers and generating maps of such active enhancers across spatiotemporal axis might improve understanding of the molecular events governing cortical patterning and connectivity (Markenscoff-Papadimitriou et al. 2020; Pattabiraman et al. 2014; Silberberg et al. 2016; Visel et al. 2013). Characterization of the cortical *Fezf2* enhancer also identified sequence changes within the enhancer along evolutionary lines that create binding sites for SOX4 and SOX11, and which may underlie evolutionary origins of the subcerebral projections including the corticospinal tract (Shim et al. 2012).

Other relevant studies of evolutionary specification of projection neuron laminar organization have revealed Hominini-specific deletions in an otherwise conserved cortical enhancer of the gene encoding the synaptic organizer *Cbln2* (Shibata et al. 2021b). These regulatory deletions prevent SOX5 from repressing the expression of *Cbln2* in human L5 pyramidal neurons. This leads to increased expression of *Cbln2* and formation of dendritic spines in L5 corticospinal neurons.

Critical transcriptional regulators of IT neurons have also been identified. CUX1 and CUX2, are both selectively expressed by upper layer IT neurons, and some scattered IT neurons in the deeper layers, as well as their progenitor cells in the SVZ (Arion et al. 2007; Nieto et al. 2004; Zimmer et al. 2004). Both *Cux1* and *Cux2* knockout mice show defects in cell proliferation of the SVZ, and in the development of dendrites and dendritic spines, but not in the laminar identity or callosal connectivity of IT neurons (Cubelos et al. 2010; Li et al. 2010). This indicates that CUX1 and CUX2 play important roles in the development of this class of neurons but do not function as essential determinants driving their cell fate and callosal projections. Similarly, although the analyses of mice lacking both *Pou3f3* and *Pou3f2* (*Brn1* and *Brn2*, respectively) and *Zbtb18* (*Rp58*) revealed decreases in callosal axons, these genes likely play a broader role in the development of neocortical projection neurons, as evidenced by the reduced generation and migration of projection neurons in L5 through L2 (McEvilly et al. 2002; Oishi et al. 2016; Sugitani et al. 2002). Similarly, the chromatin remodeling protein SATB2, which becomes progressively enriched in IT neurons as neocortical development progresses, regulates IT neuron migration and callosal projections (Alcamo et al. 2008;

Britanova et al. 2008). However, a recent study of conditional *Satb2* knockout mice revealed that this protein broadly regulates differentiation and axonal projections of both IT and ET neurons (Leone et al. 2015). Together, these studies have identified essential components of gene regulatory networks directing cell fate specification of cortical projection neurons and their connection patterns. It also identifies key evolutionary changes in this regulatory network that generate variations in cortical circuits across species.

13.4 Molecular Mechanisms Governing the Areal Identity of Cortical Projection Neurons

Differences in long-range connectivity of excitatory projection neurons provide the basis for functional specification of cortical areas and information integration. Cortical wiring patterns also may vary across species, individuals, and disorders. Thus, understanding how areal distinctions in the properties and connectivity of projection neurons are generated is essential for discerning how larger cortical maps are formed. During the early stages of forebrain development, patterning centers and gradients of morphogens and signaling molecules, including BMP, WNT, and SHH, emerge. These gradients direct the graded expression of TFs in cortical progenitors to guide early regional and areal patterning of the cerebral cortex (Armentano et al. 2007; Bhaduri et al., 2021; Bishop et al. 2002; Borello et al. 2014; Cadwell et al. 2019; Cholfin and Rubenstein 2007; Fukuchi-Shimogori and Grove 2001; Kim et al. 2001; O'Leary et al. 2007; Rash and Grove 2011; Sur and Rubenstein 2005). In addition to these early gene expression gradients within cortical progenitors, distinct regional gradients and compartments of gene expression are present within the forming cortical plate, reflecting the prospective areal patterning across the fronto-temporal axis of the cortex (Bhaduri et al. 2021; Johnson et al. 2009; Kang et al. 2011; Lambert et al. 2011; Miller et al. 2014; Pletikos et al. 2014).

Interrogation of human and macaque transcriptomic data revealed that the genes encoding proteins involved in retinoic acid (RA) signaling or regulated by RA are enriched in the early and mid-fetal macaque and human frontal cortex (Johnson et al. 2009; Kang et al. 2011; Pletikos et al. 2014; Shibata et al. 2021a; Shibata et al. 2021b; Ziffra et al. 2021). Consistent with these findings, quantification of RA concentrations in the mid-fetal cortex identified a conserved, PFC-enriched, anterior-to-posterior gradient of RA that is more pronounced in the developing human cortex compared to the macaque or mouse cortices (Shibata et al. 2021a). Intriguingly, multiple risk genes linked to autism spectrum disorder, schizophrenia, and intellectual disability (ID) were among the genes upregulated in the mid-fetal human PFC (Shibata et al. 2021a; Willsey et al. 2013; Gulsuner et al. 2013). Deletion of the murine RA receptors, RARB and RXRG attenuates RA signaling in the developing mPFC and diminishes expression of other genes that also are enriched in the human and macaque mid-fetal frontal cortex and for encoding axon and synapse development (Shibata et al., 2021a). Furthermore, the majority of altered genes related to axon and synapse development showed the presence of RA receptor binding sites in their associated regulatory elements (promoters and enhancers); and genes with reduced expression in the *Rarb* and *Rxrg* were more likely to have at least one RA receptor binding site (For extended data see figure 5 in Shibata et al. 2019). This suggests that RA can directly regulate their expression in cortical neurons, as demonstrated for *Cbln2* (Shibata et al. 2021b). Consistent with these findings, treatment of primary human mid-fetal cortical neurons or human iPSC-derived cerebral organoids with RA or vitamin A (the precursor for RA synthesis) increased the expression of frontally enriched marker genes, *Cbln2*, *Meis2*, and *Auts2* (Shibata et al. 2021a; Ziffra et al. 2021) that also have been implicated in several neuropsychiatric disorders.

The establishment of the mid-fetal cortical RA gradient was proposed to be by a species-specific pattern involving expanded frontal expression of the RA-synthesizing enzymes, ALDH1A1 and ALDH1A3, compared to the mouse frontal cortex (Johnson et al. 2009; Ma et al. 2022; Shibata et al. 2021a; Wagner et al. 2002), and enrichment of the RA-degrading enzyme, CYP26B1, in the adjacent prospective motor and anterior insular cortices (Johnson et al. 2009; Larsen et al. 2019; Shibata et al. 2021a). Disruption of the RA signaling in the mPFC of neonatal *Rarb;Rxrg* double knockout mice at developmental stages equivalent to human mid-fetal development led to reduction of excitatory synapses in the rostral cortex and selective disruption of reciprocal connections between the MD-PFC. Alteration of this connectivity underlies risk for neuropsychiatric disorders including schizophrenia and autism spectrum disorder (Giraldo-Chica et al. 2018; Nair et al. 2015; Reay et al. 2020). In neonatal mice lacking *Cyp26b1*, RA signaling expands into the lateral frontal cortex and is associated with precocious and ectopic innervation of axons from the medial thalamus. Together, these findings show that RA signaling plays a critical role in the molecular patterning and connectivity of the PFC and, potentially, in its evolutionary expansion (see Wallace and Pollen 2021).

13.5 Human Specializations of Cortical Projection Neurons and their Circuitry

The human cerebral cortex contains approximately 16.3 billion neurons (Azevedo et al. 2009; Silbereis et al. 2016), 164 trillion synapses, and 160,000 km of white-matter myelinated axons (Pattabiraman et al. 2020; Silbereis et al. 2016), surpassing that of our closest living relative, the chimpanzee which has roughly 7.4 billion neurons (Collins et al. 2016). While the remarkable evolution of cellular, structural, and functional complexity of the human brain may be inseparable from our success in the world, the same features may also leave us susceptible to neurodevelopmental and neuropsychiatric disorders. Understanding how and why the brain has changed throughout evolution, and identifying such features that are human specific, may be a throughline to greater knowledge of our humanity and most challenging diseases.

This is especially true when considering the protracted development of the human cortex, its complex connectivity, and its refinement through experience-dependent mechanisms (Figure 13.2). Yet identifying human-specific molecular, cellular, developmental, and circuit features is particularly challenging experimentally. Many of the approaches used in standard biological research are not applicable to human studies due to ethical and legal limitations (Farahany et al. 2018). Thus, evaluation of comparative cortical expansion and language function across primates provides natural experiments with great insight.

Although humans do not have the largest brain or the greatest number of cortical neurons across animals (Sousa et al. 2017a), our cognitive abilities are remarkable. Compared with our closest primate relatives, the association areas of the frontal, parietal, and temporal cortices have expanded (Hill et al. 2010; Van Essen and Dierker 2007; Yeo et al. 2011) and are postulated to involve a more elaborate cortico-cortical connections in humans (Sherwood et al. 2012; Sousa et al. 2017a; van den Heuvel et al. 2019). The uniquely extensive development of language and speech abilities in humans also coincides with the elaboration of specialized perisylvian cortical areas and long-range connectivity (Figure 13.3) (Catani et al. 2005; Geschwind 1965).

Amongst cortical regions, anthropoid primates exhibit prominent lateral expansion of the prefrontal (PFC) and the parieto-temporal association areas that are thought to be important for higher order cognitive functions (Molnar et al. 2019). Although it is still unclear whether the human PFC falls within the expected size range for primates or is slightly disproportionately

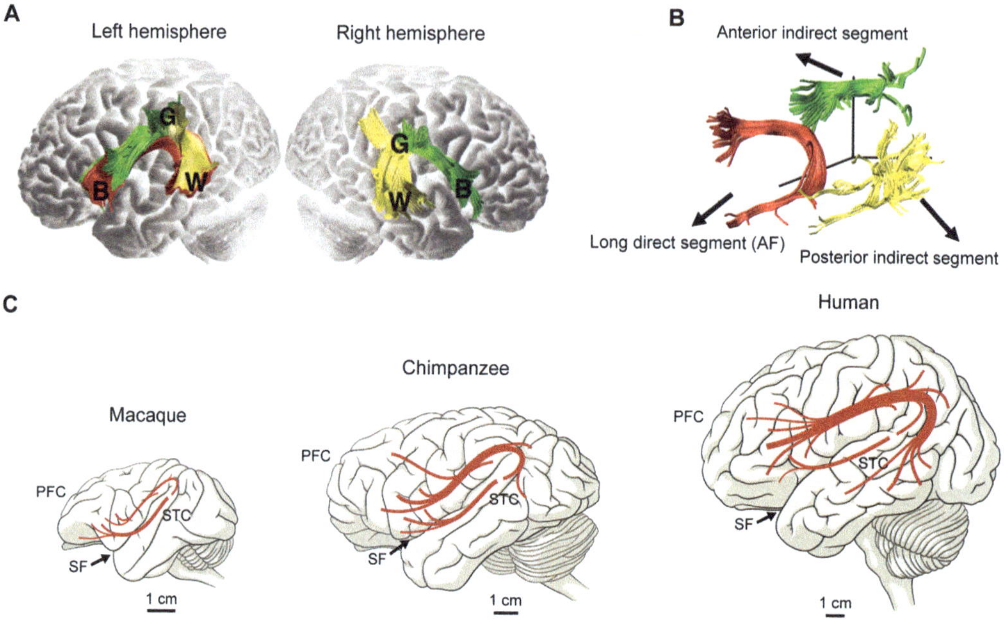

Figure 13.3 Language-related pathways in humans (A and B) Language-related pathways connecting Broca's – B, Geschwind's – G, and Wernicke's – W neocortical territories, reconstructed based on diffusion tensor imaging data. Both hemispheres share the long direct segment and the posterior indirect segments. (C) Comparison of arcuate fasciculus projections in humans and nonhuman primates. In humans, projections extend far into the medial and inferior temporal gyri, whereas projections to the chimpanzee temporal lobe are less extensive into the inferior temporal gyrus. In macaques, the projection into the inferior temporal gyrus appears to be completely absent. PFC, prefrontal cortex; SF, Sylvian fissure; STC, superior temporal cortex. Adapted from Sousa et al. (2017a).

larger, there are many features that are divergent compared to our closest living relatives, chimpanzees (Preuss and Wise 2022; Sherwood et al. 2012; Sousa et al. 2017a; Teffer and Semendeferi, 2012). A recent single cell transcriptomic analysis of the adult dlPFC in humans, chimpanzees, macaque, and marmosets, revealed that human PFC has 113 transcriptomically defined cell types: 40 glutamatergic excitatory neuron subtypes, 45 GABAergic inhibitory neuron, 13 glial, and 15 nonneural cell subtypes (Ma et al. 2022). Interestingly, at the cellular level, the human PFC has a lower neuronal density as well as increased spacing of mini-columns compared to nonhuman primates, which may be due to increased neuropil content and cortico-cortical connectivity (Elston 2003; Teffer and Semendeferi 2012). Pyramidal cells within the human PFC also display greater dendritic complexity and synaptic spine density as compared to the nonhuman primates (Elston 2003; Teffer and Semendeferi 2012).

Various comparative studies across species suggest that the overall number of neurons and glia follow the same isometric and allometric scaling as brain size and brain region size. This suggests that absolute cell number, like brain or region size, may be just one of several factors underlying human cognition and that our unique mental abilities may also be driven by more subtle brain characteristics. Since brain size or neuronal/glial cell numbers may not explain human cortical uniqueness, new studies are exploring the emergence of human-specific cell types, the molecular reorganization of conserved cell types, and the unique electrophysiological properties of these cells (Kanton et al. 2019; Muchnik et al. 2019; Pollen et al. 2019; Shibata et al. 2021a, 2021b; Zhu et al. 2018). For example, it has been observed that rare cortical GABAergic inhibitory interneurons exhibit human-specific switching between expression of the neuropeptide somatostatin (SST) and tyrosine hydroxylase (TH), the rate-limiting enzyme in dopamine production (Ma et al. 2022; Sousa et al. 2017b). These interneurons originate from the ganglionic eminences and were found to be depleted in Parkinson's disease or Lewy body dementia, suggesting an association with disease (Sousa et al. 2017b). Other studies have characterized the emergence of unique cell types in primates, for example, the TAC3-expressing striatal neuron (Krienen et al. 2020), which is expressed in primates but not rodents or ferrets, and the distinct "rosehip" neuron with unique morphology and physiological properties in humans (Boldog et al. 2018). Although there is evidence of these unique subtypes of microglia within the human cortex, most of the profiled cells in these studies have homologous cell types in other primates (Bakken et al. 2021; Franjic et al. 2022; Krienen et al. 2020; Ma et al. 2022; Zhu et al. 2018). The observed differences primarily lie in the expression levels of specific groups of genes within these homologous cell types, suggesting that even more nuanced changes besides cell number and cell type may drive the brain structure changes associated with human cognition.

In addition to the appearance of newer areas and cell types in humans, there are also human-specific genomic features (Dennis and Eichler 2016; Muchnik et al. 2019; Reilly and Noonan 2016; Whalen and Pollard 2022) that include gene duplications, deletions, indels, and mutations. For example, segmental duplications resulted in three human gene paralogs of the NOTCH2 receptor that are expressed in human fetal RGCs and oRGCs. Amongst the NOTCH2 gene paralogs, NOTCH2NLB is the essential clonal expansion of the progenitors in human and thus, underlie the increase in numbers of glutamatergic neurons seen in humans (Fiddes et al. 2018; Sousa et al. 2017a). Similarly, partial gene duplication of SRGAP2 has been implicated in human brain development. Over-expression of human paralog for SRGAP2 during mouse brain development led to the protraction of spinogenesis, mirroring that of human spinogenesis, resulting in increased spine density (Dennis et al. 2012). Another human-specific gene duplication is for the gene ARHGAP11B and is seen in chromosome 15q13.3, which is one of the most unstable loci associated with several developmental disorders. Ectopic expression of the human specific expression of ARHGAP11B, which was also present in Neanderthals and Denisovan, in the mouse and marmosets results in the expansion of the oRGC pool causing an increase in the number of upper layer neurons and the folding of the otherwise lissencephalic mouse and marmoset brain (Florio et al. 2015; Heide et al. 2020). Due to their human-specific evolution at the genomic level, along with their phenotypic characterization in mouse, SRGAP2 and ARHGAP11B likely play an important role in contributing to the differences in human brain development that occurred after the split of human and chimpanzees.

Another driver of phenotypic change is the genetic differences in protein-coding regions caused by missense mutation that result in amino acid substitutions and affect the functionality of the protein. Such genes are under positive selection pressure and are of special interest because they may regulate specific features of human brain development and functioning. For example, mutations in FOXP2 gene have been previously linked to speech and language disorders and two amino acid substitutions have been suggested to have occurred in the human FOXP2 after the divergence from the chimpanzee lineage, leading to speculation about its role in human evolution (Fisher et al. 2003). However, a recent study has found no evidence of recent adaptive evolution at the human FOXP2 (Atkinson et al. 2018). Another example is of the NOVA1 gene, which plays a regulatory role in neurodevelopment and functioning. NOVA1 undergoes amino acid substitution at the divergent point between the extant humans and the Neanderthal and Denisovan genomes. By reintroducing the archaic allele into human iPSCs and generating organoids, researchers identified alterations in the neurodevelopment and synaptic complexity that were reflected by changes in electrophysiological properties (Trujillo et al. 2021).

In addition to the differences in the coding domains, genetic variations in regulatory domains encompassing noncoding intergenic and intragenic regions, can also underlie the phenotypic differences between the extant humans and NHPs. Genome-wide association studies (GWAS) have revealed noncoding genetic domains that undergo human-specific substitutions that are otherwise conserved in other species, many of which are associated with neurodevelopmental and neuropsychiatric disorders also called as human accelerated regions (HARs) (Doan et al. 2016; Hubisz and Pollard 2014; Lindblad-Toh et al. 2011; Meyer et al. 2017; Prabhakar et al. 2006). The greatest density of HARs is observed within the intronic regions of the gene NPAS3, which has 14 HARs. Out of the 14, 11 act as transcriptional enhancers to drive the expression of NPAS3, as tested by *Lacz* expression in zebrafish (Kamm et al. 2013a; Kamm et al. 2013b). These HARs drive the expression of NPAS3 specifically in the anterior telencephalon (Kamm et al. 2013a; Kamm et al. 2013b). Many studies have identified the accelerated regions within the human genome and postulated the nearby gene regulation by these regions (Hubisz and Pollard 2014; Lindblad-Toh et al. 2011). Until recently, testing the gene regulation by these HARs was not feasible. However, the massive parallel reporter assay (MPRA) has made testing multiple accelerated regions possible. Ten thousand barcoded HARs can be expressed in iPSC-derived neurons from different species and the differential regulation by each of these HARs is quantified by performing RNA-seq and DNA-seq, which allows for evolutionary divergent points of regulatory elements and disease-associated copy number variants to be tested. Recently, 3100 HARs active during human neurodevelopment were tested using MPRA and a HAR, they underwent massive rearrangement, which was identified to regulate the expression of PPP1R17. PPP1R17 slowed the rate of progenitor cell division, matching that of nonhuman primates and humans (Girskis et al. 2021). Similar studies have helped to establish the enhancer landscape of human neurodevelopment and have identified the role of HARs as a key component in the rewiring of human-specific neurodevelopmental regulatory programs.

Overall, these data demonstrate that humans have changes in their genome, which may underlie an expanded and enhanced proliferative zone, a great diversity of neural stem cells and progenitor cells that facilitate brain expansion, and that ultimately lead to human-specific brain features and likely underly our remarkable cognitive abilities. As psychiatric and neurodevelopmental disorders are associated with alterations across specific brain circuits, cells, and genes, such studies can point to precisely timed and spatially specific mechanisms that may go awry and contribute to disease.

13.6 Human Neurodevelopmental and Neuropsychiatric Disorders

Understanding human-specific features of brain development has strong clinical relevance for identifying the molecular antecedents of neurodevelopmental and neuropsychiatric disorders. An important and often unappreciated feature of these disorders is their emergence early in life, hinting that environmental and genetic perturbations especially during early development are key to understanding their etiology (Figure 13.4). Most of these disorders are complex and polygenic, with multiple genes contributing to disease risk. This risk can be comprised of both common and rare variants, and similar genes may underly risk across different disorders. For example, a large GWAS study recently revealed pleotropic single nucleotide polymorphisms (SNPs) that explained 51 percent of the genetic variation across eight neuropsychiatric disorders and demonstrated that many of the identified SNPs overlap across disorders (Cross Disorder Group of the Psychiatric Genomics Consortium, J.W.S. 2019). Importantly, pleiotropic loci are found within genes playing prominent roles in neurodevelopmental processes and that show heightened expression in the brain beginning prenatally and continuing across the lifespan (Cross Disorder Group of the

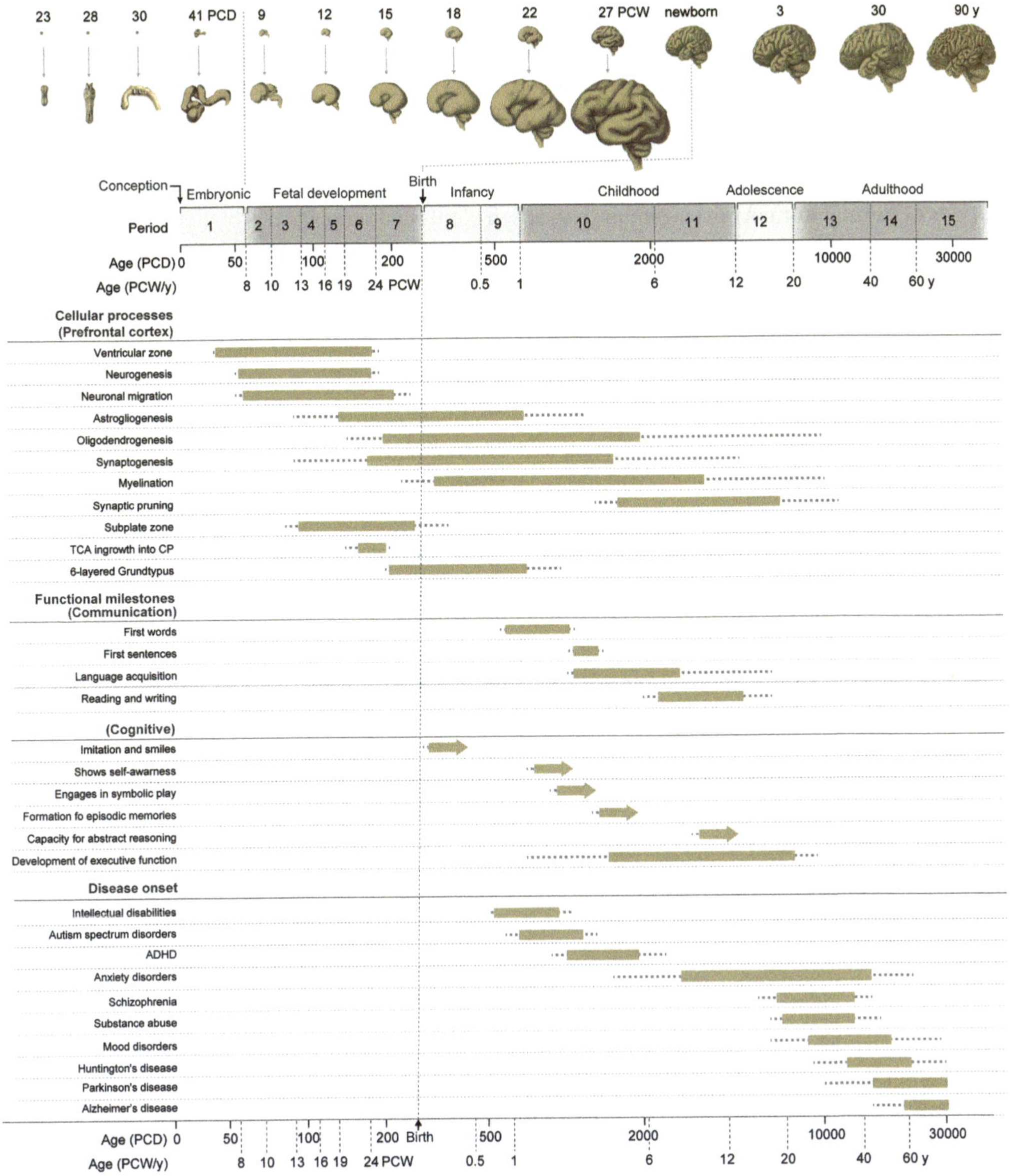

Figure 13.4 Timeline of key human neurodevelopmental processes, functional milestones, and neurological disorders. Illustrations in the top panel show the gross anatomical features of the developing and adult CNS, with prenatal brain features magnified. The second panel, which is duplicated at the bottom of the figure, provides a timeline of human development and the associated periods (Kang et al. 2011), and age in postconceptional days (PCD), postconceptional weeks (PCW), and postnatal years (y). The schematic below details the approximate timing and sequence of key cellular processes and developmental milestones. Bars indicate the peak developmental period in which each feature is acquired; dotted lines indicate that feature acquisition occurs at these ages, though to a relatively minor degree. In the lowest panel the bars indicate age range during which the neurodevelopmental and neuropsychiatric disorders manifest, with less-frequent ages of diagnosis denoted as dotted lines. Note that the age of diagnosis is highly variable between brain disorders. Many psychiatric disorders emerge in adolescence and early adulthood. This variability is indicative of dysregulation of tightly controlled developmental processes. Adapted from Kang et al. (2011); Lee et al. (2014); Silbereis et al. (2016).

Psychiatric Genomics Consortium, J.W.S. 2019). Similarly, more nuanced polygenic or multifactorial dysregulation of neurodevelopmental processes can confer risk for neuropsychiatric disease syndromes such as schizophrenia, depression, autism spectrum disorders, and others (Gleeson and Walsh 2000; Sullivan and Geschwind 2019; Weinberger 1995; Willsey et al. 2022). Therefore, studying neurotypical development will identify mechanisms that are important in mediating neurodevelopmental and neuropsychiatric diseases. In this section, we describe studies that focus on periods of normal human development that, when combined with studies on neurodevelopmental and psychiatric diseases, identify disease mechanisms in terms of specific genes, time periods, and brain regions where these mechanisms are likely to be important.

Fragile X syndrome (FXS) is an example of a neurodevelopmental disorder with a clear genetic link in which a mutation in a single gene (FMR1) causes a broad range of symptoms due to the loss of function of the RNA-binding protein FMRP during neurodevelopment. It causes ID, and often manifests with autistic-like features, anxiety, hyperactivity, aggression, attention deficits, and delays in speech and language development (Bagni and Greenough 2005). The FMRP protein is involved in mRNA localization, stability, and translation. As a result, when FMRP is lost, there are broad consequences impacting translation and gene expression. FMRP regulates the translation of the neuronal nitric oxide synthase 1 (NOS1) gene in the developing human neocortex. Although the mRNA for *Nos1* is widely expressed, the NOS1 protein is transiently translated by FMRP during early synaptogenesis within the human mid-fetal L5 projection neurons that are arranged into alternating columns in the primordium of the Broca's area and orofacial motor cortex (Kwan et al. 2012a).

In contrast to FXS, Down syndrome (DS) represents a neurodevelopmental disorder in which the source is from a large polygenic disruption, trisomy 21, which manifests with delayed growth, mild to moderate ID, and characteristic facial features. While its well established that trisomy 21 is the genetic cause of DS, the biological processes associated with trisomy 21 have only recently been discovered. Trisomy 21 causes widespread disruptions in gene expression and although it is not fatal, transcriptomic analysis of the developing frontal cortex and cerebellum with DS found that between 3–5 percent of genes across all chromosomes were dysregulated during development (Olmos-Serrano et al. 2016). Additionally, many genes were related to myelination and oligodendrocyte development. Further analysis of postmortem human DS brains revealed lower levels of myelination and associated decreases in conduction velocity during infancy and adolescence (Olmos-Serrano et al. 2016), suggesting that a possible pathway underlying DS is an early function of oligodendrocytes. This was especially prominent in the dlPFC, which undergoes late myelination and performs critical functions related to behavior and cognitive functions.

Autism spectrum disorder (ASD) is a one of the most studied neurodevelopmental disorders (An et al. 2018; Garcia-Forn et al. 2020; Tebbenkamp et al. 2014), yet its causes remain mysterious. ASD involves multiple brain regions and variable etiologies, making it difficult to implicate any specific brain region or cellular/molecular process (Carroll et al. 2021; Sestan and State 2018). ASD is a highly heritable disorder that typically manifests during early childhood at the age of one to three and is comorbid with many other neuropsychiatric disorders, like ID, attention-deficit hyperactivity disorder (ADHD), and other neurological disorders (Figure 13.4). It manifests with variable impairments in three main domains: reciprocal social interactions (verbal and nonverbal); communication; and restrictive, repetitive, and stereotyped patterns of behavior, interests, or activities (Carroll et al. 2021; Garcia-Forn et al. 2020).In recent years research involving genomic studies of healthy and ASD postmortem brain, cell-lines, and animal models systems have investigated genetic and biological processes underlying ASD (Cotney et al. 2015; D'Gama and Walsh 2018; Garcia-Forn et al. 2020; Jin et al. 2020; Kelley and Pasca 2022; Paulsen et al. 2022; Sestan and State 2018; State and Sestan 2012; Tebbenkamp et al. 2014; Walsh et al. 2008).

Postmortem molecular, cellular, and genetic evidence shows that ASD-specific genetic disruptions converge upon features of prenatal neurodevelopment and affect multiple stages and processes involving one or more genetic variants or somatic mutations in subsets of patients (Courchesne et al. 2020; Garcia-Forn et al. 2020; Li et al. 2018; Tebbenkamp et al. 2014; Werling et al. 2020). These studies revealed that there are excess neurons in the cerebral cortex of autistic brain (30% more), with the PFC (67% more) and von Economo neurons (57% more) leading these numbers (Santos et al. 2011). High throughput genomic studies involving ever-increasing sample size have now proposed more than 100 genes to be strongly implicated as a risk factor for ASD, with 63 genes designated as "high-risk" variants (https://gene.sfari.org/database/gene-scoring). Since most neurons are born within the first and second trimester, genetic risk variants involving neurodevelopmental processes of cell division, cell-type specification, and DNA damage repair fall in the first risk category of genes associated with ASD. This group contain ASD risk genes broadly clustered into the category of gene expression regulators, and especially chromatin modifiers, transcription factors, and proteins assisting with RNA and protein expression (Courchesne et al. 2020; Parikshak et al. 2013; Werling et al. 2020; Willsey et al. 2013). Disruption of neurodevelopment during the third trimester involves genetic risk variants involving neuronal migration and related functions, and their disruption causes multifocal cerebral dysplasia due to dysregulated axon elongation, migration, and maturation of neurons. These neurons have reduced dendritic arbors and smaller axons. Thus, this category genes that are heavily implicated in ASD are axon guidance and synapse associated proteins that modulate the electrophysiological properties of neurons (Courchesne et al. 2019, 2020; Parikshak et al. 2013; Willsey et al. 2013). Future studies on ASD should focus on connecting the insights from genes to molecular mechanisms, neural circuits, behavior, and therapeutics.

Other recent studies utilizing ASD subject-derived iPSC cells may provide insights into the prenatal origins of ASD (Carroll et al. 2021). Compared to the control brains, ASD iPSC-derived neuronal cultures displayed increased rates of proliferation, shorter G1/S phase transitions, impaired differentiation, abnormal excitatory/inhibitory neuronal ratio, and reduced neuronal maturation with reduced dendrites and axons, leading to reduced neuronal activity (Amiri et al. 2018; Garcia-Forn et al. 2020; Jin et al. 2020; Mariani et al. 2015; Paulsen et al. 2022). Further, using CRISPR-Cas9 technology, in vitro iPSC cell-based models can be generated that carry proposed ASD-related mutations. These iPSC cells are used to generate 3D-cerebral organoids that partially mimic human cortical neurodevelopmental processes (Kanton et al. 2019; Mariani et al. 2015; Paulsen et al. 2022; Uzquiano and Arlotta 2022). Mutant organoids carrying ASD-related mutations then can be used to characterize and compare cellular and molecular features observed in ASD cells or tissues directly (Amiri et al. 2018; Garcia-Forn et al. 2020; Jin et al. 2020; Mariani et al. 2015; Paulsen et al. 2022). However, the cell-based models used cannot determine the effect of the axon guidance cue disruptions, circuit-based alterations, and other substrate- or system-level dysfunction seen in ASD.

Some neurodevelopmental disorders arise during prenatal or early postnatal stages; however, other neuropsychiatric disorders like schizophrenia, anxiety, depression, and substance abuse disorder emerge during early childhood through adolescence (Lee et al. 2014; Sestan and State 2018; Silbereis et al. 2016). Although it is unclear how early prenatal development underlies these disorders, a hypothesis increasingly gaining traction outlines a sequence that pathogenesis includes a strong genetic component, emerges postnatally, and is more likely to arise under certain environmental conditions (Lee et al. 2014). Schizophrenia is one such debilitating disorder. Schizophrenia often emerges during adolescence and is characterized by positive symptoms like delusions, hallucinations, disorganized speech, and disorganized or catatonic behavior, and by negative symptoms that include affective flattening, avolition, alogia, or diminished vocal/emotional expression, and an absence/paucity of thoughts leading to significant cognitive impairment. The heritability of schizophrenia may be as high as 60–80 percent, which would suggest a very strong genetic contribution for such a multifactorial, polygenic syndrome (Trubetskoy et al. 2022). Although the genetic component of schizophrenia is not as extensively studied as ASD, a recent GWAS estimated that at least 108 genetic loci are associated with schizophrenia (Schizophrenia Working Group of the Psychiatric Genomics, C 2014), many of which are associated with synapse properties, cell migration, and development (Selemon and Zecevic 2015). This pattern is noteworthy, since schizophrenia symptoms often appear during adolescence, when the cortex (and especially the PFC) matures and when synapses are being pruned and refined. In normative brain development, the number of synapses peak before puberty, and then are trimmed and strengthened, allowing for the refinement of brain connectivity (Trubetskoy et al. 2022). Individuals with schizophrenia often present with reduced gray matter within the medial, lateral, and inferior PFC, superior temporal gyrus, and parietal cortex. Postmortem studies show evidence of reduced spine density on PFC excitatory neurons (Sakurai and Gamo 2019; Selemon et al. 2003), suggesting that synaptic pruning mechanisms maybe overactive in these patients and may contribute to the decrease in gray matter volume. Another area with significant alterations in connectivity in schizophrenia is the thalamus. Normally, dorso-medial thalamic nuclei form reciprocal connections with the dlPFC, and alterations in this circuitry may be implicated in schizophrenia (Giraldo-Chica et al. 2018; Tan et al. 2007). However, in this relationship and others, the causal vs. consequential pattern remains difficult to determine.

Like schizophrenia, other neuropsychiatric disorders such as anxiety, depression, and posttraumatic stress disorder often emerge during late childhood and adolescence (Paus et al. 2008). Multiple experimental modalities suggest that these disorders have a shared neural circuit that includes cortical regions like the insula and PFC, as well as cortex-like regions such as the amygdala (Etkin and Wager 2007; Fox et al. 2015; Gogtay et al. 2004; Goodkind et al. 2015; Meyer and Lee 2019; Villard et al. 2021; Zhu et al. 2018). These disorders are strongly to moderately heritable, with estimates ranging from 20–49 percent (Polderman et al. 2015; Purves et al. 2020; Sullivan et al. 2000), pointing to a substantial genetic contribution to their pathoetiology. More specifically, studies have found that these disorders are highly polygenic, with many common genetic variants of small effect sizes contributing to the emergence of these disorders (Martin et al. 2019). Large-scale GWAS studies have identified several common variants associated with depression, anxiety, posttraumatic stress disorder, and bipolar disorder. Of the genes identified, MAD1L1 may be especially notable due to its presumed function and timing of expression. As a regulator of cell cycling that may have human-specific features, MAD1L1 may be an important gene to study in normative brain development with respect to timing, broad activity, or specification in certain cell populations.

13.7 Conclusions

High-throughput functional genomic studies have helped to elucidate the molecular and cellular networks active during neurodevelopment, and especially those that are most elaborated in primates and humans or that may be associated with neuropsychiatric disorders. However, more work is needed to understand the mechanisms behind how brain regions take shape during development, how genetic and somatic variations cause disease, why certain therapeutic approaches fail to work, and even what features make us uniquely human. To accomplish this, alternative models that can elucidate functions of human-specific sequence variants and gene expression differences observed in neurodevelopmental disorders are still needed, as are ways to model human-specific regions and neuronal circuits. These goals can be achieved by employing methodologies for better and faster tissue procurement, addressing the ethical concerns related to work on human and nonhuman primate specimens, and by developing better in vitro model systems.

Acknowledgments

We would like to acknowledge Dr Marcel Oberlander for providing us with the file to adapt the figure from their manuscript that we have used in Figure 13.1. We would like to acknowledge colleagues in laboratories for their useful inputs and discussions. We apologize to all colleagues whose relevant studies were not cited because of space limitations, the broad scope of this review, and the emphasis on recent studies. Work in our laboratory was supported by grants from the National Institutes of Health and the Simons Foundation.

References

Alcamo, E.A. et al. (2008). Satb2 regulates callosal projection neuron identity in the developing cerebral cortex. *Neuron* 57: 364–377. doi: 10.1016/j.neuron.2007.12.012.

Amiri, A. et al. (2018). Transcriptome and epigenome landscape of human cortical development modeled in organoids. *Science* 362: eaat6720. doi: 10.1126/science.aat6720.

An, J.Y. et al. (2018). Genome-wide de novo risk score implicates promoter variation in autism spectrum disorder. *Science* 362: eaat6576. doi: 10.1126/science.aat6576.

Arion, D. et al. (2007). Molecular markers distinguishing supragranular and infragranular layers in the human prefrontal cortex. *Eur J Neurosci* 25 (6): 1843–1854. doi: 10.1111/j.1460-9568.2007.05396.x.

Armentano, M. et al. (2007). COUP-TFI regulates the balance of cortical patterning between frontal/motor and sensory areas. *Nat Neurosci* 10 (10): 1277–1286. doi: 10.1038/nn1958.

Atkinson, E.G. et al. (2018). No evidence for recent selection at FOXP2 among diverse human populations. *Cell* 174 (6): 1424–1435 e1415. doi: 10.1016/j.cell.2018.06.048.

Azevedo, F.A. et al. (2009). Equal numbers of neuronal and nonneuronal cells make the human brain an isometrically scaled-up primate brain. *J Comp Neurol* 513: 532–541. doi: 10.1002/cne.21974.

Bagni, C. and Greenough, W.T. (2005). From mRNP trafficking to spine dysmorphogenesis. *Nat Rev Neurosci* 6: 376–387. doi: 10.1038/nrn1667.

Bakken, T.E. et al. (2021). Comparative cellular analysis of motor cortex in human, marmoset and mouse. *Nature* 598: 111–119. doi: 10.1038/s41586-021-03465-8.

Bhaduri, A. et al. (2021). An atlas of cortical arealization identifies dynamic molecular signatures. *Nature* 598 (7879): 200–204. doi: 10.1038/s41586-021-03910-8.

Bishop, K.M. et al. (2002). Distinct actions of Emx1, Emx2, and Pax6 in regulating the specification of areas in the developing neocortex. *J Neurosci* 22: 7627–7638.

Boldog, E. et al. (2018). Transcriptomic and morphophysiological evidence for a specialized human cortical GABAergic cell type. *Nat Neurosci* 21: 1185–1195. doi: 10.1038/s41593-018-0205-2.

Borello, U. et al. (2014). Sp8 and COUP-TF1 reciprocally regulate patterning and Fgf signaling in cortical progenitors. *Cereb Cortex* 24: 1409–1421. doi: 10.1093/cercor/bhs412.

Breunig, J.J. et al. (2011). Neural stem cells. *Neuron* 70: 614–625. doi: 10.1016/j.neuron.2011.05.005.

Britanova, O. et al. (2008). Satb2 is a postmitotic determinant for upper-layer neuron specification in the neocortex. *Neuron* 57: 378–392. doi: 10.1016/j.neuron.2007.12.028.

Cadwell, C.R. et al. (2019). Development and arealization of the cerebral cortex. *Neuron* 103: 980–1004. doi: 10.1016/j.neuron.2019.07.009.

Carroll, L. et al. (2021). Autism spectrum disorders. *Neuroscientist* 27: 10–29. doi: 10.1177/1073858420921378.

Catani, M. et al. (2005). Perisylvian language networks of the human brain. *Ann Neurol* 57: 8–16. doi: 10.1002/ana.20319.

Chen, B. et al. (2005a). Fezl regulates the differentiation and axon targeting of layer 5 subcortical projection neurons in cerebral cortex. *Proc Natl Acad Sci USA* 102: 17184–17189. doi: 10.1073/pnas.0508732102.

Chen, J.G. et al. (2005b). Zfp312 is required for subcortical axonal projections and dendritic morphology of deep-layer pyramidal neurons of the cerebral cortex. *Proc Natl Acad Sci USA* 102: 17792–17797. doi: 10.1073/pnas.0509032102.

Cholfin, J.A. and Rubenstein, J.L. (2007). Patterning of frontal cortex subdivisions by Fgf17. *Proc Natl Acad Sci USA* 104: 7652–7657. doi: 10.1073/pnas.0702225104.

Collins, C.E. et al. (2016). Cortical cell and neuron density estimates in one chimpanzee hemisphere. *Proc Natl Acad Sci USA* 113: 740–745. doi: 10.1073/pnas.1524208113.

Cotney, J. et al. (2015). The autism-associated chromatin modifier CHD8 regulates other autism risk genes during human neurodevelopment. *Nat Commun* 6: 6404. doi: 10.1038/ncomms7404.

Courchesne, E. et al. (2020). Prenatal origins of ASD. *Trends Neurosci* 43: 326–342. doi: 10.1016/j.tins.2020.03.005.

Courchesne, E. et al. (2019). The ASD living biology. *Mol Psychiatry* 24: 88–107. doi: 10.1038/s41380-018-0056-y.

Cross Disorder Group of the Psychiatric Genomics Consortium, J.W.S. (2019). Genomic relationships, novel loci, and pleiotropic mechanisms across eight psychiatric disorders. *Cell* 179: 1469–1482 e1411. doi: 10.1016/j.cell.2019.11.020.

Cubelos, B. et al. (2010). Cux1 and Cux2 regulate dendritic branching, spine morphology, and synapses of the upper layer neurons of the cortex. *Neuron* 66 (4): 523–535. doi: 10.1016/j.neuron.2010.04.038.

D'Gama, A.M. and Walsh, C.A. (2018). Somatic mosaicism and neurodevelopmental disease. *Nat Neurosci* 21: 1504–1514. doi: 10.1038/s41593-018-0257-3.

DeFelipe, J. et al. (2013). New insights into the classification and nomenclature of cortical GABAergic interneurons. *Nat Rev Neurosci* 14: 202–216. doi: 10.1038/nrn3444.

Dennis, M.Y. and Eichler, E.E. (2016). Human adaptation and evolution by segmental duplication. *Curr Opin Genet Dev* 41: 44–52. doi: 10.1016/j.gde.2016.08.001.

Dennis, M.Y. et al. (2012). Evolution of human-specific neural SRGAP2 genes by incomplete segmental duplication. *Cell* 149: 912–922. doi: 10.1016/j.cell.2012.03.033.

Doan, R.N. et al. (2016). Mutations in human accelerated regions disrupt cognition and social behavior. *Cell* 167: 341–354 e312. doi: 10.1016/j.cell.2016.08.071.

Elston, G.N. (2003). Cortex, cognition and the cell: new insights into the pyramidal neuron and prefrontal function. *Cereb Cortex* 13: 1124–1138. doi: 10.1093/cercor/bhg093.

Etkin, A. and Wager, T.D. (2007). Functional neuroimaging of anxiety: a meta-analysis of emotional processing in PTSD, social anxiety disorder, and specific phobia. *Am J Psych* 164: 1476–1488. doi: 10.1176/appi.ajp.2007.07030504.

Farahany, N.A. et al. (2018). The ethics of experimenting with human brain tissue. *Nature* 556: 429–432. doi: 10.1038/d41586-018-04813-x.

Fazel Darbandi, S. et al. (2018). Neonatal Tbr1 dosage controls cortical layer 6 connectivity. *Neuron* 100 (4): 831–845.e7. doi: 10.1016/j.neuron.2018.09.027.

Fiddes, I.T. et al. (2018). Human-specific NOTCH2NL genes affect notch signaling and cortical neurogenesis. *Cell* 173: 1356–1369 e1322. doi: 10.1016/j.cell.2018.03.051.

Fisher, S.E. et al. (2003). Deciphering the genetic basis of speech and language disorders. *Ann Rev Neurosci* 26: 57–80. doi: 10.1146/annurev.neuro.26.041002.131144.

Florio, M. et al. (2015). Human-specific gene ARHGAP11B promotes basal progenitor amplification and neocortex expansion. *Science* 347: 1465–1470. doi: 10.1126/science.aaa1975.

Fox, A.S. et al. (2015). Intergenerational neural mediators of early-life anxious temperament. *Proc Natl Acad Sci USA* 112: 9118–9122. doi: 10.1073/pnas.1508593112.

Franjic, D. et al. (2022). Transcriptomic taxonomy and neurogenic trajectories of adult human, macaque, and pig hippocampal and entorhinal cells. *Neuron* 110: 452–469 e414. doi: 10.1016/j.neuron.2021.10.036.

Fukuchi-Shimogori, T. and Grove, E.A. (2001). Neocortex patterning by the secreted signaling molecule FGF8. *Science* 294: 1071–1074. doi: 10.1126/science.1064252.

Garcia-Forn, M. et al. (2020). Linking autism risk genes to disruption of cortical development. *Cells* 9: 2500. doi: 10.3390/cells9112500.

Geschwind, N. (1965). Disconnexion syndromes in animals and man. II. *Brain* 88: 585–644. doi: 10.1093/brain/88.3.585.

Giraldo-Chica, M. et al. (2018). Prefrontal-thalamic anatomical connectivity and executive cognitive function in schizophrenia. *Biol Psych* 83: 509–517. doi: 10.1016/j.biopsych.2017.09.022.

Girskis, K.M. et al. (2021). Rewiring of human neurodevelopmental gene regulatory programs by human accelerated regions. *Neuron* 109: 3239–3251 e3237. doi: 10.1016/j.neuron.2021.08.005.

Gleeson, J.G. and Walsh, C.A. (2000). Neuronal migration disorders: from genetic diseases to developmental mechanisms. *Trends Neurosci* 23: 352–359. doi: 10.1016/s0166-2236(00)01607-6.

Gogtay, N. et al. (2004). Dynamic mapping of human cortical development during childhood through early adulthood. *Proc Natl Acad Sci USA* 101: 8174–8179. doi: 10.1073/pnas.0402680101.

Goodkind, M. et al. (2015). Identification of a common neurobiological substrate for mental illness. *JAMA Psych* 72: 305–315. doi: 10.1001/jamapsychiatry.2014.2206.

Gray, P.A. et al. (2004). Mouse brain organization revealed through direct genome-scale TF expression analysis. *Science* 306: 2255–2257. doi: 10.1126/science.1104935.

Gulsuner, S. et al. (2013). Spatial and temporal mapping of de novo mutations in schizophrenia to a fetal prefrontal cortical network. *Cell* 154 (3): 518–529. doi: 10.1016/j.cell.2013.06.049.

Han, W. et al. (2011). TBR1 directly represses Fezf2 to control the laminar origin and development of the corticospinal tract. *Proc Natl Acad Sci USA* 108: 3041–3046. doi: 10.1073/pnas.1016723108.

Heide, M. et al. (2020). Human-specific ARHGAP11B increases size and folding of primate neocortex in the fetal marmoset. *Science* 369: 546–550. doi: 10.1126/science.abb2401.

Hevner, R.F. et al. (2001). Tbr1 regulates differentiation of the preplate and layer 6. *Neuron* 29: 353–366. doi: 10.1016/s0896-6273(01)00211-2.

Hill, J. et al. (2010). Similar patterns of cortical expansion during human development and evolution. *Proc Natl Acad Sci USA* 107: 13135–13140. doi: 10.1073/pnas.1001229107.

Hirata, T. et al. (2004). Zinc finger gene fez-like functions in the formation of subplate neurons and thalamocortical axons. *Dev Dyn* 230: 546–556. doi: 10.1002/dvdy.20068.

Hoerder-Suabedissen, A. and Molnar, Z. (2015). Development, evolution and pathology of neocortical subplate neurons. *Nat Rev Neurosci* 16: 133–146. doi: 10.1038/nrn3915.

Hu, J.S. et al. (2017). Cortical interneuron development. *Development* 144: 3867–3878. doi: 10.1242/dev.132852.

Hubisz, M.J. and Pollard, K.S. (2014). Exploring the genesis and functions of Human Accelerated Regions sheds light on their role in human evolution. *Curr Opin Genet Dev* 29: 15–21. doi: 10.1016/j.gde.2014.07.005.

Inoue, K. et al. (2004). Fezl is layer-specifically expressed in the adult mouse neocortex. *Eur J Neurosci* 20: 2909–2916. doi: 10.1111/j.1460-9568.2004.03763.x.

Jin, X. et al. (2020). In vivo Perturb-Seq reveals neuronal and glial abnormalities associated with autism risk genes. *Science* 370 (6520): eaaz6063. doi: 10.1126/science.aaz6063.

Johnson, M.B. et al. (2009). Functional and evolutionary insights into human brain development through global transcriptome analysis. *Neuron* 62 (4): 494–509. doi: 10.1016/j.neuron.2009.03.027.

Juric-Sekhar, G. and Hevner, R.F. (2019). Malformations of cerebral cortex development. *Ann Rev Pathol* 14: 293–318. doi: 10.1146/annurev-pathmechdis-012418-012927.

Kaas, J.H. (2019). The origin and evolution of neocortex. *Prog Brain Res* 250: 61–81. doi: 10.1016/bs.pbr.2019.03.017.

Kamm, G.B. et al. (2013a). A fast-evolving human NPAS3 enhancer gained reporter expression in the developing forebrain of transgenic mice. *Philos Trans Royal Soc London. Series B, Biol Sci* 368: 20130019. doi: 10.1098/rstb.2013.0019.

Kamm, G.B. et al. (2013b). The developmental brain gene NPAS3 contains the largest number of accelerated regulatory sequences in the human genome. *Mol Biol Evol* 30: 1088–1102. doi: 10.1093/molbev/mst023.

Kang, H.J. et al. (2011). Spatio-temporal transcriptome of the human brain. *Nature* 478 (7370): 483–489. doi: 10.1038/nature10523.

Kanton, S. et al. (2019). Organoid single-cell genomic atlas uncovers human-specific features of brain development. *Nature* 574: 418–422. doi: 10.1038/s41586-019-1654-9.

Kaur, N. et al. (2020). Neural stem cells direct axon guidance via their radial fiber scaffold. *Neuron* 107: 1197–1211 e1199. doi: 10.1016/j.neuron.2020.06.035.

Kelley, K.W. and Pasca, S.P. (2022). Human brain organogenesis. *Cell* 185: 42–61. doi: 10.1016/j.cell.2021.10.003.

Kim, A.S. et al. (2001). Pax-6 regulates expression of SFRP-2 and Wnt-7b in the developing CNS. *J Neurosci* 21: RC132.

Kostovic, I. et al. (2019). Sublaminar organization of the human subplate. *J Anat* 235: 481–506. doi: 10.1111/joa.12920.

Kostovic, I. and Rakic, P. (1980). Cytology and time of origin of interstitial neurons in the white matter in infant and adult human and monkey telencephalon. *J Neurocytol* 9: 219–242. doi: 10.1007/BF01205159.

Kriegstein, A. and Alvarez-Buylla, A. (2009). The glial nature of embryonic and adult neural stem cells. *Ann Rev Neurosci* 32: 149–184. doi: 10.1146/annurev.neuro.051508.135600.

Krienen, F.M. et al. (2020). Innovations present in the primate interneuron repertoire. *Nature* 586: 262–269. doi: 10.1038/s41586-020-2781-z.

Kumamoto, T. and Hanashima, C. (2014). Neuronal subtype specification in establishing mammalian neocortical circuits. *Neurosci Res* 86: 37–49. doi: 10.1016/j.neures.2014.07.002.

Kwan, K.Y. et al. (2012a). Species-dependent posttranscriptional regulation of NOS1 by FMRP in the developing cerebral cortex. *Cell* 149: 899–911. doi: 10.1016/j.cell.2012.02.060.

Kwan, K.Y. et al. (2008). SOX5 postmitotically regulates migration, postmigratory differentiation, and projections of subplate and deep-layer neocortical neurons. *Proc Natl Acad Sci USA* 105: 16021–16026. doi: 10.1073/pnas.0806791105.

Kwan, K.Y. et al. (2012b). Transcriptional co-regulation of neuronal migration and laminar identity in the neocortex. *Development* 139: 1535–1546. doi: 10.1242/dev.069963.

Lai, T. et al. (2008). SOX5 controls the sequential generation of distinct corticofugal neuron subtypes. *Neuron* 57: 232–247. doi: 10.1016/j.neuron.2007.12.023.

Lambert, N. et al. (2011). Genes expressed in specific areas of the human fetal cerebral cortex display distinct patterns of evolution. *PLoS One* 6 (3): e17753. doi: 10.1371/journal.pone.0017753.

Larsen, R. et al. (2019). The thalamus regulates retinoic acid signaling and development of parvalbumin interneurons in postnatal mouse prefrontal cortex. *eNeuro* 6 (1): ENEURO.0018-19.2019. doi: 10.1523/ENEURO.0018-19.2019.

Lee, F.S. et al. (2014). Mental health. Adolescent mental health – opportunity and obligation. *Science* 346: 547–549. doi: 10.1126/science.1260497.

Leone, D.P. et al. (2015). Satb2 regulates the differentiation of both callosal and subcerebral projection neurons in the developing cerebral cortex. *Cereb Cortex* 25 (10): 3406–3419. doi: 10.1093/cercor/bhu156.

Leone, D.P. et al. (2008). The determination of projection neuron identity in the developing cerebral cortex. *Curr Opin Neurobiol* 18: 28–35. doi: 10.1016/j.conb.2008.05.006.

Li, M. et al. (2018). Integrative functional genomic analysis of human brain development and neuropsychiatric risks. *Science* 362 (6420): eaat7615. doi: 10.1126/science.aat7615.

Li, N. et al. (2010). The transcription factor Cux1 regulates dendritic morphology of cortical pyramidal neurons. *PLoS One* 5: e10596. doi: 10.1371/journal.pone.0010596.

Lindblad-Toh, K. et al. (2011). A high-resolution map of human evolutionary constraint using 29 mammals. *Nature* 478: 476–482. doi: 10.1038/nature10530.

Lindwall, C. et al. (2007). Commissure formation in the mammalian forebrain. *Curr Opin Neurobiol* 17 (1): 3–14. doi: 10.1016/j.conb.2007.01.008.

Lui, J.H. et al. (2011). Development and evolution of the human neocortex. *Cell* 146: 18–36. doi: 10.1016/j.cell.2011.06.030.

Ma, S. et al. (2022). Molecular and cellular evolution of the primate dorsolateral prefrontal cortex. *Science* 377 (6614): eabo7257. doi: 10.1126/science.abo7257.

Mariani, J. et al. (2015). FOXG1-dependent dysregulation of GABA/glutamate neuron differentiation in autism spectrum disorders. *Cell* 162: 375–390. doi: 10.1016/j.cell.2015.06.034.

Marin, O. et al. (2002). Patterning of the basal telencephalon and hypothalamus is essential for guidance of cortical projections. *Development* 129: 761–773. doi: 10.1242/dev.129.3.761.

Markenscoff-Papadimitriou, E. et al. (2020). A chromatin accessibility atlas of the developing human telencephalon. *Cell* 182: 754–769 e718. doi: 10.1016/j.cell.2020.06.002.

Martin, A.R. et al. (2019). Predicting polygenic risk of psychiatric disorders. *Biol Psych* 86: 97–109. doi: 10.1016/j.biopsych.2018.12.015.

McConnell, S.K. et al. (1994). Subplate pioneers and the formation of descending connections from cerebral cortex. *J Neurosci* 14: 1892–1907.

McEvilly, R.J. et al. (2002). Transcriptional regulation of cortical neuron migration by POU domain factors. *Science* 295 (5559): 1528–1532. doi: 10.1126/science.1067132.

McKenna, W.L. et al. (2011). Tbr1 and Fezf2 regulate alternate corticofugal neuronal identities during neocortical development. *J Neurosci* 31: 549–564. doi: 10.1523/JNEUROSCI.4131-10.2011.

Meyer, H.C. and Lee, F.S. (2019). Translating developmental neuroscience to understand risk for psychiatric disorders. *Am J Psych* 176: 179–185. doi: 10.1176/appi.ajp.2019.19010091.

Meyer, K.A. et al. (2017). Differential gene expression in the human brain is associated with conserved, but not accelerated, noncoding sequences. *Mol Biol Evol* 34: 1217–1229. doi: 10.1093/molbev/msx076.

Mi, D. et al. (2018). Early emergence of cortical interneuron diversity in the mouse embryo. *Science* 360: 81–85. doi: 10.1126/science.aar6821.

Miller, D.J. et al. (2019). Shared and derived features of cellular diversity in the human cerebral cortex. *Curr Opin Neurobiol* 56: 117–124. doi: 10.1016/j.conb.2018.12.005.

Miller, J.A. et al. (2014). Transcriptional landscape of the prenatal human brain. *Nature* 508 (7495): 199–206. doi: 10.1038/nature13185.

Molnar, Z. et al. (2019). New insights into the development of the human cerebral cortex. *J Anat* 235: 432–451. doi: 10.1111/joa.13055.

Molyneaux, B.J. et al. (2009). Novel subtype-specific genes identify distinct subpopulations of callosal projection neurons. *J Neurosci* 29: 12343–12354. doi: 10.1523/JNEUROSCI.6108-08.2009.

Molyneaux, B.J. et al. (2005). Fezl is required for the birth and specification of corticospinal motor neurons. *Neuron* 47: 817–831. doi: 10.1016/j.neuron.2005.08.030.

Molyneaux, B.J. et al. (2007). Neuronal subtype specification in the cerebral cortex. *Nat Rev Neurosci* 8: 427–437. doi: 10.1038/nrn2151.

Muchnik, S.K. et al. (2019). Modeling the evolution of human brain development using organoids. *Cell* 179: 1250–1253. doi: 10.1016/j.cell.2019.10.041.

Nair, A. et al. (2015). Regional specificity of aberrant thalamocortical connectivity in autism. *Hum Brain Mapp* 36: 4497–4511. doi: 10.1002/hbm.22938.

Nieto, M. et al. (2004). Expression of Cux-1 and Cux-2 in the subventricular zone and upper layers II-IV of the cerebral cortex. *J Comp Neurol* 479 (2): 168–180. doi: 10.1002/cne.20322.

Nimchinsky, E.A. et al. (1999). A neuronal morphologic type unique to humans and great apes. *Proc Natl Acad Sci USA* 96: 5268–5273. doi: 10.1073/pnas.96.9.5268.

O'Leary, D.D. et al. (2007). Area patterning of the mammalian cortex. *Neuron* 56: 252–269. doi: 10.1016/j.neuron.2007.10.010.

Oberlaender, M. et al. (2012). Cell type-specific three-dimensional structure of thalamocortical circuits in a column of rat vibrissal cortex. *Cereb Cortex* 22: 2375–2391. doi: 10.1093/cercor/bhr317.

Oishi, K. et al. (2016). Mutually repressive interaction between Brn1/2 and Rorb contributes to the establishment of neocortical layer 2/3 and layer 4. *Proc Natl Acad Sci USA* 113 (12): 3371–3376. doi: 10.1073/pnas.1515949113.

Olmos-Serrano, J.L. et al. (2016). Down syndrome developmental brain transcriptome reveals defective oligodendrocyte differentiation and myelination. *Neuron* 89: 1208–1222. doi: 10.1016/j.neuron.2016.01.042.

Oswald, M.J. et al. (2013). Diversity of layer 5 projection neurons in the mouse motor cortex. *Front Cell Neurosci* 7: 174. doi: 10.3389/fncel.2013.00174.

Parikshak, N.N. et al. (2013). Integrative functional genomic analyses implicate specific molecular pathways and circuits in autism. *Cell* 155: 1008–1021. doi: 10.1016/j.cell.2013.10.031.

Pattabiraman, K. et al. (2014). Transcriptional regulation of enhancers active in protodomains of the developing cerebral cortex. *Neuron* 82: 989–1003. doi: 10.1016/j.neuron.2014.04.014.

Pattabiraman, K. et al. (2020). The evolution of the human brain and disease susceptibility. *Curr Opin Genet Dev* 65: 91–97. doi: 10.1016/j.gde.2020.05.004.

Paulsen, B. et al. (2022). Autism genes converge on asynchronous development of shared neuron classes. *Nature* 602: 268–273. doi: 10.1038/s41586-021-04358-6.

Paus, T. et al. (2008). Why do many psychiatric disorders emerge during adolescence? *Nat Rev Neurosci* 9: 947–957. doi: 10.1038/nrn2513.

Pletikos, M. et al. (2014). Temporal specification and bilaterality of human neocortical topographic gene expression. *Neuron* 81 (2): 321–332. doi: 10.1016/j.neuron.2013.11.018.

Polderman, T.J. et al. (2015). Meta-analysis of the heritability of human traits based on fifty years of twin studies. *Nat Genet* 47: 702–709. doi: 10.1038/ng.3285.

Pollen, A.A. et al. (2019). Establishing cerebral organoids as models of human-specific brain evolution. *Cell* 176: 743–756 e717. doi: 10.1016/j.cell.2019.01.017.

Prabhakar, S. et al. (2006). Accelerated evolution of conserved noncoding sequences in humans. *Science* 314: 786. doi: 10.1126/science.1130738.

Preuss, T.M. and Wise, S.P. (2022). Evolution of prefrontal cortex. *Neuropsychopharmacology* 47: 3–19. doi: 10.1038/s41386-021-01076-5.

Purves, K.L. et al. (2020). A major role for common genetic variation in anxiety disorders. *Mol Psych* 25: 3292–3303. doi: 10.1038/s41380-019-0559-1.

Rakic, P. (1971). Guidance of neurons migrating to the fetal monkey neocortex. *Brain Res* 33: 471–476. doi: 10.1016/0006-8993(71)90119-3.

Rakic, P. (1988). Specification of cerebral cortical areas. *Science* 241: 170–176. doi: 10.1126/science.3291116.

Rash, B.G. and Grove, E.A. (2011). Shh and Gli3 regulate formation of the telencephalic-diencephalic junction and suppress an isthmus-like signaling source in the forebrain. *Dev Biol* 359: 242–250. doi: 10.1016/j.ydbio.2011.08.026.

Rasin, M.R. et al. (2007). Numb and Numbl are required for maintenance of cadherin-based adhesion and polarity of neural progenitors. *Nat Neurosci* 10: 819–827. doi: 10.1038/nn1924.

Reay, W.R. et al. (2020). Polygenic disruption of retinoid signalling in schizophrenia and a severe cognitive deficit subtype. *Mol Psych* 25: 719–731. doi: 10.1038/s41380-018-0305-0.

Reilly, S.K. and Noonan, J.P. (2016). Evolution of gene regulation in humans. *Ann Rev Genom Hum Genet* 17: 45–67. doi: 10.1146/annurev-genom-090314-045935.

Rivara, C.B. et al. (2003). Stereologic characterization and spatial distribution patterns of Betz cells in the human primary motor cortex. *Anat Rec Part A, Discov Mol Cell Evol Biol* 270: 137–151. doi: 10.1002/ar.a.10015.

Rouaux, C. and Arlotta, P. (2013). Direct lineage reprogramming of post-mitotic callosal neurons into corticofugal neurons in vivo. *Nat Cell Biol* 15: 214–221. doi: 10.1038/ncb2660.

Rudy, B. et al. (2011). Three groups of interneurons account for nearly 100% of neocortical GABAergic neurons. *Dev Neurobiol* 71: 45–61. doi: 10.1002/dneu.20853.

Sakurai, T. and Gamo, N.J. (2019). Cognitive functions associated with developing prefrontal cortex during adolescence and developmental neuropsychiatric disorders. *Neurobiol Dis* 131: 104322. doi: 10.1016/j.nbd.2018.11.007.

Santos, M. et al. (2011). von Economo neurons in autism. *Brain Res* 1380: 206–217. doi: 10.1016/j.brainres.2010.08.067.

Scala, F. et al. (2019). Layer 4 of mouse neocortex differs in cell types and circuit organization between sensory areas. *Nat Commun* 10: 4174. doi: 10.1038/s41467-019-12058-z.

Schizophrenia Working Group of the Psychiatric Genomics (2014). Biological insights from 108 schizophrenia-associated genetic loci. *Nature* 511: 421–427. doi: 10.1038/nature13595.

Seeley, W.W. et al. (2012). Distinctive neurons of the anterior cingulate and frontoinsular cortex. *Cereb Cortex* 22: 245–250. doi: 10.1093/cercor/bhr005.

Selemon, L.D. et al. (2003). Regional specificity in the neuropathologic substrates of schizophrenia. *Arch Gen Psych* 60: 69–77. doi: 10.1001/archpsyc.60.1.69.

Selemon, L.D. and Zecevic, N. (2015). Schizophrenia: a tale of two critical periods for prefrontal cortical development. *Trans Psych* 5: e623. doi: 10.1038/tp.2015.115.

Sestan, N. and State, M.W. (2018). Lost in translation. *Neuron* 100: 406–423. doi: 10.1016/j.neuron.2018.10.015.

Sherwood, C.C. et al. (2012). Human brain evolution writ large and small. *Prog Brain Res* 195: 237–254. doi: 10.1016/B978-0-444-53860-4.00011-8.

Shibata, M. et al. (2015). From trans to cis: transcriptional regulatory networks in neocortical development. *Trends Genet* 31: 77–87. doi: 10.1016/j.tig.2014.12.004.

Shibata, M. et al. (2019). Regulation of prefrontal patterning, connectivity and synaptogenesis by retinoic acid. *BioRxiv*: 2019.2012.2031.891036. doi: 10.1101/2019.12.31.891036.

Shibata, M. et al. (2021a). Regulation of prefrontal patterning and connectivity by retinoic acid. *Nature* 598: 483–488. doi: 10.1038/s41586-021-03953-x.

Shibata, M. et al. (2021b). Hominini-specific regulation of CBLN2 increases prefrontal spinogenesis. *Nature* 598: 489–494. doi: 10.1038/s41586-021-03952-y.

Shim, S. et al. (2012). Cis-regulatory control of corticospinal system development and evolution. *Nature* 486: 74–79. doi: 10.1038/nature11094.

Silberberg, S.N. et al. (2016). Subpallial enhancer transgenic lines. *Neuron* 92: 59–74. doi: 10.1016/j.neuron.2016.09.027.

Silbereis, J.C. et al. (2016). The cellular and molecular landscapes of the developing human central nervous system. *Neuron* 89: 248–268. doi: 10.1016/j.neuron.2015.12.008.

Sousa, A.M.M. et al. (2017a). Evolution of the human nervous system function, structure, and development. *Cell* 170: 226–247. doi: 10.1016/j.cell.2017.06.036.

Sousa, A.M.M. et al. (2017b). Molecular and cellular reorganization of neural circuits in the human lineage. *Science* 358: 1027–1032. doi: 10.1126/science.aan3456.

State, M.W. and Sestan, N. (2012). Neuroscience. The emerging biology of autism spectrum disorders. *Science* 337: 1301–1303. doi: 10.1126/science.1224989.

Sugitani, Y. et al. (2002). Brn-1 and Brn-2 share crucial roles in the production and positioning of mouse neocortical neurons. *Genes Dev* 16: 1760–1765. doi: 10.1101/gad.978002.

Sullivan, P.F. and Geschwind, D.H. (2019). Defining the genetic, genomic, cellular, and diagnostic architectures of psychiatric disorders. *Cell* 177: 162–183. doi: 10.1016/j.cell.2019.01.015.

Sullivan, P.F. et al. (2000). Genetic epidemiology of major depression: review and meta-analysis. *Am J Psych* 157: 1552–1562. doi: 10.1176/appi.ajp.157.10.1552.

Sur, M., and Rubenstein, J.L. (2005). Patterning and plasticity of the cerebral cortex. *Science* 310 (5749): 805–810. doi: 10.1126/science.1112070.

Taverna, E. et al. (2014). The cell biology of neurogenesis. *Ann Rev Cell Dev Biol* 30: 465–502. doi: 10.1146/annurev-cellbio-101011-155801.

Tan, H.Y. et al. (2007). Dysfunctional and compensatory prefrontal cortical systems, genes and the pathogenesis of schizophrenia. *Cereb Cortex* 17 (Suppl 1): i171–181. doi: 10.1093/cercor/bhm069.

Tebbenkamp, A.T. et al. (2014). The developmental transcriptome of the human brain: implications for neurodevelopmental disorders. *Curr Opin Neurol* 27: 149–156. doi: 10.1097/WCO.0000000000000069.

Teffer, K. and Semendeferi, K. (2012). Human prefrontal cortex. *Prog Brain Res* 195: 191–218. doi: 10.1016/B978-0-444-53860-4.00009-X.

Thomson, A.M. (2010). Neocortical layer 6, a review. *Front Neuroanat* 4: 13. doi: 10.3389/fnana.2010.00013.

Tissir, F. and Goffinet, A.M. (2003). Reelin and brain development. *Nat Rev Neurosci* 4: 496–505. doi: 10.1038/nrn1113.

Trubetskoy, V. et al. (2022). Mapping genomic loci implicates genes and synaptic biology in schizophrenia. *Nature* 604: 502–508. doi: 10.1038/s41586-022-04434-5.

Trujillo, C.A. et al. (2021). Reintroduction of the archaic variant of NOVA1 in cortical organoids alters neurodevelopment. *Science* 371 (6530): eaax2537. doi: 10.1126/science.aax2537.

Tsyporin, J. et al. (2021). Transcriptional repression by FEZF2 restricts alternative identities of cortical projection neurons. *Cell Rep* 35: 109269. doi: 10.1016/j.celrep.2021.109269.

Uzquiano, A. and Arlotta, P. (2022). Brain organoids: the quest to decipher human-specific features of brain development. *Curr Opin Genet Dev* 75: 101955. doi: 10.1016/j.gde.2022.101955.

van den Heuvel, M.P. et al. (2019). Evolutionary modifications in human brain connectivity associated with schizophrenia. *Brain* 142 (12): 3991–4002. doi: 10.1093/brain/awz330.

Van Essen, D.C. and Dierker, D.L. (2007). Surface-based and probabilistic atlases of primate cerebral cortex. *Neuron* 56: 209–225. doi: 10.1016/j.neuron.2007.10.015.

Villard, J. et al. (2021). Structural differences in the hippocampus and amygdala of behaviorally inhibited macaque monkeys. *Hippocampus* 31: 858–868. doi: 10.1002/hipo.23329.

Visel, A. et al. (2013). A high-resolution enhancer atlas of the developing telencephalon. *Cell* 152: 895–908. doi: 10.1016/j.cell.2012.12.041.

Wagner, E. et al. (2002). Retinoic acid synthesis in the postnatal mouse brain marks distinct developmental stages and functional systems. *Cereb Cortex* 12 (12): 1244–1253. doi: 10.1093/cercor/12.12.1244.

Wallace, J.L. and Pollen, A.A. (2021). The genetic symphony underlying evolution of the brain's prefrontal cortex. *Nature* 598 (7881): 417–418. doi: 10.1038/d41586-021-02460-3.

Walsh, C.A. et al. (2008). Autism and brain development. *Cell* 135: 396–400. doi: 10.1016/j.cell.2008.10.015.

Weinberger, D.R. (1995). From neuropathology to neurodevelopment. *Lancet* 346: 552–557. doi: 10.1016/s0140-6736(95)91386-6.

Werling, D.M. et al. (2020). Whole-genome and RNA sequencing reveal variation and transcriptomic coordination in the developing human prefrontal cortex. *Cell Rep* 31: 107489. doi: 10.1016/j.celrep.2020.03.053.

Whalen, S. and Pollard, K.S. (2022). Enhancer function and evolutionary roles of human accelerated regions. *Ann Rev Genet* 56: 423–439. doi: 10.1146/annurev-genet-071819-103933.

Willsey, A.J. et al. (2013). Coexpression networks implicate human midfetal deep cortical projection neurons in the pathogenesis of autism. *Cell* 155: 997–1007. doi: 10.1016/j.cell.2013.10.020.

Willsey, H.R. et al. (2022). Genomics, convergent neuroscience and progress in understanding autism spectrum disorder. *Nat Rev Neurosci* 23 (6): 323–341. doi: 10.1038/s41583-022-00576-7.

Yeo, B.T. et al. (2011). The organization of the human cerebral cortex estimated by intrinsic functional connectivity. *J Neurophysiol* 106: 1125–1165. doi: 10.1152/jn.00338.2011.

Zhu, Y. et al. (2018). Spatiotemporal transcriptomic divergence across human and macaque brain development. *Science* 362 (6420): eaat8077. doi: 10.1126/science.aat8077.

Ziffra, R.S. et al. (2021). Single-cell epigenomics reveals mechanisms of human cortical development. *Nature* 598 (7879): 205–213. doi: 10.1038/s41586-021-03209-8.

Zimmer, C. et al. (2004). Dynamics of Cux2 expression suggests that an early pool of SVZ precursors is fated to become upper cortical layer neurons. *Cereb Cortex* 14 (12): 1408–1420. doi: 10.1093/cercor/bhh102.

14

Intrinsic and Input-dependent Development of Cortical Neuron Types

Esther Klingler[1], *Sergi Roig Puiggros*[1], *and Denis Jabaudon*[1,2]

[1] *Department of Basic Neurosciences, University of Geneva, Geneva, Switzerland*
[2] *Clinic of Neurology, Geneva University Hospital, Geneva, Switzerland*

Neuronal diversity sets the frame for the combination of connections that can be made within the brain, which in turn determines behavioral complexity and flexibility. Within a given organism, neuron type diversity reflects two primary and opposing developmental and evolutionary forces. First, reproducibility: cell-type generation should be reliable enough to guarantee essential functions across individuals and generations. Second, flexibility: developing organisms should be able to adapt to their surroundings when circumstances change durably. In other words, to increase the evolutionary fitness of the organism that harbors them, neurons must be able, to some extent, to diverge from their cell-intrinsically encoded fate in a manner directed by environmental signals.

Reproducibility requires developmental programs that are largely shielded from environmental conditions, that is, cell-intrinsic processes that unfold intracellularly *no matter what*. Strictly cell-intrinsic processes are probably rare in multicellular organisms since cell-to-cell contacts and interactions with the extracellular matrix are essential for organogenesis. Still, for all practical purposes, strongly genetically determined cellular programs form the backbone of corticogenesis, as detailed in Chapters 10, 11, 13, and 22. Cell-extrinsic (i.e., input-dependent) programs instead are initiated or predominantly driven by extracellular signals from various sources, including the extracellular matrix, the cerebrospinal fluid (see Chapter 32), and other cells. Cell–cell interactions can occur through diffusible molecules or actual physical contact (e.g., during cell migration and axonal guidance, dendritogenesis, and synaptogenesis) and through synaptic input, that is, through the release of neurotransmitters by evoked or spontaneous electrical activity (Figure 14.1).

The division of developmental processes into cell-intrinsic and cell-extrinsic is a convenient conceptual framework to dissect temporal sequences and tackle causality. However, these two processes are not independent and co-occur during corticogenesis. As will be highlighted by several examples in this chapter, intrinsic cell properties determine the ability of cells to respond to input, and brief extrinsic events can trigger long-lasting intrinsic processes. Intrinsic and extrinsic processes are thus intertwined and dynamically developmentally regulated.

This chapter reviews the literature on how intrinsic and extrinsic processes interact to generate diverse cortical neuron types. Since cell-intrinsic genetic processes are covered in detail in several other chapters (see Chapters 10, 11, 13, and 22), we focus primarily on cell-extrinsic processes, emphasizing cell-type-specific susceptibilities to input. In the first section, we provide a macroscopic, classical description of cortical areas and of the role of thalamocortical input in their emergence and plasticity, which is foundational to our understanding of this field. In the second section, we provide what we feel is a more modern, still-emerging view of how intrinsic and extrinsic signals interact to drive neuronal differentiation and diversity by providing a cell-type-specific

Neocortical Neurogenesis in Development and Evolution, First Edition. Edited by Wieland B. Huttner.

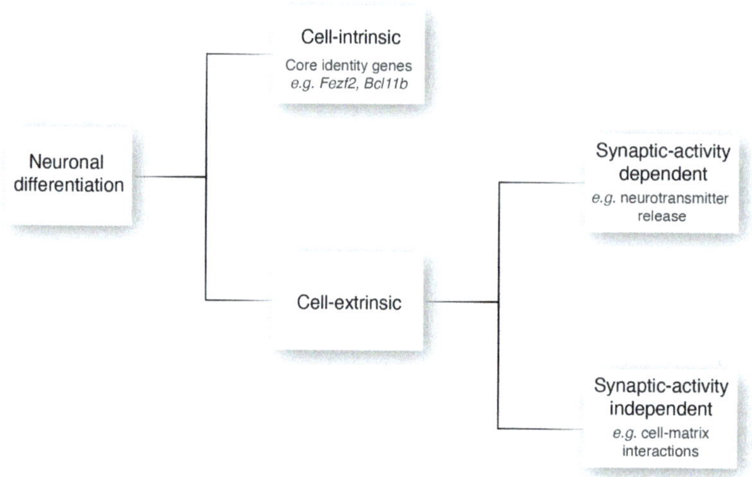

Figure 14.1 Cell-intrinsic and extrinsic mechanisms of neuronal differentiation. Adapted from Pouchelon and Jabaudon (2014).

account of the role of input in the acquisition of cellular identity in various types of excitatory and inhibitory interneurons, and progenitors. In both sections, most of the citations refer to work performed in mice, which provides the most detailed mechanistic molecular insights, but these findings will be put in an evolutionary context when possible.

14.1 Developmental Emergence of Neocortical Areas

Layer size and composition are not homogenous across the tangential surface of the neocortex. Instead, local cytoarchitecture varies rostro-caudally and medio-laterally, defining distinct cortical areas (see Cadwell et al. (2019); Sydnor et al. (2021) for comprehensive reviews of cortical arealization in mouse and human). The different cortical areas are classically divided into primary areas, secondary areas, and associative areas (Figure 14.2a–b). Primary areas comprise sensory (i.e., somatosensory, S1; auditory, A1; visual, V1) and motor areas that either receive input from exteroceptive, first-order thalamic nuclei (for sensory areas) or contain the bulk of the neurons projecting directly to lower motor neurons in the brainstem and spinal cord (for the motor cortex). Secondary cortical areas (S2, A2, V2, and supplementary motor cortex), receive input from the corresponding primary areas and process higher-order features (e.g., roughness in the case of S2, or motion in the case of V2 – which comprises a number of subregions – For the motor cortex, secondary areas contain subregions that coordinate sequences of movements). Finally, associative cortex contains neurons that establish associations between distinct sensory modalities (e.g., auditory-visual) or are involved in inner states and executive functions (e.g., prefrontal cortex). Interestingly, while primary and secondary sensory cortices comprise a large fraction of the total cortical surface in rodents, in primates, the proportion of associative cortex expands, consistent with an increased level of sensory processing and associative processes in these species (see also Section 14.1.2.1).

Histological discontinuities between cortical areas can be quite abrupt, such as in the barrel cortex of mice, which is sharply delineated, while transitions are more progressive in other areas. In humans, differences in local cytoarchitecture form the basis of the Brodmann

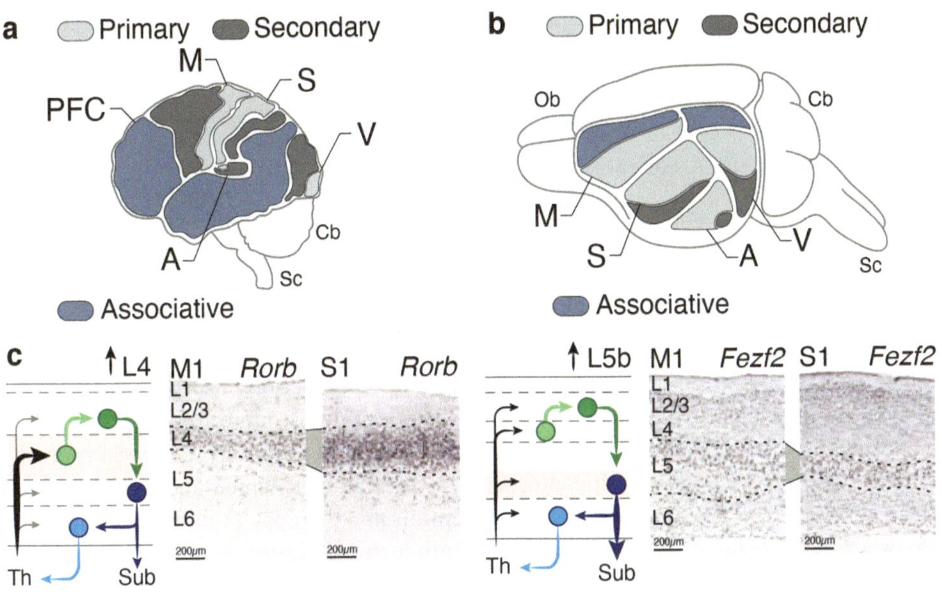

Figure 14.2 Expansion of cortical areas and layers depends on connectivity and function. (a–b) Primary, secondary, and associative areas in the human (a) and mouse (b) cortex. (c) Left, input from the thalamus to the sensory cortex and expansion of Rorb-positive layer 4 cortical neurons, recipient of thalamus input, in S1. Right, output from the primary motor cortex and expansion of Fezf2-positive layer 5 output neurons in M1. In situ hybridizations are from the Allen Brain Atlas. A, auditory cortex; Br, Broadmann area; Cb, cerebellum; Hi, hippocampus; L, layer; M1, primary motor cortex; Ob, olfactory bulb; Sc, spinal cord; S1, primary somatosensory cortex; Sub, subcortical; Th, thalamus.

classification of cortical areas (Zilles and Amunts 2010). While such areas may, in some cases, appear arbitrarily defined, cytoarchitectural differences are genuine and local cytoarchitecture corresponds to functional requirements. For example, layer (L) 4, which contains the neurons that are the primary recipients of sensory thalamic input, is particularly prominent in the primary somatosensory (S1), visual (V1), and auditory (A1) cortices, while L5b, which contains corticospinal neurons underlying motor control is the thickest in the motor cortex (Amunts and Zilles 2015; Sydnor et al. 2021) (Figure 14.2c).

How inter-areal differences emerge during development is still poorly understood since a quantitative account of inter-areal differences and similarities is only beginning to emerge. Two main explanations have, however, been put forward to account for the emergence of distinct cortical areas: the protomap hypothesis and the protocortex hypothesis (Sur and Rubenstein 2005). The protomap hypothesis posits that cortical area identity is molecularly pre-patterned within neuronal progenitors through rostro-caudal and medio-lateral gradients of gene expression. Such prepatterning would give rise to region-specific daughter neurons with distinctive molecular features, resulting in distinct physiological and connectivity properties (Bishop et al. 2000; Rakic 1988; Rubenstein 1999). The protocortex hypothesis, in contrast, proposes that the cortex is initially homogeneous (a "*tabula rasa*" (Bienenstock 1996)), that is, that progenitors and neurons across cortical areas initially have similar molecular properties and that region-specific features are only later imparted by cortex-extrinsic signals, in particular by thalamic input (O'Leary 1989; Van der Loos and Woolsey 1973). In other words, while the protomap hypothesis proposes that cortical arealization is largely input-independent, in the protocortex hypothesis, input-dependence is primordial. As illustrated later, these two hypotheses are not mutually exclusive, and both processes are likely at play (reviewed in Cadwell et al. 2019). For example, initial differences in cellular molecular features across areas may impart distinct susceptibilities to later-occurring input-dependent signals.

14.1.1 Input-independent Arealization

As discussed in detail in Chapter 32, several genes are expressed along tangential spatial gradients during corticogenesis and act as determinants of area identity; they will thus only be briefly covered here. Such genes positionally define progenitors and their daughter neurons to drive their differentiation towards area-specific functions. For example, the orphan nuclear receptor COUP-TF1 (officially called *Nr2f1*) is expressed in a high caudo-lateral to low rostro-medial gradient (Liu et al. 2000; Zhou et al. 2001), which is critical for the emergence of sensory areas by repression of frontal cortical identity. Accordingly, molecularly-defined frontal areas expand when NR2F1 is specifically ablated from the cortex, and sensory areas shift posteriorly and are atrophied, together with their corresponding thalamocortical innervation (Armentano et al. 2007). Remarkably, although *Nr2f1* is expressed both in progenitors and their daughter neurons, ablation of *Nr2f1* expression limited to neurons is sufficient to mimic the full knockout phenotype (Alfano et al. 2014). These findings not only suggest a critical role for this transcription factor in postmitotic neuronal differentiation, but also that the protomap hypothesis needs to be examined on a cell-type by cell-type basis. Understanding the cell-type-specific effects of classical cortical patterning genes such as *Nr2f1*, *Sp8*, *Pax6*, and *Emx2* will thus likely be a key area of research in the years to come. Interaction between patterning genes and activity-dependent processes will also have to be considered: for example, NR2F1 regulates the expression of genes coding for voltage-gated ion channels in S1 L5 neurons, which control their electrophysiological properties, but which can also affect their synaptic partners within and beyond the cortex (Del Pino et al. 2020).

14.1.2 Input-dependent Arealization

The role of sensory input has been best studied in the somatosensory and visual cortices, which are the primary cortical recipients of pathways originating on the body surface. Such pathways lend themselves well to experimental manipulations such as infraorbital nerve section (section of the nerve conveying input from the whiskers) or enucleation (removal of the eyes), making them powerful study models. In particular, in the mouse, the whisker somatosensory cortex, with its patterned cytoarchitecture into macroscopic barrels (Figure 14.3), has provided major insights into our understanding of how manipulation of peripheral input affects cortical organization, since manipulations of whiskers or their input pathways during early postnatal life lead to disruption of the barrel organization (see later).

14.1.2.1 Thalamic Input-dependent Emergence of Cortical Areas

Except for olfaction (Bekkers and Suzuki 2013), sensory information transits through the thalamus before reaching the cortex (Figure 14.4a). Thalamocortical input is thus considered the key pathway for input-dependent control of cortical neuron properties. Although not the focus of the present review, thalamic neurons themselves differentiate in an input-dependent manner, and changes occurring at the thalamic level are typically reflected in the cortical areas they project to (Chou et al. 2013; Frangeul et al. 2016; Vue et al. 2013). When referring to thalamic input, most studies refer to first-order thalamic input (i.e., exteroceptive thalamic input, which relays input from the sense organs). However, for each sensory modality, higher-order nuclei, which are driven

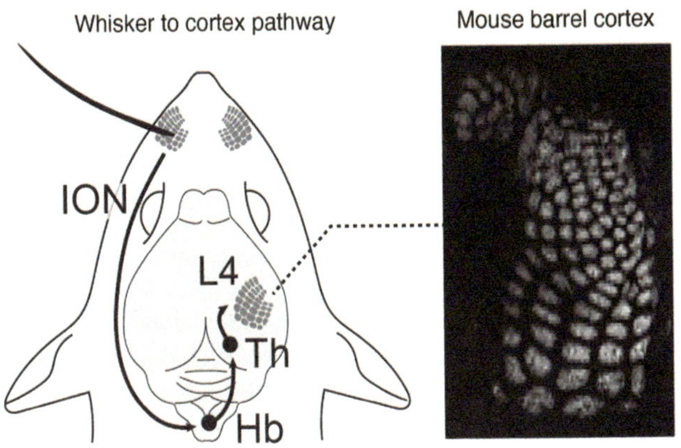

Figure 14.3 Organization of the whisker primary somatosensory cortex into barrels. Left, Whisker to cortex circuit. Right, vesicular glutamate transporter 2 (VGluT2) staining of thalamic afferences to the layer 4. Hb, hindbrain; ION, infraorbital nerve; L, layer; Th, thalamus. Adapted from Pouchelon and Jabaudon (2014).

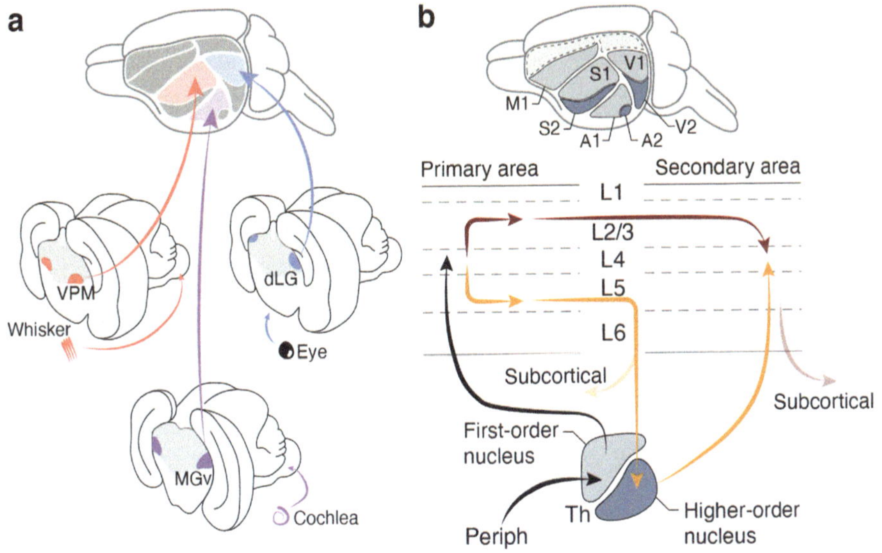

Figure 14.4 Sensory information reaches the cortex via specific thalamic nuclei. (a) First-order thalamic nuclei and their projections to cortical areas. (b) Connectivity of first- and higher-order thalamic nuclei with primary and secondary cortical sensory areas. A1, primary auditory cortex; A2, secondary auditory cortex; dLG, dorsal lateral geniculate thalamic nucleus; L, layer; MGv, medial geniculate thalamic nucleus ventral part; S1, primary somatosensory cortex; S2 secondary somatosensory cortex; Th, thalamus; V1, primary visual cortex; V2, secondary visual cortex; VPM, ventroposterior medial thalamic nucleus. Adapted from Jabaudon, 2017 and Nakagawa and Shimogori, 2012.

by descending corticothalamic inputs, also project to the cortex, although their role in cortical patterning, if any, is less well understood (Halassa and Sherman 2019; Miller-Hansen and Sherman 2022). Similarly, the developmental role of non-sensory thalamic nuclei, such as the ventrolateral nucleus (which projects to the primary motor cortex) in the acquisition of cortical neuron identity is unknown. Cross-talks between first- and higher-order nuclei are, however, important, and their role in cortical patterning and evolution is discussed later. Finally, input-dependent processes are likely at play beyond thalamocortical pathways, including, for instance, within intracortical pathways, which develop during the first postnatal week (Klingler et al. 2021; Rodríguez-Tornos et al. 2016). Interactions between primary and secondary sensory areas may be particularly relevant in this respect, for example, between V1 and secondary visual cortices (V2) (Dong et al. 2004; Imam and Finlay 2020). Of note, interactions between cortical areas can occur not only through cortico-cortical connections, but also through cortico-thalamo-cortical pathways, which earlier in evolution may have been the primary mode of communications between different parts of the pallium (Figure 14.4b).

In an evolutionary perspective, neurons of primary cortical areas and first-order thalamic nuclei may have arisen from higher-order type neurons, based on their ability to convey high-resolution signals generated by body sensory receptors thanks to specific metabolic, electrophysiological, and connectivity features (Frangeul et al. 2016) (Figure 14.5). The distributed projections of higher-order nuclei and areas may then have acquired a new role by allowing for multisensory integration. Along this line of thought, the expansion of associative cortex in humans and primates has been proposed to be a consequence of "untethering" from thalamocortical input during evolutionary enlargement of the brain (Buckner and Krienen 2013).

14.1.2.2 Spontaneous Activity

Early in development, thalamic activity does not necessarily reflect events occurring in sense organs. Instead, early spontaneous thalamic calcium waves ("spontaneous activity") occur before sensory-evoked activity, which acts at least in part to pre-pattern cortical cytoarchitecture and molecular identity in specific areas for later-occurring sensory experience-evoked activity (see Martini et al. (2021) for a recent review). Interestingly, such pre-patterning does not appear to be modality-specific since seemingly spontaneous gap-junction-mediated calcium waves initially propagate across somatosensory, auditory, and visual thalamic nuclei, which only later become segregated into distinct sensory channels (Moreno-Juan et al. 2017) (Figure 14.6).

There appears to be some level of competition across sensory modalities at the level of the thalamus for cortical functional space, as blocking thalamic spontaneous calcium waves in the auditory nucleus alters activity and gene expression in the somatosensory thalamus, ultimately enlarging the barrel field in S1 (Moreno-Juan et al. 2017). Hence, within the thalamus and cortex, sensory input may initially be treated in a modality-independent way and only later become specific as sensory experience occurs. Supporting this view, the molecular identity of all primary sensory

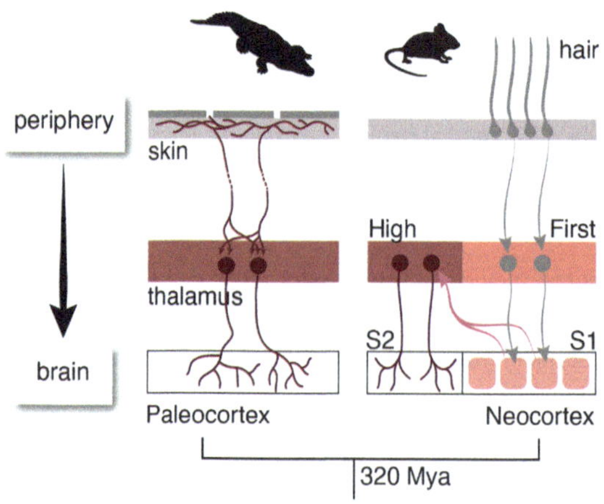

Figure 14.5 Emergence of first-order types of neurons from higher-order neurons. Comparison of the somatosensory system in crocodile and mouse. Mya, millions years ago; S1, primary somatosensory cortex; S2, secondary somatosensory cortex; Th, thalamus.

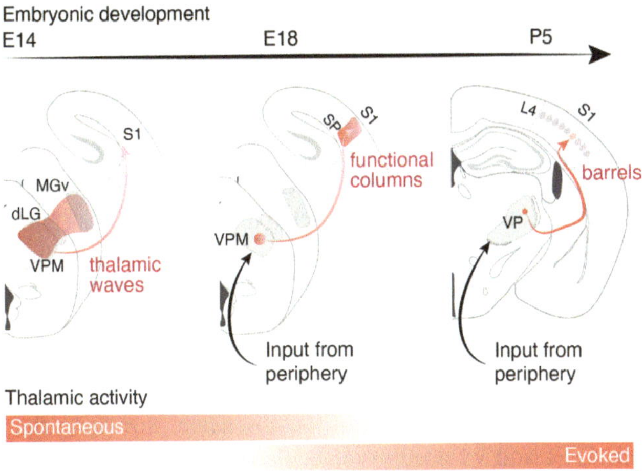

Figure 14.6 Thalamic activity shapes the emergence of functional cortical columns. Before birth, spontaneous thalamic waves of activity spread from one to another thalamic nucleus, which is important for the development of thalamocortical connectivity. After birth, thalamic activity evoked by sensory experience allows the emergence of functional columns and later barrels in S1. dLG, dorsal lateral geniculate thalamic nucleus; E, embryonic day; L, layer; MGv, medial geniculate thalamic nucleus ventral part; P, postnatal day; S1, primary somatosensory cortex; VPM, ventroposterior medial thalamic nucleus. Adapted from Martini et al. (2021).

areas is initially relatively homogenous and yet distinct from non-sensory areas, and only later does the molecular distinction between somatosensory, visual, and auditory thalamic nuclei and areas emerge (Chou et al. 2013; Frangeul et al. 2016; Vue et al. 2013). Spontaneous activity also plays a critical role at the level of the sense organs themselves, as has been well studied for the visual system, where the emergence of binocular vision requires "retinal waves" before eye opening, which trigger activity in the midbrain and primary visual cortex and modulate activity in secondary visual areas (Ackman et al. 2012; Shatz 1996). These waves topographically pattern various target structures during brain development, including in the superior colliculus, the dorso-lateral geniculate nucleus (dLGN) of the thalamus (Burbridge et al. 2014) and, indirectly, the visual cortex.

Calcium waves are transmitted by proximity from one cell to another via gap junctions. Hence, such waves represent a convenient way to translate spatial proximity into a temporal electrical code (i.e., spatially adjacent cells depolarize with temporal contiguity). However, how this activity translates into the emergence of specific, spatially-appropriate cellular molecular features remains poorly understood. Ca^{2+}-dependent signals and immediate-early genes such as c-fos are involved in such cellular response, but precisely how this translates in cellular properties remains unknown (Chen et al. 2020; Hrvatin et al. 2018; Tyssowski et al. 2018; and see Section 14.2).

14.1.2.3 Sensory Activity Sculpts Cortical Differentiation

Whether activity evoked from the sense organs plays a permissive or instructive role in neuronal differentiation is unclear. If permissive, input "only" acts as a trigger for cell-intrinsic differentiation programs. In contrast, for input to be instructive, specific patterns of activity are required to induce and sustain particular programs of differentiation. Both situations probably exist, but examples of instructive signals are harder to demonstrate. For instance, following the loss of exteroceptive somatosensory input from the ventroposterior medial thalamic nucleus (VPM), acquisition input from another somatosensory nucleus (the posterior thalamic nucleus (Po)) is not sufficient to rescue L4 neuron differentiation in S1; VPM information thus appears to be instructive for these neurons (Pouchelon et al. 2014). Similarly, specific patterns of optogenetic activation are required to instruct eye-specific segregation in the visual system (Zhang et al. 2012). Again, here molecular mechanisms through which specific activity patterns would impart specific cellular features remain elusive.

Lesioning of sensory input pathways (e.g., sectioning of the infraorbital nerve to remove whisker input or enucleation to remove retinal input) is not equivalent to silencing neurons along that pathway (Frangeul et al. 2017), such that care should be taken in comparing results obtained through different experimental paradigms. In contrast to lesion-based experiments, genetic ablation and electrical silencing experiments allow insights into cell type-specific, activity-dependent effects on differentiation within defined developmental periods (De León Reyes et al. 2019; Pouchelon et al. 2014; Vue et al. 2013). Typically, such genetic studies have shown that primary sensory areas emerge input-dependently from a genetically relatively uniform cortex. In the absence of first-order thalamic input, primary cortical areas such as S1 and V1 acquire molecular identities of secondary associative cortical areas, that is, S2 and V2 (Chou et al. 2013; Pouchelon et al. 2014; Vue et al. 2013) (Figure 14.7). In the case of the somatosensory cortex, input-deprived S1 circuits acquire S2-like properties (i.e. they increase their excitatory/inhibitory ratio), suggesting that thalamic input also affects cortical circuit assembly (Pouchelon et al. 2014). Higher-order cortical identity is, therefore, a ground-state feature, as is the case for higher-order thalamic nucleus identity (Frangeul et al. 2016), and acquisition of primary cortical area circuit properties requires first-order thalamic input.

14.1.2.4 Critical Periods of Plasticity

The susceptibility of neurons to changes in input varies with age. Critical periods of plasticity have been defined as developmental periods in which changes in the environment (e.g., dark housing) or manipulation of sense organs (e.g., enucleation, infraorbital nerve section) lead to drastic and long-lasting changes in function and behavior (see Hooks and Chen (2020) for the visual system and Erzurumlu and Gaspar (2012) for the barrel cortex critical periods). While this concept is important at the level of sensory function and behavior (e.g., critical periods for binocular vision,

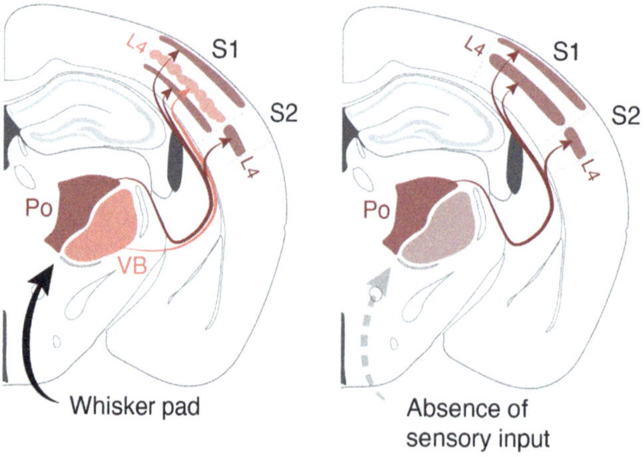

Figure 14.7 Input deprivation prevents first-order identity to emerge. Patterning of the primary and secondary sensory cortex by first- and higher-order thalamic input in normal condition (left) and after input ablation (right). L, layer; Po, posterior thalamic nucleus; S1, primary somatosensory cortex; S2, secondary somatosensory cortex; Th, thalamus; VPM, ventroposterior medial thalamic nucleus. Adapted from Pouchelon et al. (2014).

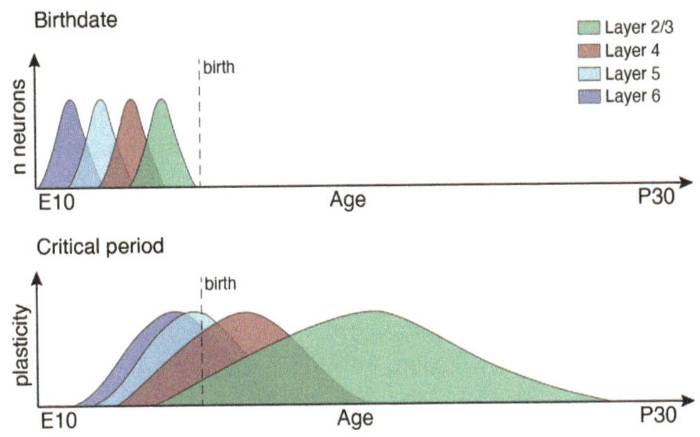

Figure 14.8 Relationships between cortical neuron birthdate and critical periods of plasticity. Different cell types may have different, sequential critical periods that at least in part reflect their birth order. E, embryonic day; P, postnatal day.

barrel cortex formation, socialization), whether it reflects a developmental window of molecular processes that are genuinely distinct from what occurs later in life in response to learning and experience is unclear. Instead, developmental periods during which specific systems are susceptible to input may reflect distinct birth orders and levels of maturation of the cells that compose it (Figure 14.8). Namely, because of the sequential birth of cortical neuron types over a week or so in the mouse (~15 weeks in humans), neurons at distinct maturation levels coexist within a cortical column. For example, in the mouse, L2/3 neurons are still migrating during the first postnatal days (Hippenmeyer 2014), while deep layer neurons are already more than a week old and are establishing connections with target regions.

Consequently, sensory manipulations have cell-type-specific effects that reflect their level of maturation, such that critical periods may be best understood on a cell-type by cell-type basis and likely reflect the progressive fading-off of multipotent cellular fates with time rather than privileged windows of extraordinary plasticity. Supporting this possibility, the human cerebral cortex has a prolonged developmental timing compared with other species, including protracted maturation of neurons and glia, axonal and dendritic growth, and synapse formation and refinement (see Libé-Philippot and Vanderhaeghen 2021). Since humans are born in a relatively immature state, the slowly differentiating young cells of their brains may be particularly susceptible to environmental conditions and such neoteny may contribute to our species' diversity in behavioral and social features.

14.2 Cell-type Specific Input-dependent Differentiation

As introduced earlier, until recently, input-dependent controls over cortical development could only be studied with relatively low resolution through changes in the spatial distribution of expression "areal" genes and markers (e.g., *Fgf8*, cytochrome oxidase) or in salient cytoarchitecture features (e.g., barrel cortex of mice). Thanks to the ability to optogenetically manipulate specific cell types and to the advent of single-cell/nucleus RNA sequencing, the question of intrinsic vs. extrinsic controls over brain development can now be studied with single-cell resolution. These approaches have begun to reveal dynamic cell-type-specific developmental susceptibilities to extrinsic signals, as described later. In this section we start by outlining generic effects of input on cortical neurons and then review recent findings relating to specific subtypes of neurons and non-neuronal cells.

14.2.1 Generic Effects of Input/Activity on Neuronal Differentiation

Following their birth from progenitors in cortical germinal zones (see Chapters 3, 5, 24, and 25), neurons radially migrate to the cortical plate to reach their proper laminar location, extend axons and dendrites, contact and are contacted by diverse types of neurons through synaptic connections, which together determines the extent to which they will integrate circuits and survive or will undergo programmed cell death (Wang et al. 2021). Each of these developmental steps is, in principle, susceptible to modulation by input and activity-dependent processes. Early in corticogenesis, before mature synapses are present (i.e., before embryonic day (E)13.5 in the mouse, the time at which thalamocortical axons invade the cortical plate), intrinsic spontaneous activity plays a predominant role. For example, disrupting spontaneous Ca^{2+} activity by deleting the voltage-gated Ca^{2+} channel gene *Cacna1* causes abnormal brain development (Smedler et al. 2022). Migration itself is susceptible to activity-dependent modulation since optogenetic/chemogenetic activation of neurons in vivo induces premature branching and migration arrest of superficial layer neurons (Hurni et al. 2017).

Because of the timing of synaptogenesis in the cortex, events occurring before E13.5 in the mouse are thus presumably relatively synaptic input independent, while later-occurring ones are potentially susceptible to input. Deep-layer neurons in L6 and L5, which are born earlier than that, may thus have relatively cell-intrinsic developmental trajectories until this time point and be affected by input mostly in terms of dendritic extension or synaptogenesis. In contrast, later-born neurons in superficial layers 4 and 2/3 may be affected from their birth on, including in their migration and early differentiation. In addition, as discussed earlier and in more detail later, there might be cell-type-specific periods of plasticity in which the latest-born, least-mature neurons may be most susceptible to postnatal experience, emphasizing the importance of identifying cell-type-specific critical periods of plasticity (Cheng et al. 2022). Consistent with this possibility, in the whisker-to-barrel pathway, synaptic plasticity (e.g., as assessed by the ability to induce synaptic long-term potentiation) decreases postnatally in a sequence corresponding to the date of birth of the neurons (Fox and Wong 2005). Similarly, transcriptomic analysis of single cells from distinct adult neocortical areas showed that L2/3 neurons are transcriptionally more diverse between areas than deep-layer neurons, consistent with a stronger degree of experience-dependent controls over their differentiation (Tasic et al. 2018).

In contrast, however, the gross formation of the cortex is relatively normal in mutant mice lacking a protein essential for evoked synaptic vesicular release (*Snap25*), as is the growth of thalamocortical fibers or corticofugal projections (Miyashita-Lin et al. 1999; Molnár et al. 2002). *Celsr3/Dlx* mutant mice, which lack extrinsic neocortical connections, survive until P20 and have normal gross behavior (although finer cortex-dependent skills are expected to be affected). Despite the disruption of the barrel field and global cortical atrophy, lamination and arealization are roughly normal (Zhou et al. 2008, 2010).

Sensory experience appears to regulate common gene programs across cell types, for example, involving *Fos*, *Egr1*, or *Npas4* genes, whose expressions increase in all visual cortical neurons upon light exposure in dark-housed mice (Spiegel et al. 2014). However, cell-type-specific programs are also regulated and induce cell-type-specific responses to sensory experience. For example, the expressions of *Adcyap1*, *Bdnf*, or *Nrn1* increase specifically in excitatory neurons, while the expressions of *Prss23*, *Serpin1*, and *Igf1* increase in Parvalbumin-, Somatostatin- and Vasoactive intestinal peptide (VIP)-expressing inhibitory neurons, respectively (Mardinly et al. 2016; Spiegel et al. 2014). How such gene expression regulations relate to the emergence of specific circuit properties and cellular identities is still largely unknown.

14.2.2 L4 Neurons

L4 neurons of primary sensory areas are the immediate postsynaptic targets of thalamocortical afferents and the poster child for input-dependent differentiation. Much more is known about them than other cortical cell types on this topic. L4 neurons of S1 have been particularly extensively characterized and are described in detail later.

The whisker-to-barrel system and its characteristic topographic organization have been well described by Woolsey and van der Loos (1970): inputs from the whiskers reach the brainstem principal trigeminal nucleus (PrV) via trigeminal ganglion neurons and are relayed in the contralateral thalamus VPM, to reach S1 layer 4. At each level, clear anatomical structures are organized into a somatotopic map reflecting the whisker pad: barrelettes, barreloids, and barrels with neighboring barrellettes, barreloids, and barrels representing neighboring whiskers. One whisker activates one barrelette of the PrV, which activates one barreloid of the VPM, to finally activate one cortical barrel, such that each barrel responds to a single principal whisker (Figure 14.3).

In L4, excitatory spiny stellate neurons (SSN) orient their dendrites towards bundled thalamocortical axons (Nakazawa et al. 2018). At birth, "SSN" have a pyramidal morphology, and it is only around postnatal day (P) 5 in the mouse that they acquire a stellate morphology through retraction of their apical dendrite and dendritic polarization (Callaway and Borrell 2011) (Figure 14.9). In addition to their initial pyramidal morphology L4 S1 neurons initially transiently project an axon across the corpus callosum, which retracts upon acquisition of thalamocortical input (Figure 14.9), suggesting that L4 and L2/3 neurons bear an ontogenic relationship (De León Reyes et al. 2019; and see later).

Synaptic release of glutamate from thalamocortical axons is the main driver for patterning SSN somas into barrels and polarizing their dendrites towards thalamic input. For example, in mice lacking vesicular glutamate transporters in thalamocortical axons (i.e., where thalamocortical neurotransmission is abolished), barrels are disrupted, and L4 neurons abnormally retain a pyramidal morphology (Li et al. 2013). Likewise, thalamic deletion of Rab3-interacting molecules 1 and 2 (RIM1/2), which are involved in neurotransmitter release, alters barrel formation and L4 neuron dendritic polarization (Lu et al. 2006; Narboux-Neme et al. 2012). Interestingly, pre- or postsynaptic loss of the same gene does not equivalently affect cortical patterning. For example, thalamic inactivation of adenylyl cyclase 1 (AC1) impairs barrel formation (Suzuki et al. 2015). In contrast, its cortical inactivation only results in minor L4 neuron dendritic orientation defects (Iwasato et al. 2008), and RIM1/2 loss in the cortex

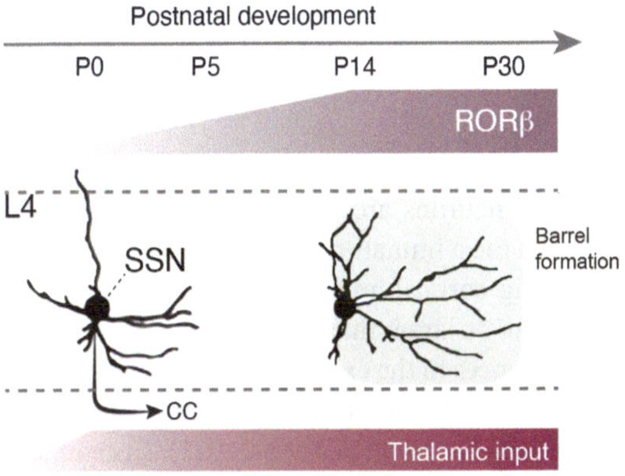

Figure 14.9 Layer 4 spiny stellate morphology and connectivity relies on thalamic input. CC, corpus callosum; L, layer; P, postnatal day. SSN reconstructions are from Nakazawa et al. (2018).

does not affect barrel formation and L4 neuron polarization (Narboux-Neme et al. 2012). Consistent with a critical role for glutamate in L4 neuron differentiation, loss of N-methyl-D-aspartate receptors (NMDAR) or of the metabotropic glutamate receptor mGluR5 affects dendritic polarization of L4 neurons and barrel cortex patterning (Mizuno et al. 2014; Wijetunge et al. 2008).

Before the arrival of thalamocortical afferents, L4 S1 neurons must become intrinsically competent to respond to input-dependent signals. For example, the transcription factor LHX2 is required for L4 neurons to form barrels and develop dendritic polarization through regulation of excitability (Shetty et al. 2013). In the absence of cortical LHX2, thalamic axons do not arborize, suggesting feedback processes through which the properties of L4 neurons condition the properties of thalamocortical axons (Wang et al. 2017, 2022; Zembrzycki et al. 2015). Other transcriptional programs also contribute to the ability of L4 neurons to respond to thalamic input, including the transcription factors NPAS4, ZBZB20, and the GPI-linked semaphorin member Sema7a (Carcea et al. 2014; Pouchelon et al. 2014; Shetty et al. 2013; Wang et al. 2017). Of note, polarization of dendrites towards thalamocortical afferents is not restricted to L4 S1 neurons, as the transcription factor BTBD3, whose nuclear localization requires neuronal activity, has a similar role in L4 neurons in V1 (Matsui et al. 2013). Whether distinct transcriptional programs are generally at play in V1 vs. S1 neuron dendritic polarization is, however, unknown.

Amongst genes associated with L4 neuron identity, RORB is arguably best known. Expression of this orphan nuclear receptor increases in L4 neurons when thalamocortical input synapses form and decreases in the absence of thalamic input (Jabaudon et al. 2012; Pouchelon et al. 2014) (Figure 14.9). RORB is sufficient to impart spiny stellate neuron-type morphology, electrical properties, and connectivity to L2/3 neurons when misexpressed in these cells (Klingler et al. 2019; Oishi et al. 2016). Interestingly, RORB overexpression early in development leads to mismigration of new-born neurons, perhaps reflecting premature differentiation, and ectopically located neurons form barrel-like structures through innervation by thalamocortical axons (Jabaudon et al. 2012). Similarly, ectopically located neurons in cortical heterotopias can receive thalamocortical innervation and display barrel-like patterns (Cappello et al. 2012). Ectopically located L5 neurons following *Fezf2* overexpression (a critical determinant of L5 identity) project to the spinal cord (Molyneaux et al., 2005) (De la Rossa et al. 2013) and receive the proper complement of input from inhibitory interneurons (Lodato et al. 2011). Hence, neuronal location is not a strict determinant of neuronal identity, and even ectopically located neurons can display coherent, if not appropriate, patterns of input and output connectivity. This is for example the case in the Reeler mice, which lack a layer organization but present relatively conserved input-output properties (Guy and Staiger 2017). Related to this observation is the "equivalent circuit hypothesis," whereby across species, and in particular in birds and reptiles vs. mammals, cells expressing equivalent complements of genes might establish similar circuits regardless of the spatial layout of the neurons of these circuits (Dugas-Ford et al. 2012; Karten 2013; see Chapters 5 and 15 for more insight into these evolutionary considerations).

14.2.3 L2/3 Neurons

Layer 2/3 neurons are the latest-generated cortical neuron type during embryogenesis and are hence the most immature at the time when pups are born. Given the role of these neurons in interconnecting cortical areas, the input-dependent component of these neurons' differentiation is expected to be larger than that of early-born neuronal types. Accordingly, although there are laminar differences in the expression of specific genes within layer 2/3 (Molyneaux et al. 2007), specific subtypes of S2 and M1 projecting-neurons in S1 do not display salient function-related differential gene expression (Klingler et al. 2021). Instead, differences in the temporality of gene expression seem to be the primary driver of differences in connectivity.

Consistent with a significant input-dependent identity component, diminishing L2/3 neuron excitability by overexpressing the inward-rectifying potassium ion channel *Kir2.1* (which hyperpolarizes neurons) significantly reduces axonal branching and changes the columnar patterns of callosal innervation in the contralateral hemisphere both in S1 and V1 (Mizuno et al. 2010; Suárez et al. 2014; Wang et al. 2007). Accordingly, transcriptional regulation of *Kv1.1* and *Kv1.3* potassium channel genes by CUX1, a transcription factor highly expressed in intracortically-projecting neurons, seems to play a critical role in the action of this gene (Rodríguez-Tornos et al. 2016). Furthermore, unilateral whisker cauterization disrupts S1 L2/3 neurons projections to the opposite hemisphere, while bilateral cauterization results in a partial rescue of the phenotype (Suárez et al. 2014), suggesting that callosal projections require a balance of endogenous activity between hemispheres (Figure 14.10). Finally, as recently shown, visual cortical L2/3 neurons refine their identities after birth, whereas deep-layer neurons do not, demonstrating that different types of visual cortical neurons have various sensitivities to visual experience, with intracortically projecting neurons being most sensitive (Cheng et al. 2022; Puiggros and Jabaudon 2022).

14.2.4 Deep-layer Neurons

Relatively little is known about the input dependence of the differentiation of L5 and L6 neurons. While they receive thalamocortical input (Constantinople and Bruno 2013), these are some of the earliest-born cells of the cortex, and they are already 2–3 days old at the time thalamocortical axons contact them. Hence, a significant part of their initial differentiation is likely independent of thalamocortical input. L5 and L6 neurons strongly project to the thalamus, with L5 neurons projecting specifically to higher-order nuclei (Grant et al. 2016). Upon monocular or binocular enucleation in young postnatal mice, Rbp4^{+} L5 neurons of the primary visual cortex (V1) rewire to contact the first-order nucleus dLGN, which loses its first-order genetic identity to resemble that of higher-order LP nucleus (Frangeul et al. 2016; Giasafaki et al. 2022; Grant et al. 2016). L6 axons reach the dLGN at postnatal days 3–4, after retinal afferents, and innervation is not complete before P12 (corresponding to eye opening), while adult-like synapse responses start from two weeks of age. Eliminating retinal input accelerates this innervation, which is complete at P8–10, although the synapses mature at the same rate as in normal conditions (Grant et al. 2016; Seabrook et al. 2013). Of note, S1 Rbp4^{+} L5 neurons also project to the medial auditory thalamus, where they modulate auditory responses (Lohse et al. 2021).

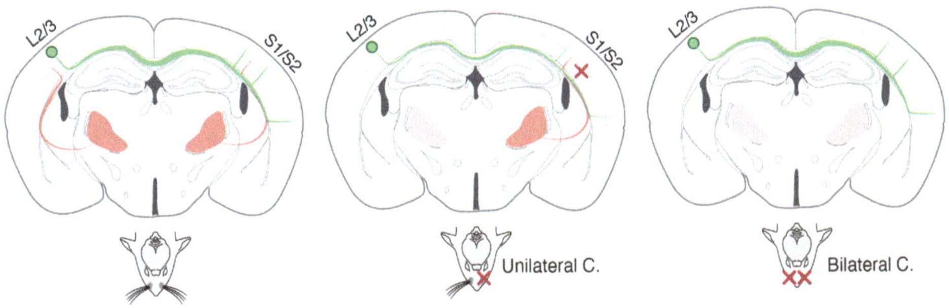

Figure 14.10 Balanced activity is required for proper corpus callosum development. Development of the corpus callosum in normal condition (left), unilateral whisker cauterization (middle), or bilateral whisker cauterization (right). Red shows the thalamic input to the cortex. L, layer; S1, primary somatosensory cortex; S2, secondary somatosensory cortex; Th, thalamus.

14.2.5 Cajal–Retzius and Subplate Neurons

The correct establishment of the cortical circuit properties relies on two early-generated (from E9 to E12 in mice) and transient neuronal populations: the Cajal–Retzius (CR) cells, located in the marginal zone (Barber and Pierani 2016; Genescu and Garel 2021), and subplate neurons, located in deep layer 6, which are essential for the correct establishment of thalamocortical connections and cortical columns architecture (Kanold and Luhmann 2010). These cell types are discussed in detail in Chapter 16 and will only be briefly covered by select examples here.

CR neurons produce Reelin, a secreted glycoprotein essential for cortical lamination, whose absence prevents the formation of cortical layers in a cell-extrinsic manner (Ogawa et al. 1995; Sekine et al. 2014). CR neurons are a heterogeneous population, with distinct subtypes generated in distinct brain regions. The elimination of one or the other of these subtypes affects their respective distribution across the cortex, which in turn disrupts cortical arealization (Griveau et al. 2010). Although CR neurons die during the first two postnatal week, they are embedded into functional circuits, and receive serotonergic and noradrenergic inputs, and GABAergic inputs postnatally. The position and later death of CR neurons is, at least partially, activity dependent. The distribution of distinct subtypes of CR neurons across the cortex is regulated by NMDA receptors (de Frutos et al. 2016). CR neuron activity mediated by NKCC1 Na-K-Cl transporter, via $GABA_A$ receptor-mediated membrane depolarization, is critical for their postnatal apoptosis, and CR neuron hyperpolarization or NKCC1 deletion prevents their elimination resulting in aberrant electrically active CR neurons in layer 1 (Blanquie et al. 2016; Riva et al. 2019). Reduction in CR neuron numbers result in an increased density of interneurons originating from the caudal ganglionic eminence (CGE) or the pre-optic area (POA) and decreased axonal collaterals and apical dendrite complexity (de Frutos et al. 2016). When CR neurons are not properly eliminated, and stay in the superficial layer circuits, their apical dendrites display an increased branching, spine numbers and excitatory/inhibitory ratio (Ledonne et al. 2016; Riva et al. 2019). Hence, although the exact mechanisms remain to be elucidated, CR neurons seem to play an important transient role in cortical wiring.

Subplate neurons send their axons toward the thalamus around E12.5. Thalamic projections invade the cortex at E15–16 but they first accumulate in the subplate until the cortex becomes mature enough (Allendoerfer and Shatz 1994). Within the subplate, thalamocortical axons develop transient axonal branches allowing activity-dependent interactions with subplate cells, which may lead to their realignment before they enter the cortex (Catalano and Shatz 1998; Krug et al. 1998). In an in vitro system, the thalamus provides trophic factors for the survival of subplate neurons, which is not the case for cortical plate neurons) (Price and Lotto 1996); loss of these factors once the thalamic axons invade the cortical plate may contribute to subplate neuron death. In mice lacking LHX2 in cortical progenitors giving rise to subplate neurons, the later cells are present but have abnormal molecular identities and electrophysiological properties, and thalamocortical axons display a premature and exuberant growth into the cortex at E15.5, resulting in the elimination of sensory input from the thalamus and loss of somatosensory barrels in the mature cortex (Pal et al. 2021).

14.2.6 Inhibitory Interneurons

Inhibitory interneurons undergo massive apoptosis during postnatal periods (Wong and Marín 2019), in a manner that tightly relies on input. During the second postnatal week, L2/3 callosal and retinal inputs drive the apoptosis of GABAergic chandelier cells in V1, which is critical for correct binocular vision (Wang et al. 2021); whisker trimming at P7 (but not 15) decreases the level of parvalbumin protein in L4 parvalbumin-expressing interneurons and reduces their perisomatic inhibition onto spiny stellate neurons (Jiao 2006); the activity-dependent transcription factor NPAS4 increases inhibition of excitatory neurons specifically (Spiegel et al. 2014; Wamsley and Fishell 2017).

Moreover, adult parvalbumin$^+$ interneurons can be rejuvenated by transplantation of embryonic interneurons: they become re-sensitized to sensory experience, which can rescue visual impairment caused by deprivation during the juvenile critical period (Davis et al. 2015; Zheng et al. 2021). This reopening of critical period induced by young transplanted neurons may be mediated by their release of factors, although those remain to be identified.

The examples above suggest that interneurons are programmed to be functionally plastic and adapt their behavior to the environment to control the excitatory/inhibitory balance. However, in some cases, interneurons are remarkably unaffected by changes in environmental conditions. For example, light deprivation does not affect the transcriptional signatures of inhibitory neurons of the visual cortex (Cheng et al. 2022), and interneuron subtypes seem to be relatively homogeneous across cortical areas (which is not the case for excitatory neurons) (Tasic et al. 2018). This relative transcriptional stability in face of a striking functional plasticity suggests that key properties of cortical interneurons may be regulated at the post-transcriptional level.

14.2.7 Non-neuronal Cells

Cortical neurons are born from progenitors located at the ventricular wall, which divide during corticogenesis to give rise to successive types of cells (see Chapter 2). Single-cell RNA sequencing of ventricular zone progenitors (i.e., radial glia, or apical progenitors) has revealed sequential waves of gene expression that are transmitted to the daughter neurons for further (input-dependent) postmitotic refinement in gene expression (Telley et al. 2019). Hence, whereas environment does not appear to affect the transmission of transcriptional ground states from mother cells to daughter neurons (i.e., this is a largely cell-autonomous process), cell-extrinsic processes come into play at later stages for the acquisition of fine-grained type-specific neuronal identity. This is demonstrated by the progressive loss of apical progenitor-derived molecular birthmarks and the emergence of input-dependent transcriptional programs. The temporal progression in apical progenitor states is itself likely largely cell-autonomous. It is epigenetically regulated by molecules such as the Polycomb repressor complex PRC2, whose loss accelerates apical progenitor neurogenic competencies (Telley et al. 2019).

Extrinsic factors, however, also come into play, as progressive changes in the membrane potential progenitors during corticogenesis coordinate the successive generation of distinct neuronal subtypes and manipulations of membrane potential affect progenitor neurogenic properties (Vitali et al. 2018). Similarly, thalamocortical input has a mitogenic effect on neuronal progenitors in vitro (Dehay et al. 2001). Also, Ephrin A5, expressed by thalamocortical axons, binds to EphA4 on apical progenitors to regulate the generation of intermediate progenitors and, therefore, the neuronal output for cortical layers (Gerstmann et al. 2015). Consistent with some level of extrinsic drive over apical progenitor identity, recent transplantation experiments have shown that contrary to what had been previously thought, these cells can normally generate earlier-born neurons when transplanted into a younger host, in a process driven by extracellular WNT levels. By contrast, intermediate progenitors are committed progenitors that lack such retrograde fate plasticity, emphasizing the importance of a cell-type-specific understanding of extrinsic and intrinsic drivers of cellular identity (Oberst et al. 2019).

Although out of the scope of this chapter, the development of cortical astrocytes and oligodendrocytes also relies heavily on interactions with their environment and activity-dependent processes. Astrocytes are generated after cortical neurons but play an important role in synapse formation and function (for a review on astrocyte role in cortical circuit development, see Farhy-Tselnicker and Allen 2018). For example, increased neuronal activity extends the astrocyte coverage of dendritic spines and the number of spines contacted by astrocyte processes (Bernardinelli et al. 2014; Genoud et al. 2006), while deleting the glutamate transporter VGLUT1 results in fewer contacts between astrocytes and synapses (Morel et al. 2014). Likewise, neuronal activity regulates oligodendrocyte progenitor proliferation, differentiation and myelin remodeling; and glutamatergic signaling through AMPA receptors from active axons influences the survival of pre-myelinating oligodendrocytes (Gibson et al. 2014; Kougioumtzidou et al. 2017).

14.3 Outstanding Questions and Perspectives

The past ten years have seen a shift in our approach to studying input-dependent differentiation. While historically, experiments involving lesions or environmental deprivation have been used to assess macroscopic effects on brain structure and patterning, we are now in the position to interrogate circuit formation and transcriptional controls with cell-type specificity using spatially and temporally constrained manipulations of specific circuits. Further insights into the relationship between spontaneous activity and experience-dependent activity are required; how activity patterns can be engineered ex-vivo to pattern cells in vitro is critical too, and the potential for plasticity to define the identity of mature neurons and cell types remains poorly explored and understood. In this context, the extent to which circuits in novel in vitro systems, such as organoids, recapitulate what is found in vivo is still unclear. However, basic wiring patterns seem preserved (e.g., in assembloids, cortex projects to striatum and not vice versa, as is the case in vivo; Miura et al. 2020). Reverse engineering of developing cortical circuits in vitro through combinations of genetic strategies and optogenetic emulation of activity patterns will be an exciting challenge for the years to come.

References

Ackman, J.B. et al. (2012). Retinal waves coordinate patterned activity throughout the developing visual system. *Nature* 490: 219–225. doi: 10.1038/nature11529.

Alfano, C. et al. (2014). Postmitotic control of sensory area specification during neocortical development. *Nat Commun* 5: 5632. doi: 10.1038/ncomms6632.

Allendoerfer, K.L. and Shatz, C.J. (1994). The subplate, a transient neocortical structure. *Ann Rev Neurosci* 17: 185–218.

Amunts, K. and Zilles, K. (2015). Architectonic mapping of the human brain beyond brodmann. *Neuron* 88: 1086–1107. doi: 10.1016/j.neuron.2015.12.001.

Armentano, M. et al. (2007). COUP-TFI regulates the balance of cortical patterning between frontal/motor and sensory areas. *Nat Neurosci* 10: 1277–1286. doi: 10.1038/nn1958.

Barber, M. and Pierani, A. (2016). Tangential migration of glutamatergic neurons and cortical patterning during development: lessons from Cajal-Retzius cells. *Dev Neurobiol* 76: 847–881. doi: 10.1002/dneu.22363.

Bekkers, J.M. and Suzuki, N. (2013). Neurons and circuits for odor processing in the piriform cortex. *Trends Neurosci* 36: 429–438. doi: 10.1016/j.tins.2013.04.005.

Bernardinelli, Y. et al. (2014). Activity-dependent structural plasticity of perisynaptic astrocytic domains promotes excitatory synapse stability. *Curr Biol* 24: 1679–1688. doi: 10.1016/j.cub.2014.06.025.

Bienenstock, E. (1996). On the dimensionality of cortical graphs. *J Physiol-Paris* 90: 251–256. doi: 10.1016/S0928-4257(97)81434-9.

Bishop, K.M. et al. (2000). Regulation of area identity in the mammalian neocortex by *Emx2* and *Pax6*. *Science* 288: 344–349. doi: 10.1126/science.288.5464.344.

Blanquie, O. et al. (2016). NKCC1-mediated GABAergic signaling promotes postnatal cell death in neocortical Cajal–Retzius cells. *Cereb Cortex* 27 (2): 1644–1659. doi: 10.1093/cercor/bhw004.

Buckner, R.L. and Krienen, F.M. (2013). The evolution of distributed association networks in the human brain. *Trends Cogn Sci* 17: 648–665. doi: 10.1016/j.tics.2013.09.017.

Burbridge, T.J. et al. (2014). Visual circuit development requires patterned activity mediated by retinal acetylcholine receptors. *Neuron* 84: 1049–1064. doi: 10.1016/j.neuron.2014.10.051.

Cadwell, C.R. et al. (2019). Development and arealization of the cerebral cortex. *Neuron* 103: 980–1004. doi: 10.1016/j.neuron.2019.07.009.

Callaway, E.M. and Borrell, V. (2011). Developmental sculpting of dendritic morphology of layer 4 neurons in visual cortex. *J Neurosci* 31: 7456–7470. doi: 10.1523/JNEUROSCI.5222-10.2011.

Cappello, S. et al. (2012). A radial glia-specific role of Rhoa in double cortex formation. *Neuron* 73: 911–924. doi: 10.1016/j.neuron.2011.12.030.

Carcea, I. et al. (2014). Maturation of cortical circuits requires Semaphorin 7A. *Proc Natl Acad Sci USA* 111: 13978–13983. doi: 10.1073/pnas.1408680111.

Catalano, S.M. and Shatz, C.J. (1998). Activity-dependent cortical target selection by thalamic axons. *Science* 281: 559–562. doi: 10.1126/science.281.5376.559.

Chen, M.B. et al. (2020). Persistent transcriptional programmes are associated with remote memory. *Nature* 587: 437–442. doi: 10.1038/s41586-020-2905-5.

Cheng, S. et al. (2022). Vision-dependent specification of cell types and function in the developing cortex. *Cell* 185: 311–327.e24. doi: 10.1016/j.cell.2021.12.022.

Chou, S.-J. et al. (2013). Geniculocortical input drives genetic distinctions between primary and higher-order visual areas. *Science* 340: 1239–1242. doi: 10.1126/science.1232806.

Constantinople, C.M. and Bruno, R.M. (2013). Deep cortical layers are activated directly by thalamus. *Science* 340: 1591–1594. doi: 10.1126/science.1236425.

Davis, M.F. et al. (2015). Inhibitory neuron transplantation into adult visual cortex creates a new critical period that rescues impaired vision. *Neuron* 86: 1055–1066. doi: 10.1016/j.neuron.2015.03.062.

de Frutos, C.A. et al. (2016). Reallocation of olfactory Cajal-Retzius cells shapes neocortex architecture. *Neuron* 92: 435–448. doi: 10.1016/j.neuron.2016.09.020.

De la Rossa, A. et al. (2013 February). In vivo reprogramming of circuit connectivity in postmitotic neocortical neurons. *Nat Neurosci* 16 (2): 193–200. doi: 10.1038/nn.3299. Epub 2013 Jan 6. PMID: 23292682.

De León Reyes, N.S. et al. (2019). Transient callosal projections of L4 neurons are eliminated for the acquisition of local connectivity. *Nat Commun* 10: 4549. doi: 10.1038/s41467-019-12495-w.

Dehay, C. et al. (2001). Cell-cycle kinetics of neocortical precursors are influenced by embryonic thalamic axons. *J Neurosci* 21: 201–214. doi: 10.1523/JNEUROSCI.21-01-00201.2001.

Del Pino, I. et al. (2020). COUP-TFI/Nr2f1 orchestrates intrinsic neuronal activity during development of the somatosensory cortex. *Cereb Cortex* 30: 5667–5685. doi: 10.1093/cercor/bhaa137.

Dong, H. et al. (2004). Experience-dependent development of feedforward and feedback circuits between lower and higher areas of mouse visual cortex. *Vision Res* 44: 3389–3400. doi: 10.1016/j.visres.2004.09.007.

Dugas-Ford, J. et al. (2012). Cell-type homologies and the origins of the neocortex. *Proc Natl Acad Sci USA* 109: 16974–16979. doi: 10.1073/pnas.1204773109.

Erzurumlu, R.S. and Gaspar, P. (2012). Development and critical period plasticity of the barrel cortex: barrel cortex plasticity. *Eur J Neurosci* 35: 1540–1553. doi: 10.1111/j.1460-9568.2012.08075.x.

Farhy-Tselnicker, I. and Allen, N.J. (2018). Astrocytes, neurons, synapses. *Neural Dev* 13 (1): 7. doi: 10.1186/s13064-018-0104-y.

Fox, K. and Wong, R.O.L. (2005). A comparison of experience-dependent plasticity in the visual and somatosensory systems. *Neuron* 48: 465–477. doi: 10.1016/j.neuron.2005.10.013.

Frangeul, L. et al. (2017). Input-dependent regulation of excitability controls dendritic maturation in somatosensory thalamocortical neurons. *Nat Commun* 8 (1): 2015. doi: 10.1038/s41467-017-02172-1.

Frangeul, L. et al. (2016). A cross-modal genetic framework for the development and plasticity of sensory pathways. *Nature* 538: 96–98. doi: 10.1038/nature19770.

Genescu, I. and Garel, S. (2021). Being superficial. *Curr Opin Neurobiol* 66: 125–134. doi: 10.1016/j.conb.2020.10.003.

Genoud, C. et al. (2006). Plasticity of astrocytic coverage and glutamate transporter expression in adult mouse cortex. *PLoS Biol* 4: e343. doi: 10.1371/journal.pbio.0040343.

Gerstmann, K. et al. (2015). Thalamic afferents influence cortical progenitors via ephrin A5-EphA4 interactions. *Development* 142: 140–150. doi: 10.1242/dev.104927.

Giasafaki, C. et al. (2022). Cross-hierarchical plasticity of corticofugal projections to dLGN after neonatal monocular enucleation. *J Comp Neurol* 530: 978–997. doi: 10.1002/cne.25304.

Gibson, E.M. et al. (2014). Neuronal activity promotes oligodendrogenesis and adaptive myelination in the mammalian brain. *Science* 344: 1252304. doi: 10.1126/science.1252304.

Grant, E. (2016). The regulation of corticofugal fiber targeting by retinal inputs. *Cereb Cortex* 26: 1336–1348. doi: 10.1093/cercor/bhv315.

Griveau, A. et al. (2010). A novel role for Dbx1-derived cajal-retzius cells in early regionalization of the cerebral cortical neuroepithelium. *PLoS Biol* 8: e1000440. doi: 10.1371/journal.pbio.1000440.

Guy, J. and Staiger, J.F. (2017). The functioning of a cortex without layers. *Front Neuroanat* 11: 54. doi: 10.3389/fnana.2017.00054.

Halassa, M.M. and Sherman, S.M. (2019). Thalamocortical circuit motifs. *Neuron* 103: 762–770. doi: 10.1016/j.neuron.2019.06.005.

Hippenmeyer, S. (2014). Molecular pathways controlling the sequential steps of cortical projection neuron migration. In: *Cellular and Molecular Control of Neuronal Migration, Advances in Experimental Medicine and Biology* (ed. L. Nguyen and S. Hippenmeyer), 1–24. Netherlands, Dordrecht: Springer. doi: 10.1007/978-94-007-7687-6_1.

Hooks, B.M. and Chen, C. (2020). Circuitry underlying experience-dependent plasticity in the mouse visual system. *Neuron* 106: 21–36. doi: 10.1016/j.neuron.2020.01.031.

Hrvatin, S. et al. (2018). Single-cell analysis of experience-dependent transcriptomic states in the mouse visual cortex. *Nat Neurosci* 21: 120–129. doi: 10.1038/s41593-017-0029-5.

Hurni, N. et al. (2017). Transient cell-intrinsic activity regulates the migration and laminar positioning of cortical projection neurons. *Cereb Cortex* 27: 3052–3063. doi: 10.1093/cercor/bhx059.

Imam, N. and Finlay, B.L. (2020). Self-organization of cortical areas in the development and evolution of neocortex. *Procee Natl Acad Sci USA* 117: 29212–29220. doi: 10.1073/pnas.2011724117.

Iwasato, T. et al. (2008). Cortical adenylyl cyclase 1 is required for thalamocortical synapse maturation and aspects of layer IV barrel Development. *J Neurosci* 28: 5931–5943. doi: 10.1523/JNEUROSCI.0815-08.2008.

Jabaudon, D. et al. (2012). RORβ induces barrel-like neuronal clusters in the developing neocortex. *Cereb Cortex* 22: 996–1006. doi: 10.1093/cercor/bhr182.

Jiao, Y. (2006). Major effects of sensory experiences on the neocortical inhibitory circuits. *J Neurosci* 26: 8691–8701. doi: 10.1523/JNEUROSCI.2478-06.2006.

Kanold, P.O. and Luhmann, H.J. (2010). The subplate and early cortical circuits. *Ann Rev Neurosci* 33: 23–48.

Karten, H.J. (2013). Neocortical evolution. *Curr Biol* 23: R12–R15. doi: 10.1016/j.cub.2012.11.013.

Klingler, E. et al. (2019). A translaminar genetic logic for the circuit identity of intracortically projecting neurons. *Curr Biol* 29: 332–339.e5. doi: 10.1016/j.cub.2018.11.071.

Klingler, E. et al. (2021). Temporal controls over inter-areal cortical projection neuron fate diversity. *Nature* 599: 453–457. doi: 10.1038/s41586-021-04048-3.

Kougioumtzidou, E. et al. (2017). Signalling through AMPA receptors on oligodendrocyte precursors promotes myelination by enhancing oligodendrocyte survival. *Elife* 6: e28080. doi: 10.7554/eLife.28080.

Krug, K. et al. (1998). The development of topography in the hamster geniculo-cortical projection. *J Neurosci* 18: 5766–5776. doi: 10.1523/JNEUROSCI.18-15-05766.1998.

Ledonne, F. et al. (2016). Targeted inactivation of Bax reveals a subtype-specific mechanism of Cajal-Retzius neuron death in the postnatal cerebral cortex. *Cell Rep* 17: 3133–3141. doi: 10.1016/j.celrep.2016.11.074.

Li, H. et al. (2013). Laminar and columnar development of barrel cortex relies on thalamocortical neurotransmission. *Neuron* 79: 970–986. doi: 10.1016/j.neuron.2013.06.043.

Libé-Philippot, B. and Vanderhaeghen, P. (2021). Cellular and molecular mechanisms linking human cortical development and evolution. *Annu Rev Genet* 55: 555–581.

Liu, Q. et al. (2000). Differential expression of COUP-TFI, CHL1, and two novel genes in developing neocortex identified by differential display PCR. *J Neurosci* 20: 7682–7690. doi: 10.1523/JNEUROSCI.20-20-07682.2000.

Lodato, S. et al. (2011). Excitatory projection neuron subtypes control the distribution of local inhibitory interneurons in the cerebral cortex. *Neuron* 69: 763–779. doi: 10.1016/j.neuron.2011.01.015.

Lohse, M. et al. (2021). Subcortical circuits mediate communication between primary sensory cortical areas in mice. *Nat Commun* 12: 3916. doi: 10.1038/s41467-021-24200-x.

Lu, H.-C. et al. (2006). Role of efficient neurotransmitter release in barrel map development. *J Neurosci* 26: 2692–2703. doi: 10.1523/JNEUROSCI.3956-05.2006.

Mardinly, A.R. et al. (2016). Sensory experience regulates cortical inhibition by inducing IGF1 in VIP neurons. *Nature* 531: 371–375. doi: 10.1038/nature17187.

Martini, F.J. et al. (2021). Spontaneous activity in developing thalamic and cortical sensory networks. *Neuron* 109: 2519–2534. doi: 10.1016/j.neuron.2021.06.026.

Matsui, A. et al. (2013). BTBD3 controls dendrite orientation toward active axons in mammalian neocortex. *Science* 342: 1114–1118. doi: 10.1126/science.1244505.

Miller-Hansen, A.J. and Sherman, S.M. (2022). Conserved patterns of functional organization between cortex and thalamus in mice. *Proc Natl Acad Sci USA* 119: e2201481119. doi: 10.1073/pnas.2201481119.

Miura, Y. et al. (2020). Generation of human striatal organoids and cortico-striatal assembloids from human pluripotent stem cells. *Nat Biotechnol* 38: 1421–1430. doi: 10.1038/s41587-020-00763-w.

Miyashita-Lin, E.M. et al. (1999). Early neocortical regionalization in the absence of thalamic innervation. *Science* 285: 906–909. doi: 10.1126/science.285.5429.906.

Mizuno, H. et al. (2010). Pre-synaptic and post-synaptic neuronal activity supports the axon development of callosal projection neurons during different post-natal periods in the mouse cerebral cortex. *Eur J Neurosci* 31: 410–424. doi: 10.1111/j.1460-9568.2009.07070.x.

Mizuno, H. et al. (2014). NMDAR-regulated dynamics of layer 4 neuronal dendrites during thalamocortical reorganization in neonates. *Neuron* 82: 365–379. doi: 10.1016/j.neuron.2014.02.026.

Molnár, Z. et al. (2002). Normal development of embryonic thalamocortical connectivity in the absence of evoked synaptic activity. *J Neurosci* 22: 10313–10323. doi: 10.1523/JNEUROSCI.22-23-10313.2002.

Molyneaux, B.J. et al. (2005 September 15). Fezl is required for the birth and specification of corticospinal motor neurons. *Neuron* 47 (6): 817–831. doi: 10.1016/j.neuron.2005.08.030. PMID: 16157277.

Molyneaux, B.J. et al. (2007). Neuronal subtype specification in the cerebral cortex. *Nat Rev Neurosci* 8: 427–437. doi: 10.1038/nrn2151.

Morel, L. et al. (2014). VGluT1+ neuronal glutamatergic signaling regulates postnatal developmental maturation of cortical protoplasmic astroglia. *J Neurosci* 34: 10950–10962. doi: 10.1523/JNEUROSCI.1167-14.2014.

Moreno-Juan, V. et al. (2017). Prenatal thalamic waves regulate cortical area size prior to sensory processing. *Nat Commun* 8: 14172. doi: 10.1038/ncomms14172.

Nakazawa, S. et al. (2018). Differential dynamics of cortical neuron dendritic trees revealed by long-term in vivo imaging in neonates. *Nat Commun* 9: 3106. doi: 10.1038/s41467-018-05563-0.

Narboux-Neme, N. et al. (2012). Neurotransmitter release at the thalamocortical synapse instructs barrel formation but not axon patterning in the somatosensory cortex. *J Neurosci* 32: 6183–6196. doi: 10.1523/JNEUROSCI.0343-12.2012.

O'Leary, D.D.M. (1989). Do cortical areas emerge from a protocortex. *Trends Neurosci* 12 (10): 400–406.

Oberst, P. et al. (2019). Temporal plasticity of apical progenitors in the developing mouse neocortex. *Nature* 573: 370–374. doi: 10.1038/s41586-019-1515-6.

Ogawa, M. et al. (1995). The Reeler gene-associated antigen on Cajal-Retzius neurons is a crucial molecule for laminar organization of cortical neurons. *Neuron* 14: 14.

Oishi, K. et al. (2016). Mutually repressive interaction between Brn1/2 and Rorb contributes to the establishment of neocortical layer 2/3 and layer 4. *Proc Natl Acad Sci USA* 113: 3371–3376. doi: 10.1073/pnas.1515949113.

Pal, S. et al. (2021). An early cortical progenitor-specific mechanism regulates thalamocortical innervation. *J Neurosci* 41: 6822–6835. doi: 10.1523/JNEUROSCI.0226-21.2021.

Pouchelon, G. et al. (2014). Modality-specific thalamocortical inputs instruct the identity of postsynaptic L4 neurons. *Nature* 511: 471–474. doi: 10.1038/nature13390.

Pouchelon, G. and Jabaudon, D. (2014). Nurturing the cortex's thalamic nature. *Curr Opin Neurol* 27: 142–148. doi: 10.1097/WCO.0000000000000070.

Price, D.J. and Lotto, R.B. (1996). Influences of the thalamus on the survival of subplate and cortical plate cells in cultured embryonic mouse brain. *J Neurosci* 16: 3247–3255. doi: 10.1523/JNEUROSCI.16-10-03247.1996.

Puiggros, S.R. and Jabaudon, D. (2022). Visual identity isn't a light decision for all neurons. *Nature* 37–38. doi: 10.1038/d41586-022-00463-2.

Rakic, P. (1988). Specification of cerebral cortical areas. *Science* 241: 170–176. doi: 10.1126/science.3291116.

Riva, M. et al. (2019). Activity-dependent death of transient Cajal-Retzius neurons is required for functional cortical wiring. *Elife* 8: e50503. doi: 10.7554/eLife.50503.

Rodríguez-Tornos, F.M. et al. (2016). Cux1 enables interhemispheric connections of layer II/III neurons by regulating Kv1-dependent firing. *Neuron* 89: 494–506. doi: 10.1016/j.neuron.2015.12.020.

Rubenstein, J.L.R. (1999). Genetic control of cortical development. *Cereb Cortex* 9: 521–523. doi: 10.1093/cercor/9.6.521.

Seabrook, T.A. et al. (2013). Retinal input regulates the timing of corticogeniculate innervation. *J Neurosci* 33: 10085–10097. doi: 10.1523/JNEUROSCI.5271-12.2013.

Sekine, K. et al. (2014). How does Reelin control neuronal migration and layer formation in the developing mammalian neocortex? *Neurosci Res* 86: 50–58. doi: 10.1016/j.neures.2014.06.004.

Shatz, C.J. (1996). Emergence of order in visual system development. *Proc Natl Acad Sci USA* 93 (2): 602–608. doi: 10.1073/pnas.93.2.602.

Shetty, A.S. et al. (2013). Lhx2 regulates a cortex-specific mechanism for barrel formation. *Proc Natl Acad Sci USA* 110 (50): E4913–21. doi: 10.1073/pnas.1311158110.

Smedler, E. et al. (2022). Disrupted Cacna1c gene expression perturbs spontaneous Ca2+ activity causing abnormal brain development and increased anxiety. *Proc Natl Acad Sci USA* 119: e2108768119. doi: 10.1073/pnas.2108768119.

Spiegel, I. et al. (2014). Npas4 regulates excitatory-inhibitory balance within neural circuits through cell-type-specific gene programs. *Cell* 157: 1216–1229. doi: 10.1016/j.cell.2014.03.058.

Suárez, R. et al. (2014). Balanced interhemispheric cortical activity is required for correct targeting of the corpus callosum. *Neuron* 82: 1289–1298. doi: 10.1016/j.neuron.2014.04.040.

Sur, M. and Rubenstein, J.L.R. (2005). Patterning and plasticity of the cerebral cortex. *Science* 310: 805–810. doi: 10.1126/science.1112070.

Suzuki, A. et al. (2015). Thalamic adenylyl cyclase 1 is required for barrel formation in the somatosensory cortex. *Neuroscience* 290: 518–529. doi: 10.1016/j.neuroscience.2015.01.043.

Sydnor, V.J. et al. (2021). Neurodevelopment of the association cortices. *Neuron* 109: 2820–2846. doi: 10.1016/j.neuron.2021.06.016.

Tasic, B. et al. (2018). Shared and distinct transcriptomic cell types across neocortical areas. *Nature* 563: 72–78. doi: 10.1038/s41586-018-0654-5.

Telley, L. et al. (2019). Temporal patterning of apical progenitors and their daughter neurons in the developing neocortex. *Science* 364: eaav2522. doi: 10.1126/science.aav2522.

Tyssowski, K.M. et al. (2018). Different neuronal activity patterns induce different gene expression programs. *Neuron* 98: 530–546.e11. doi: 10.1016/j.neuron.2018.04.001.

Van der Loos, H. and Woolsey, T.A. (1973). Somatosensory cortex. *Science* 179: 395–398. doi: 10.1126/science.179.4071.395.

Vitali, I. et al. (2018). Progenitor hyperpolarization regulates the sequential generation of neuronal subtypes in the developing neocortex. *Cell* 174: 1264–1276.e15. doi: 10.1016/j.cell.2018.06.036.

Vue, T.Y. et al. (2013). Thalamic control of neocortical area formation in mice. *J Neurosci* 33: 8442–8453. doi: 10.1523/JNEUROSCI.5786-12.2013.

Wamsley, B. and Fishell, G. (2017). Genetic and activity-dependent mechanisms underlying interneuron diversity. *Nat Rev Neurosci* 18: 299–309. doi: 10.1038/nrn.2017.30.

Wang, B.-S. et al. (2021). Retinal and callosal activity-dependent chandelier cell elimination shapes binocularity in primary visual cortex. *Neuron* 109: 502–515.e7. doi: 10.1016/j.neuron.2020.11.004.

Wang, C.-F. et al. (2017). Lhx2 expression in postmitotic cortical neurons initiates assembly of the thalamocortical somatosensory circuit. *Cell Rep* 18: 849–856. doi: 10.1016/j.celrep.2017.01.001.

Wang, C.-F. et al. (2023). Activity-dependent feedback regulation of thalamocortical axon development by Lhx2 in cortical layer 4 neurons. *Cereb Cortex* 33 (5): 1693–1707. doi: 10.1093/cercor/bhac166.

Wang, C.-L. et al. (2007). Activity-dependent development of callosal projections in the somatosensory cortex. *J Neurosci* 27: 11334–11342. doi: 10.1523/JNEUROSCI.3380-07.2007.

Wijetunge, L.S. et al. (2008). mGluR5 regulates glutamate-dependent development of the mouse somatosensory cortex. *J Neurosci* 28: 13028–13037. doi: 10.1523/JNEUROSCI.2600-08.2008.

Wong, F.K. and Marín, O. (2019). Developmental cell death in the cerebral cortex. *Ann Rev Cell Dev Biol* 35: 523–542. doi: 10.1146/annurev-cellbio-100818-125204.

Woolsey, T.A. and Van der Loos, H. (1970). The structural organization of layer IV in the somatosensory region (SI) of mouse cerebral cortex. The description of a cortical field composed of discrete cytoarchitectonic units. *Brain Res* 17 (2): 205–242. doi: 10.1016/0006-8993(70)90079-x.

Zembrzycki, A. et al. (2015). Postmitotic regulation of sensory area patterning in the mammalian neocortex by Lhx2. *Proc Natl Acad Sci USA* 112: 6736–6741. doi: 10.1073/pnas.1424440112.

Zhang, J. et al. (2012). Visual map development depends on the temporal pattern of binocular activity in mice. *Nat Neurosci* 15: 298–307. doi: 10.1038/nn.3007.

Zheng, X. et al. (2021). Host interneurons mediate plasticity reactivated by embryonic inhibitory cell transplantation in mouse visual cortex. *Nat Commun* 12: 862. doi: 10.1038/s41467-021-21097-4.

Zhou, C. et al. (2001). COUP-TFI: an intrinsic factor for early regionalization of the neocortex. *Genes Dev* 15: 2054–2059. doi: 10.1101/gad.913601.

Zhou, L. et al. (2008). Early forebrain wiring: genetic dissection using conditional *Celsr3* mutant mice. *Science* 320: 946–949. doi: 10.1126/science.1155244.

Zhou, L. et al. (2010). Maturation of "neocortex isole" in vivo in mice. *J Neurosci* 30: 7928–7939. doi: 10.1523/JNEUROSCI.6005-09.2010.

Zilles, K. and Amunts, K. (2010). Centenary of Brodmann's map — conception and fate. *Nat Rev Neurosci* 11: 139–145. doi: 10.1038/nrn2776.

15

Corpus Callosum Evolution and Development

Catarina Martins-Costa[1,2] *and Jürgen A. Knoblich*[1,3,*]

[1] *IMBA – Institute of Molecular Biotechnology of the Austrian Academy of Sciences, Vienna Biocenter (VBC), Vienna, Austria*
[2] *Vienna BioCenter PhD Program, Doctoral School of the University of Vienna and Medical University of Vienna, Vienna, Austria*
[3] *Medical University of Vienna, Department of Neurology, Vienna, Austria*
[*] *Corresponding author*

All animals belonging to the *bilateria* clade present a near-symmetry about the midsagittal body plane, including in the nervous system (Arendt et al. 2008; Semmler et al. 2010). A key feature of bilaterally symmetrical bodies is coordinated contralateral communication. This function is carried out by axon tracts that cross the body midline at different levels of the CNS axis, called commissures. The importance of these structures is showcased by the cruciality of contralateral coordination in mobility, locomotion, and posture, largely mediated by the spinal commissural system (Maxwell and Soteropoulos 2020). Similarly, integration of information across distant brain regions relies on interhemispheric routes of communication. In this chapter, we focus on the evolution and development of the main brain commissure of eutherian mammals, the corpus callosum (CC). We start by giving a broad overview on commissure evolution in vertebrates, which culminated with the emergence of the CC. Thereafter, the chapter follows the temporal sequence of CC development: generation of callosal projection neurons (CPNs), axon guidance mechanisms, and establishment of contralateral connections. Finally, we examine the properties of the adult human CC and the implications of its loss in disease. Throughout, we draw parallels between CC development and that of other commissures, especially focusing on events that reflect evolution and neuronal plasticity.

15.1 Evolution of Telencephalic Commissures

15.1.1 Interhemispheric Connections in Vertebrates

Telencephalic commissures have undergone drastic changes during vertebrate evolution. Commissural innovations include axon rerouting through preexistent pathways and appearance of entirely new tracts (Suárez 2017; Suárez et al. 2014b; Suárez et al. 2018) (Figure 15.1A). The anterior commissure (AC) is the most ancient interhemispheric connection route in vertebrates. It is already present in non-tetrapods, travelling through the subpallium and interconnecting regions related to universal basic functions, like olfaction and survival (Fenlon et al. 2021; Shang et al. 1997; Wullimann et al. 1996). Dorsal to the AC, sauropsids (reptiles and birds) evolved the hippocampal commissure (HC), which connects the hippocampi and projects to the septum and parahippocampal areas (Abellán and Medina 2009; Cui et al. 2013; Ebner 1969; Nomura et al. 2013, 2018; Osborn 1886; Silver et al. 1982; Tosches et al. 2018). Connections through the AC and HC are evolutionarily maintained thereafter, including in non-eutherian mammals, such as monotremes

Neocortical Neurogenesis in Development and Evolution, First Edition. Edited by Wieland B. Huttner.

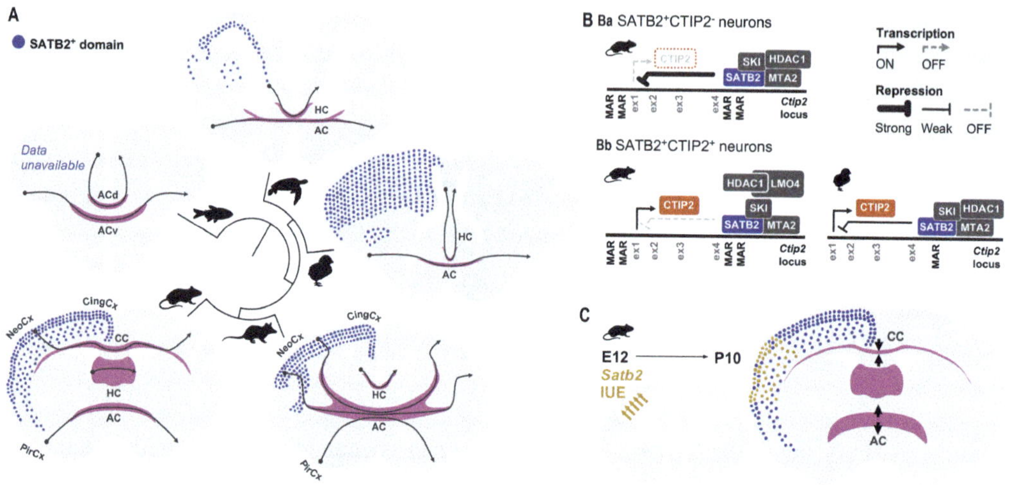

Figure 15.1 Evolution of telencephalic commissures and gene regulatory networks. (A) Diagram of the telencephalic commissures and domain of SATB2^{+} neurons in the adult brain of the fish (Wullimann et al. 1996), turtle (Nomura et al. 2013; Osborn 1886; Tosches et al. 2018), chicken (Abellán and Medina 2009; Nomura et al. 2018), dunnart (Paolino et al. 2020), and mouse (Paolino et al. 2020). The AC is the most ancient commissure, already present in non-tetrapods. In addition, sauropsids evolved the HC. Although SATB2^{+} neurons are seen across vertebrates and a six-layered neocortex is present in most mammals, the CC is an evolutionary innovation in eutherian mammals. (B) Modulation of *Ctip2* transcription by SATB2. (Ba) In the mouse, layer II/III CPNs (SATB2^{+}CTIP2^{-}) are generated by assembly of a NurD complex – SATB2, MTA2, SKI and HDAC1 – at several MARs of the *Ctip2* locus, leading to deacetylation and silencing (Alcamo et al. 2008; Baranek et al. 2012; Nomura et al. 2018). (Bb) In contrast, generation of SATB2^{+}CTIP2^{+} neurons in layer V depends on sequestration of HDAC1 by LMO4, leading to de-repression and transcriptional activation of the *Ctip2* locus (Harb et al. 2016). In the chicken, however, extensive SATB2 and CTIP2 co-expression is possible given the presence of only one MAR with attenuated transcription suppression activity at the *Ctip2* locus (Nomura et al. 2018). (C) *Satb2* expression onset occurs at stage 20 (S20) in the dunnart, but not until S22 (E14) in the mouse. Over-expression of *Satb2* in the mouse at stage 20 (E12) via in utero electroporation leads to decreased projections through the CC and increased projections through the AC, mimicking the non-eutherian connectome (Paolino et al. 2020). AC, anterior commissure (ACd, dorsal AC; ACv, ventral AC); CC, corpus callosum; CingCx, cingulate cortex; ex, exon; HC, hippocampal commissure; IUE, *in utero* electroporation; MAR, matrix attachment region; NeoCx, neocortex; PirCx, piriform cortex.

and marsupials (Paolino et al. 2020; Suárez et al. 2018). The CC, however, is an evolutionary innovation exclusive to eutherian mammals. It is located dorsally to the hippocampal commissure and connects most areas of the neocortex, the cingulate cortex, and the claustrum (Aboitiz and Montiel 2003; Ebner 1969; Paolino et al. 2020; Rakic and Yakovlev 1968; Silver et al. 1982). In eutherian development, the AC is the first commissure to appear, followed by the HC and finally the CC (Ashwell et al. 1996). Notably, the development of different clades of mammals occurs in dramatically different environments: monotremes hatch from eggs, non-eutherians are born underdeveloped and continue to mature outside the mother's body, and eutherians undergo prolonged intrauterine gestation (Abbot and Capra 2017; Guernsey et al. 2017). Thus, it is not surprising that such dramatic differences led to significant changes in brain development. Interestingly, though, global features of interhemispheric connectivity, including layered organization of commissural neurons and connections between similar regions of each hemisphere, span all mammals, having arisen at least 80 million years before the CC (Suárez et al. 2018). Ultimately, the emergence of such a prominent structure raises the question: which events mediated CC evolution?

15.1.2 Evolutionary Appearance of the CC

The appearance of the CC has been linked to broad and profound anatomical and cellular innovations that arose during evolution. In fact, significant structural novelties are exclusively observed in eutherian mammals, such as the closure of the septum along the interhemispheric fissure (Gobius et al. 2016; Katz et al. 1983; Silver et al. 1982; Suárez 2017) (see Section 15.4.4.1). Another contribution comes from the different developmental timings in eutherian compared to non-eutherian mammals – a phenomenon known as heterochronicity (Kozulin et al. 2022; Paolino et al. 2020) (see Section 15.2.3). At the cellular and molecular level, protracted neuronal development resulted in expansion of the upper cortical layers, leading to increased number and complexity of cell types, including CPNs (Berg et al. 2021; Fame et al. 2017; Smart 2002) (see Section 15.2.5). Finally, at the functional level, connection through the CC presents advantages in wiring of larger brains – it allows fast interhemispheric transfer of information while minimizing volume, total wiring length, and conduction delay (Ashwell 2016; Neves et al. 2017; Wang et al. 2008) (see Section 15.6.1). Overall, these studies highlight how adaptation to distinct brain topographies, developmental timing, and novel cell populations correlate with the evolutionary emergence of the CC. What remains unclear, however, is which (if any) of these processes was causative, or if, instead, the combination of multiple factors culminated in CC evolution.

15.2 Molecular Characterization of Callosal Projection Neurons

15.2.1 SATB2, a Marker of CPNs

CPNs are found in the cingulate cortex, derived from the medial pallium, and in the neocortex, part of the dorso-lateral pallium (García-Moreno and Molnár 2015; Medina and Abellán 2009). Their cell bodies reside in layers II through VI of the cortex, with the majority in layer II/III (80 percent in the mouse) (Alcamo et al. 2008; Britanova et al. 2008; Molyneaux et al. 2009). In 2008, the studies of Olga Britanova and Elisabeth Alcamo spearheaded the identification of the transcription factor (TF) AT-rich sequence-binding protein 2 (SATB2) as a determinant of CPN identity in the mouse cortex (Alcamo et al. 2008; Britanova et al. 2008). Both studies found that *Satb2*$^{-/-}$ mice presented agenesis (absence) of the corpus callosum (ACC). Remarkably, SATB2$^{-/-}$ axons were found redirected to the internal capsule, projecting along the path of normal corticospinal axons, as well as to the AC (Figure 15.2B, the phenotypes of several mouse mutants described throughout this chapter are depicted in Figure 15.2B–D). Thus, loss of *Satb2* not only precluded CC formation, but also seemed to impact global fate-acquisition dynamics in the cerebral cortex, eliminating the callosal projection neuron population. These findings marked a crucial turning point that opened way to entirely new experimental possibilities in the study of the CC and, more generally, corticogenesis. Since then, a vast repertoire of SATB2 functions and interactors has been described.

15.2.2 Gene Regulatory Networks in the Differentiation of Projection Neurons

During corticogenesis, early-born deep-layer (DL) neurons mainly project subcortically; and late-born upper-layer (UL) neurons mainly project contralaterally. Notably, however, CPN specification spans different developmental stages, happening in two main waves in the mouse: a minority of CPNs are born early (E11.5–E13.5) from progenitors located in the ventricular zone underlying the neocortex and occupy the deep layers; and the majority of CPNs are born later (peak at

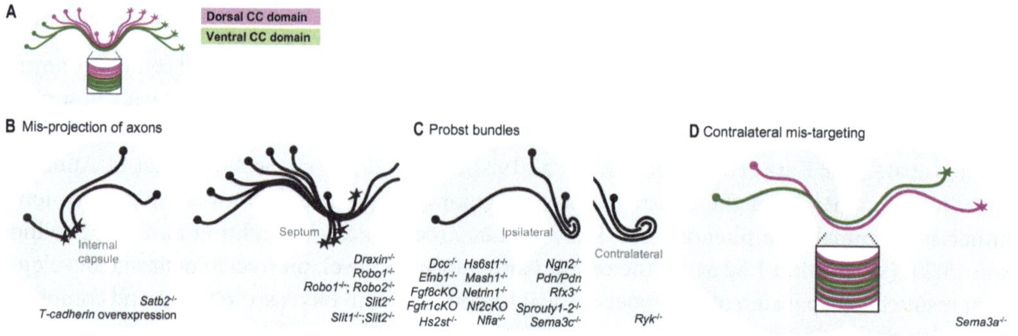

Figure 15.2 Mouse models of CC defects. (A) In the wild-type mouse brain, there is orderly projection of callosal axons across the midline and formation of mostly homotopic contralateral connections. Phenotypes seen in mutants include misprojection of axons to ectopic regions, such as the internal capsule (B, left) or the septum (B, right); formation of Probst bundles either in the ipsilateral (C, left) or in the contralateral (C, right) hemisphere; and loss of CC domains, with disorganized axonal crossing and mistargeting on the contralateral hemisphere (D). Some of these models present a mixture of phenotypes; the predominant one is depicted here. cHet, conditional heterozygous mutation; cKO, conditional knockout. **References:** *Satb2*$^{-/-}$ (Alcamo et al. 2008; Britanova et al. 2008), T-cadherin over-expression in UL CPNs (Hayano et al. 2014), *Draxin*$^{-/-}$ (Islam et al. 2009), *Robo1*$^{-/-}$ (Andrews et al. 2006; López-Bendito et al. 2007), *Robo1*$^{-/-}$; *Robo2*$^{-/-}$ (López-Bendito et al. 2007), *Slit2*$^{-/-}$ and *Slit1*$^{-/-}$;*Slit2*$^{-/-}$ (Bagri et al. 2002; Unni et al. 2012), *Dcc*$^{-/-}$ (Fazeli et al. 1997; Fothergill et al. 2014; Ren et al. 2007), *Efnb1*$^{-/-}$ (Bush and Soriano 2009; Mendes 2006), *Fgf8*$^{fl/fl}$; *Emx1-Cre* (*Fgf8cKO*) (Gobius et al. 2016), *Fgfr1*$^{fl/fl}$;*hGFAP-Cre* (*Fgfr1cKO*) (Smith et al. 2006), *Hs2st*$^{-/-}$ and *Hs6st1*$^{-/-}$ (Clegg et al. 2014; Conway et al. 2011), *Mash1*$^{-/-}$ (Niquille et al. 2009), *Netrin1*$^{-/-}$ (Fothergill et al. 2014; Hakanen and Salminen 2015; Ren et al. 2007; Serafini et al. 1996), *Nf2*$^{fl/fl}$;*Emx1-Cre* (*Nf2cKO*) (Lavado et al. 2014), *Nfia*$^{-/-}$ (Shu et al. 2003a), *Ngn2*$^{-/-}$ (Hand and Polleux 2011), *Pdn/Pdn* (Magnani et al. 2014), *Rfx3*$^{-/-}$ (Benadiba et al. 2012), *Sprouty1-2*$^{-/-}$ (Magnani et al. 2014), *Sema3c*$^{-/-}$ (Niquille et al. 2009), *Ryk*$^{-/-}$ (Keeble et al. 2006), *Sema3a*$^{-/-}$ (Zhou et al. 2013).

approximately E15.5), mostly from a second pool of progenitors located in the subventricular zone and occupy the upper layers (Huang et al. 2013; Molyneaux et al. 2009). Fate-specification dynamics in the cortex are controlled by a set of genes whose expression defines distinct cortical projection neuron (PN) identities, most importantly *Satb2*, *Ctip2* (also known as *Bcl11b*), *Fezf2* (*Fezl* or *Zfp312*), *Sox5*, and *Tbr1*. Their interplay is temporally and spatially regulated, on par with the stepwise progression of cortical development.

15.2.2.1 Specification of Subcortical Projection Neurons

The deep cortical layers are the first to be generated and predominantly contain subcortical projection neurons (SCPNs) that extend axons towards the thalamus and spinal cord. Initially, the development of corticothalamic projections from layer VI neurons is regulated by SOX5 (Kwan et al. 2008; Lai et al. 2008) and TBR1 (Han et al. 2011; McKenna et al. 2011); their concerted action blocks corticospinal fate through direct repression of *Fezf2* (Lai et al. 2008). Later, downregulation of *Sox5* allows expression of *Fezf2* in cycling progenitors and layer V and VI neurons (B. Chen et al. 2005; Molyneaux et al. 2005). At this stage, co-expression of *Fezf2*, *Ctip2* (Arlotta et al. 2005), and *Ctip1* (Canovas et al. 2015) marks the transition to a corticospinal-projection program. Accordingly, corticothalamic projections are lost in *Sox5*$^{-/-}$ mice (Lai et al. 2008), and subcerebral projections are disrupted in *Fezf2*$^{-/-}$ (B. Chen et al. 2005, 2008; Molyneaux et al. 2005) and *Ctip2*$^{-/-}$ mice (Arlotta et al. 2005). Conversely, over-expression of *Sox5* (Lai et al. 2008), *Fezf2*, or *Ctip2* (B. Chen et al. 2008) can asynchronously and ectopically activate their respective genetic programs, leading to abnormal projection patterns. Interestingly, more recent studies using conditional *Satb2* knockout

(KO) in the mouse confirmed the aforementioned callosal phenotypes but also found additional roles of SATB2 in the regulation of thalamocortical (Zhang et al. 2019) and subcortical connections (Leone et al. 2015; McKenna et al. 2015). Indeed, *Satb2* is expressed in SCPNs and activates *Sox5*, *Tbr1*, and *Fezf2*, but is in turn repressed by FEZF2; as such, SATB2 protein levels are low enough to create an environment that is permissive of a subcortical-projection genetic program but not sufficient to elicit a callosal-projection genetic program (McKenna et al. 2011, 2015; Srinivasan et al. 2012). This balance changes in CPNs.

15.2.2.2 Generation of SATB2$^+$CTIP2$^-$ Neurons

From mid-gestation, the mouse neocortex globally switches from production of CTIP2$^+$ to SATB2$^+$ neurons in a lateral-to-medial graded fashion (Dominguez et al. 2013), starting laterally at around E12, and medially one or two days thereafter (Takahashi et al. 1999). As layer II/III begins to form, the downregulation of *Fezf2* in cortical progenitors allows their progeny to express *Satb2* at higher levels. SATB2, in turn, activates an UL genetic program, including high *Sip1* and low *Tbr1* expression, and repression of DL genes, such as *Ctip2* (McKenna et al. 2011, 2015; Srinivasan et al. 2012). In the upper layers, the repression of *Ctip2* is mediated by recruitment of SKI to several matrix attachment regions (MARs) in the *Ctip2* locus (Alcamo et al. 2008; Baranek et al. 2012; Cera et al. 2019; Nomura et al. 2018). SKI is required to assemble a functional Nucleosome Remodeling and Deacetylase (NuRD) repressor complex containing SATB2, MTA2, and histone deacetylase 1 (HDAC1), which together mediate deacetylation (inactivation) of the *Ctip2* locus (Alcamo et al. 2008; Baranek et al. 2012; Britanova et al. 2008; Cera et al. 2019) (Figure 15.1Ba). As detailed in Section 15.2.3, this mechanism has been postulated as an evolutionary novelty absent in the avian and reptilian pallia (Nomura et al. 2018). In deep layers, however, *Satb2* and *Ski* co-expression occurs to a much lower extent and, instead, *Ski* and *Ctip2* co-expression is preponderant (Baranek et al. 2012). As SATB2$^+$CTIP2$^-$ cells are still found in layer V, this indicates that *Ski* expression might be transient during initiation of callosal identity, or that SATB2 is able to repress *Ctip2* independently of SKI in this layer. As expected, this network is perturbed in *Satb2*$^{-/-}$ (Alcamo et al. 2008; Britanova et al. 2008) and *Ski*$^{-/-}$ mice (Baranek et al. 2012), in which loss of SATB2 leads to ectopic activation of *Ctip2* and expansion of the normal layer V domain into the upper layers of the cortex. The callosal agenesis phenotype of these mice can be partially rescued with concomitant loss of *Ctip2* (Srinivasan et al. 2012), suggesting that neurons that would normally express *Satb2* regain the ability to enter a callosal-projection program. Ultimately, depending on the developmental time, different molecular mechanisms converge towards the differentiation of SATB2$^+$CTIP2$^-$ cells with callosal-projection potential.

15.2.2.3 Generation of SATB2$^+$CTIP2$^+$ Neurons

Although SATB2 and CTIP2 protein expression is largely mutually exclusive in the mammalian brain, SATB2$^+$CTIP2$^+$ neurons exist and are a stable population. In the mouse, they are established at around E13 in layer V, when there is a switch from predominant production of CTIP2$^+$ to SATB2$^+$ neurons (Lickiss et al. 2012). Within this layer, different subpopulations have been identified, such as CPNs co-expressing *Er81* (Harb et al. 2016; Lickiss et al. 2012), and cortico-brainstem PNs co-expressing *Bhlhb5* and/or *Sox5* (Harb et al. 2016). In these cells, LMO4 sequesters HDAC1, thus de-repressing the *Ctip2* locus and allowing *Satb2* and *Ctip2* co-expression (Harb et al. 2016) (Figure 15.1Bb, mouse). Therefore, the interplay between CTIP2 and SATB2 can be modulated by the presence of other proteins, contributing to further diversification of projection neuron subpopulations.

15.2.2.4 BRN1/2 as Upstream Regulators of SATB2

Adding to the intricacy of these networks, corticogenesis involves the action of many other TFs. For example, new-born neurons switching from *Ctip2* to *Satb2* expression show mutual repression between Brain-1/Brain-2 (BRN1/2) and RAR-related orphan receptor beta (RORβ). Consequently, BRN1/2 becomes restricted to layer II/III and some layer V neurons, being excluded from most CTIP2$^+$ neurons, as seen in the mouse (Dominguez et al. 2013; Oishi et al. 2016; Sugitani et al. 2002) and the rhesus monkey (Dominguez et al. 2013). Accordingly, *Brn1;Brn2* double-KO severely affects cortical progenitor cells and migration of UL neurons, leading to disorganization and thinning of the cortex (Sugitani et al. 2002). Conversely, early over-expression of either *Brn1* or *Brn2* at around E12 promotes premature production of CUX1$^+$ and SATB2$^+$ neurons, which migrate to the upper layers and project through the CC, at the expense of CTIP2$^+$ cells projecting into the internal capsule (Dominguez et al. 2013). Thus, although SATB2 is a master regulator, a cascade of upstream and downstream factors is indispensable for CPN fate acquisition.

15.2.2.5 Developmental Regulation of SATB2 Functions

Notably, in the mouse, not all retrogradely labelled CPNs express *Satb2* at E18.5 (Alcamo et al. 2008; Lickiss et al. 2012); and, after knockdown of *Satb2* in UL neurons at E15.5, projection across the CC is unaffected (Zhang et al. 2012). These observations suggest that a subpopulation of CPNs do not require SATB2 to form callosal connections; or that, in some cells, SATB2 might be required only at early stages of fate specification and can later be lost without affecting projection patterns. Also, there is re-location of SATB2 from superficial layers at E14.5 to all cortical layers at P0 (Britanova et al. 2008; Dominguez et al. 2013; Jaitner et al. 2016), possibly reflecting a functional switch from transcriptional repression during development, when it is involved in fate acquisition, to organization of chromatin superstructure in the adult, when it may play a role in cognition (Cera et al. 2019).

In summary, SATB2 is a multifaceted transcription factor. Besides its main function of *Ctip2* repression, SATB2 takes on broad roles during corticogenesis, modulated by the developmental stage and interactions with other proteins.

15.2.3 *Satb2* Expression in Acallosal Species

15.2.3.1 Evolving Functions of SATB2 and CTIP2

Despite the absence of a CC, most aforementioned genes are expressed in the avian, reptilian and non-eutherian pallia (Kozulin et al. 2022; Naumann and Laurent 2017; Nomura et al. 2013; Paolino et al. 2020; Suzuki and Hirata 2014; Suzuki et al. 2012), including *Satb2* (Figure 15.1A, SATB2$^+$ domains). Initial comparative studies in chick and turtle postulated that in these species neurogenesis would be spatially (and not temporally) regulated, such that CTIP2-positive neurons would be generated from progenitors in the medial pallium and SATB2-positive neurons from the lateral pallium (Suzuki and Hirata 2012, 2014; Suzuki et al. 2012). This would contrast with the largely homogenous medial-to-lateral domains of the mammalian neocortex. However, subsequent studies questioned this hypothesis (Belgard et al. 2013; García-Moreno and Molnár 2020; Nomura et al. 2018; Puelles et al. 2016). In fact, broad transcriptomic analysis challenged predicted anatomical homologies between mouse and chick pallia (Belgard et al. 2013), favoring a scenario in which there are divergent and species-specific functions of the same TFs. Accordingly, the comparison of *Satb2* and *Ctip2* expression patterns in the avian, reptilian, and murine dorsal pallia revealed striking species differences (Nomura et al. 2018). The predominant SATB2$^+$CTIP2$^-$ population found in upper cortical layers in the mouse is absent from the chicken and gecko dorsal pallia, where instead $SATB2^{+}CTIP2^{+}$ and $SATB2^{-}CTIP2^{+}$ neurons are abundant (Nomura et al. 2018). In chicken, extensive *Satb2* and *Ctip2* co-expression is possible due to the presence of only one MAR with attenuated transcription suppression activity at the *Ctip2* locus (Nomura et al. 2018) (Figure 15.1Bb, chicken). This mechanism differs from the one postulated to specify $SATB2^{+}CTIP2^{+}$ neurons in the mouse (Harb et al. 2016), showcasing how distinct mechanisms of transcriptional regulation can give rise to similar patterns of expression. However, identical combinatorial marker expression does not always translate into identical projection patterns. In the turtle, domains expressing the equivalent layer II/III markers of mouse project to the thalamus (Suzuki and Hirata 2014); whereas, in the gecko, $SATB2^{-}CTIP2^{+}$ neurons form interhemispheric projections (Nomura et al. 2018). These studies show that TF function is variable across evolution, giving rise to species-specific populations of PNs.

15.2.3.2 Heterochronicity of Neurogenesis and Onset of Satb2 Expression

The heterochronicity of developmental processes adds another layer of complexity to evolutionary differences. Firstly, heterochronic onset of neurogenesis might contribute to distinct differentiation potential of cortical progenitors. In fact, in the mouse, a subset of cycling progenitors is not neurogenic at early stages, later becoming fate-restricted and generating only upper-layer CPNs and glia; however, the homologous population is neither delayed nor fate-restricted in the chicken (García-Moreno and Molnár 2015). Secondly, studies comparing the mouse and the marsupial fat-tailed dunnart showed that non-eutherians achieve higher neuronal maturation earlier in development (Kozulin et al. 2022), including earlier onset of *Satb2* expression (Paolino et al. 2020). Remarkably, premature SATB2 over-expression in mice to match the expression onset stage seen in the dunnart results in an ectopic marsupial-like projection fate via the AC, leading to enlargement of this commissure at the expense of the CC (Paolino et al. 2020) (Figure 15.1C). Furthermore, the ability of SATB2 to repress *Ctip2* seems to be maintained in the dunnart, as evidenced by the decrease in CTIP2 upon ectopic *Satb2* expression, as well as an increase in subcerebral fate of cortical axons following *Satb2* knockdown (Paolino et al. 2020). This emphasizes that central mechanisms of transcriptional regulation known in eutherians still precede CC appearance and are, therefore, not sufficient to explain it.

Overall, these studies highlight not only that a single gene is not sufficient to define a cell type, but also that *Satb2* expression can be independent from the generation of callosal connections. Interspecies differences are influenced by several elements, including evolving functions of a core networks of TFs, as well as timing of neurogenesis onset and subsequent *Satb2* expression, relative to other developmental milestones.

15.2.4 Temporal and Spatial Regulation of Gene Expression in CPNs

Dynamic gene expression allows CPNs to arise, adequately respond to changing environmental cues, and ultimately establish functional connections. Therefore, although reliant on a core gene-expression program, the broad transcriptome of CPNs varies across three axes: time, space, and evolution. CPN subpopulations are marked by unique molecular signatures that have been extensively characterized, mostly resorting to transcriptomic and proteomic assays in the mouse.

15.2.4.1 Temporal Regulation of CPN Identity

Important temporal milestones in CC development include specification of layer V CPNs (in the mouse, at E11.5–E13.5), specification of layer II/III CPNs (E15.5), complete crossing of callosal axons from layer II/III (around P3), and postnatal onset of myelination (around P10). As a result,

CPNs first express genes that globally control neuronal subtype specification, differentiation, migration, and initial axonal extension[1] (Molyneaux et al. 2009). This is followed by a second set of genes at early postnatal stages (P3–P6) that regulates neuronal maturation, axon guidance, and establishment of contralateral connectivity (Molyneaux et al. 2009; A. I. Son et al. 2017).[2] After P7, a third set of genes is required to regulate the final stages of CPN maturation and axonal pruning, refinement, and maintenance[3] (Molyneaux et al. 2009; A. I. Son et al. 2017). Finally, the late postnatal period between P10 and P15 is marked by an increase of astrocyte,[4] late neuronal,[5] and myelination[6] markers that account for the axonal maturation and myelination of the CC (Son et al. 2017).

15.2.4.2 Spatial Regulation of CPN Identity

Besides temporal control, CPN identity is spatially regulated. Genes common to most CPNs, such as *Satb2, Hspb3, Cited2,* and *Lpl*, are expressed in upper and deeper layers at E18 and generally absent from SCPNs (Alcamo et al. 2008; Britanova et al. 2008; Fame et al. 2016; Molyneaux et al. 2009). However, there are also signatures characteristic of CPNs from the cingulate cortex[7] (Leone et al. 2015), and deep[8] and upper layers[9] (Cubelos et al. 2010; Molyneaux et al. 2009; Rodríguez-Tornos et al. 2016). Superficial layers can be further subdivided according to gene expression in upper lamina,[10] middle lamina,[11] and deeper lamina[12] (Molyneaux et al. 2009). Importantly, unique molecular signatures are reflected in topographic and functional differences. For instance, in layer Va, PLXND1 and GFRA2 mark CPNs that maintain collateral projections to ipsilateral and/or contralateral striatum (Molyneaux et al. 2009); whereas CAV1 identifies dual-projecting CPNs extending axons both contralaterally and to ipsilateral frontal areas (MacDonald et al. 2018). Additionally, the layer distribution of certain marker genes varies across functional cortical areas. For example, *Lmo4* is highly expressed by all CPNs in the motor cortex, but exclusive to layer II/III CPNs in the somatosensory cortex (Azim et al. 2009), a pattern conserved between mouse and macaque (Fame et al. 2017); and *Lhx2* shows a lateral-high to medial-low expression pattern in layer II/III, distinguishing adjacent motor cortex areas (Azim et al. 2009). Conversely, intralayer temporal dynamics are also common. *Lmo4* and *Clim1* are co-expressed at E15.5 in presumptive layer V CPNs, the majority of which become CLIM1$^-$ at P6 (Azim et al. 2009).

15.2.4.3 Spatial Segregation of Callosal Axons

Moreover, markers of callosal axons include L1CAM (A. I. Son et al. 2017), Neuropilin-1 (NRP1) (Piper et al. 2009b), NF2 (Lavado et al. 2014), Nectin-3 (Fame et al. 2017; Molyneaux et al. 2009), TAG1 (or CNTN2) (Kastriti et al. 2019; Nishikimi et al. 2011), EPHA3 (Nishikimi et al. 2011), NEFM, MBP, and Plexin-A1 (Son et al. 2017). Notably, marker expression can be used to distinguish pioneering axons (NRP1$^+$), and dorsal and ventral CC domains (TAG1$^+$ and EPHA3$^+$, respectively) (Nishikimi et al. 2011; Zhou et al. 2013) (see Section 15.4.1.2). However, some of these proteins take on broad roles in axonogenesis, rather than CC-specific functions. Such is the case of TAG1, expressed by both SATB2$^+$ and CTIP2$^+$ neurons (Kastriti et al. 2019; Nishikimi et al. 2011), and whose loss has been associated to general defects in axon fasciculation affecting several axons tracts (Bormuth et al. 2013).

Together, these studies highlight the complex regulatory programs involved in CPN identity during development, providing numerous markers that can be informative of CPN location, projection pattern, and maturation stage.

15.2.5 Evolutionary Regulation of Gene Expression in CPNs

Most of our understanding about the molecular signatures of CPNs is derived from studies of the mouse brain. However, primates show a dramatic expansion of the upper cortical layers and the volume of white matter in the CC. Comparative studies have begun to shed light onto the implications of these events in gene expression patterns.

15.2.5.1 Evolution of CPN Populations

The initial stages of corticogenesis are greatly conserved across species, in agreement with the similar expression of *Ptn*, *Lmo4*, *Inhba*, and *Cited2* in the E14 mouse and the E94 macaque brain. Similarly, in P3 mouse and E108/113 macaque, there is conservation of genes that are expressed across all cortical layers, including *Cited2*, *Chn2*, *EphA3*, and *Limch1*; as well as DL expression of *Dkk3*, *Plexin-D1*, and *Gfra2*. Also, expression of genes like *Nkk3* and *Nnmt* is conserved in early and late corticogenesis stages (Fame et al. 2017). However, differences become apparent in ULs. At the histological level, the indivisible layer II/III of rodents laminates into architecturally distinct sublayers II, IIIa, and IIIb in the primate cerebral cortex (Berg et al. 2021; Smart 2002). Furthermore, whereas in mice 80 percent of CPNs reside in ULs, 90 percent do so in primates. Additionally, laminar organization differs, as CPNs are evenly distributed throughout layer II/III in mice, but essentially restricted to layer III and more specifically concentrated in the deeper part of layer III (IIIb) in the primate sensorimotor cortex (Fame et al. 2017). Unsurprisingly, comparison of the P3 mouse and the E108/113 macaque brain revealed differences in molecular signatures of UL CPNs (Fame et al. 2017) (summarized in Table 15.1). Notably, even when the layer expression is similar, some populations show expanded domains in macaque. For instance, the expansion of *Gfra2* from layers Va and VI in the mouse to ULs in the macaque implies that a new population of UL CPNs acquired genetic controls first employed by DL CPNs (Fame et al. 2017). Accordingly, neuronal diversification has also been described in the upper cortical layers of the human brain, compared to the mouse (Berg et al. 2021). These studies suggest an elaboration of CPN populations along evolution, likely translating to functional processing differences between species.

Table 15.1 Cortical location of CPN markers in the mouse and macaque brains.

Gene	Mouse	Macaque
	E14	**E94**
Conserved	*Ptn, Lmo4, Inhba, Cited2, Nkk3, Nnmt, Gfra2*	
Plexin-D1	Immature CP neurons	Not expressed
	P3	**E108/113**
Conserved	*Cited2, Chn2, EphA3, Limch1, Plexin-D1, Dkk3, Nkk3, Nnmt*	
EphA3	Restricted to the most superficial cells of layer II/III	Broad distribution in layer II/III
Limch1	Broad distribution in layer II/III	Restricted to the most superficial cells of layer II
Inhba	Broad distribution in layer II/III	Layer II
Gfr2	Layers Va and VI only	Layers Va and VI UL neurons

(Adapted from Fame et al. 2017)

Previous sections summarized the complex gene regulatory networks involved in the generation of callosal projection neurons. Given the complex dynamics of gene expression, a global map of CPN identities across brain regions, developmental times, and species is still missing, and that will likely be the case for years to come. Perhaps even more relevant, the mechanisms that govern the specification of CPN subpopulations, as well as their functional significance in brain wiring, are only beginning to be understood (Oran et al. 2021). After CPN differentiation, a series of events leads to the formation of contralateral connections.

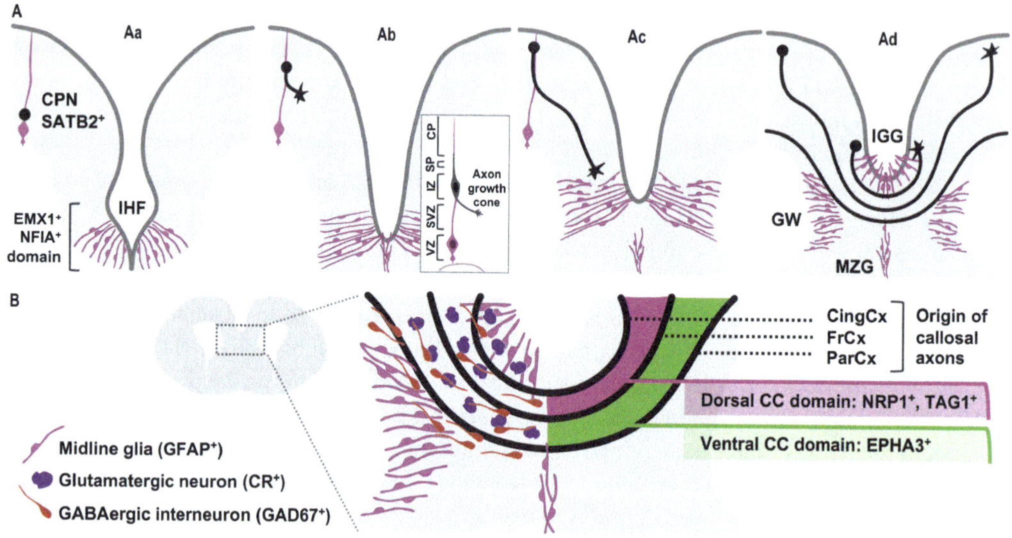

Figure 15.3 Stages of callosal axon projection and guidepost populations. (A) Stages of axonal projection during CC formation. (Aa) The initial stages of CC formation involve CPN differentiation (SATB2$^+$; DL-CPNs at E11.5–13.5, UL-CPNs at E15.5 (Huang et al. 2013; Molyneaux et al. 2009)). After commissural plate regionalization, callosal axons cross an EMX1$^+$NFIA$^+$ domain (Moldrich et al. 2010). Following fusion of the septal halves at E15, the IHF progressively retracts until E18, by action of MZG (Ab–Ad) (Gobius et al. 2016). (Ab) CPNs migrate through the VZ/SVZ towards the CP and, as they enter the IZ, axonal projection starts. Sensing of environmental cues is carried out by the axon growth cone. (Ac) When axons approach the midline, glia cells transecting their path translocate, creating space for crossing and segregating into GW and IGG populations (Clegg et al. 2014; Conway et al. 2011; Magnani et al. 2014; Smith et al. 2006). (Ad) The final stages of CC formation involve midline crossing, extension to the contralateral hemisphere, and establishment of connections, which are mostly homotopic (Yang et al. 2022). (B) Midline guideposts include GFAP$^+$ glia populations surrounding the CC, as well as CR$^+$ glutamatergic neurons and GAD67$^+$ GABAergic interneurons intermingled with the white matter (Niquille et al. 2009, 2013; Shu et al. 2003b). Pioneering NRP1$^+$ callosal axons originating from the cingulate cortex are the first to cross and occupy the dorsal-most domain of the CC; TAG1$^+$ axons from the frontal cortex cross afterwards and occupy the middle CC domain; finally, EPHA3$^+$ axons from parietal cortex are the last and most ventral. These axonal domains are separated by three stripes of glutamatergic guidepost neurons (Niquille et al. 2009; Nishikimi et al. 2011; Zhou et al. 2013). CC, corpus callosum; Cing/Fr/ParCx, cingulate, frontal and parietal cortex; CP, cortical plate; CPN, callosal projection neuron; GW, glia wedge; IGG, glia within the indusium griseum; IHF, interhemispheric fissure; IZ, intermediate zone; MZG, midline zipper glia; SP, subplate; SVZ, subventricular zone; VZ, ventricular zone.

15.3 Patterning of the Commissural Plate

One of the first steps required for CC development is the formation and patterning of the commissural plate. These events start at post-conception week (PCW) 10 in the human (Reyes et al. 2020) and E11.5 in the mouse (Suárez et al. 2014b) when a new structure named *massa commissuralis* forms after fusion of the two hemispheres. The commissural plate is then regionalized into distinct anatomical regions that are crossed by specific commissures (reviewed in Suárez et al. 2014b). First, morphogenic signaling of bone morphogenic proteins (BMPs), WNT, and Sonic hedgehog (SHH) defines pallial and subpallial territories. Next, the subpallium is refined into septal and preoptic regions through concerted action of SHH and fibroblast growth factor 8 (FGF8) expressed between the *massa commissuralis* and the septum (Gobius et al. 2016; Moldrich et al. 2010; Storm et al. 2006). After regionalization, CC axons transverse an EMX1$^+$NFIA$^+$ domain

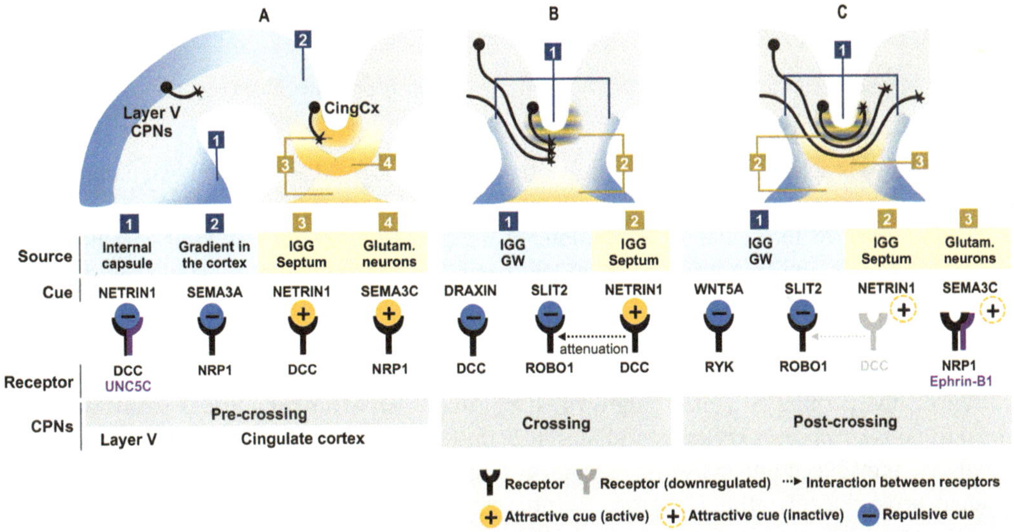

Figure 15.4 Axon guidance mechanisms of CC development during midline approach, crossing, and exit. (A) The mechanisms of medial axonal turn differ between classes of CPNs. In layer V CPNs, high expression of *Unc5d* leads to the formation of a UNC5C/DCC heterodimer receptor and a repulsive response to NETRIN1 expressed laterally in the internal capsule (Fothergill et al. 2014; Morcom et al. 2016; Srivatsa et al. 2014). In pioneering neurons from the cingulate cortex (CingCx), UNC5D levels are low, leading to formation of a DCC homodimer and consequent attractive response towards NETRIN1 produced at the brain midline by IGG and septum cells (Fothergill et al. 2014; Serafini et al. 1996). Furthermore, NRP1 levels are high in pioneering axons, mediating repulsion from SEMA3A expressed at high levels in the lateral cortex (Zhao et al. 2011; Zhou et al. 2013), and attraction to SEMA3C produced by midline glutamatergic guidepost neurons (Hossain et al. 2019; Piper et al. 2009b; Ren et al. 2006). (B) During midline crossing, IGG and GW cells generate different chemorepulsive cues that channel axons across. Two important repulsive pathways are DRAXIN/DCC (Ahmed et al. 2011; Islam et al. 2009) and SLIT2/ROBO1 (Fothergill et al. 2014; Lavado et al. 2014; López-Bendito et al. 2007; Shu and Richards 2001; Shu et al. 2003d; Unni et al. 2012). Notably, signaling of NETRIN1 through the DCC receptor, present in all crossing axons, leads to interaction between DCC and ROBO1, attenuating repulsion and allowing crossing (Fothergill et al. 2014). (C) Finally, repulsion from the midline depends on RYK/WNT5A signaling (Hutchins et al. 2011; Keeble et al. 2006) and DCC downregulation, which prevents attraction to NETRIN1 and increases the strength of ROBO1/SLIT2-mediated repulsion (Fothergill et al. 2014). From E17.5, Ephrin-B1 interacts with NRP1 and switches off the attraction to SEMA3C (Mire et al. 2018).

(Figure 15.3Aa); HC axons an NFIA$^+$ZIC2$^+$SIX3$^+$ domain; and AC axons a SIX3$^+$ domain (Lavado et al. 2014; Moldrich et al. 2010). Perturbation of this organization has profound effects on commissural development. For instance, *Rfx3*$^{-/-}$ mice present a mild expansion of *Fgf8* expression at E12.5 (Benadiba et al. 2012); and *Gli3* hypomorphic (*Pdn/Pdn*) and *Sprouty1/2*$^{-/-}$ mice show upregulation of FGF and downregulation of W/β-catenin signaling (Magnani et al. 2014). In these mouse models, abnormal commissural plate regionalization leads to severe disorganization of corticoseptal guidepost cells and, ultimately, CC agenesis with formation of ipsilateral Probst bundles (Figure 15.2C). These are large bilateral, barrel-shaped axonal structures that form longitudinal intrahemispheric bundles situated in both hemispheres (Probst 1901); they are a hallmark of CC agenesis that occurs after axons approach the midline but are unable to cross it. Overall, these studies show that the commissural plate forms an indispensable substrate for later crossing of callosal axons.

15.4 Axon Guidance Mechanisms of CC Development

15.4.1 Molecular Machinery and Developmental Timing of Axonogenesis

15.4.1.1 Axon Growth Cone of CPNs

Axon guidance is achieved through a motile sensing device located at the tip of extending axons, termed growth cone. Analysis of the transcriptome and proteome of CPN growth cones and parent cell bodies revealed molecular specializations of the growth cone, such as local enrichment of mTOR machinery and transcripts with mTOR-dependent translation (Poulopoulos et al. 2019). Accordingly, *mTOR*-KO in the mouse leads to CC agenesis due to failure of axon extension (Poulopoulos et al. 2019). Upon establishment of this specialized local machinery, receptors at the growth cone bind to chemotactic (diffusible) or haptotactic (substrate-bound) cues, sensing a permissive or non-permissive axonal outgrowth signal that leads to an attractive or repulsive directional response, respectively (Raper and Mason 2016; Tessier-Lavigne and Goodman 1996). These signals are transduced into cytoskeletal changes that direct axonogenesis (Kahn and Baas 2016). Gradual projection of callosal neurons towards and across the brain midline is mediated by response to guidance cues generated by specialized populations.

15.4.1.2 Timing of CPN Axonal Projection

At PCW11-12 in the human and E15.5 in the mouse, NRP1$^+$ pioneering axons from CPNs of the cingulate cortex begin crossing the midline and make up the dorsal-most domain of the CC (Ozaki and Wahlsten 1998; Rash and Richards 2001; Ren et al. 2006; Reyes et al. 2020; Wahlsten 1981). Increasing numbers of callosal fibers establish the callosal plate, distinct and independent from the AC and HC (Rakic and Yakovlev 1968; Ren et al. 2006). By PCW17/E16.5, axons from neocortical CPNs follow the path set by pioneering axons, with dorsal fronto-cingulate axons (TAG1$^+$) projecting first through the dorsal CC, and parietal axons (EPHA3$^+$) projecting afterwards through the ventral CC (Nishikimi et al. 2011; Zhou et al. 2013) (Figure 15.3B). All callosal axons extend medially, turn and cross to the contralateral hemisphere. Contralateral growth involves several shifts in the sensing of environmental cues, such that midline attraction is switched off, at the same time as midline repulsion is increased (Fothergill et al. 2014; Mire et al. 2018). All these processes are described in following sections.

15.4.2 Initiation of Axon Projection

Callosal axons start extending in a direction-selective manner while CPNs migrate radially along the intermediate zone (IZ), before their cell body has reached the final position in the cortical plate (CP) (Figure 15.3Ab, inset). Thus, a key feature of these migrating neurons is a medial-lateral polarized morphology, consisting of a unipolar leading process (apical dendrite) and a trailing process (axon) (Hand and Polleux 2011; Lickiss et al. 2012; Polleux 2013). The timing of axon initiation and establishment of correct polarity are mediated by response to chemotactic cues.

15.4.2.1 Initiation of Pioneering Axons from the Cingulate Cortex

CPNs from the cingulate cortex are the first to project pioneering axons towards and across the midline, relying on unique chemotactic responses (Figure 15.4A). Initially, precocious axon outgrowth is inhibited by BMP7 secreted by the meninges; this signal is overcome at around E15.5, upon onset of *Wnt3* expression (Choe et al. 2012). After axon initiation, high expression of NRP1 instructs medial turn via repulsion from a lateral-high to medial-low cortical gradient of SEMA3A

(Zhao et al. 2011; Zhou et al. 2013), and attraction to a source of SEMA3C at the midline (Hossain et al. 2019; Piper et al. 2009b; Ren et al. 2006). In these neurons, response to NETRIN1 is also crucial. NETRIN1 can induce chemoattraction, if signaling through a DCC homodimer, or chemorepulsion, if signaling through a DCC/UNC5 heterodimer (Finci et al. 2014). Pioneering axons have high-DCC/low-UNC5C levels, which mediate attraction to a source of NETRIN1 at the brain midline (Fothergill et al. 2014; Serafini et al. 1996). Showing the importance of this mechanism, mutations that disrupt NETRIN1/DCC signaling are among the most well-studied in the context of CC agenesis in the mouse (Fazeli et al. 1997; Fothergill et al. 2014; Hakanen and Salminen 2015; Ren et al. 2007; Serafini et al. 1996) (Figure 15.2C) and human (Finci et al. 2014; Jamuar et al. 2017; Marsh et al. 2017). Ultimately, initiation of pioneering axons marks the start of the CC tract and sets a path for neocortical axons to follow, making it one of the most vital events in CC development.

15.4.2.2 Differential Response to Chemotactic Cues in Early-born PNs

Although layer V subcortical and callosal projection neurons are born simultaneously, they project in opposite directions (SCPNs laterally, CPNs medially). Several receptor/ligand interactions account for their differential perception of the same environmental cues. T-cadherin (also known as Cadherin 13) is selectively expressed by SCPNs, but not by CPNs; whereas suppressing T-cadherin causes SCPNs to incorrectly project medially, over-expressing it in upper layer CPNs causes some lateral projections (Hayano et al. 2014) (Figure 15.2B). Also, there is opposite response to a NETRIN1 gradient surrounding the internal capsule. In layer V CPNs, SATB2 represses *Dcc* and activates *Unc5c*; a DCC/UNC5D receptor promotes chemorepulsion and medial projection (Figure 15.4A). Conversely, in SCPNs, CTIP2 represses *Unc5c*, resulting in DCC-mediated attraction to NETRIN1 and lateral projection (Fothergill et al. 2014; Morcom et al. 2016; Srivatsa et al. 2014). Remarkably, over-expressing *Satb2* or *Unc5c*, or knocking down *Dcc*, in deep layers of *Satb2*$^{-/-}$ brains partially rescues the callosal agenesis (Srinivasan et al. 2012; Srivatsa et al. 2014).

15.4.2.3 Medial Turn of Upper-layer CPNs

Regarding upper-layer CPNs, late onset of expression of Neurogenin2 (NGN2) in intermediate progenitor cells is involved in medial turn (Hand et al. 2005; Hand and Polleux 2011). Genetic loss of *Ngn2* results in ACC with the formation of Probst bundles and mis-projecting axons; and knockdown of *Ngn2* in layer II/III neurons leads to aberrant lateral projections towards cortical and subcortical targets (Hand and Polleux 2011).

Overall, early guidance decisions involve timely outgrowth of pioneering axons, opposite responses of CPNs and SCPNs to a shared environment, and unique molecular features of CPN subpopulations.

15.4.3 Guidance in the Subplate Compartment

The subplate (SP) is a transient neuronal compartment between the CP and the IZ, at the interface of gray and white matter. It contains various cell populations, including glutamatergic neurons and GABAergic interneurons, and exists in all eutherian mammals, although molecular and morphological characteristics and persistence into adulthood vary (Bystron et al. 2008; Hoerder-Suabedissen and Molnár 2013, 2015; Kostović 2020). Mutations in members of the multi-subunit mammalian SWItch/Sucrose Non-fermentable (mSWI/SNF) complex have been associated with profound neurodevelopmental defects in humans, including high penetrance of ACC (Kosho et al. 2013, 2014; Santen et al. 2013; Son and Crabtree 2014). A mouse KO for one of the complex components, AT-rich interactive domain-containing protein 1A (*Arid1a*), revealed that selective loss of SP neuron function impairs axon pathfinding and is responsible for complete AC and CC agenesis with extensive axonal mistargeting (Doyle et al. 2021). This expanded the known function of the SP in thalamocortical wiring (Kanold and Luhmann 2010) to establishment of interhemispheric connections. The terminal arborizations of callosal, thalamocortical and associative axons undergo a prolonged waiting period in the SP (Kostović 2020), indicating that it may similarly instruct different wiring routes. However, the precise molecular mechanisms of callosal guidance remain unexplored. Importantly, subplate expansion is one of the most dramatic events in cortical evolution (Hoerder-Suabedissen and Molnár 2015); the human SP is four times ticker than the CP (Kostović 2020), in striking contrast with the two-cell-layer thickness in the mouse (Hoerder-Suabedissen et al. 2009). Thus, it is likely that it takes on even more prominent functions in higher mammals and a possible involvement in ACC should be considered in future studies.

15.4.4 Guidepost Populations at the Brain Midline

With continued axon outgrowth, a mix of transient glial and neuronal cells at the brain midline (Figure 15.3B) act as guideposts for axon attraction, channeling, and repulsion into the contralateral hemisphere. This section gives an overview on the generation and functions of these guidepost populations, as well as examples of the impact of their loss in disease.

15.4.4.1 Midline Glia

Arguably the most prominent guidepost cells required for CC formation are midline glia, in particular three populations: midline zipper glia (MZG), glia wedge (GW), and glia within the indusium griseum (IGG) (Shu et al. 2003c). The importance of midline glial guideposts was discovered when providing a glia-covered scaffold spanning the hemispheres restored callosal crossing in brains where the midline had been cut at pre-callosal stages (Silver and Ogawa 1983). Since then, these cell populations have been extensively studied in mouse models and confirmed to be conserved in the human (Ren et al. 2006), although a detailed molecular characterization in the latter is still missing.

The role of NFI TFs in midline glia development. Even though most cortical astrocytes are generated postnatally, midline glia populations differentiate during development and their maturation is required for proper callosal guidance. Nuclear factor one (NFI) transcription factors A and B act in the transition of radial glia progenitors into the mature astroglial cells in the embryonic telencephalon (Lu et al. 2007; Piper et al. 2010; Shu et al. 2003a); this transition is accompanied by morphological and molecular changes, such as onset of expression of *Gfap* (Piper et al. 2010; Shu et al. 2003a). Due to various defects in all midline glia populations, *Nfia* and *Nfib* mutations lead to CC abnormalities, both in the human (Chen et al. 2011; Gobius et al. 2016; Sajan et al. 2013) and mouse (Piper et al. 2009a; Shu et al. 2003a; Steele-Perkins et al. 2005) (Figure 15.2C). Interestingly, the hippocampal commissure is always affected (Gobius et al. 2016; Lu et al. 2007; Steele-Perkins et al. 2005), suggesting the need of a common dorsal midline niche for HC and CC development. Orchestrated by NFI TFs, different classes of midline glia execute specific functions that ensure CC formation.

MZG function in IHF remodeling in eutherian mammals. A prerequisite for CC development is the closure of the interhemispheric fissure (IHF) in the septum area (Figure 15.3Aa–d), which depends on removal of leptomeningeal fibroblasts and extracellular matrix from the septal midline (Donahoo and Richards 2009). The IHF is formed between E9 and E12, at which point the two hemispheres are connected only by a small hinge of tissue; then, the bilateral expansion of the septum culminates in the fusion of the septal halves at E15 (Gobius et al. 2016). Thereafter, the IHF progressively retracts from E15 to E18, starting at the ventro-caudal base of the septum and ending at the dorso-rostral apex of the septum (Gobius et al. 2016). This process is largely mediated by MZG. At early stages, MZG cells serve as substrate for pioneering callosal axons to cross (Gobius et al. 2016). Later, radial MZG transition into multipolar astroglia, as they intercalate around leptomeningeal inclusions and actively degrade the leptomeninges (Bremer et al. 2001; Gobius et al. 2016). Unsurprisingly, failure of septal fusion is a common finding in complete ACC, as seen in *Netrin1* (Hakanen and Salminen 2015) and *Fgf8* mouse mutants (Gobius et al. 2016). The latter study revealed that the levels and timing of *Fgf8* expression regulate MZG maturation, including translocation of the pial surface and transition to a multipolar morphology (Gobius et al. 2016). Importantly, failure of IHF remodeling in the developing human brain is always observed in isolated cases of ACC (Gobius et al. 2016), where it can be either cause or consequence of the agenesis. Together, these studies show that a mechanism of IHF closure governed by MZG and unique to eutherian mammals is critical for CC development.

Guidance of callosal axons by GW and IGG. As initially postulated based on morphological and molecular similarities (Shu et al. 2003c), GW and IGG start as a common population that becomes spatially segregated during CC formation (Figure 15.3Ab–d). In fact, the IGG is formed from the GW, when radial glia in dorso-medial ventricular zone retract their apical-endfeet and translocate to the to the subpial region of the dorso-medial pallium (Smith et al. 2006), a process that depends on FGF/ERK signaling (Clegg et al. 2014; Conway et al. 2011; Magnani et al. 2014; Smith et al. 2006). Thereafter, GW and IGG promote the channeling of callosal axons across the midline through diverse ligand/receptor signaling cascades, including SLIT/ROBO (Fothergill et al. 2014; Lavado et al. 2014; López-Bendito et al. 2007; Shu and Richards 2001; Shu et al. 2003d; Unni et al. 2012), Ephrin/Eph (Bush and Soriano 2009), DRAXIN/DCC (Ahmed et al. 2011; Islam et al. 2009), and WNT5A/RYK (Hutchins et al. 2011; Keeble et al. 2006) (Figure 15.4). The importance of these populations is showcased by the vast array of mouse models that present CC defects alongside impaired GW to IG glial movement (Clegg et al. 2014; Conway et al. 2011; Islam et al. 2009; Lavado et al. 2014; Magnani et al. 2014; Mendes 2006; Smith et al. 2006; Unni et al. 2012). The phenotype can be due to the physical boundary that non-translocated glial cells impose in the path crossed by callosal axons, as well as to abnormal chemical guidance. In *Nf2* mutants (Figure 15.2C), for instance, the two factors seem to contribute to the callosal agenesis (Lavado et al. 2014): non-translocated GW fibers transect and block the path of extending axons, and *Slit2* over-expression promotes repulsive signaling (Fothergill et al. 2014; Shu and Richards 2001; Unni et al. 2012). Strikingly, when *Nf2* deletion is restricted to the dorsal cortex (*Nf2*$^{fl/fl}$;*Emx1-Cre*), CC and HC are absent, but the AC is normal; however, full brain deletion (*Nf2*$^{fl/fl}$;*Nestin-Cre*) results in CC, HC, and AC agenesis (Lavado et al. 2014). Similarly, *Fgfr1* mutants show HC and CC defects, but the AC is spared (Smith et al. 2006). Contrasting with other mutations, even when the AC is present, callosal axons are not rerouted towards that path, showing that they are not responsive to more ventral midline guideposts, or that the anatomical distance is too great for a response to be elicited. Altogether, these observations demonstrate how non-cell autonomous defects can singlehandedly disturb commissure formation, and clearly disentangle the dorsal and ventral midline niches as necessary for the formation of different commissures.

Modulation of SLIT2/ROBO1 during and after midline crossing. The interaction between SLIT family members and their receptors, roundabout homologs (ROBO), is crucial for several axon guidance mechanisms. During CC development, all *Slit* ligands (*Slit1*, *Slit2*, and *Slit3*) are expressed at the brain midline, whereas *Robo1* and low levels of *Robo2*, but not *Robo3*, are expressed by CPNs (Andrews et al. 2006; Shu and Richards 2001). In particular, GW and IGG cells express *Slit2*, repulsing *Robo1/2*-expressing callosal axons and channeling them across the midline to prevent projections to the septum (Fothergill et al. 2014; López-Bendito et al. 2007; Shu and Richards 2001; Shu et al. 2003d; Unni et al. 2012). The effects of SLIT2/ROBO1 signaling are modulated along the different stages of axon crossing. Initially, NETRIN1 produced by IGG and septum cells attracts pioneering callosal axons that express high-DCC/low-UNC5C levels at E15.5 (Fothergill et al. 2014; Serafini et al. 1996) (Figure 15.4A). Later, upregulation of DCC in all crossing axons allows its interaction with ROBO1, leading to attenuation of SLIT2/ROBO1-mediated repulsion (Fothergill et al. 2014) (Figure 15.4B). Finally, in post-crossing axons, downregulation of DCC amplifies the repulsive effect of SLIT2 and facilitates contralateral outgrowth (Fothergill et al. 2014) (Figure 15.4C). This process is impaired in *Robo1*$^{-/-}$ (Andrews et al. 2006; López-Bendito et al. 2007), *Robo1*$^{-/-}$;*Robo2*$^{-/-}$ (López-Bendito et al. 2007), *Slit2*$^{-/-}$ (Bagri et al. 2002; Unni et al. 2012), and *Slit1*$^{-/-}$;*Slit2*$^{-/-}$ mouse mutants (Unni et al. 2012), which present mis-placement of midline glia and a severe thinning of the CC with ectopic projections into the septum (Figure 15.2B). Notably, as SLIT ligands and ROBO receptors co-evolved (Yu et al. 2014), pairwise interactions seem to have gained commissure specificity. In fact, there are HC defects in *Slit2*$^{-/-}$ (Bagri et al. 2002) and *Robo1*$^{-/-}$ mutants (Andrews et al. 2006; Unni et al. 2012), namely ectopic projections and intermingling of HC and CC axons, indicating that SLIT2/ROBO1 signaling is needed to separate the two commissural paths; in contrast, the AC is grossly normal in these mutants. Together, these studies show how CC formation relies on modulation of SLIT2/ROBO1 interactions across axonogenesis stages.

15.4.4.2 Midline Neurons

In addition to glia populations, other midline guideposts are composed of neurons. These are transiently found within or around the CC white matter and can be excitatory (glutamatergic), as seen in the subcallosal sling (SS), or inhibitory (GABAergic) (Bielle and Garel 2013; Niquille et al. 2009, 2013) (Figure 15.3B). Such populations have been extensively studied in mouse models and identified in the human brain (Jovanov-Milošević et al. 2010; Ren et al. 2006).

Glutamatergic neurons. Present from E12.5 to P2, the subcallosal sling (SS) is a migratory pathway for Calretinin-positive (CR^{+}) glutamatergic immature neurons in the rostral forebrain, which migrate medially from the ventricular zone (Niquille et al. 2009; Shu et al. 2003b). From E18.5 to P3, the SS splits into three stripes of neurons located at the ventral, middle, and dorsal boundary of the white matter bundle. Importantly, the middle stripe separates two distinct topographic domains of the CC: the dorsal fronto-cingulate pathway (NRP1^{+}TAG1^{+}), which includes pioneering axons, and the ventral parietal pathway (EPHA3^{+}) (Niquille et al. 2009; Nishikimi et al. 2011; Zhou et al. 2013) (Figure 15.3B). SS neurons produce SEMA3C, which attracts NRP1^{+} pioneering axons (Hossain et al. 2019; Piper et al. 2009b; Ren et al. 2006) (Figure 15.4A). The attractive signal is turned off in post-crossing axons upon *EfnB1* upregulation from E17.5 (Mire et al. 2018) (Figure 15.4C). This process is impaired in mutants and leads to CC defects, such as callosal agenesis with formation of Probst bundles (Bush and Soriano 2009; Mendes 2006; Niquille et al. 2009; Piper et al. 2009b) (Figure 15.2C).

GABAergic interneurons. GABAergic guidepost interneurons are a heterogenous population generated between E12.5 and E14.5 from the medial and lateral ganglionic eminences. Concomitantly with callosal axon ingrowth, they migrate tangentially from the ventral telencephalon into the CC (Niquille et al. 2013) and, from E15.5 to E18.5, invade the CC white matter and surround callosal axons. These interneurons are marked by GAD67 and produce guidance factors that help direct outgrowth (Niquille et al. 2013). From P7 to P14, they disappear in a spatiotemporal gradient from the medial to the lateral CC regions (Niquille et al. 2013). Strikingly, mutations affecting global interneuron production, such as those in Aristaless-related homeobox (*Arx*)

(Ffrench-Constant et al. 2019; Hartmann et al. 2004; Kitamura et al. 2002; Shoubridge et al. 2010; Takeshita et al. 2020) or *Mash1* (Niquille et al. 2009) (Figure 15.2C) result in CC defects in the mouse and human. It is likely that this phenotype is, at least in part, mediated by non-cell autonomous guidance impairment upon loss of GABAergic guideposts.

Taken together, these studies show that CC development critically depends on a finely orchestrated series of guidance responses. Although there are important differences, many of these are shared with those of other commissural axons. Thus, on the one hand, fundamentals of callosal development reflect general principles of axon guidance; and, on the other hand, the differential impact of genetic mutations on HC, AC, and CC development (Donahoo and Richards 2009; Fenlon et al. 2021) can provide valuable insights on brain evolution. Still, the study of axon guidance is challenging and ever ongoing. It involves non-cell autonomous effects, numerous ligand/receptor interactions, molecular switches, and brief windows of response. The combination of mouse models with in vitro systems will continue to shed light onto these mechanisms, and genetic studies of ACC patients can help in understanding their conservation and significance in human health.

15.5 Connection to the Contralateral Hemisphere

After midline crossing, callosal axons go on to establish functional connections in the contralateral hemisphere (reviewed in Fenlon and Richards 2015). Most of this process occurs postnatally. In the mouse, tracing of somatosensory callosal axons labelled at E15.5 revealed that axons terminate midline crossing at P3, extend beneath the gray matter of the contralateral cortex at P5, penetrate the gray matter at P6, reach the upper cortical layers at P7, and finally gradually arborize in layer II/III of the cortex from P9, reaching at P12 a state similar to that observed at P60 (Wang et al. 2007). The final stages of profuse branching in a layer-specific manner culminate with the establishment of synaptic contacts both with pyramidal neurons and interneurons (Suárez et al. 2014a), which are later refined (Innocenti and Price 2005).

15.5.1 Determination of Connection Partners

During normal development, callosal axons connect mostly homotopic (bilateral homologous) regions of opposing hemispheres (Yang et al. 2022; Yorke and Caviness 1976), and, to a much lesser extent, heterotopic (non-homologous) regions (Cauller et al. 1998; Mitchell and Macklis 2005). Failure in this process is a hallmark of CC defects. Indeed, diffusion magnetic resonance imaging (dMRI) and tractography studies revealed that CC defects in humans are often accompanied by variable and disturbed contralateral callosal targeting (Bénézit et al. 2015; Tovar-Moll et al. 2007; Wahl et al. 2009), which often correlates with the degree of neurological impairment (Tovar-Moll et al. 2007).

15.5.1.1 Topographic Organization of Callosal Axons

As described previously, callosal axons from different cortical areas are segregated within the corpus callosum tract, such that the first axons to project are found dorsally and the last ones ventrally (Piper et al. 2009b; Zhou et al. 2013). This topography is thought to be achieved via repulsive Eph interactions between axons originating from different regions of the cortex (Nishikimi et al. 2011), as well as SEMA3A/NRP1 signaling (Zhou et al. 2013). Accordingly, genetic KO of *Sema3a* or overexpression of *Nrp1* (Zhou et al. 2013) disrupt axon order. However, interestingly, the position within the CC still determines projection targets, resulting in many abnormal heterotopic contralateral projections that fail to be refined (Zhou et al. 2013) (Figure 15.2D).

15.5.1.2 Electrophysiological properties of CPNs

Correct targeting of callosal axons also requires spontaneous and sensory-evoked neuronal activity, depending on a balance of intrinsic (endogenous cortical activity) and extrinsic (from the sensory periphery) stimuli between ipsilateral and contralateral areas (Huang et al. 2013; Mizuno et al. 2010; Suárez et al. 2014a). On the one hand, mature CPNs possess unique electrophysiological properties that distinguish them from other projection neuron classes (Hattox and Nelson 2007). The transcription factor CUX1 is involved in CPN electrical maturation. It regulates the expression of KV1 voltage-dependent potassium channels, resulting in a postnatal switch to a KV1-dependent firing mode; thus, loss of CUX1 leads to aberrant firing and defective contralateral innervation (Rodríguez-Tornos et al. 2016). Similarly, selective silencing of pre- or post-synaptic UL neurons leads to defects in axon projections (Mizuno et al. 2010). Furthermore, several studies found that disruption of sensory activity in one hemisphere can disrupt projections from homotopic regions in the contralateral hemisphere (Huang et al. 2013; Mizuno et al. 2010; Suárez et al. 2014a). Importantly, this phenotype can be partially rescued by bilateral disruption of sensory input or endogenous cortical activity, showing that appropriate callosal targeting relies on spatially symmetric interhemispheric activity (Huang et al. 2013; Suárez et al. 2014a). Currently, the molecular mechanisms regulating activity-dependent axon targeting and functional stabilization remain largely unknown.

Overall, orderly axonal organization within the CC, intrinsic electrophysiological properties of CPNs, and balanced interhemispheric activity are required for the generation of the stereotypical map of mostly homotopic callosal connections. Postnatally, these undergo selection to establish the final network.

15.5.2 Developmental Exuberance and Pruning of Connections

One of the hallmarks of cortical development is an overproduction of axons, axonal branches, and synapses – the so-called developmental exuberance (reviewed in Innocenti and Price 2005). Upon innervating target regions, callosal axons undergo selective branching and pruning, gradually shaping the axonal routes that define adult connectivity patterns. Although the degree and specificity of exuberance-selection is likely to have evolved significantly, this process has been identified across different species, including mouse, cat, monkey, and human, leading to loss of as much as 70 percent of callosal axons (Berbel and Innocenti 1988; Jovanov-Milosevic 2009; LaMantia and Rakic 1990). Specifically, humans show a decrease in size of the midsagittal cross-sectional area of the corpus callosum from 32PCW to the second postnatal month (Jovanov-Milosevic 2009). This process mainly occurs by axonal retraction, relying on the combination of activity-dependent mechanisms, sensory and hormonal inputs, as well as axon-axon competition dynamics (Innocenti and Price 2005).

15.5.2.1 Selective Pruning of Layer IV Contralateral Axons

The degree and rate of refinement of callosal axons depend on the layer and area of the cortex (De León Reyes et al. 2019). An example is layer IV excitatory neurons of the primary somatosensory (S1) barrel, which were long thought to project only ipsilaterally. A recent study has shown, however, that RORβ^+ layer IV neurons develop transient interhemispheric axons that are refined only postnatally, following thalamocortical input (De León Reyes et al. 2019). As such, layer IV neurons present an initial potential for callosal connectivity that is later lost. This study illustrates how neuron fate is neither fixed at birth nor even set prior to axonal extension, but rather gradually restricted across development downstream of cell-intrinsic properties and environmental inputs.

15.6 The Adult Corpus Callosum

In humans, at 18–20 PCW, the CC assumes a form and place essentially indistinguishable from that of the CC in the adult brain, except for its rostro-caudal portions, which continue to extend and thicken (Rakic and Yakovlev 1968). In its final form, the human CC yields about 200 million fibers (Aboitiz et al. 1992), and can be divided into seven antero-posterior segments: rostrum, genu, rostral body, anterior midbody, posterior midbody, isthmus, and splenium (Edwards et al. 2014; Mancuso et al. 2019; Rakic and Yakovlev 1968; Witelson 1989) (Figure 15.5A). Studies of patients that underwent partial callosotomy revealed functional specificity of segments, such that, for example, transfer of word-, but not color-, shape, or size-information occurs through splenial callosal fibers (Funnell et al. 2000).

15.6.1 Histological and Functional Properties of Callosal Fibers

In large brains, the length of fibers involved in circuits is increased, leading to conduction delay and slower transfer of information. And although increasing axonal myelination/diameter leads to higher conduction velocity, it cannot be applied to every fiber tract equally, due to spatial limitations (Ashwell 2016; Neves et al. 2017; Wang et al. 2008). Therefore, there needs to be a trade-off of axon properties, such that unmyelinated axons are compact but slow-conducting and energetically expensive; whereas myelinated and giant-myelinated axons are fast-conducting and energetically inexpensive, but large (Aboitiz et al. 1992; Wang et al. 2008). Overall, the CC is 30–40 percent myelinated (Mack et al. 1995) and axonal function is mainly maintained by glucose supply from

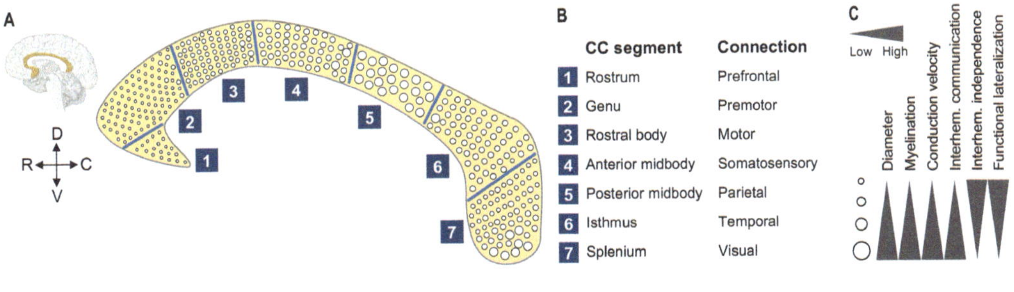

Figure 15.5 The adult human CC. A. The human CC can be divided into seven segments along the rostral–caudal axis: rostrum, genu, rostral body, anterior midbody, posterior midbody, isthmus, and splenium (Edwards et al. 2014; Mancuso et al. 2019; Rakic and Yakovlev 1968; Witelson 1989). (B) CC segments are structurally and functionally distinct, connecting different cortical areas. (C) Increased axon myelination/diameter leads to higher conduction velocity and interhemispheric communication; these properties are preferred in the body of the CC and gain particular relevance in the fast connection of motor and somatosensory areas. On the other hand, decreased axon myelination/diameter is associated with a delay in conduction velocity; these properties are preferred in areas such as the prefrontal cortex, where the human brain shows a higher degree of interhemispheric independence and functional lateralization (Aboitiz and Montiel 2003; Aboitiz et al. 1992; Hofman et al. 2014; Karolis et al. 2019; Mancuso et al. 2019; Phillips et al. 2015; Yang et al. 2022).

oligodendrocytes to axons via gap-junction-coupled glial networks (Meyer et al. 2018). Both the diameter and length of callosal fibers vary between species and along the antero-posterior axis of the CC, corresponding to the connection of specific cortical regions (Aboitiz and Montiel 2003; Aboitiz et al. 1992; Caminiti et al. 2013; Yang et al. 2022) (Figure 15.5B). Thus, the analysis of fiber properties can uncover important differences in evolutionary or developmental demand for fast interhemispheric communication (Figure 15.5C).

15.6.1.1 Connection of Motor and Sensory Cortices

The largest and fastest conducting axons in the human CC can reach up to 15 μm in diameter, an upper limit that is lower in the macaque (Aboitiz et al. 1992), and even lower in the mouse (Jerison 1992). These giant myelinated fibers are enriched in the midbody, corresponding to connections of motor and somatosensory areas (Aboitiz and Montiel 2003; Aboitiz et al. 1992; Mancuso et al. 2019). In addition to myelination status, a recent study used dMRI tractography to evaluate the scaling of callosal fiber length in relation to scaling of brain size in humans; some fibers were found to scale equally with brain size (iso-scaling), while others scaled less (under-scaling) or more (over-scaling) (Yang et al. 2022). Notably, fibers connecting the precentral gyrus and parietal cortices are under-scaled, preferably maintaining shorter fiber length (Yang et al. 2022). Therefore, the human brain evolved to increase myelination and decrease connection distance between motor and sensory areas, resulting in shorter connection delays and safeguarding basic functions needed for survival.

15.6.1.2 Evolution of Brain Lateralization

Small-diameter fibers connecting higher-order processing areas, such as the prefrontal cortex, make up a higher proportion of the total fibers in the human than in the macaque (Aboitiz et al. 1992; LaMantia and Rakic 1990), and in the macaque than in the mouse (Jerison 1992). Also, the prefrontal cortices are preferably connected by callosal fibers with over-scaling of length (Yang et al. 2022), and therefore larger delays in conduction (Caminiti et al. 2013; Yang et al. 2022). As initially proposed by James Ringo (Ringo et al. 1994), transfer delays produced by slow and long fibers may have promoted hemispheric computational independence and, consequently, forced lateral compartmentalization of networks (Aboitiz and Montiel 2003; Karolis et al. 2019; Phillips et al. 2015). In fact, specialized functions of the human brain, such as linguistic communication, require a high degree of local processing and sequential control, being therefore under selective pressure to develop locally in one hemisphere (Hofman et al. 2014; Karolis et al. 2019).

Together, these studies demonstrate that changing properties of callosal fibers may be at the core of brain evolution. Two critical determinants of conduction speed can be adjusted to achieve functional and structural efficacy, namely fiber myelination and length. Highly myelinated fibers with under-scaled length, on one hand, maintain fast sensory and motor responses despite cortical expansion; whereas less myelinated and lengthier fibers, on the other hand, potentially promoted a selective pressure towards lateralization of brain functions and development of higher-order local processing centers.

15.6.2 Excitatory and Inhibitory Roles of the CC

The understanding of the functions carried out by the CC has changed significantly since the 1950s. Pioneering studies by Roger Myers showed that, following sectioning of the optic chiasma and the CC, cats trained to perform a task with one eye masked were unable to remember with the second eye what had been learned (Myers 1956). These results led to the model proposed by Roger

Sperry in 1962 (Sperry 1962), which favored that the CC takes on an excitatory role in interhemispheric communication. This was supported by similar observations in humans that had undergone callosotomy (Gazzaniga 1995), by the fact that most callosal neurons are glutamatergic (Alcamo et al. 2008; Britanova et al. 2008; Conti and Manzoni 1994), and the use of callosotomy to prevent the interhemispheric propagation of seizures (Devinsky and Laff 2003). However, callosotomy was later shown to disrupt not only positive but also negative functional connectivity (Johnston et al. 2008), a finding that is consistent with the idea that the CC supports both excitatory and inhibitory functions (Bloom and Hynd 2005; Cook 1984; Mancuso et al. 2019). In fact, GABAergic CPNs have been described in layer V and postulated to respond to a strong stimulus by inhibiting postsynaptic targets (Zurita et al. 2018). Altogether, these studies support the hypothesis that communication through the CC is carried out both by excitatory and inhibitory synapses, depending on the task that is being performed.

15.7 CC Agenesis and Developmental Plasticity in the Human Brain

Several human neurodevelopmental defects involve agenesis of the CC, a congenital condition marked by complete or partial absence of the corpus callosum, either in isolation or associated with other neurodevelopmental anomalies (Edwards et al. 2014; Leyva-Díaz and López-Bendito 2013; Raybaud 2010; Warkany 1971). The study of patients with congenital CC defects has been crucial to further the understanding of the brain in clinical, evolutionary, and developmental biology perspectives.

15.7.1 Etiology of CC Agenesis

ACC affects approximately 1 in 4,000 newborns and 3–5 percent of children with intellectual disability (Marsh et al. 2017). It can be associated with a broad variety of symptoms, ranging from mild motor incoordination to language dysfunction, abnormal social interaction, and attention deficits (Edwards et al. 2014; Leyva-Díaz and López-Bendito 2013). In accordance with the intricacies of CC development, ACC is an extremely heterogeneous condition. It can arise from defects in neuronal specification or migration, neuronal or glial generation, midline patterning, axonal growth or guidance, or post-guidance development (reviewed in Edwards et al. 2014). Adding to its complexity, of the 30–45 percent ACC cases with an identifiable genetic root, only 20–35 percent are caused by a mutation affecting a single gene, and thus amenable for studies using mouse models (Donahoo and Richards 2009). However, the majority of ACC arises from unknown reasons, such as yet unidentified genetic mutations, or putative environmental factors like maternal malnutritional, prenatal alcohol exposure, or infections (Bhambal et al. 2015; Edwards et al. 2014; Paul et al. 2007). When the defect is due to general causes, timing of malformation onset determines whether other commissures are affected: before PCW10, formation of all forebrain commissures can fail; between PCW10 and 11, the AC may be normal (most common type of ACC); and from PCW11 both the AC and HC can be preserved (Cesaretti et al. 2016; Mancuso et al. 2019).

15.7.2 CC Agenesis in Autism Spectrum Disorder and Intellectual Disability

CC abnormalities are the most consistent finding in autism spectrum disorder (ASD) (Haar et al. 2016; Valenti et al. 2019) and constitute a major risk factor for developing ASD (Paul et al. 2014). Also, co-existence of CC agenesis and intellectual disability (ACC-ID) is common. *ARID1B* is the most frequently mutated gene in idiopathic ID (E. Y. Son and Crabtree 2014) and the main causal genetic link for ACC-ID (Edwards et al. 2016; Mignot et al. 2016; van der Sluijs et al. 2019); up to one-third of *ARID1B* patients present ACC, and a large fraction are diagnosed with ASD (Bögershausen and Wollnik 2018). However, the cellular origin and relationship between these phenotypes remains unclear. Several hypotheses have been formulated, from a theory of general underconnectivity, to combination of reduced long-distance and increased local connectivity (Valenti et al. 2019). In support of this, ASD patients have an increased percentage of small-diameter axons and a decreased percentage of large-diameter axons, suggestive of focal inter-hemispheric disconnection and diffuse underconnectivity (Wegiel et al. 2018). However, general corticogenesis defects might underlie some of the phenotypes. For instance, Timothy syndrome, a form of ASD caused by *Cav1/2* mutations, presents with a decrease in $SATB2^+$ and an increase in $CTIP2^+$ neurons (Paşca et al. 2011). And mutations in *Auts2*, a downstream target of TBR1 and, indirectly, SATB2, cause ASD (Srinivasan et al. 2012). Together, these studies show how both structural and behavioral phenotypes can arise from failure of common genetic programs.

15.7.3 Developmental Plasticity in CC Agenesis

Publications by Roger Sperry in the 1960s reported the remarkable identification of ACC patients by accident, following brain imaging for other purposes (Sperry 1968). In fact, subjects with congenital ACC often present no clinical manifestation at all (reviewed in Mancuso et al. 2019). Instead, compensatory wiring routes make up for the loss of the CC, such as ectopic tracts or enlargement of naturally occurring ones, like the anterior commissure (Barr and Corballis 2002; Bénézit et al. 2015; Tovar-Moll et al. 2007, 2014). These novel networks connect homotopic cortical regions, possibly compensating at least in part for the lack of interhemispheric connectivity normally mediated by the CC (Tovar-Moll et al. 2014). Such a phenomenon is also observed in other species, as seen with rerouting through the AC in *Satb2*$^{-/-}$ mice (Alcamo et al. 2008; Britanova et al. 2008) and in surgically induced acallosal hamsters (Lent and Guimarães 1990). Interestingly, in such cases, the compensatory rewiring can resemble the non-eutherian connectome (large AC, no CC), suggesting that under certain developmental conditions neocortical commissural neurons may exploit developmental plasticity of ancient mechanisms of axon guidance. Therefore, callosal neurons are likely to retain an intrinsic ability to employ of alternative axon pathfinding mechanisms when unable to project through the CC, leading to developmental adaptative reorganizations that, in some cases, are sufficient to safeguard brain function.

Overall, we are still far from being able to predict when the absence of the CC might, or not, lead to cognitive impairment. Ultimately, a continued investigation of the developmental basis of CC malformations will improve our fundamental understanding of brain wiring and can provide significant benefits for patients by improving diagnosis and management of conditions from early stages of life (Virues-Ortega et al. 2022).

15.8 Conclusion

Investigation on the corpus callosum has come a long way since the early studies in the first half of the twentieth century. Nowadays, it is undeniable that this field of research unifies central aspects of neurobiology. On an evolutionary perspective, it answers questions pertaining to structural innovations in the brain, cortical expansion, and emergence of higher-order cognition. Developmentally, it reflects basic conserved principles of axon guidance, as well as novelties unique to eutherian mammals and with particular relevance in humans. Finally, while some cases of CC agenesis show the devastating effects of impaired interhemispheric communication, others constitute prime examples of neuronal plasticity, showcasing the astounding capability of the brain to adapt to perturbations. Nevertheless, after almost a century of research, we are still far from understanding the functional relevance of the CC to the fullest, and exciting questions with translational relevance remain unsolved. But something has become clear: once adjectivized as the "largest, most useless" part of the brain (Sperry 1962), the corpus callosum is now recognized as an essential structure and an enabler of the human condition itself.

Acknowledgments

The animal silhouettes in Figure 15.1 and sagittal scheme of the brain in Figure 15.5 were generated with BioRender.com.

Notes

1. *Cux2, Btg1, EphA3, Frmd4b, Inhba, Ptn.*
2. *Cav1, Cntn2, ChL1, Chn2, Cpne4, Gap43, Gm879, L1cam, Nectin-3, Neo1, Nnmt, Tmtc4.*
3. *Add1, Add3, Camk2, Dkk3, Gfra2, Gsk3b, PlxnA1, PlxA4, PlxnD1, TcrB.*
4. *GFAP.*
5. *Nefl, Nefm, Thy1.*
6. *MAB, Plp1.*
7. *Fog-2.*
8. *Dkk3, Gfra2, Plexin-D1, Tcrb.*
9. *Btg1, Cpne4, Cux1, Cux2, Inhba, Tmtc4.*
10. *EphA3, Frmd4b, Nnmt.*
11. *Chn2, Nectin-3.*
12. *Cav1, Gm879, Ptn.*

References

Abbot, P. and Capra, J.A. (2017). What is a placental mammal anyway? many developmental functions in marsupials and eutherian mammals are accomplished by different tissues, but similar genes. *Elife* 6: 1–3. doi: 10.7554/eLife.30994.

Abellán, A. and Medina, L. (2009). Subdivisions and derivatives of the chicken subpallium based on expression of LIM and other regulatory genes and markers of neuron subpopulations during development. *J Comp Neurol* 515 (4): 465–501. doi: 10.1002/cne.22083.

Aboitiz, F. and Montiel, J. (2003). One hundred million years of interhemispheric communication: the history of the corpus callosum. *Braz J Med Biol Res* 36 (4): 409–420. doi: 10.1590/S0100-879X2003 000400002.

Aboitiz, F. et al. (1992). Fiber composition of the human corpus callosum. *Brain Res* 598: 143–153.

Ahmed, G. et al. (2011). Draxin inhibits axonal outgrowth through the netrin receptor dcc. *J Neurosci* 31 (39): 14018–14023. doi: 10.1523/JNEUROSCI.0943-11.2011.

Alcamo, E.A. et al. (2008). Satb2 regulates callosal projection neuron identity in the developing cerebral cortex. *Neuron* 57 (3): 364–377. doi: 10.1016/j.neuron.2007.12.012.

Andrews, W. et al. (2006). Robo1 regulates the development of major axon tracts and interneuron migration in the forebrain. *Development* 133 (11): 2243–2252. doi: 10.1242/dev.02379.

Arendt, D. et al. (2008). The evolution of nervous system centralization. *Philos Trans R Soc B: Biol Sci* 363 (1496): 1523–1528. doi: 10.1098/rstb.2007.2242.

Arlotta, P. et al. (2005). Neuronal subtype-specific genes that control corticospinal motor neuron development in vivo. *Neuron* 45 (2): 207–221. doi: 10.1016/j.neuron.2004.12.036.

Ashwell, K.W.S. (2016). Anterior commissure versus corpus callosum: a quantitative comparison across mammals. *Zoology* 119 (2): 126–136. doi: 10.1016/j.zool.2016.02.004.

Ashwell, K.W.S. et al. (1996). Ontogeny of the projection tracts and commissural fibres in the forebrain of the Tammar Wallaby (Macropus eugenii): timing in comparison with other mammals. *Brain, Behav Evol* 47: 8–22.

Azim, E. et al. (2009). Lmo4 and Clim1 progressively delineate cortical projection neuron subtypes during development. *Cereb Cortex* 19 (Suppl. 1): 62–69. doi: 10.1093/cercor/bhp030.

Bagri, A. et al. (2002). Slit proteins prevent midline crossing and determine the dorsoventral position of major axonal pathways in the mammalian forebrain. *Neuron* 33 (2): 233–248. doi: 10.1016/S0896-6273(02)00561-5.

Baranek, C. et al. (2012). Protooncogene Ski cooperates with the chromatin-remodeling factor Satb2 in specifying callosal neurons. *Proc Natl Acad Sci* 109 (9): 3546–3551. doi: 10.1073/pnas.1108718109.

Barr, M.S. and Corballis, M.C. (2002). The role of the anterior commissure in callosal agenesis. *Neuropsychology* 16 (4): 459–471. doi: 10.1037/0894-4105.16.4.459.

Belgard, T.G. et al. (2013). Adult pallium transcriptomes surprise in not reflecting predicted homologies across diverse chicken and mouse pallial sectors. *Proc Natl Acad Sci USA* 110 (32): 13150–13155. doi: 10.1073/pnas.1307444110.

Benadiba, C. et al. (2012). The ciliogenic transcription factor RFX3 regulates early midline distribution of guidepost neurons required for corpus callosum development. *PLoS Genet* 8 (3): e1002606. doi: 10.1371/journal.pgen.1002606.

Bénézit, A. et al. (2015). Organising white matter in a brain without corpus callosum fibres. *Cortex* 63: 155–171. doi: 10.1016/j.cortex.2014.08.022.

Berbel, P. and Innocenti, G.M. (1988). The development of the corpus callosum in cats: a light- and electron-microscopic study. *J Comp Neurol* 276 (1): 132–156. doi: 10.1002/cne.902760109.

Berg, J. et al. (2021). Human neocortical expansion involves glutamatergic neuron diversification. *Nature* 598 (7879): 151–158. doi: 10.1038/s41586-021-03813-8.

Bhambal, A.M. et al. (2015). Orodental manifestations in cases with partial agenesis of corpus callosum-rare phenomena. *J Oral Biol Craniofac Res* 5 (2): 106–111. doi: 10.1016/j.jobcr.2015.04.003.

Bielle, F. and Garel, S. (2013). Neuronal migration of guidepost cells. In: *Cellular Migration and Formation of Neuronal Connections*, vol. 2 (ed. J.L.R Rubenstein and P. Rakic), 457–479. doi: 10.1016/B978-0-12-397266-8.00037-5.

Bloom, J.S. and Hynd, G.W. (2005). The role of the corpus callosum in interhemispheric transfer of information: excitation or inhibition? *Neuropsychol Rev* 15 (2): 59–71. doi: 10.1007/s11065-005-6252-y.

Bögershausen, N. and Wollnik, B. (2018 August). Mutational landscapes and phenotypic spectrum of SWI/SNF-related intellectual disability disorders. *Front Mol Neurosci* 11: 1–18. doi: 10.3389/fnmol.2018.00252.

Bormuth, I. et al. (2013). Neuronal basic helix-loop-helix proteins neurod2/6 regulate cortical commissure formation before midline interactions. *J Neurosci* 33 (2): 641–651. doi: 10.1523/JNEUROSCI.0899-12.2013.

Bremer, C. et al. (2001). In vivo molecular target assessment of matrix metalloproteinase inhibition. *Nat Med* 7 (6): 743–748. doi: 10.1038/89126.

Britanova, O. et al. (2008). Satb2 is a postmitotic determinant for upper-layer neuron specification in the neocortex. *Neuron* 57 (3): 378–392. doi: 10.1016/j.neuron.2007.12.028.

Bush, J.O. and Soriano, P. (2009). Ephrin-B1 regulates axon guidance by reverse signaling through a PDZ-dependent mechanism. *Genes Dev* 23 (13): 1586–1599. doi: 10.1101/gad.1807209.

Bystron, I. et al. (2008). Development of the human cerebral cortex. *Nat Rev Neurosci* 9: 110–122. doi: 10.1038/nrn2252.

Caminiti, R. et al. (2013). Diameter, length, speed, and conduction delay of callosal axons in macaque monkeys and humans. *J Neurosci* 33 (36): 14501–14511. doi: 10.1523/JNEUROSCI.0761-13.2013.

Canovas, J. et al. (2015). The specification of cortical subcerebral projection neurons depends on the direct repression of TBR1 by CTIP1/BCL11a. *J Neurosci* 35 (19): 7552–7564. doi: 10.1523/JNEUROSCI.0169-15.2015.

Cauller, L.J. et al. (1998). Backward cortical projections to primary somatosensory cortex in rats extend long horizontal axons in layer I. *J Comp Neurol* 390 (2): 297–310. doi: 10.1002/(SICI)1096-9861(19980112)390:2<297::AID-CNE11>3.0.CO;2-V.

Cera, I. et al. (2019). Genes encoding SATB2-interacting proteins in adult cerebral cortex contribute to human cognitive ability. *PLoS Genet* 15 (2): 1–21. doi: 10.1371/journal.pgen.1007890.

Cesaretti, C. et al. (2016). Variability of forebrain commissures in callosal agenesis. *Am J Neuroradiol* 37 (3): 521–527. doi: 10.3174/ajnr.A4570.

Chen, B. et al. (2005). Fezl regulates the differentiation and axon targeting of layer 5 subcortical projection neurons in cerebral cortex. *Proc Natl Acad Sci USA* 102 (47): 17184–17189. doi: 10.1073/pnas.0508732102.

Chen, B. et al. (2008). The Fezf2-Ctip2 genetic pathway regulates the fate choice of subcortical projection neurons in the developing cerebral cortex. *Proc Natl Acad Sci USA* 105 (32): 11382–11387. doi: 10.1073/pnas.0804918105.

Chen, C.P. et al. (2011). Chromosome 1p32-p31 deletion syndrome. *Taiwan J Obstet Gynecol* 50 (3): 345–352. doi: 10.1016/j.tjog.2011.07.014.

Choe, Y. et al. (2012). A cascade of morphogenic signaling initiated by the meninges controls corpus callosum formation. *Neuron* 73 (4): 698–712. doi: 10.1016/j.neuron.2011.11.036.

Clegg, J.M. et al. (2014). Heparan sulfotransferases Hs6st1 and Hs2st keep Erk in check for mouse corpus callosum development. *J Neurosci* 34 (6): 2389–2401. doi: 10.1523/JNEUROSCI.3157-13.2014.

Conti, F. and Manzoni, T. (1994). The neurotransmitters and postsynaptic actions of callosally projecting neurons. *Behav Brain Res* 64 (1–2): 37–53. doi: 10.1016/0166-4328(94)90117-1.

Conway, C.D. et al. (2011). Heparan sulfate sugar modifications mediate the functions of Slits and other factors needed for mouse forebrain commissure development. *J Neurosci* 31 (6): 1955–1970. doi: 10.1523/JNEUROSCI.2579-10.2011.

Cook, N.D. (1984). Homotopic callosal inhibition. *Brain Lang* 23 (1): 116–125. doi: 10.1016/0093-934X(84)90010-5.

Cubelos, B. et al. (2010). Cux1 and Cux2 regulate dendritic branching, spine morphology, and synapses of the upper layer neurons of the cortex. *Neuron* 66 (4): 523–535. doi: 10.1016/j.neuron.2010.04.038.

Cui, Z. et al. (2013). Hypothalamic and other connections with dorsal CA2 area of the mouse hippocampus. *J Comp Neurol* 521 (8): 1844–1866. doi: 10.1002/cne.23263.

De León Reyes, N.S. et al. (2019). Transient callosal projections of L4 neurons are eliminated for the acquisition of local connectivity. *Nat Commun* 10 (1): 1–15. doi: 10.1038/s41467-019-12495-w.

Devinsky, O. and Laff, R. (2003). Callosal lesions and behavior. *Epilepsy Behav* 4 (6): 607–617. doi: 10.1016/j.yebeh.2003.08.029.

Dominguez, M.H. et al. (2013). POU-III transcription factors (Brn1, Brn2, and Oct6) influence neurogenesis, molecular identity, and migratory destination of upper-layer cells of the cerebral cortex. *Cereb Cortex* 23 (11): 2632–2643. doi: 10.1093/cercor/bhs252.

Donahoo, A.L.S. and Richards, L.J. (2009). Understanding the mechanisms of callosal development through the use of transgenic mouse models. *Semin Pediatr Neurol* 16 (3): 127–142. doi: 10.1016/j.spen.2009.07.003.

Doyle, D.Z. et al. (2021). Chromatin remodeler Arid1a regulates subplate neuron identity and wiring of cortical connectivity. *Proc Natl Acad Sci USA* 118: 21. doi: 10.1073/pnas.2100686118.

Ebner, F.F. (1969). A comparison of primitive forebrain organization in metatherian and eutherian mammals. *Ann N Y Acad Sci* 167 (1): 241–257. doi: 10.1111/j.1749-6632.1969.tb20447.x.

Edwards, T.J. et al. (2014). Clinical, genetic and imaging findings identify new causes for corpus callosum development syndromes. *Brain* 137 (6): 1579–1613. doi: 10.1093/brain/awt358.

Edwards, T.J. et al. (2016). Reply. *Brain* 139 (11): e65. doi: 10.1093/brain/aww171.

Fame, R.M. et al. (2017). Subtype-specific genes that characterize subpopulations of callosal projection neurons in mouse identify molecularly homologous populations in macaque cortex. *Cereb Cortex* 27 (3): 1817–1830. doi: 10.1093/cercor/bhw023.

Fame, R.M. et al. (2016). Cited2 regulates neocortical layer II/III generation and somatosensory callosal projection neuron development and connectivity. *J Neurosci* 36 (24): 6403–6419. doi: 10.1523/JNEUROSCI.4067-15.2016.

Fazeli, A. et al. (1997). Phenotype of mice lacking functional Deleted in colorectal cancer (Dec) gene. *Nature* 386 (6627): 796–804. doi: 10.1038/386796a0.

Fenlon, L.R. and Richards, L.J. (2015). Contralateral targeting of the corpus callosum in normal and pathological brain function. *Trends Neurosci* 38 (5): 264–272. doi: 10.1016/j.tins.2015.02.007.

Fenlon, L.R. et al. (2021). The evolution, formation and connectivity of the anterior commissure. *Semin Cell Dev Biol* 118: 50–59. doi: 10.1016/j.semcdb.2021.04.009.

Ffrench-Constant, S. et al. (2019). Fetal and neonatal MRI features of ARX-related lissencephaly presenting with neonatal refractory seizure disorder. *Quant Imaging Med Surg* 9 (11): 1767–1772. doi: 10.21037/qims.2019.10.14.

Finci, L.I. et al. (2014). The crystal structure of netrin-1 in complex with DCC reveals the bifunctionality of netrin-1 as a guidance cue. *Neuron* 83 (4): 839–849. doi: 10.1016/j.neuron.2014.07.010.

Fothergill, T. et al. (2014). Netrin-DCC signaling regulates corpus callosum formation through attraction of pioneering axons and by modulating slit2-mediated repulsion. *Cereb Cortex* 24 (5): 1138–1151. doi: 10.1093/cercor/bhs395.

Funnell, M.G. et al. (2000). Insights into the functional specificity of the human corpus callosum. *Brain* 123 (Pt 5): 920–926. doi: 10.1093/brain/123.5.920.

García-Moreno, F. and Molnár, Z. (2015). Subset of early radial glial progenitors that contribute to the development of callosal neurons is absent from avian brain. *Proc Natl Acad Sci* 112 (36): E5058–E5067. doi: 10.1073/pnas.1506377112.

García-Moreno, F. and Molnár, Z. (2020). Variations of telencephalic development that paved the way for neocortical evolution. *Prog Neurobiol* 194: 101865. doi: 10.1016/j.pneurobio.2020.101865.

Gazzaniga, M.S. (1995). Principles of human brain organization derived from split-brain studies. *Neuron* 14 (2): 217–228. doi: 10.1016/0896-6273(95)90280-5.

Gobius, I. et al. (2016). Astroglial-mediated remodeling of the interhemispheric midline is required for the formation of the corpus callosum. *Cell Rep* 17 (3): 735–747. doi: 10.1016/j.celrep.2016.09.033.

Guernsey, M.W. et al. (2017). Molecular conservation of marsupial and eutherian placentation and lactation. *Elife* 6: 1–19. doi: 10.7554/eLife.27450.

Haar, S. et al. (2016). Anatomical abnormalities in autism? *Cereb Cortex* 26 (4): 1440–1452. doi: 10.1093/cercor/bhu242.

Hakanen, J. and Salminen, M. (2015). Defects in neural guidepost structures and failure to remove leptomeningeal cells from the septal midline behind the interhemispheric fusion defects in Netrin1 deficient mice. *Int J Dev Neurosci* 47: 206–215. doi: 10.1016/j.ijdevneu.2015.08.005.

Han, W. et al. (2011). TBR1 directly represses Fezf2 to control the laminar origin and development of the corticospinal tract. *Proc Natl Acad Sci USA* 108 (7): 3041–3046. doi: 10.1073/pnas.1016723108.

Hand, R. et al. (2005). Phosphorylation of neurogenin2 specifies the migration properties and the dendritic morphology of pyramidal neurons in the neocortex. *Neuron* 48 (1): 45–62. doi: 10.1016/j.neuron.2005.08.032.

Hand, R. and Polleux, F. (2011). Neurogenin2 regulates the initial axon guidance of cortical pyramidal neurons projecting medially to the corpus callosum. *Neural Dev* 6: 1. doi: 10.1186/1749-8104-6-30.

Harb, K. et al. (2016). Area-specific development of distinct projection neuron subclasses is regulated by postnatal epigenetic modifications. *Elife* 5: 1–25. doi: 10.7554/eLife.09531.

Hartmann, H. et al. (2004). Agenesis of the corpus callosum, abnormal genitalia and intractable epilepsy due to a novel familial mutation in the aristaless-related homeobox gene. *Neuropediatrics* 35 (3): 157–160. doi: 10.1055/s-2004-817919.

Hattox, A.M. and Nelson, S.B. (2007). Layer V neurons in mouse cortex projecting to different targets have distinct physiological properties. *J Neurophysiol* 98 (6): 3330–3340. doi: 10.1152/jn.00397.2007.

Hayano, Y. et al. (2014). The role of T-cadherin in axonal pathway formation in neocortical circuits. *Development* 141 (24): 4784–4793. doi: 10.1242/dev.108290.

Hoerder-Suabedissen, A. and Molnár, Z. (2013). Molecular diversity of early-born subplate neurons. *Cereb Cortex* 23 (6): 1473–1483. doi: 10.1093/cercor/bhs137.

Hoerder-Suabedissen, A. and Molnár, Z. (2015). Development, evolution and pathology of neocortical subplate neurons. *Nat Rev Neurosci* 16 (3): 133–146. doi: 10.1038/nrn3915.

Hoerder-Suabedissen, A. et al. (2009). Novel markers reveal subpopulations of subplate neurons in the murine cerebral cortex. *Cereb Cortex* 19 (8): 1738–1750. doi: 10.1093/cercor/bhn195.

Hofman, M.A. et al. (2014). Evolution of the human brain. *Front Neuroanat* 8: 15. doi: 10.3389/fnana.2014.00015.

Hossain, Md.M. et al. (2019). PlexinA1 is crucial for the midline crossing of callosal axons during corpus callosum development in BALB/cAJ mice. *Plos One* 14 (8): e0221440. doi: 10.1371/journal.pone.0221440.

Huang, Y. et al. (2013). Sensory input is required for callosal axon targeting in the somatosensory cortex. *Mol Brain* 6 (1): 1–12. doi: 10.1186/1756-6606-6-53.

Hutchins, B.I. et al. (2011). Wnt/calcium signaling mediates axon growth and guidance in the developing corpus callosum. *Dev Neurobiol* 71 (4): 269–283. doi: 10.1002/dneu.20846.

Innocenti, G.M. and Price, D.J. (2005). Exuberance in the development of cortical networks. *Nat Rev Neurosci* 6 (12): 955–965. doi: 10.1038/nrn1790.

Islam, S.M. et al. (2009). Draxin, a repulsive guidance protein for spinal cord and forebrain commissures. *Science* 323 (5912): 388–393. doi: 10.1126/science.1165187.

Jaitner, C. et al. (2016). Satb2 determines miRNA expression and long-term memory in the adult central nervous system. *Elife* 5: 1–24. doi: 10.7554/eLife.17361.

Jamuar, S.S. et al. (2017). Biallelic mutations in human DCC cause developmental split-brain syndrome. *Nat Genet* 49 (4): 606–612. doi: 10.1038/ng.3804.

Jerison, H.J. (1992). Brain size and the evolution of mind. The 59th James Arthur lecture on the evolution of the human brain. *Brain, Behav Evol* 39: 195–196.

Johnston, J.M. et al. (2008). Loss of resting interhemispheric functional connectivity after complete section of the corpus callosum. *J Neurosci* 28 (25): 6453–6458. doi: 10.1523/JNEUROSCI.0573-08.2008.

Jovanov-Milosevic, N. (2009 June). Growth of the human corpus callosum. *Front Neuroanat* 3: 1–10. doi: 10.3389/neuro.05.006.2009.

Jovanov-Milošević, N. et al. (2010). Morphology, molecular phenotypes and distribution of neurons in developing human corpus callosum. *Eur J Neurosci* 32 (9): 1423–1432. doi: 10.1111/j.1460-9568.2010.07400.x.

Kahn, O.I. and Baas, P.W. (2016). Microtubules and growth cones. *Trends Neurosci* 39 (7): 433–440. doi: 10.1016/j.tins.2016.04.009.

Kanold, P.O. and Luhmann, H.J. (2010). The subplate and early cortical circuits. *Ann Rev Neurosci* 33: 23–48. doi: 10.1146/annurev-neuro-060909-153244.

Karolis, V.R. et al. (2019). The architecture of functional lateralisation and its relationship to callosal connectivity in the human brain. *Nat Commun* 10 (1): 1–9. doi: 10.1038/s41467-019-09344-1.

Kastriti, M.E. et al. (2019 November). Ablation of CNTN2+ pyramidal neurons during development results in defects in neocortical size and axonal tract formation. *Front Cell Neurosci* 13: 1–19. doi: 10.3389/fncel.2019.00454.

Katz, M.J. (1983). Ontophyletics of the nervous system. *Proc Natl Acad Sci USA* 80 (19): 5936–5940.

Keeble, T.R. et al. (2006). The Wnt receptor Ryk is required for Wnt5a-mediated axon guidance on the contralateral side of the corpus callosum. *J Neurosci* 26 (21): 5840–5848. doi: 10.1523/JNEUROSCI.1175-06.2006.

Kitamura, K. et al. (2002). Mutation of ARX causes abnormal development of forebrain and testes in mice and X-linked lissencephaly with abnormal genitalia in humans. *Nat Genet* 32 (3): 359–369. doi: 10.1038/ng1009.

Kosho, T. et al. (2014). Genotype-phenotype correlation of coffin-siris syndrome caused by mutations in SMARCB1, SMARCA4, SMARCE1, and ARID1A. *Am J Med Genet Part C, Semin Med Genet* 166 (3): 262–275. doi: 10.1002/ajmg.c.31407.

Kosho, T. et al. (2013). Clinical correlations of mutations affecting six components of the SWI/SNF complex. *Am J Med Genet Part A* 161 (6): 1221–1237. doi: 10.1002/ajmg.a.35933.

Kostović, I. (2020). The enigmatic fetal subplate compartment forms an early tangential cortical nexus and provides the framework for construction of cortical connectivity. *Prog Neurobiol* 194: 101883. doi: 10.1016/j.pneurobio.2020.101883.

Kozulin, P. et al. (2022). Divergent evolution of developmental timing in the neocortex revealed by marsupial and eutherian transcriptomes. *Development* 149 (3): dev200212. doi: 10.1242/dev.200212.

Kwan, K.Y. et al. (2008). SOX5 postmitotically regulates migration, postmigratory differentiation, and projections of subplate and deep-layer neocortical neurons. *Proc Natl Acad Sci USA* 105 (41): 16021–16026. doi: 10.1073/pnas.0806791105.

Lai, T. et al. (2008). SOX5 controls the sequential generation of distinct corticofugal neuron subtypes. *Neuron* 57 (2): 232–247. doi: 10.1016/j.neuron.2007.12.023.

LaMantia, A.S. and Rakic, P. (1990). Axon overproduction and elimination in the corpus callosum of the developing rhesus monkey. *J Neurosci* 10 (7): 2156–2175. doi: 10.1523/jneurosci.10-07-02156.1990.

Lavado, A. et al. (2014). The tumor suppressor Nf2 regulates corpus callosum development by inhibiting the transcriptional coactivator Yap. *Development* 141 (21): 4182-4193. doi: 10.1242/dev.111260.

Lent, R. and Guimarães, R.Z. (1990). Development of interhemispheric connections through the anterior commissure in hamsters. *Braz J Med Biol Res* 23 (8): 671–675.

Leone, D.P. et al. (2015). Satb2 regulates the differentiation of both callosal and subcerebral projection neurons in the developing cerebral cortex. *Cereb Cortex* 25 (10): 3406–3419. doi: 10.1093/cercor/bhu156.

Leyva-Díaz, E. and López-Bendito, G. (2013). In and out from the cortex. *Neuroscience* 254: 26–44. doi: 10.1016/j.neuroscience.2013.08.070.

Lickiss, T. et al. (2012). Examining the relationship between early axon growth and transcription factor expression in the developing cerebral cortex. *J Anat* 220 (3): 201–211. doi: 10.1111/j.1469-7580.2011.01466.x.

López-Bendito, G. et al. (2007). Robo1 and Robo2 cooperate to control the guidance of major axonal tracts in the mammalian forebrain. *J Neurosci* 27 (13): 3395–3407. doi: 10.1523/JNEUROSCI.4605-06.2007.

Lu, W. et al. (2007). NFIA haploinsufficiency is associated with a CNS malformation syndrome and urinary tract defects. *PLoS Genet* 3 (5): 830–843. doi: 10.1371/journal.pgen.0030080.

MacDonald, J.L. et al. (2018). Caveolin1 identifies a specific subpopulation of cerebral cortex callosal projection neurons (CPN) including dual projecting cortical callosal/frontal projection neurons (CPN/FPN). *eNeuro* 5 (1): ENEURO.0234-17.2017. doi: 10.1523/ENEURO.0234-17.2017.

Mack, C.M. et al. (1995). Sex differences in the distribution of axon types within the genu of the rat corpus callosum. *Brain Res* 697 (1–2): 152–156. doi: 10.1016/0006-8993(95)00804-Y.

Magnani, D. et al. (2014). Gli3 controls corpus callosum formation by positioning midline guideposts during telencephalic patterning. *Cereb Cortex* 24 (1): 186–198. doi: 10.1093/cercor/bhs303.

Mancuso, L. et al. (2019). Brain functional connectivity in individuals with callosotomy and agenesis of the corpus callosum: a systematic review. *Neurosci Biobehav Rev* 105: 231–248. doi: 10.1016/j.neubiorev.2019.07.004.

Marsh, A.P.L. et al. (2017). Mutations in DCC cause isolated agenesis of the corpus callosum with incomplete penetrance. *Nat Genet* 49 (4): 511–514. doi: 10.1038/ng.3794.

Maxwell, D.J. and Soteropoulos, D.S. (2020). The mammalian spinal commissural system: properties and functions. *J Neurophysiol* 123 (1): 4–21. doi: 10.1152/jn.00347.2019.

McKenna, W.L. et al. (2011). Tbr1 and Fezf2 regulate alternate corticofugal neuronal identities during neocortical development. *J Neurosci* 31 (2): 549–564. doi: 10.1523/JNEUROSCI.4131-10.2011.

McKenna, W.L. et al. (2015). Mutual regulation between *Satb2* and *Fezf2* promotes subcerebral projection neuron identity in the developing cerebral cortex. *Proc Natl Acad Sci* 112 (37): 11702–11707. doi: 10.1073/pnas.1504144112.

Medina, L. and Abellán, A. (2009). Development and evolution of the pallium. *Semin Cell Dev Biol* 20 (6): 698–711. doi: 10.1016/j.semcdb.2009.04.008.

Mendes, S.W. (2006). Multiple Eph receptors and B-class ephrins regulate midline crossing of corpus callosum fibers in the developing mouse forebrain. *J Neurosci* 26 (3): 882–892. doi: 10.1523/JNEUROSCI.3162-05.2006.

Meyer, N. et al. (2018). Oligodendrocytes in the mouse corpus callosum maintain axonal function by delivery of glucose. *Cell Rep* 22 (9): 2455–2468. doi: 10.1016/j.celrep.2018.02.022.

Mignot, C. et al. (2016). ARID1B mutations are the major genetic cause of corpus callosum anomalies in patients with intellectual disability. *Brain* 139 (11): e64. doi: 10.1093/brain/aww181.

Mire, E. et al. (2018). Developmental upregulation of Ephrin-B1 silences Sema3c/Neuropilin-1 signaling during post-crossing navigation of corpus callosum axons. *Curr Biol* 28 (11): 1768–1782.e4. doi: 10.1016/j.cub.2018.04.026.

Mitchell, B.D. and Macklis, J.D. (2005). Large-scale maintenance of dual projections by callosal and frontal cortical projection neurons in adult mice. *J Comp Neurol* 482 (1): 17–32. doi: 10.1002/cne.20428.

Mizuno, H. et al. (2010). Pre-synaptic and post-synaptic neuronal activity supports the axon development of callosal projection neurons during different post-natal periods in the mouse cerebral cortex. *Eur J Neurosci* 31 (3): 410–424. doi: 10.1111/j.1460-9568.2009.07070.x.

Moldrich, R.X. et al. (2010). Molecular regulation of the developing commissural plate. *J Comp Neurol* 518 (18): 3645–3661. doi: 10.1002/cne.22445.

Molyneaux, B.J. et al. (2009). Novel subtype-specific genes identify distinct subpopulations of callosal projection neurons. *J Neurosci* 29 (39): 12343–12354. doi: 10.1523/JNEUROSCI.6108-08.2009.

Molyneaux, B.J. et al. (2005). Fezl is required for the birth and specification of corticospinal motor neurons. *Neuron* 47 (6): 817–831. doi: 10.1016/j.neuron.2005.08.030.

Morcom, L.R. et al. (2016). Cortical architecture, midline guidance, and tractography of 3D white matter tracts. In: *Axons and Brain Architecture* (ed. K.S. Rockland), 289–313. doi: 10.1016/b978-0-12-801393-9.00014-1.

Myers, R.E. (1956). Function of corpus callosum in interocular transfer. *Brain* 79 (2): 358–363. doi: 10.1093/brain/79.2.358.

Naumann, R.K. and Laurent, G. (2017). Function and evolution of the reptilian cerebral cortex. In: *Evolution of Nervous Systems*, 2e, vol. 1 (ed. J.H. Kass), 491–518. Amsterdam: Elsevier. doi: 10.1016/B978-0-12-804042-3.00022-1.

Neves, K. et al. (2017). White matter expansion. In: *Evolution of Nervous Systems*, 2e, vol. 2 (ed. J.H. Kass, 291–308. Amsterdam: Elsevier.

Niquille, M. et al. (2009). Transient neuronal populations are required to guide callosal axons. *PLoS Biology* 7: 10. doi: 10.1371/journal.pbio.1000230.

Niquille, M. et al. (2013). Two specific populations of GABAergic neurons originating from the medial and the caudal ganglionic eminences aid in proper navigation of callosal axons. *Dev Neurobiol* 73 (9): 647–672. doi: 10.1002/dneu.22075.

Nishikimi, M. et al. (2011). Segregation and pathfinding of callosal axons through EphA3 signaling. *J Neurosci* 31 (45): 16251–16260. doi: 10.1523/JNEUROSCI.3303-11.2011.

Nomura, T. et al. (2013). Changes in the regulation of cortical neurogenesis contribute to encephalization during amniote brain evolution. *Nat Commun* 4: 2206. doi: 10.1038/ncomms3206.

Nomura, T. et al. (2018). Species-specific mechanisms of neuron subtype specification reveal evolutionary plasticity of amniote brain development. *Cell Rep* 22 (12): 3142–3151. doi: 10.1016/j.celrep.2018.02.086.

Oishi, K. et al. (2016). Mutually repressive interaction between Brn1/2 and Rorb contributes to the establishment of neocortical layer 2/3 and layer 4. *Proc Natl Acad Sci USA* 113 (12): 3371–3376. doi: 10.1073/pnas.1515949113.

Oran, Y. et al. (2021). Reduction of corpus callosum activity during whisking leads to interhemispheric decorrelation. *Nat Commun* 12 (1): 4095. doi: 10.1038/s41467-021-24310-6.

Osborn, H.F. (1886). The corpus callosum in lower vertebrates. *Science* 8 (185): 167–168.

Ozaki, H.S. and Wahlsten, D. (1998). Timing and origin of the first cortical axons to project through the corpus callosum and the subsequent emergence of callosal projection cells in mouse. *J Comp Neurol* 400 (2): 197–206. doi: 10.1002/(SICI)1096-9861(19981019)400:2<197::AID-CNE3>3.0.CO;2-4.

Paolino, A. et al. (2020). Differential timing of a conserved transcriptional network underlies divergent cortical projection routes across mammalian brain evolution. *Proc Natl Acad Sci USA* 117 (19): 10554–10564. doi: 10.1073/pnas.1922422117.

Paşca, S.P. et al. (2011). Using iPSC-derived neurons to uncover cellular phenotypes associated with Timothy syndrome. *Nat Med* 17 (12): 1657–1662. doi: 10.1038/nm.2576.

Paul, L.K. et al. (2007). Agenesis of the corpus callosum. *Nat Rev Neurosci* 8 (4): 287–299. doi: 10.1038/nrn2107.

Paul, L.K. et al. (2014). Agenesis of the corpus callosum and autism. *Brain* 137 (6): 1813–1829. doi: 10.1093/brain/awu070.

Phillips, K.A. et al. (2015). The corpus callosum in primates. *Proc R Soc B: Biol Sci* 282 (1818): 20151535. doi: 10.1098/rspb.2015.1535.

Piper, M. et al. (2010). NFIA controls telencephalic progenitor cell differentiation through repression of the Notch effector Hes1. *J Neurosci* 30 (27): 9127–9139. doi: 10.1523/JNEUROSCI.6167-09.2010.

Piper, M. et al. (2009a). Multiple non-cell-autonomous defects underlie neocortical callosal dysgenesis in Nfib-deficient mice. *Neural Dev* 4 (1): 1–16. doi: 10.1186/1749-8104-4-43.

Piper, M. et al. (2009b). Neuropilin 1-sema signaling regulates crossing of cingulate pioneering axons during development of the corpus callosum. *Cereb Cortex* 19 (Suppl 1): i11–21. doi: 10.1093/cercor/bhp027.

Polleux, F. (2013). Development of neuronal polarity in vivo. In: *Cellular Migration and Formation of Neuronal Connections* (ed. J.L.R. Rubenstein and P. Rakoc), 3–18. San Diego: Academic Press. doi: 10.1016/B978-0-12-397266-8.00123-X.

Poulopoulos, A. et al. (2019). Subcellular transcriptomes and proteomes of developing axon projections in the cerebral cortex. *Nature* 565 (7739): 356–360. doi: 10.1038/s41586-018-0847-y.

Probst, M. (1901). Über den Bau des vollständigen balkenlosen Groβhirns sowie über Microgyrie und Heterotopie den Grauen Substanz. *Archiv furPsychiatrie und Nervenkrankheiten* 34: 709–786.

Puelles, L. et al. (2016). Selective early expression of the orphan nuclear receptor Nr4a2 identifies the claustrum homolog in the avian mesopallium: impact on sauropsidian/mammalian pallium comparisons. *J Comp Neurol* 524 (3): 665–703. doi: 10.1002/cne.23902.

Rakic, P. and Yakovlev, P.I. (1968). Development of the corpus callosum and cavum septi in man. *J Comp Neurol* 132 (1): 45–72. doi: 10.1002/cne.901320103.

Raper, J. and Mason, C. (2016). Cellular strategies of axonal pathfinding. *Cold Spring Harb Perspect Biol* 2 (9): 1–22. doi: 10.1101/cshperspect.a001933.

Rash, B.G. and Richards, L.J. (2001). A role for cingulate pioneering axons in the development of the corpus callosum. *J Comp Neurol* 434 (2): 147–157. doi: 10.1002/cne.1170.

Raybaud, C. (2010). The corpus callosum, the other great forebrain commissures, and the septum pellucidum. *Neuroradiology* 52 (6): 447–477. doi: 10.1007/s00234-010-0696-3.

Ren, T. et al. (2006). Imaging, anatomical, and molecular analysis of callosal formation in the developing human fetal brain. *Anat Rec – Part A Discov Mol, Cel, Evol Biol* 288 (2): 191–204. doi: 10.1002/ar.a.20282.

Ren, T. et al. (2007). Diffusion tensor magnetic resonance imaging and tract-tracing analysis of probst bundle structure in netrin1- and DCC-deficient mice. *J Neurosci* 27 (39): 10345–10349. doi: 10.1523/JNEUROSCI.2787-07.2007.

Reyes, N.S.D.L. et al. (2020). Development and plasticity of the corpus callosum. *Development* 147 (18): dev189738. doi: 10.1242/dev.189738.

Ringo, J.L. et al. (1994). Time is of the essence: a conjecture that hemispheric specialization arises from interhemispheric conduction delay. *Cereb Cortex* 4 (4): 331–343.

Rodríguez-Tornos, F.M. et al. (2016). Cux1 enables interhemispheric connections of layer II/III neurons by regulating Kv1-dependent firing. *Neuron* 89 (3): 494–506. doi: 10.1016/j.neuron.2015.12.020.

Sajan, S.A. et al. (2013). Both rare and De Novo copy number variants are prevalent in agenesis of the corpus callosum but not in cerebellar hypoplasia or polymicrogyria. *PLoS Genet* 9: 10. doi: 10.1371/journal.pgen.1003823.

Santen, G.W.E. et al. (2013). Coffin-siris syndrome and the BAF complex: genotype-phenotype study in 63 patients. *Hum Mutat* 34 (11): 1519–1528. doi: 10.1002/humu.22394.

Semmler, H. et al. (2010). Steps towards a centralized nervous system in basal bilaterians. *Dev, Growth Diff* 52 (8): 701–713. doi: 10.1111/j.1440-169X.2010.01207.x.

Serafini, T. et al. (1996). Netrin-1 is required for commissural axon guidance in the developing vertebrate nervous system. *Cell* 87: 1001–1014. doi: 10.1523/jneurosci.22-01-00239.2002.

Shang, F. et al. (1997). Development of commissural neurons in the wallaby (Macropus eugenii). *J Comp Neurol* 387 (4): 507–523. doi: 10.1002/(SICI)1096-9861(19971103)387:4<507::AID-CNE3>3.0.CO;2-6.

Shoubridge, C. et al. (2010). ARX spectrum disorders. *Hum Mutat* 31 (8): 889–900. doi: 10.1002/humu.21288.

Shu, T. et al. (2003a). Abnormal development of forebrain midline glia and commissural projections in Nfia knock-out mice. *J Neurosci* 23 (1): 203–212.

Shu, T. et al. (2003b). The glial sling is a migratory population of developing neurons. *Development* 130 (13): 2929–2937. doi: 10.1242/dev.00514.

Shu, T. et al. (2003c). Development of midline glial populations at the corticoseptal boundary. *J Neurobiol* 57 (1): 81–94. doi: 10.1002/neu.10252.

Shu, T. and Richards, L.J. (2001). Cortical axon guidance by the glial wedge during the development of the corpus callosum. *J Neurosci* (8): 2749–2758. doi: 10.1523/JNEUROSCI.21-08-02749.2001.

Shu, T. et al. (2003d). Slit2 guides both precrossing and postcrossing callosal axons at the midline in vivo. *J Neurosci* 23 (22): 8176–8184. doi: 10.1523/jneurosci.23-22-08176.2003.

Silver, J. et al. (1982). Axonal guidance during development of the great cerebral commissures. *J Comp Neurol* 210 (1): 10–29. doi: 10.1002/cne.902100103.

Silver, J. and Ogawa, M.Y. (1983). Postnatally induced formation of the corpus callosum in acallosal mice on glia-coated cellulose bridges. *Science* 220 (4601): 1067–1069. doi: 10.1126/science.6844928.

Smart, I.H.M. (2002). Unique morphological features of the proliferative zones and postmitotic compartments of the neural epithelium giving rise to striate and extrastriate cortex in the monkey. *Cereb Cortex* 12 (1): 37–53. doi: 10.1093/cercor/12.1.37.

Smith, K.M. et al. (2006). Midline radial glia translocation and corpus callosum formation require FGF signaling. *Nat Neurosci* 9 (6): 787–797. doi: 10.1038/nn1705.

Son, A.I. et al. (2017). Proteome dynamics during postnatal mouse corpus callosum development. *Sci Rep* 7: 1–14. doi: 10.1038/srep45359.

Son, E.Y. and Crabtree, G.R. (2014). The role of BAF (mSWI/SNF) complexes in mammalian neural development. *Am J Med Genet Part C, Semin Med Genet* 166 (3): 333–349. doi: 10.1002/ajmg.c.31416.

Sperry, R.W. (1962). Some general aspects of interhemispheric integration. In: *Interhemispheric Relations and Cerebral Dominance* (ed. V.B. Mountcastle). Baltimore: Johns Hopkins Press.

Sperry, R.W. (1968). Plasticity of neural maturation. In: *The Emergency of Order in Developing Systems*, vol. 7 (ed. M. Locke), 306–327. New York: Academic Press Inc.

Srinivasan, K. et al. (2012). A network of genetic repression and derepression specifies projection fates in the developing neocortex. *Proc Natl Acad Sci USA* 109 (47): 19071–19078. doi: 10.1073/pnas.1216793109.

Srivatsa, S. et al. (2014). Unc5C and DCC act downstream of Ctip2 and Satb2 and contribute to corpus callosum formation. *Nat Commun* 5: 1–15. doi: 10.1038/ncomms4708.

Steele-Perkins, G. et al. (2005). The transcription factor gene Nfib is essential for both lung maturation and brain development. *Mol Cell Biol* 25 (2): 685–698. doi: 10.1128/mcb.25.2.685-698.2005.

Storm, E.E. et al. (2006). Dose-dependent functions fo Fgf8 in regulating telencephalic patterning centers. *Development* 133 (9): 1831–1844. doi: 10.1242/dev.02324.

Suárez, R. (2017). Evolution of telencephalic commissures: conservation and change of developmental systems in the origin of brain wiring novelties. In: *Evolution of Nervous Systems*, 2e, vol. 2 (ed. J.H. Kass), 205–223. Amsterdam: Elsevier. doi: 10.1016/B978-0-12-804042-3.00042-7.

Suárez, R. et al. (2014a). Balanced interhemispheric cortical activity is required for correct targeting of the corpus callosum. *Neuron* 82 (6): 1289–1298. doi: 10.1016/j.neuron.2014.04.040.

Suárez, R. et al. (2014b July). Evolution and development of interhemispheric connections in the vertebrate forebrain. *Front Hum Neurosci* 8: 1–14. doi: 10.3389/fnhum.2014.00497.

Suárez, R. et al. (2018). A pan-mammalian map of interhemispheric brain connections predates the evolution of the corpus callosum. *Proc Nat Acad Sci* 115 (38): 9622–9627. doi: 10.1073/pnas.1808262115.

Sugitani, Y. et al. (2002). Brn-1 and Brn-2 share crucial roles in the production and positioning of mouse neocortical neurons. *Genes Dev* 16 (14): 1760–1765. doi: 10.1101/gad.978002.

Suzuki, I.K. and Hirata, T. (2012). Evolutionary conservation of neocortical neurogenetic program in the mammals and birds. *Bioarchitecture* 2 (4): 124–129. doi: 10.4161/bioa.21032.

Suzuki, I.K. and Hirata, T. (2014). A common developmental plan for neocortical gene-expressing neurons in the pallium of the domestic chicken gallus gallus domesticus and the Chinese softshell turtle pelodiscus sinensis. *Front Neuroanat* 8: 1–17. doi: 10.3389/fnana.2014.00020.

Suzuki, I.K. et al. (2012). The temporal sequence of the mammalian neocortical neurogenetic program drives mediolateral pattern in the chick pallium. *Dev Cell* 22 (4): 863–870. doi: 10.1016/j.devcel.2012.01.004.

Takahashi, T. et al. (1999). Sequence of neuron origin and neocortical laminar fate. *J Neurosci* 19 (23): 10357–10371. doi: 10.1523/jneurosci.19-23-10357.1999.

Takeshita, Y. et al. (2020). Novel ARX mutation identified in infantile spasm syndrome patient. *Hum Genome Var* 7 (1): 7–9. doi: 10.1038/s41439-020-0094-2.

Tessier-Lavigne, M. and Goodman, C.S. (1996). The molecular biology of axon guidance. *Science* 274 (5290): 1123–1133. doi: 10.1126/science.274.5290.1123.

Tosches, M.A. et al. (2018). Evolution of pallium, hippocampus, and cortical cell types revealed by single-cell transcriptomics in reptiles. *Science* 360 (6391): 881–888. doi: 10.1126/science.aar4237.

Tovar-Moll, F. et al. (2007). Neuroplasticity in human callosal dysgenesis. *Cereb Cortex* 17 (3): 531–541. doi: 10.1093/cercor/bhj178.

Tovar-Moll, F. et al. (2014). Structural and functional brain rewiring clarifies preserved interhemispheric transfer in humans born without the corpus callosum. *Proc Natl Acad Sci* 111 (21): 7843–7848. doi: 10.1073/pnas.1400806111.

Unni, D.K. et al. (2012). Multiple Slits regulate the development of midline glial populations and the corpus callosum. *Dev Biol* 365 (1): 36–49. doi: 10.1016/j.ydbio.2012.02.004.

Valenti, M. et al. (2019). Abnormal structural and functional connectivity of the corpus callosum in autism spectrum disorders: a review. *Rev J Autism Dev Disord* 7 (1): 46–62. doi: 10.1007/s40489-019-00176-9.

van der Sluijs, P.J. et al. (2019). The ARID1B spectrum in 143 patients. *Genet Med* 21 (6): 1295–1307. doi: 10.1038/s41436-018-0330-z.

Virues-Ortega, J. et al. (2022 February 2). A callosal biomarker of behavioral intervention outcomes for autism spectrum disorder? A case-control feasibility study with diffusion tensor imaging. *PLoS ONE* 17: 1–14. doi: 10.1371/journal.pone.0262563.

Wahl, M. et al. (2009). Variability of homotopic and heterotopic callosal connectivity in partial agenesis of the corpus callosum. *Am J Neuroradiol* 30 (2): 282–289. doi: 10.3174/ajnr.A1361.

Wahlsten, D. (1981). Prenatal schedule of appearance of mouse brain commissures. *Dev Brain Res* 1 (4): 461–473. doi: 10.1016/0165-3806(81).

Wang, C.-L. et al. (2007). Activity-dependent development of callosal projections in the somatosensory cortex. *J Neurosci* 27 (42): 11334–11342. doi: 10.1523/JNEUROSCI.3380-07.2007.

Wang, S.S.H. et al. (2008). Functional trade-offs in white matter axonal scaling. *J Neurosci* 28 (15): 4047–4056. doi: 10.1523/JNEUROSCI.5559-05.2008.

Warkany, J. (1971). *Congenital Malformations; Notes and Comments*. Chicago: Year Book Medical Publishers.

Wegiel, J. et al. (2018). Deficit of corpus callosum axons, reduced axon diameter and decreased area are markers of abnormal development of interhemispheric connections in autistic subjects. *Acta Neuropathol Commun* 6 (1): 143. doi: 10.1186/s40478-018-0645-7.

Witelson, S.F. (1989). Hand and sex differences in the isthmus and genu of the human corpus callosum. *Brain* 112 (3): 799–835. doi: 10.1093/brain/112.3.799.

Wullimann, M.F. et al. (1996). *Neuroanatomy of the Zebrafish Brain: A Topological Atlas*. http://libproxy.mit.edu/login?url=http://search.ebscohost.com/login.aspx?direct=true&db=cat00916a&AN=mit.002257818&site=eds-live%5Cnhttp://grammy.mit.edu/F/?func=service-sfx&doc_number=002257818&line_number=0000&service_type=RECORD.

Yang, L. et al. (2022). Callosal fiber length scales with brain size according to functional lateralization, evolution, and development. *J Neurosci* 42 (17): 3599–3610. doi: 10.1523/JNEUROSCI.1510-21.2022.

Yorke, C.H. and Caviness, V.S. (1976). Interhemispheric neocortical connections of the corpus callosum in the Reeler mutant mouse. *J Comp Neurol* 164: 233–246. doi: 10.1002/cne.901700405.

Yu, Q. et al. (2014). Coevolution of axon guidance molecule slit and its receptor robo. *PLoS ONE* 9 (5): 1–6. doi: 10.1371/journal.pone.0094970.

Zhang, L. et al. (2012). Satb2 is required for dendritic arborization and soma spacing in mouse cerebral cortex. *Cereb Cortex* 22 (7): 1510–1519. doi: 10.1093/cercor/bhr215.

Zhang, Q. et al. (2019 February). Loss of satb2 in the cortex and hippocampus leads to abnormal behaviors in mice. *Front Mol Neurosci* 12: 1–12. doi: 10.3389/fnmol.2019.00033.

Zhao, H. et al. (2011). A molecular mechanism that regulates medially oriented axonal growth of upper layer neurons in the developing neocortex. *J Comp Neurol* 519 (5): 834–848. doi: 10.1002/cne.22536.

Zhou, J. et al. (2013). Axon position within the corpus callosum determines contralateral cortical projection. *Proc Natl Acad Sci* 110 (29): E2714–E2723. doi: 10.1073/pnas.1310233110.

Zurita, H. et al. (2018). Layer 5 callosal parvalbumin-expressing neurons. *Front Cell Neurosci* 12: 1–14. doi: 10.3389/fncel.2018.00053.

16

Towards the Transcriptionally based Classification of L6b in the Adult Mouse Brain

Thomas Henning Sara Bandiera, and Zoltán Molnár

Department of Physiology, Anatomy and Genetics, Sherrington Building, Parks Road, Oxford, OX1 3PT, UK

16.1 Introduction

One of the major goals of neuroscience is to understand the cellular constituents of the nervous system, classified according to their parameters such as position, orientation, somatodendritic morphology, connectivity, birthdate, lineage, and physiological properties (Ramón y Cajal 1909; Yao et al. 2021a; Yao et al. 2021b). Their diversity is what drives the computational capacity of the brain. The better we can group and subsequently type the cells into clusters, the closer we would come to understanding circuit properties and these complex computations. Therefore, the endeavor to produce a coherent classification and, by extension, the generation of a cell type is very topical (Lein et al. 2017; Yuste et al. 2020).

Such an effort could be of importance in Layer 6b (L6b), which contains some of the least investigated neurons in the cortex (Zolnik et al. 2020). L6b develops from the early-born (Price et al. 1997) cortical subplate zone in mouse (Marx and Feldmeyer 2013; Marx et al. 2017; Woo et al. 1991), which has multiple places of origins and is heterogenous in birthdates (Hoerder-Suabedissen and Molnár 2013; Pedraza et al. 2014). This structure was first described in human (Kostovic and Molliver 1974), then in macaque (Rakic 1977), and rat (Rickmann et al. 1977). It forms widespread but transient intra- and extracortical connections, notably with the thalamus (Allendoerfer and Shatz 1994; Ghosh et al. 1990; Liao and Lee 2012), but also contributes to thalamus development by guiding and reinforcing thalamocortical and long-range cortical projections (Ayoub and Kostovic 2009; Ghosh et al. 1990). Interestingly, thalamic axons accumulate in the subplate before synapsing onto their ultimate target neurons mostly in L4 of the neocortex (Ghosh et al. 1990). The transient circuits established by the subplate link the early spontaneous activity patterns with the sensory driven activity of the cerebral cortex (Kanold et al. 2020).

The subplate displays a postnatal decrease in its number of cells and a large part of the rodent subplate disappears by postnatal day 8 (P8) (Price et al. 1997), with this phenomenon being even more striking in the carnivore and human brain. Currently it is not known which subplate neurons are transient although histological evaluations of some markers of these cells (Ctgf, Cplx3, Nurr1) in the mouse cortex revealed L6b populations that have a lower apoptotic rate between P2 and 8 compared to the average NeuN positive neuron in L6b (Hoerder-Suabedissen and Molnár 2013). The cells constituting L6b neurons remain (Duque et al. 2016; Hoerder-Suabedissen and Molnár 2013), forming a cytoarchitectonically separate layer between the underlying white matter and the neocortex, clearly distinguishable from cortical L6 (Reep and Goodwin 1988). They still comprise a heterogenous cell population based on their origin, gene expression (Hoerder-Suabedissen et al.

Neocortical Neurogenesis in Development and Evolution, First Edition. Edited by Wieland B. Huttner.

2009), morphology, and electrophysiology (Marx and Feldmeyer 2013; Scala et al. 2021), with some cells maintaining rich cortico-cortical (Friedlander and Torres-Reveron 2009; Kostovic and Rakic 1990; Suarez-Sola et al. 2009; Zolnik et al. 2020) as well as cortico-thalamic connections (Hoerder-Suabedissen et al. 2018; Molnár 1998).

Recently, L6b populations have received more attention because of their presumed role in regulating brain state control and cognition (Zolnik et al. 2020) due to their unique sensitivity to neuromodulators such as orexin (Bayer et al. 2004), cholecystokinin (CCK) (Chung et al. 2009), oxytocin (Newmaster et al. 2020), and neurexophilin (Beglopoulos et al. 2005). Furthermore, histopathological findings revealed altered distribution and numbers of interstitial white matter neurons and subplate / L6b to occur in schizophrenia, for example, in the latter, a larger density of cells is found in subplate of the prefrontal and lateral temporal cortex (Akbarian et al. 1993a, 1993b). Several microarray- and sequencing-based studies provided the first lists of L6b enriched genes during development (Oeschger et al. 2012) and in the adult (Belgard et al. 2011; Hoerder-Suabedissen et al. 2009; Osheroff and Hatten 2009). In line with this finding, in 2013 Hoerder-Suabedissen and colleagues pointed out the overlap between subplate-/L6b-enriched gene expressions during development to susceptibility genes implicated in schizophrenia and autism (Hoerder-Suabedissen et al. 2013).

Hence, a comprehensive classification of L6b neuron subtypes, and a characterization of their roles in the different physiological and pathological processes is crucial in understanding the mechanisms linking alterations in the number and distribution of these neurons and cognitive conditions. Unfortunately, not much is known about how cells grouped through one form of investigations is consistent with subpopulations of another, for example, which group of neuromodulator-sensitive cells receive thalamic input, which could tell us more about their computational functionality.

High-throughput methodologies such as whole brain sequencing identifying layer-specific (Belgard et al. 2011) or area-specific (Hawrylycz et al. 2012) RNA profiles have since added weight to this inquiry. Nowadays, single cell throughput of large sample sizes is possible, and allows a comparison across species in a unified molecular landscape (BRAIN Initiative Cell Census Network (BICCN) 2021). Moreover, the expectation arose that cell types could be formed based on this industrial-scale effort (Zeisel et al. 2015), as the high-throughput measurements of cortical cells and generation of datasets are considered "complete, accurate and permanent" (Yuste et al. 2020).

There are well-established computational methodologies of transcriptomic clustering (Figure 16.1). Cells, identified with transgenic mouse driver lines are identified and, in the case of mouse studies, the whole-cell data read out. Each cell is then placed in a multidimensional map according to how its overall RNA expression levels compare to other cells. The map is algorithmically condensed into a two-dimensional (2D) space. Cells are then assigned to branches and clusters of a tree structure by a second algorithm, which separates groups of cells by introducing threshold values of RNA concentrations. One or two genes are later attached as a label for a branch or class by an external investigator (=superclass).

Single cell transcriptomics has become important clinically in neuropathological investigations (Akbarian et al. 1993a, 1993b; Hoerder-Suabedissen et al. 2013), since comparative transcriptomics can show us how expression levels may change between two populations, as has been shown in autism (Velmeshev et al. 2019). Regionally specific transcriptomic studies by Tasic and colleagues from the Allen Institute for Brain Science (AIBS) in the mouse primary visual cortex (Tasic et al. 2016), and additionally anterolateral motor cortex (Tasic et al. 2018) provided novel markers, and genetic tools allowing manipulations of target areas (Zhang et al. 2014). In 2021, Yao et al. published a study where they had performed a transcriptomic analysis on the entire mouse neocortex and the hippocampus (Yao et al. 2021b). Here clusters were linked to cortical location (Figure 16.2A). Identifiable as cortical superclasses are Clic5 (303–307; 311–316) and the single cluster Slc17a8 (317). According to the study, the Clic5 types 306, 312, and 314 identify the visual, posterior

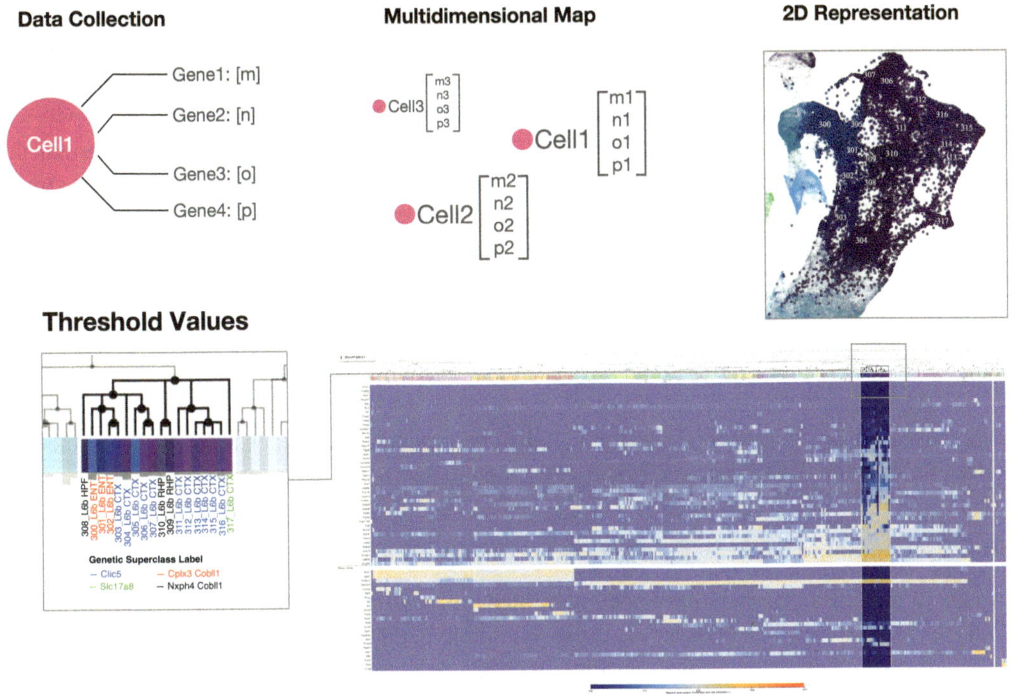

Figure 16.1 Overview of computational methodology of transcriptomic clustering. *Source:* Adapted from Allen Institute for Brain Science (2004). Allen Brain Map [Mouse Whole Cortex and Hippocampus (10xChromium v3)]. [https://celltypes.brain-map.org/rnaseq/mouse_ctxhpf_10x?selectedVisualization = Scatter + Plot&colorByFeature = Cell + Type&colorByFeatureValue = Gad1] State: 11 November 2021.

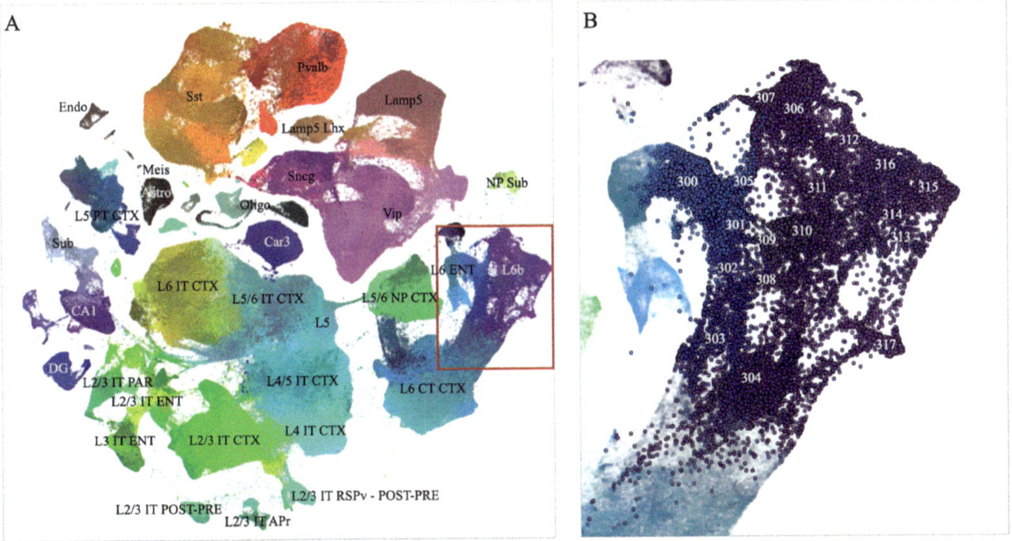

Figure 16.2 (A) Transcriptomic 2D map of the cortex and hippocampal formation with annotated clustering. (B) High power view of cell clustering of L6. *Source:* Allen Institute for Brain Science (2004). Allen Brain Map [Mouse Whole Cortex and Hippocampus (10xChromium v3)]. [https://celltypes.brain-map.org/rnaseq/mouse_ctx hpf_10x?selectedVisualization = Scatter + Plot&colorByFeature = Cell + Type&colorByFeatureValue = Gad1] State: 11 November 2021.

parietal, and auditory cortex L6b cells respectively while 307, 311, 315, and 316 are found in the somatosensory, motor, frontal, and anterior cingulate cortex. Clic5 types 303 and 305 mark the temporal association (TEa), perirhinal (PERI), and ectorhinal (ECT) areas, while 317 is expressed throughout all cortical areas and in parts of the entorhinal cortex (Figure 16.2B).

Ideally, linking transcriptomic data in L6b with previous investigations will lead to the establishment of a cell card, forming a community-based standard of a cell type (Yuste et al. 2020) as aimed at by the BRAIN initiative (BRAIN Initiative Cell Census Network (BICCN) 2021; Tasic et al. 2018). However, there are considerable challenges to link the single cell transcriptomics of L6b with other anatomical and physiological parameters due to the high complexity of the data.

16.2 Traditional Literature Data

When investigating different cell features in L6b, it becomes clear that each is very well established in its own individual confines.

16.2.1 Traditional Markers Identified by Layer-specific Gene Expression Analysis:

In L6b 47 molecular markers have been identified, one of the first being Nurr1 (Watakabe et al. 2007). Bayer and colleagues (Bayer et al. 2004) found hypocretin receptor 2 (Hcrtr2) to be present in L6b through pharmacological application of orexin-receptor active compounds. Later, a microarray study (Hoerder-Suabedissen et al., 2009; Hoerder-Suabedissen et al., 2013) identified also Cplx3, CTGF, MoxD1, Tmem163, Nurr1, and DDC to be selectively enriched compared with L6 at P8 and to be continuously expressed in the adult. Lpar1 (Hoerder-Suabedissen and Molnár 2013), Trh (Wang et al. 2011), and Nxph3 (Beglopoulos et al. 2005) followed. Newer markers have emerged by combining gene expression analysis with other methods such as tracing, like in the case of Kcnab1 in unilaterally projecting neurons in L6b (Tiong et al. 2019). There are very few studies that specifically address how these markers overlap (Hoerder-Suabedissen and Molnár 2013), with a focus on the level of the layer rather than neuronal populations (Table 16.1).

Table 16.1 Available data on the overlap of gene expression in L6b neuronal populations (Bayer et al. 2004; Beglopoulos et al. 2005; Bruguier et al. 2020; Hoerder-Suabedissen et al. 2009; Hoerder-Suabedissen and Molnár 2013; Wang et al. 2011; Watakabe et al. 2007; Tiong et al. 2019).

	Cplx3 (%)	CTGF (%)	MoxD1 (%)	Tmem163 (%)	Nurr1 (%)	DDC (%)	Lpar1 (%)	Trh (%)	Drd1 (%)	NeuN (P8) (%)
Cplx3	-	-	-	-	-	-	87	-	-	43
CTGF	-	-	-	-	-	-		-	-	66
MoxD1	-	-	-	-	-	-		-	-	-
Tmem163	-	-	-	-	-	-		-	-	-
Nurr1 (NR4A2)	-	-	-	-	-	-	6	-	-	34
DDC	-	-	-	-	-	-	-	-	-	-
Lpar1	0	-	-	-	8	-	-	-	0	-
Trh	-	-	-	-	-	-	-	-	-	33
Drd1	33.0 ± 2.2	34	-	-	-	-	-	-	-	-
Kcnab1	78.7 ± 0.02	87.8 ± 0.02	-	-	57.7 ± 0.04	-	-	-	-	-

16.2.2 Morphology and Electrophysiology

The morphology and electrophysiology of L6b DRD1 neurons was assessed by Marx and Feldmeyer (Marx and Feldmeyer 2013) by patch-clamping and filling them with biocytin. They identified three primary subtypes of morphology, which they named C1 (pyramidal), C2 (non-pyramidal), and C3 (multipolar). The C2 type was subdivided into three further types: inverted, tangential, and horizontal morphology (Figure 16.3). C1 can also be divided in two subtypes according to axonal field span: a columnar and a trans-columnar type. Pyramidal neurons make up between 31.7 percent and 45 percent of L6b cell (Marx and Feldmeyer 2013; Zolnik et al. 2020), multipolar neurons about 35.6 percent (Marx and Feldmeyer 2013), non-pyramidal classes between 10.3 percent and 11.5 percent each (Marx and Feldmeyer 2013).

The study found no significant difference between the resting membrane potential, the half-width, and the amplitude of the action potential (Marx and Feldmeyer 2013).

The effect of neuromodulators on selected subtypes of L6b cells is profound: Orexin can act on Orexin-2 receptors across the rostro-caudal axis of the brain and create a depolarizing block in potassium currents (Bayer et al. 2004; Radnikow and Feldmeyer 2018; Wenger Combremont et al. 2016a).

Acetylcholine may act on these same cells, but not exclusively (Bayer et al. 2004). Extraordinary nicotinic receptors with an alpha-5 subunit are found in L6b that induce slow desensitization (Radnikow and Feldmeyer 2018), and in orexin sensitive cells potentiate depolarization. Other layers either did not express this receptor or only showed weak expression (Radnikow and Feldmeyer 2018).

CCK acts on the CCK-B receptor to induce strong depolarization by suppressing leak potassium channels (Chung et al. 2009). Neurotensin in the somatosensory cortex has a varied response in L6b and some L6a neurons, ranging from depolarization from quiescence to rhythmic bistability, transient depolarization, or a biphasic response (depolarization followed by hyperpolarization) (Case et al. 2017; Wenger Combremont et al. 2016a, b).

Noradrenaline, acetylcholine, orexin, and neurotensin all appear to affect high-frequency cortical activity (Wenger Combremont et al. 2016b), noradrenaline and acetylcholine through direct

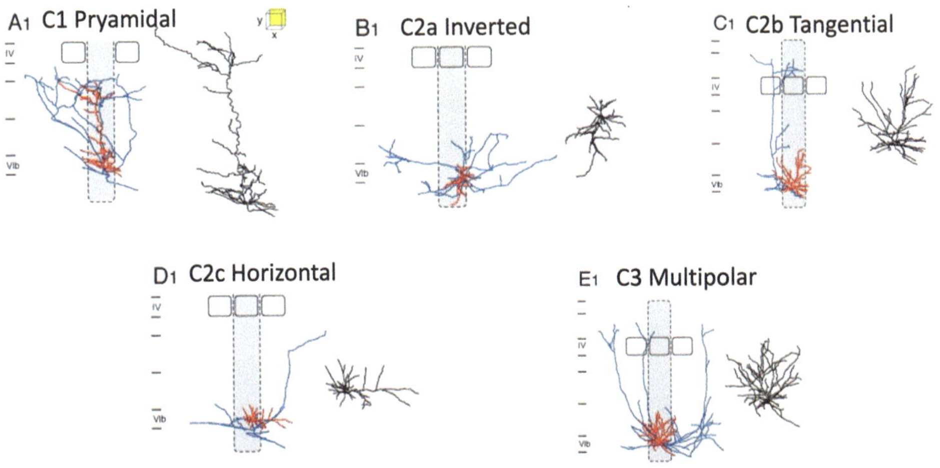

Figure 16.3 Graphical reproduction of cell type morphology C1–C3 A = Pyramidal (C1), B = Inverted (C2a), C = Tangential (Cb), D = Horizontal (C2c), E = Multipolar (C3), respectively. *Source:* Marx, M., and Feldmeyer, D. (2013). Morphology and physiology of excitatory neurons in layer 6b of the somatosensory rat barrel. *Cerebral Cortex* 23 (12): 2803–2817 (Marx and Feldmeyer 2013).

action, orexin and neurotensin by indirect action on fast spiking GABAergic parvalbumin cells by affecting presynaptic connections of neighboring neurons (Wenger Combremont et al. 2016a).

16.2.3 Connectivity

Input:
L6b cells have a varying array of intracortical, intercortical, and subcortical inputs (Hoerder-Suabedissen et al. 2018; Killackey and Sherman 2003; Marx and Feldmeyer 2013; Munoz-Castaneda et al. 2021; Viswanathan et al. 2017; Zolnik et al. 2020). When L6b connectivity is investigated in the somatosensory cortex, the largest intracortical input comes from non-pyramidal L6 cells, while ipsilateral intracortical input stems primarily from motor cortex (95.1%), specifically from L5 cells. Of contralateral input, the majority comes from L6 of the contralateral somatosensory cortex. Subcortical input is dominated by thalamic input, however, that represents only a minority of all input into L6b (Figure 16.4). Overall, cortical inputs dominate over subcortical, which suggests L6b to play a role in integration of perceptual information that has already been manipulated by other cortical layers and areas.

Output:
Projection sites of subpopulations of layer 6b neurons were identified in Cre-expressing mouse lines (Drd1a-Cre and Ctgf-Cre) crossed to reporter lines (Hoerder-Suabedissen et al. 2018) with retrograde tracers and anterograde cre-dependent AAV tracing (Hoerder-Suabedissen et al. 2018; Zolnik et al. 2020). Multiple projections connect the cortex to higher order thalamic areas, as well as thalamo-recipient cortical layers (L1, L4, L5a) (Hoerder-Suabedissen et al. 2018; Viswanathan et al. 2017).

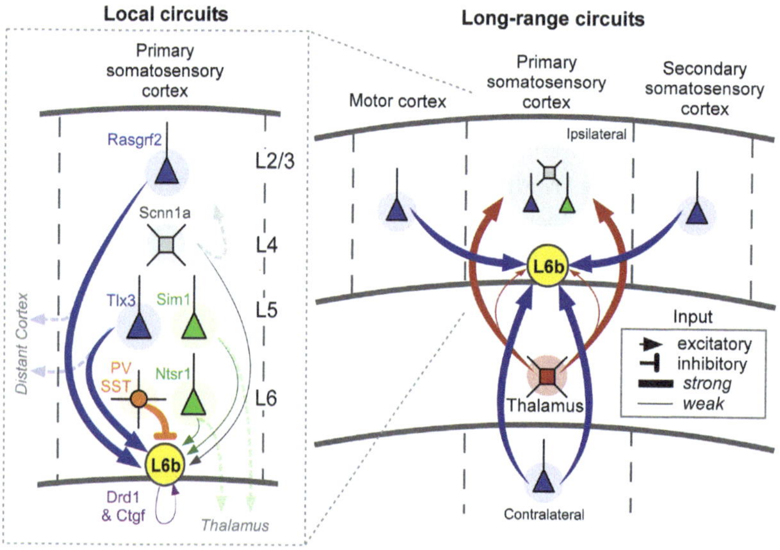

Figure 16.4 Overview of input to somatosensory cortex L6b in primary somatosensory cortex of the mouse. Somatosensory cortex L6b receives short-range input from within the ipsilateral somatosensory cortex, specifically from L2/3 and L5, and long-range input from related cortices ipsilaterally (e.g., motor cortex, S2) and the contralateral homologue. *Source:* Zolnik, T.A., Ledderose, J., Toumazou, M. et al. (2020). Layer 6b is driven by intracortical long-range projection neurons. *Cell Reports* 30 (10): 3492–3505. (Zolnik et al. 2020).

16.3 The Problem of Biological Classification

When we explore the integration of transcriptomic datasets into this structure, this effort of classification comes to a standstill, as we are faced with a problem of classification.

Genetic superclass separation (i.e., by genetic label) is not always mirrored in structural analytical separation (i.e., overall genetic relatedness). The tree structure of glutamatergic L6b cells is split in four large branches consisting of one branch of entorhinal and cortical cells, one retrohippocampal group, one pure cortical group, and the single group 317 (Figure 16.2b). Yet, cells belonging to a single superclass (e.g., Clic5) may be found in the subbranches of either of these groups. In short, just because two cell groups belong to the same superclass, that is, are grouped together by a label, they do not appear next to each other in the tree structure. Vice versa, the superclass labels do not follow the separation shown by the branching of the tree structure, that is, because cell groups are genetically similar as they are next to each other in the branching of the tree structure, does not mean they received the same genetic superclass label.

Furthermore, despite having received a gene as a superclass label, transcriptomic clusters of glutamatergic cells do not always express the gene with which they have been labelled.

Case 1:
Cplx3 and Cobll1 (300–302), and Nxph4 and Cobll1 (308–310) identify entorhinal cortical area and the retrohippocampal regions respectively (Figure 16.2b). *Nxph4* was expressed in all L6b labelled cells except 302, at high levels (central tendency >6) in 306–308 and 311–316. *Cobll1* was expressed in 300–303, 305, 306, 308–310. Double labelling of cells 308–310 as Nxph4 Cobll1 cells therefore does not hold up as 309 would be excluded.

Case 2:
Clic5 has been used as a label for the cell clusters 303–307 and 311–316. What we can clearly tell from the scatterplot view shown below is that Clic5 does not label cluster 303 (Figure 16.5).

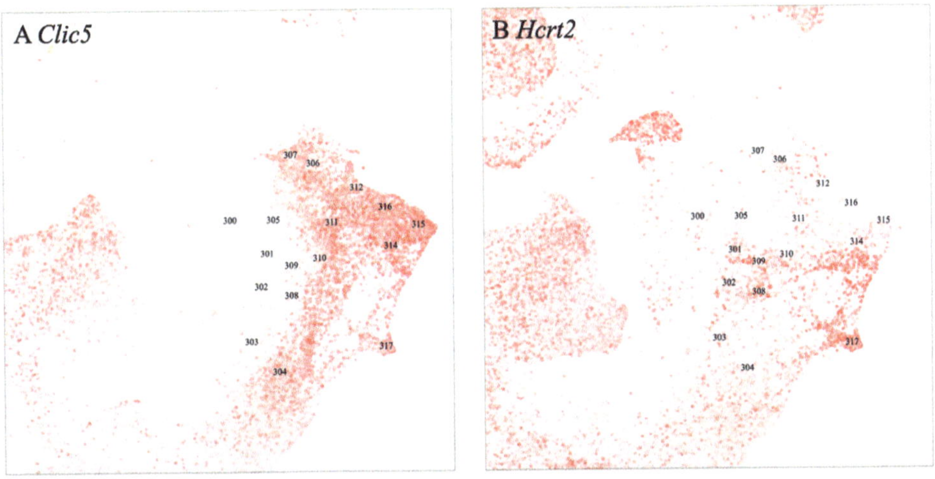

Figure 16.5 Expression of (A) Clic5 and (B) Hcrtr2 in the scatterplot view of different cells of L6b. Individual cells are displayed in their relatedness (see Figure 16.1), then expression levels of the selected RNA are shown for each cell via the strength of coloring. *Source:* Allen Institute for Brain Science (2004). Allen Brain Map [Mouse Whole Cortex and Hippocampus (10xChromium v3)]. [https://celltypes.brain-map.org/rnaseq/mouse_ctx hpf_10x?selectedVisualization = Scatter + Plot&colorByFeature = Cell + Type&colorByFeatureValue = Gad1] State: 11 November 2021.

16.4 Analysis of Classical Markers in Global Transcriptomic

In the Heatmap representation, some markers (*Glra1, Hspa1l, Tle1, Rgs1, Pde6g, DDC, Chrna5*) do not appear in any cell types, while others label all types of glutamatergic L6b cells consistently (*Satb2, Cdh11, Cdh18, Gng12, Usp46, Tmem163, Rai14, Pcsk5, Mmp16*), but may span a wider number of cells than those solely in L6b (*Mmp16, Cdh18, Cdh11, Pcsk5, CCKBR*). Typically, when not all clusters are labelled, a gradient of expression can be observed (*Hpcal1, Galnt10, Chst11, Lpar1, Moxd1*) (Figure 16.6).

We can observe a similar range of graded responses when the markers are displayed in the single-cell scatterplot representation (Figure 16.7).

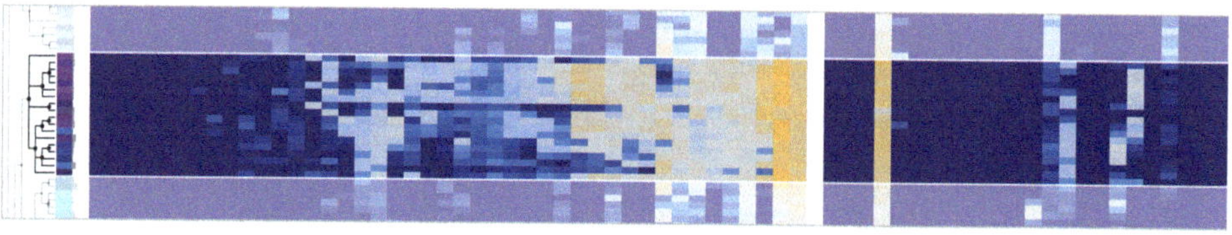

Figure 16.6 Representation of L6b in Heatmap view exposing the division of L6b into subclasses by genetic similarity (left). Traditional markers (middle) show gradients of expression across divisions of cell groups. General transcriptomic markers identified as key markers (right) also show a gradient. *Source:* Adapted from Allen Institute for Brain Science (2004). Allen Brain Map [Mouse Whole Cortex and Hippocampus (10xChromium v3)]. https://celltypes.brain-map.org/rnaseq/mouse_ctx-hpf_10x?selectedVisualization=Heatmap&colorByFeature=Cell+Type&colorByFeatureValue=Gad1 State: 11 November 2021

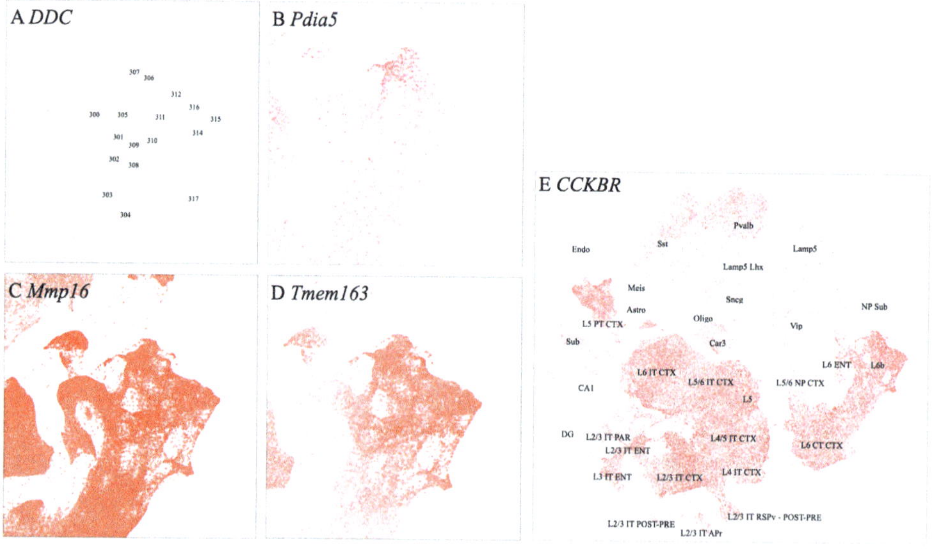

Figure 16.7 Traditional markers in transcriptomic scatterplot (A–E) focus on L6b (A: DDC; B: Pdia5; C: Mmp16; D: Tmem163); E: Global visualization of L6b-specific marker CCKB. Source: Adapted from Allen Institute for Brain Science (2004). Allen Brain Map [Mouse Whole Cortex and Hippocampus (10xChromium v3)]. [https://celltypes.brain-map.org/rnaseq/mouse_ctx hpf_10x?selectedVisualization = Scatter + Plot&colorByFeature = Cell + Type&colorByFeatureValue = Gad1] State: 11 November 2021.

16.5 The Use of Transcriptomics as a Classing Factor

Considering these factors we must reevaluate the reliability of transcriptomic readouts as the basis of definitive cell clustering. The problems outlined earlier are explained and can be expanded when we explore how diversity affects the idea of cluster-based cell typing.

When one attempts to merge data to form a cell type, it is inherently biased towards the clustering method used to set the first framework basis. By using transcriptomics as the cell type defining factor, we use a high-resolution but microlevel of information processing to infer global computation. Giving transcriptomics such a large weight, due to its comprehensiveness and the vast availability of its data, has distorted the view on the integration of features. It is believed that the clustering of cells according to transcriptomic readouts is absolute and other features are dependent on this. Yet, there are overlapping features indistinct of one singular cluster.

It is generally assumed that transcriptomics reveals ideas about different properties beyond intracellular or intranuclear processes, disregarding that, a particular transcriptomic readout represents only a momentous image of a dynamic process. For example, morphology reflects how a cell connects earlier in development; the morphological make-up of L6b does not change from that of the "precursor," the subplate (Marx et al. 2017) while its transcriptome will (BRAIN Initiative Cell Census Network (BICCN) 2021). Some of the signals and receptors are only expressed during development when these connections are established, but not present at adulthood. There are very few genes that have constant expression within subplate and layer 6b (Hoerder-Suabedissen et al., 2009, 2013).

Furthermore, a cell's electrophysiological property is dependent on the ratio of specific receptors and ion channels expressed in its membrane. While determined by the transcription of these proteins, it is not directly causative. The recycling of membrane proteins and the overall proteome of the cell are factors affecting cell electrophysiology that are not measured in the transcriptome. The transcripts important in these fate restrictions are only present during development and might not be present in the adult. It is therefore reductive to assume the function of the cell to be solely dependent or correlated with the transcriptome at adult stages.

Next to the problem of level differences, the mere need to compress the multidimensional map of cells to 2D poses distortions. While Yao and colleagues (Yao et al. 2021a, Yao et al. 2021b) compared the sequencing and clustering results of different platforms and showed large similarity, which makes one hopeful for a consensus based on this differentially acquired data, the usefulness of unsupervised transcriptomic clustering, as conducted in the papers analyzed for transcriptomic classes (Scala et al. 2021; Tasic et al. 2016, 2018; Yao et al. 2021a, Yao et al. 2021b), has been questioned recently (Chari et al. 2021). Large distortions of data, when compressed into a 2D space, limit their visual usefulness in subtype assignment (Chari et al. 2021). Instead of an algorithm that is solely biased depending on the mathematical reduction, biasing this process knowingly using key biological properties as a reference was suggested.

Lastly, the clustering process conducted by the second algorithm is truly destructive. In theory, a cell's overall transcriptomic relationship to the other cells identifies a single cell as part of its cluster, and a cluster as part of a superclass. Because cells do not form separate groups in their multidimensional or reduced representation, which we can see in the fluid representation of cells in the scatterplot, a hard threshold must be used to separate clusters from each other. This means separate algorithms create a hard threshold for different input values (i.e., expressed genes) to distinguish them, despite them having a continuous, gradually changing value, which creates the issues we have seen above in the discrepancies of transcriptomic classification.

The strict distinction in cell clustering is therefore not representative of the gradient of genetic expression of the gene used to label this specific superclass. This is visible in the scatterplot representation of transcriptomic data. It can be shown that the expression of transcriptomic markers does not conform to the clustering, as identifying genes of a cluster do not stain all cells of this group, but only gradually distinguishes few cells at a much higher strength. This mirrors the stark discrepancies of genetic, algorithmic, and labelling separation.

The aim of the BRAIN initiative cell consensus network is to produce a comprehensive view of morphological, neurophysiological, and molecular properties (BRAIN Initiative Cell Census Network (BICCN) 2021; Tasic et al. 2018), as these categories have traditionally contributed to the definition of a cell type, either of their own accord (Marx and Feldmeyer 2013) or in conjunction (Miller et al. 2020). They support the idea of a simplified Cell Card. This chapter should have demonstrated that this is difficult to achieve and has opened many new questions about how we define a cell type.

It would be unwise to dismiss this diversity of neurons. Rather, we should embrace it. In biology, we like to show this diversity in two ways: through separate clusters or via the absence of structure. While our results show that there is an absence of clear clustering as RNA expression is graded, there remains structure, visible in the transcriptomic map. It is therefore not unreasonable to assume that L6b and, by extension, the cortex, represents a structural multidimensional continuum of multiple gradients, not an assortment of definitive cell types.

16.6 Orexin Receptor Expressing L6b Superclass

Despite the challenges described, one transcriptomic superclass in L6b proves to be interesting. The Slc17a8 class (Neuron 317) is shown to be expressed across the entirety of L6b of the neocortex (Figures 16.2b and 16.5b) (Yao et al. 2021a, Yao et al. 2021b). This class clusters separately from all other clusters of L6b early on within the tree structure of L6b and does not divide further into any subclasses, furthermore, in the scatterplot it forms a clear evagination of the continuous structure that L6b forms, suggesting it evades the fluid structure of L6b and does indeed form a group of cells that is continuous with yet different from L6b (Figure 16.2b). Therefore, we can assume it to be more isolated, even in an algorithm that clusters through hard thresholds. It is consistent with previous investigations in regionally specific transcriptomic analyses, namely the Hsd17b2 superclass in the visual cortex and the anterolateral motor cortex (ALM) (Tasic et al. 2018) as well as the superclass Kcnip1 in the motor cortex (Scala et al. 2021; Yao et al. 2021a, Yao et al. 2021b). Assuming that the data on the Kcnip1 class is generalizable to the global class of Slc17a8, this group of neurons has one of the highest input resistances across L6b cells (400 Mohm), as well as the highest time constant (32 ms) (Scala et al. 2021). In the motor cortex, the cells are either pyramidal or horizontal in shape (Scala et al. 2021). In the whole-brain analysis, they do not express common traditional markers (*Cplx3, Ctgf, Lpar1*) or express these markers at lower levels than the other cells in the L6b cluster yet express Hcrtr2 as one of three clusters (Figure 16.5b) (Yao et al. 2021a, Yao et al. 2021b). It would be interesting to know how this class of cells connects to other cells, as the orexin receptor has a stereotypical function in cognition and specifically activates L6b cells (Bayer et al. 2004; Radnikow and Feldmeyer 2018; Wenger Combremont et al. 2016a).

16.7 Conclusions

Transcriptomic analyses allow us to explore a large set of data with more information than foregone methods of cell investigation, helping us interpret a cell's function in a more comprehensive manner. However, it does so only on a microlevel (Chari et al., 2021). While being able to highlight starkly different sets of cells (e.g., Slc17a8), they should not be used as the sole basis of cellular identification. Rather the future of cell typing is dependent on a sufficient quantitative integration of cellular properties into an expanded multidimensional structural continuum of multiple gradients. Patch-sequencing, which establishes electrophysiological recordings, morphology, and transcriptomic identity via scRNA-seq (Scala et al. 2021), is a particularly valuable large-scale technique for establishing links between different clustering methods. Combining Patch-sequencing with large-scale tracing efforts as presented by Winnubst and colleagues (Winnubst et al. 2019) would advance the field extraordinarily. However, this is only achievable if the functional importance of the structures is respected, for example, by introducing a semi-supervised reduction of a multidimensional map that includes these different types of data. We must investigate how we approach this diversity of neurons. One approach could be to identify the slopes with which the structure of this continuum changes, as was described in a very simple way on the evagination of Slc17a8 earlier. It is then that the identity of L6b, the knowledge about their behavior both in development and in adult will give us insight into alterations and dysfunctions.

Acknowledgments

The work in the laboratory of Zoltán Molnár was supported by Medical Research Council (G00900901), Biotechnology and Biological Sciences Research Council (BB/X008711/1), The Anatomical Society, The Wellcome Trust, The Royal Society, and Einstein Stiftung. Sara Bandiera was supported by a Medical Research Council Graduate Studentship. Thomas Henning is Scholar of St Edmund Hall, Oxford. We thank Professor Chiaki Maruyama, Miss Hitomi Achiwa, and Professor David Dupret for their very helpful comments on an earlier version of this manuscript.

References

Akbarian, S. et al. (1993a). Altered distribution of nicotinamide-adenine dinucleotide phosphate-diaphorase cells in frontal lobe of schizophrenics implies disturbances of cortical development. *Arch Gen Psychiatry* 50 (3): 169–177.

Akbarian, S. et al. (1993b). Distorted distribution of nicotinamide-adenine dinucleotide phosphate-diaphorase neurons in temporal lobe of schizophrenics implies anomalous cortical development. *Arch Gen Psychiatry* 50 (3): 178–187.

Allendoerfer, K.L. and Shatz, C.J. (1994). The subplate, a transient neocortical structure. *Ann Rev Neurosci* 17: 185–218.

Ayoub, A.E. and Kostovic, I. (2009). New horizons for the subplate zone and its pioneering neurons. *Cereb Cortex* 19 (8): 1705–1707.

Bayer, L. et al. (2004). Exclusive postsynaptic action of hypocretin-orexin on sublayer 6b cortical neurons. *J Neurosci* 24 (30): 6760–6764.

Beglopoulos, V. et al. (2005). Neurexophilin 3 is highly localized in cortical and cerebellar regions and is functionally important for sensorimotor gating and motor coordination. *Mol Cell Biol* 25 (16): 7278–7288.

Belgard, T.G. et al. (2011). A transcriptomic atlas of mouse neocortical layers. *Neuron* 71 (4): 605–616.

BRAIN Initiative Cell Census Network (BICCN) (2021). A multimodal cell census and atlas of the mammalian primary motor cortex. *Nature* 598 (7879): 86–102.

Bruguier, H. et al. (2020). In search of common developmental and evolutionary origin of the claustrum and subplate. *J Comp Neurol* 528 (17): 2956–2977.

Case, L. et al. (2017). Desynchronization of the rat cortical network and excitation of white matter neurons by neurotensin. *Cereb Cortex* 27 (4): 2671–2685.

Chari, T. et al. (2021). The specious art of single-cell genomics. *BioRxiv* doi: 10.1101/2021.08.25.457696.

Chung, L. et al. (2009). Cholecystokinin action on layer 6b neurons in somatosensory cortex. *Brain Res* 1282: 10–19.

Duque, A. et al. (2016). Secondary expansion of the transient subplate zone in the developing cerebrum of human and nonhuman primates. *Proc Natl Acad Sci USA* 113 (35): 9892–9897.

Friedlander, M.J. and Torres-Reveron, J. (2009). The changing roles of neurons in the cortical subplate. *Front Neuroanat* 3: 15.

Ghosh, A. et al. (1990). Requirement for subplate neurons in the formation of thalamocortical connections. *Nature* 347 (6289): 179–181.

Hawrylycz, M.J. et al. (2012). An anatomically comprehensive atlas of the adult human brain transcriptome. *Nature* 489 (7416): 391–399.

Hoerder-Suabedissen, A. et al. (2018). Subset of cortical layer 6b neurons selectively innervates higher order thalamic nuclei in mice. *Cereb Cortex* 28 (5): 1882–1897.

Hoerder-Suabedissen, A. and Molnár, Z. (2013). Molecular diversity of early-born subplate neurons. *Cereb Cortex* 23 (6): 1473–1483.

Hoerder-Suabedissen, A. et al. (2013). Expression profiling of mouse subplate reveals a dynamic gene network and disease association with autism and schizophrenia. *Proc Natl Acad Sci USA* 110 (9): 3555–3560.

Hoerder-Suabedissen, A. et al. (2009). Novel markers reveal subpopulations of subplate neurons in the murine cerebral cortex. *Cereb Cortex* 19 (8): 1738–1750.

Kanold, P.O. et al. (2020). Transient cortical circuits match spontaneous and sensory-driven activity during development. *Science* 370 (6514): eabb2153.

Killackey, H.P. and Sherman, S.M. (2003). Corticothalamic projections from the rat primary somatosensory cortex. *J Neurosci* 23 (19): 7381–7384.

Kostovic, I. and Molliver, M.E. (1974). New interpretation of laminar development of cerebral-cortex-synaptogenesis in different layers of neopallium in human fetus. *Anat Rec* 176.

Kostovic, I. and Rakic, P. (1990). Developmental history of the transient subplate zone in the visual and somatosensory cortex of the macaque monkey and human brain. *J Comp Neurol* 297 (3): 441–470.

Lein, E. et al. (2017). The promise of spatial transcriptomics for neuroscience in the era of molecular cell typing. *Science* 358 (6359): 64–69.

Liao, C.C. and Lee, L.J. (2012). Evidence for structural and functional changes of subplate neurons in developing rat barrel cortex. *Brain Struct Funct* 217 (2): 275–292.

Marx, M. and Feldmeyer, D. (2013). Morphology and physiology of excitatory neurons in layer 6b of the somatosensory rat barrel cortex. *Cereb Cortex* 23 (12): 2803–2817.

Marx, M. et al. (2017). Neocortical layer 6B as a remnant of the subplate – a morphological comparison. *Cereb Cortex* 27 (2): 1011–1026.

Miller, J.A. et al. (2020). Common cell type nomenclature for the mammalian brain. *Elife* 9 (10): 7554/eLife.59928.

Molnár, Z. (1998). *Development of Thalamocortical Connections.* Berlin: Springer. ISBN-10 3540642250.

Munoz-Castaneda, R. et al. (2021). Cellular anatomy of the mouse primary motor cortex. *Nature* 598 (7879): 159–166.

Newmaster, K.T. et al. (2020). Quantitative cellular-resolution map of the oxytocin receptor in postnatally developing mouse brains. *Nat Commun* 11 (1): 1885–1.

Oeschger, F.M. et al. (2012). Gene expression analysis of the embryonic subplate. *Cereb Cortex* 22 (6): 1343–1359.

Osheroff, H. and Hatten, M.E. (2009). Gene expression profiling of preplate neurons destined for the subplate. *Cereb Cortex* 19 (Suppl1): 126.

Pedraza, M. et al. (2014). Extracortical origin of some murine subplate cell populations. *Proc Natl Acad Sci USA* 111 (23): 8613–8618.

Price, D.J. et al. (1997). Fates of the earliest generated cells in the developing murine neocortex. *J Comp Neurol* 377 (3): 414–422.

Radnikow, G. and Feldmeyer, D. (2018). Layer- and cell type-specific modulation of excitatory neuronal activity in the neocortex. *Front Neuroanat* 12: 1.

Rakic, P. (1977). Prenatal development of the visual system in rhesus monkey. *Philos Trans R Soc B: Biol Sci* 278 (961): 245–260.

Ramón y Cajal, S. (1909). *Histologie du système nerveux de l'homme & des vertébrés.* Paris: Maloine.

Reep, R.L. and Goodwin, G.S. (1988). Layer VII of rodent cerebral cortex. *Neurosci Lett* 90 (1–2): 15–20.

Rickmann, M. et al. (1977). On the development of non-pyramidal neurons and axons outside the cortical plate. *Anat Embryol* 151 (3): 285–307.

Scala, F. et al. (2021). Phenotypic variation of transcriptomic cell types in mouse motor cortex. *Nature* 598 (7879): 144–150.

Suarez-Sola, M.L. et al. (2009). Neurons in the white matter of the adult human neocortex. *Front Neuroanat* 3: 7.

Tasic, B. et al. (2016). Adult mouse cortical cell taxonomy revealed by single cell transcriptomics. *Nat Neurosci* 19 (2): 335–346.

Tasic, B. et al. (2018). Shared and distinct transcriptomic cell types across neocortical areas. *Nature* 563 (7729): 72–78.

Tiong, S.Y.X. et al. (2019). Kcnab1 is expressed in subplate neurons with unilateral long-range inter-areal projections. *Front Neuroanat* 13: 39.

Velmeshev, D. et al. (2019). Single-cell genomics identifies cell type-specific molecular changes in autism. *Science* 364 (6441): 685–689.

Viswanathan, S. et al. (2017). Molecularly defined subplate neurons project both to thalamocortical recipient layers and thalamus. *Cereb Cortex* 27 (10): 4759–4768.

Wang, W.Z. et al. (2011). Comparative aspects of subplate zone studied with gene expression in sauropsids and mammals. *Cereb Cortex* 21 (10): 2187–2203.

Watakabe, A. et al. (2007). Comparative analysis of layer-specific genes in mammalian neocortex. *Cereb Cortex* 17 (8): 1918–1933.

Wenger Combremont, A.L. et al. (2016a). Slow bursting neurons of mouse cortical layer 6b are depolarized by hypocretin/orexin and major transmitters of arousal. *Front Neurol* 7: 88.

Wenger Combremont, A.L. et al. (2016b). Effects of hypocretin/orexin and major transmitters of arousal on fast spiking neurons in mouse cortical layer 6B. *Cereb Cortex* 26 (8): 3553–3562.

Winnubst, J. et al. (2019). Reconstruction of 1,000 projection neurons reveals new cell types and organization of long-range connectivity in the mouse brain. *Cell* 179 (1): 268–281.e13.

Woo, T.U. et al. (1991). Dual fate of subplate neurons in a rodent. *Cereb Cortex* 1 (5): 433–443.

Yao, Z. et al. (2021a). A transcriptomic and epigenomic cell atlas of the mouse primary motor cortex. *Nature* 598 (7879): 103–110.

Yao, Z. et al. (2021b). A taxonomy of transcriptomic cell types across the isocortex and hippocampal formation. *Cell* 184 (12): 3222–3241.e26.

Yuste, R. et al. (2020). A community-based transcriptomics classification and nomenclature of neocortical cell types. *Nat Neurosci* 23 (12): 1456–1468.

Zeisel, A. et al. (2015). Brain structure. Cell types in the mouse cortex and hippocampus revealed by single-cell RNA-seq. *Science* 347 (6226): 1138–1142.

Zhang, Y. et al. (2014). An RNA-sequencing transcriptome and splicing database of glia, neurons, and vascular cells of the cerebral cortex. *J Neurosci* 34 (36): 11929–11947.

Zolnik, T.A. et al. (2020). Layer 6b is driven by intracortical long-range projection neurons. *Cell Rep* 30 (10): 3492–3505.

Part 4

Neuron Migration

17

Cortical Neuron Migration in Health and Disease

*Míriam Javier-Torrent and Laurent Nguyen**

GIGA Stem Cells, GIGA-Neurosciences, University of Liège, CHU Sart Tilman, Liège 4000, Belgium
** Corresponding author*

17.1 Modes of Cell Migration in the Forebrain: From Rodents to Primates

17.1.1 Projection Neurons

The cerebral cortex is a complex structure mostly composed of PNs and cINs that organize into functional neuronal circuits. The initial histological observations by Ramón y Cajal revealed a great diversity of cell shapes and types (Ramón y Cajal 1909). The position of these cells in the cortex is not random, but rather depends on a tightly regulated process to which both intrinsic and extrinsic migration mechanisms contribute. Furthermore, cell migration within the forebrain favors dynamic cellular crosstalk, which is necessary for the formation of the cerebral cortex (reviewed in Silva et al. 2019). Once mature, the neocortex displays unique cytoarchitectural features, including the distribution of interconnected neurons into six horizontal layers (reviewed in Lodato and Arlotta 2015).

The formation of cortical layers involves the migration and settlement of PNs that are born from progenitors that reside in the cortical wall. In mouse, these progenitors are called apical progenitors (APs) or basal (BPs) progenitors, according to their location and their division that occurs either at the surface of the ventricular zone (VZ) for APs, or in the basal part of the VZ/subventricular zone (SVZ) for BPs (Götz and Huttner 2005; Laguesse et al. 2015; Malatesta et al. 2000; Noctor et al. 2001a). APs include neuroepithelial cells (NEs), apical radial glial cells (aRGs) and short neural precursors (SNPs). Two types of BPs can be distinguished: the intermediate progenitors (IPs) and the outer radial glial cells (oRGs) (Wang et al. 2011a). The forebrain is initially populated by polarized NEs that proliferate using symmetric (also termed proliferative) divisions, contributing to the lateral expansion of the cerebral cortex (Rakic 1995). At the onset of corticogenesis, around embryonic day (E) 12 in mice and gestational week (GW) 5–6 in humans, NEs differentiate into aRGs progenitors (also known as ventricular vRGs) (Hartfuss et al. 2001; Howard et al. 2008; Mo et al. 2007; Zecevic 2004). The aRGs exhibit an elongated morphology that consists in a cell body in the VZ, a short apical process (also termed radial glia process) that reaches the ventricle and a long basal process that contacts the pial surface of the cortex and which is essential in neuronal locomotion (discussed later). The aRGs can undergo two modes of cell division: proliferative division or asymmetric (also termed differentiative division) that occurs later during corticogenesis to give birth to a neuron directly or indirectly, via the generation of BPs (Haubensak et al. 2004; Miyata et al. 2001; Noctor et al. 2001a; Wu et al. 2005). During the

Neocortical Neurogenesis in Development and Evolution, First Edition. Edited by Wieland B. Huttner.

division of APs (both NEs and aRGs), the nucleus moves between the apical and basal parts of the VZ in close coordination with cell cycle progression, a process termed interkinetic nuclear migration (INM) (Ueno et al. 2006 and reviewed in Taverna and Huttner 2010). This process, initially described by Hesse, is responsible for the pseudostratified appearance of the neuroepithelium and later the VZ (Hesse et al. 2012). INM limits cell soma crowding above the ventricular surface where cell mitosis occurs. The regulation of this process is thus important for the balance between the progenitor pool and its neuronal output (Xie et al. 2007). The bidirectional nuclear movement underlying INM in aRG cells depends on distinct microtubule motors whose recruitment is responsible for the cell-cycle control of INM in rodents (Hu et al. 2013; Tsai et al. 2010). Along this line, a study performed in the zebrafish retina shows that the impairment of INM, resulting from the disruption of the motor protein Dynactin-1, leads to an increased number of progenitors exiting the cell cycle (Del Bene et al. 2008). Importantly, the apical to basal migration of the nucleus also relies on actomyosin contractions and its inhibition impairs the fate of VZ/SVZ progenitors (Schenk et al. 2009).

In the cortex, the first wave of postmitotic neurons leaving the VZ is observed between E11 and E13 in mice, and they populate a transient layer called the preplate (PP), which later splits under the migration of PNs into the marginal zone (MZ), mainly consisting in Cajal–Retzius cells, and the subplate (SP) populated by subplate neurons. Successive waves of PNs are generated and arrange themselves into the cortical plate following an inside-out pattern (Ayala et al. 2007; Hoerder-Suabedissen and Molnár 2015). Around E17.5, neurogenesis shifts progressively to gliogenesis to produce astrocytes and oligodendrocytes also derived from aRG cells (Clavreul et al. 2019; Guo et al. 2013; Magavi et al. 2012; Shen et al. 2021).

In primates including humans, the SVZ is compartmentalized into an inner and outer SVZ (iSVZ and oSVZ, respectively) which are divided by an inner fiber layer (iFL) (Smart 2002). Besides the iFL, there is a second fiber layer (outer fiber layer; oFL) that limits the upper side of the oSVZ. After the gestational week (GW) 16.5, aRGs generate oRGs and truncated radial glial cells (tRGs) (Nowakowski et al. 2016). While oRGs mainly contribute to the generation of deep and upper layer PNs (Hansen et al. 2010; Pollen et al. 2015), a recent work suggests that tRGs may be responsible for cortical gliogenesis via the generation of basal multipotent intermediate progenitors (bMIPC) around GW23 (Yang et al. 2022). In humans, the PP appears between GW5 and GW8 and is followed by the emergence of the cortical plate that splits it into the MZ and the SP layers. While in mouse the SP is composed of early-born neocortical cells, a birth dating study showed that SP neurons are continuously migrating throughout cortical neurogenesis in primates (Duque et al. 2016). After the colonization of the SP by early-born neurons (around E54), it undergoes a secondary expansion that causes a spreading of these cells by the ingrowth of axons from neurons of cortical and subcortical origins (by E83). The SP thickness thus differs considerably between species, being smaller in rodents than in primates (Kostovic and Rakic 1990; Smart 2002). Moreover, another distinctive feature considered as being primate specific, is the existence between GW 11 and GW29 of a transient cell layer located below the pia and above the MZ, which is named subpial granular layer (SGL) (Brun 1965; Gadisseux et al. 1992; Meyer et al. 1998).

Live imaging of the radial migration of PNs revealed that this process is discontinuous and breaks down into three contiguous migration modes: multipolar, locomotion, and somal translocation. Shortly after birth, PNs display a transient multipolar morphology and time-lapse experiments on organotypic slices of embryonic mouse brains indicate that multipolar cells contain highly dynamic processes that undergo continuous extension and retraction steps (Tabata and Nakajima 2003). In contrast, during glia-dependent locomotion, neurons adopt a bipolar shape with an apical leading process and a thin basal trailing one (Kawauchi 2015; Nadarajah et al. 2001; Nishimura et al. 2010) to cross the cortical wall. Once their leading process approaches the MZ and reaches the pial surface, locomoting PNs attach their apical process to the pial surface and initiate somal translocation to their final position in ad hoc cortical layer. As the leading process shortens, the cell soma is progressively pulled causing the neurons to undergo continuous forward migration (Nadarajah et al. 2001). The exact molecular signals that underlie the transition between these modes of migration are not fully understood and likely involve crosstalk between environmental factors and cell intrinsic signaling. The secretion of Reelin by Cajal–Retzius cells located in the MZ (Alcántara et al. 1998; Ogawa et al. 1995) may act as a stop signal for migrating neurons. An initial study showed that while neurons approach the MZ, Reelin induces the phosphorylation of n-cofilin, an actin depolymerizing protein, in the leading process of migrating neurons thereby stabilizing their actin cytoskeleton (Chai et al. 2009). In addition, by acting on the Rap1-NCad pathway, it contributes to the repolarization of multipolar PNs, allowing them to undergo locomotion (Jossin and Cooper 2011). Another study also indicated que Dab1-mediated Reelin signaling is essential later for somal translocation (Franco et al. 2011).

17.1.2 Interneurons

In rodents, GABAergic cINs are born in the subpallium (Figure 17.1). Most of them are generated within the proliferative zones of the medial ganglionic eminence (MGE), while some are born in the caudal ganglionic eminence (CGE) and preoptic area (POA) (Anderson et al. 2001; Gelman et al. 2009; Nery et al. 2002; Tamamaki et al. 1997). After their generation, cINs migrate

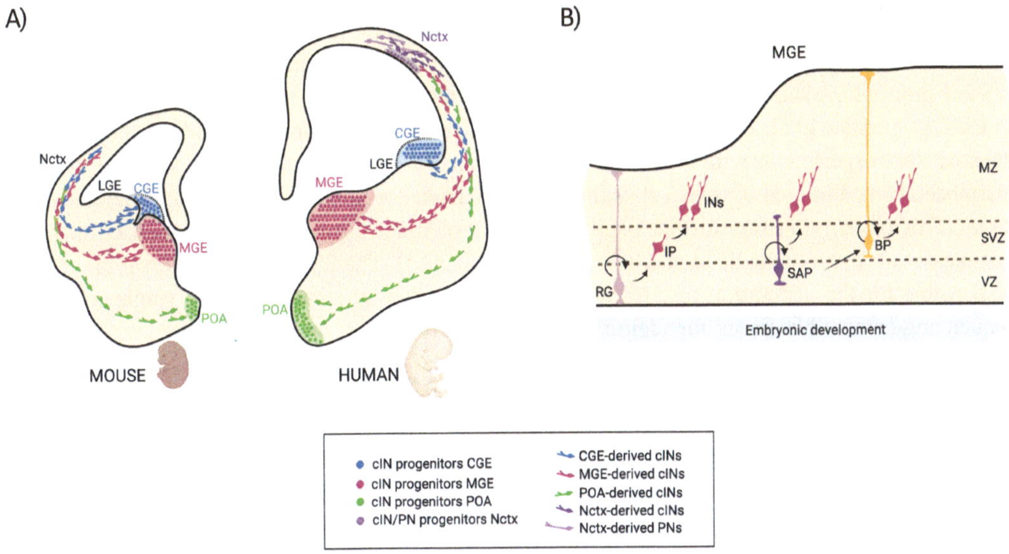

Figure 17.1 Neurogenesis and migration processes of cINs during mouse and human cerebral cortex development. (A) Schematic illustration of half-coronal sections of mouse (left) and human (right) forebrains depicting the main proliferative regions from where cortical interneurons (cINs) are born. Mouse cINs are generated in three regions in the subpallium: caudal ganglionic eminence (CGE; in blue), medial ganglionic eminence (MGE; in pink), and preoptic area (POA; in green); from where they migrate tangentially to reach the cortex. In humans, a subpopulation of neuronal progenitors in the neocortex generates both projection neurons (PNs; in light purple) and cINs (in dark purple). In addition, similar to mouse, human cINs are also born in the subpallium. (B) Schematic illustration of the distinct progenitors dividing in the MGE in mouse. Apical progenitors reside in the ventricular zone (VZ) and include radial glia (RG; light pink) and subapical progenitors (SAP; purple). Intermediate progenitors (IP) localize mainly in the subventricular zone (SVZ) together with the basal progenitors (BPs; yellow). Migrating cINs mostly appear in the marginal zone (MZ) from where they start to migrate toward the cortex. The potential result after the division of each progenitor cell is indicated by an arrow. Circular arrows represent the self-renewal capacity of the progenitors. Nctx: neocortex. Created with BioRender.com.

tangentially long distances to reach the cortex (Anderson et al. 1997; Corbin et al. 2001; Métin et al. 2007; Tamamaki et al. 1997; Tanaka et al. 2003). Here, we focus on cINs born in MGE and CGE since the lateral ganglionic eminence (LGE) mainly contributes to the generation of GABAergic neurons that will incorporate the striatum and the olfactory bulbs (Deacon et al. 1994; Olsson et al. 1998, 1995). The MGE contains two different proliferating domains, the VZ and SVZ where radial glia (RG) cells and BPs are dividing, respectively (Flames et al. 2007; Petros et al. 2015; Turrero García and Harwell 2017). A study showed that most progenitor cells divide in the apical zone of the MGE at E12, while the proportion of mitotic progenitors increases in the basal region (SVZ) as embryogenesis proceeds (E14–E16) (Pilz et al. 2013). This study also highlights a new progenitor type that divides at subapical position (i.e., subapical progenitors; SAPs). Of interest, SAP divisions at the MGE represent half of the mitoses occurring in the VZ, evidencing a notable difference with the dorsal telencephalon, where most progenitor divisions occur at apical positions (Pilz et al. 2013).

In humans and nonhuman primates, most cINs are also born in the ganglionic eminences (GEs) (Al-Jaberi et al. 2015; Letinic et al. 2002; Ma et al. 2013a; Petanjek et al. 2009). Single cell RNA sequencing (scRNAseq) performed on human fetal brain samples identified two distinct populations of cIN progenitors that are located in the VZ and SVZ of the GEs (Yu et al. 2021). Several transcription factors and gene regulatory networks that underly cIN specification are conserved in mice and primates (Flames et al. 2007; Ma et al. 2013a; Shi et al. 2021). Indeed, comparative scRNAseq analyses performed on mouse and human GEs suggest an overall evolutionary-conserved transcriptional control of cIN specification and diversity (Shi et al. 2021). However, the cortical distribution and number of some cINs are unique to primates (Krienen et al. 2020; Shi et al. 2021).

Some groups have shown strong evidence in favor of a model where most human cINs are produced in the GEs (Arshad et al. 2016; Hansen et al. 2013; Ma et al. 2013b). However, this has been largely debated since experiments with retroviral labeling performed on human fetal brain slices suggest the existence of an additional source of cINs that originate from dorsal cortical progenitors (Letinic et al. 2002). This observation was further back up by data obtained in monkeys (Al-Jaberi et al. 2015; Petanjek et al. 2009; Radonjić et al. 2014; Zecevic et al. 2011). The identity of the dorsal progenitor responsible for the generation of cINs was recently unveiled by clonal analysis (single-cell-RNA-sequencing-compatible tracer for identifying clonal relationships, or STICR), demonstrating that some human cortical progenitors can generate both PNs and cINs (Delgado et al. 2022) (Figure 17.1).

When ventrally born cINs exit the GEs, they invade the cortical wall via two main tangential routes located in the intermediate zone (IZ) and the MZ (Anderson et al. 2001). These cells then undergo intracortical dispersion by exiting the streams via radial or oblique migration (reviewed in Kriegstein and Noctor 2004). During this process, some cINs also adopt a ventricle-directed migration (Nadarajah et al. 2002). MGE-derived cINs populate the cortex following an inside-out pattern with early-born MGE cells mainly colonizing the deep layer V and the majority of late-born cells settling in layers II and III (Valcanis and Tan 2003). Similar results were obtained by another group using GAD65-GFP transgenic mice, who showed that late-born GAD65-GFP cINs prefer to occupy upper cortical layers (López-Bendito et al. 2004). Heterochronic brain transplantation of MGE progenitors switches the cortical destination of their cIN progeny (Valcanis and Tan 2003) highlighting a critical role for some extrinsic factors in the positioning of cINs. CGE-derived cINs migrate to the cortex where they populate almost exclusively the layer V at more caudal levels (Nery et al. 2002; Yozu et al. 2005). It is worth noting that some apparent contradictions exist as to whether cell fate also "instructs" positioning in the cortex. On the one hand, early studies in mouse indicate that MGE-derived clonally related cINs tend to cluster in the neocortex (Brown et al. 2011; Ciceri et al. 2013), while later clonal studies using barcoded viral libraries suggested that such lineage-related cINs can populate distant regions of the pallium (Harwell et al. 2015; Mayer et al. 2015). Subtype specification of cINs is acquired before or just after cell cycle exit but their final identity is only unfolded when they settle into the cortex (Bandler et al. 2022; Mayer et al. 2018; Mi et al. 2018). There is a correlation between the birth place in the subpallium and the identity that cINs adopt in the cortex. MGE and adjacent POA mostly produce somatostatin (SST) + and paravalbumine (PV) + cINs, while CGE generates vasoactive intestinal peptide (VIP) +, cholecystokinin (CCK) + and other less abundant cIN subtypes (Butt et al. 2005; D. Gelman et al. 2011; Lavdas et al. 1999; Niquille et al. 2018; Wichterle et al. 2001; Xu et al. 2004). Recent transcriptomic analyses also indicate that most SST + cINs that migrate within the MZ will become Martinotti cells (Lim et al. 2018), suggesting a link between their migratory route and identity.

The tangential migration of cINs is discontinuous (saltatory) and relies on repetitive cycles including the growth and dynamic branching of a leading process together with nuclear motions (i.e., nucleokinesis) that alternate phases of movement and pause (Bellion et al. 2005). The migratory cycle can be broken down into three sequential steps: formation and forward displacement of a cytoplasmic bulge encompassing the centrosome and Golgi apparatus, followed by the elongation and branching of the leading process, and nucleokinesis that depends on the contraction of polarized actomyosin fibers to propel the nucleus towards the centrosome/Golgi apparatus (Bellion et al. 2005; Martini and Valdeolmillos 2010). The migration cycle is not synchronized among moving cINs, which allows proper sorting of cINs in streams, from the subpallium to the pallium (Silva et al. 2018). Recent technologic development in organoids allowed the analysis of the migration of human cIN-like cells by real-time imaging. These studies have confirmed that human cINs also undergo unsynchronized saltatory migration in ventral-dorsal fused organoids (i.e., assembloids) derived from human pluripotent stem cells (hPSCs) (Bagley et al. 2017; Birey et al. 2017; Xiang et al. 2017). The molecular mechanism that underlies neuronal migration will be discussed in more detail in the following sections.

17.2 Prototypic Neuronal Migration Disorders

Most cortical neurons have to travel long distances to reach their ad hoc position in the cortex where they functionally integrate into neuronal circuits. Disruption of this process can lead to a broad array of cortical malformation in humans. Therefore, the cellular and molecular investigation of these genetic disorders is key to identify important molecular drivers that underlie different stages of neuronal migration.

17.2.1 Lissencephaly

Lissencephaly, which literally means "smooth brain," includes a group of disorders characterized by the absence or reduction of folding of the cerebral cortex. This cortical malformation has been divided into classic lissencephaly (or type I) and cobblestone dysplasia (or type II). However, cobblestone dysplasia was recently recognized as a distinct syndrome with a different etiology (Severino et al. 2020). In patients suffering from type I lissencephaly, the cortical wall is subdivided into three or four layers instead of six, and the brain shows agyria and/or pachygyria, depending on whether the gyri are totally absent or only reduced in number, respectively. In general terms, individuals suffering from lissencephaly present intellectual disability often accompanied by epilepsy and usually they have a poor prognosis due to severe seizures or respiratory disease (Dobyns 2010). The patients' symptoms depend therefore on the degree of brain malformation, and the less severe malformations involve subcortical band heterotopia (SBH). Mutations in *LIS1* have been associated with type I lissencephaly and include two clinical conditions: isolated lissencephaly sequence (ILS) and Miller-Dieker syndrome (MDS) (Reiner et al. 1995, 1993). MDS patients present distinctive facial features and visceral abnormalities at birth that accompany lissencephaly (Dobyns et al. 1991). Together with *LIS1*, mutations in X-linked gene doublecortin (*DCX*) account for most cases of type I lissencephaly (Dobyns et al. 1993; Gleeson et al. 1998; Pilz et al. 1999). Interestingly, mutations in the *DCX* gene present sex-specific differences: while 38 percent of male patients with ILS without deletions in *LIS1* present mutations in this gene, more females rather develop SBH (D'Agostino et al. 2002; Gleeson et al. 1999; Pilz et al. 1999). In addition to *LIS1* and *DCX*, several genes whose mutation underlie lissencephaly have been discovered over the past years and include *ARX, RELN, TUBA1A, VLDLR*, and *YWHAE* (Boycott et al. 2005; Hong et al. 2000; Keays et al. 2007; Kitamura et al. 2002; Nagamani et al. 2009). MDS is caused by larger deletions in chromosome 17p13.3, a region that in addition to *LIS1* encompass other 25 genes, including *CRK* and *YWHAE* that have been related to the more severe forms of the disease (Cardoso et al. 2003). In addition to type I, lissencephaly with cerebellar hypoplasia (LCH) and X-linked lissencephaly with abnormal genitalia (XLAG) have recently been described. One of the main features that characterizes LCH is the underdevelopment of the cerebellum due to mutations in *RELN* or *TUBA1A* genes, which are involved in the control of neuronal migration (Hong et al. 2000; Keays et al. 2007; Kumar et al. 2010). XLAG occurs exclusively in males due to mutations in the X-linked *ARX* gene, which encode a transcription factor that controls specification and migration of cINs (Dobyns et al. 1999; Friocourt and Parnavelas 2010a; Kitamura et al. 2009, 2002).

Lissencephaly is mostly characterized by neuronal migration defects (Kato and Dobyns 2003), but recent studies using human cerebral organoids derived from MDS iPSc-neurons showed that divisions of oRG are also impaired (Bershteyn et al. 2017). The role of these genes has been extensively studied in different animal models and cell types. Complete deletion of *Lis1* in mice is embryonically lethal, while reduced dosage of this gene results in disorganization of the cerebral cortex, hippocampus, and olfactory bulbs (Hirotsune et al. 1998). A reduced *Lis1* expression level also results in shorter distance travelled and reduced speed of migration by postmitotic neurons (Hirotsune et al. 1998; Youn et al. 2009). At the molecular level, *Lis1* is a microtubule associated protein (MAP), which regulates nuclear movements in migrating neurons. This protein is also expressed by NEs and RG progenitors where it plays key roles to support INM as well as control the orientation of the mitotic spindle (Tsai et al. 2005; Yingling et al. 2008). At a cellular level, in addition to impairing migration, *Lis1* disruption alters the organization of both RG cells and pyramidal neurons, with the latest presenting less dendritic branches (Cahana et al. 2001; Fleck et al. 2000). Cerebral organoids generated from MDS patient-derived iPSC show that the radial migration of PNs is also impaired in humans, which present less elongated nuclei and migrate slower than controls. Furthermore, the migration of MDS iPSC-derived PNs is also disrupted when using control human cortical tissue at GW18.5 as a migration substrate (Bershteyn et al. 2017), suggesting that their defects in migration are mostly cell autonomous. In contrast, transplantation assays in mouse in which the GEs are cultured "en face" to control or *Lis1*$^{-/-}$ cortex showed that *Lis1* deficient cINs migrate shorter distances when exiting the GE due to both cell autonomous and nonautonomous cell defects (McManus et al. 2004). Moreover, time-lapse video microscopy demonstrated that *Lis1* +/− migrating cINs have reduced nucleokinesis speed and increased nuclear pausing, as well as increased average length of the leading process, which also presents fewer branches (Nasrallah et al. 2006). These results are consistent with the localization of Lis1 in the centrosome where it colocalizes with the dynein-dynactin complex and its role as a microtubule-organizing center (MTOC) (Feng et al. 2000; Sasaki et al. 2000; Smith et al. 2000).

17.2.2 Cobblestone Dysplasia

Cobblestone dysplasia was formerly known as "type II lissencephaly" (Dobyns et al. 1985). In cobblestone dysplasia, neurons migrate too much and overshoot the pial surface, leading to the formation of an extracortical layer beyond the MZ and the disorganization of the cortical layering with ectopic neurons and glia (i.e., heterotopia) (Muntoni and Voit 2004; Olson and Walsh 2002). Imaging studies reveal cases of pachygyria, agyria (as in classical lissencephaly) as well as polymicrogyria, which consists of an excessive number of small gyri in the cerebral cortex. These defects are usually accompanied by malformations of the cerebellum. Cobblestone dysplasia includes three autosomal recessive disorders characterized for presenting brain, ocular, and muscular anomalies: Fukuyama congenital muscular dystrophy (FCMD), Walker-Warburg syndrome (WWS), and muscle-eye-brain disease (MEB), albeit some histological features can be differentiated among them. In general terms, FCMD is characterized by polymicrogyria in the frontal lobe, while clinical features of MEB and WWS are more dramatic with extended areas of agyria or pachygyria (van der Knaap et al. 1997). In some patients suffering from cobblestone dysplasia the hypoglycosylation of α-dystroglycan has been reported (Muntoni et al. 2002; Waite et al. 2012). The functional importance of α-dystroglycan lies on its interaction with both the extracellular matrix (ECM) and the intracellular cytoskeleton (Ibraghimov-Beskrovnaya et al. 1992). The α-dystroglycan works as an ECM receptor and thus interacts with ligands, such as laminin and agrin. Its proper activity requires posttranslational processing, including glycosyltransferase-mediated glycosylation (Yoshida-Moriguchi et al. 2010). Thus, mutations in genes that encode for glycosyltransferases or related accessory proteins (*FKTN, FKRP, POMT1, POMT2, POMGNT1, LARGE*), have been associated with cobblestone disorders (Beltrán-valero de Bernabé et al. 2002; Brockington et al. 2001; Inamori et al. 2012; Longman et al. 2003; Toda 1999; van Reeuwijk et al. 2005; Yoshida et al. 2001). Nonetheless, the pathomechanisms triggered by these mutations are not fully understood. In the case of the *FKTN* gene, mouse models that have been generated were embryonically lethal (Kurahashi et al. 2005) or failed to recreate the brain or muscle defects observed in patients (Kanagawa et al. 2009). Recently, *fukutin* (*fktn*)-conditional knockout mice under the Emx1 promoter have been generated. In this mouse model, glycosylation of α-dystroglycan is impaired leading to loss of integrity of the glia limitans-basement membrane, which can be partially restored by in utero electroporation of *fktn* at early stages of development (Myshrall et al. 2012; Sudo et al. 2018). However, the above-mentioned *fktn* mouse models only partially mimic patient phenotype, further suggesting interspecies functional differences. In contrast, cortical brain organoids derived from FCMD patient iPSCs recapitulate a cobblestone-like surface and disorganization of RG fibers that leads to a higher ratio of breaches extruding from the surface of the organoid as observed in human patients (Taniguchi-Ikeda et al. 2021). This defect in RG fiber migration can be partially restored by administration of Mannan-007, which enhances the glycosylation of α-dystroglycan in vitro (Lv et al. 2015; Taniguchi-Ikeda et al. 2021). Interestingly, a downregulation of the gene encoding for fukutin-related protein *FKRP* in zebrafish embryos leads to morphological defects in eye and neuronal structures (Thornhill et al. 2008). In support of these findings, mice carrying a missense mutation in the *Fkrp* gene present impaired glycosylation of α-dystroglycan and brain defects that suggest disrupted neuronal migration and fusion of the interhemispheric fissure, which is characteristic of human polymicrogyria (Chan et al. 2010). Glycosylated α-dystroglycan is expressed by migrating neurons in the developing and adult cerebral cortex (Ohtsuka-Tsurumi et al. 2004). Impairment of the dystroglycan encoding gene *Dag1* in the mouse brain causes gaps in the glial limiting membrane and the appearance of neuronal/glial heterotopia, which mirrors the defects observed in the brains of cobblestone lissencephaly patients (Moore et al. 2002; Satz et al. 2008).

The conditional knockout of *Dag1* under the postmitotic neuronal promoter NEX-Cre fails to induce heterotopia, suggesting an important role of glial dystroglycan during development of the forebrain (Satz et al. 2010). In fact, dystroglycan protein localizes at the endfeet of RG that contacts with the glial limiting membrane in the developing brain (Myshrall et al. 2012). Along this line, Myshrall et al. also studied the nature of these ectopic neurons and found that in *Dag1* cKO mice CR cells, PNs and cINs accumulated above those breaches of the glial limiting membrane, leading to meningeal heterotopia. Besides neuronal ectopy, IP and RG progenitors also display ectopic mitosis above the subplate and far from their proliferative niches in *Dag1* cKO mice (Myshrall et al. 2012). Taken together, these results reinforce the idea that the glial limiting membrane acts as a spatial boundary for neuronal migration. Of interest, experiments done in *Drosophila* indicate that dystroglycan levels are tightly controlled during development via posttranscriptional mechanisms that involve miRNA regulation and that dysregulation of those mechanisms is associated with defects in brain morphology (Yatsenko et al. 2014). Collectively, these results show the importance of glycosylated α-dystroglycan in the correct development of the cerebral cortex.

17.2.3 Periventricular Nodular Heterotopia

Periventricular nodular heterotopia (PNH) is characterized by the presence of single or multiple aggregates of neuronal and glial cells that fail to migrate to the cerebral cortex and remain adjacent to the ventricles. PNH can affect one or both hemispheres, leading to different clinical outcomes, which frequently include focal epilepsy.

Bilateral PNH is related to loss-of-function mutations in the *FLNA* gene that encodes filamin A, located in the Xq28 chromosome in humans. This type of PNH has a X chromosome-linked dominant inheritance and is usually lethal for males, which explain the higher prevalence in females who often exhibit a mosaic phenotype due to random X inactivation (Eks¸iog et al. 1996; Parrini et al. 2006). Filamin A is an actin-binding protein that links the actin cytoskeleton to cell membranes and provides mechanical protection to cells from the surrounding physical forces (Glogauer et al. 1998). Apart from its interaction with filamentous actin several filamin-binding partners have been reported, including integrins and presenilins, coupling receptor signal transduction to the actin cytoskeleton involved in the regulation of cell-adhesion-mediated processes (Stossel et al. 2001). Initial studies showed that *FLNA* is expressed in migrating and settled neurons in the human embryonic brain (Fox et al. 1998). In the mouse brain, Filamin A localizes at the cell soma and the leading processes of migratory neurons at early stages, while it becomes more restricted to the cell body as neuronal differentiation proceeds, suggesting a role in neuronal migration (Sheen et al. 2002). This was further confirmed by disruption of *FlnA* gene, which resulted in impaired neuronal migration and accumulation of PNs in the VZ, SVZ, and IZ (Nagano et al. 2004; Zhang et al. 2013). This phenotype likely results from defects in filopodia formation in neuronal progenitors that are indeed also observed in *FlnA* knockout mice (Zhang et al. 2013). Although the pathogenic mechanisms underlying the mutations of *FLNA* are not fully understood, the Filamin A-interacting protein (FILIP), which induces Filamin A degradation, might play an important role in this process. FILIP inhibition increases the abundance of Filamin A, that in turn influences neuronal morphology and thus multipolar or bipolar orientation (Nagano et al. 2004). Histological samples from PNH patients also show a disruption in the integrity of the neuroependyma along the ventricle. Similarly, loss of *FlnA* function in mice leads to disruption of the neuroependymal lining and loss of cell-to-cell contacts (Ferland et al. 2009). Since the apical endfeet of RG extend their processes to reach the VZ forming the adherent lining, one may think that RG function is relevant for this process. Consistently ß1-integrins, a known binding partner of Filamin A, are involved in the anchoring of radial glial endfeet to the ventricle surface (Graus-Porta et al. 2001). It is worth noting that knocking down *FlnA* in rats impairs both the orientation of the apical processes of RG that leads to impairment of RG scaffold that neurons use during radial migration, and reduction of cell-cycle proliferation of neural progenitors (Carabalona et al. 2012). Later studies showed that loss of *FlnA* impairs degradation of cyclin B1 leading to a prolonged cell cycle in neural progenitors (Lian et al. 2012). Taken together, these results suggest that PNH may result as a combination of defects in radial glia scaffolding, neuronal migration and proliferation of neural progenitors.

PNH also exists as an autosomal recessive form caused by mutations in the ADP Ribosylation Factor Guanine Nucleotide Exchange Factor 2 (*ARFGEF2*) gene, localized at 20q13.13 (Sheen et al. 2004). *ARFGEF2* encodes for the protein brefeldin-inhibited GEF2 (BIG2), which is involved in vesicle and membrane trafficking from the trans-Golgi network to endosomes (Shin et al. 2004). Of interest, disruption of *ARFGEF2* homologs impairs cell division and adhesion in plants (Shevell 1994). Inhibition of Big2 also disrupts E-cadherin-catenin complexes that mediate cell-cell adhesions in MDCK cells (Sheen et al. 2004). Moreover, treatment with brefeldin A, which inhibits the membrane-associated ARF GEF activity, impairs the development of neuronal polarity and blocks axon formation in cultured mouse hippocampal neurons (Jareb and Banker 1997). Similar to the *FlnA* expression pattern, *Arfgef2* mRNA levels are enriched in the VZ and in the cerebral cortex in mouse (Sheen et al. 2004), suggesting that an interplay between the two gene products is possible. Indeed, immunolabeling of brain slices from both mouse and human embryos showed a colocalization between BIG2 and Filamin A in neuroependymal progenitors (Lu et al. 2006; Zhang et al. 2012) and further in vitro studies confirmed their interaction in cell lines (Zhang et al. 2012). In mice, intraventricular injection of brefeldin-A disrupts the neuroependymal lining and induces the formation of neuronal nodules around the ventricle as was previously seen with altered *FlnA* activity (Ferland et al. 2009). Similar results were found in *Arfgef2* knockout mice, who exhibit an increase in the proportion of migrating neurons in the VZ and SVZ, at expense of the CP (Zhang et al. 2012). Moreover, inhibition of Big2 function disrupts the Golgi complex (Sheen et al. 2004) and induces the translocation of Filamin A from the cell surface to the cytoplasm (Lu et al. 2006), suggesting that Big2-mediated transport of Filamin A may contribute to the pathogenic mechanisms underlying PNH. Big2 regulates indirectly Filamin A phosphorylation, thereby modifying its affinity for actin filaments and leading to changes in focal adhesion size and number (Zhang et al. 2012). Likewise, Filamin A phosphorylation induces Big2 subcellular relocation from the Golgi to the cell membrane, which impacts the activation of Arf1 proteins (Zhang et al. 2013). Thus, disruption of the feedback between Filamin A and Big2 may result in alteration of vesicle trafficking leading to recruitment of proteins to adhesions sites. Taken together this suggest that neuronal migration defects observed in PHN may result from defects in both cell-autonomous (vesicle trafficking) and nonautonomous processes (integrity of RG scaffold).

So far, even though mutations in *FLNA* and *ARFGEF2* have been identified as causatives of PNH, the etiology of most clinical cases remains unknown. Compelling efforts have identified de novo missense mutation in *C6orf70* gene in one PNH patient (Conti et al. 2013). Silencing of *C6orf70* in neuronal progenitors in the embryonic rat neocortex results in extensive neuronal migration defects with the presence of heterotopic nodules along the ventricles. C6orf70 protein shows a punctuate distribution that decorates the endoplasmic reticulum, which suggests that it may also function as a vesicle-associated protein (Conti et al. 2013). More recent studies have also identified missense mutations in *NEDD4L* gene, an E3 ubiquitin ligase, in 11 patients with PNH, cleft palate, and syndactyly. Most of those mutations map to the catalytic HECT domain of *NEDD4L* and lead to protein instability (Broix et al. 2016; Elbracht et al. 2018; Kato et al. 2017), although mutations in the WW domain have also been detected (Stouffs et al. 2020). In vivo studies performed in mice show that over-expression of wild-type *Nedd4l* or PNH-related mutants induce a significant arrest of neurons within the VZ, SVZ, and IZ and increase the proliferation of APs (Broix et al. 2016; Hsia et al. 2014).

17.2.4 Subcortical Band Heterotopia

SBH, also known as band heterotopia or double cortex, is a migration disorder characterized by the presence of heterotopic neurons that form a thick band below the neocortex. In the majority of cases, bands are bilateral and symmetric, and their size is associated with the severity of the clinical features that include intellectual disability and epilepsy. In females, heterozygous mutations in the *DCX* brain-specific gene cause SBH in females (Des Portes et al. 1998). In contrast, males with mutations in *DCX* usually develop lissencephaly, albeit an association with SBH has also been reported (D'Agostino et al. 2002; Gleeson et al. 1998). Mutations in *Lis1* gene have been also shown as causative of SBH, although it is less frequent (D'Agostino et al. 2002; Pilz et al. 1999). *DCX* is a MAP expressed in the cell soma and in the leading process of migrating neurons and the axon of differentiated neurons (Francis et al. 1999; Gleeson et al. 1999). Cortical organization is well preserved in constitutive *Dcx*-knockout mouse brains (Corbo et al. 2002), but *Dcx*-knockout migrating neurons have abnormal morphology and increased branching, defects that are aggravated by *Lis1* inactivation, suggesting that a genetic interaction may exist between these two genes (Pramparo et al. 2010). In contrast, *knocking down Dcx* (*Dcx* RNAi) specifically in migrating PNs inhibits radial migration, and leads to heterotopic accumulation of cells around the IZ at embryonic stages in rats and the formation of subcortical bands below the cortex at postnatal stages (Bai et al. 2003). Interestingly, temporally controlled reexpression of *Dcx* in the *Dcx* RNAi rats reduces the size of SBH malformations, being more effective early in postnatal stages (Manent et al. 2009). However, the same experimental approach fails to reproduce the subcortical bands in mouse (Ramos et al. 2006), highlighting that some species-difference between rats and mouse may exist regarding *Dcx* function. The phenotypical differences between the *Dcx knockout* and *knockdown* models may rely on the inequal temporal disruption or total inhibition of the first model that could lead to activation of compensatory mechanisms. In fact, some works indicate that this may be the case for doublecortin-like kinase (*Dclk*), which may share overlapping functions with *Dcx* (Deuel et al. 2006; Koizumi et al. 2006b). Another important point to keep in mind is the existing differences in terms of distance and time window that underlie cortical migration in humans and rodents. Olfactory bulb interneurons are generated during embryogenesis and throughout adult stages (Batista-Brito et al. 2008). Postnatally, they are born in the anterior subventricular zone (SVZa) and they migrate long distances through the rostral migratory stream (RMS) to reach the olfactory bulbs (Alvarez-Buylla and Garcia-Verdugo 2002). Of interest, *Dcx knockout* mice in adult stages present an enlargement of the RMS and a reduced number of calbindin and calretinin-positive interneurons in the glomerular layer of the olfactory bulbs (Koizumi et al. 2006a). *Dcx knockout* neurons also display a lower frequency of nucleokinesis, reduction of the average length of leading processes, and increased percentage of secondary branches per cell (Koizumi et al. 2006a). Similar observations were made with *Dcx knockout* MGE cINs that suffer from reduced frequency of swelling formation and various branching abnormalities, such as their shortening, the higher frequency of secondary branching, and more frequency of growth cone splitting and formation at the leading edge than control cells (Kappeler et al. 2006). Similarly, inactivation of *Dcx* through injection of RNA in the GE of rat causes migration delay of cINs and increased frequency of branching (Friocourt et al. 2007). Branching formation appears to be tightly regulated by MTs remodeling, which is consistent with the requirement of *Dcx* function to maintain the bipolar morphology that interneurons exhibit during the dynamics of nucleokinesis to ensure their correct migration.

17.3 Molecular Mechanisms Regulating Neuronal Migration

The functional connectivity of the cerebral cortex relies on two main processes: migration of neurons to their final position and acquisition of their identity. Due to its importance, neuronal migration during neocortical development must be highly regulated through the coordination of several molecular mechanisms including transcriptional programs, cytoskeletal modulators, and environmental factors.

17.3.1 Transcriptional Programs

Transcriptional programs control not only neuronal migration but also several events involved in cerebral cortex formation such as neurogenesis, cell fate acquisition, and positioning of PNs within cortical layers (Benamer et al. 2020; Leone et al. 2008; Mancinelli and Lodato 2018; Nóbrega-Pereira and Marín 2009). A recent study has shown that the fate of PNs relies on their APs, which show temporal changes throughout corticogenesis. The identity of early-born PNs (E12/E13) strongly depends on cell-intrinsic transcriptional programs encoded in APs, whereas the fate of later-born PNs (E14/E15) relies more on their ability to sense environmental signals (Telley et al. 2019). It remains to be deciphered whether the migration mode of early-born (somal translocation) and late-born (locomotion) PNs is also partly encoded in APs and whether their specificity relies on temporal changes of molecular signaling occurring in these progenitors.

17.3.1.1 Proneural bHLH Genes

Proneural bHLH genes such as neurogenin 1 and 2 (*Neurog1/2)* and achaete-scute-complex-homolog-like-1 (*Ascl1*, previously named *Mash1)*, are a family of transcription factors necessary and sufficient to promote neuronal specification to progenitor cells, a function that is evolutionary conserved (reviewed in Bertrand et al. 2002; Dennis et al. 2019). In order to act as transcriptional activators or repressors, bHLH proteins must bind to the E-boxes of the DNA after their heterodimerization with E proteins (Murre et al. 1989). Beyond their role helping bHLH proteins to bind to the DNA, E proteins also modulate the activity of proneural proteins based on their preference for the E-box (le Dréau et al. 2018).

Neurog1 is expressed mainly by dorsal telencephalic progenitors in the VZ from early neurogenesis but its expression declines after E15.5. In contrast, *Neurog2* is also expressed in the VZ but throughout neurogenesis in the dorsal telencephalon. Beyond its proneural function, *Neurog2* also participates in the choice of the initial axon guidance and specifies the projection of thalamocortical axons, while its disruption in mouse leads to pathfinding defects in the ventral telencephalon (Hand and Polleux 2011; Seibt et al. 2003). Similarly, ectopic expression of *Neurog2* in progenitors outside their normal temporal window also induces abnormal axonal projection to the ventral telencephalon (Dennis et al. 2017). Although initial studies showed that loss of *Neurog2* does not affect the laminar fate of cortical neurons (Hand and Polleux 2011), a more recent work indicates that both *Neurog2* and *Ascl1* are required to promote the cell identity of layer V (Dennis et al. 2017). *Neurog2* also promotes the formation of the leading process that pyramidal neurons need to initiate radial migration (Hand et al. 2005). Mechanistically, evidence indicates that Neurog1/2 bind and activate the promoter of *Dcx* by recruiting the transcriptional coactivator CBP (Ge et al. 2006). Moreover, Neurog2 also directly promotes the transcription of the Rho GTPAse *Rnd2* in PNs to allow their proper migration (Heng et al. 2008).

Ascl1 is the main proneural bHLH gene found in the subpallium. In mouse, it is expressed in the VZ and SVZ of the GEs, in the POA and in the ventral thalamus during neurogenesis (Horton et al. 1999).

Ascl1 is also transiently expressed at a low level by progenitors of the cerebral cortex. Its expression is important as it initiates the migration of PNs by regulating the expression of *Rnd3*, an atypical Rho GTPase (Pacary et al. 2011). A recent study indicates that Rnd3 may also interact with Plexin B2, which activates RhoA in part by inhibiting Rnd3 (Azzarelli et al. 2014). These results suggest the coordination of both cell intrinsic programs (through *Ascl1*) and cell-extrinsic signals (via interaction with PlexinB2) regulates the activation level of *Rnd3*, thereby contributing to radial migration. Another transcriptional target of Ascl1 is the microencephaly associated gene *Cenpj/CPAP*. Silencing *Cenpj*/CPAP in post-mitotic neurons in mouse slows down radial migration and leads to neuronal morphology defects and abnormal centrosome position, as a result of higher MTs stability (Garcez et al. 2015).

17.3.1.2 Homeobox Transcription Factors

The DLX family includes homeodomain transcription factors that are central players for regulating the fate and migration of cINs (Anderson et al. 1997; Cobos et al. 2007). In human and mouse, the Dlx family includes six members (Dlx1 to Dlx6). The first assumption that some *Dlx* genes were required for tangential migration of cINs came from immunohistochemical experiments in which co-expression of GABA or calbindin and Dlx1 was observed (Anderson et al. 1997). At early stages these transcription factors are expressed in the proliferative zones of the MGE and LGE, and the septum, whereas at later stages they are detected in migrating cINs. Specifically, *Dlx1* and *Dlx2* are expressed in the VZ in NEs, while *Dlx5* is mostly expressed in the SVZ and migrating cINs (Bulfone et al. 1993; Eisenstat et al. 1999; Porteus et al. 1994; Simeone et al. 1994). *Dlx1* and *Dlx2* are necessary to drive expression of *Dlx5* and *Dlx6* (Long et al. 2009).

Mutations in both *Dlx1/Dlx2* in mouse impairs the migration of cINs from the GEs to the neocortex (Anderson et al. 1997). Furthermore, *Dlx1/Dlx2* double mutant cINs exhibit longer dendrites and axons due in part to premature activation of PAK3 and MAP2 (Cobos et al. 2007). These results indicate that in normal conditions, *Dlx1* and *Dlx2* must repress the expression of *Pak3* and *Map2* in migrating cINs until they reach the cortex. *Dlx1* and *Dlx2* might also act as transcriptional repressors of *Neuropilin-2* to promote cIN migration from the basal forebrain (Le et al. 2007). Of interest, neuropilin-2 is a receptor for Sema3A and Sema3F, which act as chemorepulsive signals directing the migration of cINs to the cortex (Marín et al. 2001). Notably, selected *Dlx* transcription factors regulate dendrite formation in some cIN subtypes. For instance, *Dlx1* modulates dendrite differentiation of somatostatin, calretinin and Npy-expressing cINs (Cobos et al. 2005b), whereas Dlx5/Dlx6 promote dendritogenesis of parvalbumin cINs (Y. Wang et al. 2010). Along this line, mouse lacking *Dlx5* and *Dlx6* genes display migration defects specifically in Lhx6 + and Mafb + cINs (Y. Wang et al. 2010).

The aristaless-related homeobox (*Arx*) gene is widely expressed in the cortex and the subpallium. In the ventral telencephalon, Arx is enriched in the SVZ of the GEs, whereas in the pallium it is expressed in progenitors in the VZ and in migrating cINs that invade the cortex (Cobos et al. 2005a; Colombo et al. 2004; Poirier et al. 2004). Expression of *Arx* is directly controlled by Dlx transcription factors and thus, disruption of both *Dlx1/Dlx2* impairs *Arx* expression in mouse (Cobos et al. 2005a; Colasante et al. 2008). Further studies demonstrate that Arx activity is involved in the Dlx-dependent migration of cINs but not in their subtype specification (Colasante et al. 2008). Indeed, loss of *Arx* disrupts the migration of GABAergic cINs from the MGE to the cortical IZ in mouse (Kitamura et al. 2002). In this regard, Arx is considered as a causative gene for X-linked lissencephaly and several mutations in this gene have been reported (Kitamura et al. 2009, 2002). Accordingly, *ARX* mutations found in patients also lead to defects in neuronal migration (reviewed in Friocourt and Parnavelas 2010a). Despite the fact that we do not know much about how its mutations lead to cIN migration defects, transcriptomic analysis revealed the existence of common gene regulatory networks between the targets of *Arx* and *Dlx* transcription factors (Fulp et al. 2008).

The LIM homeobox transcription factor 6 (*Lhx6)* is expressed by SVZ and MZ progenitors of the MGE (Grigoriou et al. 1998). Between E15.5 and E17.5, *Lhx6* expression is also detected in cINs that invade the developing cerebral cortex (Lavdas et al. 1999). During early development, Lhx6 is preferentially expressed in parvalbumin and somatostatin-expressing cINs and it is required for their proper tangential migration and cortical layering (Liodis et al. 2007). Focal electroporation of *Lhx6* siRNA in E13.5 organotypic brain slices disrupts specifically tangential migration of cINs without affecting the movement of cells within the GEs (Alifragis et al. 2004). Accordingly, mice expressing truncated *Lhx6* display a delay in cIN migration with reduced numbers of GAD67 cells in the MZ and CP (Liodis et al. 2007). Furthermore, MGE-explant cultures of Lhx6-deficient mouse embryos also exhibit migration defects, suggesting that they are likely cell intrinsically driven (Liodis et al. 2007). Importantly, *Lhx6* mutant mice display a reduced expression of some receptors such as Cxcr4, Cxcr7, and ErbB4 and the transcription factor *Arx*, which are involved in the regulation of cIN migration, suggesting a complex molecular mechanism acting downstream of *Lhx6* (Vogt et al. 2014; Zhao et al. 2008). Similar to the defects observed in mouse, *LHX6*-knockout cINs derived from hESC also exhibit reduced migratory behavior while over-expression of *LHX6* enhances their migration ability (Yuan et al. 2020).

17.3.2 Unconventional Cytoskeletal Modulators

During migration, cINs adopt a bipolar shape with a branched leading process forming ahead of the soma followed by a trailing process. The base of the leading process is characterized by a motile cytoplasmic bulge that encompasses the centrosome (MTOC) and the Golgi apparatus (Bellion et al. 2005; Gomes et al. 2005; Yanagida et al. 2012). Neuronal migration is a highly dynamic process driven by the coordination of actomyosin and microtubule cytoskeletons. Over the years, many cytoskeletal modulators have been demonstrated as key for proper cIN migration. Among them, two classical ones are *Lis1* and *Dcx*, whose roles have been discussed in the previous section. Therefore, in this section we will focus on three unconventional cytoskeleton modulators, whose implication in neuronal migration has been discovered over the recent years.

The Cip/kip protein $p27^{Kip1}$ (further termed p27) is encoded by *cdkn1b*. This protein acts as a master regulator of cell cycle progression by promoting cell cycle exit via blocking of the activity of the cyclin-dependent kinases Cdk1 and 2. p27-deficient mice suffer from enhanced proliferation that leads to an overall increased body size and brain hyperplasia (Fero et al. 1996). Recently, the contribution of p27 in multiple cellular processes beyond cell cycle regulation has been reported (reviewed in Besson et al. 2008). In this regard, p27 has de ability to bind and stabilize Neurogenin-2, thus regulating its expression and promoting the differentiation of PNs in the cerebral cortex (Nguyen et al. 2006). p27 whose stabilization depends on Cdk5-induced phosphorylation also regulates radial migration of PNs via its direct binding to RhoA, thereby inhibiting the RhoA signaling pathway and ultimately modulating actomyosin contractions that drive cell movement (Besson et al. 2004; Itoh et al. 2007; Kawauchi et al. 2006; Nguyen et al. 2006). In addition, a recent study demonstrated that p27 also controls the tangential migration of cINs by acting on both the actin and the MT cytoskeletons. This protein act as a "chef d'orchestre" by: 1) promoting nucleokinesis via a fine regulation of actomyosin contractions polarizing behind the nucleus; 2) regulating branch formation at the extremity of the leading process upon actomyosin-dependent splitting of the growth cone like structure; and 3) promoting the extension of newly formed leading process branches, via promotion of MT polymerization (Godin et al. 2012).

Another unconventional regulator of neuronal migration is the Elongator complex that is formed by two copies of six subunits (Elp1–Elp6). This complex was first identified for its role in transcription elongation through its association with RNA polymerase II (Kim et al. 2002). Nuclear Elp3 encodes for the catalytic subunit of the complex, it has histone acetyltransferase activity and mediates paternal genome demethylation (Okada et al. 2010; Winkler et al. 2002). Besides those nuclear functions, some independent cytoplasmic roles such as polarized exocytosis, tRNA modification, and cell motility have been associated with the elongator complex (Close et al. 2006; Esberg et al. 2006; Huang et al. 2005; Rahl et al. 2005). However, it is now well accepted that the direct role of Elongator is to promote tRNA modifications (Glatt et al. 2016; Huang et al. 2005; Selvadurai et al. 2014). During cerebral cortex development, loss of *Elp3* triggers the activation of unfolded protein response impairing the balance between direct and indirect neurogenesis in favor of the direct one, and leading to microcephaly (Laguesse et al. 2015). Elongator is expressed in the cytoplasm of cortical neurons where it acts as an indirect cytoskeletal modulator during neuronal migration. Indeed, deficiency of Elongator in PNs is associated with reduced levels of acetylated α-tubulin, which results in slow radial migration and defects in branching (Creppe et al. 2009). This defect likely arises from a decrease of MT-associated transport of Atat1-enriched vesicles as well as an impaired stability of Acly upon loss of Elongator activity (Even et al. 2019, 2021). Besides a role in neuronal migration, Elongator is also important for the morphological differentiation of PNs (Creppe et al. 2009). Elp1, Elp3, Elp4, and Elp5 proteins are also detected in the GEs (Creppe et al. 2009). A closer look on the distribution of *Elp3* mRNA in E12.5 mouse brains revealed the presence of a ventral gradient from the VZ to the MZ in the MGE, suggesting a potential role of Elongator in new-born cINs. Deletion of *Elp3* in cINs indeed reduces the number of cells that migrate tangentially to the cortex. In agreement, time-lapse experiments of *Elp3*-deficient MGE explants or brain slices of E13.5 mouse show defects in several migration parameters: reduced speed, frequency, amplitude of nucleokinesis, and directional persistence (Tielens et al. 2016). Further experiments indicate that those migration defects result from disruption of actomyosin dynamics rather than disruption of acetylation of α-tubulin in MTs as it occurs in PNs (Creppe et al. 2009; Tielens et al. 2016). Such discrepancy may reflect different requirements for MT-depend transport during the migration of cINs and PNs.

The important role played by MT acetylation in cell migration led to the investigation of other enzymes that induce post-translational modifications such as polyglutamylation. Polyglutamylation consists in the addition of glutamate residues and therefore extending the length of the polyglutamate chain, which modulates the binding affinity of MT-associated proteins and hence their function (Bonnet et al. 2001). Polyglutamylation is a reversible post-translational modification promoted by proteins that glutamylate (tubulin tyrosine ligase-like, TTLL) or (de)glutamylate (cytosolic carboxypeptidases, CCPs) (Janke et al. 2005; van Dijk et al. 2007). Several TTLLs and CCPs are expressed in the subpallium, with *Ccp1* being enriched in the SVZ and the mantle zone of GEs (Silva et al. 2018). Migration of cINs is characterized by alternating phases of movement and pause. Postmitotic cINs deficient for *Ccp1* display a significant reduction of the migratory pausing time that induce changes in the mode of migration from saltatory to slithery. It is striking that while the average migration speed remains unaffected, reduction of "migratory pauses" enhances cortical invasion by cINs. This can be explained by the resulting increase of movement synchronization at the cIN population level (Silva et al. 2018). At molecular level, Ccp1 (de)glutamylates myosin light-chain kinase (MLCK) controlling its activity and thereby regulating the levels of myosin light chain (MLC) phosphorylation, which is required during actomyosin contraction processes (Silva et al. 2018).

17.3.3 Environmental Factors

17.3.3.1 Secreted Factors

Throughout this chapter, we have discussed some of the fundamental differences between the progenitors of PNs and cINs, which migrate through very different environments and therefore must cope and integrate with various extracellular signals that modulate their migration. In the case of cINs, after being born in the GEs, they migrate towards the cortex where they settle in their final position. As soon as they are generated, they begin their migration towards the cortex guided by chemorepulsive cues and motogenic factors, such as Netrin1, Slit1/2, and ephrin A5 (Hamasaki et al. 2001; Marín et al. 2003; Zimmer et al. 2008). In contrast, the cortex contains an attractive activity for tangentially migrating cINs. Neuregulin 1 (*Nrg1*) is expressed in the proliferative zones of the cortex, and in vitro experiments indicated that it mediates chemoattractive signals through the ErbB4 receptors expressed by cINs (Flames et al. 2004; Yau et al. 2003), although more recent studies indicate that Neuregulins may also mediate repulsive signals for MGE-derived cINs (H. Li et al. 2012a). The migration stream is also determined to a great extent by gradients of chemoattract cues, such as Cxcl12 produced by IPs but also secreted by the meninges (Borrell and Marín 2006; G. Li et al. 2008; López-Bendito et al. 2008; Stumm et al. 2003; Tiveron et al. 2006). The presence of Cxcl12 in turn activates the receptors Cxcr4 and Cxcr7, which are co-expressed in cINs, and regulate their migration via activation of distinct signaling pathways (Stumm et al. 2003; Y. Wang et al. 2011b). Conditional deletion of Cxcr7 from mouse migrating cINs abrogates their response to Cxcl12 through regulation of the expression levels of Cxcr4 receptors, thereby modulating the Cxcl12 responsiveness of cINs (Sánchez-Alcañiz et al. 2011). It is important to note that Cxcl12 also promotes the migration of other cell types including Cajal–Retzius cells (Borrell and Marín 2006; Paredes et al. 2006).

17.3.3.2 Extracellular Matrix

As mentioned above, Cajal–Retzius cells located in the MZ secrete the extracellular matrix (ECM) protein reelin, which is one of the most studied molecular mechanisms underlying neuronal migration. Disruption of reelin in mouse (i.e., *Reeler* mice) results in abnormal neuronal migration leading to inverted cortical lamination (Ogawa et al. 1995; reviewed in D'Arcangelo 2006). Beyond the role of reelin controlling the multipolar to bipolar transition before initiation of locomotion in radial migrating PNs (Franco et al. 2011; Jossin and Cooper 2011), two main roles have been attributed to reelin as a regulator of neuronal migration. First, reelin may act as a "stop" signal as PNs approach the CP, inhibiting their migration and promoting their detachment from RG (Dulabon et al. 2000; Hack et al. 2002; Sanada et al. 2004). Second, reelin may promote both cell-matrix adhesion and transient neuronal aggregation during cortical neuronal positioning (Matsunaga et al. 2017; Sekine et al. 2012). In order to initiate the signaling cascade, reelin binds to the lipoprotein receptors Apoer2 and Vldl that are expressed by migrating neurons and RG cells. Of interest, even though mice lacking both receptors display a *Reeler*-like phenotype, disruption of only one gene leads to a milder phenotype (Benhayon et al. 2003). Fate mapping experiments in mouse after deletion of ApoER2 and/or Vldlr receptors indicate that they may play distinct functions: while activation of ApoER2 favors migration of late born PNs, activation of Vldlr receptors induce a stop signal for migrating PNs (Hack et al. 2007). While both ApoER2 and Vldlr can bind to the cytoplasmic adaptor protein disabled-1 (Dab1), mice lacking both reelin receptors induce upregulation of Dab1 (Trommsdorff et al. 1999). Finally, mice lacking *Dab1* or with mutations in all potential tyrosine phosphorylation sites also exhibit *Reeler*-like phenotypes, suggesting that Dab1 must be phosphorylated in order to initiate reelin signaling (Howell et al. 2000; Sheldon et al. 1997; Sweet et al. 1996).

17.3.3.3 Extracellular Vesicles

As cerebral cortex gains in complexity, the transfer of cellular content through extracellular vesicles (EVs) may represent another layer of regulation of neural migration in the cortex. EVs are heterogeneous lipid bilayer vesicles that contain RNA and proteins, which are released from cells into the ECM and that participate in intercellular communication (Skog et al. 2008; Valadi et al. 2007). Depending on whether they are directly secreted from the plasma membrane or via multivesicular bodies (MVBs), they are classified as microvesicles and exosomes, respectively (reviewed in Kalluri and LeBleu 2020). Moreover, MVBs can also be fused to lysosomes, which will then degrade their content. An increasing number of studies show the involvement of EVs in motility in different cell types, especially in cancer cells (He et al. 2019; Sung and Weaver 2017). Microglia starts populating the forebrain as neurogenesis begins where they play essential roles in cortical morphogenesis (reviewed in Ginhoux et al. 2010; Squarzoni et al. 2015). Some extracellular cues such as ATP activate microglia, inducing the release of the EV contents and stimulating their migration (Dou et al. 2012). In this regard, a recent study indicates that by exposing Oligodendrocyte precursor cell (OPC) cultures to microglia-derived EVs for 24 hours, sphingosine 1 phosphate *(Sip1)*, which is expressed on the surface of the microglial EVs, acts as an attractive cue for OPCs, and thereby promotes their migration (Lombardi et al. 2019). This highlights the importance of the microglia-EVs beyond the regulation of their own migration. In the context of neuronal migration not much is known. Initial work evidenced that suppression of *Rab5*, a crucial regulator of endosome fusion, blocks endocytosis by regulating the trafficking of N-cadherin thereby leading to impaired neuronal migration during cerebral cortex development in mouse (Kawauchi et al. 2010). Other studies also showed the role of vacuole protein sorting 18 (Vps18), which is involved in intracellular vesicle transport, in neuronal migration as *Vps18* deficiency leads to neuronal migration defects in the cerebral cortex and cerebellum (Peng et al. 2012). A recent work indicates that the addition of EVs extracted from culture medium of three glioblastoma cell lines promotes the migration of mouse neural progenitor cells through the activation of the PI3K-Akt pathway. This suggest that exosome may be used for molecular signaling between neural progenitor cells and glioblastoma cells in the brain environment (Pan et al. 2022). Another study combining human brain organoids and scRNAseq showed the involvement of LGALS3BP, a molecule transported and secreted by EVs, in the anchoring of neural progenitor cells to the ECM and their migration (Kyrousi et al. 2021). Although this field is only at the beginning of its development, EVs may represent a key layer of extrinsic regulation for the fine control of neuron migration in the brain. However, more work needs to be done to shed light on the mechanisms (recognition signal, specific receptors etc.) that regulate specificity between EVs donor and acceptor neural cells.

17.4 Crosstalk between Migrating Cells to Control Cortex Morphogenesis

As neurogenesis occurs, multiple cellular crosstalk between new-born migrating cells takes place in the neocortex. In fact, once cINs cross the pallium-subpallium boundary, they continue to migrate within the neocortex in coexistence with PNs. Local microcircuits between these two neuronal populations are then assembled, which require a precise excitatory–inhibitory balance (Liu 2004). One way to control this process is via the establishment of contacts and crosstalk between PNs and cINs. Initial work indicates that PNs regulate the position adopted by cINs in the cerebral cortex through non-cell autonomous mechanism (Lodato et al. 2011). *Fezf2* is a transcription factor that controls neurogenesis and specification of subcerebral PNs (Chen et al. 2005, 2008; Molyneaux et al. 2005). Furthermore, by affecting PNs, cINs also acquired abnormal laminar distribution through the cerebral cortex, while their generation and migration remain unaffected (Lodato et al. 2011). The excitatory/inhibitory ratio in the cerebral cortex must be regulated throughout space and time (Xue et al. 2014). Along this line, cINs are initially generated in too great amount (around 30%) and their final number is later regulated via apoptosis (Southwell et al. 2012). Early studies indicate that IPs modulate the amount of cINs in the SVZ via cell-extrinsic mechanisms (Sessa et al. 2010; Tiveron et al. 2006). Furthermore, the activity of excitatory PNs during the period when cIN undergo cell death also controls the survival of cINs (Wong et al. 2018). A recent study showed that the asynchronicity of movement among cINs governs how they invade the cortex, which in turn controls the proliferation of IPs and thereby the generation of age-matched excitatory PNs (Silva et al. 2018). This work thus highlights how an extrinsic mechanism (i.e., crosstalk between cINs and PNs) relies on an earlier intrinsic mechanism (i.e., regulation of pausing time during cIN nucleokinesis), to model the cerebral corticogenesis during brain development.

Microglia invades the brain at early embryonic stages and thus is also present during the formation of the neuronal circuitry (Ginhoux et al. 2010; Schulz et al. 2012). Recent works indicate that microglia mediates multiple functions beyond its immune role, including formation of synapses and regulation of neuronal activity (Hoshiko et al. 2012; Y. Li et al. 2012b; Parkhurst et al. 2013; Schafer et al. 2012), neurogenesis (Cunningham et al. 2013; Sierra et al. 2010), and neuronal survival (Ueno et al. 2013). Moreover, disruption of microglia leads to defects in axon outgrowth of dopaminergic neurons and the laminar neocortical distribution of a subset of cINs (Squarzoni et al. 2014), pointing out the role of non-neuronal cells in shaping the cortical morphogenesis.

During cortex morphogenesis, neurons also establish transient synapses with OPCs (Bergles et al. 2000; Orduz et al. 2015; Zonouzi et al. 2015). OPCs are generated in three successive "spatiotemporal waves" and the first wave gives rise to OPCs that are born embryonically in the ventral forebrain, migrate to the cortex, and then most of them undergo cell death early postnatally (Marques et al. 2018). Since cINs and OPCs coexist and interact in the same space within a temporal window, potential functions for the cIN-OPC interaction have been speculated over the years (reviewed in Benamer et al. 2020). As a proof of concept, a crosstalk between cINs and first-wave OPCs has been recently discovered in mouse. First-wave OPCs guide cINs migration by preventing them aggregating around blood vessels via a unidirectional contact repulsion (UCoRe) mechanism (Lepiemme et al. 2022). Accordingly, depletion of these OPCs impairs the migration of cINs within their migratory cortical streams. At the cellular level, time-lapse experiments in mouse, both in vitro and in vivo, show that OPCs migrate along blood vessels from where they repel cINs by UCoRe, leading to cIN polarity reversal and migration "away" via an unconventional semaphorin/plexin-based mechanism (Lepiemme et al. 2022).

Cerebral corticogenesis is a tightly regulated process where not only cell intrinsic and extrinsic factors are important, but also where cellular communication plays a central role. There is a growing body of evidence supporting the existence of various relevant cellular crosstalk for cortical morphogenesis. However, how this crosstalk is integrated and coordinated by migrating cells with their genetic and molecular environmental signals remain elusive. Future studies are thus required to shed further light on how those distinct cellular and molecular mechanisms are spatially and temporally regulated to shape and fine tune cerebral cortical morphogenesis. Such information will be essential to understand the mechanisms underlying neurodevelopmental disorders better, which as we have discussed, have severe neurological consequences for humans.

Acknowledgments

Míriam Javier-Torrent and Laurent Nguyen are postdoctoral fellow and Research Director of the F.R.S.-F.N.R.S., respectively. The work performed in the Nguyen laboratory is supported by ULiège (Crédit Classique), the F.R.S.-F.N.R.S. (PDR T.0185.20; EOS 0019118F-RG36), WELBIO (CR-2022A-12), the Fonds Leon Fredericq, the Fondation Médicale Reine Elisabeth, the Fondation Simone et Pierre Clerdent, the Belgian Science Policy (IAP-VII network P7/20), the ERANET Neuron (STEM-MCD and NeuroTalk), and the Win2Wal (ChipOmics; #2010126).

References

Alcántara, S. et al. (1998). Regional and cellular patterns of reelin mRNA expression in the forebrain of the developing and adult mouse. *J Neurosci* 18 (19): 7779–7799.

Alifragis, P. et al. (2004). Lhx6 regulates the migration of cortical interneurons from the ventral telencephalon but does not specify their GABA phenotype. *J Neurosci* 24 (24): 5643–5648.

Al-Jaberi, N. et al. (2015). The early fetal development of human neocortical GABAergic interneurons. *Cereb Cortex* 25 (3): 631–645.

Alvarez-Buylla, A. and Garcia-Verdugo, J.M. (2002). Neurogenesis in adult subventricular zone. *J Neurosci* 22 (3): 629–634.

Anderson, S.A. et al. (1997). Interneuron migration from basal forebrain to neocortex. *Science* 278 (5337): 474–476.

Anderson, S.A. et al. (2001). Distinct cortical migrations from the medial and lateral ganglionic eminences. *Development* 128 (3): 353–363.

Arshad, A. et al. (2016). Extended production of cortical interneurons into the third trimester of human gestation. *Cereb Cortex* 26 (5): 2242–2256.

Ayala, R. et al. (2007). Trekking across the brain. *Cell* 128 (1): 29–43.

Azzarelli, R. et al. (2014). An antagonistic interaction between PlexinB2 and Rnd3 controls RhoA activity and cortical neuron migration. *Nat Commun* 5: 3405.

Bagley, J.A. et al. (2017). Fused cerebral organoids model interactions between brain regions. *Nat Methods* 14 (7): 743–751.

Bai, J. et al. (2003). RNAi reveals doublecortin is required for radial migration in rat neocortex. *Nat Neurosci* 6 (12): 1277–1283.

Bandler, R.C. et al. (2022). Single-cell delineation of lineage and genetic identity in the mouse brain. *Nature* 601 (7893): 404–409.

Batista-Brito, R. et al. (2008). The distinct temporal origins of olfactory bulb interneuron subtypes. *J Neurosci* 28 (15): 3966–3975.

Bellion, A. et al. (2005). Nucleokinesis in tangentially migrating neurons comprises two alternating phases. *J Neurosci* 25 (24): 5691–5699.

Beltrán-valero de Bernabé, D. et al. (2002). Mutations in the O-mannosyltransferase gene POMT1 give rise to the severe neuronal migration disorder Walker-Warburg syndrome. *Am J Hum Genet* 71 (5): 1033–1043.

Benamer, N. et al. (2020). The cerebral cortex is a substrate of multiple interactions between GABAergic interneurons and oligodendrocyte lineage cells. *Neurosci Lett* 715: 134615.

Benhayon, D. et al. (2003). Binding of purified Reelin to ApoER2 and VLDLR mediates tyrosine phosphorylation of Disabled-1. *Mol Brain Res* 112 (1–2): 33–45.

Bergles, D.E. et al. (2000). Glutamatergic synapses on oligodendrocyte precursor cells in the hippocampus. *Nature* 405 (6783): 187–191.

Bershteyn, M. et al. (2017). Human iPSC-derived cerebral organoids model cellular features of lissencephaly and reveal prolonged mitosis of outer radial glia. *Cell Stem Cell* 20 (4): 435–449.e4.

Bertrand, N. et al. (2002). Proneural genes and the specification of neural cell types. *Nat Rev Neurosci* 3 (7): 517–530.

Besson, A. et al. (2008). CDK inhibitors. *Dev Cell* 14 (2): 159–169.

Besson, A. et al. (2004). p27Kip1 modulates cell migration through the regulation of RhoA activation. *Genes Dev* 18 (8): 862–876.

Birey, F. et al. (2017). Assembly of functionally integrated human forebrain spheroids. *Nature* 545 (7652): 54–59.

Bonnet, C. et al. (2001). Differential binding regulation of microtubule-associated proteins MAP1A, MAP1B, and MAP2 by tubulin polyglutamylation. *J Biol Chem* 276 (16): 12839–12848.

Borrell, V. and Marín, O. (2006). Meninges control tangential migration of hem-derived Cajal-Retzius cells via CXCL12/CXCR4 signaling. *Nat Neurosci* 9 (10): 1284–1293.

Boycott, K.M. et al. (2005). Homozygous deletion of the very low-density lipoprotein receptor gene causes autosomal recessive cerebellar hypoplasia with cerebral gyral simplification. *Am J Hum Genet* 77 (3): 477–483.

Brockington, M. et al. (2001). Mutations in the fukutin-related protein gene (FKRP) cause a form of congenital muscular dystrophy with secondary laminin a2 deficiency and abnormal glycosylation of a-dystroglycan. *Am J Hum Genet* 69 (6): 1198–1209.

Broix, L. et al. (2016). Mutations in the HECT domain of NEDD4L lead to AKT-mTOR pathway deregulation and cause periventricular nodular heterotopia. *Nat Genet* 48 (11): 1349–1358.

Brown, K.N. et al. (2011). Clonal production and organization of inhibitory interneurons in the neocortex. *Science* 334 (6055): 480–486.

Brun, A. (1965). The subpial granular layer of the foetal cerebral cortex in man. Its ontogeny and significance in congenital cortical malformations. *Acta Pathol et Microbiol Scand* Suppl 179: 3–98.

Bulfone, A. et al. (1993). Spatially restricted expression of D/x-1, D/x-Z (Tes-I), Gbx-2, and Writ-3 in the embryonic day 12.5 mouse forebrain defines potential transverse and longitudinal segmental boundaries. *J Neurosci* 13 (7): 3315–3172.

Butt, S.J.B. et al. (2005). The temporal and spatial origins of cortical interneurons predict their physiological subtype. *Neuron* 48 (4): 591–604.

Cahana, A. et al. (2001). Targeted mutagenesis of Lis1 disrupts cortical development and LIS1 homodimerization. *Proc Natl Acad Sci USA* 98 (11): 6429–6434.

Carabalona, A. et al. (2012). A glial origin for periventricular nodular heterotopia caused by impaired expression of Filamin-A. *Hum Mol Genet* 21 (5): 1004–1017.

Cardoso, C. et al. (2003). Refinement of a 400-kb critical region allows genotypic differentiation between isolated lissencephaly, Miller-Dieker syndrome, and other phenotypes secondary to deletions of 17p13.3. *Am J Hum Genet* 72 (4): 918–930.

Chai, X. et al. (2009). Reelin stabilizes the actin cytoskeleton of neuronal processes by inducing n-cofilin phosphorylation at serine. *J Neurosci* 29 (1): 288–299.

Chan, Y.M. et al. (2010). Fukutin-related protein is essential for mouse muscle, brain and eye development and mutation recapitulates the wide clinical spectrums of dystroglycanopathies. *Hum Mol Genet* 19 (20): 3995–4006.

Chen, B. et al. (2005). Fezl regulates the differentiation and axon targeting of layer 5 subcortical projection neurons in cerebral cortex. *Proc Natl Acad Sci USA* 102 (47): 17184–17189.

Chen, B. et al. (2008). The Fezf2-Ctip2 genetic pathway regulates the fate choice of subcortical projection neurons in the developing cerebral cortex. *Proc Natl Acad Sci USA* 105 (32): 11382–11387.

Ciceri, G. et al. (2013). Lineage-specific laminar organization of cortical GABAergic interneurons. *Nat Neurosci* 16 (9): 1199–1210.

Clavreul, S. et al. (2019). Cortical astrocytes develop in a plastic manner at both clonal and cellular levels. *Nat Commun* 10 (1): 4884.

Close, P. et al. (2006). Transcription impairment and cell migration defects in elongator-depleted cells. *Mol Cell* 22 (4): 521–531.

Cobos, I. et al. (2007). Dlx transcription factors promote migration through repression of axon and dendrite growth. *Neuron* 54 (6): 873–888.

Cobos, I. et al. (2005a). The vertebrate ortholog of Aristaless is regulated by Dlx genes in the developing forebrain. *J Comp Neurol* 483 (3): 292–303.

Cobos, I. et al. (2005b). Mice lacking Dlx1 show subtype-specific loss of interneurons, reduced inhibition and epilepsy. *Nat Neurosci* 8 (8): 1059–1068.

Colasante, G. et al. (2008). Arx is a direct target of Dlx2 and thereby contributes to the tangential migration of GABAergic interneurons. *J Neurosci* 28 (42): 10674–10686.

Colombo, E. et al. (2004). Mouse orthologue of ARX, a gene mutated in several X-linked forms of mental retardation and epilepsy, is a marker of adult neural stem cells and forebrain GABAergic neurons. *Dev Dyn* 231 (3): 631–639.

Conti, V. et al. (2013). Periventricular heterotopia in 6q terminal deletion syndrome. *Brain* 136 (11): 3378–3394.

Corbin, J.G. et al. (2001). Telencephalic cells take a tangent. *Nat Neurosci* 4 (11s): 1177–1182.

Corbo, J.C. et al. (2002). Doublecortin is required in mice for lamination of the hippocampus but not the neocortex. *J Neurosci* 22 (17): 7548–7557.

Creppe, C. et al. (2009). Elongator controls the migration and differentiation of cortical neurons through acetylation of α-tubulin. *Cell* 136 (3): 551–564.

Cunningham, C.L. et al. (2013). Microglia regulate the number of neural precursor cells in the developing cerebral cortex. *J Neurosci* 33 (10): 4216–4233.

D'Agostino, M.D. et al. (2002). Subcortical band heterotopia (SBH) in males. *Brain* 125 (Pt11): 2507–2522.

D'Arcangelo, G. (2006). Reelin mouse mutants as models of cortical development disorders. *Epilepsy Behav* 8 (1): 81–90.

Deacon, T.W. et al. (1994). The lateral ganglionic eminence is the origin of cells committed to striatal phenotypes. *Brain Res* 668 (1–2): 211–219.

Del Bene, F. et al. (2008). Regulation of neurogenesis by interkinetic nuclear migration through an apical-basal notch gradient. *Cell* 134 (6): 1055–1065.

Delgado, R.N. et al. (2022). Individual human cortical progenitors can produce excitatory and inhibitory neurons. *Nature* 601 (7893): 397–403.

Dennis, D.J. et al. (2019). bHLH transcription factors in neural development, disease, and reprogramming. *Brain Res* 1705: 48–65.

Dennis, D.J. et al. (2017). Neurog2 and Ascl1 together regulate a postmitotic derepression circuit to govern laminar fate specification in the murine neocortex. *Proc Natl Acad Sci USA* 114 (25): E4934–E4943.

Des Portes, V. et al. (1998). doublecortin is the major gene causing X-linked subcortical laminar heterotopia (SCLH). *Hum Mol Genet* 7 (7): 1063–1070.

Deuel, T.A.S. et al. (2006). Genetic interactions between doublecortin and doublecortin-like kinase in neuronal migration and axon outgrowth. *Neuron* 49 (1): 41–53.

Dobyns, W.B. (2010). The clinical patterns and molecular genetics of lissencephaly and subcortical band heterotopia. *Epilepsia* 51 (Suppl. 1): 5–9.

Dobyns, W.B. et al. (1999). X-linked lissencephaly with absent corpus callosum and ambiguous genitalia. *Am J Med Genet* 86 (4): 331–337.

Dobyns, W.B. et al. (1991). Clinical and molecular diagnosis of Miller-Dieker syndrome. *Am J Hum Genet* 48 (3): 584–594.

Dobyns, W.B. et al. (1985). Syndromes with lissencephaly. *Am J Med Genet* 22 (1): 157–195.

Dobyns, W.B. et al. (1993). Lissencephaly. A human brain malformation associated with deletion of the LIS1 gene located at chromosome 17p13. *JAMA* 270 (23): 2838–2842.

Dou, Y. et al. (2012). Microglial migration mediated by ATP-induced ATP release from lysosomes. *Cell Res* 22 (6): 1022–1033.

Dulabon, L. et al. (2000). Reelin binds 31 integrin and inhibits neuronal migration three mutant mice show a remarkably similar cellular phenotype, suggesting that the corresponding proteins represent a biochemical pathway that mediates proper formation of cerebral cortical lamination. *Neuron* 27 (1): 33–44.

Duque, A. et al. (2016). Secondary expansion of the transient subplate zone in the developing cerebrum of human and nonhuman primates. *Proc Natl Acad Sci USA* 113 (35): 9892–9897.

Eisenstat, D.D. et al. (1999). DLX-1, DLX-2, and DLX-5 expression define distinct stages of basal forebrain differentiation. *J Comp Neurol* 414 (2): 217–237.

Ekşioğlu, Y.Z. et al. (1996). Periventricular heterotopia. *Neuron* 16 (1): 77–87.

Elbracht, M. et al. (2018). Familial NEDD4L variant in periventricular nodular heterotopia and in a fetus with hypokinesia and flexion contractures. *Mol Genet Genom Med* 6 (6): 1255–1260.

Esberg, A. et al. (2006). Elevated levels of two tRNA species bypass the requirement for elongator complex in transcription and exocytosis. *Mol Cell* 24 (1): 139–148.

Even, A. et al. (2019). ATAT1-enriched vesicles promote microtubule acetylation via axonal transport. *Sci Adv* 5 (12): eaax2705.

Even, A. et al. (2021). ATP-citrate lyase promotes axonal transport across species. *Nat Commun* 12 (1): 5878.

Feng, Y. et al. (2000). LIS1 regulates CNS lamination by interacting with mNudE, a central component of the centrosome. *Neuron* 28 (3): 665–679.

Ferland, R.J. et al. (2009). Disruption of neural progenitors along the ventricular and subventricular zones in periventricular heterotopia. *Hum Mol Genet* 18 (3): 497–516.

Fero, M.L. et al. (1996). A syndrome of multiorgan hyperplasia with features of gigantism, tumorigenesis, and female sterility in p27 Kip1-deficient mice. *Cell* 8 (5): 733–744.

Flames, N. et al. (2004). Short-and long-range attraction of cortical GABAergic interneurons by Neuregulin-1. *Neuron* 44 (2): 251–261.

Flames, N. et al. (2007). Delineation of multiple subpallial progenitor domains by the combinatorial expression of transcriptional codes. *J Neurosci* 27 (36): 9682–9695.

Fleck, M.W. et al. (2000). Hippocampal abnormalities and enhanced excitability in a murine model of human lissencephaly. *J Neurosci* 20 (7): 2439–2450.

Fox, J.W. et al. (1998). Mutations in filamin 1 prevent migration of cerebral cortical neurons in human periventricular heterotopia. *Neuron* 21 (6): 1315–1325.

Francis, F. et al. (1999). Doublecortin is a developmentally regulated, microtubule-associated protein expressed in migrating and differentiating neurons. *Neuron* 23 (2): 247–256.

Franco, S.J. et al. (2011). Reelin regulates cadherin function via Dab1/Rap1 to control neuronal migration and lamination in the neocortex. *Neuron* 69 (3): 482–497.

Friocourt, G. et al. (2007). Both doublecortin and doublecortin-like kinase play a role in cortical interneuron migration. *J Neurosci* 27 (14): 3875–3883.
Friocourt, G. and Parnavelas, J.G. (2010a March). Mutations in ARX result in several defects involving GABAergic neurons. *Front Cell Neurosci* 4: 4.
Fulp, C.T. et al. (2008). Identification of Arx transcriptional targets in the developing basal forebrain. *Hum Mol Genet* 17 (23): 3740–3760.
Gadisseux, J.F. et al. (1992). The human transient subpial granular layer. *J Comp Neurol* 324 (1): 94–114.
Garcez, P.P. et al. (2015). Cenpj/CPAP regulates progenitor divisions and neuronal migration in the cerebral cortex downstream of Ascl1. *Nat Commun* 6: 6474.
Ge, W. et al. (2006). Coupling of cell migration with neurogenesis by proneural bHLH factors. *Proc Natl Acad Sci USA* 103 (5): 1319–1324.
Gelman, D. et al. (2011). A wide diversity of cortical GABAergic interneurons derives from the embryonic preoptic area. *J Neurosci* 31 (46): 16570–16580.
Gelman, D.M. et al. (2009). The embryonic preoptic area is a novel source of cortical GABAergic interneurons. *J Neurosci* 29 (29): 9380–9389.
Ginhoux, F. et al. (2010). Fate mapping analysis reveals that adult microglia derive from primitive macrophages. *Science* 330 (6005): 841–845.
Glatt, S. et al. (2016). Structural basis for tRNA modification by Elp3 from Dehalococcoides mccartyi. *Nat Struct Mol Biol* 23 (9): 794–802.
Gleeson, J.G. et al. (1998). Doublecortin, a brain-specific gene mutated in human X-linked lissencephaly and double cortex syndrome, encodes a putative signaling protein. *Cell* 92 (1): 63–72.
Gleeson, J.G. et al. (1999). Doublecortin is a microtubule-associated protein and is expressed widely by migrating neurons. *Neuron* 23 (2): 257–271.
Glogauer, M. et al. (1998). The role of actin-binding protein 280 in integrin-dependent mechanoprotection. *J Biol Chem* 273 (3): 1689–1698.
Godin, J.D. et al. (2012). P27Kip1 is a microtubule-associated protein that promotes microtubule polymerization during neuron migration. *Dev Cell* 23 (4): 729–744.
Gomes, E.R. et al. (2005). Nuclear movement regulated by Cdc42, MRCK, myosin, and actin flow establishes MTOC polarization in migrating cells. *Cell* 121 (3): 451–463.
Götz, M. and Huttner, W.B. (2005). The cell biology of neurogenesis. *Nat Rev Mol Cell Biol* 6 (10): 777–788.
Graus-Porta, D. et al. (2001). Beta1-class integrins regulate the development of laminae and folia in the cerebral and cerebellar cortex. *Neuron* 31 (3): 367–379.
Grigoriou, M. et al. (1998). Expression and regulation of Lhx6 and Lhx7, a novel subfamily of LIM homeodomain encoding genes, suggests a role in mammalian head development. *Development* 125 (11): 2063–2074.
Guo, C. et al. (2013). Fezf2 expression identifies a multipotent progenitor for neocortical projection neurons, astrocytes, and oligodendrocytes. *Neuron* 80 (5): 1167–1174.
Hack, I. et al. (2002). Reelin is a detachment signal in tangential chain-migration during postnatal neurogenesis. *Nat Neurosci* 5 (10): 939–945.
Hack, I. et al. (2007). Divergent roles of ApoER2 and Vldlr in the migration of cortical neurons. *Development* 134 (21): 3883–3891.
Hamasaki, T. et al. (2001). A role of netrin-1 in the formation of the subcortical structure striatum. *J Neurosci* 21 (12): 4272–4280.
Hand, R. et al. (2005). Phosphorylation of neurogenin2 specifies the migration properties and the dendritic morphology of pyramidal neurons in the neocortex. *Neuron* 48 (1): 45–62.
Hand, R. and Polleux, F. (2011). Neurogenin2 regulates the initial axon guidance of cortical pyramidal neurons projecting medially to the corpus callosum. *Neural Dev* 6 (1): 30.

Hansen, D.V. et al. (2013). Non-epithelial stem cells and cortical interneuron production in the human ganglionic eminences. *Nat Neurosci* 16 (11): 1576–1587.

Hansen, D.V. et al. (2010). Neurogenic radial glia in the outer subventricular zone of human neocortex. *Nature* 464 (7288): 554–561.

Hartfuss, E. et al. (2001). Characterization of CNS precursor subtypes and radial glia. *Dev Biol* 229 (1): 15–30.

Harwell, C.C. et al. (2015). Wide dispersion and diversity of clonally related inhibitory interneurons. *Neuron* 87 (5): 999–1007.

Haubensak, W. et al. (2004). Neurons arise in the basal neuroepithelium of the early mammalian telencephalon. *Proc Natl Acad Sci USA* 101 (9): 3196–201.

He, S. et al. (2019). Exosomal miR-499a-5p promotes cell proliferation, migration and EMT via mTOR signaling pathway in lung adenocarcinoma. *Exp Cell Res* 379 (2): 203–213.

Heng, J.I.T. et al. (2008). Neurogenin 2 controls cortical neuron migration through regulation of Rnd2. *Nature* 455 (7209): 114–118.

Hesse, M. et al. (2012). Direct visualization of cell division using high-resolution imaging of M-phase of the cell cycle. *Nat Commun* 3: 1076.

Hirotsune, S. et al. (1998). Graded reduction of Pafah1b1 (Lis1) activity results in neuronal migration defects and early embryonic lethality. *Nat Genet* 19 (4): 333–339.

Hoerder-Suabedissen, A. and Molnár, Z. (2015). Development, evolution and pathology of neocortical subplate neurons. *Nat Rev Neurosci* 16 (3): 133–146.

Hong, S.E. et al. (2000). Autosomal recessive lissencephaly with cerebellar hypoplasia is associated with human RELN mutations. *Nat Genet* 26 (1): 93–96.

Horton, S. et al. (1999). Correct coordination of neuronal differentiation events in ventral forebrain requires the bHLH factor MASH1. *Mol Cell Neurosci* 14 (4–5): 355–369.

Hoshiko, M. et al. (2012). Deficiency of the microglial receptor CX3CR1 impairs postnatal functional development of thalamocortical synapses in the barrel cortex. *J Neurosci* 32 (43): 15106–15111.

Howard, B.M. et al. (2008). Radial glia cells in the developing human brain. *Neuroscientist* 14 (5): 459–473.

Howell, B.W. et al. (2000). Dab1 tyrosine phosphorylation sites relay positional signals during mouse brain development. *Curr Biol* 10 (15): 877–885.

Hsia, H.E. et al. (2014). Ubiquitin E3 ligase Nedd4-1 acts as a downstream target of PI3K/PTEN-mTORC1 signaling to promote neurite growth. *Proc Natl Acad Sci USA* 111 (36): 13205–13210.

Hu, D.J.K. et al. (2013). Dynein recruitment to nuclear pores activates apical nuclear migration and mitotic entry in brain progenitor cells. *Cell* 154 (6): 1300.

Huang, B. et al. (2005). An early step in wobble uridine tRNA modification requires the Elongator complex. *RNA* 11 (4): 424–436.

Ibraghimov-Beskrovnaya, O. et al. (1992). Primary structure of dystrophin-associated glycoproteins linking dystrophin to the extracellular matrix. *Nature* 355 (6362): 696–702.

Inamori, K. et al. (2012). Dystroglycan function requires xylosyl- and glucuronyltransferase activities of LARGE. *Science* 335 (6064): 93–96.

Itoh, Y. et al. (2007). The cyclin-dependent kinase inhibitors p57 and p27 regulate neuronal migration in the developing mouse neocortex. *J Biol Chem* 282 (1): 390–396.

Janke, C. et al. (2005). Tubulin polyglutamylase enzymes are members of the TTL domain protein family. *Science* 308 (5729): 1758–1762.

Jareb, M. and Banker, G. (1997). Inhibition of axonal growth by brefeldin A in hippocampal neurons in culture. *J Neurosci* 17 (23): 8955–8963.

Jossin, Y. and Cooper, J.A. (2011). Reelin, Rap1 and N-cadherin orient the migration of multipolar neurons in the developing neocortex. *Nat Neurosci* 14 (6): 697–703.

Kalluri, R. and LeBleu, V.S. (2020). The biology, function, and biomedical applications of exosomes. *Science* 367 (6478): eaau6977.

Kanagawa, M. et al. (2009). Residual laminin-binding activity and enhanced dystroglycan glycosylation by LARGE in novel model mice to dystroglycanopathy. *Hum Mol Genet* 18 (4): 621–631.

Kappeler, C. et al. (2006). Branching and nucleokinesis defects in migrating interneurons derived from doublecortin knockout mice. *Hum Mol Genet* 15 (9): 1387–1400.

Kato, K. et al. (2017). A novel missense mutation in the HECT domain of NEDD4L identified in a girl with periventricular nodular heterotopia, polymicrogyria and cleft palate. *J Hum Genet* 62 (9): 861–863.

Kato, M. and Dobyns, W.B. (2003). Lissencephaly and the molecular basis of neuronal migration. *Hum Mol Genet* 12 (Special issue 1): R89–96.

Kawauchi, T. (2015 October 7). Cellular insights into cerebral cortical development. *Front Cell Neurosci* 9: 394.

Kawauchi, T. et al. (2006). Cdk5 phosphorylates and stabilizes p27kip1 contributing to actin organization and cortical neuronal migration. *Nat Cell Biol* 8 (1): 17–26.

Kawauchi, T. et al. (2010). Rab GTPases-dependent endocytic pathways regulate neuronal migration and maturation through N-cadherin trafficking. *Neuron* 67 (4): 588–602.

Keays, D.A. et al. (2007). Mutations in alpha-tubulin cause abnormal neuronal migration in mice and lissencephaly in humans. *Cell* 128 (1): 45–57.

Kim, J.-H. et al. (2002). Human Elongator facilitates RNA polymerase II transcription through chromatin. *Proc Natl Acad Sci USA* 99 (3): 1241–1246.

Kitamura, K. et al. (2009). Three human ARX mutations cause the lissencephaly-like and mental retardation with epilepsy-like pleiotropic phenotypes in mice. *Hum Mol Genet* 18 (19): 3708–3724.

Kitamura, K. et al. (2002). Mutation of ARX causes abnormal development of forebrain and testes in mice and X-linked lissencephaly with abnormal genitalia in humans. *Nat Genet* 32 (3): 359–369.

Koizumi, H. et al. (2006a). Doublecortin maintains bipolar shape and nuclear translocation during migration in the adult forebrain. *Nat Neurosci* 9 (6): 779–786.

Koizumi, H. et al. (2006b). Doublecortin-like kinase functions with doublecortin to mediate fiber tract decussation and neuronal migration. *Neuron* 49 (1): 55–66.

Kostovic, I. and Rakic, P. (1990). Developmental history of the transient subplate zone in the visual and somatosensory cortex of the macaque monkey and human brain. *J Comp Neurol* 297 (3): 441–470.

Kriegstein, A.R. and Noctor, S.C. (2004). Patterns of neuronal migration in the embryonic cortex. *Trends Neurosci* 27 (7): 392–399.

Krienen, F.M. et al. (2020). Innovations present in the primate interneuron repertoire. *Nature* 586 (7828): 262–269.

Kumar, R.A. et al. (2010). TUBA1A mutations cause wide spectrum lissencephaly (smooth brain) and suggest that multiple neuronal migration pathways converge on alpha tubulins. *Hum Mol Genet* 19 (14): 2817–2827.

Kurahashi, H. et al. (2005). Basement membrane fragility underlies embryonic lethality in fukutin-null mice. *Neurobiol Dis* 19 (1–2): 208–217.

Kyrousi, C. et al. (2021). Extracellular LGALS3BP regulates neural progenitor position and relates to human cortical complexity. *Nat Commun* 12 (1): 6298.

Laguesse, S. et al. (2015). Progenitor genealogy in the developing cerebral cortex. *Cell Tissue Res* 359 (1): 17–32.

Lavdas, A.A. et al. (1999). The medial ganglionic eminence gives rise to a population of early neurons in the developing cerebral cortex. *J Neurosci* 19 (18): 7881–7888.

le Dréau, G. et al. (2018). E proteins sharpen neurogenesis by modulating proneural bHLH transcription factors' activity in an E-box-dependent manner. *Elife* 7: e37267.

Le, T.N. et al. (2007). Dlx homeobox genes promote cortical interneuron migration from the basal forebrain by direct repression of the semaphorin receptor neuropilin-2. *J Biol Chem* 282 (26): 19071–19081.

Leone, D.P. et al. (2008). The determination of projection neuron identity in the developing cerebral cortex. *Curr Opin Neurobiol* 18 (1): 28–35.

Lepiemme, F. et al. (2022). Oligodendrocyte precursors guide interneuron migration by unidirectional contact repulsion. *Science* 376 (6595): eabn6204.

Letinic, K. et al. (2002). Origin of GABAergic neurons in the human neocortex. *Nature* 417 (6889): 645–649.

Li, G. et al. (2008). Regional distribution of cortical interneurons and development of inhibitory tone are regulated by Cxcl12/Cxcr4 signaling. *J Neurosci* 28 (5): 1085–1098.

Li, H. et al. (2012a). Neuregulin repellent signaling via ErbB4 restricts GABAergic interneurons to migratory paths from ganglionic eminence to cortical destinations. *Neural Dev* 7: 10.

Li, Y. et al. (2012b). Reciprocal regulation between resting microglial dynamics and neuronal activity in vivo. *Dev Cell* 23 (6): 1189–1202.

Lian, G. et al. (2012). Filamin a regulates neural progenitor proliferation and cortical size through Wee1-dependent Cdk1 phosphorylation. *J Neurosci* 32 (22): 7672–7684.

Lim, L. et al. (2018). Optimization of interneuron function by direct coupling of cell migration and axonal targeting. *Nat Neurosci* 21 (7): 920–931.

Liodis, P. et al. (2007). Lhx6 activity is required for the normal migration and specification of cortical interneuron subtypes. *J Neurosci* 27 (12): 3078–3089.

Liu, G. (2004). Local structural balance and functional interaction of excitatory and inhibitory synapses in hippocampal dendrites. *Nat Neurosci* 7 (4): 373–379.

Lodato, S. and Arlotta, P. (2015). Generating neuronal diversity in the mammalian cerebral cortex. *Ann Rev Cell Dev Biol* 31: 699–720.

Lodato, S. et al. (2011). Excitatory projection neuron subtypes control the distribution of local inhibitory interneurons in the cerebral cortex. *Neuron* 69 (4): 763–779.

Lombardi, M. et al. (2019). Detrimental and protective action of microglial extracellular vesicles on myelin lesions. *Acta Neuropathol* 138 (6): 987–1012.

Long, J.E. et al. (2009). Dlx1&2 and Mash1 transcription factors control MGE and CGE patterning and differentiation through parallel and overlapping pathways. *Cereb Cortex* 19 (Suppl. 1): i96–i106.

Longman, C. et al. (2003). Mutations in the human LARGE gene cause MDC1D, a novel form of congenital muscular dystrophy with severe mental retardation and abnormal glycosylation of alpha-dystroglycan. *Hum Mol Genet* 12 (21): 2853–2861.

López-Bendito, G. et al. (2008). Chemokine signaling controls intracortical migration and final distribution of GABAergic interneurons. *J Neurosci* 28 (7): 1613–1624.

López-Bendito, G. et al. (2004). Preferential origin and layer destination of GAD65-GFP cortical interneurons. *Cereb Cortex* 14 (10): 1122–1133.

Lu, J. et al. (2006). Overlapping expression of ARFGEF2 and filamin A in the neuroependymal lining of the lateral ventricles. *J Comp Neurol* 494 (3): 476–484.

Lv, F. et al. (2015). Small molecules enhance functional O-mannosylation of Alpha-dystroglycan. *Bioorg Med Chem* 23 (24): 7661–7670.

Ma, T. et al. (2013). Subcortical origins of human and monkey neocortical interneurons. *Nat Neurosci* 16 (11): 1588–1597.

Magavi, S. et al. (2012). Coincident generation of pyramidal neurons and protoplasmic astrocytes in neocortical columns. *J Neurosci* 32 (14): 4762–4772.

Malatesta, P. et al. (2000). Isolation of radial glial cells by fluorescent-activated cell sorting reveals a neuronal lineage. *Development* 127 (24): 5253–5263.

Mancinelli, S. and Lodato, S. (2018). Decoding neuronal diversity in the developing cerebral cortex. *Curr Opin Neurobiol* 53: 146–155.

Manent, J.B. et al. (2009). Dcx reexpression reduces subcortical band heterotopia and seizure threshold in an animal model of neuronal migration disorder. *Nat Med* 15 (1): 84–90.

Marín, O. et al. (2003). Directional guidance of interneuron migration to the cerebral cortex relies on subcortical Slit1/2-independent repulsion and cortical attraction. *Development* 130 (9): 1889–1901.

Marín, O. et al. (2001). Sorting of striatal and cortical interneurons regulated by semaphorin-neuropilin interactions. *Science* 293 (5531): 872–875.

Marques, S. et al. (2018). Transcriptional convergence of oligodendrocyte lineage progenitors during development. *Dev Cell* 46 (4): 504–517.e7.

Martini, F.J. and Valdeolmillos, M. (2010). Actomyosin contraction at the cell rear drives nuclear translocation in migrating cortical interneurons. *J Neurosci* 30 (25): 8660–8670.

Matsunaga, Y. et al. (2017). Reelin transiently promotes N-cadherin-dependent neuronal adhesion during mouse cortical development. *Proc Natl Acad Sci USA* 114 (8): 2048–2053.

Mayer, C. et al. (2018). Developmental diversification of cortical inhibitory interneurons. *Nature* 555 (7697): 457–462.

Mayer, C. et al. (2015). Clonally related forebrain interneurons disperse broadly across both functional areas and structural boundaries. *Neuron* 87 (5): 989–998.

McManus, M.F. et al. (2004). Lis1 is necessary for normal non-radial migration of inhibitory interneurons. *Am J Pathol* 165 (3): 775–784.

Métin, C. et al. (2007). Conserved pattern of tangential neuronal migration during forebrain development. *Development* 134 (15): 2815–2827.

Meyer, G. et al. (1998). Different origins and developmental histories of transient neurons in the marginal zone of the fetal and neonatal rat cortex. *J Comp Neurol* 397 (4): 493–518.

Mi, D. et al. (2018). Early emergence of cortical interneuron diversity in the mouse embryo. *Science* 360 (6384): 81–85.

Miyata, T. et al. (2001). Asymmetric inheritance of radial glial fibers by cortical neurons. *Neuron* 31: 727–741.

Mo, Z. et al. (2007). Human cortical neurons originate from radial glia and neuron-restricted progenitors. *J Neurosci* 27 (15): 4132–4145.

Molyneaux, B.J. et al. (2005). Fezl is required for the birth and specification of corticospinal motor neurons. *Neuron* 47 (6): 817–831.

Moore, S.A. et al. (2002). Deletion of brain dystroglycan recapitulates aspects of congenital muscular dystrophy. *Nature* 418 (6896): 422–425.

Muntoni, F. et al. (2002). Defective glycosylation in muscular dystrophy. *Lancet* 360 (9343): 1419–1421.

Muntoni, F. and Voit, T. (2004). The congenital muscular dystrophies in 2004. *Neuromuscul Disord* 14 (10): 635–649.

Murre, C. et al. (1989). Interactions between heterologous helix-loop-helix proteins generate complexes that bind specifically to a common DNA sequence. *Cell* 58 (3): 537–544.

Myshrall, T.D. et al. (2012). Dystroglycan on radial glia end feet is required for pial basement membrane integrity and columnar organization of the developing cerebral cortex. *J Neuropathol Exp Neurol* 71 (12): 1047–1063.

Nadarajah, B. et al. (2002). Ventricle-directed migration in the developing cerebral cortex. *Nat Neurosci* 5 (3): 218–224.

Nadarajah, B. et al. (2001). Two modes of radial migration in early development of the cerebral cortex. *Nat Neurosci* 4 (2): 143–150.

Nagamani, S.C.S. et al. (2009). Microdeletions including YWHAE in the Miller-Dieker syndrome region on chromosome 17p13.3 result in facial dysmorphisms, growth restriction, and cognitive impairment. *J Med Genet* 46 (12): 825–833.

Nagano, T. et al. (2004). Filamin A and FILIP (Filamin A-interacting protein) regulate cell polarity and motility in neocortical subventricular and intermediate zones during radial migration. *J Neurosci* 24 (43): 9648–9657.

Nasrallah, I.M. et al. (2006). Analysis of non-radial interneuron migration dynamics and its disruption in Lis1± mice. *J Comp Neurol* 496 (6): 847–858.

Nery, S. et al. (2002). The caudal ganglionic eminence is a source of distinct cortical and subcortical cell populations. *Nat Neurosci* 5 (12): 1279–1287.

Nguyen, L. et al. (2006). p27kip1 independently promotes neuronal differentiation and migration in the cerebral cortex. *Genes Dev* 20 (11): 1511–1524.

Niquille, M. et al. (2018). Neurogliaform cortical interneurons derive from cells in the preoptic area. *Elife* 7: e32017.

Nishimura, Y.V. et al. (2010). Dissecting the factors involved in the locomotion mode of neuronal migration in the developing cerebral cortex. *J Biol Chem* 285 (8): 5878–5887.

Nóbrega-Pereira, S. and Marín, O. (2009). Transcriptional control of neuronal migration in the developing mouse brain. *Cereb Cortex* 19 (Suppl. 1): 107–113.

Noctor, S.C. et al. (2001a). Neurons derived from radial glial cells establish radial units in neocortex. *Nature* 409 (6821): 714–720.

Nowakowski, T.J. et al. (2016). Transformation of the radial glia scaffold demarcates two stages of human cerebral cortex development. *Neuron* 91 (6): 1219–1227.

Ogawa, M. et al. (1995). The reeler gene-associated antigen on Cajal-Retzius neurons is a crucial molecule for laminar organization of cortical neurons. *Neuron* 14 (5): 899–912.

Ohtsuka-Tsurumi, E. et al. (2004). Co-localization of fukutin and α-dystroglycan in the mouse central nervous system. *Dev Brain Res* 152 (2): 121–127.

Okada, Y. et al. (2010). A role for the elongator complex in zygotic paternal genome demethylation. *Nature* 463 (7280): 554–558.

Olson, E.C. and Walsh, C.A. (2002). Smooth, rough and upside-down neocortical development. *Curr Opin Genet Dev* 12 (3): 320–327.

Olsson, M. et al. (1998). Early specification of striatal projection neurons and interneuronal subtypes in the lateral and medial ganglionic eminence. *Neuroscience* 84 (3): 867–876.

Olsson, M. et al. (1995). Projection neurons in fetal striatal transplants are predominantly derived from the lateral ganglionic eminence. *Neuroscience* 69 (4): 1169–1182.

Orduz, D. et al. (2015). Interneurons and oligodendrocyte progenitors form a structured synaptic network in the developing neocortex. *Elife* 4: e06953.

Pacary, E. et al. (2011). Proneural transcription factors regulate different steps of cortical neuron migration through Rnd-mediated inhibition of RhoA signaling. *Neuron* 69 (6): 1069–1084.

Pan, J. et al. (2022). Extracellular vesicles derived from glioblastoma promote proliferation and migration of neural progenitor cells via PI3K-Akt pathway. *Cell Commun Signal* 20 (1): 7.

Paredes, M.F. et al. (2006). Stromal-derived factor-1 (CXCL12) regulates laminar position of Cajal-Retzius cells in normal and dysplastic brains. *J Neurosci* 26 (37): 9404–9412.

Parkhurst, C.N. et al. (2013). Microglia promote learning-dependent synapse formation through brain-derived neurotrophic factor. *Cell* 155 (7): 1596–1609.

Parrini, E. et al. (2006). Periventricular heterotopia. *Brain* 129 (Pt 7): 1892–1906.

Peng, C. et al. (2012). Ablation of vacuole protein sorting 18 (Vps18) gene leads to neurodegeneration and impaired neuronal migration by disrupting multiple vesicle transport pathways to lysosomes. *J Biol Chem* 287 (39): 32861–32873.

Petanjek, Z. et al. (2009). Origins of cortical GABAergic neurons in the cynomolgus monkey. *Cereb Cortex* 19 (2): 249–262.

Petros, T.J. et al. (2015). Apical versus basal neurogenesis directs cortical interneuron subclass fate. *Cell Rep* 13 (6): 1090–1095.

Pilz, D.T. et al. (1999). Subcortical band heterotopia in rare affected males can be caused by missense mutations in DCX (XLIS) or LIS1. *Hum Mol Genet* 8 (9): 1757–1760.

Pilz, G.A. et al. (2013). Amplification of progenitors in the mammalian telencephalon includes a new radial glial cell type. *Nat Commun* 4: 2125.

Poirier, K. et al. (2004). Neuroanatomical distribution of ARX in brain and its localisation in GABAergic neurons. *Mol Brain Res* 122 (1): 35–46.

Pollen, A.A. et al. (2015). Molecular identity of human outer radial glia during cortical development. *Cell* 163 (1): 55–67.

Porteus, M.H. et al. (1994). DLX-2, MASH-1, and MAP-2 expression and bromodeoxyuridine incorporation define molecularly distinct cell populations in the embryonic mouse forebrain. *J Neurosci* 14 (11): 6370–6383.

Pramparo, T. et al. (2010). Novel embryonic neuronal migration and proliferation defects in Dcx mutant mice are exacerbated by Lis1 reduction. *J Neurosci* 30 (8): 3002–3012.

Radonjić, N.V. et al. (2014). Diversity of cortical interneurons in primates. *Cell Rep* 9 (6): 2139–2151.

Rahl, P.B. et al. (2005). Elp1p, the yeast homolog of the FD disease syndrome protein, negatively regulates exocytosis independently of transcriptional elongation. *Mol Cell* 17 (6): 841–853.

Rakic, P. (1995). A small step for the cell, a giant leap for mankind. *Trends Neurosci* 18 (9): 383–388.

Ramón y Cajal, S. (1909). *Histologie du système nerveux de l'homme & des vertébrés*. Paris: Maloine.

Ramos, R.L. et al. (2006). Heterotopia formation in rat but not mouse neocortex after RNA interference knockdown of DCX. *Cereb Cortex* 16 (9): 1323–1331.

Reiner, O. et al. (1995). Lissencephaly gene (LISI) expression in the CNS suggests a role in neuronal migration. *J Neurosci* 15 (5): 3730–3738.

Reiner, O. et al. (1993). Isolation of a Miller-Dieker lissencephaly gene containing G protein beta-subunit-like repeats. *Nature* 364 (6439): 717–721.

Sanada, K. et al. (2004). Disabled-1-regulated adhesion of migrating neurons to radial glial fiber contributes to neuronal positioning during early corticogenesis. *Neuron* 42 (2): 197–211.

Sánchez-Alcañiz, J.A. et al. (2011). Cxcr7 controls neuronal migration by regulating chemokine responsiveness. *Neuron* 69 (1): 77–90.

Sasaki, S. et al. (2000). A LIS1/NUDEL/cytoplasmic dynein heavy chain complex in the developing and adult nervous system. *Neuron* 28 (3): 681–696.

Satz, J.S. et al. (2008). Brain and eye malformations resembling Walker-Warburg syndrome are recapitulated in mice by dystroglycan deletion in the epiblast. *J Neurosci* 28 (42): 10567–10575.

Satz, J.S. et al. (2010). Distinct functions of glial and neuronal dystroglycan in the developing and adult mouse brain. *J Neurosci* 30 (43): 14560–14572.

Schafer, D.P. et al. (2012). Microglia sculpt postnatal neural circuits in an activity and complement-dependent manner. *Neuron* 74 (4): 691–705.

Schenk, J. et al. (2009). Myosin II is required for interkinetic nuclear migration of neural progenitors. *Proc Natl Acad Sci USA* 106 (38): 16487–16492.

Schulz, C. et al. (2012). A lineage of myeloid cells independent of Myb and hematopoietic stem cells. *Science* 336 (6077): 86–90.

Seibt, J. et al. (2003). Neurogenin2 specifies the connectivity of thalamic neurons by controlling axon responsiveness to intermediate target cues. *Neuron* 39 (3): 439–452.

Sekine, K. et al. (2012). Reelin controls neuronal positioning by promoting cell-matrix adhesion via inside-out activation of integrin α5β1. *Neuron* 76 (2): 353–369.

Selvadurai, K. et al. (2014). Archaeal Elp3 catalyzes tRNA wobble uridine modification at C5 via a radical mechanism. *Nat Chem Biol* 10 (10): 810–812.

Sessa, A. et al. (2010). Tbr2-positive intermediate (basal) neuronal progenitors safeguard cerebral cortex expansion by controlling amplification of pallial glutamatergic neurons and attraction of subpallial GABAergic interneurons. *Genes Dev* 24 (16): 1816–1826.

Severino, M. et al. (2020). Definitions and classification of malformations of cortical development. *Brain* 143 (10): 2874–2894.

Sheen, V.L. et al. (2002). Filamin A and Filamin B are co-expressed within neurons during periods of neuronal migration and can physically interact. *Hum Mol Genet* 11 (23): 2845–2854.

Sheen, V.L. et al. (2004). Mutations in ARFGEF2 implicate vesicle trafficking in neural progenitor proliferation and migration in the human cerebral cortex. *Nat Genet* 36 (1): 69–76.

Sheldon, M. et al. (1997). *Scrambler* and *yotari* disrupt the *disabled* gene and produce a *reeler*-like phenotype in mice. *Nature* 389 (6652): 730–733.

Shen, Z. et al. (2021). Distinct progenitor behavior underlying neocortical gliogenesis related to tumorigenesis. *Cell Rep* 34 (11): 108853.

Shevell, D. (1994). EMB30 is essential for normal cell division, cell expansion, and cell adhesion in Arabidopsis and encodes a protein that has similarity to Sec7. *Cell* 77 (7): 1051–1062.

Shi, Y. et al. (2021). Mouse and human share conserved transcriptional programs for interneuron development. *Science* 374 (6573): eabj6641.

Shin, H.-W. et al. (2004). BIG2, a guanine nucleotide exchange factor for ADP-ribosylation factors. *Mol Biol Cell* 15 (12): 5283–5294.

Sierra, A. et al. (2010). Microglia shape adult hippocampal neurogenesis through apoptosis-coupled phagocytosis. *Cell Stem Cell* 7 (4): 483–495.

Silva, C.G. et al. (2018). Cell-intrinsic control of interneuron migration drives cortical morphogenesis. *Cell* 172 (5): 1063–1078.e19.

Silva, C.G. et al. (2019). Cell migration promotes dynamic cellular interactions to control cerebral cortex morphogenesis. *Nat Rev Neurosci* 20 (6): 318–329.

Simeone, A. et al. (1994). Cloning and characterization of two members of the vertebrate Dlx gene family. *Dev Biol* 91 (6): 2250–2254.

Skog, J. et al. (2008). Glioblastoma microvesicles transport RNA and proteins that promote tumour growth and provide diagnostic biomarkers. *Nat Cell Biol* 10 (12): 1470–1476.

Smart, I.H.M. (2002). Unique morphological features of the proliferative zones and postmitotic compartments of the neural epithelium giving rise to striate and extrastriate cortex in the monkey. *Cereb Cortex* 12 (1): 37–53.

Smith, D.S. et al. (2000). Regulation of cytoplasmic dynein behaviour and microtubule organization by mammalian Lis1. *Nat Cell Biol* 2: 767–775.

Southwell, D.G. et al. (2012). Intrinsically determined cell death of developing cortical interneurons. *Nature* 491 (7422): 109–113.

Squarzoni, P. et al. (2014). Microglia modulate wiring of the embryonic forebrain. *Cell Rep* 8 (5): 1271–1279.

Squarzoni, P. et al. (2015 June). Neuronal and microglial regulators of cortical wiring. *Front Neurosci* 9: 248.

Stossel, T.P. et al. (2001). Filamins as integrators of cell mechanics and signalling. *Nat Rev Mol Cell Biol* 2 (2): 138–145.

Stouffs, K. et al. (2020). Recurrent NEDD4L variant in periventricular nodular heterotopia, polymicrogyria and syndactyly. *Front Genet* 11: 26.

Stumm, R.K. et al. (2003). CXCR4 regulates interneuron migration in the developing neocortex. *J Neurosci* 23 (12): 5123–5130.

Sudo, A. et al. (2018). Temporal requirement of dystroglycan glycosylation during brain development and rescue of severe cortical dysplasia via gene delivery in the fetal stage. *Hum Mol Genet* 27 (7): 1174–1185.

Sung, B.H. and Weaver, A.M. (2017). Exosome secretion promotes chemotaxis of cancer cells. *Cell Adh Mig* 11 (2): 187–195.

Sweet, H.O. et al. (1996). Scrambler, a new neurological mutation of the mouse with abnormalities of neuronal migration. *Mamm Genome* 7 (11): 798–802.

Tabata, H. and Nakajima, K. (2003). Multipolar migration. *J Neurosci* 23 (31): 9996–10001.

Tamamaki, N. et al. (1997). Origin and route of tangentially migrating neurons in the developing neocortical intermediate zone. *J Neurosci* 17 (21): 8313–8323.

Tanaka, D. et al. (2003). Multimodal tangential migration of neocortical GABAergic neurons independent of GPI-anchored proteins. *Development* 130 (23): 5803–5813.

Taniguchi-Ikeda, M. et al. (2021). Restoration of the defect in radial glial fiber migration and cortical plate organization in a brain organoid model of Fukuyama muscular dystrophy. *IScience* 24 (10): 103140.

Taverna, E. and Huttner, W.B. (2010). Neural progenitor nuclei IN motion. *Neuron* 67 (6): 906–914.

Telley, L. et al. (2019). Temporal patterning of apical progenitors and their daughter neurons in the developing neocortex. *Science* 364 (6440).

Thornhill, P. et al. (2008). Developmental defects in a zebrafish model for muscular dystrophies associated with the loss of fukutin-related protein (FKRP). *Brain* 131 (6): 1551–1561.

Tielens, S. et al. (2016). Elongator controls cortical interneuron migration by regulating actomyosin dynamics. *Cell Res* 26 (10): 1131–1148.

Tiveron, M.C. et al. (2006). Molecular interaction between projection neuron precursors and invading interneurons via stromal-derived factor 1 (CXCL12)/CXCR4 signaling in the cortical subventricular zone/intermediate zone. *J Neurosci* 26 (51): 13273–13278.

Toda, T. (1999). Fukutin, a novel protein product responsible for Fukuyama-type congenital muscular dystrophy. *Seikagaku. J Jpn Biochem Soc* 71 (1): 55–61.

Trommsdorff, M. et al. (1999). Reeler/disabled-like disruption of neuronal migration in knockout mice lacking the VLDL receptor and ApoE receptor 2. *Cell* 97 (6): 689–701.

Tsai, J.W. et al. (2005). LIS1 RNA interference blocks neural stem cell division, morphogenesis, and motility at multiple stages. *J Cell Biol* 170 (6): 935–945.

Tsai, J.W. et al. (2010). Kinesin 3 and cytoplasmic dynein mediate interkinetic nuclear migration in neural stem cells. *Nat Neurosci* 13 (12): 1463–1472.

Turrero García, M. and Harwell, C.C. (2017). Radial glia in the ventral telencephalon. *FEBS Lett* 591 (24): 3942–3959.

Ueno, M. et al. (2013). Layer V cortical neurons require microglial support for survival during postnatal development. *Nat Neurosci* 16 (5): 543–551.

Ueno, M. et al. (2006). Cell cycle progression is required for nuclear migration of neural progenitor cells. *Brain Res* 1088 (1): 57–67.

Valadi, H. et al. (2007). Exosome-mediated transfer of mRNAs and microRNAs is a novel mechanism of genetic exchange between cells. *Nature Cell Biology* 9 (6): 654–659.

Valcanis, H. and Tan, -S.-S. (2003). Layer specification of transplanted interneurons in developing mouse neocortex. *J Neurosci* 23 (12): 5113–5122.

van der Knaap, M.S. et al. (1997). Magnetic resonance imaging in classification of congenital muscular dystrophies with brain abnormalities. *Ann Neurol* 42 (1): 50–59.

van Dijk, J. et al. (2007). A targeted multienzyme mechanism for selective microtubule polyglutamylation. *Mol Cell* 26 (3): 437–448.

van Reeuwijk, J. et al. (2005). POMT2 mutations cause alpha-dystroglycan hypoglycosylation and Walker-Warburg syndrome. *J Med Genet* 42 (12): 907–912.

Vogt, D. et al. (2014). Lhx6 directly regulates Arx and CXCR7 to determine cortical interneuron fate and laminar position. *Neuron* 82 (2): 350–364.

Waite, A. et al. (2012). The dystrophin-glycoprotein complex in brain development and disease. *Trends Neurosci* 35 (8): 487–496.

Wang, X. et al. (2011a). A new subtype of progenitor cell in the mouse embryonic neocortex. *Nat Neurosci* 14 (5): 555–562.

Wang, Y. et al. (2010). Dlx5 and Dlx6 regulate the development of parvalbumin-expressing cortical interneurons. *J Neurosci* 30 (15): 5334–5345.

Wang, Y. et al. (2011b). CXCR4 and CXCR7 have distinct functions in regulating interneuron migration. *Neuron* 69 (1): 61–76.

Wichterle, H. et al. (2001). In utero fate mapping reveals distinct migratory pathways and fates of neurons born in the mammalian basal forebrain. *Development* 128 (19): 3759–3771.

Winkler, G.S. et al. (2002). Elongator is a histone H3 and H4 acetyltransferase important for normal histone acetylation levels in vivo. *Proc Natl Acad Sci USA* 99 (6): 3517–3522.

Wong, F.K. et al. (2018). Pyramidal cell regulation of interneuron survival sculpts cortical networks. *Nature* 557 (7707): 668–673.

Wu, S.-X. et al. (2005). Pyramidal neurons of upper cortical layers generated by NEX-positive progenitor cells in the subventricular zone. *Proc Natl Acad Sci USA* 102 (47): 17172–17177.

Xiang, Y. et al. (2017). Fusion of regionally specified hPSC-derived organoids models human brain development and interneuron migration. *Cell Stem Cell* 21 (3): 383–398.e7.

Xie, Z. et al. (2007). Cep120 and TACCs control interkinetic nuclear migration and the neural progenitor pool. *Neuron* 56 (1): 79–93.

Xu, Q. et al. (2004). Origins of cortical interneuron subtypes. *J Neurosci* 24 (11): 2612–2622.

Xue, M. et al. (2014). Equalizing excitation-inhibition ratios across visual cortical neurons. *Nature* 511 (7511): 596–600.

Yanagida, M. et al. (2012). Dynamics of the leading process, nucleus, and Golgi apparatus of migrating cortical interneurons in living mouse embryos. *Proc Natl Acad Sci USA* 109 (41): 16737–16742.

Yang, L. et al. (2022). Developmental origins of human cortical oligodendrocytes and astrocytes. *Neurosci Bulletin* 38 (1): 47–68.

Yatsenko, A.S. et al. (2014). miRNA-based buffering of the cobblestone-lissencephaly-associated extracellular matrix receptor dystroglycan via its alternative 3′-UTR. *Nat Commun* 5: 4906.

Yau, H.-J. et al. (2003). Neural development of the neuregulin receptor ErbB4 in the cerebral cortex and the hippocampus. *Cereb Cortex* 13 (3): 252–264.

Yingling, J. et al. (2008). Neuroepithelial stem cell proliferation requires LIS1 for precise spindle orientation and symmetric division. *Cell* 132 (3): 474–486.

Yoshida, A. et al. (2001). Muscular dystrophy and neuronal migration disorder caused by mutations in a glycosyltransferase, POMGnT1. *Dev Cell* 1 (5): 717–724.

Yoshida-Moriguchi, T. et al. (2010). O-mannosyl phosphorylation of alpha-dystroglycan is required for laminin binding. *Science* 327 (5961): 88–92.

Youn, Y.H. et al. (2009). Distinct dose-dependent cortical neuronal migration and neurite extension defects in Lis1 and Ndel1 mutant mice. *J Neurosci* 29 (49): 15520–15530.

Yozu, M. et al. (2005). The caudal migratory stream. *J Neurosci* 25 (31): 7268–7277.
Yu, Y. et al. (2021). Interneuron origin and molecular diversity in the human fetal brain. *Nat Neurosci* 24 (12): 1745–1756.
Yuan, F. et al. (2020). LHX6 is essential for the migration of human pluripotent stem cell-derived GABAergic interneurons. *Protein and Cell* 11 (4): 286–291.
Zecevic, N. (2004). Specific characteristic of radial glia in the human fetal telencephalon. *GLIA* 48 (1): 27–35.
Zecevic, N. et al. (2011). Interneurons in the developing human neocortex. *Dev Neurobiol* 71 (1): 18–33.
Zhang, J. et al. (2013). Filamin a regulates neuronal migration through brefeldin a-inhibited guanine exchange factor 2-dependent Arf1 activation. *J Neurosci* 33 (40): 15735–15746.
Zhang, J. et al. (2012). Brefeldin A-inhibited guanine exchange factor 2 regulates Filamin a phosphorylation and neuronal migration. *J Neurosci* 32 (36): 12619–12629.
Zhao, Y. et al. (2008). Distinct molecular pathways of development of telencephalic interneuron subtypes revealed through analysis of Lhx6 mutants. *J Comp Neurol* 510 (1): 79–99.
Zimmer, G. et al. (2008). Ephrin-A5 acts as a repulsive cue for migrating cortical interneurons. *Eur J Neurosci* 28 (1): 62–73.
Zonouzi, M. et al. (2015). GABAergic regulation of cerebellar NG2 cell development is altered in perinatal white matter injury. *Nat Neurosci* 18 (5): 674–682.

18

The Emerging Roles of LIS1 Biomechanics in Cellular and Cortical Homeostasis

Aditya Kshirsagar and Orly Reiner

Departments of Molecular Genetics and Molecular Neuroscience, Weizmann Institute of Science, Rehovot, Israel

18.1 LIS1 and Brain Structure, an Introduction

Folds in the cerebral cortex, the sulci, and the gyri, are the most striking feature of the human brain. Disruption of the biochemical signals and mechanical forces driving neuronal migration and developing brain tissue mechanics are thought to be involved in forming abnormal folds and cortical malformation (Varner et al. 2010; Welker 1990). Malformations of the cerebral cortex folding are often categorized as being on the lissencephaly and pachygyria spectrum of disorders. These spectra of diseases include lissencephaly (smooth surface area of the brain), agyria (lack of gyri), pachygyria (thick and broadened gyri), polymicrogyria, and heterotopias (Di Donato et al. 2017). *LIS1* (*LISSENCEPHALY-1*, also known as *PAFAH1B1*) was the first gene identified and reported to be involved in neuronal migration disorders (Brock et al. 1993; Dobyns et al. 1993; Reiner et al. 1993, 1995).

Multiple studies have reported that *LIS1* is engaged in organizing cortical layers and patterning the mammalian cerebral cortex (Gambello et al. 2003; Hirotsune et al. 1998; Pawlisz et al. 2008; Shu et al. 2004). De novo mutations during fetal development in the *PAFAH1B1* gene locus (chromosome 17p13.3) involving deletions, duplications, or triplications cause developmental delay and cortical defects in humans (Avela et al. 2011; Bi et al. 2009; Classen et al. 2013; Farris et al. 2018; Henry et al. 2016; Hyon et al. 2011; Roos et al. 2009; Stutterd et al. 2020). Patients with small deletions in the gene or point mutations usually present with lissencephaly, generalized hypotonia, central visual impairment, developmental delay, and epilepsy ranging from infantile spasms to severe drug-resistant epilepsy (Brock et al. 1993). Affected individuals may develop moderate spastic quadriplegia and scoliosis. Seizures occur in >90 percent of the patients, and the majority (65%) are drug resistant. Rare mosaic mutations in *PAFAH1B1* result in subcortical band heterotopic (SBH) or doublecortex (Gilliam et al. 2021; Gonzalez-Moron et al. 2017). Large hemizygous deletions, unbalanced translocations of a chromosomal segment involving *PAFAH1B1* and *YAWHAE*, and sometimes aneuploidy due to the ring chromosome have been reported in cases of Miller-Dieker syndrome (MDS), a severe form of lissencephaly with devastating neurological consequences (Atwal and Macmurdo 2015; Bellucco et al. 2017; Blazejewski et al. 2018; Brock et al. 1993;

Neocortical Neurogenesis in Development and Evolution, First Edition. Edited by Wieland B. Huttner.

Kim et al. 2014; Mishima et al. 2017; Shi et al. 2021). Affected individuals typically have severe lissencephaly, characteristic facial changes, other more variable malformations, and severe neurologic and developmental abnormalities (Brock et al. 1993). The developmental prognosis is poor for all children with MDS. Patients with duplications, including the *PAFAH1B1* locus, present with mild-to-severe developmental and psychomotor delay, hypotonia, and growth restriction. Brain malformations include hypoplasia/dysgenesis of the corpus callosum, mild cerebellar volume loss, mildly reduced brain volume, often with a posterior-to-anterior gradient, and microcephaly (Brock et al. 1993). One affected individual with bilateral perisylvian polymicrogyria (extra brain folds) has been reported (Stutterd et al. 2020). A detailed classification and clinical perspective on LIS1-associated lissencephaly and cortical anomalies is a recurrent collective effort (Brock et al. 1993; Oegema et al. 2020).

18.2 LIS1, the Protein

LIS1 is a well-conserved, highly phosphorylated, multifaceted protein known for interacting with microtubules and associated proteins (Reiner and Sapir 2013). LIS1 structurally resembles G-beta proteins with a LisH N-terminal domain and a C-terminal part composed of seven tryptophan-aspartic acids (WD) repeats imparting beta-propeller structure (Gerlitz et al. 2005; Kim et al. 2004; Mateja et al. 2006; Reiner et al. 1993). Biochemical studies and the crystal structures of the N- and C- terminals parts suggest that the N-terminal LisH domain generally tends to form a dimer with a flexible scaffold for macromolecular assembly (Garcia-Higuera et al. 1996; Gerlitz et al. 2005; Kim et al. 2004; Sapir et al. 1999).

18.3 Known LIS1 Functions

The most extensively studied and evolutionary conserved LIS1 role involves its structural interaction and regulation of the molecular motor cytoplasmic dynein, which may act as a clutch (Huang et al. 2012). It facilitates the motility of cytoplasmic dynein for dynein–dynactin–adapter high-load cargo complexes (Baumbach et al. 2017; Elshenawy et al. 2020). Its function in spindle orientation and microtubule dynamics is well studied (Moon et al. 2020; Sapir et al. 1997; Schwamborn and Knoblich 2008; Yingling et al. 2008). One of the recent in vitro studies provided the 3Å structure of the LIS1-dynein complex in yeast and human, revealing the binding sites between LIS1 beta-propellers to four different positions in the molecular motor AAA5 of the ATPase domain to regulate its activity (Gillies et al. 2022; Zhuang et al. 2007). Cytoplasmic dynein transports cargo in different subcellular localizations. It recruits large macromolecular assemblies with dynactin-adaptor complexes on microtubules in its active "open" state (Xiang and Qiu 2020). LIS1 and its interacting partners in the cytoplasmic dynein complex define its affinity towards microtubules and the gliding velocity for the transport (Elshenawy et al. 2020; Reddy et al. 2016; Schmidt 2015). The stochastic transition from the recently proposed cytoplasmic dynein autoinhibitory "phi" conformation to the active state is also driven by LIS1's ability to promote the assembly of dynein–dynactin–adaptor complexes (Elshenawy et al. 2020; Gillies et al. 2022; Qiu et al. 2019). LIS1/NDE1/NDEL1 complex is one of the most significant regulators of cytoplasmic dynein binding to the microtubules (Kuijpers et al. 2016; Lam et al. 2010; Reddy et al. 2016; Shmueli et al. 2010). LIS1-NDE1 complex competes with dynactin and thus supervises cytoplasmic dynein activity in a dual-way (Elshenawy et al. 2020; McKenney et al. 2011). NDE1 facilitates the recruitment of LIS1 to cytoplasmic dynein heavy chain, and then dynein affiliates with the microtubules in a ternary complex with NDEL1 (Kuijpers et al. 2016; Lam et al. 2010). NDEL1 post-translational modifications, including phosphorylation and palmitoylation, regulate retrograde trafficking of the cytoplasmic dynein puncta and neuronal migration (Shmueli et al. 2010; Toba and Hirotsune 2012). Cytoplasmic dynein-mediated activation of CDK5-dependent phosphorylation of NDEL1, together with LIS1, at the axon-initial segment prevents the entry of KIF17-coupled dendritic cargoes in the axons (Chapman et al. 2019; Franker et al. 2016; Klinman et al. 2017; Kuijpers et al. 2016).

The LIS1 protein plays a crucial role in various brain regions during development in a dose-dependent manner (Gambello et al. 2003; Hippenmeyer et al. 2010; Youn et al. 2009). Copy number variations (CNVs) with duplication or triplication of the LIS1 chromosomal fragment at 17p13.3 in patients lead to developmental defects with a decrease in the size of the brain, affecting splenium due to dysgenesis in the corpus callosum (Avela et al. 2011; Bi et al. 2009; Curry et al. 2013). Reduction and over-expression of LIS1 in mice cause defects in non-radially or tangentially migrating GABAergic neuronal progenitors from the ganglionic eminences into the neocortex (Bi et al. 2009; Dominguez-Sala et al. 2022a, 2022b; Garcia-Lopez et al. 2021; Gopal et al. 2010). *Lis1* adult heterozygotes mice have disorganized layers in the cerebral cortex, causing hyperexcitability with defects in the hippocampal dentate gyrus pyramidal neurons (Wang and Baraban 2008). *Lis1* heterozygosity also affects the GABAergic or inhibitory responses in the pyramidal neurons (Valdes-Sanchez et al. 2007). The genetic insult by LIS1 reduction also exerts its effects on adult neurogenesis in the dentate gyrus, reducing glial and neuronal progenitors (Wang and Baraban 2008). The septohippocampal region in *Lis1/sLis1* mice was afflicted with aggrandized calbindin, calretinin, and GAD67 neurons in the perinatal stage (Garcia-Lopez et al. 2021). The cholinergic septohippocampal projections in *Lis1* mutants were found to have receded (Garcia-Lopez et al. 2015). Some conditional knockout studies of *Lis1* in the adult stage also reveal that the reduction of LIS1 alters short-term synaptic plasticity and leads to ectopic positioning of newly formed granule cells (Hunt et al. 2012; Wang and Baraban 2007). LIS1 deficits in neurons affect synaptogenesis and social behavior by reducing RhoA activity-dependent change in dendritic filopodia dynamics (Sudarov et al. 2013). LIS1 ablation imbalances excitatory and inhibitory synapses by affecting the microtubule-mediated PSD-95 mobility and distribution in interneuron dendrites (Kawabata et al. 2012).

LIS1 is known to syndicate many complexes in different compartments of biological cells. LIS1 interacts with PAFAH1B catalytic subunits α1 and α2 in the cytoplasm to form a catalytic complex, crucial for blood platelet functioning, thus the name platelet-activating factor acetylhydrolase (PAFAH) complex (Hattori et al. 1994). It serves as a non-catalytic subunit and forms a complex with α1 or α2 homodimers and α1-α2 heterodimers (Ho et al. 1997). Truncated LIS1 fails to create the PAFAH1B catalytic complex (Ho et al. 1997; Tarricone et al. 2004). PAFAH1B α1 & α2 (PAFAH1B2 and PAFAH1B3) subunits are essential for modulation of the Wnt pathway in developing GABAergic neurons (Livnat et al. 2010). REELIN is another molecule that, when mutated, leads to pachygyria and lissencephaly in human patients (Balza et al. 2021; Chang et al. 2007; Clark et al. 1997; Di Donato et al. 2022; Eriksson et al. 2001; Hong et al. 2000). Reeler mice have an inverted cortical organization, that is, abnormally located subplate cells above the cortical plate in the subpial zone with altered thalamocortical innervations and decreased cerebellum size (Badea et al. 2007; D'Arcangelo 2006; Lossi et al. 2019). LIS1 also interacts with Dab1 and mediators of the Reelin signaling pathway. Hemizygous *Lis1* mice develop hydrocephalus during the neonatal stages, and mutants of Dab1, VLDLR, and ApoeR2 in the Reelin signaling pathway show enhanced and progressive neonatal hydrocephalus (Assadi et al. 2003; Zhang et al. 2007, 2009). Conditional knockout of *Ndel1* mice that allowed to bypass the early embryonic lethality affected postnatal hippocampal organization (Jiang et al. 2016). These mice exhibited reduced NDE1, NDEL1, and Reelin levels but increased expression of LIS1 and cytoplasmic dynein heavy chain (Gavrilovici et al. 2021; Jiang et al. 2016). Reelin injections normalized the LIS1 levels in *Ndel1* conditional knockout hippocampi and improved cognitive functions and behavior (Gavrilovici et al. 2021; Jiang et al. 2016; Kiroski et al. 2020). Furthermore, the addition of Reelin extended the lifespan of the *Ndel1* conditional knockout mice by reducing epileptic seizures (Kiroski et al. 2020).

LIS1 expression is constitutively maintained and regulated in several cell types, and its role is highly relevant to and is not limited to the developing brain. Most of these studies were limited to rodent models due to LIS1's complexity and fundamental role in homeostasis. Correspondingly, studies suggest the crucial role of LIS1 in the myeloid lineage. Depleting levels of LIS1 in bone marrow cells indicate its involvement in the NFKB ligand RANKL pathway, which affects the formation of osteoclasts and leads to bone deformity (Ye et al. 2016). Conditional deletion of *Lis1* in hematopoietic stem cells, using Cre expressed using the *Vav1* promoter, impersonates the bloodless phenotype in the developing mouse embryo, including the brain (Zimdahl et al. 2014). The phenotype observed is similar to that observed in neuroepithelial stem cells (Yingling et al. 2008). LIS1 reduction affects the distribution of NUMB, a cell fate determinant of the NOTCH pathway, in daughter cells of myeloid origin. The spindle fails to orient perpendicular to the polarization axis, marking it as a critical regulator for hematopoiesis and leukemogenesis.

An extensive CRISPR screen performed in mice identified LIS1 as one of the essential regulators of aggressive myeloid leukemia progression (Bajaj et al. 2020). LIS1 is a critical gene identified in all CRISPR and RNAi screens collected in cancer-related cell lines data analyzed in depmap.org (Tsherniak et al. 2017). To understand better the vital functions of LIS1, we have undertaken a multi-omics approach.

18.4 LIS1 is an RNA Binding Protein

Recent findings show the importance of LIS1 as a premium RNA binding protein (RBP) in several post-transcriptional and RNA metabolic processes (Kshirsagar et al. 2022). Biochemically, around 30 percent of the LIS1 protein is nuclear in multiple cell types, including mouse blastocysts, embryonic stem cells (ESCs), neurons, and glia, implying that the LIS1 protein may also function in the nucleus. We found that LIS1 binds RNA as well as multiple RBPs, and, therefore, can participate in ribonucleoprotein (RNP) complexes. RNP granules are non-membrane-bound compartments that form from RNA molecules and RNA-binding proteins. Many of these interactions are conserved in evolution. A high throughput proteomic study conducted in *Drosophila* showed an overlap with many orthologs in mice, including the Argonaute complex, heat shock proteins, and several SNRNP and HNRNP splicing factors (Guruharsha et al. 2011). The different RBP complexes LIS1 may participate in are shown in Table 18.1. We highlight several RBP-related processes in which LIS1 may be involved Figure 18.1.

RBPs are vital in gene expression regulation, RNA localization and metabolism, and mechanotransduction (Lunde et al. 2007; Mitchell and Parker 2014; Zhang and Li 2021). The ability of these proteins to form complexes allows high fidelity, efficiency, and spatial precision to maintain a dynamic cellular state through post-transcriptional mechanisms (Bhat et al. 2021). These events include nuclear splicing, polyadenylation, reading and editing epitranscriptomic modifications to cytoplasmic transport, stability, localization, and translation (Das et al. 2021; Frye et al. 2018; Passmore and Coller 2022; Suzuki 2021; Wiener and Schwartz 2021). All these functions put RBPs in a unique position to influence neuronal progenitor proliferation, differentiation, migration, and

Table 18.1 LIS1-RNP complexes. The LIS1 interactome was sorted to RBPs. The functional complexes are indicated by the type of the RNP complex, the intracellular compartment, the number of proteins detected, and the names of the related genes.

RNP complex	Compartment	N	Genes
spliceosomal complex	Nucleus	75	Api5,Clns1a,Dhx15,Ddx5,Frg1,Hnrnpc,Hnrnpa1, Hnrnpk,Hspa8,Lgals3,Magoh,Ncl,Pabpc1,Rbm3, Rbmxl1,Srsf2,Tra2b,Eftud2,Snrnp70,Snrpb,Snrpb2, Snrpd1,Snrpe,Alyref,U2af2,Sf1,Ik,Txnl4a,Lsm2,Prpf19, Usp39,Srrm1,Hnrnpu,Plrg1,Hnrnpa2b1,Snrpa,Ddx39b, Syncrip,Hnrnph1,Sf3b5,Snw1,Snrnp40,Gemin2,Crnkl1, Snrpd3,Sf3a1,Snrpg,Bcas2,Rbm28,Ppil1,Prpf6,Snrpa1, Snrpf,Prpf4,Zcchc8,Prpf3,Cdc5l,Sf3a3,Srrm2,Lsm8, Rbmxl2,Hnrnpm,Rbm17,Sf3b1,Hnrnpf,Tra2a,Sf3b3, Snrpd2,Sf3b4,U2af1,Srsf1,Prpf8,Hnrnpa3,Sf3b2,Snrnp200
catalytic step 2 spliceosome	Nucleus	52	Ddx5,Frg1,Hnrnpc,Hnrnpa1,Hnrnpk,Magoh,Pabpc1,Eftud2,Snrpb, Snrpb2,Snrpd1,Snrpe,Alyref,Lsm2,Prpf19,Srrm1,Hnrnpu,Plrg1, Hnrnpa2b1,Syncrip,Hnrnph1,Rbm8a,Snw1,Snrnp40,Crnkl1, Cwc27,Snrpd3,Sf3a1,Snrpg,Bcas2,Ppil1,Prpf6,Snrpa1,Snrpf, Zcchc8,Cdc5l,Hnrnpr,Ddx23,Sf3a3,Srrm2,Hnrnpm,Sf3b1, Hnrnpf,Sf3b3,Snrpd2,U2af1,Srsf1,Prpf8,Eif4a3,Hnrnpa3, Sf3b2,Snrnp200
nuclear envelope	Nucleus	29	Parp1,Anxa11,Anxa7,Apoe,Bax,Calr,Cbx3,Dync1h1,Faf1, Kpnb1,Lmnb1,Nup62,Pafah1b1,Ran,Ranbp2,Rrm1,Rrm2, S100a6,Tmpo,Rtcb,Chmp2a,Nup93,Sirt1,Tpr,Cse1l,Clic1, Abcf1,Ipo7,Gpx4
fibrillar center	Nucleus	29	Coil,Fbl,Ncl,Snrpb2,Ubtf,Tcof1,Top1,Sumo1,Ezr,Txnrd1, Plrg1,Nono,Nop58,Uso1,Pspc1,Eef1d,Nop56,Mri1,Rnmt, Gar1,Nolc1,Rai14,Sirt1,Smarca5,Ube2n,Acaca,Ddx46,Eif3l,Dkc1
U2-type precatalytic spliceosome	Nucleus	28	Eftud2,Snrpb,Snrpb2,Snrpd1,Snrpe,Ik,Txnl4a,Lsm2, Sf3b5,Cwc27,Snrpd3,Sf3a1,Snrpg,Prpf6,Snrpa1,Snrpf, Prpf4,Prpf3,Sf3a3,Srrm2,Lsm8,Sf3b1,Sf3b3,Snrpd2,Sf3b4, Prpf8,Sf3b2,Snrnp200
nuclear matrix	Nucleus	25	Anp32a,Csnk2b,Smc3,Lmnb1,Matr3,Uhrf1,Npm1,Smc1a, Psma6,Srrm1,Hnrnpu,Hnrnpa2b1,Nono,Ddx39b,Tcerg1, Prpf40a,Ruvbl1,Snw1,Cad,Basp1,Sfpq,Hnrnpm,Sf3b1,Numa1,Ppig
nuclear membrane	Nucleus	22	Ctnnb1,Gapdh,Kpnb1,Lmnb1,Myo6,Nup50,Nup62,Lypla1, Ranbp2,Tmpo,Sumo1,Ybx1,Txnl4a,Rif1,Plrg1,Gtpbp4, Nup93,Cenpv,Rcc1,Xpo1,Tpr,Zc3hc1
U2-type catalytic step 2 spliceosome	Nucleus	20	Eftud2,Snrpb,Snrpb2,Snrpd1,Snrpe,Prpf19,Plrg1, Snw1,Snrnp40,Crnkl1,Snrpd3,Snrpg,Bcas2,Ppil1,Snrpa1, Snrpf,Cdc5l,Srrm2,Snrpd2,Prpf8
U4/U6 x U5 tri-snRNP complex	Nucleus	19	Eftud2,Snrpb,Snrpd1,Snrpe,Txnl4a,Lsm2,Usp39,Ppih, Snrpd3,Snrpg,Prpf6,Snrpf,Prpf4,Prpf3,Ddx23,Lsm8, Snrpd2,Prpf8,Snrnp200
Cajal body	Nucleus	17	Cdk2,Coil,Ewsr1,Fbl,Smn1,Eftud2,Snrpc,Zpr1, Hnrnpa2b1,Sart3,Nop58,Prpf4,Prpf3,Nolc1,Srrm2,Dkc1,Gemin4

(Continued)

Table 18.1 (Continued)

RNP complex	Compartment	N	Genes
U2 snRNP	Nucleus	15	Snrpb,Snrpb2,Snrpd1,Snrpe,Sf3b5,Snrpd3,Sf3a1, U2surp,Snrpg,Snrpa1,Sf3a3,Sf3b1,Sf3b3,Snrpd2,Sf3b2
U1 snRNP	Nucleus	15	Snrpc,Snrnp70,Snrpb,Snrpb2,Snrpd1,Snrpe,Snrpa, Prpf40a,Luc7l,Snrpd3,Luc7l3,Snrpg,Snrpf,Snrpd2,Luc7l2
U12-type spliceosomal complex	Nucleus	14	Dhx15,Snrpb,Snrpd1,Snrpe,Ybx1,Sf3b5,Snrpd3, Snrpg,Snrpf,Sf3b1,Sf3b3,Snrpd2,Sf3b4,Sf3b2
U5 snRNP	Nucleus	11	Snrpb,Snrpd1,Snrpe,Txnl4a,Snrpd3,Snrpg,Prpf6,Ddx23,Snrpd2, Prpf8,Snrnp200
nuclear pore	Nucleus	11	Kpnb1,Myo1c,Nup50,Nup62,Ran,Ranbp1,Ranbp2, Xpo7,Nup93,Tpr,Eif5a
U2-type prespliceosome	Nucleus	10	Snrnp70,Snrpb,U2af2,Prpf40a,Luc7l,Sf3a1,Luc7l3,Snrpg,Sf3b1, Luc7l2
telomerase holoenzyme complex	Nucleus	10	Hnrnpc,Snrpb,Snrpe,Hnrnpu,Nhp2,Ptges3,Snrpd3,Gar1,Nat10, Dkc1
precatalytic spliceosome	Nucleus	9	Snrpd1,Snrpe,Lsm2,Sf3b5,Snrpd3,Snrpg, Lsm8,Snrpd2,Sf3b2
U4 snRNP	Nucleus	8	Snrpb,Snrpd1,Snrpe,Ddx39b,Snrpd3,Snrpg,Snrpf,Snrpd2
PML body	Nucleus	8	Eif3e,Rpa2,Ube2i,Sumo1,Park7,Rpa1,Basp1,Sirt1
nuclear chromosome	Nucleus	8	Smc2,H3f3a,Hmga2,Top1,Top2a,Ik,Hnrnpu,Ncapd2
exon–exon junction complex	Nucleus	8	Magoh,Upf1,Alyref,Acin1,Rbm8a,Srsf1,Eif4a3,Thrap3
RNA polymerase II transcription regulator complex	Nucleus	7	Cbx3,Hmga1,Hnrnpab,Trim28,Hnrnpu,Nono,Sfpq
MLL1 complex	Nucleus	7	Hcfc1,Ruvbl2,Ash2l,Ruvbl1,Pelp1,Senp3,Wdr5
transcription export complex	Nucleus	6	Alyref,Ddx39b,Sarnp,Chtop,Zc3h11a,Thoc6
small nuclear ribonucleoprotein complex	Nucleus	6	Snrpb2,Snrpf,Nolc1,Sf3b1,Snrpd2,Prpf8
Paraspeckles	Nucleus	6	Nono,Pspc1,Nudt21,Sfpq,Hnrnpm,Cpsf6
mRNA cleavage and polyadenylation specificity factor complex	Nucleus	6	Fip1l1,Nudt21,Ssu72,Cpsf1,Cpsf7,Cpsf6
condensed nuclear chromosome	Nucleus	6	Ttn,Dnmt3l,Brd4,Rpa1,Rcc1,Ago3
U7 snRNP	Nucleus	5	Snrpb,Snrpe,Snrpd3,Snrpg,Snrpf
U2-type catalytic step 1 spliceosome	Nucleus	5	Prpf19,Rbm8a,Prpf8,Eif4a3,Snrnp200

Table 18.1 (Continued)

RNP complex	Compartment	N	Genes
histone deacetylase complex	Nucleus	5	Rbbp4,Tbl1x,Mta2,Rbbp7,Hdac1
Set1C/COMPASS complex	Nucleus	4	Hcfc1,Ash2l,Dpy30,Wdr5
pronucleus	Nucleus	4	Eed,Hnrnpc,Hnrnpl,Ncapd2
nuclear inner membrane	Nucleus	4	Lmnb1,Tra2b,Tmpo,Sirt1
histone methyltransferase complex	Nucleus	4	Hcfc1,Ash2l,Dpy30,Wdr5
box H/ACA snoRNP complex	Nucleus	4	Nhp2,Gar1,Nolc1,Dkc1
U6 snRNP	Nucleus	3	Lsm2,Ddx39b,Lsm8
U4/U6 snRNP	Nucleus	3	Sart3,Ppih,Prpf4
spliceosomal tri-snRNP complex	Nucleus	3	Snrpd1,Snrpd3,Snrpg
post-mRNA release spliceosomal complex	Nucleus	3	Myef2,Crnkl1,Hnrnpm
perichromatin fibrils	Nucleus	3	Dhx9,Tardbp,Cpsf6
nuclear exosome (RNase complex)	Nucleus	3	Exosc6,Dis3,Exosc4
NuA4 histone acetyltransferase complex	Nucleus	3	Ruvbl2,Actl6a,Ruvbl1
nBAF complex	Nucleus	3	Smarcc1,Smarce1,Smarcd1
mRNA cleavage factor complex	Nucleus	3	Nudt21,Cpsf7,Cpsf6
MLL3/4 complex	Nucleus	3	Ash2l,Dpy30,Wdr5
interchromatin granule	Nucleus	3	Srsf2,Tardbp,Cpsf6
histone pre-mRNA 3′-end processing complex	Nucleus	3	Snrpb,Ybx1,Syncrip
histone acetyltransferase complex	Nucleus	3	Hcfc1,Ogt,Wdr5
delta DNA polymerase complex	Nucleus	3	Pold1,Pold2,Pold3
commitment complex	Nucleus	3	Snrpd1,U2af2,Snrpd3

(Continued)

Table 18.1 (Continued)

RNP complex	Compartment	N	Genes
chromatin silencing complex	Nucleus	3	Eed,Sirt1,Smarca5
box H/ACA telomerase RNP complex	Nucleus	3	Nhp2,Gar1,Dkc1
U2AF complex	Nucleus	2	U2af2,U2af1
U2-type spliceosomal complex	Nucleus	2	Sf3a1,Sf3b2
supraspliceosomal complex	Nucleus	2	Rbmxl1,Upf1
RNA polymerase III complex	Nucleus	2	Polr1c,Polr2e
RNA polymerase II, core complex	Nucleus	2	Polr2c,Polr2e
RNA polymerase I complex	Nucleus	2	Polr1c,Polr2e
NURF complex	Nucleus	2	Rbbp4,Smarca5
nucleoplasmic periphery of the nuclear pore complex	Nucleus	2	Hnrnpc,Hnrnpa1
cyclin/CDK positive transcription elongation factor complex	Nucleus	2	Brd4,Snw1
U2-type post-mRNA release spliceosomal complex	Nucleus	1	Dhx15
transcription factor TFIIH holo complex	Nucleus	1	Psmc5
transcription factor TFIID complex	Nucleus	1	Tceal
TRAMP complex	Nucleus	1	Zcchc8
THO complex part of transcription export complex	Nucleus	1	Thoc6
RNA polymerase II, holoenzyme	Nucleus	1	Myo6
RNA polymerase II transcription repressor complex	Nucleus	1	Ddx20
nucleolar ribonuclease P complex	Nucleus	1	Pop1

Table 18.1 (Continued)

RNP complex	Compartment	N	Genes
mRNA cleavage stimulating factor complex	Nucleus	1	Cstf1
mRNA cap methyltransferase complex	Nucleus	1	Rnmt
VCP-NPL4-UFD1 AAA ATPase complex	Endoplasmic Reticulum	5	Faf1,Nploc4,Ubxn7,Ubxn1,Vcp
cytosolic large ribosomal subunit	Cytoplasm	38	Rplp0,Rpl10a,Rpl18,Rpl21,Rpl26,Rpl27,Rpl28,Rpl30,Rpl32,Rpl37a,Rpl36a,Rpl6,Rpl7,Rpl9,Rps12,Rpl13a,Rpl27a,Rpl8,Rpl7a,Rpl3,Rpl36,Rplp1,Rpl35a,Rpl23,Rpl35,Rpl14,Rplp2,Rpl38,Rpl4,Rpl24,Rpl18a,Rpl10,Rpl31,Rpl23a,Rpl12,Rpl13,Rpl17,Rpl5
cytosolic small ribosomal subunit	Cytoplasm	31	Ddx3x,Rpsa,Rps2,Rps12,Rps14,Rps15,Rps16,Rps17,Rps19,Rps24,Rps4x,Rps5,Rps6,Rps7,Rps8,Rps3,Rps11,Rps26,Rps28,Rps27,Rps23,Rps21,Rps10,Rps20,Rps27l,Rps13,Rps9,Rps27a,D1Pas1,Eif2a,Rps15a
cytoplasmic ribonucleoprotein granule	Cytoplasm	29	Rplp0,Ddx6,Dhx9,Eif4e,Fxr1,Mov10,Ncl,Pabpc1,Psmc2,Rac1,Rpl28,Rpl6,Rps4x,Rps6,Smn1,Snrpb2,Tuba1a,Tubb5,Fxr2,Pcbp1,Iqgap1,Hnrnpu,Sarnp,Chtop,Poldip3,Ago3,Edc4,Ago1,Ago2
polysomal ribosome	Cytoplasm	24	Dhx9,Eef2,Rpl10a,Rpl18,Rpl30,Rpl32,Rpl36a,Rpl6,Rpl8,Rpl7a,Rps26,Rps28,Rpl36,Rps23,Rps21,Rpl38,Eif3h,Rpl24,Nufip2,Larp1,Rpl18a,Rpl31,Btf3,Abcf1
cytoplasmic stress granule	Cytoplasm	22	Ddx3x,Ddx6,Eif2s1,Ddx19a,Eif4e,Hnrnpk,Elavl1,Kpnb1,Khsrp,Kpna2,Pabpc1,Rbpms,Ybx1,G3bp2,G3bp1,Caprin1,Nufip2,Larp1,Ddx1,D1Pas1,Igf2bp1,Vcp
P-body	Cytoplasm	19	Ddx6,Eif4e,Mov10,Psma2,Psmc2,Psmc3,Top1,Psma4,Psma6,Lsm2,Caprin1,Dcps,Tnrc6b,Tnrc6c,Tnrc6a,Cnot1,Edc4,Ago1,Ago2
SMN-Sm protein complex	Cytoplasm	15	Smn1,Snrpb,Snrpd1,Snrpe,Strap,Ddx20,Gemin2,Gemin6,Snrpd3,Snrpg,Gemin7,Snrpf,Snrpd2,Gemin5,Gemin4
eukaryotic translation initiation factor 3 complex	Cytoplasm	15	Ddx3x,Eif3a,Eif3e,Eif3b,Eif3g,Eif3i,Eif3d,Eif3c,Eif3f,Eif3h,Eif3k,Eif3m,D1Pas1,Eif3l,Eif3j2
Methylosome	Cytoplasm	11	Clns1a,Erh,Prmt1,Snrpb,Snrpd1,Snrpe,Snrpd3,Snrpg,Snrpf,Wdr77,Snrpd2
endoplasmic reticulum-Golgi intermediate compartment	Cytoplasm	9	Fn1,Hspa5,Lrpap1,Nucb1,P4hb,Pdia6,Erp44,Rab1b,Dicer1
SMN complex	Cytoplasm	8	Smn1,Strap,Ddx20,Gemin2,Gemin6,Gemin7,Gemin5,Gemin4

(Continued)

Table 18.1 (Continued)

RNP complex	Compartment	N	Genes
eukaryotic translation initiation factor 3 complex, eIF3m	Cytoplasm	8	Eif3a,Eif3b,Eif3i,Eif3d,Eif3c,Eif3f,Eif3h,Eif3m
pICln-Sm protein complex	Cytoplasm	6	Clns1a,Snrpd1,Snrpe,Snrpd3,Snrpf,Snrpd2
CRD-mediated mRNA stability complex	Cytoplasm	6	Dhx9,Ybx1,Hnrnpu,Syncrip,Igf2bp1,Csde1
P granule	Cytoplasm	4	Ddx3x,Mov10,Snrpg,D1Pas1
eukaryotic translation initiation factor 2 complex	Cytoplasm	4	Eif2s1,Eif2s3x,Eif2s2,Eif2a
signal recognition particle, endoplasmic reticulum targeting	Cytoplasm	3	Srp14,Srp72,Srp68
cytoplasmic exosome (RNase complex)	Cytoplasm	3	Exosc6,Dis3,Exosc4
chromatoid body	Cytoplasm	3	Ddx6,Eif4e,Nsun2
ribonucleoside-diphosphate reductase complex	Cytoplasm	2	Rrm1,Rrm2
phenylalanine-tRNA ligase complex	Cytoplasm	2	Farsb,Farsa
neuronal ribonucleoprotein granule	Cytoplasm	2	Hnrnpa2b1,Ckap5
nascent polypeptide-associated complex	Cytoplasm	2	Naca,Btf3
eukaryotic translation initiation factor 4F complex	Cytoplasm	2	Eif4e,Eif4g1
eukaryotic translation initiation factor 2B complex	Cytoplasm	2	Eif2s1,Eif2b4
eukaryotic 43S preinitiation complex	Cytoplasm	2	Eif1,Eif3h

Table 18.1 (Continued)

RNP complex	Compartment	N	Genes
eukaryotic translation initiation factor 3 complex, eIF3e	Cytoplasm	1	Eif3a
eukaryotic translation elongation factor 1 complex	Cytoplasm	1	Eef1d
eukaryotic 80S initiation complex	Cytoplasm	1	Rpl38
eukaryotic 48S preinitiation complex	Cytoplasm	1	Eif2s1
extracellular exosome	Extracellular region	25	Actg1,Alb,Aldoa,Anxa2,Cd9,Fn1,Hspa8,Hspd1, Hspa4,Ide,Anxa1,Pdcd6ip,Plaa,Tfrc,Tsg101,Ybx1, Nsun2,Hnrnpa2b1,Ahnak,Acy1,Clic1,Dicer1, Bag6,Ago2,Gars
catalytic step 2 spliceosome	Nucleus	52	Ddx5,Frg1,Hnrnpc,Hnrnpa1,Hnrnpk,Magoh, Pabpc1,Eftud2,Snrpb,Snrpb2,Snrpd1,Snrpe, Alyref,Lsm2,Prpf19,Srrm1,Hnrnpu,Plrg1, Hnrnpa2b1,Syncrip,Hnrnph1,Rbm8a,Snw1, Snrnp40,Crnkl1,Cwc27,Snrpd3,Sf3a1,Snrpg, Bcas2,Ppil1,Prpf6,Snrpa1,Snrpf,Zcchc8,Cdc5l, Hnrnpr,Ddx23,Sf3a3,Srrm2,Hnrnpm,Sf3b1, Hnrnpf,Sf3b3,Snrpd2,U2af1,Srsf1,Prpf8,Eif4a3, Hnrnpa3,Sf3b2,Snrnp200
nuclear envelope	Nucleus	29	Parp1,Anxa11,Anxa7,Apoe,Bax,Calr,Cbx3,Dync1h1, Faf1,Kpnb1,Lmnb1,Nup62,Pafah1b1,Ran,Ranbp2, Rrm1,Rrm2,S100a6,Tmpo,Rtcb,Chmp2a, Nup93,Sirt1,Tpr,Cse1l,Clic1,Abcf1,Ipo7,Gpx4

axon development (Livneh et al. 2020; Salamon and Rasin 2021; Szeto et al. 2021). RBPs and their role in energy metabolic and enzymatic pathways have also been highlighted, and numerous possible links are to be investigated (Castello et al. 2015; Ho et al. 2020). The primary and abundant classes of known RNA types in eukaryotes include tRNAs, ribosomal RNAs, small nuclear RNAs (snRNAs), small nucleolar RNAs (snoRNAs), mRNAs, small noncoding RNAs (sRNAs), and long noncoding RNAs (lncRNAs). RNA Polymerase (Pol) I controls rRNA transcription, whereas Pol III controls tRNAs, snRNAs, and snoRNAs (Lesniewska and Boguta 2017; Scull and Schneider 2019). The RNA-Pol II complex in the form of a membrane-less organelle regulates the transcription of mRNAs, miRNAs, and lncRNAs, followed by capping, splicing, editing, and polyadenylation in the nucleus (Girbig et al. 2022; Rippe and Papantonis 2022).

The Argonaute complex composes a significant portion of the LIS1-RBP-interactome. MicroRNAs and miRNPs coordinate pleiotropic functions in the early stages and nervous system development (Cho et al. 2019; Kosik and Nowakowski 2018; Prieto-Colomina et al. 2021; Zolboot et al. 2021). It

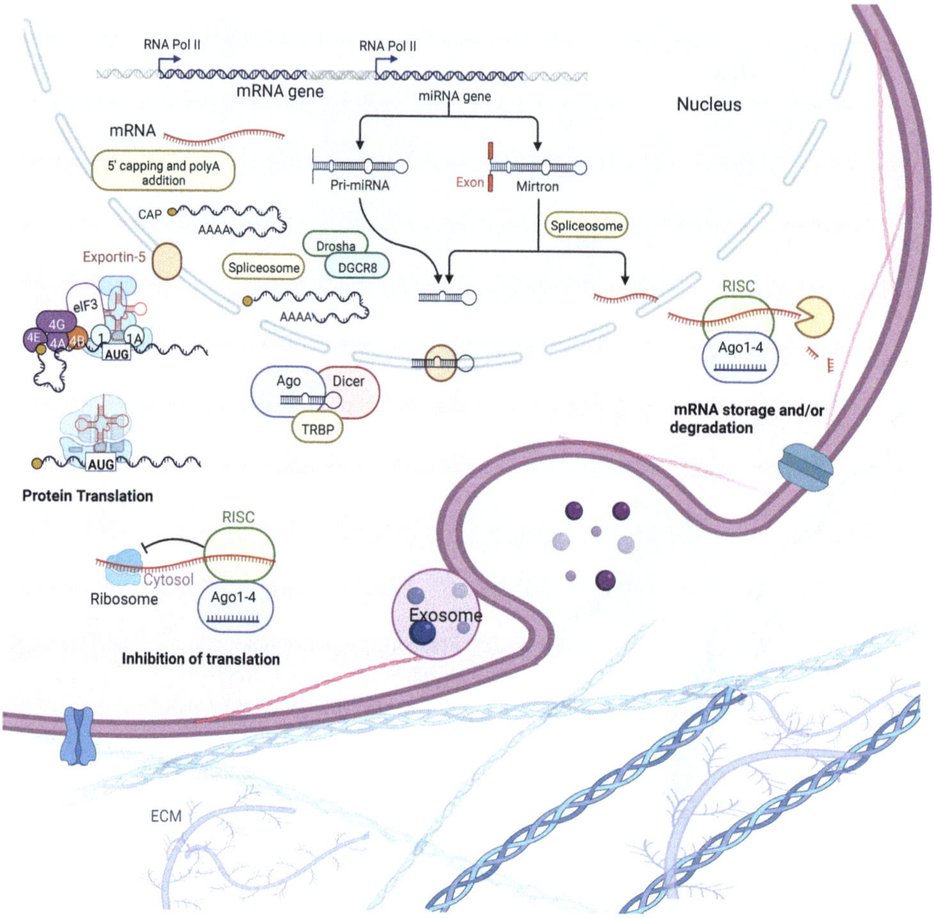

Figure 18.1 Schematic presentation of the processes LIS1 associated RBPs and RNA binding functions in different cellular compartments. LIS1 can be detected in the nucleus, affecting mRNA and small RNA transcription and splicing. LIS1 can be seen in the cytoplasm with the Dicer and RISC complexes and in association with many eukaryotic initiation factors (eIFs) and ribosomal proteins, among others. In addition, LIS1 can be detected in complex with exosomal proteins and affects the composition of the extracellular matrix (ECM). The figure was created with BioRender.com.

is conspicuous that the ablation of *Ago2, Dicer1*, and *Dgcr8* shows a dosage effect in gene expression, and complete knockout results in early embryonic lethality (Bernstein et al. 2003; Liu et al. 2004; Wang et al. 2007). Mutations in the genes involved in the machinery of microRNA processing and RNA-inducing silencing complexes like MECP2, DGCR8, DROSHA, DICER, and AGO2 are also associated with developmental and neurological defects (Barish et al. 2022; Cheng et al. 2014; Huang et al. 2022; Karayiorgou et al. 2010; Luhur et al. 2014; Urdinguio et al. 2010). They are known to regulate neurogenesis in miRNA-dependent and independent ways. RBPs like FMRP, SMAUG2, PTBP1, ARPP21, LIN28, PUMILIO2, STAUFEN2, ELAVL4, YTHDF, and FMRP are associated with neurodevelopmental disorders (Schieweck et al. 2021). Splicing factors like HNRNPU and RBFOX1 have been recognized as necessary for maintaining progenitor niche during neurogenesis (Du et al. 2014; Sapir et al. 2022).

18.4.1 RNA Transcription and Splicing

Initiation of transcription and formation of nascent or pre-mRNAs are mediated by DNA templated translocation of RNA polymerase II together with a 5'-end cap-binding complex and 3′-end polyadenylation complex. LIS1 interacts with several proteins of the RNA polymerase II transcription regulator complex, suggesting that LIS1 dosage may affect gene transcription (Table 18.1 and Figure 18.1), which was evident in our findings (Kshirsagar et al. 2022). DNA topoisomerases create transient double-stranded breaks during the transcriptional cycle to relieve supercoiling, which facilitates RNA Pol II occupancy and reduces torsional stress promoting efficient transcription continuation. Following transcription initiation, RNA:DNA hybrids induce pausing of RNA Pol II, and the pause release includes the recruitment of the PAF1 complex and others (Abuhashem et al. 2022; Chen et al. 2018). The resulting RNA polymerase activity at promoters has a proclivity to generate small RNAs through DGCR8/DROSHA independent and DICER/AGO2 dependent mechanisms (Zamudio et al. 2014). LIS1 interacts with most of the proteins in the Argonaute complex, and LIS1 dosage affects the expression of multiple miRs. Many LIS1 binding sites were nearby and enriched with highly expressed miRNA in the genome (Kshirsagar et al. 2022). The AGO-TNRC6-DDX21 complex may help release paused Pol II and miRNA-mediated transcription activation (Ohno et al. 2022).

The pre-mRNAs contain introns removed by a supramacromolecular RNP spliceosome assembly and are marked by an exon junction complex. The spliceosome assembly is sequential and directed by the intron's 5′ and 3′ ends, followed by a two-step transesterification catalysis. The U1, U2, U4, U5, and U6 snRNPs are five components of the spliceosome assembly. LIS1 strongly interacts with the many U-snRNPs (Table 18.1). Catalytic activity directs the ligation of the 5′ exon to the 3′ exon and the excised intron lariat with post-catalytic spliceosome complex P and intron lariat spliceosome (Bertram et al. 2017; Haselbach et al. 2018; Herzel et al. 2017; Zhan et al. 2022; Zhang et al. 2019). LIS1 binds RNA mainly in introns, and the RNA-binding mapping is strongly enriched for U1-binding sites (Kshirsagar et al. 2022). LIS1 binds to RNA in the intronic regions like RBFOX2 and QKI towards the exon donor site regulating splicing. We further detected that LIS1 dosage affects RNA splicing, including intron retention events. Intron retention is a specific mechanism that correlates with reduced gene expression (Pimentel et al. 2016; Yap et al. 2012). RNA Pol II pausing and processing speed at various sites throughout the genome are known to influence the intron-exon splicing and polyadenylation (polyA) outcome (Muniz et al. 2021). DNA methylation levels and CTCF and MECP2 occupancy also control the kinetics of RNA polymerase II stalling to regulate exon-intron skipping or inclusion (Maunakea et al. 2013; Shukla et al. 2011; Wong et al. 2017). MECP2, another LIS1-binding protein, is a methyl CpG DNA binding protein, and mutations in *MECP2* cause RETT syndrome (Keidar et al. 2019). MECP2 is highly expressed in differentiated neurons compared to ESCs and is essential for neuronal activity. The deposition of m6A modifications by the METTL3-METTL14 complex influences transcript stability. The binding of YTHDC1 at m6A sites in intronic splice junctions contributes to faster splicing and regulates alternative splicing through SRSF factors (Gehring and Roignant 2021). mRNAs with retained intron undergo rapid nuclear degradation through not well-known mechanisms and may involve independent quality-control mechanisms through the 5′ and 3′ decay due to XRN1 and XRN2 exonucleases, TRAMP complex, and RNA exosomes, which are strongly present in the LIS1 interactome (Table 18.1 and Figure 18.1) (Vanacova and Stefl 2007; Zinder and Lima 2017).

18.4.2 RNA Polyadenylation and Export

The first step in mRNA packaging is the addition of a 5′ cap. The 5′ cap is a modified guanosine nucleotide that is added to the 5′ end of the mRNA. The 5′ cap protects the mRNA from degradation by exonucleases and helps to ensure that it is adequately localized within cells (Galloway and Cowling 2019). Adding a 5′ cap also affects the stability of an mRNA. After being capped, the mRNA is polyadenylated at the 3′ end. The 3′ end of the newly formed transcript is processed by adding a string of adenosines called polyadenylation. The poly(A) tail protects the mRNA from degradation by exonucleases and helps to ensure that it is appropriately localized within the cell. This event is catalyzed by enzymes called polyA polymerases. LIS1 interacts with several components of the poly(A)-binding proteins (PABP) complex that binds to the template RNA near the polyadenylation site and helps stabilize the interaction between the RNA and the polymerase. LIS1 also interacts with cleavage and polyadenylation specificity factor (CPSF) components. The binding of CPSF also helps to recruit other factors needed for cleavage and polyadenylation, including cleavage factor (CF) and cleavage stimulation factor (CstF). The binding of these proteins leads to a conformational change in CPSF that allows it to cleave the phosphodiester bond between the penultimate adenosine nucleotide and the 3′ end of the mRNA. This cleavage step is essential for releasing the newly processed mRNA from the template RNA (Casanal et al. 2017; Clerici et al. 2018; Passmore and Coller 2022; Stewart 2019).

The LIS1 interactome also implies that it may be involved in mRNA and mRNPs export. The export of mRNA from the nucleus is highly coordinated and consists of the transport by Exportin-5 through the nuclear pore complex (NPC) into the cytoplasm. The NPC is a large complex of proteins that forms a channel through which proteins and RNAs can move between the nucleus and the cytoplasm. The binding of Exportin-5 to an mRNA promotes the release of Ran-GTP, which is thought to help disassemble the mRNP and allow it to pass through the NPC for translation or degradation (De Magistris 2021).

18.4.3 Protein Translation

We further detected the interaction of LIS1 with multiple ribosomal subunits, tRNA synthetases, and the translation initiation complex (Table 18.1 and Figure 18.1). Future experiments are directed to test the role of LIS1 in these processes. Translation initiation is a complex process that occurs when the small subunit of the ribosome binds to the start codon of an mRNA molecule. The ribosome comprises two subunits, the large subunit and the small subunit. The small subunit contains peptidyl transferase activity, which catalyzes the formation of peptide bonds between amino acids. The large subunit contains the binding sites for tRNA molecules and the start codon of the mRNA. The initiator tRNA is the most important factor in translation initiation. This tRNA binds to the start codon of the mRNA and delivers the first amino acid to the ribosome. tRNA molecules during translation initiation carry amino acids to the small subunit of the ribosome, where they are incorporated into the nascent peptide chain. This process is mediated by enzymes called aminoacyl-tRNA synthetases (aaRSs). These enzymes attach the correct amino acid to its cognate tRNA. The aaRS enzymes recognize the correct amino acid by its chemical structure and then attach it to the 3′ ends of the appropriate tRNA molecule via an ester bond. The aaRS enzymes play a crucial role in protein synthesis, ensuring that the correct amino acid is attached to the tRNA molecule. Without these enzymes, the translation would be inaccurate, and proteins would not be able to function correctly. There are 20 different aaRS enzymes, each responsible for attaching a specific amino acid to its cognate tRNA. The aaRS enzymes are divided into two groups: class I and class II. Class I aaRS enzymes are responsible for attaching amino acids with a hydrophobic side chain, while class II aaRS enzymes are responsible for attaching amino acids with a charged side chain (Ibba and Söll 2000; Musier-Forsyth 2019). In addition to the aaRS enzymes, several other proteins are involved in protein synthesis. There are two types of translation initiation: cap-dependent and cap-independent. In general, eukaryotic cells prefer cap-dependent translation initiation. Cap-dependent translation initiation requires the presence of a 7-methylguanosine (m7G) cap at the 5′ end of the mRNA. The m7G cap is recognized by a protein complex called the eukaryotic initiation factor 4F (eIF4F), which then recruits the small ribosomal subunit to the mRNA. Cap-independent translation initiation does not require the presence of an m7G cap. Instead, this type of translation initiation relies on the presence of specific sequence elements, called internal ribosome entry sites (IRESs), in the mRNA. IRESs are recognized by IRES-binding proteins (IBPs), which then recruit the small ribosomal subunit to the mRNA. While cap-independent translation initiation is less efficient than cap-dependent, it can be used when the m7G cap is absent or damaged (Merrick and Pavitt 2018). The translation initiation complex is assembled on the mRNA in a stepwise fashion. The eIF3 complex is a large protein complex that helps to recruit the ribosome to the mRNA. This complex consists of 11 subunits: eIF3a, eIF3b, eIF3c, eIF3d, eIF3e, eIF3f, eIF3g, eIF3h, eIF3i, eIF3j, and PRP4. eIF3a binds to the small subunit, while eIF3b, eIF3c, eIF3d, and eIF3e bind to the large subunit. eIF3f, eIF3g, and eIF3h are required to bind tRNA to the ribosome. Finally, eIF3i and eIF3j are regulatory subunits that modulate the activity of the complex (Aitken and Lorsch 2012; Guca and Hashem 2018). The eukaryotic translation initiation factor 2 subunit 1 (eIF2S1) and eIF2S2 are GTPase-activating proteins (GAPs) that regulate the activity of the translation initiation factor 2 (eIF2). This factor is a key player in protein synthesis, as it helps to position the initiator tRNA at the start codon of the mRNA. eIF2S1 and eIF2S2 act as GAPs by hydrolyzing GTP to GDP. This process reduces the activity of eIF2 and slows down protein synthesis. In addition, eIF2S1 and eIF2S2 also help to keep the ribosome in its inactive state. The eIF4A /eIF4B-RNA helicases are involved in the unwinding of structured mRNAs. The eukaryotic translation initiation factor 4A (eIF4A) and eIF4B are RNA helicases that play a role in protein synthesis by unwinding structured mRNAs, thus enabling the ribosome to access the start codon. eIF4A and eIF4B work together to form a complex that can bind to and unwind double-stranded RNAs. In addition, eIF4A can bind to and unwind single-stranded RNAs. The eukaryotic translation initiation factor 4G (eIF4G) is a protein scaffold required to assemble the translation initiation complex. This complex consists of the initiator tRNA, the translation factors eIF2 and eIF4F. Without eIF4G this complex would not be able to form correctly, and protein synthesis would be disrupted. The eukaryotic translation initiation factor 5B (eIF5B) is an ATPase that provides the energy needed to recycle translation factors. This process is necessary for the translation factor eIF2 to be reused. In addition to the proteins mentioned above, several other factors play a role in translation initiation (Jackson et al. 2010).

18.4.4 mRNA Stability and Degradation

mRNA stability affects gene expression. The half-life of an mRNA can range from minutes to hours, depending on the particular transcript. Several factors have been shown to affect mRNA stability, including the length of the polyA tail, the sequence of the 3′ UTR (untranslated region), and the presence of modifications (Menezes et al. 2018; Passmore and Coller 2022). Adding a polyA tail to the 3′ end of an mRNA increases its stability by protecting it from degradation by exonucleases. In general, mRNAs with long 3′ UTRs are more stable than mRNAs with short 3′ UTRs. This is because mRNAs with long 3′ UTRs have more opportunities to form secondary structures that protect them from degradation (Wu and Bartel 2017). Another modification that can occur at the 3′ end of an mRNA is the addition of a uridine nucleotide (U) to the 3′ end of the transcript. This modification is known as U-tailoring and typically occurs in mRNAs destined for export from the nucleus to the cytoplasm. U-tailoring has been shown to affect mRNAs' localization, translation, and stability (Lee et al. 2014). mRNA decay is a highly regulated process that is essential for the proper control of gene expression. All major mRNA decay pathways characterized thus far in eukaryotes are initiated by deadenylation, that is, shortening of the mRNA 3′ poly(A) tail by PAN2-PAN3 and CCR4-NOT complexes (Chen et al. 2009; Inada and Makino 2014; Takahashi et al. 2020; Wahle and Winkler 2013; Yi et al. 2018). Our data suggest that LIS1 may participate in the three major pathways of mRNA decay. The three pathways are the exosome-mediated pathway, the microRNA-mediated pathway, and the nonsense-mediated pathway (Schoenberg and Maquat 2012). All three pathways play essential roles in mRNA decay, depending on the particular cell type and context. The exosome-mediated pathway is the most well-characterized primary pathway responsible for the degradation of mRNAs in cells. This pathway involves mRNA degradation by a complex of proteins called the exosome. The exosome is a large complex of proteins responsible for the degradation of various RNA molecules, including mRNAs. The exosome recognizes and binds to mRNAs that contain specific sequence motifs, such as AU-rich elements (AREs). Once attached to an mRNA, the exosome degrades the transcript by cleaving it at particular sites. The exosome proteins responsible for degrading mRNAs are distinct in nuclear and cytoplasmic exosomes (Houseley et al. 2006; Kilchert et al. 2016; Vanacova and Stefl 2007). LIS1 is also identified as a constituent of exosome or extracellular vesicles (Kugeratski et al. 2021). Association with RBPs, such as Annexin A1 and A2, MVP, ELAVL1 (HuR), HNRNPA2B1, YBX1, SYNCRIP, and lupus La protein can affect the packaging of RNAs into exosome- or endosome-derived extracellular vesicles (O'Brien et al. 2020). Several studies have indicated that miRNAs and AGO2 processing machinery are part of different classes of extracellular vesicles (Groot and Lee 2020; Jeppesen et al. 2019; Liu et al. 2021; Murillo et al. 2019). A separate study has also established that over-expression of the KRAS oncogene promotes the sorting of AGO2-associated miRNAs into extracellular vesicles downstream of ERK signaling (McKenzie et al. 2016). The microRNA-mediated pathway involves the degradation of mRNA by small RNA molecules called microRNAs (miRNAs). MiRNAs are short (~22 nucleotides long) RNA molecules that bind to mRNAs and target them for degradation. The microRNA-mediated pathway of mRNA decay involves binding microRNAs (miRNAs) to mRNAs. miRNAs are small RNA molecules that play essential roles in regulating gene expression. miRNAs typically bind to mRNAs that contain complementary sequences and inhibit their translation. However, in some cases, miRNAs can also promote the degradation of mRNAs. The binding of a miRNA to an mRNA encourages the recruitment of proteins that degrade the transcript. The best-characterized proteins involved in this process are the Argonautes (AGO1-4) and TNRC6A-C (Jonas and Izaurralde 2015; Pawlica et al. 2020). The nonsense-mediated decay (NMD) pathway involves mRNA degradation by a protein called UPF1. UPF1, with SMG1, SMG8, SMG9, and RNPS1, forms the NMD complex. The function of the NMD complex is to recognize and bind to mRNAs that contain premature stop codons. Once attached to an mRNA, the NMD complex initiates transcript degradation (Kurosaki et al. 2019; Lykke-Andersen and Jensen 2015). Mammalian mRNA degradation occurs in both the nucleus and cytoplasm (Schoenberg and Maquat 2012; Stavast and Erkeland 2019). In the nucleus, mRNA degradation is primarily mediated by the exosome-mediated pathway (Kilchert et al. 2016). In the cytoplasm, mRNA degradation is mediated mainly by the microRNA-mediated pathway (Jonas and Izaurralde 2015; Leung 2015). The different mechanisms of mRNA degradation in the nucleus and cytoplasm are thought to be due to the various roles of these two compartments in gene expression and protein synthesis.

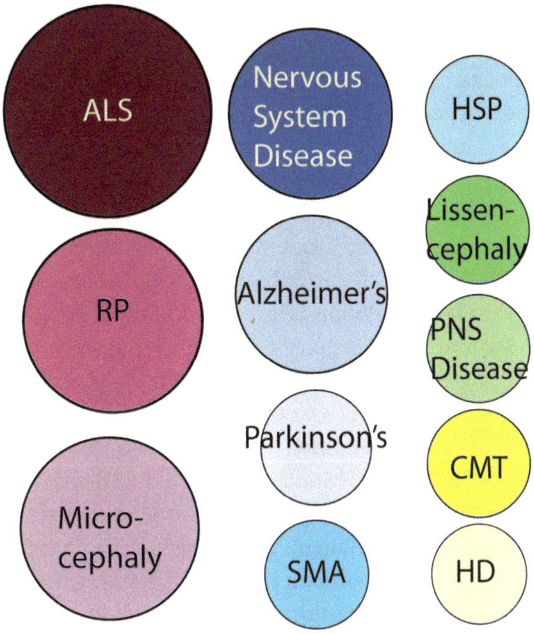

Figure 18.2 The LIS1 interactome and nervous system-related diseases. The LIS1 interactome was subjected to GeneAnalytics analysis, and the disease output was plotted according to the relative scores. The top scores revealed relatedness to ALS (Amyotrophic lateral sclerosis), RP (Retinitis pigmentosa), and microcephaly. The LIS1 interactome was associated in general with nervous system diseases, including Alzheimer's, Parkinson's, SMA (spinal muscular atrophy), HSP (hereditary spastic paraplegia), lissencephaly, PNS (peripheral nervous system disease), CMT (Charcot-Marie-Tooth), and HD (Huntington disease).

We next mapped the LIS1 interactome to known nervous-system-related diseases using GeneAnalytics (Ben-Ari Fuchs et al. 2016) (Figure 18.2). The LIS1 interactome was highly enriched in nervous system disease-associated genes. These diseases include developmental diseases such as lissencephaly and microcephaly, early onset neurodegenerative diseases such as spinal muscular atrophy (SMA), and late onset neurodegenerative diseases such as Alzheimer's and Parkinson's disease.

18.5 LIS1 and Mechanotransduction

Human *LIS1* mutations were generated using CRISPR-based strategies or by reprogramming lissencephaly or MDS patient fibroblast (Bershteyn et al. 2017; Iefremova et al. 2017; Karzbrun et al. 2018; Kim et al. 2014; Kshirsagar et al. 2022). Though difficult to achieve, studies show that it is possible to rescue the ring chromosome or large chromosomal deletion defects by reprogramming MDS patients' fibroblasts to iPSCs with the occurrence of uniparental disomy (Bershteyn et al. 2014).

Mechanotransduction refers to the processes through which cells sense and respond to mechanical stimuli by converting them to biochemical signals that elicit specific cellular responses. During vertebrate development, signaling is mediated through extracellular morphogens like Wnts, FGFs, Hedgehog proteins, and TGFβ superfamily of ligands such as BMP and ACTIVIN/NODAL factors (Hill 2022; Ingham 2022; Mittermeier and Virshup 2022; Ornitz and Itoh 2022). Canonical and non-canonical Wnt signaling show a mechanotransductive effect via mechanically responsive elements downstream of Wnt signaling in early embryo lineage specification and brain development. In canonical Wnt signaling, the β-catenin translocation from the membrane to the nucleus activates downstream genes and depends on Wnt (Albrecht et al. 2021). E-cadherin-based cell adhesion can regulate the expression and translocation of membrane-bound β-catenin for its transcriptional activity (Bhattacharyya et al. 2022; Stockinger et al. 2001). A physical or mechanical strain can regulate β-catenin translocation activity in tissue deformations (Bhattacharyya et al.

2022). In contrast, non-canonical Wnt signaling is directed by the planar cell polarity (PCP) pathway independent of β-catenin through atypical cadherins of PCP components (Humphries and Mlodzik 2018; Koca et al. 2022). Embryonic stem cells (ESCs) have immense potential for sensing morphogen gradients such as Wnt, enabling them as miniature-organ and disease models.

β-catenin viscoelastic mechanics and cadherin-mediated cell crowding are critical in guiding embryonic cell division, peri-implantation, and gastrulation (Alikani 2005; Benham-Pyle et al. 2015; Lecuit and Yap 2015; Valet et al. 2022). Cadherins directed persistent collective cell migration, and sustained β-catenin alters the neuroepithelium emergence (Hari et al. 2002; Herrera et al. 2014; Masek et al. 2016). In the developing brain, loss of E-cadherin in RGs disrupts mitotic cleavage plane orientation affecting adherence junctions of RGs and neuronal migration (Itoh et al. 2013; Martinez-Martinez et al. 2016). In human naïve pluripotent conditions with Wnt inhibition, *LIS1* heterozygous shows increased translocation of B-catenin in the nucleus. *LIS1* +/– compared to control, and over-expression of LIS1 showed a stark change in morphology of ESC colonies and loss of epithelial markers such as E-cadherin. Counter polarized expression of LEFTY genes in LIS1 mutants ESCs indicates that reduced adhesive intensity of the intercellular adhesion has a more substantial influence on cell–cell coordination and a more considerable impact on cell migration persistence. With different levels of LIS1, dose-dependent transcriptomic studies conducted in naïve mouse and human ESCs emphasize the involvement in various regulatory pathways crucial for stem cell homeostasis and differentiation. Approaches taken to model the LIS1 dosage effect in mouse and human ESCs also highlight the importance of LIS1 in cell mechanics coupled to fate (Kshirsagar et al. 2022) (Figure 18.3).

LIS1 is connected to mechanotransduction also through interacting with the Argonaute complex and affecting miRNA expression. The interaction with Argonaute proteins is consistent in mouse ESCs, human ESCs, and the developing mouse brain.

miRNAs have the potential to control the mechanical properties directly or by AGO2 influencing the YAP-Hippo Pathway or the levels of the cytoskeleton-adhesion-ECM regulatory network (Moro et al. 2019). The miRNA 302a/b/c/d-367 cluster is specifically known to regulate the expression of LEFTY and YAP signaling. It is essential in embryogenesis, mammalian ESC pluripotency, and reprogramming (Anokye-Danso et al. 2011; Du et al. 2018; Lipchina et al. 2011; Tian et al. 2015). Mammalian miRNA clusters from DLK1-GTL2 (MEG3-MIRG) imprinted locus play a crucial role in energy homeostasis, cytoskeletal-ECM remodeling, pluripotency, reprogramming, neuronal differentiation, and homeostasis (Benetatos et al. 2013; Huang et al. 2018; Kameswaran et al. 2014; Lin et al. 2003; Mondal et al. 2015; Sanli et al. 2018; Shen et al. 2018; Whipple et al. 2020). LIS1

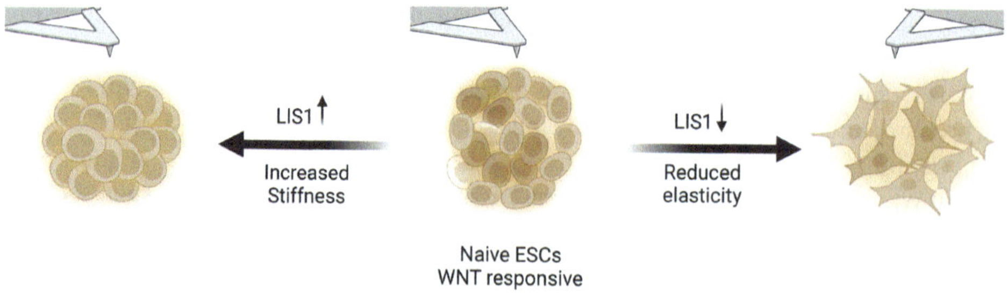

Figure 18.3 LIS1 dosage influences the fates of ESCs. Schematics for measuring physical properties of ESCs with different expression levels of LIS1 using atomic force microscopy (AFM). Modulations in LIS1 dosage and factors influencing Wnt signaling to affect the mechanical fate of ESCs. Created with BioRender.com.

over-expression rescues the mechanical elastic defects and expression of a subset of miRNA from the MEG3-MIRG locus in AGO null ESCs.

18.6 Modeling Cortical Folds and Lissencephaly in Human Brain Organoid Models

Conventionally, LIS1 knockout mice are embryonic lethal around implantation, but a vast amount of our understanding regarding LIS1 in early development and neuronal functions is from studies conducted in mice models (Bi et al. 2009; Cahana et al. 2001, 2003; Dominguez-Sala et al. 2022b; Garcia-Lopez et al. 2021; Hirotsune et al. 1998; Moore et al. 2012; Penisson et al. 2022; Valdes-Sanchez et al. 2007). The neuroepithelial cells, also called neural stem cells (NESCs) of the developing central nervous system, proliferate through symmetric divisions to form daughter cells. These daughter cells undergo several rounds of self-renewing divisions, ultimately differentiating into apical radial glia (aRGs). These aRGs undergo symmetric and asymmetric divisions with apical-basal interkinetic nuclear movement (INM), contributing to the basal radial glial (bRGs) populations and neuronal progenitors in the ventricular zone. Neurons generated through asymmetric divisions migrate in parallel trajectories along radial glia processes/extensions to situate in different cortical layers (Reiner 2013) (Figure 18.4A). LIS1 is also crucial for defining neuroepithelial

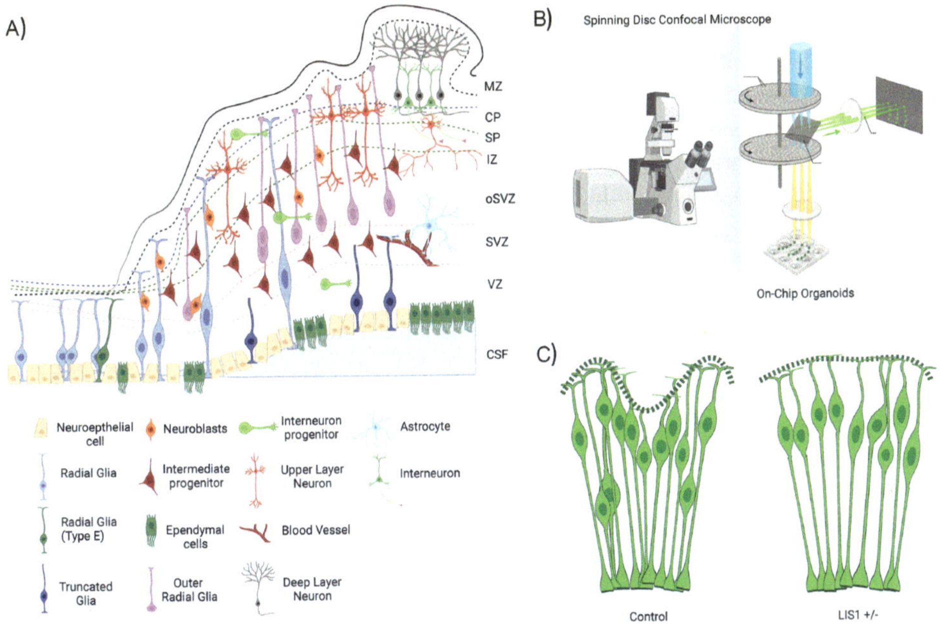

Figure 18.4 (A) Cell lineages during early cortical neurogenesis. Neuroepithelium expansion leads to the generation of several subtypes of radial glia, which undergo symmetric or asymmetric divisions to form intermediate progenitors (IPCs) or neuroblasts involved in cortical layering and growth. The neuroblasts can also be generated from IPCs, which migrate along the glial fibers extending to the pial surface, contributing to the diverse composition of different cell types in the cortex. CSF, Cerebrospinal fluid, VZ, ventricular zone; ISVZ, inner subventricular zone; OSVZ, outer subventricular zone; IZ, intermediate zone; SP, subplate; CP, cortical plate; MZ, marginal zone. (B) Schematics of the microfluidic system generated by Karzbrun et al. (2018) for live imaging of organoids. (C) Arrangement of radial glia-like cells in control and *LIS1* +/− organoids modeling induction of folds due to nuclear density and growth gradients. Created with BioRender.com.

fate; conditional deletion of *Lis1* in mice with Wnt1-Cre causes defects in the induction and subsequently fails in correctly forming the telencephalon. During NESCs division, in the absence of LIS1, the dysfunctional cortical dynein fails to capture the microtubules, resulting in an inability to pivot the apical mitotic spindle in cell bodies of aRGs, thus leading to the chromosome congregational defects and apoptosis (Moon et al. 2014; Yingling et al. 2008). This role of LIS1 in survival and involvement in multiple profound molecular tasks throughout the development makes understanding the etiology of lissencephaly complex.

The human brain is gyrencephalic and has unique folding characteristics. The most prevalent theory so far relates to the increase in size and occurrence of folding in the human brain concordance with tangential expansion (Budday et al. 2015; Reillo et al. 2011; Tallinen et al. 2014). The sublayers of the cortex generate compressive stress, leading to the mechanical folding of the cortex arising from dynamics within the cortical layers. In contrast, the embryonic or adult mouse brain is lissencephalic, which poses a fundamental problem in studying the etiology of lissencephaly in rodent models. In lissencephalic species like the mouse, bRGs are limited in numbers compared to aRGs and intermediate progenitors (IPs) in the subventricular zone (SVZ). Both bRGs and IPs form the progenitor population arising from the division of aRGs, expressing PAX6 and EOMES, respectively (Li et al. 2020; Pollen et al. 2015; Sansom et al. 2009; Sessa et al. 2008; Wong et al. 2015). Whereas in gyrencephalic species, like humans, the SVZ is expanded during the development into inner SVZ (ISVZ) and outer SVZ (OSVZ) enriched with subapical RGs and subtypes of basal progenitors constituting bRG, respectively. The oRGs having high levels of STAT3 and HOPX divide differently than the apical radial glia, and the resulting progenitor pool has a typical gene signature (Pollen et al. 2015). aRGs and bRGs both extend their process along the apicobasal axis and are defined by the presence of cell bodies on either of the surfaces. bRGs comprise one or two basal processes with a single or no apically directed processes (Kalebic et al. 2019; Kalebic and Huttner 2020).

Different morphological subtypes of RGs in humans are critical for neuroepithelium-neocortical expansion and define the brain topology. A subset of aRGs in the human cerebral cortex extend their basal processes by wrapping endothelial cells without connecting to the pial surface. They are defined as truncated radial glia (tRGs). These tRGs allow bRGs to develop their processes to create a much larger fiber scaffold for tangential dispersion of radially migrating neurons (Nowakowski et al. 2016). The expression of SATB2, TBR1, and WNT7B is evident in the resulting neuronal population of sub-plate and deep cortical neurons in both mice and humans (Bedogni et al. 2010; Britanova et al. 2008; Eze et al. 2021; Roberts et al. 2021; Rubenstein et al. 1999). Microdissection of progenitor population in the human fetal cortical layers with single-cell transcriptomics confirmed the RGs diversity contributes to patterned transcriptional programs and a large subset of cells enriched on several genes related to stemness and ECM (Güven et al. 2020; Long et al. 2018; Nowakowski et al. 2017). The resting membrane potential of RGs rapidly changes during the neurogenic niche and becomes increasingly hyperpolarized to define neuronal fate. Voltage-gated ion channels such as SCN3A and Wnt signaling are involved in layer IV and subsequent layer II/III nascent neurons. The expansion of the upper layer surfaces, including cortical layer IV splitting in humans, is directed by the interplay of neuronal migration, cell division, and cell adhesion forces in ISVZ and OSVZ. This divergence, coupled with simultaneous neurogenesis in the neocortex and ganglionic eminences, is assumed to lead to mechanically constrained induced gyrification. In addition, elevated pressure is formed in the embryonic vesicles due to cerebrospinal fluid (CSF) accumulation by the choroid plexus or progenitors during the ventricle development. Tight junctions counterbalance the differential pressure maintained by circulating CSF in the tissue lining and emerging angiogenesis. The counterbalanced surface tension across the diffusion barrier is also thought to promote the outward bulging of epithelium.

The information about MDS and lissencephaly primarily comes from analysis of MRI studies and postmortem human brains. Thus, to model the disease, human brain organoids have also been used to investigate how MDS affects human cortical progenitor subtypes, specifically the outer radial glia population. Although transgenic mouse models help understanding of neuronal migration and other developmental phenotypes, they have the disadvantage of being naturally lissencephalic and lacking the outer radial glial scaffold. Cerebral organoids derived from MDS-iPSCs showed morphological and mitotic defects in the oRGs (Bershteyn et al. 2017). The resulting cell migration defects and severe apoptosis of the neuroepithelial stem cells, accompanied by increased horizontal cell divisions in MDS organoids, were rescued by correcting the chromosomal deletion (Bershteyn et al. 2017). β-catenin is a crucial transcription factor in Wnt signaling and maintaining proliferation of the cortical progenitor pool. Loss of β-catenin leads to disruption of adherence junction and reductions in RGs number. In another study, MDS forebrain organoids showed size reduction with a change and irregularity in symmetric-asymmetric cell divisions of ventricular zone RGs dependent on Wnt signaling. Consequently, restoring active N-cadherin/β-catenin signaling with a Wnt pathway activator could rescue division modes and partially ameliorate growth defects in the organoids (Iefremova et al. 2017). Although these studies in human brain organoids have relevant cell types and partly molecular mechanisms involving the disease formation, they do not recapitulate the major gyrification defects.

The mechanical folding model hypothesis was tested with real three-dimensional (3D) fetal brain geometries in an emulated developmental setting. The studies mimicking human brain geometries in polymer gel models with differentially swelling materials suggest that wrinkling emerges spontaneously due to the development of localized compression forces (Greiner et al. 2021; Tallinen et al. 2016). Relevant cellular and molecular mechanisms occur before actual tissue folding, and the effect of mechanical factors depends on specific initial conditions that must be set in advance by early developmental processes (Costa Campos et al. 2021; Llinares-Benadero and Borrell 2019). Moreover, exogenous treatment of ECM to developing brain explants in culture conditions has been shown to modulate and induce the folding of the cortical plate (Long et al. 2018). Karzbrun et al. established an in vitro microfluidic system of brain organoids to model brain folding. In this system, the organoids can be grown over weeks, allowing the organoids' growth only in the x and y axes and limiting in the z axis, enabling live in situ imaging. This unique system allowed characterizing the interkinetic nuclear migration in RGs like cells and physical mechanisms that lead to the formation of folds in the growing organoids (Karzbrun et al. 2018) (Figure 18.4B).

The folds formed due to two opposing forces in the discoid organoid structure. On the one hand, there is cytoskeleton contraction at the organoid core, whereas, at the organoid perimeter, there is cell-cycle-dependent nuclear expansion. These two constant opposing forces result in mechanical instability and the emergence of convolutions at a critical cell density with maximal nuclear strain. Furthermore, fold wavelength exhibited linear scaling with tissue thickness and was consistent with an equilibrium between bending and stretching energies. The effect of the *LIS1* mutation during the growth of neuroepithelium-like structures was also studied, and *LIS1* +/− mutant organoids displayed reduced convolutions (Figure 18.4C). The gyrification index of these organoids showed linear scaling with an increased slope in mutants at later stages is synonymous with the human lissencephalic brain. *LIS1* +/− mutant cells showed reduced viscoelastic properties in ESCs and differentiated neuronal progenitors (Karzbrun et al. 2018). The nucleus is a mechanosensor, and reduced LIS1 levels may affect the nuclear envelope breakdown during cell division. Together mechanical instability induced by the surface tension of the organoid and the collective heterogenous INM events with cell cycle dynamics in RGs was affected in lissencephalic organoids. These findings highlight a mechanical model for folding occurring in the developing human brain through changes in cellular trajectories and differential expression of cytoskeletal and ECM-related genes. RBP *TRIM71* mutations in humans and homozygous deletion in mice affect neurogenesis-dependent biomechanics causing monogenic hydrocephalus and ventricular CSF-parenchyma defects in the absence of altered CSF flow (Duy et al. 2022). *LIS1* mutations in humans causing lissencephaly or MDLS show typical features of ventriculomegaly or hydrocephalus (Holzgreve et al. 1993; Pilz and Quarrell 1996; Zhang et al. 2022). Moreover, heterozygous *Lis1* hypomorphs and conditional knockout studies in the adult stage (unpublished data) show severe hydrocephalus phenotypes synonymous in MDS or lissencephaly patients, as seen in MRI. It can be postulated that the macroscopic stresses due to hydrocephalus, disruption of differential progenitor expansion, and neuronal migration impairments during gestation collectively influence gyrification in lissencephaly patients.

Acknowledgments

Orly Reiner is an incumbent of the Berstein-Mason professorial chair of Neurochemistry and the Head of M. Judith Ruth Institute for Preclinical Brain Research. Our research has been supported by a research grant from Ethel Lena Levy, a research grant from the Estate of Olga Klein Astrachan, the Weizmann Gladys Monroy and Larry Marks Center for Brain Disorders, the Selsky Memory Research Project, the Advantage Trust, the William and Joan Brodsky Foundation and the Edward F. Anixter Family Foundation, the Helen and Martin Kimmel Institute for Stem Cell Research, the Kekst Center, the Nella and Leon Benoziyo Center for Neurological Diseases, the David and Fela Shapell Family Center for Genetic Disorders Research, the Brenden-Mann Women's Innovation Impact Fund, The Irving B. Harris Fund for New Directions in Brain Research, the Irving Bieber, M.D. and Toby Bieber, M.D. Memorial Research Fund, The Leff Family, Barbara and Roberto Kaminitz, Sergio and Sônia Lozinsky, Debbie Koren, Jack Lowenthal, Lenore Lowenthal, and the Dears Foundation, a research grant from the Weizmann SABRA – Yeda-Sela – WRC Program, the Estate of Emile Mimran, and The Maurice and Vivienne Wohl Biology Endowment Canadian Institutes of Health Research (CIHR), the International Development Research Centre (IDRC), the Israel Science Foundation (ISF) and the Azrieli Foundation (2397/18), the ISF grant (545/21), and the United States-Israel Binational Science Foundation (BSF; Grant No. 2017006).

References

Abuhashem, A. et al. (2022). RNA polymerase II pausing in development. *Open Biol* 12: 210220.

Aitken, C.E. and Lorsch, J.R. (2012). A mechanistic overview of translation initiation in eukaryotes. *Nat Struct Mol Biol* 19: 568–576.

Albrecht, L.V. et al. (2021). Cell biology of canonical Wnt signaling. *Ann Rev Cell Dev Biol* 37: 369–389.

Alikani, M. (2005). Epithelial cadherin distribution in abnormal human pre-implantation embryos. *Hum Reprodu* 20: 3369–3375.

Anokye-Danso, F. et al. (2011). Highly efficient miRNA-mediated reprogramming of mouse and human somatic cells to pluripotency. *Cell Stem Cell* 8: 376–388.

Assadi, A.H. et al. (2003). Interaction of reelin signaling and Lis1 in brain development. *Nat Genet* 35: 270–276.

Atwal, P.S. and Macmurdo, C. (2015). A case of concurrent Miller-Dieker syndrome (17p13.3 deletion) and 22q11.2 deletion syndrome. *J Pediatr Genet* 4: 201–203.

Avela, K. et al. (2011). A microduplication on chromosome 17p13.1p13.3 including the PAFAH1B1 (LIS1) gene. *Am J Med Genet Part A* 155A: 875–879.

Badea, A. et al. (2007). Neuroanatomical phenotypes in the reeler mouse. *Neuroimage* 34: 1363–1374.

Bajaj, J. et al. (2020). An in vivo genome-wide CRISPR screen identifies the RNA-binding protein Staufen2 as a key regulator of myeloid leukemia. *Nat Cancer* 1: 410–422.

Balza, C. et al. (2021). A prenatal case of lissencephaly with cerebellar hypoplasia. *Clin Case Rep* 9: e04882.

Barish, S. et al. (2022). The microRNA processor DROSHA is a candidate gene for a severe progressive neurological disorder. *Hum Mol Genet* 31: 2934–2950.

Baumbach, J. et al. (2017). Lissencephaly-1 is a context-dependent regulator of the human dynein complex. *Elife* 6: e21768.

Bedogni, F. et al. (2010). Tbr1 regulates regional and laminar identity of postmitotic neurons in developing neocortex. *Proc Natl Acad Sci USA* 107: 13129–13134.

Bellucco, F.T. et al. (2017). Miller-Dieker syndrome due to a 5.5-Mb 17p deletion in a 17;Y pseudodicentric chromosome. *Cytogenet Genome Res* 152: 29–32.

Ben-Ari Fuchs, S. et al. (2016). GeneAnalytics. *OMICS* 20: 139–151.

Benetatos, L. et al. (2013). The microRNAs within the DLK1-DIO3 genomic region. *Cell Mol Life Sci* 70: 795–814.

Benham-Pyle, B.W. et al. (2015). Cell adhesion. Mechanical strain induces E-cadherin-dependent Yap1 and beta-catenin activation to drive cell cycle entry. *Science* 348: 1024–1027.

Bernstein, E. et al. (2003). Dicer is essential for mouse development. *Nat Genet* 35: 215–217.

Bershteyn, M. et al. (2014). Cell-autonomous correction of ring chromosomes in human induced pluripotent stem cells. *Nature* 507: 99–103.

Bershteyn, M. et al. (2017). Human iPSC-derived cerebral organoids model cellular features of lissencephaly and reveal prolonged mitosis of outer radial glia. *Cell Stem Cell* 20: 435–449 e434.

Bertram, K. et al. (2017). Cryo-EM structure of a pre-catalytic human spliceosome primed for activation. *Cell* 170: 701–713.e711.

Bhat, P. et al. (2021). Nuclear compartmentalization as a mechanism of quantitative control of gene expression. *Nat Rev Mol Cell Biol* 22: 653–670.

Bhattacharyya, S. et al. (2022). Cell-cell adhesions in embryonic stem cells regulate the stability and transcriptional activity of beta-catenin. *FEBS Lett* 596: 1647–1660.

Bi, W. et al. (2009). Increased LIS1 expression affects human and mouse brain development. *Nat Genet* 41: 168–177.

Blazejewski, S.M. et al. (2018). Neurodevelopmental genetic diseases associated with microdeletions and microduplications of chromosome 17p13.3. *Front Genet* 9: 80.

Britanova, O. et al. (2008). Satb2 is a postmitotic determinant for upper-layer neuron specification in the neocortex. *Neuron* 57: 378–392.

Brock, S. et al. (1993). PAFAH1B1-related lissencephaly/subcortical band heterotopia. In: *GeneReviews((R))* (ed. M.P. Adam, D.B. Everman, G.M. Mirzaa, R.A. Pagon, S.E. Wallace, L.J.H. Bean, K.W. Gripp, and A. Amemiya). Seattle: University of Washington.

Budday, S. et al. (2015). Physical biology of human brain development. *Front Cell Neurosci* 9: 257.

Cahana, A. et al. (2001). Targeted mutagenesis of Lis1 disrupts cortical development and LIS1 homodimerization. *Proc Natl Acad Sci USA* 98: 6429–6434.

Cahana, A. et al. (2003). A study of the nature of embryonic lethality in LIS1-/- mice. *Mol Rep Dev* 66: 134–142.

Casanal, A. et al. (2017). Architecture of eukaryotic mRNA 3′-end processing machinery. *Science* 358: 1056–1059.

Castello, A. et al. (2015). Metabolic enzymes enjoying new partnerships as RNA-binding proteins. *Trends Endocrinol Metab* 26: 746–757.

Chang, B.S. et al. (2007). The role of RELN in lissencephaly and neuropsychiatric disease. *Am J Med Genet Part B, Neuropsychiatr Genet* 144B: 58–63.

Chapman, D.E. et al. (2019). Regulation of in vivo dynein force production by CDK5 and 14-3-3epsilon and KIAA0528. *Nat Commun* 10: 228.

Chen, C.Y. et al. (2009). Ago-TNRC6 triggers microRNA-mediated decay by promoting two deadenylation steps. *Nat Struct Mol Biol* 16: 1160–1166.

Chen, F.X. et al. (2018). Born to run: control of transcription elongation by RNA polymerase II. *Nat Rev Mol Cell Biol* 19: 464–478.

Cheng, T.L. et al. (2014). MeCP2 suppresses nuclear microRNA processing and dendritic growth by regulating the DGCR8/Drosha complex. *Dev Cell* 28: 547–560.

Cho, K.H.T. et al. (2019). Emerging roles of miRNAs in brain development and perinatal brain injury. *Front Physiol* 10: 227.

Clark, G.D. et al. (1997). Predominant localization of the LIS family of gene products to Cajal-Retzius cells and ventricular neuroepithelium in the developing human cortex. *J Neuropathol Exp Neurol* 56: 1044–1052.

Classen, S. et al. (2013). A novel inverted 17p13.3 microduplication disrupting PAFAH1B1 (LIS1) in a girl with syndromic lissencephaly. *Am J Med Genet Part A* 161A: 1453–1458.

Clerici, M. et al. (2018). Structural basis of AAUAAA polyadenylation signal recognition by the human CPSF complex. *Nat Struct Mol Biol* 25: 135–138.

Costa Campos, L.D. et al. (2021). The role of thickness inhomogeneities in hierarchical cortical folding. *Neuroimage* 231: 117779.

Curry, C.J. et al. (2013). The duplication 17p13.3 phenotype. *Am J Med Genet Part A* 161A: 1833–1852.

D'Arcangelo, G. (2006). Reelin mouse mutants as models of cortical development disorders. *Epilepsy Behav* 8: 81–90.

Das, S. et al. (2021). Intracellular mRNA transport and localized translation. *Nat Rev Mol Cell Biol* 22: 483–504.

De Magistris, P. (2021). The great escape: mRNA export through the nuclear pore complex. *Int J Mol Sci* 22: 11767.

Di Donato, N. et al. (2017). Lissencephaly: expanded imaging and clinical classification. *Am J Med Genet Part A* 173: 1473–1488.

Di Donato, N. et al. (2022). Monoallelic and biallelic mutations in RELN underlie a graded series of neurodevelopmental disorders. *Brain* 145 (9): 3274–3287.

Dobyns, W.B. et al. (1993). Lissencephaly. A human brain malformation associated with deletion of the LIS1 gene located at chromosome 17p13. *JAMA* 270: 2838–2842.

Dominguez-Sala, E. et al. (2022a). Properties of the epileptiform activity in the cingulate cortex of a mouse model of LIS1 dysfunction. *Brain Struct Funct* 227: 1599–1614.

Dominguez-Sala, E. et al. (2022b). Abnormalities in cortical GABAergic interneurons of the primary motor cortex caused by Lis1 (Pafah1b1) mutation produce a non-drastic functional phenotype. *Front Cell Dev Biol* 10: 769853.

Du, P. et al. (2018). An intermediate pluripotent state controlled by MicroRNAs is required for the naive-to-primed stem cell transition. *Cell Stem Cell* 22: 851–864.e855.

Du, X. et al. (2014). A genomic copy number variant analysis implicates the MBD5 and HNRNPU genes in Chinese children with infantile spasms and expands the clinical spectrum of 2q23.1 deletion. *BMC Med Genet* 15: 62.

Duy, P.Q. et al. (2022). Impaired neurogenesis alters brain biomechanics in a neuroprogenitor-based genetic subtype of congenital hydrocephalus. *Nat Neurosci* 25: 458–473.

Elshenawy, M.M. et al. (2020). Lis1 activates dynein motility by modulating its pairing with dynactin. *Nat Cell Biol* 22: 570–578.

Eriksson, S.H. et al. (2001). Persistent reelin-expressing Cajal-Retzius cells in polymicrogyria. *Brain* 124: 1350–1361.

Eze, U.C. et al. (2021). Single-cell atlas of early human brain development highlights heterogeneity of human neuroepithelial cells and early radial glia. *Nat Neurosci* 24: 584–594.

Farris, N. et al. (2018). 17p13.3 quadruplication: a prenatal and postpartum clinical characterization of a copy number variant. *Cold Spring Harb Mol Case Stud* 4 (3): a002196.

Franker, M.A. et al. (2016). Three-step model for polarized sorting of KIF17 into dendrites. *Curr Biol* 26: 1705–1712.

Frye, M. et al. (2018). RNA modifications modulate gene expression during development. *Science* 361: 1346–1349.

Galloway, A. and Cowling, V.H. (2019). mRNA cap regulation in mammalian cell function and fate. *Biochim et Biophys Acta – Gene Regul Mech* 1862: 270–279.

Gambello, M.J. et al. (2003). Multiple dose-dependent effects of Lis1 on cerebral cortical development. *J Neurosci* 23: 1719–1729.

Garcia-Higuera, I. et al. (1996). Folding of proteins with WD-repeats: comparison of six members of the WD-repeat superfamily to the G protein ß subunit. *Biochemistry* 35: 13985–13994.

Garcia-Lopez, R. et al. (2015). Developmental alterations of the septohippocampal cholinergic projection in a lissencephalic mouse model. *Exp Neurol* 271: 215–227.

Garcia-Lopez, R. et al. (2021). Interneuron heterotopia in the Lis1 mutant mouse cortex underlies a structural and functional schizophrenia-like phenotype. *Front Cell Dev Biol* 9: 693919.

Gavrilovici, C. et al. (2021). Behavioral deficits in mice with postnatal disruption of Ndel1 in forebrain excitatory neurons: implications for epilepsy and neuropsychiatric disorders. *Cereb Cortex Commun* 2: tgaa096.

Gehring, N.H. and Roignant, J.Y. (2021). Anything but ordinary – emerging splicing mechanisms in eukaryotic gene regulation. *Trends Genet* 37: 355–372.

Gerlitz, G. et al. (2005). Novel functional features of the Lis-H domain. *Cell Cycle* 4: 1632–1640.

Gilliam, F.G. et al. (2021). Case report: PAFAH1B1 mutation and posterior band heterotopia with focal temporal lobe epilepsy treated by responsive neurostimulation. *Front Neurol* 12: 779113.

Gillies, J.P. et al. (2022). Structural basis for cytoplasmic dynein-1 regulation by Lis1. *Elife* 11: e71229.

Girbig, M. et al. (2022). Structural insights into nuclear transcription by eukaryotic DNA-dependent RNA polymerases. *Nat Rev Mol Cell Biol* 23: 603–622.

Gonzalez-Moron, D. et al. (2017). Germline and somatic mutations in cortical malformations. *PLoS One* 12: e0185103.

Gopal, P.P. et al. (2010). Leading process branch instability in Lis1+/– nonradially migrating interneurons. *Cereb Cortex* 20: 1497–1505.

Greiner, A. et al. (2021). Physical aspects of cortical folding. *Soft Matter* 17: 1210–1222.

Groot, M. and Lee, H. (2020). Sorting mechanisms for MicroRNAs into extracellular vesicles and their associated diseases. *Cells* 9 (4): 1044.

Guca, E. and Hashem, Y. (2018). Major structural rearrangements of the canonical eukaryotic translation initiation complex. *Curr Opin Struct Biol* 53: 151–158.

Guruharsha, K.G. et al. (2011). A protein complex network of Drosophila melanogaster. *Cell* 147: 690–703.

Güven, A. et al. (2020). Extracellular matrix-inducing Sox9 promotes both basal progenitor proliferation and gliogenesis in developing neocortex. *Elife* 9: e49808.

Hari, L. et al. (2002). Lineage-specific requirements of beta-catenin in neural crest development. *J Cell Biol* 159: 867–880.

Haselbach, D. et al. (2018). Structure and conformational dynamics of the human spliceosomal B(act) complex. *Cell* 172: 454–464.e411.

Hattori, M. et al. (1994). Miller-Dieker lissencephaly gene encodes a subunit of brain platelet-activating factor acetylhydrolase [corrected]. *Nature* 370: 216–218.

Henry, R.K. et al. (2016). 17p13.3 microduplication including CRK leads to overgrowth and elevated growth factors. *Eur J Med Genet* 59: 512–516.

Herrera, A. et al. (2014). Sustained Wnt/β-catenin signalling causes neuroepithelial aberrations through the accumulation of aPKC at the apical pole. *Nat Commun* 5: 4168.

Herzel, L. et al. (2017). Splicing and transcription touch base: co-transcriptional spliceosome assembly and function. *Nat Rev Mol Cell Biol* 18: 637–650.

Hill, C.S. (2022). Establishment and interpretation of NODAL and BMP signaling gradients in early vertebrate development. *Curr Topics Dev Biol* 149: 311–340.

Hippenmeyer, S. et al. (2010). Genetic mosaic dissection of Lis1 and Ndel1 in neuronal migration. *Neuron* 68: 695–709.

Hirotsune, S. et al. (1998). Graded reduction of Pafah1b1 (Lis1) activity results in neuronal migration defects and early embryonic lethality. *Nat Genet* 19: 333–339.

Ho, J.J.D. et al. (2020). A network of RNA-binding proteins controls translation efficiency to activate anaerobic metabolism. *Nat Commun* 11: 2677.

Ho, Y.S. et al. (1997). Brain acetylhydrolase that inactivates platelet-activating factor is a G-protein-like trimer. *Nature* 385: 89–93.

Holzgreve, W. et al. (1993). Prenatal diagnosis and management of fetal hydrocephaly and lissencephaly. *Child's Nerv Syst* 9: 408–412.

Hong, S.E. et al. (2000). Autosomal recessive lissencephaly with cerebellar hypoplasia is associated with human RELN mutations. *Nat Genet* 26: 93–96.

Houseley, J. et al. (2006). RNA-quality control by the exosome. *Nat Rev Mol Cell Biol* 7: 529–539.

Huang, J. et al. (2012). Lis1 acts as a "clutch" between the ATPase and microtubule-binding domains of the dynein motor. *Cell* 150: 975–986.

Huang, X. et al. (2018). The mechanism of long non-coding RNA MEG3 for hepatic ischemia-reperfusion. *J Cell Biochem* 119: 1163–1172.

Huang, Y.-S. et al. (2022). Two genetic mechanisms in two siblings with intellectual disability, autism spectrum disorder, and psychosis. *J Pers Med* 12: 1013.

Humphries, A.C. and Mlodzik, M. (2018). From instruction to output. *Curr Opin Cell Biol* 51: 110–116.

Hunt, R.F. et al. (2012). LIS1 deficiency promotes dysfunctional synaptic integration of granule cells generated in the developing and adult dentate gyrus. *J Neurosci* 32: 12862–12875.

Hyon, C. et al. (2011). A new 17p13.3 microduplication including the PAFAH1B1 and YWHAE genes resulting from an unbalanced X;17 translocation. *Eur J Med Genet* 54: 287–291.

Ibba, M. and Söll, D. (2000). Aminoacyl-tRNA Synthesis. *Ann Rev Biochem* 69: 617–650.

Iefremova, V. et al. (2017). An organoid-based model of cortical development identifies non-cell-autonomous defects in Wnt signaling contributing to Miller-Dieker syndrome. *Cell Rep* 19: 50–59.

Inada, T. and Makino, S. (2014). Novel roles of the multi-functional CCR4-NOT complex in post-transcriptional regulation. *Front Genet* 5: 135.

Ingham, P.W. (2022). Hedgehog signaling. *Curr Topics Dev Biol* 149: 1–58.

Itoh, Y. et al. (2013). Scratch regulates neuronal migration onset via an epithelial-mesenchymal transition-like mechanism. *Nat Neurosci* 16: 416–425.

Jackson, R.J. et al. (2010). The mechanism of eukaryotic translation initiation and principles of its regulation. *Nat Rev Mol Cell Biol* 11: 113–127.

Jeppesen, D.K. et al. (2019). Reassessment of exosome composition. *Cell* 177: 428–445 e418.

Jiang, Y. et al. (2016). Ndel1 and Reelin maintain postnatal CA1 hippocampus integrity. *J Neurosci* 36: 6538–6552.

Jonas, S. and Izaurralde, E. (2015). Towards a molecular understanding of microRNA-mediated gene silencing. *Nat Rev Genet* 16: 421–433.

Kalebic, N. et al. (2019). Neocortical expansion due to increased proliferation of basal progenitors is linked to changes in their morphology. *Cell Stem Cell* 24: 535–550.e539.

Kalebic, N. and Huttner, W.B. (2020). Basal progenitor morphology and neocortex evolution. *Trends Neurosci* 43: 843–853.

Kameswaran, V. et al. (2014). Epigenetic regulation of the DLK1-MEG3 microRNA cluster in human type 2 diabetic islets. *Cell Metab* 19: 135–145.

Karayiorgou, M. et al. (2010). 22q11.2 microdeletions. *Nat Rev Neurosci* 11: 402–416.

Karzbrun, E. et al. (2018). Human brain organoids on a chip reveal the physics of folding. *Nat Phys* 14: 515–522.

Kawabata, I. et al. (2012). LIS1-dependent retrograde translocation of excitatory synapses in developing interneuron dendrites. *Nat Commun* 3: 722.

Keidar, L. et al. (2019). Interplay of LIS1 and MeCP2. *Front Cell Neurosci* 13: 370.

Kilchert, C. et al. (2016). The regulation and functions of the nuclear RNA exosome complex. *Nat Rev Mol Cell Biol* 17: 227–239.

Kim, M.H. et al. (2004). The structure of the N-terminal domain of the product of the lissencephaly gene Lis1 and its functional implications. *Structure* 12: 987–998.

Kim, T. et al. (2014). Chromosome therapy. Correction of large chromosomal aberrations by inducing ring chromosomes in induced pluripotent stem cells (iPSCs). *Nucleus* 5: 391–395.

Kiroski, I. et al. (2020). Reelin improves cognition and extends the lifespan of mutant Ndel1 mice with postnatal CA1 hippocampus deterioration. *Cereb Cortex* 30: 4964–4978.

Klinman, E. et al. (2017). CDK5-dependent activation of dynein in the axon initial segment regulates polarized cargo transport in neurons. *Traffic* 18: 808–824.

Koca, Y. et al. (2022). Wnt-frizzled planar cell polarity signaling in the regulation of cell motility. *Curr Topics Dev Biol* 150: 255–297.

Kosik, K.S. and Nowakowski, T. (2018). Evolution of new miRNAs and cerebro-cortical development. *Ann Rev Neurosci* 41: 119–137.

Kshirsagar, A. et al. (2022). LIS1 RNA-binding orchestrates the mechanosensitive properties of embryonic stem cells in AGO2-dependent and independent ways. *BioRxiv*. doi: 10.1101/2022.03.08.483407.

Kugeratski, F.G. et al. (2021). Quantitative proteomics identifies the core proteome of exosomes with syntenin-1 as the highest abundant protein and a putative universal biomarker. *Nat Cell Biol* 23: 631–641.

Kuijpers, M. et al. (2016). Dynein regulator NDEL1 controls polarized cargo transport at the axon initial segment. *Neuron* 89: 461–471.

Kurosaki, T. et al. (2019). Quality and quantity control of gene expression by nonsense-mediated mRNA decay. *Nat Rev Mol Cell Biol* 20: 406–420.

Lam, C. et al. (2010). Functional interplay between LIS1, NDE1 and NDEL1 in dynein-dependent organelle positioning. *J Cell Sci* 123: 202–212.

Lecuit, T. and Yap, A.S. (2015). E-cadherin junctions as active mechanical integrators in tissue dynamics. *Nat Cell Biol* 17: 533–539.

Lee, M. et al. (2014). Emerging roles of RNA modification. *Cell* 158: 980–987.

Lesniewska, E. and Boguta, M. (2017). Novel layers of RNA polymerase III control affecting tRNA gene transcription in eukaryotes. *Open Biol* 7 (2): 170001.

Leung, A.K.L. (2015). The whereabouts of microRNA actions. *Trends Cell Biol* 25: 601–610.

Li, Z. et al. (2020). Transcriptional priming as a conserved mechanism of lineage diversification in the developing mouse and human neocortex. *Sci Adv* 6 (45): eabd2068.

Lin, S.P. et al. (2003). Asymmetric regulation of imprinting on the maternal and paternal chromosomes at the Dlk1-Gtl2 imprinted cluster on mouse chromosome 12. *Nat Genet* 35: 97–102.

Lipchina, I. et al. (2011). Genome-wide identification of microRNA targets in human ES cells reveals a role for miR-302 in modulating BMP response. *Genes Dev* 25: 2173–2186.

Liu, J. et al. (2004). Argonaute2 is the catalytic engine of mammalian RNAi. *Science* 305: 1437–1441.

Liu, X.-M. et al. (2021). Selective sorting of microRNAs into exosomes by phase-separated YBX1 condensates. *Elife* 10: e71982.

Livnat, I. et al. (2010). PAF-AH catalytic subunits modulate the Wnt pathway in developing GABAergic neurons. *Front Cell Neurosci* 4: 19.

Livneh, I. et al. (2020). The m(6)A epitranscriptome: transcriptome plasticity in brain development and function. *Nat Rev Neurosci* 21: 36–51.

Llinares-Benadero, C. and Borrell, V. (2019). Deconstructing cortical folding: genetic, cellular and mechanical determinants. *Nat Rev Neurosci* 20: 161–176.

Long, K.R. et al. (2018). Extracellular matrix components HAPLN1, lumican, and collagen I cause hyaluronic acid-dependent folding of the developing human neocortex. *Neuron* 99: 702–719.e706.

Lossi, L. et al. (2019). The reeler mouse. *J Clin Med* 8 (12): 2088.

Luhur, A. et al. (2014). Drosha-independent DGCR8/Pasha pathway regulates neuronal morphogenesis. *Proc Natl Acad Sci USA* 111: 1421–1426.

Lunde, B.M. et al. (2007). RNA-binding proteins: modular design for efficient function. *Nat Rev Mol Cell Biol* 8: 479–490.

Lykke-Andersen, S. and Jensen, T.H. (2015). Nonsense-mediated mRNA decay: an intricate machinery that shapes transcriptomes. *Nat Rev Mol Cell Biol* 16: 665–677.

Martinez-Martinez, M.A. et al. (2016). A restricted period for formation of outer subventricular zone defined by Cdh1 and Trnp1 levels. *Nat Commun* 7: 11812.

Masek, J. et al. (2016). Tcf7l1 protects the anterior neural fold from adopting the neural crest fate. *Development* 143: 2206–2216.

Mateja, A. et al. (2006). The dimerization mechanism of LIS1 and its implication for proteins containing the LisH motif. *J Mol Biol* 357: 621–631.

Maunakea, A.K. et al. (2013). Intragenic DNA methylation modulates alternative splicing by recruiting MeCP2 to promote exon recognition. *Cell Res* 23: 1256–1269.

McKenney, R.J. et al. (2011). Mutually exclusive cytoplasmic dynein regulation by NudE-Lis1 and dynactin. *J Biol Chem* 286: 39615–39622.

McKenzie, A.J. et al. (2016). KRAS-MEK signaling controls Ago2 sorting into exosomes. *Cell Rep* 15: 978–987.

Menezes, M.R. et al. (2018). 3′ RNA uridylation in epitranscriptomics, gene regulation, and disease. *Front Mol Biosci* 5: 61.

Merrick, W.C. and Pavitt, G.D. (2018). Protein synthesis initiation in eukaryotic cells. *Cold Spring Harb Perspect Biol* 10 (12): a033092.

Mishima, T. et al. (2017). Miller-Dieker syndrome with unbalanced translocation 45, X, psu dic(17;Y)(p13;p11.32) detected by fluorescence in situ hybridization and G-banding analysis using high resolution banding technique. *Congenit Anom (Kyoto)* 57: 61–63.

Mitchell, S.F. and Parker, R. (2014). Principles and properties of eukaryotic mRNPs. *Mol Cell* 54: 547–558.

Mittermeier, L. and Virshup, D.M. (2022). An itch for things remote. *Curr Top Dev Biol* 150: 91–128.

Mondal, T. et al. (2015). MEG3 long noncoding RNA regulates the TGF-β pathway genes through formation of RNA-DNA triplex structures. *Nat Commun* 6: 7743.

Moon, H.M. et al. (2020). LIS1 determines cleavage plane positioning by regulating actomyosin-mediated cell membrane contractility. *Elife* 9: e51512.

Moon, H.M. et al. (2014). LIS1 controls mitosis and mitotic spindle organization via the LIS1-NDEL1-dynein complex. *Hum Mol Genet* 23: 449–466.

Moore, K.D. et al. (2012). Lis1 reduction causes tangential migratory errors in mouse spinal cord. *J Comp Neurol* 520: 1198–1211.

Moro, A. et al. (2019). MicroRNA-dependent regulation of biomechanical genes establishes tissue stiffness homeostasis. *Nat Cell Biol* 21: 348–358.

Muniz, L. et al. (2021). RNA polymerase II speed. *EMBO J* 40: e105740.

Murillo, O.D. et al. (2019). exRNA atlas analysis reveals distinct extracellular RNA cargo types and their carriers present across human biofluids. *Cell* 177: 463–477.e415.

Musier-Forsyth, K. (2019). Aminoacyl-tRNA synthetases and tRNAs in human disease. *J Biol Chem* 294: 5292–5293.

Nowakowski, T.J. et al. (2017). Spatiotemporal gene expression trajectories reveal developmental hierarchies of the human cortex. *Science* 358: 1318–1323.

Nowakowski, T.J. et al. (2016). Transformation of the radial glia scaffold demarcates two stages of human cerebral cortex development. *Neuron* 91: 1219–1227.

O'Brien, K. et al. (2020). RNA delivery by extracellular vesicles in mammalian cells and its applications. *Nat Rev Mol Cell Biol* 21: 585–606.

Oegema, R. et al. (2020). International consensus recommendations on the diagnostic work-up for malformations of cortical development. *Nat Rev Neurol* 16: 618–635.

Ohno, S.I. et al. (2022). Nuclear microRNAs release paused Pol II via the DDX21-CDK9 complex. *Cell Rep* 39: 110673.

Ornitz, D.M. and Itoh, N. (2022). New developments in the biology of fibroblast growth factors. *WIREs Mech Dis* 14: e1549.

Passmore, L.A. and Coller, J. (2022). Roles of mRNA poly(A) tails in regulation of eukaryotic gene expression. *Nat Rev Mol Cell Biol* 23: 93–106.

Pawlica, P. et al. (2020). How complementary targets expose the microRNA 3′ end for tailing and trimming during target-directed microRNA degradation. *Cold Spring Harb Symp Quant Biol* 84: 179–183.

Pawlisz, A.S. et al. (2008). Lis1-Nde1-dependent neuronal fate control determines cerebral cortical size and lamination. *Hum Mol Genet* 17: 2441–2455.

Penisson, M. et al. (2022). Lis1 mutation prevents basal radial glia-like cell production in the mouse. *Hum Mol Genet* 31: 942–957.

Pilz, D.T. and Quarrell, O.W. (1996). Syndromes with lissencephaly. *J Med Genet* 33: 319–323.

Pimentel, H. et al. (2016). A dynamic intron retention program enriched in RNA processing genes regulates gene expression during terminal erythropoiesis. *Nucleic Acids Res* 44: 838–851.

Pollen, A.A. et al. (2015). Molecular identity of human outer radial glia during cortical development. *Cell* 163: 55–67.

Prieto-Colomina, A. et al. (2021). MiRNAs in early brain development and pediatric cancer. *BioEssays* 43: 2100073.

Qiu, R. et al. (2019). LIS1 regulates cargo-adapter-mediated activation of dynein by overcoming its autoinhibition in vivo. *J Cell Biol* 218: 3630–3646.

Reddy, B.J. et al. (2016). Load-induced enhancement of Dynein force production by LIS1-NudE in vivo and in vitro. *Nat Commun* 7: 12259.

Reillo, I. et al. (2011). A role for intermediate radial glia in the tangential expansion of the mammalian cerebral cortex. *Cereb Cortex* 21: 1674–1694.

Reiner, O. (2013). LIS1 and DCX: implications for brain development and human disease in relation to microtubules. *Scientifica (Cairo)* 2013: 393975.

Reiner, O. et al. (1995). Lissencephaly gene (LIS1) expression in the CNS suggests a role in neuronal migration. *J Neurosci* 15: 3730–3738.

Reiner, O. et al. (1993). Isolation of a Miller-Dieker lissencephaly gene containing G protein beta-subunit-like repeats. *Nature* 364: 717–721.

Reiner, O. and Sapir, T. (2013). LIS1 functions in normal development and disease. *Curr Opin Neurobiol* 23: 951–956.

Rippe, K. and Papantonis, A. (2022). Functional organization of RNA polymerase II in nuclear subcompartments. *Curr Opin Cell Biol* 74: 88–96.

Roberts, K. et al. (2021). Transcriptome-wide spatial RNA profiling maps the cellular architecture of the developing human neocortex. *BioRxiv*. doi: 10.1101/2021.03.20.436265.

Roos, L. et al. (2009). A new microduplication syndrome encompassing the region of the Miller-Dieker (17p13 deletion) syndrome. *J Med Genet* 46: 703–710.

Rubenstein, J.L. et al. (1999). Genetic control of cortical regionalization and connectivity. *Cereb Cortex* 9: 524–532.

Salamon, I. and Rasin, M.R. (2021). Evolution of the neocortex through RNA-binding proteins and post-transcriptional regulation. *Front Neurosci* 15: 803107.

Sanli, I. et al. (2018). Meg3 non-coding RNA expression controls imprinting by preventing transcriptional upregulation in cis. *Cell Rep* 23: 337–348.

Sansom, S.N. et al. (2009). The level of the transcription factor Pax6 is essential for controlling the balance between neural stem cell self-renewal and neurogenesis. *PLoS Genet* 5: e1000511.

Sapir, T. et al. (1999). LIS1 is a microtubule-associated phosphoprotein. *Eur J Biochem* 265: 181–188.

Sapir, T. et al. (1997). Reduction of microtubule catastrophe events by LIS1, platelet-activating factor acetylhydrolase subunit. *EMBO J* 16: 6977–6984.

Sapir, T. et al. (2022). Heterogeneous nuclear ribonucleoprotein U (HNRNPU) safeguards the developing mouse cortex. *Nat Commun* 13: 4209.

Schieweck, R. et al. (2021). RNA-binding proteins balance brain function in health and disease. *Physiol Rev* 101: 1309–1370.

Schmidt, H. (2015). Dynein motors. *Bioessays* 37: 532–543.

Schoenberg, D.R. and Maquat, L.E. (2012). Regulation of cytoplasmic mRNA decay. *Nat Rev Genet* 13: 246–259.

Schwamborn, J.C. and Knoblich, J.A. (2008). LIS1 and spindle orientation in neuroepithelial cells. *Cell Stem Cell* 2: 193–194.

Scull, C.E. and Schneider, D.A. (2019). Coordinated control of rRNA processing by RNA polymerase I. *Trends Genet* 35: 724–733.

Sessa, A. et al. (2008). Tbr2 directs conversion of radial glia into basal precursors and guides neuronal amplification by indirect neurogenesis in the developing neocortex. *Neuron* 60: 56–69.

Shen, S. et al. (2018). PIWIL1/piRNA-DQ593109 regulates the permeability of the blood-tumor barrier via the MEG3/miR-330-5p/RUNX3 axis. *Mol Ther Nucleic Acids* 10: 412–425.

Shi, X. et al. (2021). Prenatal diagnosis of Miller-Dieker syndrome by chromosomal microarray. *Ann Hum Genet* 85: 92–96.

Shmueli, A. et al. (2010). Ndel1 palmitoylation: a new mean to regulate cytoplasmic dynein activity. *EMBO J* 29: 107–119.

Shu, T. et al. (2004). Ndel1 operates in a common pathway with LIS1 and cytoplasmic dynein to regulate cortical neuronal positioning. *Neuron* 44: 263–277.

Shukla, S. et al. (2011). CTCF-promoted RNA polymerase II pausing links DNA methylation to splicing. *Nature* 479: 74–79.

Stavast, C.J. and Erkeland, S.J. (2019). The non-canonical aspects of MicroRNAs. *Cells* 8 (11): 1465.

Stewart, M. (2019). Polyadenylation and nuclear export of mRNAs. *J Biol Chem* 294: 2977–2987.

Stockinger, A. et al. (2001). E-cadherin regulates cell growth by modulating proliferation-dependent beta-catenin transcriptional activity. *J Cell Biol* 154: 1185–1196.

Stutterd, C.A. et al. (2020). Polymicrogyria associated with 17p13.3p13.2 duplication. *Eur J Med Genet* 63 (4): 103774.

Sudarov, A. et al. (2013). Lis1 controls dynamics of neuronal filopodia and spines to impact synaptogenesis and social behaviour. *EMBO Mol Med* 5: 591–607.

Suzuki, T. (2021). The expanding world of tRNA modifications and their disease relevance. *Nat Rev Mol Cell Biol* 22: 375–392.

Szeto, R.A. et al. (2021). RNA processing in neurological tissue: development, aging and disease. *Semin Cell Dev Biol* 114: 57–67.

Takahashi, A. et al. (2020). The CCR4-NOT complex maintains liver homeostasis through mRNA deadenylation. *Life Sci Alliance* 3 (5): e201900494.

Tallinen, T. et al. (2014). Gyrification from constrained cortical expansion. *Proc Natl Acad Sci USA* 111: 12667–12672.

Tallinen, T. et al. (2016). On the growth and form of cortical convolutions. *Nat Phys* 12: 588–593.

Tarricone, C. et al. (2004). Coupling PAF signaling to dynein regulation. *Neuron* 44: 809–821.

Tian, Y. et al. (2015). A microRNA-Hippo pathway that promotes cardiomyocyte proliferation and cardiac regeneration in mice. *Sci Transl Med* 7: 279ra238.

Toba, S. and Hirotsune, S. (2012). A unique role of dynein and nud family proteins in corticogenesis. *Neuropathol* 32: 432–439.

Tsherniak, A. et al. (2017). Defining a cancer dependency map. *Cell* 170: 564–576.e516.

Urdinguio, R.G. et al. (2010). Disrupted microRNA expression caused by Mecp2 loss in a mouse model of Rett syndrome. *Epigenetics* 5: 656–663.

Valdes-Sanchez, L. et al. (2007). Postnatal alterations of the inhibitory synaptic responses recorded from cortical pyramidal neurons in the Lis1/sLis1 mutant mouse. *Mol Cell Neurosci* 35: 220–229.

Valet, M. et al. (2022). Mechanical regulation of early vertebrate embryogenesis. *Nat Rev Mol Cell Biol* 23: 169–184.

Vanacova, S. and Stefl, R. (2007). The exosome and RNA quality control in the nucleus. *EMBO Rep* 8: 651–657.

Varner, V.D. et al. (2010). Mechanics of head fold formation. *Development* 137: 3801–3811.

Wahle, E. and Winkler, G.S. (2013). RNA decay machines. *Biochim et biophys acta* 1829: 561–570.

Wang, Y. and Baraban, S.C. (2007). Granule cell dispersion and aberrant neurogenesis in the adult hippocampus of an LIS1 mutant mouse. *Dev Neurosci* 29: 91–98.

Wang, Y. and Baraban, S.C. (2008). Aberrant dentate gyrus cytoarchitecture and fiber lamination in Lis1 mutant mice. *Hippocampus* 18: 758–765.

Wang, Y. et al. (2007). DGCR8 is essential for microRNA biogenesis and silencing of embryonic stem cell self-renewal. *Nat Genet* 39: 380–385.

Welker, W. (1990). Why does cerebral cortex fissure and fold? In: *Cerebral Cortex. Cerebral Cortex*, vol. 8B (ed. E.G. Jones and A. Peters), 3–136. Boston, MA: Springer. doi: 10.1007/978-1-4615-3824-0_1.

Whipple, A.J. et al. (2020). Imprinted maternally expressed microRNAs antagonize paternally driven gene programs in neurons. *Mol Cell* 78: 85–95 e88.

Wiener, D. and Schwartz, S. (2021). The epitranscriptome beyond m(6)A. *Nat Rev Genet* 22: 119–131.

Wong, F.K. et al. (2015). Sustained Pax6 expression generates primate-like basal radial glia in developing mouse neocortex. *PLoS Biol* 13: e1002217.

Wong, J.J.L. et al. (2017). Intron retention is regulated by altered MeCP2-mediated splicing factor recruitment. *Nat Commun* 8: 15134.

Wu, X. and Bartel, D.P. (2017). Widespread influence of 3′-end structures on mammalian mRNA processing and stability. *Cell* 169: 905–917 e911.

Xiang, X. and Qiu, R. (2020). Cargo-mediated activation of cytoplasmic dynein in vivo. *Front Cell Dev Biol* 8: 598952.

Yap, K. et al. (2012). Coordinated regulation of neuronal mRNA steady-state levels through developmentally controlled intron retention. *Genes Dev* 26: 1209–1223.

Ye, S. et al. (2016). LIS1 regulates osteoclastogenesis through modulation of M-SCF and RANKL signaling pathways and CDC42. *Int J Biol Sci* 12: 1488–1499.

Yi, H. et al. (2018). PABP cooperates with the CCR4-NOT complex to promote mRNA deadenylation and block precocious decay. *Mol Cell* 70: 1081–1088 e1085.

Yingling, J. et al. (2008). Neuroepithelial stem cell proliferation requires LIS1 for precise spindle orientation and symmetric division. *Cell* 132: 474–486.

Youn, Y.H. et al. (2009). Distinct dose-dependent cortical neuronal migration and neurite extension defects in Lis1 and Ndel1 mutant mice. *J Neurosci* 29: 15520–15530.

Zamudio, J.R. et al. (2014). Argonaute-bound small RNAs from promoter-proximal RNA polymerase II. *Cell* 156: 920–934.

Zhan, X. et al. (2022). Mechanism of exon ligation by human spliceosome. *Mol Cell* 82: 2769–2778. e2764.

Zhang, G. et al. (2007). The Pafah1b complex interacts with the reelin receptor VLDLR. *PLoS One* 2: e252.

Zhang, G. et al. (2009). Differential interaction of the Pafah1b alpha subunits with the Reelin transducer Dab1. *Brain Res* 1267: 1–8.

Zhang, X. et al. (2019). Structures of the human spliceosomes before and after release of the ligated exon. *Cell Res* 29: 274–285.

Zhang, Y. and Li, Z. (2021). RNA binding proteins. *Cancer Lett* 496: 30–40.

Zhang, Y.L. et al. (2022). Prenatal diagnosis of Miller-Dieker syndrome/PAFAH1B1-related lissencephaly. *Eur J Obstet, Gynecol, Reprod Biol* 274: 28–32.

Zhuang, L. et al. (2007). Point mutations in the stem region and the fourth AAA domain of cytoplasmic dynein heavy chain partially suppress the phenotype of NUDF/LIS1 loss in Aspergillus nidulans. *Genetics* 175: 1185–1196.

Zimdahl, B. et al. (2014). Lis1 regulates asymmetric division in hematopoietic stem cells and in leukemia. *Nat Genet* 46 (3): 245–252.

Zinder, J.C. and Lima, C.D. (2017). Targeting RNA for processing or destruction by the eukaryotic RNA exosome and its cofactors. *Genes Dev* 31: 88–100.

Zolboot, N. et al. (2021). MicroRNAs instruct and maintain cell type diversity in the nervous system. *Front Mol Neurosci* 14: 646072.

Part 5

Neural Patterning, Specification of Cortical Regions

19

Understanding Human Forebrain Morphogenesis and Early Expansion Using Organoids

Magdalena Sutcliffe and Madeline A. Lancaster

MRC Laboratory of Molecular Biology, Cambridge Biomedical Campus, Francis Crick Avenue, Cambridge, UK

19.1 Introduction

The remarkable cognitive capabilities of the human brain sets *Homo sapiens* apart as a species. The human brain stands out among our closest and smartest relatives – chimpanzees, bonobos, and gorillas – not only due to its superior performance but also its size. Although built according to the same blueprint that all primates share, our brains are larger than those of apes and contain more neurons (Herculano-Houzel 2009). To produce the extraordinary number of neurons that set us apart, human brains start their expansion early in development, prior to the onset of neurogenesis. Even before the primordial neuroepithelium (NE) has fully transitioned to neurogenic radial glia, the human telencephalon is already larger than that of a macaque (Rakic 2007). As early as gestation week 16 we outpace our closest relatives – chimpanzees, whose brains are visibly smaller on prenatal ultrasound scans (Sakai et al. 2012). In neither species is the neurogenesis complete at this stage, pointing to early expansion events as the source of evolutionary differences. In this chapter we will focus on the role of early developmental patterning, neurulation, and pre-neurogenic expansion in setting the foundations for building the enlarged human neocortex, and how neural organoids can enable us to uncover the cellular and molecular mechanisms.

Most of our understanding of human brain development and evolution comes from extrapolation of data obtained from animal models. General principles of development and body and brain segmentation are similar across vertebrate species and can be experimentally perturbed and studied in vivo. Xenopus, chick, and rodents are widely used to investigate the most fundamental principles of neural development. Studies concerning development and expansion of the neocortex utilize gyrencephalic ferret or small primate species. The monkey brain is similar to the human brain in terms of development, structure, and organization, and therefore can be used to study some human disorders (Buffalo et al. 2019). The most valuable insight into early developmental events comes from studies of human tissue; however, due to its scarcity and the limited developmental stages available, our knowledge of early development of the human nervous system is limited. Ethical and technical restrictions for culturing human embryos beyond day 14 prevent the possibility of performing studies on living embryos. Some progress has been made on early development of nonhuman primates such as macaque (Ma et al. 2019) and even chimeric monkey–human embryos (Tan et al. 2021), but, even besides the ethical concerns, ex vivo culture of such structures cannot progress long enough to study events past gastrulation. The development of brain organoids has therefore opened up new avenues of discovery, particularly in the context of human-specific biology, evolution, and disease mechanisms.

Neocortical Neurogenesis in Development and Evolution, First Edition. Edited by Wieland B. Huttner.

19.2 A Brief History of Neural Organoids

The need for more accurate models of human neural tissue that could be used to study processes where animal models were suboptimal fueled development of multiple in vitro systems. Historically, human neurons have been induced from pluripotent stem cells (PSCs) in adherent culture (Kelava and Lancaster 2016b). Later, aggregates of PSCs called embryoid bodies (EBs), were cultured in serum-free medium or treated with inhibitors of Nodal, Wnt, and BMP pathways to promote neural differentiation. When such neuralized EBs were plated on a cell culture dish, they formed neural rosettes (Zhang et al. 2001). Further work to optimize rosette culture conditions resulted in development of serum-free floating culture of EB-like aggregates (SFEB) or SFEBq (SFEB with quick aggregation) (Eiraku et al. 2008; Watanabe et al. 2005, 2007). When human SFEBq aggregates were then plated on a cell culture dish they formed larger rosette structures intermediate between 2D and 3D. Even at a relatively low level of complexity, a neural rosette could recapitulate some of the in vivo properties of neural stem cells, which cannot be achieved in dissociated progenitor culture, such as self-organization, lumen formation, and generation of intermediate progenitors (Eiraku et al. 2008; Mariani et al. 2015; Watanabe et al. 2005, 2007). Eventually, full 3D methods for human cells were developed, where a neuralized EB was continuously cultured in suspension (Kadoshima et al. 2013; Lancaster et al. 2013). Addition of extracellular matrix (ECM), either dissolved in the culture medium or provided as a gel for encapsulation, promoted in vivo-like tissue morphology with large brain tissues reminiscent of ventricles rather than rosettes (Kadoshima et al. 2013; Lancaster et al. 2013; Nasu et al. 2012).

These complex 3D in vitro neural tissues meet the criteria to be called organoids. According to the most basic definition, organoids are in vitro cultured structures that resemble an organ. More precisely, an organoid should satisfy four criteria: (1) a 3D structure containing cells that establish or retain the identity of the organ being modelled; (2) the presence of multiple cell types, as in the organ itself; (3) the tissue exhibits some aspect of the specialized function of the organ; and (4) self-organization according to the same intrinsic organizing principles as in the organ itself (Lancaster and Huch 2019). In general, organoids can be generated from cells derived from adult tissue or pluripotent stem cells (PSCs) – either embryonic stem cells (ESCs) derived from embryos or induced pluripotent stem cells (iPSC) obtained by reprogramming of adult cells (Takahashi and Yamanaka 2006; Thomson et al. 1998). Generation of organoid cultures from PSCs allows for recapitulation of the developmental processes and tissue organogenesis that occur in vivo in a dish, and is also the only way to produce organoids from tissues with limited regeneration potential such as neural tissue (Lancaster and Huch 2019).

Neural organoids can be generated from single PSCs, aggregates of dissociated PSCs or whole colonies, and the process can be either unguided or guided. Unguided methods rely on the natural propensity of PSCs to differentiate towards neural fates without extrinsic signaling cues, whereas guided methods utilize small molecules and growth factors to promote development of the desired fates and inhibition of other tissue types. Guided methods have been demonstrated to produce a narrower range of fates at the cost of complexity and regional diversity, while the benefit is improved reproducibility and more homogeneous cellular makeup (Kelava and Lancaster 2016b; Velasco et al. 2019).

In the several years since the development of the initial neural organoid methods, the field has greatly expanded in terms of application of organoid models but also their refinement and detailed characterization. It is now accepted that neural organoids constitute a valid representation of in vivo development and as such can be applied for studies of developmental mechanisms, pathogenesis, and even evolution in a setting combining the advantages of in vitro and in vivo systems

(Chiaradia and Lancaster 2020; Kelava and Lancaster 2016a). Initially, organoids were primarily applied to questions related to neurogenesis, neuronal maturation, function, and disease modelling. But more recently, neural organoid models have been employed to study much earlier events in neural development, preceding neurogenesis and spanning events from neural induction to early expansion of neuroepithelia and radial glia (Benito-Kwiecinski et al. 2021). In vitro modelling of neurulation poses significant challenges due to the transient nature of the neural tube, the complexity of its development, its large size, and its interaction with multiple tissues in the embryo. In vitro models of neural tube represent both ends of the spectrum of complexity: from minimal reductionist model of neural cyst or neurulating ectodermal cyst to almost a whole embryo-like structure that produces a self-closing neural plate (Azhar and Sonnen 2021; Karzbrun et al. 2021). The continual evolution of neural organoid methods is producing tissues with even more impressive similarity to in vivo development, and their application to early neural developmental events is beginning to uncover unique aspects of human brain patterning, morphogenesis, and expansion.

19.3 Early Forebrain Morphogenesis

19.3.1 Neural Specification and Patterning

Neocortex formation is a result of a complex sequence of developmental events in the embryo (Figure 19.1A). The development of a new organism begins with fertilization and a resulting zygote initially divides to form a mass of cells termed the morula. The morula then hollows out to form a blastocyst with surrounding trophectoderm and an inner cell mass, which in turn separates into the epiblast and the hypoblast or the primitive endoderm. The epiblast will then continue developing to form all tissues of the body (Niakan et al. 2012). The anterior neural fate is the default developmental trajectory of the epiblast. If a portion of epiblast is separated from the rest of the embryo and maintained without any signaling cues, it will develop into the anterior nervous system (Ozair et al. 2013; Stern 2005). This is reflected in the epigenetic state of the epiblast, where the pre-neural methylation and chromatin accessibility landscape are already established (Argelaguet et al. 2019). This "blank slate" state is then maintained in the rostral ectoderm through its protection from patterning signals, whereas in other parts of the embryo it is modified by a complex interplay of signaling cues such as BMP, WNT, Nodal, and FGF (fibroblast growth factor) to give rise to other germ layers through the process of gastrulation (Levine and Brivanlou 2007). These posteriorizing cues are inhibited in the anterior epiblast by the early/mid-gastrula organizer, which secretes chordin and noggin, BMP antagonists, to initiate neural induction. Later, the anterior ventral endoderm (AVE) promotes development of the anterior neural plate with supply of lefty, DKK-1, and Cerberus, which collectively inhibit Nodal, Wnt, and BMP (Levine and Brivanlou 2007), further maintaining the absence of signaling to allow anterior identity, and eventually forebrain. More posterior identities, such as spinal cord, develop through exposure to FGF and WNT during neural induction (Metzis et al. 2018).

In early development, inhibition of BMP signaling allows for specification of neuroectoderm from ectoderm, and intermediate BMP signaling determines the neural plate border (NBP). Manipulation of BMP levels in Xenopus embryos can lead to ectopic neural tissue formation, and depletion of endogenous BMP inhibitors prevents neuroectoderm formation (Bond et al. 2012). Initially, low-BMP levels are essential for forebrain specification. Mouse cephalic explants exposed to BMP downregulate anterior forebrain markers, whereas knockout of BMP antagonists chordin and noggin prevents development of anterior brain structures in embryos (Anderson et al. 2002). Later, BMPs diffusing from the roof plate and cortical hem help establish the dorsal–ventral axis of

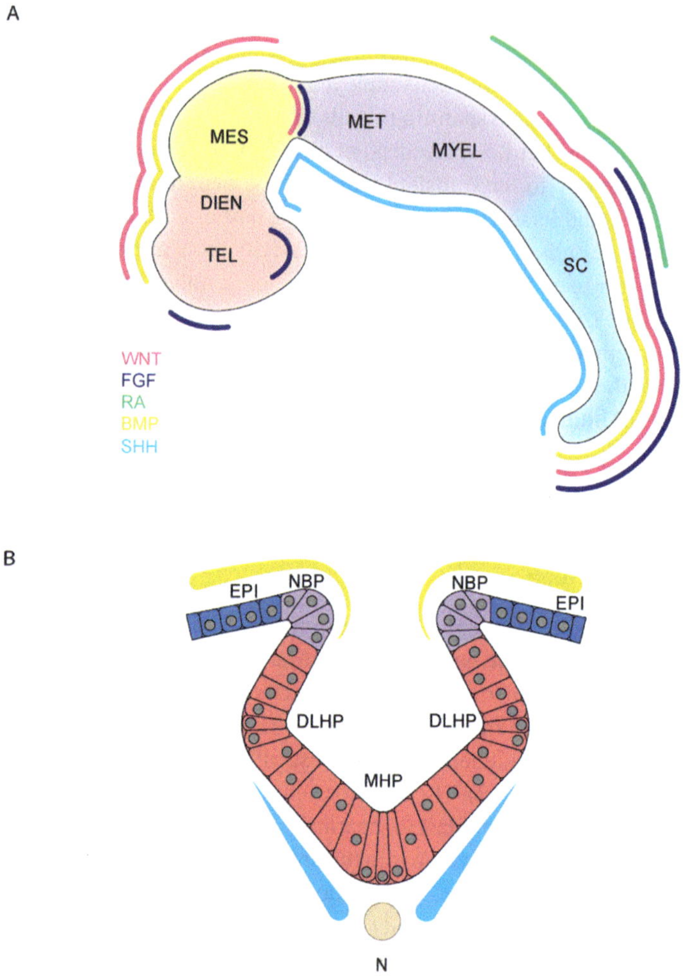

Figure 19.1 Patterning of the developing nervous system. (A) Factors in rostro-caudal and dorso-ventral patterning of the neural tube (Chiaradia and Lancaster 2020; Sanes et al. 2019). TEL, telencephalon; DIEN, diencephalon; MES, mesencephalon; MET, metencephalon; MYEL, myelencephalon, SC, spinal cord; WNT, Wingless and Int-1 ligand; FGF, fibroblast growth factor; RA, retinoic acid; BMP, bone morphogenetic protein; SHH, Sonic hedgehog. (B) Mechanisms of neural tube morphogenesis (Eom et al. 2011, 2013). EPI, epidermis; NPB, neural plate border; DLHP, dorso-lateral hinge point; MHP, medial hinge point; N, notochord.

the developing brain and are essential for formation of dorsal structures of the pallium. Knockout of BMP receptor 1a (BMPRIa) in mouse telencephalon results in loss of choroid plexus, the most dorsal–medial structure (Hébert et al. 2002). Double BMPRIa and Ib mutant shows complete loss of all dorsal midline including cortical hem, whereas ventral structures seem normal (Fernandes et al. 2007). Mice deficient in Bmpr1b constitutively and deficient in Bmpr1a conditionally in the dorsal telencephalon, display severe defects in dentate gyrus formation (Caronia et al. 2010).

Canonical WNT signaling cooperates with BMP during development and initially has an inhibitory effect on anterior neural fate formation (Kiecker and Niehrs 2001). Later, Wnt/β-catenin signaling regulates dorso-ventral patterning, as well as progenitor proliferation in the telencephalon (Chenn 2008). Different manipulations of Wnt/β-catenin can lead to either underproliferation or over-proliferation of neocortical progenitors, and inhibition of Wnt signaling from the cortical hem leads to failure of hippocampal development (Mulligan and Cheyette 2012). Thus, while a lack of BMP and WNT signaling is necessary for initial forebrain establishment, activation of these pathways is needed for patterning and expansion of dorsal telencephalic identities.

During neurulation, FGFs produced in the anterior neural ridge (ANR) induce broadly forebrain fates and promote survival and proliferation of the neural precursors (Hébert 2011). In the telencephalon, FGFs pattern and promote expansion of the neocortex. FGF8 is secreted in the commissural plate and establishes an antero-posterior gradient necessary for anterior fate specification (Fukuchi-Shimogori and Grove 2001; Toyoda et al. 2010). FGF17 determines regional specification in the dorsal rostral areas and its deletion causes loss of dorsal prefrontal cortex in mouse mutants (Cholfin and Rubenstein 2007). FGF10 is necessary for the transition of neural epithelia to radial glia specifically in the rostral forebrain (Sahara and O'Leary 2009). FGF2 drives proliferation of ventricular progenitors in the cortex (Vaccarino et al. 1999). Rat cortices injected with FGF2 showed higher proliferation of progenitors and larger number of neurons if the treatment was carried out in the neurogenic window. Mice lacking the FGF2 gene had fewer neurons and glia. FGF signaling is precisely regulated through ligand specificity and affinity to one of the four FGF receptors (FGFR), extracellular matrix components that can interact with FGFs, and intracellular modulators of signal response (Hébert 2011). FGF signaling response thus depends on the precise combination of FGFs, their receptors, and the cellular environment to regulate both patterning and proliferation in the forebrain.

Sonic hedgehog (SHH) is necessary for ventral patterning of the entire neural tube including the forebrain (Guillemot 2005). SHH in the embryo is primarily secreted from the notochord, but since the notochord does not extend as far as the developing forebrain, the dorso-ventral gradient there becomes skewed in the antero-posterior direction. However, once forebrain specification has occurred, the telencephalic anlage is patterned by the combination of SHH from the telencephalic floorplate and the BMPs, WNTs, and FGFs to form the dorsal $Pax6^{+}$ pallium and ventral $Pax6^{-}$ subpallium. Holoprosencephaly, a congenital defect caused by failure to define the midline of the forebrain, is caused by mutations in Nodal and SHH pathway components (Hong and Krauss 2018). Nodal plays a role in prechordal mesoderm specification, which in turn secretes SHH and stimulates secretion of SHH from the floor plate of the neural tube (Dubourg et al. 2007). Mutations in several genes have been identified to be causative of holoprosencephaly in humans, including SHH, ZIC2, SIX3, TGIF, PTCH, GLI2, and TDGF1; however, in 70 percent of cases the genetic causes are unknown. Affected individuals show highly variable severity of the disease suggesting that complex interaction with genetic background and environmental factors determines the phenotype (Dubourg et al. 2007). Studies in mice suggest that teratogens such as ethanol can cause more severe phenotypes in sensitive asymptomatic genotypes (Hong and Krauss 2018). Since cholesterol is needed for the SHH response, drugs or metabolic defects affecting cholesterol levels or inborn cholesterol metabolism defects can contribute to development of holoprosencephaly (Haas et al. 2007).

According to the protomap hypothesis, cortical regional identity is established early in development due to the gradient of morphogens that activate distinct gene networks depending on the position of the neural progenitor in the ventricular surface (Rakic et al. 1991). The full diversity of brain cell types is then achieved through the combination of time and the sequence of neuron generation and eventually with input from other brain parts and sensory organs. Establishment of the brain protomap could be considered a small subsection of embryonic patterning, and hence, involves the same signaling factors BMP, Shh, Wnt, and retinoic acid (RA), with local signaling centers emerging, both alongside the DV and the AP axis, leading to additional layers of patterning information (Nikolopoulou et al. 2017). Morphogens are generally thought to provide crude patterning instructions, which can be refined by gradients of concentrations of multiple signaling molecules in a so-called Turing patterning mechanism (Landge et al. 2020). A narrow range of one or more morphogen concentrations can be interpreted by the transcription factors in the underlying gene regulatory network and thus translated into sharp borders between cells that will commit to different developmental trajectories.

The brain protomap establishment most likely starts very early in development, at the point of neural induction. The anterior-most part of the neural plate is already distinct before closure due to antero-posterior patterning and the dorso-ventral patterning emerging concomitantly with neurulation (Juriloff and Harris 2018). In the anterior forebrain region in mammals the entire neural plate will become the future brain and the neural plate border (NBP) cells are not induced. This is regulated through expression of Tcf7l1, which limits activation of BMP and Wnt pathways involved in NBP specification. Overall, the same set of morphogens seem to be used throughout forebrain patterning, with the specific response being modulated at different stages so that the same molecules can be used iteratively to achieve various outcomes depending on the development time window (Bond et al. 2012; Green et al. 2020).

19.3.2 Neural Tube Formation

Once neural identity is established, the neural plate undergoes a combination of morphological changes that include elongation, bending in the middle to create the neural folds, and their elevation towards the dorsal midline (Eom et al. 2011, 2013) (Figure 19.1B). The simultaneous elongation and bending are termed convergent extension and depend upon the non-canonical Wnt/planar cell polarity (PCP) pathway. In mammals, the neuroepithelium that constitutes the neural plate and then the neural tube is polarized and pseudostratified, and displays a behavior called interkinetic nuclear migration (IKNM), where mitotic nuclei locate at the apical side and nuclei in S phase locate at the basal pole of the cells. Accumulation of cells in S phase in the middle of the neural plate, just above the notochord, permits formation of the medial hinge point (MHP). Formation of hinge points is induced by interaction of BMP4 and SHH signaling. Regions of lower BMP activity can undergo apical constriction and allow for bending either in the MHP or close to the tips of the neural folds (dorso-lateral hinge points, DLHP) of the wider anterior portion of the neural plate. High BMP activity promotes stabilization of junctional proteins and maintains width equality between the apical and basal membranes, which prevents folding. In contrast, lower BMP signaling weakens cell-to-cell junctions, which then permits apical constriction of the actomyosin network (Eom et al. 2011, 2013). The elevation of neural folds is aided by the underlying developing mesoderm and adjacent nonneural ectoderm (Araya et al. 2014). Finally, the neural fold tips meet and fuse to form the neural tube. The fusion is asynchronous and proceeds through a mechanism of multisite, progressive closure or zippering alongside the length of the neural tube (Greene and Copp 2014). In mice, neural tube closure begins on embryonic day 8.5 at the hindbrain/cervical boundary (closure 1). On embryonic day 9, closure 2 initiates in the forebrain/midbrain boundary and spreads bidirectionally from the sites of closures 1 and 2 and caudally from the rostral end of the neural tube (closure 3). In humans, closure 1 happens at approximately 21 days and the complete fusion of the neural tube by 26–28 days postfertilization. Studies of human embryos did not show evidence of closure 2 but instead closure 1 spreads all the way to the anterior neuropore. The overlying nonneural ectoderm initiates contact of the opposing neural folds and eventually separates from the neural tube upon closure (Nikolopoulou et al. 2017). Neural crest (NC) cells start to delaminate from the neural plate border just before NT closure in the anterior region, whereas in the posterior region the NC emerges after the fusion has completed. In rodents and humans, the posterior-most neural tube, beyond sacral level, forms through a process of secondary neurulation, where an initial rod of neural epithelium cells hollows out to form a lumen (Nikolopoulou et al. 2017).

Most knowledge about the mechanisms of neurulation comes from chick and rodent models. Although the general principles are similar in all vertebrates, the specific genetic mechanisms underlying pathologies differ between animals and even between different mouse strains. In mice, failure of closure 2 or incomplete fusion of neural folds between closures 1 and 2 causes anencephaly, whereas defects of closure 3 result in a phenotype of a split face usually with forebrain anencephaly (Greene and Copp 2014). In humans, anencephaly is a result of failure of neural tube closure between the hindbrain/cervical border and the rostral end of the neural tube. An open neural tube in the cranial region is termed exencephaly, and results in the exposed neuroepithelium bulging out and subsequently degenerating, which leads to anencephaly. Under such circumstances most brain structures, apart from rarely parts of the brain stem, do not develop and the defect usually results in death in utero or at birth (Greene and Copp 2014). Treatment strategies for pre- and postnatal management of caudal neural tube defects (spina bifida) already exist, either as a surgical approach or in combination with stem cell therapy, currently at the clinical trial stage (Long et al. 2019). However, the only option for anencephaly is currently prevention; therefore, accurate modelling, especially in human systems, is needed (Soltani Khaboushan et al. 2022).

Neural tube defects are understood to result from a combination of multiple genetic and environmental factors (Greene and Copp 2014). Moreover, these factors can contribute differently to abnormalities at different levels of the neural tube. Cranial neural folds are particularly large and therefore pose a challenge for successful fusion. This is reflected in a particular sensitivity of cranial neurulation to NTD-inducing agents and mutations in genes not affecting other regions of the neural tube. Apical constriction seems to be of particular importance for cranial neural tube closure (Juriloff and Harris 2018) and mutations in cytoskeletal proteins, such as vinculin or N-cofilin, are associated with isolated exencephaly (Greene and Copp 2014). In contrast, PCP pathway aberrations tend to affect the caudal neural tube more often than rostral, at least in mice (Greene and Copp 2014). Pinpointing definite genetic causes is complicated by the fact that fetuses presenting with anencephaly are often compound heterozygotes for multiple genes in one or more pathways, whereas severe mutation in single genes have pleiotropic effects and may lead to fetal death before the neural tube phenotype becomes evident. Generally, genes predisposing to anencephaly in humans can be grouped into categories of PCP pathway (CELSR1, VANGL1, VANGL2, FZD6, SCRIB1, and DVL2), actin cytoskeleton regulation (COBL, SHROOM3), RTK signaling (PDGFRa), folate one carbon metabolism (MTHFR, AMT, GLD, MTHFD1L, SLC23A32) and other metabolic genes (SOD1, SOD2, GLUT1) (Greene and Copp 2014; Ishida et al. 2018). Among environmental factors contributing are folate, vitamin B12 and inositol deficiency, maternal obesity and diabetes, maternal hyperthermia, and a range of teratogens such as the antiepileptic drug valproic acid or environmental toxins (Avagliano et al. 2019).

19.3.3 Forebrain Expansion

Upon neural tube closure, NE cells keep on dividing in a symmetric fashion to establish a founder progenitor pool. This is especially pronounced in the anterior-most part of the neural tube and contributes to lateral and radial expansion of the future neocortex (Florio and Huttner 2014). The enlarged anterior portion of the neural tube can be divided into the three primary brain vesicles: prosencephalon (forebrain), mesencephalon (midbrain), and rhombencephalon (hindbrain), which become evident at about embryonic day 29 in human. By embryonic day 49, the expanding prosencephalon further divides into telencephalon and diencephalon (Stiles and Jernigan 2010).

Eventually the NE cells lose aspects of their epithelial character and become apical radial glia (aRG) capable of producing neurons. In primates, GFAP positive radial glia emerge soon after neural tube closure. In rodents, however, neural stem cells of the brain only become GFAP positive after birth (Rakic 2007).

The initially uniform neuroepithelium of the cortex gives rise to a diverse population of radial glia (Eze et al. 2021). aRGs reside at the ventricular zone (VZ) throughout the development of the cortex and early in development they produce neurons and intermediate progenitors (IP). IPs can in turn proliferate and produce neurons, increasing both the number and the repertoire of the neurons that will eventually constitute the fully developed cortex. Initially all radial glia span the entire thickness of the developing cortical wall, with their apical processes in contact with the ventricular surface and the basal process extending towards the pial surface, whereas the soma remains relatively close to the ventricular surface. Later in development, some radial glia shift towards the margin of the proliferative zone, the subventricular zone (SVZ) and outer subventricular zone (OSVZ), and lose their apical process to become basal radial glia (bRG) (Fietz et al. 2010; Hansen et al. 2010). Others lose their basal process and transform into truncated radial glia (tRGs) (Nowakowski et al. 2016b). The fate decisions of NE and RG progenitors within the cortex are key to forebrain expansion, as they will determine how many cortical neurons and glia are made and of which types.

Once neurons are generated in the VZ and the subventricular zone (SVZ), they position themselves by using the protracted basal processes of RGs as a scaffold that guides them radially towards the basal surface (Rakic 2007). New-born neurons migrate by extension of their leading process and displacement of the nucleus, a mechanism known as nuclear and/or somal translocation. Early born neurons form a dense radial arrangement termed the cortical plate (CP). Later born neurons migrate past the earlier born cells already in the cortical plate, where they detach from the RG process and are positioned in an inside-out fashion. Finally, supportive glia of the brain including astrocytes and oligodendrocytes are generated in the final divisions of the various RG populations.

Failure of the brain to reach its normal size in the prenatal period results in a condition called microcephaly (Figure 19.2A). Clinically, microcephaly is defined as a reduction of the occipito-frontal head circumference of at least two standard deviations below the mean for a given sex and age (Severino et al. 2020). Primary microcephaly usually results from reduction of number of generated cortical neurons due to defects in progenitor proliferation, differentiation, and/or apoptosis and is already present at birth. Genetic and environmental factors alone or in combination contribute to the development of the condition (Zaqout and Kaindl 2022). The most prominent example of an environmental trigger for microcephaly is infection with Zika virus (ZIKV). In December 2016, the World Health Organization (WHO) declared ZIKV infection a public health emergency after it had been linked to development of microcephaly in babies of mothers infected with ZIKV in pregnancy (Su et al. 2022). Genes identified to date as causative for microcephaly encode for proteins involved in centrosome regulation, microtubule dynamics, mitotic spindle formation, DNA damage response, Wnt signaling, transcriptional regulation and cell cycle checkpoint control (Zaqout and Kaindl 2022). Some microcephaly related genes (MCPH1, CDK5RAP2, ASPM, and CENPJ) show evidence of positive selection in the human lineage and the eutherian lineage (Pervaiz et al. 2021). On the other hand, overgrowth of the brain leads to megalencephaly, which can be the cause of macrocephaly or abnormally enlarged head circumference (Severino et al. 2020) (Figure 19.2A). Overgrowth can affect the whole brain or only some regions or cell populations. Developmental megalencephaly is caused by disruption of signaling pathways that regulate brain cellular proliferation, differentiation, and survival (Severino et al. 2020). Mutations

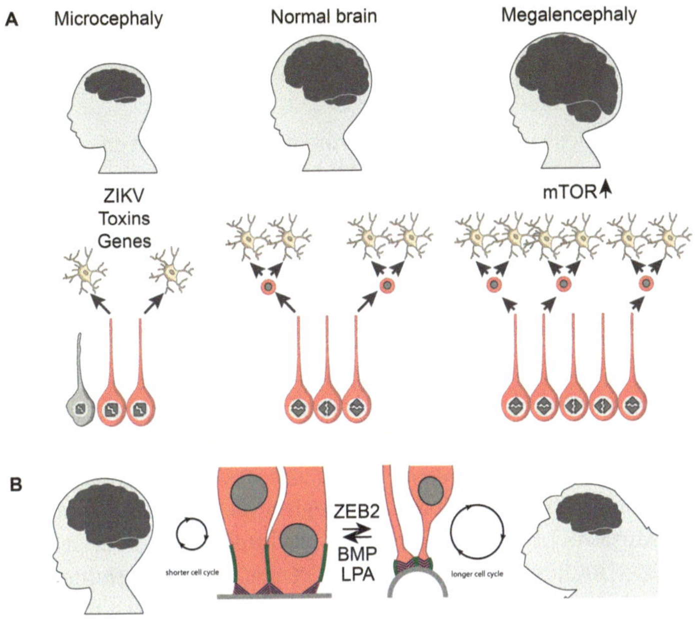

Figure 19.2 Mechanisms influencing brain size and brain size pathologies. (A) Left: genetic mutations, environmental toxins, or pathogens lead to reduced proliferation of progenitors and neuronal death leading to reduced brain size (Lancaster et al. 2013; Gabriel et al. 2016; Zhang et al. 2019; Cugola et al. 2016; Garcez et al. 2016; Qian et al. 2016). Middle: typical brain development. Right: dysregulation of mTOR pathway causes brain overgrowth (Butler 2005; Li et al. 2017; Zhang et al. 2020; Dhaliwal et al. 2021). (B) Transition between neuroepithelium and radial glia involves cell shape change and is controlled by ZEB2 (Benito-Kwiecinski et al. 2021); this transition happens earlier in nonhuman ape (right) than in human which maintains wider NE shape and divides faster for longer (left); BMP, bone morphogenetic protein; LPA, lysophosphatidic acid.

resulting in megalencephaly affect members and regulators of PI3K/PTEN/Akt/mTor signaling (Cummings et al. 2022).

All mammalian species share a general brain developmental blueprint: apicobasal organization of radial glia (RGs), sequential and timed appearance of specific cell types, and coordinated maturation of mixed-cell populations resulting in formation of functional neural circuits (Bakken et al. 2016; Campbell and Götz 2002). In some mammals this plan was further refined and elaborated in the process of evolution. Gyrencephalic brains of larger-brained mammals, such as primates and carnivores, expanded the population of outer radial glia (oRGs), which produce a larger number of neurons leading to thickening of the cortex (Kawasaki 2018; Stahl et al. 2013). Primates in particular exhibit greatly increased neuron numbers, with increased neuronal density, compared with other mammals (Herculano-Houzel 2009). Amongst primates, the human brain develops the slowest and for longest, resulting in a brain of about three times larger with twice as many cortical neurons compared to our closest living relatives, chimpanzee and gorilla (Figure 19.2B). While the slower developmental progression, or neoteny, of the human brain is widely accepted as being key to brain expansion and has been validated at morphological and transcriptional levels (Somel et al. 2009), the exact cellular and molecular mechanisms are only just beginning to be understood. Approximately 9 percent of genes in the developing brain show human specific regulation resulting in prolonged developmental trajectory when compared to rhesus monkey (Macaca mulatta) (Bakken et al. 2016). It is interesting to speculate that the vulnerability of our brains to certain human-specific disorders stems from these evolutionarily recent human-specific features of brain development (Fernandes et al. 2021).

19.4 Organoid Models

19.4.1 Neural Patterning In Vitro

Neural patterning in vivo involves a complex and beautifully coordinated dance between multiple gradients of signaling molecules, gene expression, biomechanical interactions, and tissue compartmentalization. Modelling such complexity in vitro is therefore no easy task. However, increasing understanding of the key factors from in vivo studies, combined with elegant bioengineering approaches are enabling the establishment of increasingly sophisticated models of even very complex processes, including patterning and morphogenesis.

Neuroepithelial cysts provide a reductionist model of neural tube patterning in vivo (Meinhardt et al. 2014) (Figure 19.3). They form from single PSCs seeded in Matrigel or hydrogel in N2B27 medium. After 5 days of culture the tissues hollow out to form a single lumen. The structures display striking similarities to mouse embryonic day 8 neural tube in terms of morphology and gene expression. They consist of pseudostratified, well-polarized epithelium undergoing interkinetic nuclear migration, with ZO-1 staining on the luminal side and high levels of neural stem cell markers such as SOX1, Nestin, and Musashi. Untreated neural cysts produce broadly anterior neural tissue with expression of OTX2, GBX2, and anterior-most HOX genes, demonstrating the default posterior fate in the absence of posteriorizing factors, as in vivo. However, in the presence of retinoic acid treatment they acquire more posterior identities including hindbrain and spinal cord, similar to in vivo.

Self-organizing signaling centers emerge in longer term cultures of neural cysts (Ranga et al. 2016). In synthetic matrix in medium with RA one pole of the cyst starts expressing Shh in an area similar to a floor plate. The endogenously produced Shh is then able to pattern adjacent regions of the cyst by inducing expression of Nkx-6.1 in the neighboring cells and then Olig2 beyond. The opposite pole to the cyst "floor plate" contains Pax3 cells, which in an embryonic neural tube demarcate the dorsal domain. Once established, patterning persists through neurogenesis so that daughter neurons appear near their appropriate progenitors. Thus, while neural patterning and morphogenesis is a complex process in vivo, it can be accurately accomplished in vitro by enabling tissues to self-organize and intrinsically establish complexity.

Similar evidence of self-patterning is observed in cerebral organoids generated with an unguided method (Figure 19.3). Such organoids form multiple brain regions including dorsal forebrain,

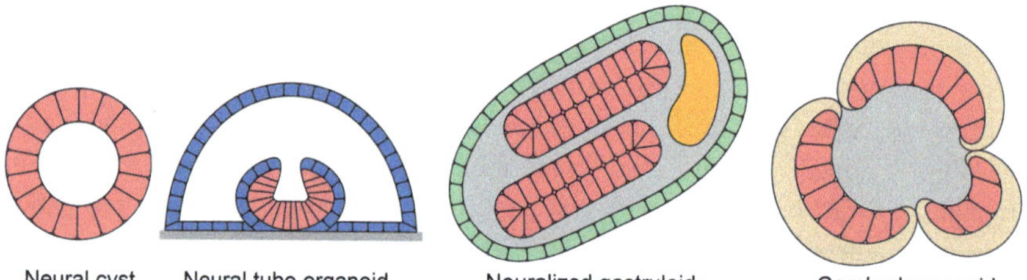

Figure 19.3 Organoid models of developing nervous system. Neural cyst – a single layer of neuroepithelial cells surrounding a lumen (Meinhardt et al. 2014; Ranga et al. 2016); neural tube organoid – a PSC-derived, self-organizing structure undergoing epidermis and neural epithelium line specification and neural tube folding and closure (Karzbrun et al. 2021); neuralized gastruloid – a coculture of a PSC-derived gastruloid and extraembryonic endoderm cells resulting in self-organization of neural tube-like structures (Bérenger-Currias et al. 2022); cerebral organoid – PSC-derived self-organizing structure that recapitulates development and architecture of the brain (Lancaster et al. 2013, 2017).

choroid plexus, ventral forebrain, and less frequently retina, arranged in discrete domains in a configuration recapitulating in vivo patterns (Lancaster et al. 2013). With organoid development the regional specification progresses and the EMX1-positive dorsal cortical areas further subdivide into prefrontal cortex (positive for AUTS2), occipital lobe (positive for TSHZ2), and frontal lobe (positive for LMO4). This suggests mutual interactions of the adjacent areas and some degree of formation of a cortical protomap that could be used for brain patterning studies.

Patterning of neural organoids is robust and easy to manipulate and therefore suitable for studies of morphogen gradients and factors that modify responsiveness to morphogens. For example, treatment of neural cysts with N-[N-(3,5-difluorophenacetyl)-1-alanyl]-S-phenylglycine t-butyl ester (DAPT, an inhibitor of γ-secretase inhibitor that abrogates Notch activity), increases intrinsic dorso-ventral patterning efficiency. Interestingly, a window of responsiveness was specified between 2 and 3 days (Ranga et al. 2016). Signaling factors can also be used to drive subregional identity within the forebrain. When exposed to BMP and Wnt agonists, forebrain organoids can be differentiated to hippocampus (Jacob et al. 2020; Sakaguchi et al. 2015) or choroid plexus (Jacob et al. 2020; Pellegrini et al. 2020). Conversely, subpallial identities can be generated to produce striatum (Miura et al. 2020), basal ganglia (Bagley et al. 2017; Birey et al. 2017; Xiang et al. 2017), hypothalamus (Qian et al. 2016), and thalamus (Xiang et al. 2019). Thus, not only can patterning factors be applied to direct initial neural differentiation and anteriorization, but they can also be used at later stages to further define which regions within the forebrain are generated.

Complex signaling molecule combinations can be studied by reduction of signaling cues to gradients of morphogens that in the embryo run alongside antero-posterior and/or dorso-ventral axes. Microfluidic devices allow formation of defined gradients of soluble factors in a controlled environment conducive to cell culture (Park et al. 2019). In a biocompatible and bioinert environment such as silicon and glass, where leaching and adsorption of molecules can be prevented, precise concentrations of morphogens leading to desired differentiation outcomes can be determined. Such a microfluidic system allowed for in vitro modelling of neural tube development in mouse ESCs embedded in natural extracellular matrix (Demers et al. 2016). Combination of a constant concentration of RA together with antiparallel gradients of pluromorphin (PM, a SHH pathway agonist) and BMP4 resulted in spatial self-organization and differentiation into motor neurons recapitulating in vivo neural tube patterning during spinal cord development. Precise and dynamic spatial and temporal microfluidic control enabled the finding that differentiating ESCs respond to a narrow range of optimal SHH concentration rather than SHH gradient or its slope. Addition of a second morphogen further defined the precise expression domain of a gene regulatory network guiding motor neuron differentiation. Microfluidic devices or "chips" can also be applied to study patterning in later development since cerebral organoids are also amenable to this type of culture (Cho et al. 2021; Karzbrun et al. 2018).

Alternatively, a source of a morphogen can be included in the organoid tissue itself. Cederquist et al. embedded a small cluster of inducible SHH (iSHH) expressing cells into embryoid bodies that were then differentiated into brain organoids (Cederquist et al. 2019). The iSHH cluster usually remained integral and localized to one pole of the organoid. Upon addition of doxycycline it started expressing soluble SHH and acted as an organizer for dorso-ventral and antero-posterior patterning of the rest of the forebrain organoid tissue. The self-patterned organoids contained diencephalon and telencephalon identities, which further subdivided into physiologically arranged areas of neocortex (FOXG1+/PAX6+), lateral ganglionic eminence (GSH2+), medial ganglionic eminence (FOXG1+/NKX2.1+), anterior hypothalamus (NKX2.2+), and ventro-posterior hypothalamus (NKX2.1+/FOXG1−). Diffusion dynamics and range of SHH in the 3D tissue were similar to in vivo models and showed sensitivity to manipulation of cholesterol synthesis.

19.4.2 Neural Tube Modelling

Cranial neurulation is not very well studied in humans or even in rodent models (Juriloff and Harris 2018) but organoid models can provide new insights for example into early patterning and hinge-point formation in the forebrain neural plate. Two-dimensional rosettes grown on patterned substrates demonstrated the intrinsic ability of these neural tube-like structures to develop with larger or smaller sized lumens depending on the anterior-posterior identity, with forebrain identity rosettes capable of forming larger individual rosettes (Knight et al. 2018). This suggests there are intrinsic differences in neuroepithelial cell shape depending on regional identity, and that these developmental programs can be recapitulated even in reductionist in vitro approaches.

Recently, complete neurulation in vitro, including neural tube folding and closure, was elegantly demonstrated through the combination of patterned substrates and Matrigel (Karzbrun et al. 2021) (Figure 19.3). By creating an elongated micropatterned surface to constrain PSCs, followed by application of Matrigel, 3D tissues formed with a fully enclosed compartment, within which neural plate-like tissue formed, elevated, and closed in a manner highly reminiscent of in vivo complete with hinge points. Substrate size manipulation of this system demonstrated how tissue size regulates the process of hinge formation in the neural plate. Wider neural tubes produced dorsolateral hinge points normally observed in the larger neural plate in the head area, whereas narrower tissues only formed medial hinge points, similar to neural tube in the upper trunk region of an embryo. Thus, organoid models could be applied for investigation of various stages of neurulation and specifically how tissue size corresponds to local regulation of signaling driving hinge-point formation.

Neurulation also involves mechanisms extrinsic to the neural tissue itself. Specifically, mesoderm is involved in neural tube formation and closure, especially in the cranial region (Araya et al. 2014; Chen and Behringer 1995). Therefore, more complex models incorporating other germ layers could be useful to model the process in vitro. Gastruloids recapitulate aspects of spatial and temporal genetics in early post-implantation development and form post-occipital patterns of neural, mesodermal, and endodermal derivatives (Beccari et al. 2018). Although gastruloids normally produce disorganized neural cells, when embedded in Matrigel or provided with extraembryonic endoderm cells (XEN), they can form neural epithelium (Bérenger-Currias et al. 2022; Veenvliet et al. 2020) (Figure 19.3). Extracellular matrix gel alone promotes maturation and organization of neuromesodermal progenitors (NMPs) and their segregation into somites and neural tube, leading to formation of trunk like structures (Veenvliet et al. 2020). On the other hand, co-culture of gastruloids with XEN cells, which provide both extracellular matrix and morphogens (Dkk1), shifts the balance of NMP maturation towards neural fate. XEN-enhanced gastruloid (XEG) neuroepithelia showed in vivo-like characteristics such as SOX1 expression, pseudostratified structure and apico-basal polarity with correct localization of aPKC and ZO-1 in the apical pole of the cells (Bérenger-Currias et al. 2022). They also displayed local self-patterning into ventral identities with Nkx6.1 expression and more dorsal ones positive for Pax6, and responded correctly to morphogens such as SHH agonist, RA, or BMP inhibitor. Interestingly, despite the initial posterior character of the structures, long exposure to Dkk1 from the XEN could shift XEG identity towards more anterior fates. Older structures showed expression of FOXG1, a fore- and midbrain marker, and produced TUJ1 and CTIP2 positive neurons characteristic to forebrain, arranged in layered structures reminiscent of cerebral cortex. This suggests some level of plasticity in the developing neural tube at least in in vitro conditions, and the possibility to use initially posteriorized systems for modelling more anterior structures.

19.4.3 Modelling Early Forebrain Expansion

Unguided or minimally guided methods of brain organoid generation allow insight into early neural specification and capture stages of neuroepithelial expansion and transition to neurogenesis. Since this process is not accelerated by exogenous morphogens, it follows developmental timing of in vivo development (Benito-Kwiecinski et al. 2021; Lancaster et al. 2013, 2017) and thus has the potential to model human-specific forebrain neuroepithelial expansion and identify regulatory mechanisms. Cerebral organoids exposed to the WNT agonist CHIR-99021 were demonstrated to exhibit increased NE expansion of neural-tube like buds (Lancaster et al. 2017), similar to the in vivo effect of Wnt activation on forebrain NE (Chenn 2008). Additionally, lysophosphatidic acid (LPA), a serum derived factor that leads to increased apical surface area and larger rosettes in 2D culture (Medelnik et al. 2018) also leads to expansion of NE buds in cerebral organoids (Benito-Kwiecinski et al. 2021). Interestingly, LPA is much more abundant in human than in nonhuman primate plasma (0.14–1.64 μM in human vs. <10nM in macaque (Michalczyk et al. 2017; Wang et al. 2019)), and could potentially reach the embryo from maternal circulation to modulate this early expansion event.

The transition of NE to aRGs proceeds in a mode similar in many aspects to epithelial to mesenchymal transition (EMT) and recent work in cerebral organoids revealed an intermediate stage of transitioning NE (tNE) in which NE cells begin to constrict their apical surface but do not yet exhibit aRG identity. At a molecular level the tNE stage is triggered by ZEB2, which inhibits SMAD signaling and determines cell shape by affecting apical constriction and regulating cell-cell junctions (Benito-Kwiecinski et al. 2021). Thus, SMAD inhibition influences not only neural induction, but also NE to aRG transition, essentially speeding up this transition and limiting NE expansion. Such extrinsic guidance would therefore override normal developmental progression, making it difficult to identify human-specific mechanisms at this key developmental stage.

19.4.4 Modelling Human Disorders of Forebrain Expansion

Neural organoids provide an excellent tool for modelling defects in neural development. Imbalances in proliferation of progenitors can lead to micro- and macrocephaly, disorders that have proven difficult to model in rodents. The 3D structure of organoids allows for studying not only cell fate and identity determination but in a context with proper tissue architecture. This enables the investigation of precise molecular mechanisms leading to the phenotype, for example mitotic spindle orientation, over-proliferation or depletion of specific progenitor populations (Krefft et al. 2021).

Mitotic spindle orientation in the neuroepithelium is generally predictive of the outcome of the cell division at early stages. Vertical mitoses with a cleavage plane perpendicular to the apical surface usually result in two NEs or RGs (a so-called proliferative division), whereas horizontal and oblique divisions tend to generate more differentiated cell types, including oRGs, IPs, and neurons (LaMonica et al. 2013). An early abundance of vertical mitoses ensures establishment of a large pool of founder progenitors that will translate into a large number of neurons in the mature brain. Therefore, precise regulation of mitotic cleavage plain is crucial for human brain growth and disruption of mitotic spindle orientation lies at the root of some forms of microcephaly. CDK5RAP2 regulates mitotic spindle orientation and, when absent, reduces the number of vertical mitoses needed for proliferative divisions. Organoids grown with iPSCs from a patient suffering from microcephaly caused by compound mutations in the CDK5RAP2 gene produced smaller neural tissues with only very few progenitor regions, which prematurely differentiated into neurons (Lancaster et al. 2013). Silencing *CDK5RAP2* in a region of a healthy organoid by shRNA showed the same phenotype of premature differentiation due to excess self-consuming neurogenic divisions.

Mutations in centrosomal P4.1-associated protein (CPAP), another centrosome regulator, are the cause of Seckel syndrome that manifests with microcephaly, amongst other symptoms. Seckel organoids grown with iPSCs from patients produced brain tissue that was smaller than that of controls, with fewer progenitors, disorganized VZ, and larger lumens (Gabriel et al. 2016). Apical progenitors lacking CPAP showed fewer vertical mitoses. Moreover, CPAP is known to participate in primary cilium disassembly and this function also contributes to the pathology of Seckel syndrome. Neural progenitor cells from Seckel patients showed longer cilia and delayed G1/S progression due to slower cilium disassembly resulting in premature differentiation (Gabriel et al. 2016). Knockout of another microcephaly associated gene WDR62 in human iPSC-derived organoids resulted in impaired primary cilium disassembly and lengthening of the cell cycle. This was particularly pronounced in human oRGs and led to drastic reduction in neuronal output and overall size of mutant organoids (Zhang et al. 2019).

Haploinsufficiency of ZEB2 causes Mowat–Wilson syndrome, a syndromic condition that often includes microcephaly. ZEB2's role in the neuroepithelium makes the effects of its reduction widespread, leading to defects not only in the brain but also neural crest derived tissues, including the enteric nervous system, heart, and face. In human organoids, heterozygous knockout led to enlarged NE, consistent with its role in NE to RG transition. The organoids displayed ballooning out of the NE with enlarged fluid-filled spaces, also consistent with the patient phenotype, which includes enlarged ventricles (Benito-Kwiecinski et al. 2021). Thus, genetic abnormalities that promote precocious developmental transitions, or delay them, can result in disrupted forebrain growth indicating a particular sensitivity of this tissue in humans.

In addition to genetic causes of microcephaly, brain organoids were employed to study the link between ZIKV infection and microcephaly and demonstrated their superiority over two-dimensional (2D) models (Qian et al. 2017). Analysis of forebrain organoids transiently exposed to ZIKV at different developmental stages confirmed the connection between ZIKV infection and microcephaly. ZIKV preferentially infected ventricular RG and oRG, where it could replicate to then release more infectious particles (Garcez et al. 2016; Qian et al. 2016). The preference of ZIKV infection was investigated through analysis of putative flavivirus entry receptor gene expression in the CNS. Especially AXL and heat shock protein genes showed strong enrichment in RG and astrocytes and were therefore hypothesized to be possible entry receptors for ZIKV (Nowakowski et al. 2016a). Apoptosis and suppression of proliferation of progenitors were proposed to be the mechanism leading to smaller organoid size and reduction of both progenitor and neuron numbers (Cugola et al. 2016; Garcez et al. 2016; Qian et al. 2016). Both apoptosis induction and lower proliferation were caused through activation of the innate immune toll-like receptor 3 (TLR3). A TLR3 competitive inhibitor attenuated the severe ZIKV-mediated apoptosis and organoid shrinkage. Treatment of organoids with TLR3 agonist produced the same gene expression changes as ZIKV infection, affecting a small subset of genes involved in neural development and synaptogenesis, in particular NTN1 and EPHB2 (Dang et al. 2016). Additionally, type I interferon signaling was shown to be a successful target for rescue of ZIKV-induced cell death (Krenn et al. 2021).

Macrocephaly can occur in various conditions and is often associated with mutations in the PI3K/Akt/mTOR pathway that plays an important role in regulating cell proliferation (Cummings et al. 2022). Mutations in the pathway regulator RAB39 are associated with X-linked macrocephaly. Cerebral organoids grown from RAB39b-deficient human iPSC cells were substantially enlarged, as a result of over-proliferation and impaired differentiation of neural progenitor cells (Zhang et al. 2020). Macrocephaly can be a feature of autism spectrum disorder (ASD) and is estimated to affect 14–34 percent of autistic patients, and mutations in genes involved in global increase of brain size often cause autism phenotypes (Cummings et al. 2022; Zhang et al. 2020). The increase in brain size in ASD is due to expansion of the surface area of the cortex rather than its thickness (Chan et al. 2020) and therefore can be attributed to early overgrowth of radial progenitors. PTEN is an inhibitor of the PI3K pathway and its mutation in patients can lead to macrocephaly with autism (Butler 2005). In organoids, deletion of PTEN leads to enlarged tissues with expanded progenitors (Li et al. 2017). On the other hand, increased expression of PTEN through a microduplication on chromosome 10 encompassing the PTEN gene instead leads to microcephaly, and over-expression of PTEN in organoids led to reduced neural precursor proliferation, premature neuronal differentiation, and overall smaller tissues (Dhaliwal et al. 2021), further confirming the role of PTEN in brain size regulation.

mTOR pathway activity in radial progenitors is also affected by extrinsic cues such as steroid hormones. Dorsal organoids treated with testosterone or its more potent form dihydrotestosterone (DHT) showed higher mTOR activation and produced more intermediate progenitors and neurons than untreated organoids or those grown with estradiol (Kelava et al. 2022). In contrast, ventralized brain organoids were not sensitive to androgens. Moreover, the mechanism of androgen regulation of cortex growth appeared to be species specific, since in mouse organoids it was estradiol, and not DHT, that led to higher abundance of intermediate progenitors.

Increased proliferation affecting only a subset of progenitors can lead to localized overgrowth or imbalances in proportions of daughter neuron populations. Tuberous sclerosis complex 1 and 2 (TSC1 and 2) are tumor suppressors involved in mTOR pathway regulation. TSC patients are usually heterozygous for mutations in either of the genes and when a second copy becomes randomly inactivated, excess cell growth and proliferation lead to development of lesions in various areas of the body including the brain (Curatolo et al. 2008). Cortical malformations result from loss of heterozygosity, however, haploinsufficiency of the TSC genes has also been proposed. Cerebral organoids deficient for TSC1 or 2 failed to downregulate mTOR signaling to enter neurogenesis, whereas heterozygous tissues developed normally. When a second allele of TSC2 was randomly inactivated in TSC2 +/− organoids, they recapitulated morphological features of cortical malformations of tuberous sclerosis patients, such as large neurons with hypertrophic dendritic arbors, giant multinucleated cells and abnormal supernumerary glia (Blair et al. 2018). The effects of biallelic inactivation were cell autonomous and phenotypic presentation depended on the timing of the second hit mutation. Rapamycin treatment rescued the neuron-astrocyte imbalance but only when applied during the neurogenic window. Recently, TSC mutant organoids revealed a specific sensitivity of late interneuron progenitors leading to increased interneurons that could be rescued through epidermal growth factor receptor inhibition (Eichmüller et al. 2022)

Faithful recapitulation of aberrant neural development in organoids grown from patient cells or carrying disease-causing mutations allows tracking imbalances between progenitors producing specific neuronal populations. Organoids from idiopathic ASD-patient iPSCs showed increased number and maturation of GABAergic neurons with no effect on excitatory neuron number (Mariani et al. 2015). This was attributed to acceleration of cell cycle due to FOXG1 over-expression observed in in vitro brain tissue. Suppression of FOXG1 expression with shRNA reduced the number of GABAergic neurons to control values. Heterozygous knockout of CHD8 in organoids produced from a genetically modified embryonic stem cell line also demonstrated increased number of GABAergic interneurons and their progenitors at 3.5 months (Paulsen et al. 2022). It was later discovered that the excess number of GABA neurons in CHD8 +/− organoids might be transient and after an initial delay the number of excitatory neurons increased and surpassed that of controls (Villa et al. 2022).

Heterozygous mutation in SUV420H1 gene showed a similar phenotype with early overabundance of GABA neurons; however, also with increased numbers of deep layer projection neurons (Paulsen et al. 2022). Although the imbalances in neuronal number reduced during in vitro development, the asynchronous maturation left a persistent effect on circuit activity. On the other hand, ARID1B +/− organoids displayed delayed progression from progenitors to deep-layer projection neurons and their delayed maturation (Paulsen et al. 2022). Interestingly, heterozygous mutations produced nonidentical phenotypes in different genetic backgrounds, analogous to variable clinical manifestations in humans carrying the same risk variants. The different genetic background could also be a reason for subtle differences reported in different studies (Paulsen et al. 2022; Villa et al. 2022).

19.4.5 Evolutionary Insight

Originally, organoids were grown from mouse or human cells and could easily be evaluated against the body of knowledge obtained from in vivo studies. Immunofluorescent, transcriptomic, and methylome analyses showed striking similarities to primary tissues (Camp et al. 2015; Lancaster et al. 2013; Luo et al. 2016; Quadrato et al. 2017). Importantly, in vitro brain tissues maintain species-specific intrinsic developmental timing and faithfully recapitulate in vivo gene networks and developmental programs (Chiaradia and Lancaster 2020; Otani et al. 2016; Pollen et al. 2019). As expected, organoids generated from mouse PSCs were smaller and contained only occasional oRGs, in contrast to primates (Lancaster et al. 2013). oRGs appeared in a scattered pattern in mouse structures and did not accumulate in an OSVZ-like region. Clonal lineage analysis of mouse and primate neural rosettes confirmed that primate cortical progenitors proliferated for longer than mouse ones and established a larger pool of stem cells that could later generate more neurons. In rodents the progenitor expansion phase ended before neurogenesis, whereas in primates early neurogenesis and expansion of the progenitor pool were not mutually exclusive (Otani et al. 2016).

Thanks to their fidelity to in vivo, organoids are an attractive opportunity to extend evolutionary studies to beyond standard model organisms to species whose embryonic tissue is difficult to obtain (Pollen et al. 2019). Through the expansion of induced pluripotent stem cell technology it is now possible to obtain iPSC lines from our closest living relatives such as chimpanzee, bonobo, gorilla, and orangutan (Pollen et al. 2019; Wunderlich et al. 2014). Generation of iPSCs and organoids from other animals could also provide important insights into mechanisms of brain evolution through evolutionary developmental biology studies.

The slower developmental progression, or neoteny, of the human brain is an accepted mechanism of brain expansion and has found validation at morphological and transcriptional levels (Somel et al. 2009). Organoids enable experimental probing of this hypothesis and offer a window into precise mechanisms of neoteny. Comparisons of human and ape organoids have revealed delayed progression at various stages of forebrain development, from pre-neurogenic NE to progression through neurogenic waves and finally neuronal maturation (Figure 19.2B). Comparative studies of human, chimpanzee, and gorilla organoids during the tNE transition revealed slower progression in human organoids (Benito-Kwiecinski et al. 2021). This was due to lower and delayed expression of ZEB2 in humans compared with gorilla, which in turn slowed down EMT-like processes of restricting cell-cell junctions and apical constriction. Because NE was shown to divide faster than the transitioning NE, this protraction allows for establishment of a larger founding progenitor population. With only a subtle extension of this faster proliferative window, the higher number of progenitors was predicted to produce about 1.9-fold more neurons, corresponding nicely to the difference observed in the in vivo mature human and gorilla brain (Benito-Kwiecinski et al. 2021). Thus, very early differences in NE expansion can explain the human-specific enlargement in forebrain size, and organoids have provided insight into the mechanisms governing this evolved trait.

Human aRGs are also slower to transition from proliferative to neurogenic divisions. In vitro studies indicated that the onset and switch from deep to upper layer neurogenesis occurred about 20 days later in humans and chimpanzees than in macaque, which resulted in their higher clonal output (Otani et al. 2016). Moreover, subtle changes in the timing of aRG mitosis are associated with further expansion. When iPSCs are differentiated to neural progenitors, the duration of their metaphase increases for as long as they undergo mostly symmetric divisions (Mora-Bermúdez et al. 2016). In human organoids at day 30 the metaphase in aRGs was 40–60 percent longer than in the same cells from chimpanzee or orangutan organoids. At day 52, when human progenitors also switched to neurogenic divisions, all analyzed species showed a similar length of metaphase.

Modern sequencing methods now allow for in-depth analysis of even a small amount of sample and analysis of whole gene regulatory networks (Pollen et al. 2019). This enables identification of evolutionary differences in either primary or in vitro tissue and further experimental validation in an organoid model. For example, comparison of human and primate organoid and brain tissue through single cell transcriptomics identified positive (INSR, ITGB8, IFNAR1) and negative (PTEN) modulators of PI3K/AKT/mTOR pathway as strongly upregulated in human in vitro RGs. Pharmacological activation of mTOR showed that mTOR target S6 was more responsive in human progenitors, especially the ones not associated with the VZ (Pollen et al. 2019). With the help of gene editing technology, such as clustered regularly interspaced short palindromic repeats (CRISPR)/Cas9, candidate genes can be inactivated or changed to ape or proto-human versions and their influence on brain development studied in vitro (Fernandes et al. 2021). Moreover, to study evolutionary changes at the level of whole genome architecture and regulation, interspecies hybrid PSCs can be generated and used for making organoids (Agoglia et al. 2021). Such hybrid organoids provide a controlled system for independent analysis of cis- and trans-acting factors contributing to divergence in cerebral cortical development.

19.5 Conclusion

The forebrain, like the rest of the central nervous system, begins as a fairly simple pseudostratified epithelium, but it must then undergo extensive, long-distance morphogenetic movements to enable closure and the formation of the large prosencephalic vesicle. This vesicle is already larger in humans compared with rodents, suggesting important evolutionary differences even at the earliest stages. These early stages are also particularly sensitive to disruption, with abnormalities having devastating consequences, such as exencephaly, while more subtle effects on early progenitors lead to disorders such as microcephaly or macrocephaly.

Neural organoids are a powerful tool to tease apart biological processes at stages that would otherwise be difficult to examine, and in species that would otherwise be impossible to study. The field of organoids has developed at a rapid pace, with more and more elegant approaches to examine early stages, including patterning and neurulation. These tools are now enabling the study of neural tube closure and neuroepithelial development. These approaches have already provided insight into how abnormalities can cause human conditions such as microcephaly, and shed light on why the human forebrain is overall enlarged compared with other apes. Future studies will continue to uncover human-specific principles and provide insight into why our brains are unique and at the same time so sensitive to disruption.

Acknowledgments

We would like to thank Joanna Westmoreland @ Visual Aids/VisLab, LMB for producing the figures for this chapter. We also thank the members of the Lancaster lab for helpful discussions. The Lancaster lab is supported by the Medical Research Council (MC_UP_1201/9) and the European Research Council (ERC STG 757710).

References

Agoglia, R.M. et al. (2021). Primate cell fusion disentangles gene regulatory divergence in neurodevelopment. *Nature* 592 (7854): 421–427. doi: 10.1038/s41586-021-03343-3.

Anderson, R.M. et al. (2002). Chordin and noggin promote organizing centers of forebrain development in the mouse. *Development* 129 (21): 4975–4987. doi: 10.1242/dev.129.21.4975.

Araya, C. et al. (2014). Mesoderm is required for coordinated cell movements within zebrafish neural plate in vivo. *Neural Dev* 9 (1): 9. doi: 10.1186/1749-8104-9-9.

Argelaguet, R. et al. (2019). Multi-omics profiling of mouse gastrulation at single-cell resolution. *Nature* 576 (7787): 487–491. doi: 10.1038/s41586-019-1825-8.

Avagliano, L. et al. (2019). Overview on neural tube defects. *Birth Defects Res* 111 (19): 1455–1467. doi: 10.1002/bdr2.1380.

Azhar, Y.E. and Sonnen, K.F. (2021). Development in a dish—in vitro models of mammalian embryonic development. *Front Cell Dev Biol* 9: 655993. doi: 10.3389/fcell.2021.655993.

Bagley, J.A. et al. (2017). Fused cerebral organoids model interactions between brain regions. *Nat Methods* 14 (7): 743–751. doi: 10.1038/nmeth.4304.

Bakken, T.E. et al. (2016). A comprehensive transcriptional map of primate brain development. *Nature* 535 (7612): 367–375. doi: 10.1038/nature18637.

Beccari, L. et al. (2018). Multi-axial self-organization properties of mouse embryonic stem cells into gastruloids. *Nature* 562 (7726): 272–276. doi: 10.1038/s41586-018-0578-0.

Benito-Kwiecinski, S. et al. (2021). An early cell shape transition drives evolutionary expansion of the human forebrain. *Cell* 184 (8): 2084–2102.e19. doi: 10.1016/j.cell.2021.02.050.

Bérenger-Currias, N.M.L.P. et al. (2022). A gastruloid model of the interaction between embryonic and extra-embryonic cell types. *J Tissue Eng* 13: 20417314221103040. doi: 10.1177/20417314221103042.

Birey, F. et al. (2017). Assembly of functionally integrated human forebrain spheroids. *Nature* 545 (7652): 54–59. doi: 10.1038/nature22330.

Blair, J.D. et al. (2018). Genetically engineered human cortical spheroid models of tuberous sclerosis. *Nat Med* 24 (10): 1568–1578. doi: 10.1038/s41591-018-0139-y.

Bond, A.M. et al. (2012). The dynamic role of bone morphogenetic proteins in neural stem cell fate and maturation. *Dev Neurobiol* 72 (7): 1068–1084. doi: 10.1002/dneu.22022.

Buffalo, E.A. et al. (2019). From basic brain research to treating human brain disorders. *Proc Natl Acad Sci* 116 (52): 26167–26172. doi: 10.1073/pnas.1919895116.

Butler, M.G. (2005). Subset of individuals with autism spectrum disorders and extreme macrocephaly associated with germline PTEN tumour suppressor gene mutations. *J Med Genet* 42 (4): 318–321. doi: 10.1136/jmg.2004.024646.

Camp, J.G. et al. (2015). Human cerebral organoids recapitulate gene expression programs of fetal neocortex development. *Proc Natl Acad Sci* 112 (51): 15672–15677. doi: 10.1073/pnas.1520760112.

Campbell, K. and Götz, M. (2002). Radial glia. *Trends Neurosci* 25 (5): 235–238. doi: 10.1016/S0166-2236(02)02156-2.

Caronia, G. et al. (2010). Bone morphogenetic protein signaling in the developing telencephalon controls formation of the hippocampal dentate gyrus and modifies fear-related behavior. *J Neurosci* 30 (18): 6291–6301. doi: 10.1523/JNEUROSCI.0550-10.2010.

Cederquist, G.Y. et al. (2019). Specification of positional identity in forebrain organoids. *Nat Biotechnol* 37 (4): 436–444. doi: 10.1038/s41587-019-0085-3.

Chan, W.K. et al. (2020). Cerebral organoids as tools to identify the developmental roots of autism. *Mol Autism* 11 (1): 58. doi: 10.1186/s13229-020-00360-3.

Chen, Z.F. and Behringer, R.R. (1995). Twist is required in head mesenchyme for cranial neural tube morphogenesis. *Genes Dev* 9 (6): 686–699. doi: 10.1101/gad.9.6.686.

Chenn, A. (2008). Wnt/β-catenin signaling in cerebral cortical development. *Organogenesis* 4 (2): 76–80. doi: 10.4161/org.4.2.5852.

Chiaradia, I. and Lancaster, M.A. (2020). Brain organoids for the study of human neurobiology at the interface of in vitro and in vivo. *Nat Neurosci* 23 (12): 1496–1508. doi: 10.1038/s41593-020-00730-3.

Cho, A.-N. et al. (2021). Microfluidic device with brain extracellular matrix promotes structural and functional maturation of human brain organoids. *Nat Commun* 12 (1): 4730. doi: 10.1038/s41467-021-24775-5.

Cholfin, J.A. and Rubenstein, J.L.R. (2007). Patterning of frontal cortex subdivisions by Fgf17. *Proc Natl Acad Sci* 104 (18): 7652–7657. doi: 10.1073/pnas.0702225104.

Cugola, F.R. et al. (2016). The Brazilian Zika virus strain causes birth defects in experimental models. *Nature* 534 (7606): 267–271. doi: 10.1038/nature18296.

Cummings, K. et al. (2022). Behavioural and psychological features of PTEN mutations. *J Neurodeve Disord* 14 (1): 1. doi: 10.1186/s11689-021-09406-w.

Curatolo, P. et al. (2008). Tuberous sclerosis. *Lancet* 372 (9639): 657–668. doi: 10.1016/S0140-6736(08)61279-9.

Dang, J. et al. (2016). Zika virus depletes neural progenitors in human cerebral organoids through activation of the innate immune receptor TLR3. *Cell Stem Cell* 19 (2): 258–265. doi: 10.1016/j.stem.2016.04.014.

Demers, C.J. et al. (2016). Development-on-chip. *Development* 143 (11): 1884–1892. doi: 10.1242/dev.126847.

Dhaliwal, N. et al. (2021). Modeling PTEN overexpression-induced microcephaly in human brain organoids. *Mol Brain* 14 (1): 131. doi: 10.1186/s13041-021-00841-3.

Dubourg, C. et al. (2007). Holoprosencephaly. *Orphanet J Rare Dis* 2 (1): 8. doi: 10.1186/1750-1172-2-8.

Eichmüller, O.L. et al. (2022). Amplification of human interneuron progenitors promotes brain tumors and neurological defects. *Science* 375 (6579): eabf5546. doi: 10.1126/science.abf5546.

Eiraku, M. et al. (2008). Self-organized formation of polarized cortical tissues from ESCs and its active manipulation by extrinsic signals. *Cell Stem Cell* 3 (5): 519–532. doi: 10.1016/j.stem.2008.09.002.

Eom, D.S. et al. (2013). Apicobasal polarity and neural tube closure. *Dev Growth Differ* 55 (1): 164–172. doi: 10.1111/dgd.12030.

Eom, D.S. et al. (2011). Bone morphogenetic proteins regulate neural tube closure by interacting with the apicobasal polarity pathway. *Development* 138 (15): 3179–3188. doi: 10.1242/dev.058602.

Eze, U.C. et al. (2021). Single-cell atlas of early human brain development highlights heterogeneity of human neuroepithelial cells and early radial glia. *Nat Neurosci* 24 (4): 584–594. doi: 10.1038/s41593-020-00794-1.

Fernandes, M. et al. (2007). Mutations in the BMP pathway in mice support the existence of two molecular classes of holoprosencephaly. *Development* 134 (21): 3789–3794. doi: 10.1242/dev.004325.

Fernandes, S. et al. (2021). Unraveling human brain development and evolution using organoid models. *Front Cell Dev Biol* 9: 737429. doi: 10.3389/fcell.2021.737429.

Fietz, S.A. et al. (2010). OSVZ progenitors of human and ferret neocortex are epithelial-like and expand by integrin signaling. *Nat Neurosci* 13 (6): 690–699. doi: 10.1038/nn.2553.

Florio, M. and Huttner, W.B. (2014). Neural progenitors, neurogenesis and the evolution of the neocortex. *Development* 141 (11): 2182–2194. doi: 10.1242/dev.090571.

Fukuchi-Shimogori, T. and Grove, E.A. (2001). Neocortex patterning by the secreted signaling molecule FGF8. *Science* 294 (5544): 1071–1074. doi: 10.1126/science.1064252.

Gabriel, E. et al. (2016). CPAP promotes timely cilium disassembly to maintain neural progenitor pool. *EMBO J* 35 (8): 803–819. doi: 10.15252/embj.201593679.

Garcez, P.P. et al. (2016). Zika virus impairs growth in human neurospheres and brain organoids. *Science* 352 (6287): 816–818. doi: 10.1126/science.aaf6116.

Green, D.G. et al. (2020). Wnt signaling regulates neural plate patterning in distinct temporal phases with dynamic transcriptional outputs. *Dev Biol* 462 (2): 152–164. doi: 10.1016/j.ydbio.2020.03.016.

Greene, N.D.E. and Copp, A.J. (2014). Neural tube defects. *Ann Rev Neurosci* 37 (1): 221–242. doi: 10.1146/annurev-neuro-062012-170354.

Guillemot, F. (2005). Cellular and molecular control of neurogenesis in the mammalian telencephalon. *Curr Opin Cell Biol* 17 (6): 639–647. doi: 10.1016/j.ceb.2005.09.006.

Haas, D. et al. (2007). Abnormal sterol metabolism in holoprosencephaly. *J Med Genet* 44 (5): 298–305. doi: 10.1136/jmg.2006.047258.

Hansen, D.V. et al. (2010). Neurogenic radial glia in the outer subventricular zone of human neocortex. *Nature* 464 (7288): 554–561. doi: 10.1038/nature08845.

Hébert, J.M. (2011). FGFs: neurodevelopment's Jack-of-all-trades – how do they do it? *Front Neurosci* 5: 133. doi: 10.3389/fnins.2011.00133.

Hébert, J.M. and Mishina, Y. (2002). BMP signaling is required locally to pattern the dorsal telencephalic midline. *Neuron* 35 (6): 1029–1041. doi: 10.1016/S0896-6273(02)00900-5.

Herculano-Houzel, S. (2009). The human brain in numbers. *Front Human Neurosci* 3: 31. doi: 10.3389/neuro.09.031.2009.

Hong, M. and Krauss, R.S. (2018). Modeling the complex etiology of holoprosencephaly in mice. *Am J Med Genet Part C: Sem Med Genet* 178 (2): 140–150. doi: 10.1002/ajmg.c.31611.

Ishida, M. et al. (2018). A targeted sequencing panel identifies rare damaging variants in multiple genes in the cranial neural tube defect, anencephaly. *Clin Genet* 93 (4): 870–879. doi: 10.1111/cge.13189.

Jacob, F. et al. (2020). Human pluripotent stem cell-derived neural cells and brain organoids reveal SARS-CoV-2 neurotropism predominates in choroid plexus epithelium. *Cell Stem Cell* 27 (6): 937–950.e9. doi: 10.1016/j.stem.2020.09.016.

Juriloff, D. and Harris, M. (2018). Insights into the etiology of mammalian neural tube closure defects from developmental, genetic and evolutionary studies. *J Dev Biol* 6 (3): 22. doi: 10.3390/jdb6030022.

Kadoshima, T. et al. (2013). Self-organization of axial polarity, inside-out layer pattern, and species-specific progenitor dynamics in human ES cell–derived neocortex. *Proc Natl Acad Sci* 110 (50): 20284–20289. doi: 10.1073/pnas.1315710110.

Karzbrun, E. et al. (2021). Human neural tube morphogenesis in vitro by geometric constraints. *Nature* 599 (7884): 268–272. doi: 10.1038/s41586-021-04026-9.

Karzbrun, E. et al. (2018). Human brain organoids on a chip reveal the physics of folding. *Nat Phys* 14 (5): 515–522. doi: 10.1038/s41567-018-0046-7.

Kawasaki, H. (2018). Molecular investigations of the development and diseases of cerebral cortex folding using gyrencephalic mammal ferrets. *Biol Pharm Bull* 41 (9): 1324–1329. doi: 10.1248/bpb.b18-00142.

Kelava, I. et al. (2022). Androgens increase excitatory neurogenic potential in human brain organoids. *Nature* 602 (7895): 112–116. doi: 10.1038/s41586-021-04330-4.

Kelava, I. and Lancaster, M.A. (2016a). Dishing out mini-brains. *Dev Biol* 420 (2): 199–209. doi: 10.1016/j.ydbio.2016.06.037.

Kelava, I. and Lancaster, M.A. (2016b). Stem cell models of human brain development. *Cell Stem Cell* 18 (6): 736–748. doi: 10.1016/j.stem.2016.05.022.

Kiecker, C. and Niehrs, C. (2001). A morphogen gradient of Wnt/β-catenin signalling regulates anteroposterior neural patterning in xenopus. *Development* 128 (21): 4189–4201. doi: 10.1242/dev.128.21.4189.

Knight, G.T. et al. (2018). Engineering induction of singular neural rosette emergence within HPSC-derived tissues. *Elife* 7: e37549. doi: 10.7554/eLife.37549.

Krefft, O. et al. (2021). Cerebral organoids to unravel the mechanisms underlying malformations of human cortical development. *Semin in Cell Dev Biol* 111: 15–22. doi: 10.1016/j.semcdb.2020.06.001.

Krenn, V. et al. (2021). Organoid modeling of Zika and herpes simplex virus 1 infections reveals virus-specific responses leading to microcephaly. *Cell Stem Cell* 28 (8): 1362–1379.e7. doi: 10.1016/j.stem.2021.03.004.

LaMonica, B.E. et al. (2013). Mitotic spindle orientation predicts outer radial glial cell generation in human neocortex. *Nat Commun* 4 (1): 1665. doi: 10.1038/ncomms2647.

Lancaster, M.A. et al. (2017). Guided self-organization and cortical plate formation in human brain organoids. *Nat Biotechnol* 35 (7): 659–666. doi: 10.1038/nbt.3906.

Lancaster, M.A. and Huch, M. (2019). Disease modelling in human organoids. *Dis Models Mechanisms* 12 (7): dmm039347. doi: 10.1242/dmm.039347.

Lancaster, M.A. et al. (2013). Cerebral organoids model human brain development and microcephaly. *Nature* 501 (7467): 373–379. doi: 10.1038/nature12517.

Landge, A.N. et al. (2020). Pattern formation mechanisms of self-organizing reaction-diffusion systems. *Dev Biol* 460 (1): 2–11. doi: 10.1016/j.ydbio.2019.10.031.

Levine, A.J. and Brivanlou, A.H. (2007). Proposal of a model of mammalian neural induction. *Dev Biol* 308 (2): 247–256. doi: 10.1016/j.ydbio.2007.05.036.

Li, Y. et al. (2017). Induction of expansion and folding in human cerebral organoids. *Cell Stem Cell* 20 (3): 385–396.e3. doi: 10.1016/j.stem.2016.11.017.

Long, C. (2019). Stem cell-based in utero therapies for spina bifida. *Neural Regen Res* 14 (2): 260. doi: 10.4103/1673-5374.244786.

Luo, C. et al. (2016). Cerebral organoids recapitulate epigenomic signatures of the human fetal brain. *Cell Rep* 17 (12): 3369–3384. doi: 10.1016/j.celrep.2016.12.001.

Ma, H. et al. (2019). In vitro culture of cynomolgus monkey embryos beyond early gastrulation. *Science* 366 (6467): eaax7890. doi: 10.1126/science.aax7890.

Mariani, J. et al. (2015). FOXG1-dependent dysregulation of GABA/glutamate neuron differentiation in autism spectrum disorders. *Cell* 162 (2): 375–390. doi: 10.1016/j.cell.2015.06.034.

Medelnik, J.-P. et al. (2018). Signaling-dependent control of apical membrane size and self-renewal in rosette-stage human neuroepithelial stem cells. *Stem Cell Rep* 10 (6): 1751–1765. doi: 10.1016/j.stemcr.2018.04.018.

Meinhardt, A. et al. (2014). 3D reconstitution of the patterned neural tube from embryonic stem cells. *Stem Cell Rep* 3 (6): 987–999. doi: 10.1016/j.stemcr.2014.09.020.

Metzis, V. et al. (2018). Nervous system regionalization entails axial allocation before neural differentiation. *Cell* 175 (4): 1105–1118.e17. doi: 10.1016/j.cell.2018.09.040.

Michalczyk, A. et al. (2017). Lysophosphatidic acid plasma concentrations in healthy subjects. *Lipids Health Dis* 16 (1): 140. doi: 10.1186/s12944-017-0536-0.

Miura, Y. et al. (2020). Generation of human striatal organoids and cortico-striatal assembloids from human pluripotent stem cells. *Nat Biotechnol* 38 (12): 1421–1430. doi: 10.1038/s41587-020-00763-w.
Mora-Bermúdez, F. et al. (2016). Differences and similarities between human and chimpanzee neural progenitors during cerebral cortex development. *Elife* 5: e18683. doi: 10.7554/eLife.18683.
Mulligan, K.A. and Cheyette, B.N.R. (2012). Wnt signaling in vertebrate neural development and function. *J Neuroimmune Pharm* 7 (4): 774–787. doi: 10.1007/s11481-012-9404-x.
Nasu, M. et al. (2012). Robust formation and maintenance of continuous stratified cortical neuroepithelium by laminin-containing matrix in mouse ES cell culture. *PLoS One* 7 (12): e53024. doi: 10.1371/journal.pone.0053024.
Niakan, K.K. et al. (2012). Human pre-implantation embryo development. *Development* 139 (5): 829–841. doi: 10.1242/dev.060426.
Nikolopoulou, E. et al. (2017). Neural tube closure. *Development* 144 (4): 552–566. doi: 10.1242/dev.145904.
Nowakowski, T.J. et al. (2016a). Expression analysis highlights AXL as a candidate Zika virus entry receptor in neural stem cells. *Cell Stem Cell* 18 (5): 591–596. doi: 10.1016/j.stem.2016.03.012.
Nowakowski, T.J. et al. (2016b). Transformation of the radial glia scaffold demarcates two stages of human cerebral cortex development. *Neuron* 91 (6): 1219–1227. doi: 10.1016/j.neuron.2016.09.005.
Otani, T. et al. (2016). 2D and 3D stem cell models of primate cortical development identify species-specific differences in progenitor behavior contributing to brain size. *Cell Stem Cell* 18 (4): 467–480. doi: 10.1016/j.stem.2016.03.003.
Ozair, M.Z. et al. (2013). Neural induction and early patterning in vertebrates. *Wiley Interdiscip Rev Deve Biol* 2 (4): 479–498. doi: 10.1002/wdev.90.
Park, S.E. (2019). Organoids-on-a-chip. *Science* 364 (6444): 960–965. doi: 10.1126/science.aaw7894.
Paulsen, B. et al. (2022). Autism genes converge on asynchronous development of shared neuron classes. *Nature* 602 (7896): 268–273. doi: 10.1038/s41586-021-04358-6.
Pellegrini, L. et al. (2020). Human CNS barrier-forming organoids with cerebrospinal fluid production. *Science* 369 (6500): eaaz5626. doi: 10.1126/science.aaz5626.
Pervaiz, N. et al. (2021). Molecular evolutionary analysis of human primary microcephaly genes. *BMC Ecol Evo* 21 (1): 76. doi: 10.1186/s12862-021-01801-0.
Pollen, A.A. et al. (2019). Establishing cerebral organoids as models of human-specific brain evolution. *Cell* 176 (4): 743–756.e17. doi: 10.1016/j.cell.2019.01.017.
Qian, X. et al. (2017). Using brain organoids to understand Zika virus-induced microcephaly. *Development* 144 (6): 952–957. doi: 10.1242/dev.140707.
Qian, X. et al. (2016). Brain-region-specific organoids using mini-bioreactors for modeling ZIKV exposure. *Cell* 165 (5): 1238–1254. doi: 10.1016/j.cell.2016.04.032.
Quadrato, G. et al. (2017). Cell diversity and network dynamics in photosensitive human brain organoids. *Nature* 545 (7652): 48–53. doi: 10.1038/nature22047.
Rakic, P. (2007). The radial edifice of cortical architecture. *Brain Res Rev* 55 (2): 204–219. doi: 10.1016/j.brainresrev.2007.02.010.
Rakic, P. et al. (1991). Experimental manipulation of cerebral cortical areas in primates. *Philo Trans R Soc London. Series B: Biol Sci* 331 (1261): 291–294. doi: 10.1098/rstb.1991.0019.
Ranga, A. et al. (2016). Neural tube morphogenesis in synthetic 3D microenvironments. *Proc Natl Acad Sci* 113 (44): E6831–6839. doi: 10.1073/pnas.1603529113.
Sahara, S. and O'Leary, D.D.M. (2009). Fgf10 regulates transition period of cortical stem cell differentiation to radial glia controlling generation of neurons and basal progenitors. *Neuron* 63 (1): 48–62. doi: 10.1016/j.neuron.2009.06.006.

Sakaguchi, H. et al. (2015). Generation of functional hippocampal neurons from self-organizing human embryonic stem cell-derived dorsomedial telencephalic tissue. *Nat Commun* 6 (1): 8896. doi: 10.1038/ncomms9896.

Sakai, T. et al. (2012). Fetal brain development in chimpanzees versus humans. *Curr Biol* 22 (18): R791–92. doi: 10.1016/j.cub.2012.06.062.

Sanes, D.H. et al. (2019). Chapter 2 - polarity and regional identity. In: *Development of the Nervous System*, 4e (ed. D.H. Sanes, T.A. Reh, W.A. Harris, and M. Landgraf), 27–54. Amsterdam: Academic Press. doi: 10.1016/B978-0-12-803996-0.00002-2.

Severino, M. et al. (2020). Definitions and classification of malformations of cortical development. *Brain* 143 (10): 2874–2894. doi: 10.1093/brain/awaa174.

Soltani Khaboushan, A. et al. (2022). Prenatal neural tube anomalies. *Stem Cell Rev Rep* 18 (2): 752–767. doi: 10.1007/s12015-021-10150-w.

Somel, M. et al. (2009). Transcriptional neoteny in the human brain. *Proc Natl Acad Sci* 106 (14): 5743–5748. doi: 10.1073/pnas.0900544106.

Stahl, R. et al. (2013). Trnp1 regulates expansion and folding of the mammalian cerebral cortex by control of radial glial fate. *Cell* 153 (3): 535–549. doi: 10.1016/j.cell.2013.03.027.

Stern, C.D. (2005). Neural induction. *Development* 132 (9): 2007–2021. doi: 10.1242/dev.01794.

Stiles, J. and Jernigan, T.L. (2010). The basics of brain development. *Neuropsychol Rev* 20 (4): 327–348. doi: 10.1007/s11065-010-9148-4.

Su, X. et al. (2022). Human brain organoids as an in vitro model system of viral infectious diseases. *Front Immunol* 12 (January): 792316. doi: 10.3389/fimmu.2021.792316.

Takahashi, K. and Yamanaka, S. (2006). Induction of pluripotent stem cells from mouse embryonic and adult fibroblast cultures by defined factors. *Cell* 126 (4): 663–676. doi: 10.1016/j.cell.2006.07.024.

Tan, T. et al. (2021). Chimeric contribution of human extended pluripotent stem cells to monkey embryos ex vivo. *Cell* 184 (8): 2020–2032.e14. doi: 10.1016/j.cell.2021.03.020.

Thomson, J.A. et al. (1998). Embryonic stem cell lines derived from human blastocysts. *Sci New Series* 282 (5391): 1145–1147.

Toyoda, R. et al. (2010). FGF8 acts as a classic diffusible morphogen to pattern the neocortex. *Development* 137 (20): 3439–3448. doi: 10.1242/dev.055392.

Vaccarino, F.M. et al. (1999). Changes in cerebral cortex size are governed by fibroblast growth factor during embryogenesis. *Nat Neurosci* 2 (3): 246–253. doi: 10.1038/6350.

Veenvliet, J.V. et al. (2020). Mouse embryonic stem cells self-organize into trunk-like structures with neural tube and somites. *Science* 370 (6522): eaba4937. doi: 10.1126/science.aba4937.

Velasco, S. et al. (2019). Individual brain organoids reproducibly form cell diversity of the human cerebral cortex. *Nature* 570 (7762): 523–527. doi: 10.1038/s41586-019-1289-x.

Villa, C.E. et al. (2022). CHD8 haploinsufficiency links autism to transient alterations in excitatory and inhibitory trajectories. *Cell Rep* 39 (1): 110615. doi: 10.1016/j.celrep.2022.110615.

Wang, J. et al. (2019). Plasma lipidomic signatures of spontaneous obese rhesus monkeys. *Lipids Health Dis* 18 (1): 8. doi: 10.1186/s12944-018-0952-9.

Watanabe, K. et al. (2005). Directed differentiation of telencephalic precursors from embryonic stem cells. *Nat Neurosci* 8 (3): 288–296. doi: 10.1038/nn1402.

Watanabe, K. et al. (2007). A ROCK inhibitor permits survival of dissociated human embryonic stem cells. *Nat Biotechnol* 25 (6): 681–686. doi: 10.1038/nbt1310.

Wunderlich, S. et al. (2014). Primate IPS cells as tools for evolutionary analyses. *Stem Cell Res* 12 (3): 622–629. doi: 10.1016/j.scr.2014.02.001.

Xiang, Y. et al. (2019). HESC-derived thalamic organoids form reciprocal projections when fused with cortical organoids. *Cell Stem Cell* 24 (3): 487–497.e7. doi: 10.1016/j.stem.2018.12.015.

Xiang, Y. et al. (2017). Fusion of regionally specified HPSC-derived organoids models human brain development and interneuron migration. *Cell Stem Cell* 21 (3): 383–398.e7. doi: 10.1016/j.stem.2017.07.007.

Zaqout, S. and Kaindl, A.M. (2022). Autosomal recessive primary microcephaly. *Front Cell Dev Biol* 9: 784700. doi: 10.3389/fcell.2021.784700.

Zhang, S.-C. et al. (2001). In vitro differentiation of transplantable neural precursors from human embryonic stem cells. *Nat Biotechnol* 19 (12): 1129–1133. doi: 10.1038/nbt1201-1129.

Zhang, W. et al. (2020). Cerebral organoid and mouse models reveal a RAB39b–PI3K–MTOR pathway-dependent dysregulation of cortical development leading to macrocephaly/autism phenotypes. *Genes Dev* 34 (7–8): 580–597. doi: 10.1101/gad.332494.119.

Zhang, W. et al. (2019). Modeling microcephaly with cerebral organoids reveals a WDR62–CEP170–KIF2A pathway promoting cilium disassembly in neural progenitors. *Nat Commun* 10 (1): 2612. doi: 10.1038/s41467-019-10497-2.

20

Early Neuronal Differentiation/patterning of the Human Pallium, Modeling by in Vitro Systems, and Disruption in Developmental Disorders

Soraya Scuderi[1], *Alexandre Jourdon*[1], *and Flora M. Vaccarino*[1,2,3,4]

[1] *Child Study Center, Yale University, New Haven, CT, USA*
[2] *Department of Neuroscience, Yale University, New Haven, CT, USA*
[3] *Yale Stem Cell Center, Yale University, New Haven, CT, USA*
[4] *Yale Kavli Institute for Neuroscience*

20.1 Regulation of Axial Development

20.1.1 Formation of Brain Regions after Neurulation

During embryonic development, the central nervous system (CNS) originates from the ectoderm in the dorso-medial region (neural plate), which progressively infolds during the neurulation process causing the neural folds to approach each other and fuse in the dorsal midline to form the neural tube. The lumen inside the primitive neural tube structure will form the future ventricles. In most vertebrates the early neural tube is a straight elongated structure, and even before its posterior portion is fully formed, its anterior portion undergoes drastic remodeling. There, the neural tube expands into three primary vesicles: the prosencephalon (forebrain), the mesencephalon (midbrain), and the rhombencephalon (hindbrain). At this three-vesicles stage, the neural tube bends on the long axis, creating the cephalic and the cervical ventral flexures (Figure 20.1A).

Subsequently, the forebrain becomes subdivided into the telencephalon anteriorly and diencephalon more posteriorly and the dorsal midline of the telencephalon invaginates to give rise to the cerebral hemispheres. The anterior diencephalon will form the hypothalamus, while the caudal diencephalon is subdivided into three prosomeres (p1–p3) and will give rise to habenula, thalamus, and prethalamus. The dorsal telencephalon or pallium will generate the cerebral cortex and hippocampus. The ventral telencephalon or subpallium is composed of lateral, medial, and caudal subdivisions of the ganglionic eminence (GE), respectively lateral ganglionic eminence (LGE), medial ganglionic eminence (MGE), and caudal ganglionic eminence (CGE), which will develop into basal ganglia (striatum and globus pallidus) and are a source of GABAergic interneurons. How and when these telencephalic subdivisions are specified in humans is still to be answered.

Different models have been proposed to explain early patterning of the nervous system. One theory is the "Activation/Transformation" hypothesis, a two-step model proposed first by Nieuwkoop (Nieuwkoop and Nigtevecht 1954), which proposes that neural cells are initially primed with an anterior identity (e.g., forebrain) and only in response to caudalizing signals do they acquire a more posterior fate (e.g., spinal cord). Other studies described the presence of different *organizers*, group of cells able to induce coordinated cell fate changes in surrounding tissue and pattern the developing neural tube in a topographically organized set of structures. Distinct organizers for the head and for most posterior regions of the CNS were described from amphibians to mouse (Figure 20.1B–C). Over a century of studies point to a mixture of both models, where the development of the vertebrate neural tube is a multi-step mechanism that involves both intrinsic

Neocortical Neurogenesis in Development and Evolution, First Edition. Edited by Wieland B. Huttner.

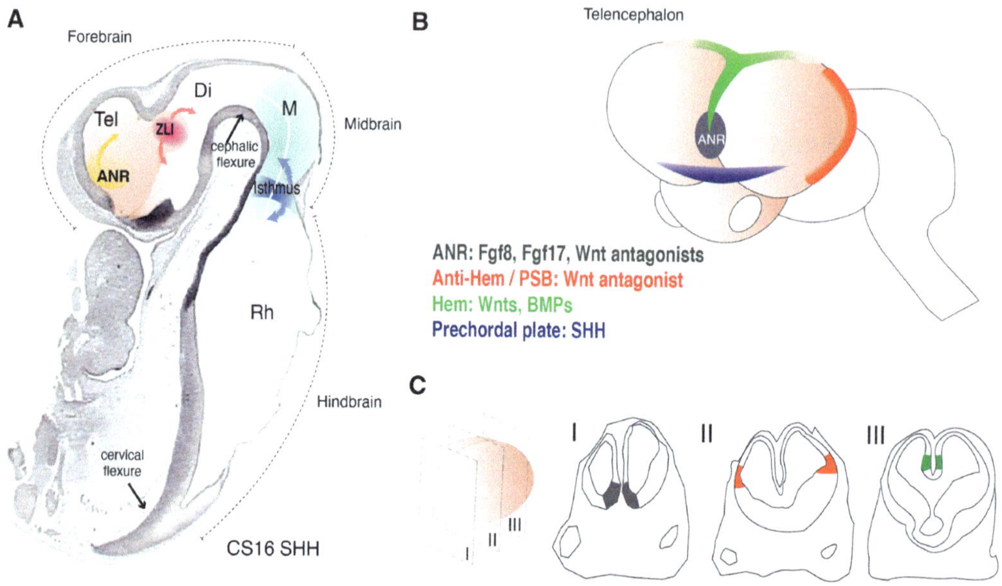

Figure 20.1 Neurulation process and dorsal-ventral patterning in the neural tube. (A) Lateral view of a CS16 human embryo, cut midsagittal, showing the lumen of the neural tube (anterior to the left) showing in situ hybridization (ISH) for SHH delineating floor and basal plate of neural tissue. Major future neural structures are indicated. Tel, Telencephalon; Di, Diencephalon; M, Mesencephalon; Rh, Rhombencephalon; ZLI, zona limitans intrathalamica. In situ hybridization (ISH) from the Joint MRC / Wellcome Trust (MR/R006237/1) Human Developmental Biology Resource (HDBR) (www.hdbr.org) (Gerrelli et al. 2015). (B) 3D rendering of main organizers and morphogenetic signals within the telencephalon and (C) their localization on transverse sections along the antero-posterior axis. Abbreviations: ANR, anterior neural ridge; PSB, pallium–subpallium boundary.

(i.e., lineage based) and extrinsic morphogenetic events (Stern 2001). The progenitor pools along the neural tube refine their identities by combinatorial spatial and temporal effect of **morphogens**, which are signaling molecules produced by localized sources (the organizers mentioned earlier) and degraded by "sink" regions, creating linear gradients (Ye et al. 1998; Yu et al. 2009).

20.1.2 Organizers: Signaling Centers Involved in Patterning

Long- and short-range diffusible morphogens help establish expression patterns of several transcription factors (TFs) that, in combination, provide positional identities and lead to the specification of discrete cell fate domains along the neural tube. How the extracellular signals are "translated" into the nuclear code of TFs is not entirely known, but recent studies point to epigenetic regulatory events that are impacted by signaling cascades and in turn regulate TF expression (Eto and Kishi 2021). Importantly, these epigenetic events must be "graded," that is, must respond to the morphogens in a concentration and time-dependent manner. TFs act by binding to cis-regulatory elements of target genes expressed in regions that often but not always coincide with the spatial coverage of the morphogen gradient. Any morphogen signal modulates information by being dynamic and varying at multiple levels – the fold change/intensity of the signal, its duration and clearance, and the rate/speed at which the signaling increases or decreases over time. Complex dynamics of morphogenetic signals occur, as morphogens interact with each other in synergistic way (e.g., WNT and bone morphogenetic proteins, or BMP) or in a competitive-repressive fashion (e.g., SHH and BMP) during neural differentiation (Manzari-Tavakoli et al. 2022; Ragsdale and Grove 2001).

Multiple signaling centers are involved in the induction and patterning of the early telencephalon: the anterior neural ridge (ANR); the "forebrain hem system" at the dorsal midline that includes cortical hem, septum, and thalamic eminence; the pallium-subpallium boundary (PSB) or antihem, and the prechordal plate ventrally (Roy et al. 2014). All of these centers have also been identified as a source of Cajal–Retzius cells (CR cells), which are thought to act as "mobile patterning units," migrating tangentially to cover the telencephalic surface, with distinct molecular profiles depending on their origin (Bielle et al. 2005; Meyer et al. 2002).

20.1.2.1 WNT, Fibroblast Growth Factors, and Bone Morphogenetic Protein

Although at gastrulation stage telencephalic territory specification requires inhibition of WNT signaling, at later stages the dorso-anterior identity requires a sequential activation of fibroblast growth factors (FGFs) followed by WNT and BMPs (Sur and Rubenstein 2005). The ANR initially secrets WNT antagonists, and later is a source of several FGFs such as FGF8, FGF15, FGF17, and FGF18, which promote rostral identity by inducing SP8 while repressing the caudalizing TFs EMX2 and COUP-TF1. FGF8 expression is reduced drastically before the beginning of cortical plate formation, in human from 7.5 postconceptional weeks (PCW).

As growth proceeds, the distance between initial signaling centers increases and additional patterning centers arise, such as the cortical hem, a dorso-medial region secreting WNT agonists (WNT8B, WNT2B, WNT3A) and members of the BMP (BMP2, 4, and 5) family with dorsalizing effects (Grove et al. 1998). The cortical hem is responsible for the specification of the hippocampus, including the dentate gyrus, and of the choroid plexus, and is itself a source of CR cells. The specification of the cortical hem occurs through joint action of FOXG1/LMX1A upstream of the LHX2 network: FOXG1 ablation in the cortical plate leads to an expansion of the cortical hem and of CR cells/hippocampal fate (Muzio and Mallamaci 2005), while the ablation of LHX2, an intrinsic determinant of cortical identity, leads to a dual expansion of both hem and antihem structures (Mangale et al. 2008).

On the opposite ventrolateral side sits the PSB or antihem more anteriorly (Assimacopoulos et al. 2003) and the thalamic eminence posteriorly, which secrete WNT antagonist like SFRP2 up to 17.5 PCW (Clowry et al. 2018). In humans, at embryonic stages preceding cortical plate formation, the PSB/antihem is characterized by PAX6-positive EMX1-negative territory, which establishes the dorsal identity of the cortical progenitors along with NEUROG1, NEUROG2, and SOX6, important regulators of pallium-subpallium segregation.

20.1.2.2 Sonic Hedgehog

Sonic hedgehog (SHH), secreted first by the notochord and later by the floor plate of the neural tube, is responsible for inducing ventral neural cell types throughout the CNS. In the telencephalon SHH induces ventral pallial identities, including the MGE, LGE, and CGE, in the mesencephalon aminergic neuron types, and posteriorly the motoneurons of the ventral cord (Brady and Vaccarino 2021; Ericson et al. 1995; Ye et al. 1998). SHH in the telencephalon is also involved in maintaining FGF8 in the ANR by inhibiting GLI3, a zinc-finger transcription factor that antagonizes the ventralizing SHH signal in the telencephalon. In humans, perturbation of the SHH pathway leads to holoprosencephaly, a condition with a defect in the formation of midline structure of the forebrain and a failure to divide into bilateral hemispheres as well as other neural tube defects (Andreu-Cervera et al. 2021).

20.1.2.3 Retinoic Acid

Retinoic acid (RA) produced by the paraxial mesoderm/meninges (Siegenthaler and Pleasure 2011) is an inducer of neural differentiation and forebrain patterning. The major role for RA in embryonic development is to promote posterior (hindbrain and spinal cord) patterning by inducing HOX TF expression (Boncinelli et al. 1991; Marshall et al. 1994) and is a potent repressor of OTX2, which is required for rostral brain development (Acampora et al. 1995; Simeone et al. 1995). However, at early to mid-fetal stage, secondary sources of RA are established in the anterior forebrain, which promote human and macaque's frontal cortex development by upregulating genes such as MEIS2 and CDH8 (Shibata et al. 2021; Ziffra et al. 2021). In the ventral telencephalon RA receptors are highly expressed in the radial glia of the LGE and regulate basal ganglia development (Chatzi et al. 2011; Rataj-Baniowska et al. 2015).

20.1.3 Translation into In Vitro Systems: Monolayers and Organoid Models

Several in vitro neural models derived from human embryonic stem cells or induced pluripotent stem cells (iPSC) have been developed over the past 15 years, either as monolayer cultures or more recently as 3D organoids (Ardhanareeswaran et al. 2017; Eiraku et al. 2008; Lancaster and Knoblich 2014; Pasca 2018; Sasai 2013). Many of those models rely on morphogens or small molecules to activate the signaling pathways that orchestrate neural differentiation with the aim of recapitulating early phases of human brain development not easily accessible via the postmortem human brain. In their more guided forms, orchestrated exposure to different morphogens has allowed several groups to reliably obtain organoid models specific to different regions of the brain, including cerebral cortex (Kadoshima et al. 2013; Mariani et al. 2012), hippocampus (Sakaguchi et al. 2015), thalamus (Xiang et al. 2019), hypothalamus (Qian et al. 2016), striatum (Bagley et al. 2017; Xiang et al. 2017), or cerebellum (Muguruma et al. 2015). The aim of many of these studies has been to recapitulate developmental processes implicated in several neurological and psychiatric disorders (Jourdon et al. 2021).

Many aspects of cortical development have been recapitulated in the pallium organoid models, including the apico-basal polarity of the neural progenitor cells surrounding a lumen-like structure, the intermediate progenitor cells that occupy the subventricular zone (SVZ), and the generation over time of deep and then upper layers cortical neurons (Qian et al. 2016). Other aspects that rely on interactions among cell types derived from multiple germ layers are more difficult to recapitulate in a simplified and largely ectodermal-derived organoid cellular system. For example, some morphogens which derive from extrinsic nonneural tissue sources could be missing and would have to be externally supplied.

All the region-specific organoid systems have relied on a single-concentration bath application of morphogens known to be involved in the development of that region in other systems, such as the mouse brain. Recent elegant studies have attempted to recapitulate morphogen concentration gradients as they occur *in vivo* in neurons derived from iPSCs. Cederquist and colleagues (Cederquist et al. 2019) developed a SHH protein gradient by placing a doxycycline inducible SHH-secreting line at one pole of developing forebrain organoids and showed the establishment of major forebrain subdivisions along the dorso-ventral and antero-posterior axis in the receiving cells, mimicking the in vivo topography. Another type of approach uses a microfluidic-controlled stem cell regionalization (MiSTR) system, where morphogen gradients are generated by external pumps over a human embryonic stem cells monolayer in a culture chamber. By generating a gradient of WNT signaling, in the presence of SHH and/or RA, this approach resulted in neural tissue exhibiting progressive caudalization from forebrain to midbrain to hindbrain, including the formation of a secondary organizer, the isthmus (Rifes et al. 2020).

In other instances, organizers are generated by intrinsic patterning and self-segregation of neural precursor cells, as in the case of the cortical hem. Micali et al. (2020), using human neural stem cells

(NSCs) *in vitro*, have shown that NSCs transition through an "organizer state" before generating neurons, and that there is variation in this early patterning states along the dorso-ventral axis, which impacts the type of neurons generated. Stem cells that transition through the cortical hem fate (marked by LMX1A expression) are biased toward dorsal lineages, whereas expression of FGF8 is biased toward ventralization (marked by SHH and GABAergic lineages). Notably, through self-patterning, organoids have been shown to generate the different major regions of the forebrain (marked by PAX6, GSX2, or TTR among others) (Renner et al. 2017). Interestingly, this ability to generate the different lineages seems to vary across individuals and to a lesser extent among replicates (Kanton et al. 2019). Extensive studies of iPSC lines and neural differentiation capacity and fate decision would help decipher how this process can be further controlled and the extent to which genetic determinants or intrinsic lineage factors are involved in fate heterogeneity (Carcamo-Orive et al. 2017).

One possibility is to guide the differentiation by reproducing the major extrinsic morphogens exposure, timed and titrated accordingly to generate the major brain subdivisions, and then rely upon secondary patterning to obtain finer refinements of such states. Some organoid models of hippocampal formation have shown a targeted reproduction of the medial fate using WNT and BMP signaling to generate hem, hippocampus (expression of ZBTB20, PROX1), or choroid plexus fate (TTR, OTX2) (Jacob et al. 2020; Pomeshchik et al. 2020; Sakaguchi et al. 2015).

20.2 Patterning of the Cortical Plate and Cell Diversity

20.2.1 Preplate and Early Neurogenesis

The development of the neocortex begins with the formation of a layer called preplate (PP) at Carnegie stages 14 (CS14) immediately above the germinal zone (Figure 20.2). The cortical plate (CP) starts forming at CS21 (7–8 PCW), when the arrival of the first cortical neurons split the preexisting preplate in two layers: marginal zone (MZ), the outermost layer above the CP, and subplate (SP), that lies between the SVZ and the CP.

CR cells first appear in the PP at CS16, shortly after the formation of the telencephalon at CS14. CR cells are the first postmitotic neuronal population and reside in the subpial region of the PP. The morphology of CR neurons in the human cortex is highly variable and age specific. From 7–12 PCW, CR cells, horizontally oriented neurons with a prominent nucleus and a large soma with a bipolar arrangement of axon and dendrites, are the only neuronal element in the PP. In humans, they are glutamatergic thus excitatory and defined by co-expression of Reelin (RELN), TBR1, and other markers (e.g., calcium binding proteins like CALB1, CALB2).

The CR population is heterogeneous with multiple origins and migratory routes, including the cortical RG cells (especially in the rostral cortex), the antihem or PSB, the olfactory plaque, the septum, and thalamic eminences (~ CS18) and, last but not least, the cortical hem complex, which is the main source of CR cells at CS21 (Bielle et al. 2005). At CS 22–23 the CR cell number in the PP continues to increase, due to a massive stream from the hem, which is especially prominent in the human cortex. Notably, human CR cells express the antiapoptotic DeltaNp73, which could be responsible for the protracted lifespan of this population in human compared to other species (Meyer 2010; Tissir et al. 2009). After the PP is split into SP and MZ by the incoming cortical plate neurons, the CR cells remain localized in the subpial region, the MZ. They secrete the extracellular glycoprotein RELN, which provides a critical signal for the control of radial migration and laminar positioning of pyramidal neurons that populate the CP. RELN mutations in humans produce lissencephaly (Hong et al. 2000). After mid-gestation, at the onset of

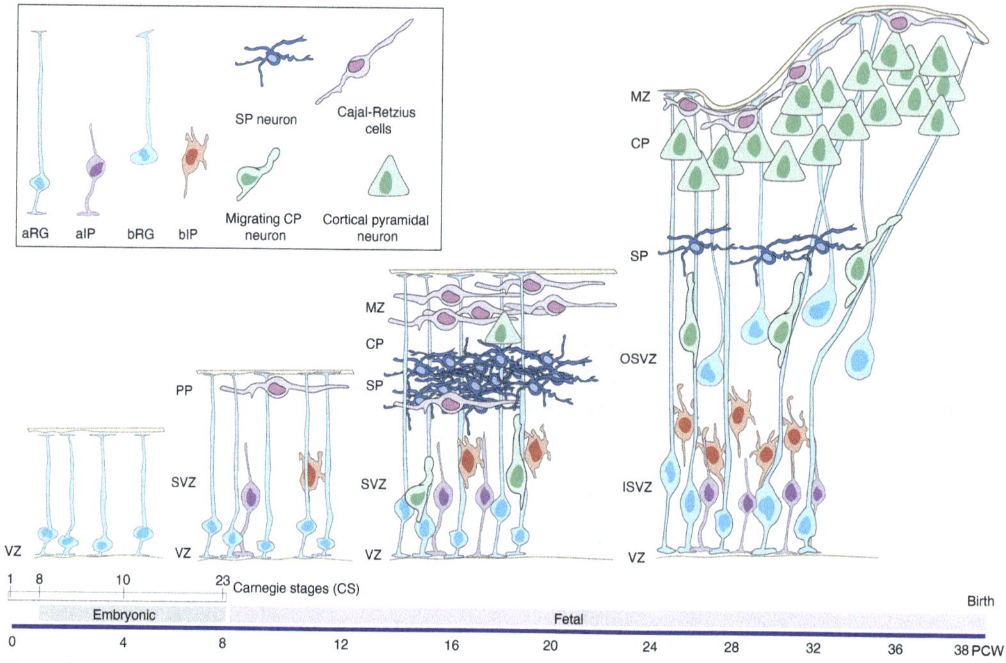

Figure 20.2 The developing human neocortex. Schematic illustration of the developing layers (VZ, ventricular zone; SVZ, subventricular zone; PP, preplate; SP, subplate; CP, cortical plate; MZ, marginal zone; ISVZ, inner subventricular zone; OSVZ, outer subventricular zone) and major cell types in the human neocortex over a timeline of human development from fertilization to birth (CS, Carnegie stages; PCW, post-conceptional weeks).

gyrification, the first-born CR cells degenerate and die and are replaced by persisting CR cells with smaller size, vertical soma, and a more local axonal field (Gonzalez-Gomez and Meyer 2014; Meyer 2010).

The SP is a highly dynamic structure that contains some of the earliest generated neurons, which are more mature than the overlying developing cortex, with distinct morphology, molecular expression profile, origin, birthdate, and cell survival time. Between 15–35 PCW in human, the SP is the most prominent embryonic zone of the telencephalon. The arrival of incoming fibers and growth of surrounding extracellular matrix are the main contributors to the expansion of the SP. It then becomes thinner over the course of development owing to programmed cell death (Kostovic 2020; Scola et al. 2018). Ablation or absence of the SP impairs the establishment of thalamocortical connections as well as inhibitory connectivity, underscoring its importance for the subsequent development of neocortical circuitry (Hoerder-Suabedissen and Molnar 2015). The SP is almost absent in marsupials, forms a distinct layer in mouse and rat, and is highly developed in human and non-human primates (Montiel et al. 2011). Analysis of prenatal human brain samples showed that the SP becomes visible only after 12 PCW, and from 15 PCW appears as the most prominent compartment of the cortical wall, consisting mostly of postmitotic NURR1 + LMO3 + neurons along with NOR1 + neurons and radially migrating immature TLE3 +, BRN2 +, and BHLHB5 + neurons. Subplate neurons in the fetal cortex express multiple markers of deep-projection neurons. By modeling SP formation in iPSC derived organoids, it was recently proposed that all classes of cortical deep-layer projection neurons can be generated from SP neurons, including TBR1 + CTIP2 + deep-layer cortical neurons (Ozair et al. 2018). In mouse, SP neurons control radial migration of cortical neurons through the formation of transient synapses on early immature neurons favoring the switch from slow multipolar to faster radial glia migration (Ohtaka-Maruyama et al. 2018). The SP layer and its neurons have been implicated in several neurodevelopmental disorders, including schizophrenia and autism (Hoerder-Suabedissen et al. 2013), as genes expressed in the SP are enriched for autism spectrum disorder (ASD) risk genes.

A general feature of MZ, CP, SP, and the early developing neural network is a sparse, spontaneous asynchronous activity. Both SP and CR neurons show relatively mature electrophysiological properties like depolarizations with action potential (Molnar et al. 2020). SP human neurons at mid-gestation (17–23 PCW) in acute cortical human slices generate spontaneous depolarization mainly by connexins hemichannels, with prolonged silent periods (Moore et al. 2014). This spontaneous neural activity may have an important role in establishing connectivity maps.

20.2.2 Dorsal Cortex Neurogenesis

20.2.2.1 Diversity of Human Radial Glial Cells

One of the most prominent features of the human brain is the larger size and folding of the cerebral cortex, a layered structure whose main function is to map and analyze sensory and motor information, integrating it with past experiences, and plan appropriate responses/actions.

In the late 1980s, Rakic and colleagues proposed the *radial unit hypothesis* to describe a common unifying mechanism that explains the generation of the neocortex. According to this model, in the embryonic/fetal period, the mammalian neocortex consists of radial proliferative columnar units that are composed of multipotent radial glial cells in the ventricular zone (VZ) and their progeny. The postmitotic cells migrate radially along the constraining glial scaffold and settle in vertical ontogenetic columns into the overlying cortical plate (Kostovic et al. 2019; Noctor et al. 2001; Rakic 1972, 2003). Cortical neurogenesis proceeds with an inside-out fashion so that early-generated neurons tend to occupy a deeper layer of the cortex, while later generated ones occupy progressively more superficial layers (Rakic 2007; Stepien et al. 2021). By retroviral gene transfer methods, which allows cell lineage analysis in vivo, it was proven that within a given column, neurons are clonally related, share connectivity, and form clusters of functionally related cells with similar tuning properties. These proliferative radial units form a proto-map, which was supported by observations of arealized expression of diffusible morphogens and their receptors (Cadwell et al. 2019), as well as differential expression of multiple transcription factors among radial glia cells in the VZ and across cortical area (Nowakowski et al. 2017). While it was shown that this primordial protomap in the proliferative layer can be established independently of thalamic innervation (Miyashita-Lin et al. 1999), evidence suggests progressive refinement during development by direct interactions with thalamic and other inputs to establish neocortical areas with specific size, cellular compositions, and functionalities (Rakic 1988, 2007).

The surface folding of the isocortex is a mechanism that begins very early in development. Alterations in cortical size or folding have been shown to lead to severe intellectual disabilities, including epilepsy (Fernandez et al. 2016; Leventer et al. 2010; Ossola and Kalebic 2021). At early embryonic stages, the cortical primordium is composed of a pseudostratified layer of neuroepithelial stem cells that maintain a direct contact with both the apical and the basal lamina, and divides symmetrically to exponentially increase the neuroepithelial precursor pool (Rakic 2009). The length of the neurogenic period differs widely among mammals, from 10 days of gestation (E10.5–E18, E19.5) in mouse to around 110 days (8–24 PCW) in humans (Rakic 1995). It has been argued that differences in the length of the neurogenic period alone, rather than any novel neurogenic progenitor lineage, are sufficient to explain variations in neuron number and neocortical size (particularly surface area) between species (Lewitus et al. 2014; Stepien et al. 2020). The size of the original pool of neuroepithelial stem cells impacts the number of progenitor cells and cortical neurons. At the onset of neurogenesis (7 PCW) neuroepithelial stem cells start to acquire apical radial glia (aRG) cell features, such as BLBP, PAX6, and VIM expression and are linked by apical junction complexes. With the initiation of neurogenesis, adherens junctions undergo constant remodeling, as new progenitors need to reestablish adhesion while the new-born neurons need to detach from the neuroepithelium (Veeraval et al. 2020).

Around 13–14 PCW aRG begin to divide asymmetrically, each cell generating a self-renewing apical progenitor and an intermediate, self-amplifying, neural progenitor cell that detaches from the apical layer and migrates basally, hence the name basal progenitor cell (BP). BPs share similarities with aRGs in terms of gene expression (SOX2, PAX6, and NESTIN), while also expressing a range of more specific genes (such as HOPX, pS6). A range of distinct BP subtypes reside in the extended SVZ comprising an inner and outer compartment (for review see Florio and Huttner 2014). The aRG contribute to deep-layer neuron formation and their overall number declines toward mid-gestation, while the number of BPs in the outer SVZ (oSVZ), also called outer radial glia (oRG), increases over the same period to become the most extensive germinal layer in primates and contributing to superficial layer neurons (Hansen et al. 2010; Kalebic et al. 2019; Reillo et al. 2011). Two major BPs have been identified in fetal human cortex: outer radial glia cells (oRGs) and truncated radial glial cells (tRGs) (LaMonica et al. 2013; Nowakowski et al. 2016). oRGs directly inherit the basal process from their aRG mother cells maintaining contact with the pial surface, but no longer contact the VZ, expand in the later part of neurogenesis and are regarded as the key drivers of the massive expansion of the human cortex (Hansen et al. 2010; Nowakowski et al. 2017, 2016; Pollen et al. 2015). On the other hand, tRGs no longer contact the pia, thus their basal processes mainly terminate in the oSVZ. The tRGs progeny was unknown until recent studies provided evidence that they generate basal multipotent intermediate progenitor cells that co-express EGFR, ASCL1, OLIG2, and OLIG1, giving rise to cortical oligodendrocytes, astrocytes, and olfactory bulb interneurons (Yang et al. 2022).

20.2.2.2 Fate Mapping and the Control of Cortical Cell Diversity

One intriguing question is how the extensive neuronal diversity within the mature cortex arises from a small progenitor population lining the embryonic lateral ventricles. To explain the emergence of such diversity, two opposite but not necessary mutually exclusive models have been proposed. In one case, distinct neuron types are gradually specified from relatively homogeneous progenitor cells (postmitotic model), while the other postulates that distinct precursors for each neuronal subtype are generated early in development (premitotic model) (Telley and Jabaudon 2018). For the postmitotic model, neuronal fate is not pre-programmed but acquired in postmitotic cells in response to extrinsic cues. Partial support for this model is the pioneer heterochronic transplantation studies in ferret as well as lineage analysis in rodents that provided evidence of multipotency of the progenitor's cells at early stage of corticogenesis, while this capacity progressively declines as development proceeds. Late-stage progenitors transplanted into the early-stage cortex were only capable of producing a superficial-layer subtype (Desai and McConnell 2000). Another study in mouse showed that during neurogenesis each radial glial progenitor cell produces around eight to nine neurons that occupy both deep and superficial layers, supporting the postmitotic model with a unitary output in neuronal production (Gao et al. 2014).

In favor of the premitotic model, other studies showed that several neuron subtype-specific transcription factors are expressed in progenitors earlier in development, suggesting that subsets of progenitors may be pre-committed to generating specific classes of projection neurons. The genetic fate-mapping study in murine cerebral cortex of Cux2-expressing cells by Franco and colleagues (Franco et al. 2012) was the first to establish that a subset of cortical progenitors, which are present from the earliest stages of corticogenesis, are committed to generating upper-layer neurons. Thus, current strong evidence of lineage-committed progenitors supports the premitotic models but does not rule out completely the existence of multipotential progenitors at the premitotic stage. Indeed, a very recent single-cell study of human mid-gestational cortical samples favors a mixed model of neurogenesis where RG progenitors are both "primed" to distinct cell fates by early expression of key TFs while also maintaining an ability to generate other subtypes, over a continuum of transcriptomic transitions tied to cell-cycle progression (Polioudakis et al. 2019). Lineage relationships among different cell types during human brain development was recently evaluated by tracking somatic mutations that occur stochastically during human development by parallel RNA and DNA analysis after deep sequencing (PRDD-seq) (Huang et al. 2020). Somatic mutation-defined clonal patterns provided independent evidence for an early divergence of precursors for lineage restricted formation of lower- and upper-layer excitatory neurons, with "inside-out" birth-dating pattern as seen previously in animal models. In addition, this analysis estimated that a founder cell population of ten precursors generate the excitatory neurons within a cortical column (Huang et al. 2020).

20.2.2.3 Regional Specification

Progenitor fate might govern not only the specification of different neuronal subtypes, but also the regional specification of the cortex, although the extent of this is debated. The cerebral cortex consists of three main regions: the neocortex, the archicortex (hippocampal formation), and the paleocortex (olfactory and some limbic areas). The boundary between archicortex and neocortex, whose positioning determines the relative size of these regions, is established early in development by reciprocal inhibitory relationships between FOXG1 and LHX2, two master regulatory genes expressed in the neocortex, and BMP/WNT signaling emanating from the hem and medial–cortical region. In the absence of FOXG1, there is a lateral-to-medial repatterning of the pallium, where the hem/hippocampal region expands dorsally, replacing the neocortex (Godbole et al. 2018; Muzio and Mallamaci 2005). LHX2 also regulates the fate decision between neocortex and paleocortex, as mice with deletion of LHX2 during a critical window exhibit a transformation of neocortex into a three-layered olfactory cortex (Chou et al. 2009).

Several functionally distinct subregions or areas exist within these broad domains, which can be distinguished from one another for their differences in cytoarchitecture, connectivity and patterns of gene expression. The process of cortical arealization has been object of debate and two opposite theories have been formulated. The *protomap* postulates that the cortical neural progenitors are prespecified and the area of origin will define the future identity even before thalamic fibers arrive. The *protocortex* instead states that the cortex is originally a *tabula rasa*, neuronal progenitors are multipotent, and only upon the arrival or afferent axons (mostly thalamic) will it start acquiring specific cortical area identities. It is now generally accepted that the layout of the cerebral cortex is initiated by morphogens expressed by telencephalic patterning centers, which drive the expression of master regulatory TFs in neocortical progenitors and postmitotic neurons that largely specify their fates, although external activity-dependent mechanisms, like thalamocortical axons, may fine tune cortex arealization (reviewed in Cadwell et al. 2019). A recent paper from Alzu'bi et al. (2019) demonstrates that in primates (human and marmoset), thalamocortical afferents innervate the cortical preplate-subplate at earlier stages than previously demonstrated in rodent studies, suggesting that pioneer thalamic afferents may participate in defining cortical neuron phenotypes.

Four primary functional subdivisions can be identified in the neocortex, one frontal motor area and three sensory areas for processing auditory, tactile, and visual stimuli (Bishop et al. 2000;

O'Leary and Sahara 2008; Simi and Studer 2018). Despite general conservation of the role of genetic factors on cortical arealization, several species-specific differences in neuronal proportions, laminar distributions, gene expression, and morphology between human and other mammals have been observed (Hodge et al. 2019). Within the neocortex of human fetal brain specimens (GW14–GW25) during the peak of neurogenesis and beginning of gliogenesis, many TF genes are differentially expressed in progenitors across distinct cortical areas, providing direct evidence for the intrinsic genetic control of area identities in cortical progenitors (e.g., EXM1/2, PAX6, NR2F1, FGFR3) (Bishop et al. 2002; Pattabiraman et al. 2014; Ypsilanti et al. 2021; Zhou et al. 2001). Importantly, the level of expression of an individual TF is a defining parameter that specifies the area identity of a cortical progenitor and its progeny. The amplitude of areal transcriptomic signatures increases over time, as radial glial cells differentiate into intermediate progenitor cells and later give rise to excitatory neurons (Bhaduri et al. 2021). Area patterning is a critical event during development and could vary across individuals within a species. This is consistent with reports that within the normal human population there is a considerable inter-individual variation in cortical area boundaries (White et al. 1997).

20.2.3 Origin of Inhibitory Neurons in Humans

Based on numerous rodent studies, it has been proposed that excitatory neurons within the cortex derive from progenitor cells in the dorsal ventricular zone of the pallium, whereas all cortical interneurons (GABAergic inhibitory neurons) are generated exclusively from the subpallial structure of the telencephalon. These interneurons first migrate tangentially into the developing neocortex and hippocampus, before shifting to radial migration to occupy the different neocortical layers (Anderson et al. 1997; Bandler et al. 2017; Lim et al. 2018). Other studies have instead suggested the possibility of a cortical origin for some interneurons. Among these, ex vivo studies in primate and human brain cortices revealed an unanticipated capacity of pallium progenitors to give rise to inhibitory neurons. Letinic et al. (2002), based on retroviral labelling of embryonic human forebrain specimens in organotypic slice cultures (10 to 25 GW), suggested the existence of two distinct lineages of neocortical GABAergic neurons. The DLX1/2$^+$/ASCL1$^+$ lineage, constituting 65 percent of cortical GABAergic neurons in humans, originated from ASCL1-expressing progenitors within the dorsal forebrain VZ/SVZ. The DLX1/2$^+$/ASCL1$^-$ lineage, constituting around the 35 percent of the cortical GABAergic neurons, originated from the GE of the ventral forebrain. The study could not exclude the possibility that some of the ASCL1$^+$ progenitors migrated from the GE at earlier embryonic stages and that the destination for some of these interneurons was the olfactory bulb. Similar findings were described for cynomolgus monkey fetal cortical samples (Petanjek et al. 2009), where ASCL1$^+$ GABAergic neurons were generated from the dorsal pallium with a temporal delay compared to the lineage coming from the GE. The ventral and dorsal GABAergic lineages displayed different distribution: lineage from the GE mostly populated the marginal zone and subplate, while the cortical plate was populated from both GABAergic lineages. Other studies in human and non-human primate forebrain tissue identified ASCL1$^+$, NKX2.1$^+$, and DLX$^+$ neuronal progenitors in the cortical VZ/SVZ niche (Alzu'bi and Clowry 2019; Radonjic et al. 2014). However, evidence provided by all these studies was circumstantial because it was essentially based on the one-time identification of these putative interneuron progenitors in the cortex by immunocytochemistry and provided no indication of their origin or their ability to generate excitatory neurons.

Recently Delgado and colleagues (Delgado et al. 2021) performed a high-throughput clonal lineage analysis and provided evidence for the existence of multipotent human cortical progenitor cells producing both excitatory and inhibitory neurons. They performed lineage tracing by using a cellular barcoding tool called single-cell-RNA-sequencing compatible tracer for identifying clonal relationships (STICR) in human progenitor cells from the cortical germinal zones of GW15 and GW18 human specimens as well as from the MGE of GW18 specimens. They confirmed the transcriptional profiles of major cell types but, more importantly, the clonal relationships among progenitors and their daughter cells. All principal cortical cell types (excitatory glutamatergic neurons, GABAergic interneurons, and glia) were observed in most multicellular clones (79%) coming from cortical germinal zones at both GW15 and GW18, revealing clonal relationships for all these cell types. Of note, the GABAergic interneurons lineage originating from cortical progenitors showed a transcriptional profile similar to CGE-derived cortical and olfactory bulb interneurons, and distinct from MGE-derived interneurons. One caveat of this study was the ex-vivo approach, where progenitors were extracted from the tissue, infected with the STICR, and cultured for several weeks. However, it seems clear from this study that dorsal cortical progenitors have at least the potential to generate both excitatory projection neurons and inhibitory interneurons.

The STICR approach was used in a parallel mouse study by Bandler and colleagues (Bandler et al. 2021) where, in contrast to the human findings, there was no evidence for shared lineages of excitatory and inhibitory cortical neurons in mice. Considering that the STICR results in mouse were limited to two developmental stages (E10, E14), this still leaves open the question as to whether the dorsal telencephalic origin of neocortical GABAergic neurons is truly a human specific phenomenon or more of a boosting of preexisting developmental mechanisms. In fact, knockout mice studies of ventral telencephalon-specific transcription factors, like Dlx1/Dlx2 or Nkx2.1 knockouts (Anderson et al. 1997, 1999; Sussel et al. 1999) showed a striking (50–75%) decrease of cortical GABAergic neurons, but never a total absence, leaving open the option of an alternative origin for this cell type in mice.

20.3 Modeling Disorders of Cortical Development In Vitro

Cortical organoids have demonstrated tremendous promise in recapitulating human-specific developmental features making them an attractive system to study disorders of human cortical development. This stem cell- or pluripotent cell-derived self-organizing 3D tissue recapitulates the architecture of the embryonic brain. It consists of progenitor zones, composed of various types of RG, at the apical side, and of newborn neurons at the basal side, forming the PP. Between those, a structure similar to an SVZ can be observed, populated by TBR2 + intermediate progenitor cells, and notably an oSVZ-like progenitor layer containing oRGs, characterized by HOPX, tenascin C, and FAM107a expression. Among other features of human cortical development, RG polarity, interkinetic nuclear migration, symmetric and asymmetric divisions, and cell migration have been recapitulated and studied in human brain organoids (Birey et al. 2017; Eiraku et al. 2008; Kadoshima et al. 2013; Lancaster et al. 2013; Mariani et al. 2012; Quadrato et al. 2017). Importantly, organoids show a correct progression of PP, with CR cells expressing Reelin, followed by cortical plate development over culture time (Lancaster et al. 2017). Early studies have directly compared bulk transcriptomes and enhancer element activity between iPSC-derived organoids (derived from reprogrammed skull fibroblasts) and postmortem isogenic human cerebral cortex, which suggested that organoids reproduce the very early stages of human corticogenesis (matching 8–16 PCW stages) (Amiri et al. 2018).

Cortical organoids contain the major types of human cortical progenitors, including neuroepithelial cells, aRG, BPs, and oRG (Bershteyn et al. 2017; Camp et al. 2015; Nowakowski et al. 2017) and display lineage restriction among different classes of progenitors (He et al. 2022). In addition to excitatory cortical neurons, various subtypes of GABAergic neurons are commonly found, including calretinin- and somatostatin-expressing neurons, however it is currently unclear whether these GABAergic interneurons are generated from a common progenitor (i.e., a single RG cell that generates both excitatory and inhibitory neurons) or from a ventral pallium-like area within the organoids, generating exclusively inhibitory neurons. Recent single-cell RNA-seq analyses (Bhaduri et al. 2020) of cortical organoids and developing human brains confirmed earlier reports of the presence of the main developing cortical cell types within organoids, with their transcriptomic and epigenetic signatures mostly conserved between organoids and human brains (Pollen et al. 2019).

However, despite recapitulation of early telencephalic layer architecture with polarized aRG, SVZ, and oRG, it is unclear whether organoid's precursor cell pool is sufficient to generate the full repertoire of cortical neurons. Cortical organoids do not contain all cell subtypes identified in cortical human samples, they show less cell type specificity at the transcriptomic level and lack many cell-type-specific open chromatin regions found in vivo (Ziffra et al. 2021). This is particularly relevant for excitatory neurons, as upper-layer excitatory neurons have increased in complexity in humans (Berg et al. 2021). There could be multiple reasons why a full recapitulation of neuronal identities is not achieved in vitro, at least with current technologies. One recently proposed theory is metabolic stress (Bhaduri et al. 2020), but there could be others, including lack of morphogenetic factors emanating from adjacent mesodermal cells, absence of vasculature and associated cell types, and mechanical stress.

20.3.1 Altered Brain Growth

Organoids have been used as a platform to model disorders of brain growth, leading to increased or decreased brain size (respectively, macrocephaly and microcephaly). Lancaster and colleagues (Lancaster et al. 2013) modeled microcephaly in cerebral organoids. Cortical regions in patient-derived cerebral organoids showed smaller progenitor zones ($SOX2^+$ cells) compared to control. The hypoplasia, reminiscent of reduced brain size observed in patients, was the result of decreased RG lateral expansion due to premature differentiation. Cortical organoids also modeled cellular features of lissencephaly in Miller-Dieker syndrome (deletion on chromosome 17) associated with mitotic defects in outer radial glia and increased apoptosis of RG cells (Bershteyn et al. 2017).

Cortical organoids provided a platform to study early disruptions in brain development in patients with ASD with disorders of cortical growth due to rare genetic mutations. For instance, in patients with 16p11.2 copy number variants (CNV), organoid size recapitulated the macrocephaly and microcephaly phenotypes observed in patients with 16p11.2 deletions and duplications, respectively. In addition, the CNV dosage affected neuronal maturation, proliferation, and synapse number (Urresti et al. 2021). Other rare syndromic forms of ASD with generalized cortical overgrowth studied in organoids include homozygous mutations in RAB39b and CNTNAP2 (de Jong et al. 2021; Zhang et al. 2020).

Disorders of the tuberous sclerosis complex (TSC), which are due to hyperactivity of the target of rapamycin (mTOR) signaling pathway, are collectively called mTORopathies and comprise a number of syndromes characterized by cortical dysplasia, hemimegalencephaly, and megalencephaly, accompanied by intellectual disability, epilepsy, and ASD comorbidity (Winden et al. 2018). Organoid-based studies of these syndromes have shown impaired differentiation of neural progenitor cells and increased proliferation, particularly for oRGs. This group of disorders often manifests with focal malformations of cortical development caused by germline mutations, for example, in TSC1/2, STRADA, and DEPDC5 genes, combined with a second hit somatic mutation in the affected cells (Dang et al. 2021; Klofas et al. 2020). Analysis of human cerebral organoid from TSC patients led to the identification of a specific neural cell subtype, called a caudal late interneuron progenitor (CLIP) cell, that over-proliferates in TSC, generating interneuron clonal expansion, which in vivo might lead to brain tumors and tuber-like cortical malformations (Eichmuller et al. 2022).

Finally, a study used iPSC lines from patients with ASD and cortical overgrowth to show that increased proliferation of progenitors resulted in increased susceptibility to double-strand DNA breaks at vulnerable gene loci (Wang et al. 2020).

20.3.2 Excitatory/inhibitory Lineage Imbalance

Given that organoids recapitulate brain development starting from the earliest phases, when neuroepithelial cells are regionally patterned and specified into various neuronal lineages, the organoid model has been instrumental in demonstrating alterations in cell fate specification in several neurodevelopmental disorders. In particular, an imbalance in excitatory vs. inhibitory neuronal lineages has been described in organoids generated from patients with both idiopathic and syndromic ASD (Mariani et al. 2015; Paulsen et al. 2022; Villa et al. 2022) and in patients with SCZ (Sawada et al. 2020), supporting the existence of shared biologic pathways between these two neurodevelopmental disorders (Gao and Penzes 2015). There is such a delicate balance between excitatory and inhibitory neurons in the cortex, that alterations in either direction seem associated with developmental neuropsychiatric diseases. At the circuit level, the numbers of excitatory and inhibitory synapses on individual cortical pyramidal neurons is highly regulated by a process that reproducibly generates a relatively invariant ratio of excitatory to inhibitory synapses (E/I ratio) across dendritic segments (Iascone et al. 2020; Loomba et al. 2022). Several developmental and genetic mechanisms can lead to an altered E/I ratio and subsequent compensatory phenomena, including altered neural lineage specification, altered progenitor proliferation, and synaptic maturation (Mariani et al. 2015; Patriarchi et al. 2015; Pizzarelli and Cherubini 2011; Sohal and Rubenstein 2019; Terauchi et al. 2010).

20.3.3 Human-specific Features

Organoids have also shown to be a good platform for investigating the functions of human-specific genes at different stages of human neurogenesis, disease pathology, and evolution. Human neural progenitor cells exhibit species-specific differences in cell shape, interkinetic nuclear migration, and cell cycle length (Benito-Kwiecinski et al. 2021). Neurogenesis is significantly longer in humans than in nonhuman primates and this is recapitulated in both organoid and monolayer culture systems, where human neural cells undergo more rounds of cell division, show a lower rate of migration and maturation, and a delayed onset of neural activity (Benito-Kwiecinski et al. 2021; Kanton et al. 2019; Marchetto et al. 2019). Transcriptome and epigenome analyses of humans', chimpanzees', and macaques' organoids revealed human-specific changes in gene expression and chromatin accessibility (Kanton et al. 2019). Even at the epitranscriptomic level (e.g., N6-methyladenosine mRNA modifications) differences were identified between mouse and human during early cortical neurogenesis using the organoid model, suggesting an enrichment of human-specific m6A tagging of transcripts related to neurogenesis and involving genes associated with genetic risk for mental disorders, such as SCZ and ASD (Yoon et al. 2017). A screen of human specific genes expressed in neuronal progenitors (Florio et al. 2018) revealed ~ 50 protein-coding genes preferentially expressed in the developing human neocortex compared to mouse, 35 of which had orthologs only in primates. One of these, NOTCH2NL, was enriched in radial glia cells, and activates NOTCH signaling in organoids, expanding the progenitor population. NOTCH2NL's function in human organoids limits direct neurogenesis and promotes instead IPC generation, SVZ expansion, and increases the size of the neuronal pool (Fiddes et al. 2018). Therefore, analysis of the specific functions of these genes and their interactions in organoids systems would provide significant insights into the mechanisms underlying cortical brain development and notably human evolution.

References

Acampora, D. et al. (1995). Forebrain and midbrain regions are deleted in $Otx2^{-/-}$ mutants due to a defective anterior neuroectoderm specification during gastrulation. *Development* 121: 3279–3290.

Alzu'bi, A. and Clowry, G.J. (2019). Expression of ventral telencephalon transcription factors ASCL1 and DLX2 in the early fetal human cerebral cortex. *J Anat* 235: 555–568.

Alzu'bi, A. et al. (2019). Thalamocortical afferents innervate the cortical subplate much earlier in development in primate than in rodent. *Cereb Cortex* 29: 1706–1718.

Amiri, A. et al. (2018). Transcriptome and epigenome landscape of human cortical development modeled in organoids. *Science* 362 (6420): eaat6720.

Anderson, S. et al. (1999). Differential origins of neocortical projection and local circuit neurons. *Cereb Cortex* 9: 646–654.

Anderson, S.A. et al. (1997). Interneuron migration from basal forebrain to neocortex: dependence on Dlx genes. *Science* 278: 474–476.

Andreu-Cervera, A. et al. (2021). Cilia, ciliopathies and hedgehog-related forebrain developmental disorders. *Neurobiol Dis* 150: 105236.

Ardhanareeswaran, K. et al. (2017). Human induced pluripotent stem cells for modelling neurodevelopmental disorders. *Nat Rev Neurol* 13: 265–278.

Assimacopoulos, S. et al. (2003). Identification of a Pax6-dependent epidermal growth factor family signaling source at the lateral edge of the embryonic cerebral cortex. *J Neurosci* 23: 6399–6403.

Bagley, J.A. et al. (2017). Fused cerebral organoids model interactions between brain regions. *Nat Methods* 14: 743–751.

Bandler, R.C. et al. (2017). Cortical interneuron specification. *Curr Opin Neurobiol* 42: 17–24.

Bandler, R.C. et al. (2021). Single-cell delineation of lineage and genetic identity in the mouse brain. *Nature* 601 (7893): 404–409.

Benito-Kwiecinski, S. et al. (2021). An early cell shape transition drives evolutionary expansion of the human forebrain. *Cell* 184: 2084–2102.e2019.

Berg, J. et al. (2021). Human neocortical expansion involves glutamatergic neuron diversification. *Nature* 598: 151–158.

Bershteyn, M. et al. (2017). Human iPSC-derived cerebral organoids model cellular features of lissencephaly and reveal prolonged mitosis of outer radial glia. *Cell Stem Cell* 20: 435–449.e434.

Bhaduri, A. et al. (2020). Cell stress in cortical organoids impairs molecular subtype specification. *Nature* 578: 142–148.

Bhaduri, A. et al. (2021). An atlas of cortical arealization identifies dynamic molecular signatures. *Nature* 598: 200–204.

Bielle, F. et al. (2005). Multiple origins of Cajal-Retzius cells at the borders of the developing pallium. *Nat Neurosci* 8: 1002–1012.

Birey, F. et al. (2017). Assembly of functionally integrated human forebrain spheroids. *Nature* 545: 54–59.

Bishop, K.M. et al. (2000). Regulation of area identity in the mammalian neocortex by Emx2 and Pax6. *Science* 288: 344–349.

Bishop, K.M. et al. (2002). Distinct actions of Emx1, Emx2, and Pax6 in regulating the specification of areas in the developing neocortex. *J Neurosci* 22: 7627–7638.

Boncinelli, E. et al. (1991). HOX gene activation by retinoic acid. *Trends Genet* 7 (10): 329–334.

Brady, M.V. and Vaccarino, F.M. (2021). Role of SHH in patterning human pluripotent cells towards ventral forebrain fates. *Cells* 10 (4): 914

Cadwell, C.R. et al. (2019). Development and arealization of the cerebral cortex. *Neuron* 103: 980–1004.

Camp, J.G. et al. (2015). Human cerebral organoids recapitulate gene expression programs of fetal neocortex development. *Proc Natl Acad Sci USA* 112: 15672–15677.

Carcamo-Orive, I. et al. (2017). Analysis of transcriptional variability in a large human iPSC library reveals genetic and non-genetic determinants of heterogeneity. *Cell Stem Cell* 20: 518–532.e519.

Cederquist, G.Y. et al. (2019). Specification of positional identity in forebrain organoids. *Nat Biotechnol* 37: 436–444.

Chatzi, C. (2011). Retinoic acid functions as a key GABAergic differentiation signal in the basal ganglia. *PLoS Biol* 9: e1000609.

Chou, S.J. et al. (2009). Lhx2 specifies regional fate in Emx1 lineage of telencephalic progenitors generating cerebral cortex. *Nat Neurosci* 12: 1381–1389.

Clowry, G.J. et al. (2018). Charting the protomap of the human telencephalon. *Semin Cell Dev Biol* 76: 3–14.

Dang, L.T. et al. (2021). STRADA-mutant human cortical organoids model megalencephaly and exhibit delayed neuronal differentiation. *Dev Neurobiol* 81: 696–709.

de Jong, J.O. et al. (2021). Cortical overgrowth in a preclinical forebrain organoid model of CNTNAP2-associated autism spectrum disorder. *Nat Commun* 12: 4087.

Delgado, R.N. et al. (2021). Individual human cortical progenitors can produce excitatory and inhibitory neurons. *Nature* 601 (7893): 397–403.

Desai, A.R. and McConnell, S.K. (2000). Progressive restriction in fate potential by neural progenitors during cerebral cortical development. *Development* 127: 2863–2872.

Eichmuller, O.L. et al. (2022). Amplification of human interneuron progenitors promotes brain tumors and neurological defects. *Science* 375: eabf5546.

Eiraku, M. et al. (2008). Self-organized formation of polarized cortical tissues from ESCs and its active manipulation by extrinsic signals. *Cell Stem Cell* 3: 519–532.

Ericson, J. et al. (1995). Sonic hedgehog induces the differentiation of ventral forebrain neurons. *Cell* 81: 747–756.

Eto, H. and Kishi, Y. (2021). Brain regionalization by polycomb-group proteins and chromatin accessibility. *Bioessays* 43: e2100155.

Fernandez, V. et al. (2016). Cerebral cortex expansion and folding. *EMBO J* 35: 1021–1044.

Fiddes, I.T. et al. (2018). Human-specific NOTCH2NL genes affect notch signaling and cortical neurogenesis. *Cell* 173: 1356–1369.e1322.

Florio, M. et al. (2018). Evolution and cell-type specificity of human-specific genes preferentially expressed in progenitors of fetal neocortex. *Elife* 7: e32332.

Florio, M. and Huttner, W.B. (2014). Neural progenitors, neurogenesis and the evolution of the neocortex. *Development* 141: 2182–2194.

Franco, S.J. et al. (2012). Fate-restricted neural progenitors in the mammalian cerebral cortex. *Science* 337: 746–749.

Gao, P. et al. (2014). Deterministic progenitor behavior and unitary production of neurons in the neocortex. *Cell* 159: 775–788.

Gao, R. and Penzes, P. (2015). Common mechanisms of excitatory and inhibitory imbalance in schizophrenia and autism spectrum disorders. *Curr Mol Med* 15: 146–167.

Gerrelli, D. et al. (2015). Enabling research with human embryonic and fetal tissue resources. *Development* 142: 3073–3076.

Godbole, G. et al. (2018). Hierarchical genetic interactions between FOXG1 and LHX2 regulate the formation of the cortical hem in the developing telencephalon. *Development* 145 (1): dev154583.

Gonzalez-Gomez, M. and Meyer, G. (2014). Dynamic expression of calretinin in embryonic and early fetal human cortex. *Front Neuroanat* 8: 41.

Grove, E.A. et al. (1998). The hem of the embryonic cerebral cortex is defined by the expression of multiple Wnt genes and is compromised in Gli3-deficient mice. *Development* 125: 2315–2325.

Hansen, D.V. et al. (2010). Neurogenic radial glia in the outer subventricular zone of human neocortex. *Nature* 464: 554–561.

He, Z. et al. (2022). Lineage recording in human cerebral organoids. *Nat Methods* 19: 90–99.

Hodge, R.D. et al. (2019). Conserved cell types with divergent features in human versus mouse cortex. *Nature* 573 (7772): 61–68.

Hoerder-Suabedissen, A. and Molnar, Z. (2015). Development, evolution and pathology of neocortical subplate neurons. *Nat Rev Neurosci* 16: 133–146.

Hoerder-Suabedissen, A. et al. (2013). Expression profiling of mouse subplate reveals a dynamic gene network and disease association with autism and schizophrenia. *Proc Natl Acad Sci USA* 110: 3555–3560.

Hong, S.E. et al. (2000). Autosomal recessive lissencephaly with cerebellar hypoplasia is associated with human RELN mutations. *Nat Genet* 26: 93–96.

Huang, A.Y. et al. (2020). Parallel RNA and DNA analysis after deep sequencing (PRDD-seq) reveals cell type-specific lineage patterns in human brain. *Proc Natl Acad Sci USA* 117: 13886–13895.

Iascone, D.M. et al. (2020). Whole-neuron synaptic mapping reveals spatially precise excitatory/inhibitory balance limiting dendritic and somatic spiking. *Neuron* 106: 566–578.e568.

Jacob, F. et al. (2020). Human pluripotent stem cell-derived neural cells and brain organoids reveal SARS-CoV-2 neurotropism predominates in choroid plexus epithelium. *Cell Stem Cell* 27: 937–950.e939.

Jourdon, A. et al. (2021). PsychENCODE and beyond: transcriptomics and epigenomics of brain development and organoids. *Neuropsychopharmacology* 46: 70–85.

Kadoshima, T. et al. (2013). Self-organization of axial polarity, inside-out layer pattern, and species-specific progenitor dynamics in human ES cell-derived neocortex. *Proc Natl Acad Sci USA* 110: 20284–20289.

Kalebic, N. et al. (2019). Neocortical expansion due to increased proliferation of basal progenitors is linked to changes in their morphology. *Cell Stem Cell* 24: 535–550.e539.

Kanton, S.et al. (2019). Organoid single-cell genomic atlas uncovers human-specific features of brain development. *Nature* 574: 418–422.

Klofas, L.K. et al. (2020). DEPDC5 haploinsufficiency drives increased mTORC1 signaling and abnormal morphology in human iPSC-derived cortical neurons. *Neurobiol Dis* 143: 104975.

Kostovic, I. (2020). The enigmatic fetal subplate compartment forms an early tangential cortical nexus and provides the framework for construction of cortical connectivity. *Prog Neurobiol* 194: 101883.

Kostovic, I. et al. (2019). Neural histology and neurogenesis of the human fetal and infant brain. *NeuroImage* 188: 743–773.

LaMonica, B.E. et al. (2013). Mitotic spindle orientation predicts outer radial glial cell generation in human neocortex. *Nat Commun* 4: 1665.

Lancaster, M.A. et al. (2017). Guided self-organization and cortical plate formation in human brain organoids. *Nat Biotechnol* 35: 659–666.

Lancaster, M.A. and Knoblich, J.A. (2014). Organogenesis in a dish. *Science* 345: 1247125.

Lancaster, M.A. et al. (2013). Cerebral organoids model human brain development and microcephaly. *Nature* 501: 373–379.

Letinic, K. et al. (2002). Origin of GABAergic neurons in the human neocortex. *Nature* 417: 645–649.

Leventer, R.J. et al. (2010). Clinical and imaging heterogeneity of polymicrogyria. *Brain* 133: 1415–1427.

Lewitus, E. et al. (2014). An adaptive threshold in mammalian neocortical evolution. *PLoS Biol* 12: e1002000.

Lim, L. et al. (2018). Development and functional diversification of cortical interneurons. *Neuron* 100: 294–313.

Loomba, S. et al. (2022). Connectomic comparison of mouse and human cortex. *Science* 377: eabo0924.

Mangale, V.S. et al. (2008). Lhx2 selector activity specifies cortical identity and suppresses hippocampal organizer fate. *Science* 319: 304–309.

Manzari-Tavakoli, A. et al. (2022). The cross-talks among bone morphogenetic protein (BMP) signaling and other prominent pathways involved in neural differentiation. *Front Mol Neurosci* 15: 827275.

Marchetto, M.C. et al. (2019). Species-specific maturation profiles of human, chimpanzee and bonobo neural cells. *Elife* 8: e37527.

Mariani, J. et al. (2015). FOXG1-dependent dysregulation of GABA/glutamate neuron differentiation in autism spectrum disorders. *Cell* 162: 375–390.

Mariani, J. et al. (2012). Modeling human cortical development in vitro using induced pluripotent stem cells. *Proc Natl Acad Sci USA* 109: 12770–12775.

Marshall, H. et al. (1994). A conserved retinoic acid response element required for early expression of the homeobox gene Hoxb-1. *Nature* 370: 567–571.

Meyer, G. (2010). Building a human cortex. *J Anat* 217: 334–343.

Meyer, G. et al. (2002). Expression of p73 and Reelin in the developing human cortex. *J Neurosci* 22: 4973–4986.

Micali, N. et al. (2020). Variation of human neural stem cells generating organizer states in vitro before committing to cortical excitatory or inhibitory neuronal fates. *Cell Rep* 31: 107599.

Miyashita-Lin, E. et al. (1999). Early neocortical regionalization in the absence of thalamic innervation. *Science* 285: 906–909.

Molnar, Z. et al. (2020). Transient cortical circuits match spontaneous and sensory-driven activity during development. *Science* 370 (6514): eabb2153.

Montiel, J.F. et al. (2011). Hypothesis on the dual origin of the Mammalian subplate. *Front Neuroanat* 5: 25.

Moore, A.R. et al. (2014). Connexin hemichannels contribute to spontaneous electrical activity in the human fetal cortex. *Proc Natl Acad Sci USA* 111: E3919–3928.

Muguruma, K. et al. (2015). Self-organization of polarized cerebellar tissue in 3D culture of human pluripotent stem cells. *Cell Rep* 10: 537–550.

Muzio, L. and Mallamaci, A. (2005). Foxg1 confines Cajal-Retzius neuronogenesis and hippocampal morphogenesis to the dorsomedial pallium. *J Neurosci* 25: 4435–4441.

Nieuwkoop, P.D. and Nigtevecht, G. (1954). Neural activation and transformation in explants of competent ectoderm under the influence of fragments of anterior notochord in urodeles. *Development* 2: 175–193.

Noctor, S.C. et al. (2001). Neurons derived from radial glial cells establish radial units in neocortex. *Nature* 409: 714–720.

Nowakowski, T.J. et al. (2017). Spatiotemporal gene expression trajectories reveal developmental hierarchies of the human cortex. *Science* 358: 1318–1323.

Nowakowski, T.J. et al. (2016). Transformation of the radial glia scaffold demarcates two stages of human cerebral cortex development. *Neuron* 91: 1219–1227.

O'Leary, D.D. and Sahara, S. (2008). Genetic regulation of arealization of the neocortex. *Curr Opin Neurobiol* 18: 90–100.

Ohtaka-Maruyama, C. et al. (2018). Synaptic transmission from subplate neurons controls radial migration of neocortical neurons. *Science* 360: 313–317.

Ossola, C. and Kalebic, N. (2021). Roots of the malformations of cortical development in the cell biology of neural progenitor cells. *Front Neurosci* 15: 817218.

Ozair, M.Z. et al. (2018). hPSC modeling reveals that fate selection of cortical deep projection neurons occurs in the subplate. *Cell Stem Cell* 23: 60–73 e66.

Pasca, S.P. (2018). The rise of three-dimensional human brain cultures. *Nature* 553: 437–445.

Patriarchi, T. et al. (2015). Imbalance of excitatory/inhibitory synaptic protein expression in iPSC-derived neurons from FOXG1$^{(+/-)}$ patients and in foxg1$^{(+/-)}$ mice. *Eur J Hum Genet* 24 (6): 871–880.

Pattabiraman, K. et al. (2014). Transcriptional regulation of enhancers active in protodomains of the developing cerebral cortex. *Neuron* 82: 989–1003.

Paulsen, B. et al. (2022). Autism genes converge on asynchronous development of shared neuron classes. *Nature* 602: 268–273.

Petanjek, Z. (2009). Origins of cortical GABAergic neurons in the cynomolgus monkey. *Cereb Cortex* 19: 249–262.

Pizzarelli, R. and Cherubini, E. (2011). Alterations of GABAergic signaling in autism spectrum disorders. *Neural Plast* 2011: 297153.

Polioudakis, D. et al. (2019). A single-cell transcriptomic atlas of human neocortical development during mid-gestation. *Neuron* 103: 785–801.e788.

Pollen, A.A. et al. (2019). Establishing cerebral organoids as models of human-specific brain evolution. *Cell* 176: 743–756.e717.

Pollen, A.A. et al. (2015). Molecular identity of human outer radial glia during cortical development. *Cell* 163: 55–67.

Pomeshchik, Y. et al. (2020). Human iPSC-derived hippocampal spheroids. *Stem Cell Rep* 15: 256–273.

Qian, X. et al. (2016). Brain-region-specific organoids using mini-bioreactors for modeling ZIKV exposure. *Cell* 165: 1238–1254.

Quadrato, G. et al. (2017). Cell diversity and network dynamics in photosensitive human brain organoids. *Nature* 545: 48–53.

Radonjic, N.V. et al. (2014). Diversity of cortical interneurons in primates. *Cell Rep* 9: 2139–2151.

Ragsdale, C.W. and Grove, E.A. (2001). Patterning the mammalian cerebral cortex. *Curr Opin Neurobiol* 11: 50–58.

Rakic, P. (1972). Mode of cell migration to the superficial layers of fetal monkey cortex. *J Comp Neurol* 145: 61–84.

Rakic, P. (1988). Specification of cerebral cortical areas. *Science* 241: 170–176.

Rakic, P. (1995). A small step for the cell, a giant leap for mankind. *Trends Neurosci* 18: 383–388.

Rakic, P. (2003). Elusive radial glial cells. *Glia* 43: 19–32.

Rakic, P. (2007). The radial edifice of cortical architecture: from neuronal silhouettes to genetic engineering. *Brain Res Rev* 55: 204–219.

Rakic, P. (2009). Evolution of the neocortex: a perspective from developmental biology. *Nat Rev Neurosci* 10: 724–735.

Rataj-Baniowska, M. et al. (2015). Retinoic acid receptor beta controls development of striatonigral projection neurons through FGF-dependent and meis1-dependent mechanisms. *J Neurosci* 35: 14467–14475.

Reillo, I. et al. (2011). A role for intermediate radial glia in the tangential expansion of the mammalian cerebral cortex. *Cereb Cortex* 21: 1674–1694.

Renner, M. et al. (2017). Self-organized developmental patterning and differentiation in cerebral organoids. *EMBO J* 36: 1316–1329.

Rifes, P. et al. (2020). Modeling neural tube development by differentiation of human embryonic stem cells in a microfluidic WNT gradient. *Nat Biotechnol* 38: 1265–1273.

Roy, A. et al. (2014). Lhx2 regulates the development of the forebrain hem system. *Cereb Cortex* 24: 1361–1372.

Sakaguchi, H. et al. (2015). Generation of functional hippocampal neurons from self-organizing human embryonic stem cell-derived dorsomedial telencephalic tissue. *Nat Commun* 6: 8896.

Sasai, Y. (2013). Next-generation regenerative medicine. *Cell Stem Cell* 12: 520–530.

Sawada, T. et al. (2020). Developmental excitation-inhibition imbalance underlying psychoses revealed by single-cell analyses of discordant twins-derived cerebral organoids. *Mol Psychiatry* 25: 2695–2711.

Scola, E. et al. (2018). High resolution post-mortem MRI of non-fixed in situ foetal brain in the second trimester of gestation. *Eur Radiol* 28: 363–371.

Shibata, M. et al. (2021). Regulation of prefrontal patterning and connectivity by retinoic acid. *Nature* 598: 483–488.

Siegenthaler, J.A. and Pleasure, S.J. (2011). We have got you "covered". *Curr Opin Genet Dev* 21: 249–255.

Simeone, A. et al. (1995). Retinoic acid induces stage-specific antero-posterior transformations of rostral central nervous system. *Mech Dev* 51: 83–98.

Simi, A. and Studer, M. (2018). Developmental genetic programs and activity-dependent mechanisms instruct neocortical area mapping. *Curr Opin Neurobiol* 53: 96–102.

Sohal, V.S. and Rubenstein, J.L.R. (2019). Excitation-inhibition balance as a framework for investigating mechanisms in neuropsychiatric disorders. *Mol Psychiatry* 24: 1248–1257.

Stepien, B.K. et al. (2020). Lengthening neurogenic period during neocortical development causes a hallmark of neocortex expansion. *Curr Biol* 30: 4227–4237.e4225.

Stepien, B.K. et al. (2021). Length of the neurogenic period – a key determinant for the generation of upper-layer neurons during neocortex development and evolution. *Front Cell Dev Biol* 9: 676911.

Stern, C.D. (2001). Initial patterning of the central nervous system. *Nat Rev Neurosci* 2: 92–98.

Sur, M. and Rubenstein, J.L. (2005). Patterning and plasticity of the cerebral cortex. *Science* 310: 805–810.

Sussel, L. et al. (1999). Loss of Nkx2.1 homeobox gene function results in a ventral to dorsal molecular respecification within the basal telencephalon. *Development* 126: 3359–3370.

Telley, L. and Jabaudon, D. (2018). A mixed model of neuronal diversity. *Nature* 555: 452–454.

Terauchi, A. et al. (2010). Distinct FGFs promote differentiation of excitatory and inhibitory synapses. *Nature* 465: 783–787.

Tissir, F. et al. (2009). DeltaNp73 regulates neuronal survival in vivo. *Proc Natl Acad Sci USA* 106: 16871–16876.

Urresti, J. et al. (2021). Cortical organoids model early brain development disrupted by 16p11.2 copy number variants in autism. *Mol Psychiatry* 26 (12): 7581.

Veeraval, L. et al. (2020). Adherens junctions. *Front Cell Dev Biol* 8: 6.

Villa, C.E. et al. (2022). CHD8 haploinsufficiency links autism to transient alterations in excitatory and inhibitory trajectories. *Cell Rep* 39: 110615.

Wang, M. et al. (2020). Increased neural progenitor proliferation in a hiPSC model of autism induces replication stress-associated genome instability. *Cell Stem Cell* 26: 221–233.e226.

White, L.E. et al. (1997). Structure of the human sensorimotor system. *Cereb Cortex* 7: 18–30.

Winden, K.D. et al. (2018). Abnormal mTOR activation in autism. *Ann Rev Neurosci* 41: 1–23.

Xiang, Y. et al. (2019). hESC-derived thalamic organoids form reciprocal projections when fused with cortical organoids. *Cell Stem Cell* 24: 487–497.e487.

Xiang, Y. et al. (2017). Fusion of regionally specified hPSC-derived organoids models human brain development and interneuron migration. *Cell Stem Cell* 21: 383–398.e387.

Yang, L. et al. (2022). Developmental origins of human cortical oligodendrocytes and astrocytes. *Neurosci Bull* 38: 47–68.

Ye, W. et al. (1998). FGF and Shh signals control dopaminergic and serotonergic cell fate in the anterior neural plate. *Cell* 93: 755–766.

Yoon, K.J. et al. (2017). Temporal control of mammalian cortical neurogenesis by m(6)A methylation. *Cell* 171: 877–889.e817.

Ypsilanti, A.R. et al. (2021). Transcriptional network orchestrating regional patterning of cortical progenitors. *Proc Natl Acad Sci USA* 118 (51): e2024795118.

Yu, S.R. et al. (2009). Fgf8 morphogen gradient forms by a source-sink mechanism with freely diffusing molecules. *Nature* 461: 533–536.

Zhang, W. et al. (2020). Cerebral organoid and mouse models reveal a RAB39b-PI3K-mTOR pathway-dependent dysregulation of cortical development leading to macrocephaly/autism phenotypes. *Genes Dev* 34 (7–8): 580–597.

Zhou, C. et al. (2001). COUP-TFI: an intrinsic factor for early regionalization of the neocortex. *Genes Dev* 15: 2054–2059.

Ziffra, R.S. et al. (2021). Single-cell epigenomics reveals mechanisms of human cortical development. *Nature* 598: 205–213.

21

Mammalian Cortical Regional Specification

Athéna R. Ypsilanti and John L. Rubenstein

Rubenstein Lab, Nina Ireland Laboratory of Developmental Neurobiology, University of California San Francisco (UCSF) Rock Hall, 1550 4th Street, Room RH-282, San Francisco, CA, 94158 USA

21.1 Introduction: Embryonic Anatomy that Contributes to Early Cortical Development

The mammalian cortex (pallium) cytoarchitecture has both a regional and a laminar organization. Distinct cortical regions are characterized by their structural and functional specializations (e.g., prefrontal, motor, somatosensory, motor, visual, auditory, olfactory, and hippocampal areas), which involve precise connectivity with the thalamus and other cortical and subcortical structures. Further, these functional regions have sharp boundaries identified by a variety of cytoarchitectural differences in molecular and neuronal make-up and in connectivity. Superimposed on this regional categorization, different cortical regions have distinct laminar organization: for instance, the neocortex has six neuronal layers, whereas the hippocampus and olfactory bulb have one primary layer of excitatory neurons, and two layers of inhibitory neurons. The neurons in each layer have specific connectivity.

All cortical regions have two main types of neurons. The first are excitatory glutamatergic projection neurons that connect cortical hemispheres, cortical regions, and subcortical regions. Secondly, are the inhibitory GABAergic interneurons that regulate local circuitry within layers, regions, and some across regions. During development, excitatory neurons originate from the pallium (dorsal telencephalon) and inhibitory neurons originate from the subpallium (ganglionic eminences (GEs), ventral telencephalon). Here, we focus on the developmental mechanisms of cortical regional specification in mice.

21.1.1 Prosencephalon

Early in development, the rostral-most regions evaginates into the prosencephalon and then secondarily into bilateral telencephalic vesicles, whose dorsal regions become the pallium (cortex) and ventral regions become the subpallium. Rostro-caudal (RC) and dorso-ventral (DV) patterning of the cortex begins at this stage through the action of midline and paramedial patterning centers that secrete morphogens. A caudo-dorsal center secretes WNTs and BMPs (Chizhikov and Millen 2005; Shimogori et al. 2004); a rostral center secretes fibroblast growth factors (FGFs) (Caronia-Brown et al. 2014; Hasenpusch-Theil et al. 2017; Hoch et al. 2015a; Yabut et al. 2020); and a ventral domain secretes SHH (Rash and Grove 2007). Patterning by morphogens is fully discussed in Chapter 22.

Neocortical Neurogenesis in Development and Evolution, First Edition. Edited by Wieland B. Huttner.

In combination, these molecular cues help establish gradiential expression of transcription factors (TFs) within pallial neuroepithelial progenitors (ventricular zone, VZ). These TFs then play a central role in establishing pallial regions; from ventral to dorsal: olfactory and amygdala (lateral-ventral pallium (LVP), neocortex (dorsal pallium) and hippocampus (medial pallium) see Figure 21.1A). These regions also have distinct RC properties. The hippocampus and amygdala are caudal structures (each with substructures). Within the neocortex, the rostral-dorsal and caudal-dorsal pallium (RDP, CDP) have distinct properties that contribute to the generation of neocortical areas (discussed later).

21.1.2 Pallial Progenitors

Neural induction generates neuroepithelial stem cells (NSC). As the neural tube is generated these cells are adjacent to the ventricles, and thus are called the VZ. NSC then differentiate into radial glia stem cells, which can divide symmetrically, or asymmetrically to generate intermediate progenitors that migrate into subventricular zone (SVZ) and then sequentially generate cortical excitatory neurons, olfactory bulb GABAergic neurons and then glia (Gorski et al. 2002). Intermediate progenitors also generate neurons. Newly generated neurons migrate radially along radial glia apical processes

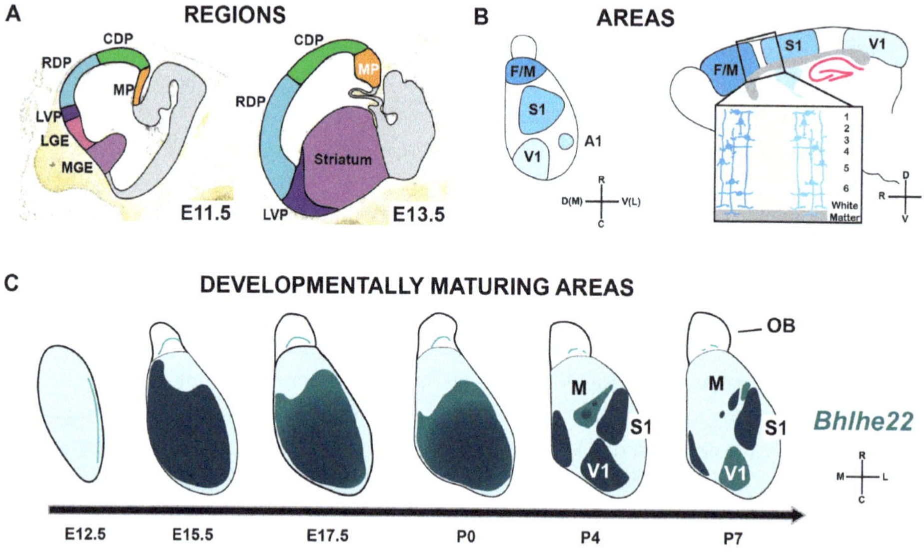

Figure 21.1 (A) Schematics of embryonic forebrains at E11.5 (left) and E13.5 (right) (sagittal planes) depicting the subregions of the developing cortex: MP: medium pallium; CDP: caudal-dorsal pallium; RDP: rostral-dorsal pallium; LVP: lateral-ventral pallium; and the basal ganglia: LGE: lateral ganglionic eminence; MGE: medial ganglionic eminence; and Striatum. (B) Schematic of principal cortical areas of the adult mouse brain including the frontal/motor (F/M), the somatosensory (S1), the auditory (A1), and the visual (V1) cortex. On the left side of the schematic is a top-down view. On the right side, the schematic depicts the primary cortical areas in a sagittal section as well as the laminar (layers 1–6) and columnar structure of the adult cortex. Spatial coordinates are shown: dorsal–(medial) D(M), ventral(lateral) V(L), rostral (R), and caudal (C). (C) Schematic of a top-down view of the mouse cortex depicting *Bhlhe22* expression during cortical development (from E12.5 to P7). These drawings are adapted from pictures of whole-mount brains from *Bhlhe22*$^{LacZ/+}$ mice after revealing β-galactosidase activity (Joshi et al. 2008). *Bhlhe22* expression during cortical development begins as a high caudo-medial graded expression that evolves into sharp borders by P7 with expression absent rostrally in the frontomotor cortex (M), and restricted to subdomains of S1 and V1, in addition to a more medial domain (perhaps retrospenial cortex). OB: olfactory bulb.

into the cortical plate (CP); this process maintains the register with the location of their generation. Thus, patterning in the VZ affects patterning in the cortical plate and eventually the mature cortex; this is the basis of the protomap model of Rakic (Rakic 1988). There is an additional type of radial glia assembly in a layer superficial to the SVZ; these are called outer radial glia (oRG). oRGs are prominent in primates and are thought to participate in the expansion of superficial cortical layers which is a characteristic of the primate cortex (Fietz et al. 2010; Hansen et al. 2010). oRGs are in part characterized by the expression of the *Hopx* TF. oRGs are also present in mouse cortex, where they are enriched in dorsal parts of the pallial progenitor zone (Vaid et al. 2018). It will be interesting to learn more about their role in specification of pallial regional differences.

21.1.3 Subpallium

The ganglionic eminences (GEs) are the subpallial structures of the developing telencephalon. They are subdivided into the medial GE (MGE), lateral GE (LGE), and caudal GE (CGE); the preoptic area (POA) and septum are additional subpallial primordia. They primarily generate GABAergic and cholinergic neurons, including projection neurons of the striatum, globus pallidus, amygdala, septum, and POA, as well as GABAergic pallial interneurons. These interneurons are initially born from progenitors located in the VZ of the MGE/CGE/POA and migrate tangentially through the subpallium to reach the cortex where they disperse and integrate into the local cortical circuitry (in a layer specific manner). Cortical interneuron development will be discussed in depth in another chapter.

21.2 Pallial Patterning

Patterning of the pallium is the process whereby the developing cortex becomes progressively subdivided into distinct regions (e.g., olfactory, neocortex, hippocampus) and areas (Figure 21.1B; e.g., neocortical frontal/motor area (M), somatosensory area (S), the auditory area (A) and the visual area (V)) reviewed by Azzarelli et al. (2015); Mallamaci and Stoykova (2006); O'Leary and Sahara (2008); O'Leary et al. (2007); Tomassy et al. (2010a)). Neocortical areas receive thalamic input from specific nuclei (López-Bendito and Martini 2020) and output to different cortical and subcortical targets (Catela 2020; Valdez 2020). For instance, layer 4 excitatory neurons in the somatosensory and visual cortex have different morphologies, transcriptomes, connectivity with the thalamus and interneurons, and electrophysiological properties (Scala et al. 2019). An example of the progression of cortical patterning can be visualized by looking at the dynamic changes in the expression of *Bhlhe22* during development; its expression progresses from a small lateral domain at E12.5, to a relatively broad pattern in late embryogenesis, to a sharply defined domains postnatally (Figure 21.1C).

As research has progressed into the development of cortical area subdivisions, it is hypothesized that patterning occurs in several stages (Cadwell et al. 2019; Tocco et al. 2022; Zembrzycki et al. 2015). First, during an early regionalization period, pallial progenitor cells are patterned by morphogen-driven combinatorial and graded expression of TFs (Grove 2020; Grove and Monuki 2020; Tole and Hébert 2020). This pre-patterning is then shaped and maintained in postmitotic neurons by the persistence of key TFs and epigenetic mechanisms in new-born neurons (Alfano et al. 2014; Golonzhka et al. 2015; Zembrzycki et al. 2015). Finally, extrinsic factors including thalamocortical inputs and activity further act to refine and preserve the boundaries of cortical areas (Chou et al. 2013; Pouchelon et al. 2014) . For early and late pre-patterning of the cortex, the precise spatiotemporal expression of cortical TFs is crucial.

21.2.1 Transcription Factors

TFs are proteins that recognize specific DNA regulatory sequences near target genes. Upon binding to their specific DNA targets, TFs act to regulate transcription of their target genes either directly by recruiting transcriptional machinery or indirectly by recruiting protein mediators that can modify the chromatin structure. TF expression levels are tightly regulated to generate spatial gradients and/or discontinuities. TF activity is regulated by controlling their distribution within cell compartments, by post-translational modifications, and by cell-signaling/activity.

TFs are classified into families of related genes that share common structural characteristics particularly their region that binds specific DNA sequences (motifs). TF families include the following: basic protein-leucine zipper, helix-loop-helix, homeodomain, and zinc fingers. For instance, the homeodomain region spans a ~ 60 amino acids helix-loop-helix-turn-helix structure (Holland et al. 2007; Leung et al. 2022). This DNA binding domain has two α-helices that recognize consensus sites in the chromatin and bind directly to the DNA: the first helix stabilizes the structure, and the second helix binds to the major groove of the DNA. Within the larger homeodomain genes, specific subfamilies can be distinguished based on molecular phylogenetic analyses of homeodomain sequences as well as by the presence of additional protein domains. For instance, many homeodomain proteins also include a POU, LIM, or zinc finger domain.

Upon binding their DNA motif, TFs recruit other TFs or mediator proteins to carry out processes such as transcription initiation or epigenetic modifications of the chromatin.

21.2.2 Patterning of the Developing Cortex by TFs

A general feature of TFs that control CNS pattering is their graded and/or sharp boundaries of expression. In the spinal cord and subpallium, TFs are expressed in clearly defined and/or overlapping regional domains. In the spinal cord, early opposing morphogen gradients set up clearly delimited regions of TF expression in neural progenitors along the dorso-ventral axis (Catela 2020). As development progresses, each progenitor domain generates distinct neuronal subtypes, which are in turn characterized by specific TF markers. In the developing pallium, by and large, only the MP has sharp TF expression boundaries (Ypsilanti et al. 2021).

21.2.2.1 A Screen to Discover New Patterning TFs

To date, several TFs have been shown to play a crucial role in patterning the developing cortex. We will discuss these known patterning TFs in more depth in the Section 21.2.2.2. Of relevance here is that a common feature of these TFs is their graded expression in the ventricular zone of the pallium along the rostro-caudal, the dorso-ventral axes (see Figure 21.2B).

To uncover new TFs with potential roles in patterning, we examined the RNA expression pattern of 700 TFs at E11.5 in the mouse developing pallium using a publicly available resource from the Allen Brain Institute (see: http://developingmouse.brain-map.org) (Ypsilanti et al. 2021). This screen identified 270 TFs that were expressed in the E11.5 pallium and 218 TFs that had expression in progenitor cells. Within this subgroup, more than half of the TFs showed ubiquitous expression (i.e., lacked a detectable regional or graded pattern). In fact, very few TFs (less than 8%) were restricted to subregions of the developing pallium (ten TFs restricted to the DP, six to the MP, and one to the LVP) and thus very few had sharp TF expression boundaries (Ypsilanti et al. 2021). Of the TFs 61 had graded expression along the rostro-caudal (n = 30) or caudo-rostral (n = 31) axes.

This systematic screen points out that adult regions of the cortex are not likely to be encoded in development by regions of TFs with sharp boundaries that specify distinct mature regions/areas.

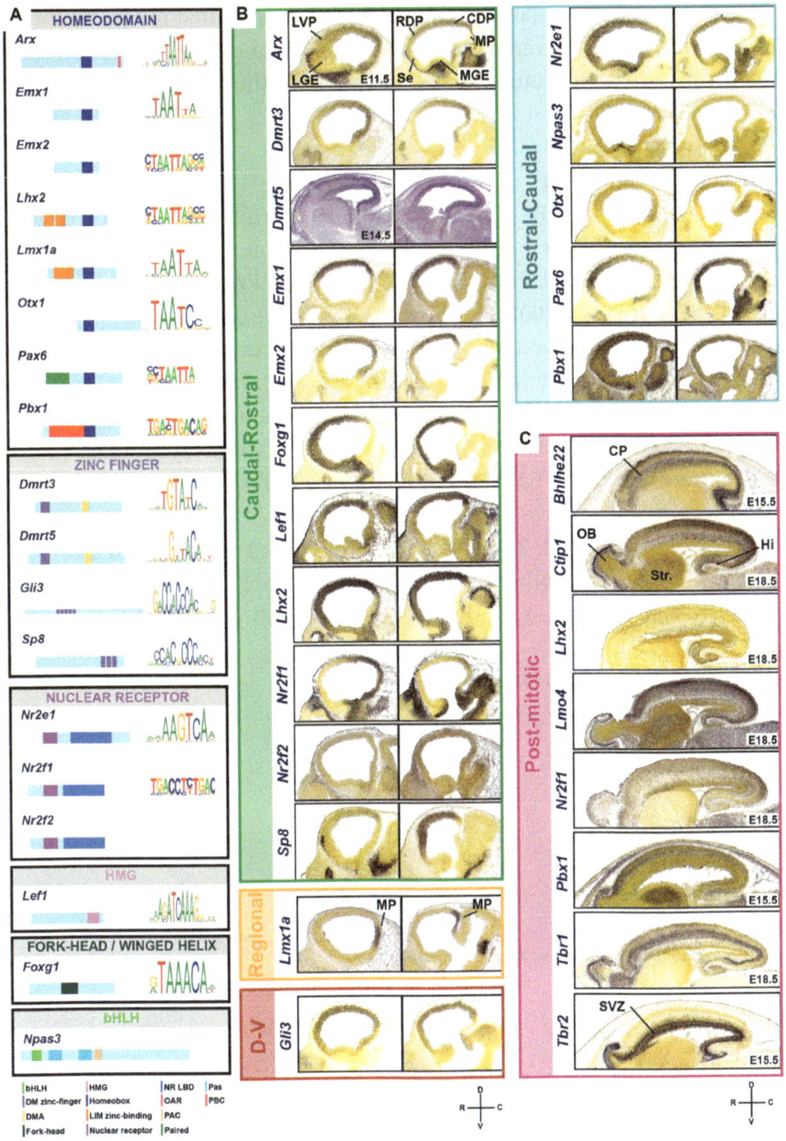

Figure 21.2 (A) Representation of the protein domains of TFs that regulate cortical patterning from the major TF families (homeodomain, zinc finger, nuclear receptor, HMG, fork head, bHLH). Color schema definition for each protein domain is indicated at the bottom. Primary DNA binding motifs were retrieved from the Jaspar database (https://jaspar.genereg.net/) or from Ypsilanti et al. (2021), when available. (B) Sagittal sections (one lateral and one medial section) at E11.5 of in situ hybridizations showing the expression of TFs that regulate regional and areal pattering in the cortical VZ (note: *Dmrt5* is at E14.5). The TFs are organized alphabetically within groups that that correspond to their VZ gradient of expression (caudo-rostral; regional [medial pallium]; dorso-ventral DV, rostro-caudal). In situ hybridizations were obtained from the Allen Developing Mouse Brain Atlas (https://developingmouse.brain-map.org/) except for *Dmrt5*, which was obtained from EurExpress (retrieved from: http://www.informatics.jax.org/). MP: medium pallium, CDP: caudal–dorsal pallium, RDP: rostral–dorsal pallium, LVP: lateral–ventral pallium; and basal ganglia: LGE: lateral ganglionic eminence, MGE: medial ganglionic eminence, Se: septum. (C) Sagittal sections (one mid-sagittal view) at either E15.5 or E18.5 of in situ hybridizations showing the expression of TFs that regulate cortical areal patterning in cortical plate postmitotic neurons, or in the SVZ (*Tbr2*). In situ hybridizations were obtained from the Allen Developing Mouse Brain Atlas (https://developingmouse.brain-map.org/). See Table 22.1 for more information about the TFs, including to which DNA binding motif family they belong. CP: cortical plate, OB: olfactory bulb; Str: striatum; SVZ; subventricular zone.

Rather, adult cortical regions/areas are more likely to emerge from a process that integrates information from the TF VZ gradients along the rostral, caudal, ventral, and dorsal axes. Therefore, graded combinatorial TFs expression appears to be a key early step in the generation of cortical regions/areas (Ypsilanti et al. 2021).

21.2.2.2 TFs that Regulate Cortical Patterning

COUPTF1, EMX2, LHX2, PAX6, PBX1, and SP8 all regulate pallial patterning. Most are expressed in graded patterns along the rostro-caudal or ventro-dorsal axes (Armentano et al. 2007; Bishop et al. 2000; Borello et al. 2014; Chou et al. 2009; Faedo et al. 2008; Golonzhka et al. 2015; Mallamaci et al. 2000; Mangale et al. 2008; Sahara et al. 2007; Yun et al. 2001) (Figure 21.2B).

Loss of *CoupTf1* or *Emx2* during embryogenesis leads to expansion of rostral regions at the expense of caudal regions (Figure 21.3B) (Armentano et al. 2007; Bishop et al. 2003, 2000; Mallamaci et al. 2000). Conversely, loss of *Pax6*, *Pbx1*, and *Sp8* leads to the expansion of caudal regions and the reduction of rostral regions (Bishop et al. 2000; O'Leary et al. 2007; Zembrzycki et al. 2007). These TFs also regulate DV patterning; loss of EMX2 leads to loss of dorsal structures, loss of PBX1 leads to expansion of dorsal structures, and loss of PAX6 and COUPTF1/2 leads to loss of ventral structures (Bishop et al. 2000; Golonzhka et al. 2015; Ypsilanti et al. 2021; Yun et al. 2001).

Besides these key patterning TFs, a host of other TFs also control pallial patterning, particularly the MP (hippocampus): ARX (Kitamura et al. 2002), DMRT3 (Saulnier et al. 2013), DMRT5 (Konno

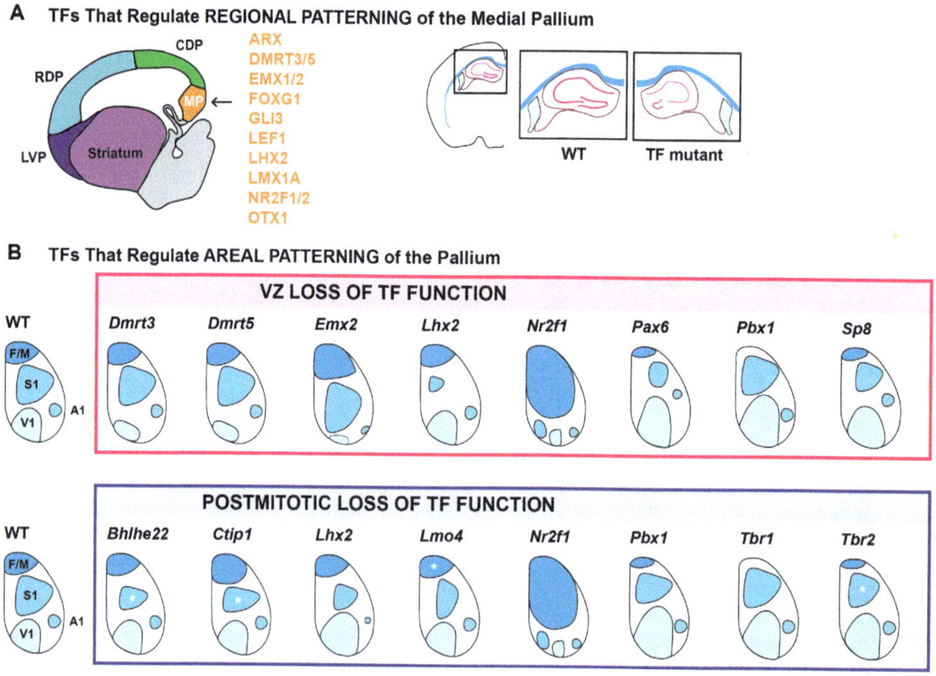

Figure 21.3 (A) Schematic indicating TFs that control regional patterning of the medial pallium (MP). In the absence of these TFs in the VZ, the size and morphology of developing hippocampus is abnormal.
(B) Schematic of a top-down view of postnatal cortex showing changes in the relative sizes and positions of cortical areas in the absence of TF mutants from the cortical plate or SVZ. The asterisk denotes that the TF loss of function mutant has histological disorganization of that particular area. The *Tbr2* loss of function has complex phenotypes with different markers of the same cortical area showing both increases and decreases; this schematic depicts our best guess of the strongest and/or most consistent phenotypes across the assayed markers.

et al. 2019), LEF1 (Galceran et al. 2000), LMX1A (Millonig et al. 2000). The pallial expression of each of these TFs is summarized in Table 22.1; their expression patterns in the E11.5 embryonic cortex can be seen in Figure 21.2B. Of note, most patterning TFs also regulate other processes, including cell proliferation, neurogenesis, neuronal migration and specification.

- ***Arx***: This homeodomain TF is expressed in a pallial CR and DV gradient where it is essential for promoting caudal/dorsal fates (Figures 21.2A/21.2B and 21.3A; Kitamura et al. 2002; Simonet et al. 2015). Inactivation of *Arx* leads to dysgenesis of the mouse hippocampus, in particular the dentate gyrus and CA3 (Kitamura et al. 2002; Lim et al. 2019). Loss of *Arx* from the embryonic mouse cortex leads to the upregulation of subpallial TFs including *Olig2* and *Gli1* and the downregulation of *Pax6* and *Tbr2* (Lim et al. 2019). Notably, in humans, mutations in *Arx* cause X-linked lissencephaly with Absent Corpus Callosum and Ambiguous Genitalia (XLAG), a severe disorder that is in part characterized by a loss of cortical gyrification, particularly in the caudal cortex (Bonneau et al. 2002; Kitamura et al. 2002).
- ***Dmrt3/Dmrt5 (Dmrta3/2):*** This pair of TFs (DM zinc finger family) are expressed in pallial CR and DV gradients (Figures 21.2A/21.2B and 21.3A). They can heterodimerize and bind similar DNA sequences (Murphy et al. 2007). Mutations in *Dmrt5* are associated with human microcephaly (Urquhart et al. 2016). *Dmrt5* deletion leads to the loss of the mouse hippocampus and a severe reduction in caudo-medial neocortical areas and in particular the V1 area (Konno et al. 2019; Saulnier et al. 2013). The absence of *Dmrt5* alters the expression of *Pax6, Emx2*, and *Lhx2* (Clercq et al. 2016). Although, *Dmrt3* has a stronger expression gradient than *Dmrt5*, its deletion leads to a milder reduction in hippocampal and caudal cortical area size (Clercq et al. 2016), suggesting compensation by *Dmrt5*.
- ***Emx1/Emx2***: These related homeodomain proteins are expressed in pallial CR and DV gradients (Figures 21.2A/21.2B and 21.3A/21.3B). Regional expression of *Emx2* is slightly more restricted than *Emx1* (except a small region in the dorsal-most MP); furthermore, its expression is largely confined to VZ progenitors, whereas *Emx1* is also expressed in the SVZ and neurons (Gulisano et al. 1996; Tole et al. 2000). *Emx2* mutants have reduced caudal and dorso-medial cortical regions (Bishop et al. 2000; Mallamaci et al. 2000). Conversely, *Emx2* over-expression in the VZ, increases caudal areas and reduces rostral areas (Hamasaki et al. 2004). In contrast, *Emx1* mutants have a subtle expansion of rostral regions and a reduction of caudal areas (Bishop et al. 2003; Stocker and O'Leary 2016; Yoshida et al. 1997). As expected *Emx1/Emx2* double mutants have more severe cortical patterning defects; both TFs act to specify caudo-dorsal patterning (Bishop et al. 2003).
- ***Foxg1 (BF1)***: *Foxg1* (winged-helix family) is expressed in the entire pallium except its dorsal-caudal midline, which has the highest expression of BMPs and WNTs (Figures 21.2A/21.2B, and 21.3A; Shimamura and Rubenstein 1997). FOXG1 represses the expression of these morphogens; in *Foxg1* mutants their expression expands more broadly into the pallium. In addition, *Foxg1*$^{-/-}$ display a loss of subpallial cell fates and an expansion of the dorsal telencephalon (Danesin et al. 2009; Dou et al. 1999; Hanashima et al. 2004). Within the pallium, loss of *Foxg1* contributes to the expansion of caudal and ventral regions at the expense of dorsal and rostral pallial regions (Hanashima et al. 2004). In humans, loss of one copy of FOXG1 is sufficient to cause a severe neurodevelopmental disorder consisting of microcephaly, developmental delay, and several structural brain abnormalities (Florian et al. 2012). Conversely, in humans, duplication of *Foxg1* has been linked to other neurodevelopmental abnormalities including developmental delay and epilepsy (but no macrocephaly) (Pontrelli et al. 2014). These syndromes illustrate the fundamental importance of tightly regulating TF dosage during pallial development.

Table 22.1 The TF that regulate pattering in the VZ and in postmitotic immature neurons, including: TF name; TF class, and TF subfamily; embryonic pallial expression pattern; VZ expression gradient; and notes about neuronal expression pattern.

TF gene name	Full name	TF class (family)	TF subfamily	Embryonic pallial expression pattern					VZ expression gradient	Neuronal expression
				VZ				Neurons		
				LVP	RDP	CDP	MP	Cx		
Arx	Aristaless related homeobox	HD	Paired Box	x	x	x	x		C-R	
Bhlhe22	Basic helix-loop-helix family member E22	Basic helix-loop-helix	Tal-related					x		Embryonically high C-R in CP. Postnatally, the expression refined to S1, V1 and A1 (Layer 2–5 neurons)
Ctip1/ Bcl11a	B-cell lymphoma/ leukemia 11A	Zinc finger	C2H2					x		Embryonically high C-R in CP. Postnatally, the expression refined to S1, V1, and A1.
Dmrt3/ Dmrta3	Doublesex and Mab-3 related TF3	Zinc finger	Dmrta	x	x	x	x		CR	
Dmrt5/ Dmrta2	Doublesex and Mab-3 related TF5	Zinc finger	Dmrta	x	x	x	x		CR	
Emx1	Empty spiracles homeobox1	HD	NK-like	x	x	x	x	x	CR	
Emx2	Empty spiracles homeobox2	HD	NK-like	x	x	x	x		CR	
Foxg1/ BF1	Forkhead box protein G1	Fork head/ winged helix factors	FOX	x	x	x	x	x	CR	

Gli3	Glioma-Associated Oncogene family zinc finger 3	Zinc Finger	C2H2	x	x	x	x		DV	
Lef1	Lymphoid enhancer binding factor 1	HMG	TCF-7 related	x	x	x	x		CR	
Lhx2	LIM homeobox 2	HD	LIM	x	x	x	x	x	CR	
Lmo4	LIM Domain Only 4		LIM					x		Its expression progressively gets restricted to rostral M1.
Lmx1a	LIM homeobox TF1 alpha	HD	LIM				x		MP	
Npas3	Neuronal Per-Arnt-Sim 3	bHLH	PAS	x	x	x	x	x	RC	
Nr2e1/ Tlx	Nuclear receptor subfamily 2 group E member 1	Nuclear receptor with C4 zinc finger	RXR-related receptors	x	x	x	x		RC	
Nr2f1/ CoupTF1	Nuclear receptor subfamily 2 group F member 1	Nuclear receptor with C4 zinc finger	RXR-related receptors		x	x	x	x	CR + LM	

(Continued)

Table 22.1 (Continued)

TF gene name	Full name	TF class (family)	TF subfamily	Embryonic pallial expression pattern					VZ expression gradient	Neuronal expression
				VZ				Neurons		
				LVP	RDP	CDP	MP	Cx		
Nr2f2/ CoupfTF2	Nuclear receptor subfamily 2 group F member 2	Nuclear receptor with C4 zinc finger	RXR-related receptors	x	x	x	x	x	CR	
Otx1	Orthodenticle homeobox 1	HD	Paired box	x	x	x	x		RC	
Pax6	Paired box 6	HD	Paired box	x	x	x	x		RC	
Pbx1	Pre-B-cell leukemia homeobox 1	HD	TALE-type	x	x	x	x	x	RC	
Sp8	Specificity Protein 8	Zinc finger	Kruppel-related	x	x	x			CR	
Tbr1	T-box brain TF1	T-box factor	Tbrain-related factors					x		Rostral = L1-6 Caudal = L6, SP, C-R
Tbr2/ Eomes	T-box brain TF2	T-Box factor	Tbrain-related factors					**SVZ**		In intermediate progenitors

Abbreviations: LVP: lateral-ventral pallium; RDP: rostral-dorsal pallium; CDP: caudal-dorsal pallium; MP: medium pallium; CR: caudo-rostral; RC: rostro-caudal; DV: dorso-ventral; S1: somatosensory area; A1: auditory area; V1: visual area; M1: motor cortex.

- ***Gli3***: This zinc finger TF has been implicated in numerous skeletal and craniofacial developmental disorders (Figures 21.2A/21.2B and 21.3A; Villavicencio et al. 2000). *Gli3*'s full-length form is as a transcriptional activator (GLI3A), whereas its truncated form functions as a repressor (GLI3R). In the developing pallium, the *Gli3* repressor is the most abundant form, and it acts as an important regulator of SHH, WNT, and FGF signaling (Grove et al. 1998; Kuschel et al. 2003; Rash and Grove 2007; Theil et al. 1999). Importantly, *Gli3* regulates the expression of other TFs that are important in pallium specification, including *Emx1* and *Emx2* (Fotaki et al. 2006; Theil et al. 1999). In the *Gli3* mutant, specification of the pallium is perturbed leading to an absence of the cortex and hippocampus. In this knockout mouse, basal ganglia and diencephalic markers are ectopically expressed by the dorsal telencephalic (Fotaki et al. 2006; Kuschel et al. 2003; Theil et al. 1999). Conditional removal of *Gli3* specifically from the developing pallium around E10.5, using *Emx1-Cre*, leads to a milder phenotype, with predominantly midline defects (Amaniti et al. 2013).
- ***Lef1***: This HMG TF is a member of the LEF1/TCF family; it is activated upon association with β-catenin, a downstream effector of *Wnt* signaling (Figures 21.2A/21.2B and 22.3A). *Lef1* is expressed in progenitors of the medial pallium and has a caudo-rostral gradient in the dorsal pallium. Mutating the *Lef1* DNA-binding domain perturbs pallial development leading to the absence of the hippocampal formation (Galceran et al. 2000). Interestingly, this *Lef1* mutant has a stronger patterning defect than the *Lef1* null, suggesting that the DNA-binding domain mutation, in which LEF1 protein is stuck in the cytoplasm, is perhaps a dominant negative repressor of WNT signaling. In fact, in this *Lef1* mutant, the expression of several other key TFs, including members of the TCF family and *Prox1* are altered, and there is loss of the *Foxg1* gradient in the MP (Galceran et al. 2000). Together, this implicated *Lef1 and* WNT-signaling, as crucial regulators of hippocampal patterning.
- ***Lhx2***: This LIM homeodomain TF is expressed in the developing pallium in a CR and DV gradient (Figures 21.2A/21.2B and 21.3A/21.3B; Mangale et al. 2008). Loss of *Lhx2* leads to suppression of cortical fate due to ventral expansion of the dorsal patterning center (cortical hem; e.g., *Wnt2b*), and dorsal expansion of properties of the pallial-subpallial boundary (antihem; e.g. *Dbx1*) (Mangale et al. 2008). Conditional deletion of *Lhx2*, using *Emx1-Cre*, removed the *Lhx2* from cortical progenitors starting at E10.5 (Chou et al. 2009). These *Lhx2* cKO (*Emx1Cre;Lhx2*$^{-/-}$) have defects in regional patterning of the ventro-lateral regions of the neocortex; this region transforming into the paleocortex (3-layer) cortex (ventro-lateral pallium). Deletion of *Lhx2* in the developing cortex beginning at ~ E11.5, showed that *Lhx2* is also essential in patterning the somatosensory cortex (Shetty et al. 2013).
- ***Lmx1a***: This LIM homeobox TF is expressed in progenitor cells of the developing medial pallium (Figures 21.2A/21.2B and 21.3A). *Lmx1a* is mutated in a spontaneous mouse missense mutant (*Dreher*), which exhibits cerebellar hypoplasia as well as cytoarchitectonic neocortical and hippocampal defects (Kuwamura et al. 2005; Millonig et al. 2000), including its invasion by choroid plexus progenitor cells (Chizhikov et al. 2010). This change in medial pallial patterning is accompanied by an increase in *Lhx2* expression in the choroid plexus indicating the *Lmx1a* might function by repressing *Lhx2*.
- ***Npas3***: Disruptions in this basic-helix-loop-helix-PAS TF are implicated in intellectual disability and schizophrenia (Figures 21.2A/21.2B; Kamnasaran et al. 2003; Rossi et al. 2021). There is evidence that *Npas3* null mice have defects in LVP development leading to piriform cortex dysmorphology (Ypsilanti et al. 2021).
- ***Nr2e1***: This orphan nuclear receptor, also known as TLX or tailless, is evolutionarily conserved in *Drosophila*, mice, and humans where it plays roles in brain and retinal development (Figures 21.2A/21.2B; Wang and Xiong 2016). Mutations in this *Nr2e1* have been implicated in several neurodevelopmental disorders including schizophrenia (Kumar et al. 2008). In the developing

cortex, it is expressed in a DV gradient (Stenman et al. 2003a, 2003b). It plays a role in patterning the pallial side of the pallial–subpallial boundary, as discussed in Section 21.2.2.4 (Stenman et al. 2003b, 2003a). Later pallial functions of *Nr2e1* include neurogenesis and laminar specification (Wang and Xiong 2016).

- ***Nr2f1/Nr2f2*:** These homologous TFs are orphan nuclear receptors (originally known as *Couptf1 & 2*), that are expressed in caudo-rostral and ventro-dorsal gradients, and play major roles in pallial patterning (Figures 21.2A/21.2B and 21.3A/21.2B; Zhou et al. 2001; Armentano et al. 2007; Faedo et al. 2008). In *Nr2f1* mutants there is a drastic loss of caudal areas (somatosensory, auditory, and visual), while rostral areas (frontal/motor) expand caudally (Armentano et al. 2007; Zhou et al. 2001). In fact, the frontal/motor cortex takes over such a large proportion of the cortex that the other sensory areas (visual, somatosensory, and auditory) are compressed into the caudal pole. Upon conditional removal of *Nr2f1* in the cortex, the mutant somatosensory area becomes "motorized" in the sense that it generates neurons with molecular and cell density more typical of motor areas in wild-type mice (Armentano et al. 2007). *Nr2f1* function in the caudal cortex includes specification of the medial entorhinal cortex and creation of boundaries via cell adhesion perhaps through *protocadherin19* (Feng et al. 2021).

  Nr2f1 also promotes cell cycle exit and neural differentiation; this regulates the balance of early- and late-born neurons and controls balanced production of different types of layer V cortical projection neurons (Faedo et al. 2008). The dosage of *Nr2f1* is implicated in a region-dependent regulation of neurogenesis (Bertacchi et al. 2020), and thus could regulate the number and type of neurons that can be produced in specific cortical locations (Borello et al. 2014; Tocco et al. 2022). Dosage of *Nr2f1* is also critically important for regulating the expression its target genes such as *Sp8*. When *Nr2f1* is constitutively over-expressed *Sp8* is repressed (Borello et al. 2014).

  Nr2f2 can compensate for loss of *Nr2f1*; *Nr2f2* expression increases in *Nr2f1* mutants (Hu et al. 2017; Tang et al. 2015, 2010). *Nr2f1/Nr2f2* and *Pax6* share ventro-dorsal expression gradients; loss of *Pax6* reduces *Nr2f1/Nr2f2* LVP expression (Ypsilanti et al. 2021). *Nr2f1* loss and gain of function mutants provide evidence that it promotes specification of LVP identity (Faedo et al. 2008). This hypothesis is strengthened by the much more severe LVP patterning defects in *Nr2f1;Nr2f2* double mutants (Ypsilanti et al. 2021). At later stages *Nr2f2* works with *Nr2f1* to regulate the switch from neurogenesis to gliogenesis (Naka et al. 2008).

  There is evidence that *Nr2f1* controls cortical development by repressing FGF/MAPK/ERK, AKT, and β-Catenin signaling (Faedo et al. 2010, 2008), and by controlling the expression of key TFs, including *Sp8* (Borello et al. 2014; Ypsilanti et al. 2021). FGF signaling, represses *Nr2f1* expression (Faedo et al. 2010; Garel et al. 2003), and conversely loss of FGF-mediated *Nr2f1* repression, in *Sprouty1/2* mutants, reduces *Nr2f1* expression. As part of this regulatory loop, *Nr2f1* promotes *Sprouty* expression (Faedo et al. 2010).

- ***Otx1*:** This paired homeobox TF is expressed in a rostro-caudal pattern that extends to the medial pallium (Figures 21.2A/21.2B and 21.3A; Frantz et al. 1994). *Otx1* null mice exhibit mispatterning of caudal domains of the pallium (Acampora et al. 1996). In $Otx1^{-/-}$; $Otx2^{+/-}$, and $Otx2^{-/-}$ mice, there is ectopic expression of mesencephalic molecular markers in the cortex (*Wnt-1* and *En2*) and septum (*En2* and *Pax3*), respectively highlighting the early functions that the *Otx* TFs have in telencephalic patterning (Acampora et al. 1999; Hoch et al. 2015b). Interestingly, when one or two alleles of *Otx1* were replaced with the *Drosophila* homolog of the TF, *Otd*, cortical defects were rescued (Acampora et al. 1999). The specification of caudal regions of the forebrain by *Otx1* happens in cooperation with *Emx2;* the *Otx1;Emx2* double mutant develops a much smaller hippocampal field and a smaller telencephalon (Kimura et al. 2005). Interestingly, in the *Emx2* mutant, there are clear epigenetic changes to the *Otx1* gene locus suggesting that *Otx1* and *Emx2* are genetically associated (Figure 21.4B).

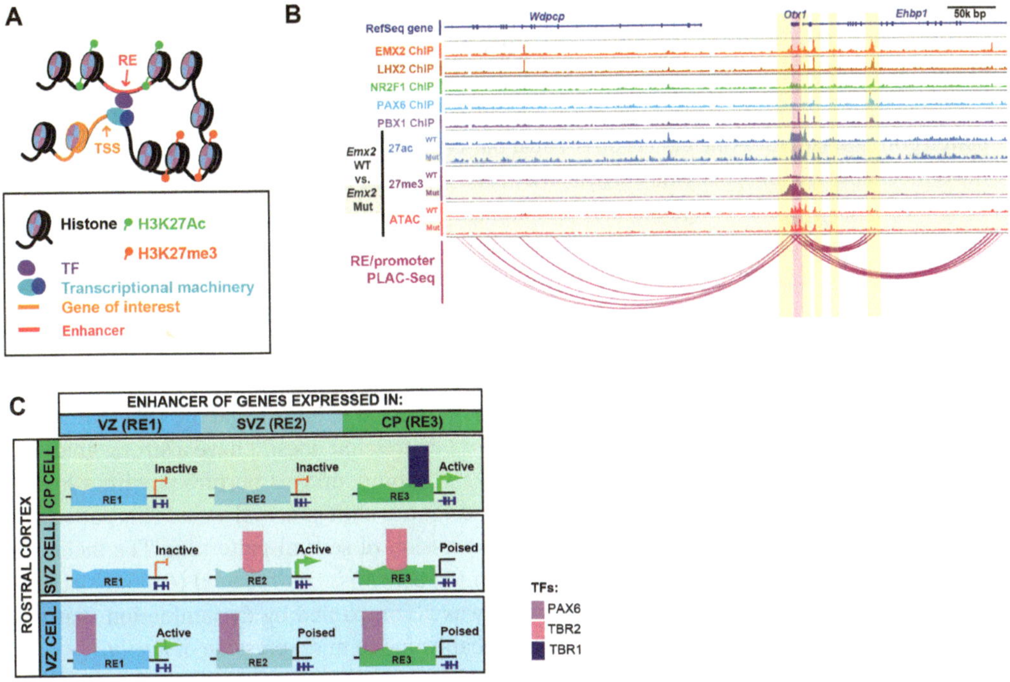

Figure 21.4 (A) Schematic of a small stretch of a chromosome that includes a region of open chromatin where an enhancer (regulatory element: RE; pink) is accessible for binding by a TF (purple). This accessible area is surrounded by histone marks with an acetylation modification on lysine 27 of histone 3 (H3K27Ac; green), which indicates an active enhancer. Other areas of the chromatin show marks of being repressed as indicated by a methylation modification on lysine 27 of histone 3 (H3K27me3; red). The transcription start site (TSS, orange) of a gene (orange) is bound by transcriptional machinery (light blue and blue) that is in contact with the enhancer; together they regulate transcription of the gene. (B) Region of the mouse genome that includes the *Otx1* locus (a small gene in the center; dark blue with pink shading). The y-axis lists TFs for which Chip-Seq was performed (EMX2, LHX2, NR2F1, PAX6, PBX1). Below the TF data are VZ epigenomic histone marks performed in wild type (WT) and *Emx2*$^{-/-}$ mutants [active: H3K27ac (27ac); repressive: H3K27me3 (27Me3); accessibility: ATAC-Seq (ATAC)] at the *Otx1* locus at E12.5. WT tracks and *Emx2*$^{-/-}$ tracks are shown. At the bottom, areas of enhancer-promoter interactions are depicted by purples arcs that are derived from PLAC-seq. Yellow vertical bars highlight regions where there are differential epigenomic marks in the *Emx2*$^{-/-}$ mutant; a pink bar highlights the *Otx1* gene body. Data from Ypsilanti et al. (2021). (C) Model postulating the activation state of three regulatory elements (REs: RE1, RE2, RE3) in the VZ, SVZ, and CP of the developing rostral cortex (modified from Ypsilanti and Rubenstein 2016). The model shows activator functions for the TFs (the repressor function is not shown). We postulate that poised epigenetic states in the VZ are transferred sequentially to the SVZ and CP (where they become active), and conversely earlier active states become repressed as differentiation proceeds.

- ***Pax6*:** This TF has a paired domain and a homeodomain; both bind DNA at different motifs (Figures 21.2A/21.2B and 21.3B; Ton et al. 1991; Yun et al. 2001). *Pax6* is expressed in a rostro-caudal and ventro-dorsal gradients (Bishop et al. 2000; Yun et al. 2001). *Pax6* has been extensively studied for its role in cortical regionalization amongst other functions in cortical development (Stoykova et al. 1996; Toresson et al. 2000; Ypsilanti and Rubenstein 2016; Yun et al. 2001).

  Pax6 confers rostral-ventral identity to the pallial VZ; in the *Pax6* mutant there is a reduction of rostral and ventral cortical regions (Bishop et al. 2000; Muzio et al. 2002; Pinon et al. 2008; Ypsilanti et al. 2021; Zembrzycki et al. 2013). Areal patterning defects can be rescued by reestablishing proper PAX6 dosage (Zembrzycki et al. 2013).

Surprisingly, over-expressing PAX6 protein does not promote rostral identity; this mutant shows a small size reduction in the somatosensory cortical area, despite having more drastic phenotypes in neurogenesis and laminar specification (Manuel et al. 2006; Sansom et al. 2009; Georgala et al. 2011). Moreover, deletion of the *Pax6* homeodomain, while maintaining the paired domain, had minimal effects on cortical patterning thus implicating the paired domain as the critical domain for specifying cortical arealization (Carbe et al. 2013).

Pax6 and *Nr2f1* are key regulators of the balance between self-renewal of cortical stem cells and neurogenesis (Sansom et al.). Early on during corticogenesis (at E13.5), loss of *Pax6* resulted in changes in cell cycling that were more pronounced in the rostral pallium indicating that proliferation was specifically affected in that region of the cortex partly through regulation of *Cdk6* (Mi et al. 2013, 2018).

- ***Pbx1***: This homeodomain is a member of the TALE family that includes the *Pbx, Meis*, and *Prep/Pknox* TFs (Figures 21.2A/21.2B and 21.3B). *Pbx1* is expressed in the VZ and the CP of the developing cortex (Golonzhka et al. 2015). Although *Pbx1* expression doesn't have a strong gradient, arealization of *Pbx1* mutants (worsened in *Pbx1/Pbx2* compound) is perturbed with a loss of rostral areas, an anterior shift of caudal regions, and ventral shift of dorsal areas. This patterning phenotype is also accompanied by changes in expression of several patterning TFs including *Emx2* and *Lhx2, a*nd over-expression of its family members *Meis2 and Pknox1* (Golonzhka et al. 2015). Interestingly, the arealization phenotype was accompanied by dyslamination that was restricted to the rostral cortex; this defect was probably due to misexpression of *Reelin.*
- ***Sp8***: This zinc-finger TF is expressed in RC and DV gradients (Figures 21.2A/21.2B and 21.3B). *Sp8* and *FGF8* induce one another in a reciprocal manner; the induction of *Fgf8* by *Sp8* is repressed by *Emx2* (Sahara et al. 2007). Expressing a *Sp8* dominant-negative reduced motor areas and had a rostral shift of somatosensory areas (Sahara et al. 2007). This caudalization of the cortex was also found in *Sp8* null mice, in part through a genetic interaction with *Emx2* (Zembrzycki et al. 2007). *Sp8* over-expression beginning at E9.5 mispatterned the ventro-lateral pallium and was associated with misexpression of *Nr2f1*, *Lhx2*, *Pax6*, and *Emx2* (Borello et al. 2014). When over-expression of *Sp8* occurs at a later stage of cortical development (at E14.5), none of these phenotypes were observed. Likewise, removal of *Sp8* early in pallial development at E9.5 using *Foxg1Cre* resulted in a rostral and dorsal expansion of *Nr2f1* expression; this did not occur when removing *Sp8* just a day later (using *Emx1Cre*) (Borello et al. 2014).

21.2.2.3 General Precepts of TF Regulation of Cortical Patterning

In summary, specific TFs each play a specific role in patterning the cortex. Together these results suggest some general principles. First, dosage of TF expression is critical (based on loss and gain of function studies, as well as studies of ectopic expression). Tight regulation of expression levels and regional expression domains are crucial in setting up a cascade of downstream molecular pathways that are essential for driving the regionalization programs. Second, TFs exert their effects by forming protein complexes that can modify the chromatin state and can interact with transcriptional machinery that either activates or represses downstream targets (D'Souza et al. 2021; Elsen et al. 2018; Muralidharan et al. 2017a; Ninkovic et al. 2013; Tuoc et al. 2013).Third, many TFs are regulators of one another's expression, as already noted *Pax6, Nr2f1*, and *Nr2f2*. In addition, the expression of *Emx2* is directly promoted by *Dmrt5* and repressed by *Emx2os*, which is the antisense transcript of *Emx2* (Saulnier et al. 2013; Spigoni et al. 2010). Fourth, beyond the crucial regulation of spatial expression, the timing of expression of these TFs is also essential. For instance, deleting *Lhx2* before cortical specification results in the absence of a neocortex whereas deleting *Lhx2* from the cortex after a certain critical period (E11.5) results in an abnormally small cortex without gross patterning defects.

Many patterning TFs play a multitude of roles during cortical development thus making their role in area specification somewhat complex to parse out. Their role in other brain regions (such as the thalamus or the subpallium) further complicates analysis of observed cortical malformations. It can sometimes be difficult to evaluate whether a cortical regional defect is due to a failure of thalamic afferents to reach their destination or whether is it due to a mispatterning of the cortical progenitors (Borello et al. 2018; Dehay et al. 1996; Monko et al. 2022; Polleux et al. 2001). To learn more about the role of thalamic afferents in the refinement of cortical area patterning, please see Chapter 22.

The histology of cortical areas differs based on their constituent neuronal subtypes (Polleux et al. 2001; Skoglund et al. 1996). Moreover, the birth date and birth rate of cortical neuronal subtypes varies between cortical areas; this has led to the idea that cell cycle parameters of progenitor proto-areas impact the generation of areal-specific features (Dehay and Kennedy 2007; Polleux et al. 2001, 1997). Several of the patterning TFs discussed earlier are also key regulators of cell cycle properties including stem-cell renewal/proliferation as well as the rate of neurogenesis. In particular, *Nr2f1* and *Pax6* regulate the cell cycle in a region-specific manner (Bertacchi et al. 2020; Mi et al. 2013). Thus, region-specific differences in cortical neuron generation are likely to create region-specific differences in the number and fate of neurons produced in cortical subregions. For instance, in the absence of *Nr2f1*, there is a region-specific deficit in the production of corticospinal motor neurons in the somatosensory area (Tomassy et al. 2010b).

21.2.2.4 Maintaining the Pallial–subpallial Boundary: An Important Role for Cortical Patterning TFs

At regional boundaries, the interplay between patterning TFs is crucial to establish and maintain the regional specification. At the pallial–subpallial boundary (PSB), *Pax6* and *Emx2* expression by cortical progenitors, and *Gsx2* and *Dlx1/2* expression by subpallial progenitors, are critical in positioning the PSB (Carney et al. 2009; Kroll and O'Leary 2005; Stoykova et al. 2000; Wang et al. 2013; Yun et al. 2001). When *Pax6* is deleted, several subpallial TF markers including *Ascl1*, *Dlx1/2*, and *Gsx2* are ectopically expressed in the pallium leading to ventralization of the dorsal telencephalon (Kroll and O'Leary 2005; Stoykova et al. 2000; Toresson et al. 2000; Yun et al. 2001). This dorsal shift of the PSB seems to be in part due to cross-repression of *Pax6* and *Gsx2* (Toresson et al. 2000; Yun et al. 2001). Interestingly, *Lhx2* deletion has no effect on the PSB (Mangale et al. 2008). However, when *Lhx2* and *Pax6* are both deleted, the PSB defect observed in *Pax6* null embryos is restored (Godbole et al. 2017). Moreover, *Emx2* also cooperates with *Pax6*, despite their opposing effects on rostral and caudal regionalization of the cortex, to prevent the ventralization of the dorsal telencephalon. Their mutual deletion leads to the suppression of pallial programs in favor of the dorsal expansion of the subpallium (Muzio et al. 2002). Additional pallial TFs that regulate the PSB include *Arx* (Lim et al. 2019), *Dmrt5;Dmrt3* (Desmaris et al. 2018; Konno et al. 2019) and *Nr2e1* (Stenman et al. 2003a). This critical role of cortical patterning TFs in controlling the integrity of the PSB, and its flanking regions, is further supported by observations that there are many enhancers that are active across the PSB and are dually regulated by pallial and subpallial TFs (Visel et al. 2013; Pattabiraman et al. 2014; Ypsilanti et al. 2021; Ypsilanti and Rubenstein, unpublished).

21.2.2.5 Uncovering Roles for Other TFs with Gradients of Expression in the VZ – Cortical Regionalization TF Network

By analyzing TF expression at E11.5 using the Allen Brain Atlas, we identified 31 TFs that are candidates for pallial patterning based on their graded VZ expression (Ypsilanti et al. 2021). We then tested their expression in *Emx2*$^{-/-}$, *Nr2f1*$^{-/-}$, and *Pax6*$^{-/-}$ mutants. Generally, caudo-rostral TFs showed decreased expression in *Emx2*$^{-/-}$ *and Nr2f1*$^{-/-}$ whereas rostro-caudal TFs were more likely to have decreased expression in *Nr2f1*$^{-/-}$ and *Pax6*$^{-/-}$. *Emx2* and *Nr2f1* have opposite dorso-ventral gradients whereas *Pax6* and *Nr2f1* have similar ventro-dorsal gradients. The TF expression differences in the mutants suggests that *Emx2 and Nr2f1* might both promote caudal pallial properties whereas *Nr2f1* and *Pax6* might both promote ventral pallial properties. In point of fact, *Pax6* promotes *Nr2f1/2* expression and, together, they co-regulate other downstream TFs that are expressed in the rostro-ventral cortex (piriform cortex and adjacent structures) (Ypsilanti et al. 2021).

21.2.2.6 TFs Involved in the Arealization of the SVZ and CP – How the Pallial Protomap is Propagated into the Maturing Cortex

As described earlier, pallial regional identity is established by TFs acting in the VZ progenitor cells. However, it remains unclear how regional identity is transferred from the VZ to secondary progenitors (SVZ), and then to immature and mature neurons. There is evidence that TF function in postmitotic neurons regulates regional/areal fate (Alfano et al. 2014; Bedogni et al. 2010; Elsen et al. 2013; Golonzhka et al. 2015; Greig et al. 2016; Joshi et al. 2008; Zembrzycki et al. 2015). There is also evidence that thalamic afferents later refine specific areal boundaries as discussed in Chapter 22 (Chou et al. 2013; Pouchelon et al. 2014). Here, we limit our discussion to TFs that have been shown to play a role in regionalization in postmitotic cortical cells.

- ***Bhlhe22:*** This basic helix-loop-helix TF is expressed in the new-born neurons of the cortical plate beginning at E12.5 at highest levels caudo-dorsally (Figures 21.1C and 21.2C and 21.3B; Joshi et al. 2008). It is expressed in a high CR and DV gradient. Postnatally, *Bhlhe22* is primarily expressed in layers 2–5. The progressive change of Bhlhe22's broad expression, to one restricted to S1 and V1, illustrates how a TF's expression can be progressively turned from gradients into sharp areal boundaries in the neonatal cortex (see Figure 21.1C). Bhlhe22 mutants have disorganization of the S1 cytoarchitecture and an alteration of the corticospinal projections (Joshi et al. 2008). The regionalization phenotypes present in the *Bhlhe22* suggest that this TF is important for translating the positional information due to VZ TF gradients into a sharper neuronal specific areal map.
- ***Ctip1 (Bcl11a):*** This zinc finger TF interacts with NR2F1 where it functions at promoters to repress transcription (Figures 21.2C and 21.3B; Avram et al. 2002). CTIP1 interacts with several corepressor complexes including the NuRD repressive chromatin modifying complex (Moody et al. 2018). In the embryonic cortex, *Ctip1* is expressed by postmitotic neurons of the cortical plate and intermediate zone in a high caudo-dorsal and low rostro-ventral gradient (Greig et al. 2016). Its expression is then progressively refined during development and in the postnatal murine cortex, *Ctip1* shows higher levels of expression in the somatosensory and visual areas in an expression pattern reminiscent of that of *Bhlhe22*. In *Ctip1* conditional knockout mice, there is an expansion of the motor area into the sensory areas. In addition, in the absence of *Ctip1*, there is a disruption of the somatosensory barrel map. Moreover, it functions to suppress sensory subcerebral projections from becoming "motorized" thus regulating sensory area identity (Greig et al. 2016).
- ***Lhx2:*** By selectively deleting *Lhx2* from postmitotic neurons, from about E11 onwards, it was shown that *Lhx2* in postmitotic neurons is crucial to regulating V1, A1, and S1 sizes and locations (Figures 21.2C and 21.3B; Zembrzycki et al. 2015). This deletion did not affect TF levels in progenitors and was consistent across all neuronal lamina of the cortical plate. Interestingly, *Lhx2* deletion in neurons causes changes to several non-progenitor TFs including *Bhlhbe22*, *Lmo4*, and *CoupTF1* as well as factors involved in epigenetic changes (i.e., methyl-CpG-binding

protein *MeCP2* and histone deacetylase *HDAC1*) and changes to methylation levels themselves (i.e., 5-methylcytosine, 5Mc) (Zembrzycki et al. 2015).

- ***Lmo4***: This LIM-domain TF contains two LIM-domains but lacks a DNA-binding domain (Figures 21.2C and 21.3B). It is expressed in the SVZ and immature and mature cortical neurons. Its neuronal expression at P0 marks rostral (motor) and caudal (visual) areas separated by an LMO4 negative (somatosensory) region (Huang et al. 2009). By P10, when the boundaries of the cortical sensory areas have been defined, *Lmo4* expression is uniform across the cortex. In *Lmo4* conditional knockout mice, the boundaries of cortical functional areas are shifted rostrally and the somatosensory cortex displays anomalies in shape and in innervation of barrel subfields (Cederquist et al. 2013; Huang et al. 2009). Interestingly, *Lmo4* has also been implicated as a TF of interest in human arealization based upon the finding that it is one of a few genes that shows asymmetrical expression between the left and the right perisylvian regions in the human embryonic brain (Sun et al. 2005).
- ***Nr2f1***: *Nr2f1* gradients in progenitors are maintained in cortical plate neurons (Figures 21.2C and 21.3B). When specifically deleted in cortical neurons, *Nr2f1* has been shown to be important in maintaining and refining areal identity (Alfano et al. 2014). Interestingly, neuronal *Nr2f1* regulation of area patterning occurs through a feedback loop that involves certain VZ patterning genes. Postmitotic *Nr2f1* was shown to be important in specifying sensory areas of the developing cortex by repressing motor identity in postmitotic neurons (Alfano et al. 2014). In fact, ectopic expression of *Nr2f1* in the rostral parts of the postmitotic cortex led to a re-specification of these frontal areas to become sensory areas. This postmitotic effect of *Nr2f1* on areal specification is distinct to the effect that *Nr2f1* has in the progenitors, thus indicating that after an initial patterning by TFs in the proliferative zones of the pallium, further areal refinement is conducted by TFs in immature postmitotic neurons. By specifically removing *Nr2f1* from layer 5 neurons, researchers were able to determine that postmitotic *Nr2f1* controls the topographic organization of somatosensory corticopontine neurons (Tocco et al. 2022). Removing *Nr2f1* from the progenitors, in contrast, leads to an increase in corticopontine innervation comparatively to corticospinal innervation (Tocco et al. 2022). This study further supports the idea that area mapping remains plastic in postmitotic neurons, and TFs play an important role in postmitotic neurons to maintain and refine cortical areal specification.
- ***Pbx1***: Loss of neuronal *Pbx1* expression using Nex-Cre resulted in a loss of the rostral cortex areas, that was less severe than in constitutive *Pbx1* mutants (Figures 21.2C and 21.3B; Golonzhka et al. 2015). Nonetheless it showed that Pbx1 is essential in immature neurons in the specification of the frontal cortex. Based on ChiP-seq and RNA expression, it was hypothesized that phenotypes arising from the VZ resulted from dysregulation of *Emx2* and *Lhx2*, whereas phenotypes arising from the cortical neurons resulted from dysregulation of genes such as *Lmo4* (Golonzhka et al. 2015).
- ***Tbr1***: This T-Box TF is expressed by postmitotic neurons and is an early postmitotic regulator layer 6 identity (Figures 21.2C and 21.3B; Hevner et al. 2001; Darbandi et al. 2018) and of gene expression gradients (Bedogni et al. 2010). *Tbr1* has a RC gradient in the cortical plate; in the null mouse, there is a loss of frontal cortex markers in all neuronal layers of the embryonic and early postnatal cortex (as well as layer 6 specification (Bedogni et al. 2010)). Further, caudal markers were also shifted rostrally. This rostral shift of cortical areas occurred without changing VZ gradients thus indicating that the loss of frontal area specification occurred in a cell autonomous manner.

- ***Tbr2 (Eomes)*:** This T-Box TF is expressed in the SVZ in a RC gradient (Figures 21.2C and 21.3B; Elsen et al. 2013). In its absence from intermediate progenitors, there is a general caudalization of the cortex with increased *Bhlhe22*. *Tbr2* functions downstream of the *Pax6* (expressed rostro-caudally in the VZ) and upstream of the *Tbr1* (expressed rostro-caudally in neurons) and is implicated in transmitting rostro-caudal maps from the VZ progenitor cells to intermediate progenitors and on to neurons of the cortex (Elsen et al. 2013; Englund et al. 2005). The *Pax6*→*Tbr2*→*Tbr1* cascade might therefore be a key constituent of the protomap theory (Rakic 1988) whereby RC gradients of the pallial VZ can be propagated to create sharp areas in the mature cortex.

21.3 Transcriptional Circuits in Pallial Patterning

Many of the TFs that have a role in patterning of the developing cortex are also expressed in other tissues. We have shown that DNA binding domains are crucial in specifying DNA targets for these TFs. So how do these TFs specifically regulate cortical targets? For instance, PAX6 is present in the developing forebrain as well as in the embryonic eye where it regulates a plethora of cell functions (Ypsilanti and Rubenstein 2016). Why doesn't PAX6 initiate retinal-specific programs in the cortex? The basic answer is that TFs can only bind their target DNA if it is readily accessible. Indeed, an important feature of coding and noncoding DNA regions is that their conformation is tightly and dynamically regulated. In eukaryotes, chromatin refers to genomic DNA that is coiled around histone proteins. Chromatin can rapidly switch from being open, a state associated with transcriptional activation, to a condensed state, which is linked with transcriptional repression (Figure 21.4A). Accessibility of chromatin at specific loci can be highly specific to particular cell types and cell states. For instance, during neural tube development, chromatin at the *Pax6* locus can be seen to progressively loosen up using fluorescence *in situ hybridization* as PAX6 expression increases (Patel et al. 2013). In addition, when comparing PAX6 binding to DNA targets in the developing forebrain and pancreas and the neonatal lens and retina, only around 20 percent of PAX6 binding targets were shared amongst the three tissue types suggesting high levels of tissue specificity for TF binding (Xie et al. 2013). Moreover, a TF can only initiate transcriptional regulation if other components of the transcriptional circuitry are available. Regardless of their expression patterns and levels, TF function is in fact constrained by the specific nuclear microenvironment in which the TF finds itself. In the cortex, besides TFs, there is a network of DNA components (e.g., enhancers, promoters, downstream transcription units), and protein components (e.g., chromatin modifiers, RNA polymerase) that are each essential in regulating cortical development.

Noncoding regions of the genome that are important for the regulation of transcription include: untranslated regions of genes (3'UTR and 5'UTR), promoters, noncoding RNAs, topologically associating domains (TADs that are the boundaries in which chromatin can form loops), and enhancers (Turner and Eichler 2019). Together with TFs, these DNA and RNA components contribute to generating cell-type specific transcriptional circuitry.

In Sections 21.3.1 and 21.3.2, we discuss some of the important features of gene regulatory elements, focusing on enhancers that are active in the developing cortex and how chromatin dynamics regulate the expression of patterning TFs. In addition, we will explore how these regulatory elements are in turn regulated by epigenetic modifiers and TFs.

21.3.1 Enhancers May Regulate the Formation of the Cortical Protomap

21.3.1.1 Defining and Identifying an Enhancer

Enhancers are noncoding DNA genomic regions that are spatial and temporal regulators of transcription. Due to the advent of next-generation sequencing technologies, and biochemical approaches to purify specific DNA domains with distinct epigenetic features, enhancers can now be readily identified (see ENCODE project and Roadmap Epigenomics project; ENCODE Project Consortium et al. 2020; Consortium 2004; Gorkin et al. 2020; Kundaje et al. 2015; Yue et al. 2014). Enhancers are regions of the genome that when active are non-compacted and possess unique molecular identifiers including chemical modifications on the histones bound to the enhancer, and its flanking region (i.e., acetylation, methylation) (Figure 21.4A; Nord and West 2020). Moreover, enhancers are genomic locations that act as a hub to bring together a number of proteins including transcriptional machinery, TFs as well as epigenomic modifiers (Figure 21.4A). Further, enhancers can be identified by probing the 3D structure of chromatin since enhancers are parts of DNA loops that form interactions with the promoter of the genes they regulate (Figure 21.4A). Finally, purely based on their sequence, enhancers tend to be conserved and genome-wide association studies (GWAS) have shown that, in humans, over 90 percent of genetic variants associated with common diseases and traits are clustered around gene regulatory elements (Cookson et al. 2009; Maurano et al. 2012).

A variety of molecular techniques can be used to identify putative gene regulatory regions based on their following properties: 1. Chromatin accessibility: ATAC-seq, which identifies regions of open chromatin; 2. DNA-protein interactions: TF ChIP-seq, which identifies regions of chromatin to which a specific TF is bound; 3. Histone modifications: Histone ChIP-seq, which is used to characterize various modifications on histones that are associated with active, repressed or poised enhancer regions; 4. Chromosomal interactions: PLAC-seq, which identifies promoter/chromatin loops and other various techniques that assess looping between chromatin regions (such as Hi-C); 5. DNA methylation: bisulfite sequencing to assess methylation profiles which usually signals an active enhancer.

Studies of many patterning TFs have examined enhancers that regulate their expression and/or identified enhancers to which they bind downstream to exert their function (see table 1 in Ypsilanti and Rubenstein 2016). Identifying these enhancers is especially informative for cortical patterning if they are bound by patterning TFs. For instance, *Dmrt3/5* have been shown to bind to *Pax6* and *Gsx2* enhancers where they act to suppress their expression (Konno et al. 2019). Another example is that *Emx2* expression is regulated by two distinct enhancers at the 5' and 3' region of the gene (García-Moreno and Molnár 2015; Suda et al. 2010; Theil et al. 2002). In turn, EMX2 has been shown to regulate two enhancers around another neurodevelopmental genes, *Sox2*, and negatively regulate its transcription both in vivo and in transfection assays (Mariani et al. 2012). Nevertheless, most of these studies provide a snapshot of the enhancer's function and activity. Indeed, a complete analysis of a cortical development enhancer would require assessment of: the gene it regulates, its spatial and temporal activity during cortical development as well as its regulation by epigenetic modifications, and TFs and noncoding RNA molecules.

In some cases, enhancers regulating patterning TFs have been linked to human diseases. For instance, an enhancer proximal to *Dmrt3* has been shown by chromosome conformation capture (hi-C) to bind to the *Dmrt3* promoter (Kubota et al. 2018). This same enhancer has been identified as a candidate for spastic cerebral palsy, a motor disorder that in some instances is associated with alterations of the motor and/or somatosensory cortex (Brun et al. 2021; Kubota et al. 2018). This *Dmrt3* enhancer contains a retinoic acid receptor/retinoid X receptor (RAR/RXR) motif, a molecule that has been shown both to regulate *Dmrt3* transcription (Kubota et al. 2018) and to be involved in patterning of the cerebral cortex (Shibata et al. 2021). Likewise, a schizophrenia-associated single polymorphism in a noncoding region (rs1191551) was shown to significantly reduce *Foxg1* expression in a reporter assay (Won et al. 2016). It is likely that mutations in many regulatory regions, which contribute to cortical patterning, will underlie risk for neuropsychiatric and neurodevelopmental disorders. For instance, two de novo autism mutations in an enhancer for *SLC6A1* negatively affected *Slc6a1* gene expression when introduced into primary mouse cortical neurons in vitro (Markenscoff-Papadimitriou et al. 2020).

To date, large-scale studies of enhancers in the developing telencephalon have demonstrated the existence of numerous enhancer regions with restricted spatial and temporal activities in the developing pallium (Nord et al. 2013; Pattabiraman et al. 2014; Visel et al. 2013; Wenger et al. 2013). In the embryonic telencephalon, a study found 145 enhancers that are active in specific regional domains (Visel et al. 2013). This enhancer encyclopedia became the foundation of the VISTA Enhancer browser, a public embryonic enhancer database in which thousands of embryonic human and mice enhancers were tested using transgenic assays in early murine development (https://enhancer.lbl.gov/). Fate-mapping of 14 of these enhancers with activity in subregion of the progenitor pallium were conducted using transgenic mice (Pattabiraman et al. 2014). This study showed that early progenitor domains give rise to distinct regions of the postnatal cortex in mice. Interestingly, in these studies, the activity pattern of enhancers generally did not replicate the expression pattern of the target gene near to the enhancer, but rather the enhancer activity was restricted to a subregion of the target gene's expression, often with sharp boundaries. Since many of the enhancers have sharp activity boundaries within the cortical VZ, they likely act as integrators of graded patterns of TF expression. Combinatorial TF binding may generate sharp regions of enhancer activity/inactivity, as is known to occur during *Drosophila* embryogenesis (Lim et al. 2018). Indeed, for a few tested enhancers, their activity was modulated in *Pax6* knockout mice suggesting that enhancers are really integrators of TF gradients in the pallial VZ (Pattabiraman et al. 2014).

21.3.1.2 Identifying Enhancers Involved in Cortical Patterning and Deciphering a TF Code for Cortical Regional/areal Specification

Major concerted efforts, such as those carried out by ENCODE project consortium and others, have been conducted to identify tissue-specific regulatory regions and characterize their epigenetic marks in different cell types at different time points in the mouse developing forebrain and cortex (Bella et al. 2021; Gorkin et al. 2020; Noack et al. 2022; Preissl et al. 2018; Takei et al. 2021; Ypsilanti et al. 2021). These studies have identified thousands of candidate regulatory elements that are associated with transcriptional activation and repression in different cortical cell types. Moreover, in the adult mouse brain, several groups have probed the epigenome/transcriptome in a region-specific manner (Bakken et al. 2021; Blankvoort et al. 2018; Tasic et al. 2018; Yao et al. 2021; Zhu et al. 2021).

However, amongst the thousands of identified regulatory regions in the embryonic cortex, only a subset is likely to be involved in cortical regionalization. To identify enhancers that participate in cortical patterning, we used TF ChIP-seq, with antibodies to EMX2, LHX2, NR2F1, PAX6, and PBX1, to identify candidate enhancers in the E12.5 cortex. This analysis in combination with ATAC-seq and Histone-Chip-seq identified candidate enhancers in the E12.5 cortex (Ypsilanti et al. 2021). Then, to identify which of these candidate enhancers is regulated by *Emx2, Nr2f1*, and *Pax6*, we studied the pallial epigenome of *Emx2*$^{-/-}$, *Nr2f1*$^{-/-}$, and *Pax6*$^{-/-}$ mice (Ypsilanti et al. 2021). We focused our analysis only on the regulatory regions within the interactome (looping region) of the 35 TFs that we identified as part of the cortical regionalization TFs network (described earlier). Within this set of TF gene loci, we found ~ 2000 putative regulatory regions, or about 20–100 candidate enhancers/locus. Of these, about 10% were sensitive to loss of EMX2, NR2F1 and/or PAX6. These ~ 200 enhancers are likely involved in regulating transcription of VZ TFs involved in patterning. Future work will likely focus on characterizing these VZ enhancers as well as identifying patterning enhancers in the developing cortical SVZ and neurons and defining their functions in the cortical VZ, SVZ, and neurons.

Figure 21.4B shows an unpublished example of the epigenetic state of a TF locus (*Otx1*) that highlights candidate enhancers (yellow vertical bars) that are likely to function in pallial patterning (data from Ypsilanti et al. 2021). These putative *Otx1* enhancers are active in the wild-type cortical progenitor cells (as indicated by H3K27Ac peaks) and repressed in the *Emx2* knockout progenitors (as indicated by H3K27me3 peaks). This illustrates the interplay of patterning TFs (*Emx2* and *Otx1*) at the genetic level. In this case, the absence of EMX2 leads to a reconfiguring of histone marks and chromatin accessibility around the *Otx1* locus.

Interestingly, studying enhancers with regional activity in subregions of the cortical VZ can also yield information about the underlying transcriptional logic implicated in regionalization. In fact, by categorizing VISTA enhancer activity along the rostro-caudal and ventro-dorsal axes of the developing pallium, we were able to determine that enhancers active in the most dorsal-caudal pallium (medial pallium) had the least binding by patterning TFs (as assessed by TF ChIP-Seq); whereas enhancers active in the most rostral ventral pallium (LVP) showed more binding by EMX2, LHX2, NR2F1, PAX6, and PBX1 (Ypsilanti et al. 2021). Depending on their spatial coordinates within the developing pallium, enhancers in progenitor cells are regulated by a dose-dependent TF combinatorial code which enables them to carry out region specific programs of gene expression.

21.3.1.3 Epigenetic Regulation of Enhancer Regions and Genes – Transcriptional Regulators

In early telencephalon development, a study found that positional identity of ventral progenitors established by SHH was then retained through epigenetic mechanisms mediated by a methyltransferase, *mixed-lineage Leukemia 1* (*Mll1*) (Delgado et al. 2020). Perturbation of *Mll1* during development leads to changes in epigenetic profiles in the neural stem cells and changes in regional cell fate from ventral to dorsal-like telencephalon progenitors. A similar mechanism that maintains regionalization within the dorsal telencephalon has yet to be found but it is known that epigenetic regulation is crucial to establishing and refining cortical regionalization.

For instance, Cited2 is a transcriptional coactivator and/or corepressor that interacts with CBP/p300 and leads to either increased or decreased transcription (Freedman et al. 2003). In the cortex, *Cited2* is expressed by SVZ progenitor cells from E15.5 onwards with expression decreasing over developmental time until its expression becomes progressively refined to neurons of the somatosensory areas postnatally (Fame et al. 2016). In *Cited2* null mice, besides other cortical phenotypes, there is a marked reduction of the somatosensory cortex that is restricted to the superficial neuronal layers. Analysis of cortical arealization in double *Lmo4;Cited2* knockouts indicate that these proteins have compensatory effects on somatosensory areal specification. Moreover, removing *Cited2* from postmitotic neurons demonstrated it did not participate in arealization in these cells, suggesting the *Cited2* regulates areal patterning in cortical progenitors (Fame et al. 2016).

Another epigenetic regulator with a role in cortical patterning is the transcriptional regulator H3K36me3 methyltransferase *Setd2* (Kizer et al. 2005). *Setd2* is expressed in progenitor and neuronal cells of the developing pallium (Xu et al. 2021). In conditional knockouts of *Setd2*, cortical areal patterning showed abnormalities with the visual area compressed caudally and several other areas exhibiting changes both in size and positioning within the postnatal cortex (Xu et al. 2021). This mispatterning was independent of changes in expression of several patterning TFs including *Emx2, Nr2f1*, *Pax6*, and *Sp8*.

Dnmt1 is an epigenetic regulator whose perturbation leads to disruption of cortical areas (Golshani et al. 2005). This enzyme is a DNA methyltransferase that is responsible for maintaining genes in a methylated state, a crucial feature of gene repression. When *Dnmt1* is conditionally ablated in the mouse cortex, the somatosensory barrel cortex fails to develop although thalamocortical axons still innervate the area (Golshani et al. 2005). A reduction in the barrel fields of *Mecp2* (a methylcytosine binding protein) null mice was also uncovered although in this case, the areal reduction might be secondary to a thalamocortical innervation defect rather than area specification (Moroto et al. 2013). Other studies have also shown the impact of DNA methylation on area-specific gene expression in the macaque (Hata et al. 2013). Specifically, promoters of genes expressed in association areas have different methylation profiles than promoters of genes expressed in V1 area. MBD4, a methyl-binding protein that acts to activate transcription of methylated genes, was also found to be differentially expressed with high expression in association areas and low expression in V1 (Hata et al. 2013). The epigenetic regulator that is responsible for the differential methylation profiles in this instance has (to our knowledge) yet to be uncovered.

The search for epigenetic factors that participate in regionalization and arealization is actively ongoing. Using RNA-Seq and ChIP-Seq assays, researchers are identifying chromatin regulators that interact with patterning TFs. For instance, TBR2 has been shown to regulate expression of *Kdm1a*, a histone lysine demethylase gene as well as *Hdac9*, encoding a histone deacetylase (Elsen et al. 2018); TBR2 can also act to recruit a histone demethylase, JMJD3, to regulate gene expression epigenetically (Sessa et al. 2016). Interestingly, PAX6, TBR2, and TBR1 all regulate switches in the composition of subunits of the BAF chromatin-remodeling complex, which is critical for neuronal differentiation (Elsen et al. 2018; Ninkovic et al. 2013; Tuoc et al. 2013). As another example, LHX2 binds several epigenetic regulators including LSD1, HDAC2, and RBBP4; LHX2's absence during cortical development leads to histone mark changes at genomic loci including *Fezf2* and *Sox11* (Muralidharan et al. 2017b).

The interplay of epigenomic regulation and TF regulation remains an active field in understanding cortical patterning. It is known that several epigenetic factors are expressed in gradients in the progenitor zone of the developing pallium (i.e., *Gadd45g* and *Chd7*; Elsen et al. 2018). Future studies on whether these gradients help establish cortical areas will be important.

21.3.1.4 Conservation and Function of Pallial Enhancers

An identifiable feature of enhancers is sequence conservation across species (Visel et al. 2007). Ultraconserved enhancers are a relatively small set of genomic elements (~500) that show near perfect conservation across vertebrate species (Snetkova et al. 2022). However, in general that degree of conservation of the roughly estimated 1 million enhancers in the genome varies greatly, as during evolution enhancers are lost and gained (Kvon et al. 2016; Thompson et al. 2018). The extent to which this sequence conservation extends to conservation of function across species has not been well characterized. One study compared the activity of zebrafish and human enhancers found that approximately 30 percent of tested conserved enhancers shared conserved activity in similar tissues/regions across those species (Ritter et al. 2010). The rest either had activity in disparate tissues or were species-specific (or negative). Further studies of pallial enhancer conservation will be required to understand whether what is learned about the regulation of cortical patterning by noncoding regions in mice and other model organisms can be applied to humans and their complex disorders.

Insights about conserved enhancers comes from studies of ultraconserved enhancers around the *Arx* locus (Snetkova et al. 2022). In the pallium, the activity of two *Arx* ultraconserved enhancers (hs122 and hs123) is very similar to *Arx* pallial expression (Pennacchio et al. 2006; Visel et al. 2013). Contrarily to $Arx^{y/-}$ mice, which die shortly after birth, deletion of either hs122 or hs123, as well as compound deletion of hs122;hs123 yielded viable and fertile mice with no gross phenotype (Dickel et al. 2018; Kitamura et al. 2002). However, detailed neuroanatomical analysis showed that $hs122^{y/-}$ and $hs122^{y/-}$;$hs123^{y/-}$ mice had decreased levels of *Arx* mRNA in the pallium and dysmorphic dentate gyri similar to (albeit less severe) hippocampal defects observed in the *Arx* conditional knockout mice (Dickel et al. 2018; Kitamura et al. 2002). Deletion of hs123 alone did not result in an observable pallial phenotype (Ahituv et al. 2007; Dickel et al. 2018). This data suggests that additional *Arx* enhancers remain in the double mutant that continue to drive *Arx* pallial expression, illustrating the redundancy that is built-into the transcriptional regulation of *Arx* gene. A subsequent mutagenesis study of these *Arx* enhancers further substantiates this redundancy (Snetkova et al. 2021). It also demonstrated that sequence conservation of some base pairs was important for enhancer activity. Mutating 5 percent of hs122's base pairs reduced enhancer activity and led to a dysmorphic dentate gyrus. Surprisingly, for other *Arx* enhancers, mutating upwards of 20 percent of their conserved base pairs did not reduce enhancer activity (Snetkova et al. 2021). This highlights that enhancer molecular biology may vary greatly between enhancers.

However, although many enhancers show sequence conservation across mammalian species, there is evidence that there are some cortical enhancers that are specific to humans (Caporale et al. 2019; Torre-Ubieta et al. 2018; Girskis et al. 2021; Luo et al. 2021; Uebbing et al. 2021; Whalen et al. 2022). In one such study, a multi-omics approach showed that around 1,200 chromatin loops were uniquely present in the human fetal cortex and not in the macaque or the mouse developing cortex at similar gestational ages (Luo et al. 2021). The human-specific interactions were enriched for enhancer–enhancer interactions and were also found to regulate genes important for regulation of the subplate, a transient developmental structure that is crucial in cortex development (Kostović et al. 2019; Molnár et al. 2019). Further studies of enhancer conservation and divergences across vertebrates will likely provide invaluable insights into disease states.

21.4 Conclusion

In this chapter we focused on the transcriptional processes that create distinct pallial regions and areas in mice. This is controlled by the graded expression of TFs in pallial progenitors. This regional, and perhaps areal, protomap is in part encoded by enhancers, with regional VZ activity, that integrate the combinatorial expression and dosage of TFs. Some of these enhancers have activities that have sharp boundaries with the pallial VZ (Pattabiraman et al. 2014). The protomap is then passed on from the VZ to daughter cells in the SVZ and then the cortical plate, where it is further refined by TFs expressed in postmitotic immature neurons. Gene expression is further regulated by chromatin-modifying enzymes that activate, repress, and/or maintain enhancer and promoter activities. Extrinsic processes such as the effect of thalamocortical and other afferent axons, membrane depolarization, and sensory input, are also implicated in shaping this process; further discussion of these points, however, is beyond the scope of this chapter.

In the cortical regionalization process, a key unanswered question is how TF gradients in the progenitor cells are translated into positional information in SVZ cells and then in immature neurons in the cortical plate, to then generate mature cortical regions and areas. Our hypothesis is that regulatory elements are epigenetically programmed to encode these positional cues and can propagate these cues as cells differentiate from progenitor cells to neurons (see Figure 21.4). We postulate that enhancers active in the VZ (RE1), SVZ (RE2), and CP (RE3) are differentially bound by TFs that drive expression of regional genes in post-mitotic cortical neurons (Ypsilanti and Rubenstein 2016). The REs are protein-binding modules that translate gradients of TF expression in cortical progenitors into region (and area)-specific expression in cortical neurons. REs active in the SVZ (RE2) and CP (RE3) are primed in the VZ by TFs. For simplicity, Figure 21.4C focuses on the role of PAX6 in the rostral cortex; analogous mechanisms would operate in the caudal cortex with TFs such as EMX2 and NR2F1. In the context of the whole pallium, binding of PAX6 in rostral VZ cells (where its concentration is highest) would preferentially activate rostral VZ REs (RE1) and not caudal VZ REs, the latter would be activated by TFs such as EMX2 and NR2F1. We postulate that PAX6, EMX2, and NR2F1 as well as other TFs discussed earlier will prime certain SVZ and CP REs (RE2 and RE3; Figure 21.4C), marking them epigenetically (e.g., modified histone marks of poised or active chromatin), thus passing on VZ positional information via these "primed" SVZ and CP REs to cells in the SVZ and CP. Propagation of the VZ protomap into the SVZ and CP would then be carried out by TFs such as BHLHE22, NR2F1, PBX1, TBR1, and TBR2 (whose regional specification functions in the SVZ and CP have been established) (Figure 21.2C) (Alfano et al. 2014; Bedogni et al. 2010; Elsen et al. 2013; Faedo et al. 2008; Golonzhka et al. 2015; Joshi et al. 2008).

As research into the role of transcriptional regulation in disease states progresses, the basic mechanisms of regionalization and of regulatory regions uncovered in mice will provide insights into the biology of human brain disorders. As multi-omic studies become more easily accessible, scientists are probing the regulatory elements of the human fetal cortex (Li et al. 2018, 2020; Mandell et al. 2020; Markenscoff-Papadimitriou et al. 2020; Song et al. 2020; Ziffra et al. 2021). In humans, a recent single cell epigenomic profiling of cortical areas in mid-gestation found that, chromatin accessibility at noncoding regions exhibited clear differences between the prefrontal cortex and the visual cortex, in contrast to smaller differences in the transcriptome (Nowakowski et al. 2017; Ziffra et al. 2021). This further supports the idea that identifying and studying enhancer states in the developing and adult cortical regions will be critical in elucidating the regulatory process that specifies cortical regionalization.

Finally, another fascinating avenue of future research will be to determine how sensory input modify and refine cortical regionalization especially in higher order mammals. In prairie voles (*Microtus ochrogaster*), the size of cortical fields and the connectivity of the somatosensory cortex differ in adults who received either high or low tactile contact from their parents (Seelke et al. 2016). Although some effects are present in the offspring of stable mating pairs soon after birth (P1), including differences in the pattern of *Id2*, other areal differences appear to develop over time and therefore may be linked to tactile stimulation (Bottom et al. 2020).

References

Acampora, D. et al. (1999). Otx genes in corticogenesis and brain development. *Cereb Cortex* 9: 533–542.

Acampora, D. et al. (1996). Epilepsy and brain abnormalities in mice lacking the Otx1 gene. *Nat Genet* 14: 218–222.

Ahituv, N. et al. (2007). Deletion of ultraconserved elements yields viable mice. *Plos Biol* 5: e234.

Alfano, C. et al. (2014). Postmitotic control of sensory area specification during neocortical development. *Nat Commun* 5: 5632.

Amaniti, E.-M. et al. (2013). Gli3 is required in Emx1+ progenitors for the development of the corpus callosum. *Dev Biol* 376: 113–124.

Armentano, M. et al. (2007). COUP-TFI regulates the balance of cortical patterning between frontal/motor and sensory areas. *Nat Neurosci* 10: 1277–1286.

Avram, D. et al. (2002). COUP-TF (chicken ovalbumin upstream promoter transcription factor)-interacting protein 1 (CTIP1) is a sequence-specific DNA binding protein. *Biochem J* 368: 555–563.

Azzarelli, R. et al. (2015). Emergence of neuronal diversity from patterning of telencephalic progenitors. *Wiley Interdiscip Rev: Dev Biol* 4: 197–214.

Bakken, T.E. et al. (2021). Comparative cellular analysis of motor cortex in human, marmoset and mouse. *Nature* 598: 111–119.

Bedogni, F. et al. (2010). Tbr1 regulates regional and laminar identity of postmitotic neurons in developing neocortex. *Proc Natl Acad Sci* 107: 13129–13134.

Bella, D.J.D. et al. (2021). Molecular logic of cellular diversification in the mouse cerebral cortex. *Nature* 595: 554–559.

Bertacchi, M. et al. (2020). NR2F1 regulates regional progenitor dynamics in the mouse neocortex and cortical gyrification in BBSOAS patients. *EMBO J* 39: e104163.

Bishop, K.M. et al. (2003). Emxl and Emx2 cooperate to regulate cortical size, lamination, neuronal differentiation, development of cortical efferents, and thalamocortical pathfinding. *J Comp Neurol* 457: 345–360.

Bishop, K.M. et al. (2000). Regulation of area identity in the mammalian neocortex by Emx2 and Pax6. *Science* 288: 344–349.

Blankvoort, S. et al. (2018). Marked diversity of unique cortical enhancers enables neuron-specific tools by enhancer-driven gene expression. *Curr Biol* 28: 2103–2114.e5.

Bonneau, D. et al. (2002). X-linked lissencephaly with absent corpus callosum and ambiguous genitalia (XLAG). *Ann Neurol* 51: 340–349.

Borello, U. et al. (2018). SP8 transcriptional regulation of cyclin D1 during mouse early corticogenesis. *Front Neurosci* 12: 119.

Borello, U. et al. (2014). Sp8 and COUP-TF1 reciprocally regulate patterning and Fgf signaling in cortical progenitors. *Cereb Cortex* 24: 1409–1421.

Bottom, R.T. et al. (2020). Early postnatal gene expression in the developing neocortex of prairie voles (Microtus ochrogaster) is related to parental rearing style. *J Comp Neurol* 528: 3008–3022.

Brun, C. et al. (2021). Somatosensory deficits and neural correlates in cerebral palsy. *Dev Med Child Neurol* 63: 1382–1393.

Cadwell, C.R. et al. (2019). Development and arealization of the cerebral cortex. *Neuron* 103: 980–1004.

Caporale, A.L. et al. (2019). Transcriptional enhancers in the FOXP2 locus underwent accelerated evolution in the human lineage. *Mol Biol Evol* 36: 2432–2450.

Carbe, C. et al. (2013). An allelic series at the paired box gene 6 (Pax6) locus reveals the functional specificity of pax genes*. *J Biol Chem* 288: 12130–12141.

Carney, R.S.E. et al. (2009). Differential regulation of telencephalic pallial–subpallial boundary patterning by Pax6 and Gsh2. *Cereb Cortex* 19: 745–759.

Caronia-Brown, G. et al. (2014). The cortical hem regulates the size and patterning of neocortex. *Development* 141: 2855–2865.

Catela, C. (2020). Patterning and generation of neural diversity in the spinal cord. In: *Patterning and Cell Type Specification in the Developing CNS and PNS*, 2e (ed. J.L.R. Rubenstein and R. Pakic), 137–155. San Diego, CA: Elsevier.

Cederquist, G.Y., Azim, E., Shnider, S.J. et al. (2013). Lmo4 establishes rostral motor cortex projection neuron subtype diversity. *J Neurosci* 33: 6321–6332.

Chizhikov, V.V. et al. (2010). Lmx1a regulates fates and location of cells originating from the cerebellar rhombic lip and telencephalic cortical hem. *Proc Natl Acad Sci* 107: 10725–10730.

Chizhikov, V.V. and Millen, K.J. (2005). Roof plate-dependent patterning of the vertebrate dorsal central nervous system. *Dev Biol* 277: 287–295.

Chou, S.-J. et al. (2013). Geniculocortical input drives genetic distinctions between primary and higher-order visual areas. *Science* 340: 1239–1242.

Chou, S.-J. et al. (2009). Lhx2 specifies regional fate in Emx1 lineage of telencephalic progenitors generating cerebral cortex. *Nat Neurosci* 12: 1381–1389.

Clercq, S.D. et al. (2016). DMRT5 together with DMRT3 directly controls hippocampus development and neocortical area map formation. *Cereb Cortex* 28: 493–509.

Consortium, E.P. (2004). The ENCODE (ENCyclopedia Of DNA elements) project. *Science* 306: 636–640.

Cookson, W. et al. (2009). Mapping complex disease traits with global gene expression. *Nat Rev Genet* 10: 184–194.

Danesin, C. et al. (2009). Integration of telencephalic Wnt and hedgehog signaling center activities by Foxg1. *Dev Cell* 16: 576–587.

Darbandi, S.F. et al. (2018). Neonatal Tbr1 dosage controls cortical layer 6 connectivity. *Neuron* 100: 831–845.e7.

Dehay, C. et al. (1996). Contribution of thalamic input to the specification of cytoarchitectonic cortical fields in the primate. *J Comp Neurol* 367: 70–89.

Dehay, C. and Kennedy, H. (2007). Cell-cycle control and cortical development. *Nat Rev Neurosci* 8: 438–450.

Delgado, R.N. et al. (2020). Maintenance of neural stem cell positional identity by mixed-lineage leukemia 1. *Science* 368: 48–53.

Desmaris, E. et al. (2018). DMRT5, DMRT3, and EMX2 cooperatively repress Gsx2 at the pallium–subpallium boundary to maintain cortical identity in dorsal telencephalic progenitors. *J Neurosci* 38: 9105–9121.

Dickel, D.E. et al. (2018). Ultraconserved enhancers are required for normal development. *Cell* 172: 491–499.e15.

Dou, C.-L. et al. (1999). Dual role of brain factor-1 in regulating growth and patterning of the cerebral hemispheres. *Cereb Cortex* 9: 543–550.

D'Souza, L. et al. (2021). Chromatin remodelling complexes in cerebral cortex development and neurodevelopmental disorders. *Neurochem Int* 147: 105055.

Elsen, G.E. et al. (2018). The epigenetic factor landscape of developing neocortex is regulated by transcription factors Pax6→ Tbr2→ Tbr1. *Front Neurosci* 12: 571.

Elsen, G.E. et al. (2013). The protomap is propagated to cortical plate neurons through an *Eomes*-dependent intermediate map. *Proc Natl Acad Sci* 110: 4081–4086.

ENCODE Project Consortium et al. (2020). Perspectives on ENCODE. *Nature* 583 (7818): 693–698.

Englund, C. et al. (2005). Pax6, Tbr2, and Tbr1 are expressed sequentially by radial glia, intermediate progenitor cells, and postmitotic neurons in developing neocortex. *J Neurosci* 25: 247–251.

Faedo, A. et al. (2010). Repression of Fgf signaling by sprouty1-2 regulates cortical patterning in two distinct regions and times. *J Neurosci* 30: 4015–4023.

Faedo, A. et al. (2008). COUP-TFI coordinates cortical patterning, neurogenesis, and laminar fate and modulates MAPK/ERK, AKT, and ß-catenin signaling. *Cereb Cortex* 18: 2117–2131.

Fame, R.M. et al. (2016). Cited2 regulates neocortical layer II/III generation and somatosensory callosal projection neuron development and connectivity. *J Neurosci* 36: 6403–6419.

Feng, J. et al. (2021). COUP-TFI specifies the medial entorhinal cortex identity and induces differential cell adhesion to determine the integrity of its boundary with neocortex. *Sci Adv* 7 (27): eabf6808.

Fietz, S.A. et al. (2010). OSVZ progenitors of human and ferret neocortex are epithelial-like and expand by integrin signaling. *Nat Neurosci* 13: 690–699.

Florian, C. (2012). FOXG1-related disorders: from clinical description to molecular genetics. *Mol Syndromol* 2: 153–163.

Fotaki, V. et al. (2006). Abnormal positioning of diencephalic cell types in neocortical tissue in the dorsal telencephalon of mice lacking functional Gli3. *J Neurosci* 26: 9282–9292.

Frantz, G. et al. (1994). Otx1 and Otx2 define layers and regions in developing cerebral cortex and cerebellum. *J Neurosci* 14: 5725–5740.

Freedman, S.J. et al. (2003). Structural basis for negative regulation of hypoxia-inducible factor-1α by CITED2. *Nat Struct Mol Biol* 10: 504–512.

Galceran, J. et al. (2000). Hippocampus development and generation of dentate gyrus granule cells is regulated by LEF1. *Development* 127: 469–482.

García-Moreno, F. and Molnár, Z. (2015). Subset of early radial glial progenitors that contribute to the development of callosal neurons is absent from avian brain. *Proc Natl Acad Sci* 112: E5058–E5067.

Garel, S. et al. (2003). Molecular regionalization of the neocortex is disrupted in Fgf8 hypomorphic mutants. *Development* 130: 1903–1914.

Georgala, P.A. et al. (2011). The generation of superficial cortical layers is regulated by levels of the transcription factor Pax6. *Cereb Cortex* 21: 81–94.

Girskis, K.M. et al. (2021). Rewiring of human neurodevelopmental gene regulatory programs by human accelerated regions. *Neuron* 109: 3239–3251.e7.

Godbole, G. et al. (2017). Novel functions of LHX2 and PAX6 in the developing telencephalon revealed upon combined loss of both genes. *Neural Dev* 12 (1): 19.

Golonzhka, O. et al. (2015). Pbx regulates patterning of the cerebral cortex in progenitors and postmitotic neurons. *Neuron* 88: 1192–1207.

Golshani, P. et al. (2005). Conditional Dnmt1 deletion in dorsal forebrain disrupts development of somatosensory barrel cortex and thalamocortical long-term potentiation. *Thalamus Related Sys* 3: 227–233.

Gorkin, D.U. et al. (2020). An atlas of dynamic chromatin landscapes in mouse fetal development. *Nature* 583: 744–751.

Gorski, J.A. et al. (2002). Cortical excitatory neurons and Glia, but not GABAergic neurons, are produced in the Emx1-expressing lineage. *J Neurosci* 22: 6309–6314.

Greig, L.C. et al. (2016). Ctip1 controls acquisition of sensory area identity and establishment of sensory input fields in the developing neocortex. *Neuron* 90 (2): 261–277.

Grove, E.A. (2020). Area patterning of the mammalian neocortex. In: *Pattern and Cell Type Specification in the Developing CNS and PNS*, 2e (ed. J.L.R. Rubenstein and R. Pakic), 49–68. San Diego, CA: Elsevier.

Grove, E.A. and Monuki, E.S. (2020). Morphogens, patterning centers, and their mechanisms of action. In: *Pattern and Cell Type Specification in the Developing CNS and PNS*, 2e (ed. J.L.R. Rubenstein and R. Pakic), 3–21. San Diego, CA: Elsevier.

Grove, E.A. et al. (1998). The hem of the embryonic cerebral cortex is defined by the expression of multiple Wnt genes and is compromised in Gli3-deficient mice. *Development* 125: 2315–2325.

Gulisano, M. et al. (1996). Emx1 and Emx2 show different patterns of expression during proliferation and differentiation of the developing cerebral cortex in the mouse. *Eur J Neurosci* 8: 1037–1050.

Hamasaki, T. et al. (2004). EMX2 regulates sizes and positioning of the primary sensory and motor areas in neocortex by direct specification of cortical progenitors. *Neuron* 43: 359–372.

Hanashima, C. et al. (2004). Foxg1 suppresses early cortical cell fate. *Science* 303: 56–59.

Hansen, D.V. et al. (2010). Neurogenic radial glia in the outer subventricular zone of human neocortex. *Nature* 464: 554–561.

Hasenpusch-Theil, K. et al. (2017). Direct interactions between Gli3, Wnt8b, and Fgfs underlie patterning of the dorsal telencephalon. *Cereb Cortex* 27: 1137–1148.

Hata, K. et al. (2013). DNA methylation and methyl-binding proteins control differential gene expression in distinct cortical areas of macaque monkey. *J Neurosci* 33: 19704–19714.

Hevner, R.F. et al. (2001). Tbr1 regulates differentiation of the preplate and layer 6. *Neuron* 29: 353–366.

Hoch, R.V. et al. (2015a). Fgf signaling controls the telencephalic distribution of Fgf-expressing progenitors generated in the rostral patterning center. *Neural Dev* 10: 8.

Hoch, R.V. et al. (2015b). OTX2 transcription factor controls regional patterning within the medial ganglionic eminence and regional identity of the septum. *Cell Rep* 12: 482–494.

Holland, P.W. et al. (2007). Classification and nomenclature of all human homeobox genes. *BMC Biol* 5: 47–47.

Hu, J.S. et al. (2017). Coup-TF1 and Coup-TF2 control subtype and laminar identity of MGE-derived neocortical interneurons. *Development* 144: 2837–2851.

Huang, Z. et al. (2009). Transcription factor Lmo4 defines the shape of functional areas in developing cortices and regulates sensorimotor control. *Devel Biol* 327: 132–142.

Joshi, P.S. et al. (2008). Bhlhb5 regulates the postmitotic acquisition of area identities in layers II–V of the developing neocortex. *Neuron* 60: 258–272.

Kamnasaran, D. et al. (2003). Disruption of the neuronal PAS3 gene in a family affected with schizophrenia. *J Med Genet* 40: 325–332.

Kimura, J. et al. (2005). Emx2 and Pax6 function in cooperation with Otx2 and Otx1 to develop caudal forebrain primordium that includes future archipallium. *J Neurosci* 25: 5097–5108.

Kitamura, K. et al. (2002). Mutation of ARX causes abnormal development of forebrain and testes in mice and X-linked lissencephaly with abnormal genitalia in humans. *Nat Genet* 32: 359–369.

Kizer, K.O. et al. (2005). A novel domain in set2 mediates RNA polymerase II interaction and couples histone H3 K36 methylation with transcript elongation. *Mol Cell Biol* 25: 3305–3316.

Konno, D. et al. (2019). Dmrt factors determine the positional information of cerebral cortical progenitors via differential suppression of homeobox genes. *Development* 146: dev174243.

Kostović, I. et al. (2019). Sublaminar organization of the human subplate. *J Anat* 235: 481–506.

Kroll, T.T. and O'Leary, D.D.M. (2005). Ventralized dorsal telencephalic progenitors in Pax6 mutant mice generate GABA interneurons of a lateral ganglionic eminence fate. *Proc Natl Acad Sci USA* 102: 7374–7379.

Kubota, N. et al. (2018). Identification of a candidate enhancer for DMRT3 involved in spastic cerebral palsy pathogenesis. *Biochem Biophys Res Commun* 496: 133–139.

Kumar, R.A. et al. (2008). Initial association of NR2E1 with bipolar disorder and identification of candidate mutations in bipolar disorder, schizophrenia, and aggression through resequencing. *Am J Med Genet Part B Neuropsychiatr Genet* 147B: 880–889.

Kundaje, A. et al. (2015). Integrative analysis of 111 reference human epigenomes. *Nature* 518: 317–330.

Kuschel, S. et al. (2003). A disrupted balance between Bmp/Wnt and Fgf signaling underlies the ventralization of the Gli3 mutant telencephalon. *Dev Biol* 260 (2): 484–495.

Kuwamura, M. et al. (2005). Mutation at the Lmx1a locus provokes aberrant brain development in the rat. *Dev Brain Res* 155: 99–106.

Kvon, E.Z. et al. (2016). Progressive loss of function in a limb enhancer during snake evolution. *Cell* 167: 633–642.e11.

Leung, R.F. et al. (2022). Genetic regulation of vertebrate forebrain development by homeobox genes. *Front Neurosci* 16: 843794.

Li, M. et al. (2018). Integrative functional genomic analysis of human brain development and neuropsychiatric risks. *Science* 362 (6420): eaat7615.

Lim, B. et al. (2018). Temporal dynamics of pair-rule stripes in living Drosophila embryos. *Proc Natl Acad Sci* 115: 8376–8381.

Lim, Y. et al. (2019). Arx expression suppresses ventralization of the developing dorsal forebrain. *Sci Rep* 9 (1): 226.

Li, Z. et al. (2020). Transcriptional priming as a conserved mechanism of lineage diversification in the developing mouse and human neocortex. *Sci Adv* 6: eabd2068.

López-Bendito, G. and Martini, F.J. (2020). Patterning of thalmus. In: *Pattern and Cell Type Specification in the Developing CNS and PNS*, 2e (ed. J.L.R. Rubenstein and R. Pakic), 69–86. San Diego, CA: Elsevier.

Luo, X. et al. (2021). 3D genome of macaque fetal brain reveals evolutionary innovations during primate corticogenesis. *Cell* 184: 723–740.e21.

Mallamaci, A. et al. (2000). Area identity shifts in the early cerebral cortex of Emx2−/− mutant mice. *Nat Neurosci* 3: 679–686.

Mallamaci, A. and Stoykova, A. (2006). Gene networks controlling early cerebral cortex arealization. *Eur J Neurosci* 23: 847–856.

Mandell, K.A.P. et al. (2020). Characterizing the dynamic and functional DNA methylation landscape in the developing human cortex. *Epigenetics* 16: 1–13.

Mangale, V.S. et al. (2008). Lhx2 selector activity specifies cortical identity and suppresses hippocampal organizer fate. *Science* 319: 304–309.

Manuel, M. et al. (2006). Controlled overexpression of Pax6 in vivo negatively autoregulates the Pax6 locus, causing cell-autonomous defects of late cortical progenitor proliferation with little effect on cortical arealization. *Development* 134: 545–555.

Mariani, J. et al. (2012). Emx2 is a dose-dependent negative regulator of Sox2 telencephalic enhancers. *Nucleic Acids Res* 40: 6461–6476.

Markenscoff-Papadimitriou, E. et al. (2020). A chromatin accessibility atlas of the developing human telencephalon. *Cell* 182: 754–769.e18.

Maurano, M.T. et al. (2012). Systematic localization of common disease-associated variation in regulatory DNA. *Science* 337: 1190–1195.

Mi, D. et al. (2013). Pax6 exerts regional control of cortical progenitor proliferation via direct repression of Cdk6 and hypophosphorylation of pRb. *Neuron* 78: 269–284.

Mi, D. et al. (2018). Pax6 lengthens G1 phase and decreases oscillating Cdk6 levels in murine embryonic cortical progenitors. *Front Cell Neurosci* 12: 419.

Millonig, J.H. et al. (2000). The mouse Dreher gene Lmx1a controls formation of the roof plate in the vertebrate CNS. *Nature* 403: 764–769.

Molnár, Z. et al. (2019). New insights into the development of the human cerebral cortex. *J Anat* 235: 432–451.

Monko, T. et al. (2022). Thalamocortical axons regulate neurogenesis and laminar fates in the early sensory cortex. *Proc Natl Acad Sci* 119: e2201355119.

Moody, R.R. et al. (2018). Probing the interaction between the histone methyltransferase/deacetylase subunit RBBP4/7 and the transcription factor BCL11A in epigenetic complexes. *J Biol Chem* 293: 2125–2136.

Moroto, M. et al. (2013). Altered somatosensory barrel cortex refinement in the developing brain of Mecp2-null mice. *Brain Res* 1537: 319–326.

Muralidharan, B. et al. (2017a). Dmrt5, a novel neurogenic factor, reciprocally regulates Lhx2 to control the neuron–glia cell-fate switch in the developing hippocampus. *J Neurosci* 37: 11245–11254.

Muralidharan, B. et al. (2017b). LHX2 interacts with the NuRD complex and regulates cortical neuron subtype determinants Fezf2 and Sox11. *J Neurosci* 37: 194–203.

Murphy, M.W. et al. (2007). Vertebrate DM domain proteins bind similar DNA sequences and can heterodimerize on DNA. *BMC Mol Biol* 8: 58.

Muzio, L. et al. (2002). Conversion of cerebral cortex into basal ganglia in Emx2−/− Pax6Sey/Sey double-mutant mice. *Nat Neurosci* 5: 737–745.

Naka, H. et al. (2008). Requirement for COUP-TFI and II in the temporal specification of neural stem cells in CNS development. *Nat Neurosci* 11 (9): 1014–1023.

Ninkovic, J. et al. (2013). The BAF complex interacts with Pax6 in adult neural progenitors to establish a neurogenic cross-regulatory transcriptional network. *Cell Stem Cell* 13: 403–418.

Noack, F. et al. (2022). Multimodal profiling of the transcriptional regulatory landscape of the developing mouse cortex identifies Neurog2 as a key epigenome remodeler. *Nat Neurosci* 25: 154–167.

Nord, A.S. et al. (2013). Rapid and pervasive changes in genome-wide enhancer usage during mammalian development. *Cell* 155: 1521–1531.

Nord, A.S. and West, A.E. (2020). Neurobiological functions of transcriptional enhancers. *Nat Neurosci* 23: 5–14.

Nowakowski, T.J. et al. (2017). Spatiotemporal gene expression trajectories reveal developmental hierarchies of the human cortex. *Science* 358: 1318–1323.

O'Leary, D.D. et al. (2007). Area patterning of the mammalian cortex. *Neuron* 56: 252–269.

O'Leary, D.D. and Sahara, S. (2008). Genetic regulation of arealization of the neocortex. *Curr Opin Neurobiol* 18: 90–100.

Patel, N.S. et al. (2013). FGF signalling regulates chromatin organisation during neural differentiation via mechanisms that can be uncoupled from transcription. *Plos Genet* 9: e1003614.

Pattabiraman, K. et al. (2014). Transcriptional regulation of enhancers active in protodomains of the developing cerebral cortex. *Neuron* 82: 989–1003.

Pennacchio, L.A. et al. (2006). In vivo enhancer analysis of human conserved non-coding sequences. *Nature* 444: 499–502.

Pinon, M.C. et al. (2008). Altered molecular regionalization and normal thalamocortical connections in cortex-specific Pax6 knock-out mice. *J Neurosci* 28: 8724–8734.

Polleux, F. et al. (2001). Pre- and post-mitotic events contribute to the progressive acquisition of area-specific connectional fate in the neocortex. *Cereb Cortex* 11: 1027–1039.

Polleux, F. et al. (1997). The timetable of laminar neurogenesis contributes to the specification of cortical areas in mouse isocortex. *J Comp Neurol* 385: 95–116.

Pontrelli, G. et al. (2014). Epilepsy in patients with duplications of chromosome 14 harboring FOXG1. *Pediatr Neurol* 50: 530–535.

Pouchelon, G. et al. (2014). Modality-specific thalamocortical inputs instruct the identity of postsynaptic L4 neurons. *Nature* 511: 471–474.

Preissl, S. et al. (2018). Single-nucleus analysis of accessible chromatin in developing mouse forebrain reveals cell-type-specific transcriptional regulation. *Nat Neurosci* 21: 432–439.

Rakic, P. (1988). Specification of cerebral cortical areas. *Science* 241: 170–176.

Rash, B.G. and Grove, E.A. (2007). Patterning the dorsal telencephalon. *J Neurosci* 27: 11595–11603.

Ritter, D.I. et al. (2010). The importance of being Cis. *Mol Biol Evol* 27: 2322–2332.

Rossi, J.J. et al. (2021). Molecular characterisation of rare loss-of-function NPAS3 and NPAS4 variants identified in individuals with neurodevelopmental disorders. *Sci Rep* 11: 6602.

Sahara, S. et al. (2007). Sp8 exhibits reciprocal induction with Fgf8 but has an opposing effect on anterior-posterior cortical area patterning. *Neural Dev* 2: 10–10.

Sansom, S.N. et al. (2009). The level of the transcription factor Pax6 is essential for controlling the balance between neural stem cell self-renewal and neurogenesis. *Plos Genet* 5: e1000511.

Saulnier, A. et al. (2013). The doublesex homolog Dmrt5 is required for the development of the caudomedial cerebral cortex in mammals. *Cereb Cortex* 23: 2552–2567.

Scala, F. et al. (2019). Layer 4 of mouse neocortex differs in cell types and circuit organization between sensory areas. *Nat Commun* 10: 4174.

Seelke, A.M.H. et al. (2016). Individual differences in cortical connections of somatosensory cortex are associated with parental rearing style in prairie voles (Microtus ochrogaster). *J Comp Neurol* 524: 564–577.

Sessa, A. et al. (2016). The Tbr2 molecular network controls cortical neuronal differentiation through complementary genetic and epigenetic pathways. *Cereb Cortex* 27 (6): 3378–3396.

Shetty, A.S. et al. (2013). Lhx2 regulates a cortex-specific mechanism for barrel formation. *Proc Natl Acad Sci* 110: E4913–E4921.

Shibata, M. et al. (2021). Regulation of prefrontal patterning and connectivity by retinoic acid. *Nature* 598: 483–488.

Shimamura, K. and Rubenstein, J.L. (1997). Inductive interactions direct early regionalization of the mouse forebrain. *Development* 124: 2709–2718.

Shimogori, T. et al. (2004). Embryonic signaling centers expressing BMP, WNT and FGF proteins interact to pattern the cerebral cortex. *Development* 131: 5639–5647.

Simonet, J.C. et al. (2015). Conditional loss of Arx from the developing dorsal telencephalon results in behavioral phenotypes resembling mild human *ARX* mutations. *Cereb Cortex* 25: 2939–2950.

Skoglund, T.S. et al. (1996). Heterogeneity in the columnar number of neurons in different neocortical areas in the rat. *Neurosci Lett* 208: 97–100.

Snetkova, V. et al. (2022). Perfect and imperfect views of ultraconserved sequences. *Nat Rev Genet* 23: 182–194.

Snetkova, V. et al. (2021). Ultraconserved enhancer function does not require perfect sequence conservation. *Nat Genet* 53: 521–528.

Song, M. et al. (2020). 3D epigenomic characterization reveals insights into gene regulation and lineage specification during corticogenesis. *BioRxiv*. doi: 10.1101/2020.02.24.963652.

Spigoni, G. et al. (2010). Regulation of Emx2 expression by antisense transcripts in murine cortico-cerebral precursors. *Plos One* 5: e8658.

Stenman, J. et al. (2003a). Tlx and Pax6 co-operate genetically to establish the pallio-subpallial boundary in the embryonic mouse telencephalon. *Development* 130: 1113–1122.

Stenman, J.M. et al. (2003b). Tlx controls proliferation and patterning of lateral telencephalic progenitor domains. *J Neurosci* 23: 10568–10576.

Stocker, A.M. and O'Leary, DDM (2016). Emx1 is required for neocortical area patterning. *Plos One* 11: e0149900.

Stoykova, A. et al. (1996). Forebrain patterning defects in small eye mutant mice. *Development* 122: 3453–3465.

Stoykova, A. et al. (2000). Pax6 modulates the dorsoventral patterning of the mammalian telencephalon. *J Neurosci* 20: 8042–8050.

Suda, Y. et al. (2010). The same enhancer regulates the earliest Emx2 expression in caudal forebrain primordium, subsequent expression in dorsal telencephalon and later expression in the cortical ventricular zone. *Development* 137: 2939–2949.

Sun, T. et al. (2005). Early asymmetry of gene transcription in embryonic human left and right cerebral cortex. *Science* 308: 1794–1798.

Takei, Y. et al. (2021). Single-cell nuclear architecture across cell types in the mouse brain. *Science* 374: 586–594.

Tang, K. et al. (2015). COUP-TFs and eye development. *Biochimica Et Biophysica Acta (BBA) – Gene Regulatory Mechanisms* 1849: 201–209.

Tang, K. et al. (2010). COUP-TFs regulate eye development by controlling factors essential for optic vesicle morphogenesis. *Development* 137: 725–734.

Tasic, B. et al. (2018). Shared and distinct transcriptomic cell types across neocortical areas. *Nature* 563 (7729): 72–78.

Theil, T. et al. (1999). Gli3 is required for Emx gene expression during dorsal telencephalon development. *Development* 126: 3561–3571.

Theil, T. et al. (2002). Wnt and Bmp signalling cooperatively regulate graded Emx 2 expression in the dorsal telencephalon. *Development* 129: 3045–3054.

Thompson, A.C. et al. (2018). A novel enhancer near the Pitx1 gene influences development and evolution of pelvic appendages in vertebrates. *Elife* 7: e38555.

Tocco, C. et al. (2022). The topography of corticopontine projections is controlled by postmitotic expression of the area-mapping gene Nr2f1. *Development* 149: dev200026.

Tole, S. et al. (2000). Emx2 is required for growth of the hippocampus but not for hippocampal field specification. *J Neurosci* 20: 2618–2625.

Tole, S. and Hébert, J. (2020). Telencepalon patterning. In: *Pattern and Cell Type Specification in the Developing CNS and PNS*, 2e (ed. J.L.R. Rubenstein and R. Pakic), 23–48. San Diego, CA: Elsevier.

Tomassy, G.S. et al. (2010a). Area-specific temporal control of corticospinal motor neuron differentiation by COUP-TFI. *Proc Natl Acad Sci* 107: 3576–3581.

Tomassy, G.S. et al. (2010b). Development and regeneration of projection neuron subtypes of the cerebral cortex. *Sci Prog* 93: 151–169.

Ton, C.C.T. et al. (1991). Positional cloning and characterization of a paired box- and homeobox-containing gene from the aniridia region. *Cell* 67: 1059–1074.

Toresson, H. et al. (2000). Genetic control of dorsal-ventral identity in the telencephalon. *Development* 127: 4361–4371.

Torre-Ubieta, L.de la. et al. (2018). The dynamic landscape of open chromatin during human cortical neurogenesis. *Cell* 172: 289–304.e18.

Tuoc, T.C. et al. (2013). Chromatin regulation by BAF170 controls cerebral cortical size and thickness. *Dev Cell* 25: 256–269.

Turner, T.N. and Eichler, E.E. (2019). The role of de novo noncoding regulatory mutations in neurodevelopmental disorders. *Trends Neurosci* 42: 115–127.

Uebbing, S. et al. (2021). Massively parallel discovery of human-specific substitutions that alter enhancer activity. *Proc Natl Acad Sci* 118: e2007049118.

Urquhart, J.E. et al. (2016). DMRTA2 (DMRT5) is mutated in a novel cortical brain malformation. *Clin Genet* 89: 724–727.

Vaid, S. et al. (2018). A novel population of Hopx-dependent basal radial glial cells in the developing mouse neocortex. *Development* 145: dev169276.

Valdez, G. (2020). Formation and maturation of neuromuscular junctions. In: *Pattern and Cell Type Specification in the Developing CNS and PNS*, 2e (ed. J.L.R. Rubenstein and R. Pakic), 157–184. San Diego, CA: Elsevier.

Villavicencio, E.H. et al. (2000). The sonic hedgehog–patched–gli pathway in human development and disease. *Am J Hum Genet* 67: 1047–1054.

Visel, A. et al. (2007). VISTA enhancer browser—a database of tissue-specific human enhancers. *Nucleic Acids Res* 35: D88–D92.

Visel, A. et al. (2013). A high-resolution enhancer atlas of the developing telencephalon. *Cell* 152: 895–908.

Wang, B. et al. (2013). Loss of Gsx1 and Gsx2 function rescues distinct phenotypes in Dlx1/2 mutants. *J Comp Neurol* 521: 1561–1584.

Wang, T. and Xiong, J.-Q. (2016). The orphan nuclear receptor TLX/NR2E1 in neural stem cells and diseases. *Neurosci Bull* 32: 108–114.

Wenger, A.M. et al. (2013). The enhancer landscape during early neocortical development reveals patterns of dense regulation and co-option. *Plos Genet* 9: e1003728.

Whalen, S. et al. (2022). Machine-learning dissection of human accelerated regions in primate neurodevelopment. *BioRxiv*. doi: 10.1101/256313.

Won, H. et al. (2016). Chromosome conformation elucidates regulatory relationships in developing human brain. *Nature* 538: 523–527.

Xie, Q. et al. (2013). Pax6 interactions with chromatin and identification of its novel direct target genes in lens and forebrain. *Plos One* 8: e54507.

Xu, L. et al. (2021). Abnormal neocortex arealization and Sotos-like syndrome–associated behavior in Setd2 mutant mice. *Sci Adv* 7: eaba1180.

Yabut, O.R. et al. (2020). The neocortical progenitor specification program is established through combined modulation of SHH and FGF signaling. *J Neurosci* 40: 6872–6887.

Yao, Z. et al. (2021). A transcriptomic and epigenomic cell atlas of the mouse primary motor cortex. *Nature* 598: 103–110.

Yoshida, M. et al. (1997). Emx1 and Emx2 functions in development of dorsal telencephalon. *Development* 124: 101–111.

Ypsilanti, A.R. et al. (2021). Transcriptional network orchestrating regional patterning of cortical progenitors. *Proc Natl Acad Sci USA* 118: e2024795118.

Ypsilanti, A.R. and Rubenstein, J.L.R. (2016). Transcriptional and epigenetic mechanisms of early cortical development. *J Comp Neurol* 524: 609–629.

Yue, F. et al. (2014). A comparative encyclopedia of DNA elements in the mouse genome. *Nature* 515: 355–364.

Yun, K. et al. (2001). Gsh2 and Pax6 play complementary roles in dorsoventral patterning of the mammalian telencephalon. *Development* 128: 193–205.

Zembrzycki, A. et al. (2013). Sensory cortex limits cortical maps and drives top-down plasticity in thalamocortical circuits. *Nat Neurosci* 16: 1060–1067.

Zembrzycki, A. et al. (2007). Genetic interplay between the transcription factors Sp8 and Emx2 in the patterning of the forebrain. *Neural Dev* 2: 8–8.

Zembrzycki, A. et al. (2015). Postmitotic regulation of sensory area patterning in the mammalian neocortex by Lhx2. *Proc Natl Acad Sci* 112: 6736–6741.

Zhou, C. et al. (2001). COUP-TFI: an intrinsic factor for early regionalization of the neocortex. *Genes Dev* 15: 2054–2059.

Zhu, C. et al. (2021). Joint profiling of histone modifications and transcriptome in single cells from mouse brain. *Nat Methods* 18: 283–292.

Ziffra, R.S. et al. (2021). Single-cell epigenomics reveals mechanisms of human cortical development. *Nature* 598: 205–213.

22

Development of the Neocortical Area Map

Elizabeth A. Grove

Department of Neurobiology and the Institute for Neuroscience, University of Chicago, Chicago, USA

22.1 Introduction

The primary functional organization of neocortex is its division into specialized areas, which form a map across the cortical sheet. To date, most studies of how the areas are positioned in the map have used mice as their model system and focused on the primary motor and sensory areas that take up most of mouse neocortex. Although carnivores, primates, and even mice have many additional prominent areas, the primary areas have strikingly similar positions in each brain (Krubitzer and Stolzenberg 2014; Nauta and Feirtag 1986). Thus, across those mammalian species examined, primary visual cortex (V1) is posterior in the cortical hemisphere, the primary somatosensory area (S1) anterior to V1, and primary motor cortex (M1) anterior to S1. Primary auditory cortex (A1) is lateral to V1. Recent studies of the human neocortex stress its much greater complexity in development, for example, a far more intricate program of neurogenesis (Cadwell et al. 2019; LaMonica et al. 2012; Lui et al. 2011). Nonetheless, similarities in the area map suggest that the most basic organization of the map and at least some mechanisms of area patterning, are conserved across mammals (Nauta and Feirtag 1986).

22.1.1 Classic Models of Neocortical Area Patterning

Two contrasting models of the development of the area map were proposed over 30 years ago, but still cause controversy. Either one could be consistent with the conserved area pattern described, as could a mix of both. In the "protomap" model, neocortex is patterned as progenitor cells are dividing in the neocortical primordium (NP). Areas are specified by "molecular determinants" in the ventricular zone (VZ), forming the template of the map. New-born neurons then migrate out of the VZ in radial arrays and carry the map with them (Rakic 1988). The orderly columns of migrating neurons seen in embryonic monkey brains, reaching from the VZ to the cortical plate, fostered this model. In the "protocortex" model, by contrast, the NP is a blank slate that is patterned into areas only by thalamic input (O'Leary 1989). This model was grounded on the relatively uniform cytoarchitecture of the prenatal neocortex, particularly in rodents, and the striking plasticity of area features caused by manipulating thalamic input (O'Leary 1989). Neither author intended the protomap and protocortex models to be as narrow as represented above; they are presented in this way to emphasize key points. Both proposals brought long-lasting attention to

Neocortical Neurogenesis in Development and Evolution, First Edition. Edited by Wieland B. Huttner.

how the neocortical area map is set up. The central questions are whether the positions and boundaries of areas in the neocortical map are determined by thalamic input, or by molecular factors intrinsic to the NP. If by both, what are their respective contributions to the area map? At present, the consensus appears to be that broad "proto-regions" (Cadwell et al. 2019) are established in the NP by intrinsic mechanisms, but that thalamocortical afferents (TCAs) initiate activity-dependent mechanisms that divide regions into areas. This chapter argues for a more prominent role for mechanisms intrinsic to the NP.

First described are studies that support the protocortex theory. It is a persuasive model given that each area is ultimately defined by its specific functions, receiving innervation from different thalamic nuclei relaying specific information. The thalamic input an area receives is therefore central to its functional identity. It is important, however, to separate the questions of how areas are specified and positioned with respect to one another in the developing mouse neocortex from how subsequent area-specific function arises.

Second is a discussion of candidate "molecular determinants" central to the protomap theory. Morphogenesis of other structures in the embryo is controlled by signaling centers that often lie at the boundaries of the tissue primordium. These centers release signaling proteins, termed morphogens, which disperse through the tissue as gradients and confer positional information (Wolpert 1996). Morphogens further regulate the spatially patterned expression of genes encoding transcription factors, continuing the patterning process. In the ventral spinal cord, in which these processes have been well studied, transcription factors activated by morphogens antagonize each other's expression, resulting in bounded regions of progenitor cells that give rise to different spinal cord cell types (Briscoe and Ericson 2001; Briscoe et al. 2000). How far development of the neocortical area map could be regulated by similar mechanisms is discussed in the second part of this chapter.

22.2 Thalamic Mechanisms of Area Development

22.2.1 Thalamic Axon Trajectories and Establishing Area Position

Gene expression patterns that demarcate areas in the postnatal mouse neocortex appear only gradually during the first week after birth in mice. By postnatal day (P)6, areas are sharply delineated (Figure 22.1). Over the same week, thalamocortical afferents (TCAs) enter, proliferate, and synapse in the neocortex. A clear possibility is that TCAs induce the expression of the gene expression patterns as well as other developmental area-specific features.

Substantial advances in understanding thalamocortical pathway development have supported the protocortex model. Major steps were the recognition of intermediate targets for thalamocortical axons, and identification of the molecular guidance molecules at work at each stage. Axons are guided out of the thalamus, through the ventral telencephalon, into and through the incipient internal capsule (IC). The cues along and adjacent to the trajectory include chemorepellant and chemoattractant axon guidance molecules, together with guidepost cells that form an essential permissive "corridor" through the otherwise nonpermissive basal telencephalon (Anton-Bolanos et al. 2018; Deck et al. 2013; Garel and Rubenstein 2004; Lopez-Bendito et al. 2006; Powell et al. 2008; Vanderhaeghen and Polleux 2004).

Thalamocortical axons are ordered from the source through the IC such that axons from different thalamic nuclei remain largely segregated and exit the IC at appropriate positions relative to the anterior/posterior (A/P) and medial/lateral (M/L) axes of the NP (Anton-Bolanos et al. 2018; Garel and Lopez-Bendito 2014; López-Bendito 2018; Powell et al. 2008). The orderliness of the thalamic axons headed for different parts of the neocortex gives a partial explanation of how a

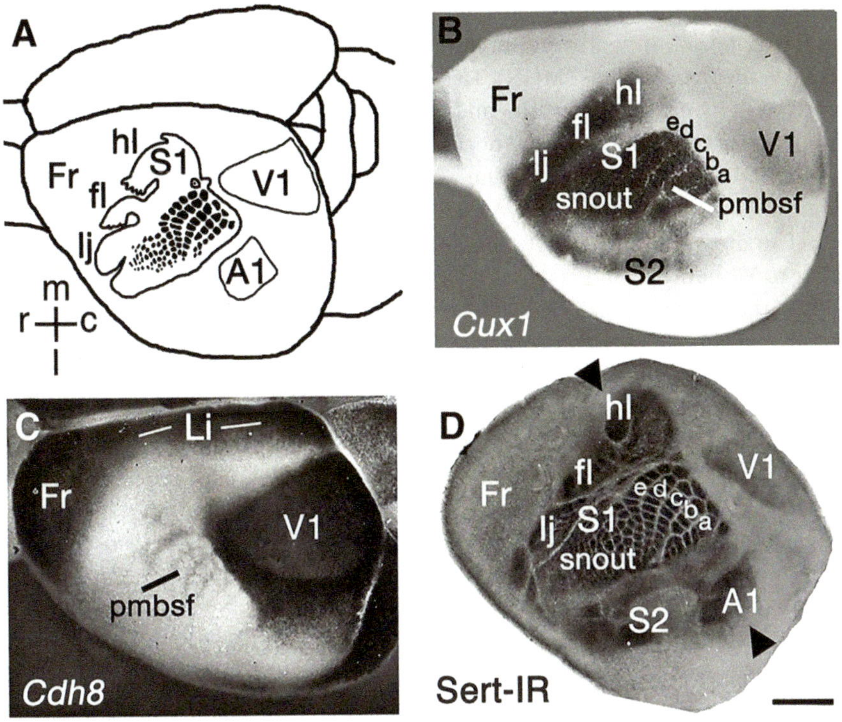

Figure 22.1 Areas are outlined by gene and protein expression by the end of first week after birth. Areas visible by the expression of a variety of genes and proteins develop during the first postnatal week in mice. Many of them are primary and secondary sensory areas; others are limbic and frontal areas. None is yet fully functional. (A) schematic of a mouse brain at P6 in a dorso-lateral view, showing positions of S1, V1, and A1. S1 hl, fl, and lj representations are rostral to the whisker barrel fields (barrels in black). Orientation of the map: rostral (r), caudal (c), medial (m), and lateral (l) indicated at lower left. (B–D) Several areas clearly delineated include S1, S2, V1, A1. (B, C) Whole P6 hemispheres processed for in situ hybridization for *Cux1* and *Cdh8*. *Cux1* is expressed in V1, S1, and S2 (B); *Cdh8* expression of different intensities distinguishes V1 from higher order visual areas lateral to V1 (C). Frontal (Fr) and limbic (Li) regions comprise areas distinguished by other markers. (D) A horizontal section through a flattened P6 cortex processed for serotonin transporter immunoreactivity (SERT-IR). Subfields of S1 and individual barrels (a–e) are clear. V1 is a triangular shape pointing toward rostral rows of the posteromedial barrel subfields (pmbsf). A1 is roughly oval, lateral to V1 and S1. Scale bar in D is 1 mm (for B–D). Arrowheads in (D) indicate rostro-medial to caudo-lateral. Abbreviations: fl, forelimb; hl, hindlimb; lj, lower jaw.

protocortex model could work in practice. Presorted thalamocortical axons arrive beneath the neocortex, interact synaptically with the subplate (SP), and require perhaps one more permissive cue to enter neocortex. Once there, thalamocortical synaptic activity could stamp an identity on each area. Other observations, however, discussed further later, indicate that the trajectories of TCAs are not so straightforward, and that final determination of where axons terminate is strongly regulated by the neocortex itself.

22.2.2 Active Thalamic Innervation Determines Function in a Cortical Area

The function of an area depends on the kind of information it receives from the thalamus, as well as from other areas of neocortex. Striking studies show that manipulating sensory modality of thalamic input that reaches a sensory area through the thalamus, can change not only its function but also induce anatomical features characteristic of a different area. In a classic study of the developing ferret, retinal inputs were forced to innervate the auditory nucleus of the thalamus, the medial geniculate nucleus (MGN). To route visual projections to auditory cortex, the retina was deprived of its major targets, the midbrain superior colliculus and the thalamic lateral geniculate nucleus (LGN). Meanwhile, normal auditory input to the MGN was interrupted surgically. Retinal afferents populated the deafferented MGN so that the MGN now relayed visual information to A1. In rewired A1 a new, systematic representation of visual space was created. The direction and orientation selectivity of visual stimuli in rewired A1 neurons was similar to V1 neurons and rewired A1 contained neurons with simple and complex receptive fields in the same proportion as V1. Remarkably, the specific sensory modality of thalamic input to rewired A1 not only controlled its function, but also its intra-area circuitry, which became more characteristic of V1. Nonetheless, rewired A1 retained its connections with other auditory areas and did not make V1-like connections with visual areas. Even visually rewired A1 maintained some of its original area identity. These findings emphasize the importance of the modality and pattern of thalamic input on the development of a neocortical area, but suggest that these factors interact with an intrinsic developmental program of area identity (Pallas and Sur 1993; Roe et al. 1990, 1992; Sur 1993; Sur et al. 1988, 1990; Sur and Rubenstein 2005).

A more recent study in mice underscores the importance of modality specific inputs (Pouchelon et al. 2014). In S1 and the secondary somatosensory area, S2, layer 4 cells normally receive mutually exclusive input from the somatosensory ventroposteromedial (VPM) relay nucleus, or the posterior nucleus of the thalamus (PO). The VPM relays tactile information from the whiskers and PO carries nociceptive input. After genetic ablation of the VPM in neonatal mice, axons from the PO innervated layer 4 cells in S2 as usual, but also invaded layer 4 of S1, the normal target of VPM. In response, layer 4 neurons in S1 downregulated genes they normally express, and upregulated expression of characteristic genes in S2. Functionally rewired S1 layer 4 neurons now responded to nociceptive input, and weakly to tactile input. Innervation by PO thus caused a convergence of normally segregated sensory modalities and gave S1 layer 4 cells a functionally hybrid identity. The findings indicate a strong influence of input modality on neocortical neurons, but again suggest an enduring underlying program of area specification.

22.2.3 Plasticity of Sensory Area Size

Classic studies in monkeys report that removing the eyes reduces the size of the LGN and causes V1 (area 17) to shrink, indicating that the size of an area depends on the volume of its thalamic innervation As V1 shrinks, adjacent neocortex increases in size. In the region lost from V1, Rakic identified an "area X," differing in cytoarchitecture from either V1 and V2 (Rakic et al. 1991). The appearance of this new region fits a modified protomap model in which an area is generated by both intrinsic and extrinsic signals (Rakic et al. 1991). Support comes from a subsequent enucleation experiment showing that in the region lost from V1, patterns of acetylcholinesterase and cytochrome oxidase reflecting functional features in visual cortex, differed from normal V1 and V2 (Dehay et al. 1996).

In both monkey and mouse, areas normally differ in progenitor cell cycle kinetics, a feature of early area differences (Dehay and Kennedy 2007; Polleux et al. 1997). Signals from thalamic axons are proposed to underlie these differences, regulating the output of neurons from both radial glial cell progenitors and the intermediate progenitor cells that amplify neuron generation (Dehay and Kennedy 2007). Thalamic signals regulating progenitor cell behavior may be more significant in primates, in which thalamocortical axons innervate the SP much earlier than in mice, providing an earlier proximity of progenitor cells to signals from TCAs (Alzu'bi et al. 2019).

Spontaneous retinal activity coordinates activity-based patterning in the visual system (Ackman et al. 2012). Retinal waves mediate the development of eye-specific layers in the dLGN and ocular dominance columns in V1. Retinal waves include the entire retinal visual field, require cholinergic neurotransmission, and exhibit spatiotemporal correlations between the two hemispheres (Ackman et al. 2012). Spontaneous activity in the somatosensory system, and its possible roles in development, have been less studied. Recently, however, spontaneous calcium waves were identified in the mouse, propagating across the sensory relay nuclei of the thalamus. The waves, which appear at late embryonic ages and last until a few days after birth, are proposed as a basis for interaction among thalamic nuclei. Manipulating wave patterns trigger changes in cortical area size and thalamic expression of activity-dependent genes, for example the TF gene *Rorb*, which plays a role in barrel-field development in S1 (Moreno-Juan et al. 2017).

22.2.4 Thalamic Activity and Somatosensory Barrel Fields

The S1 barrel fields are an example of an area-specific feature whose development appears virtually wholly controlled by thalamic afferents. Rodents display neocortical "barrels" in S1, each of which corresponds to one of the large facial whiskers, or the smaller whiskers on the snout. The layout of the barrels matches the pattern of peripheral whiskers, making the barrel fields the most visually prominent element of the rodent area map. A barrel "hollow" contains clustered thalamocortical afferents relaying input from one whisker via the somatosensory thalamic relay nucleus, which contains "barreloids" that match the peripheral whisker pattern. Layer 4 S1 neurons collect around each hollow to form the barrel "walls," and direct their dendrites inwards to receive thalamic input. Formation of the barrels is activity dependent. When glutamatergic activity is sufficiently reduced in TCA connections, barrels do not appear, and layer 4 neurons do not develop a normal morphology (Li et al. 2013).

A newer study suggests that spontaneous calcium wave activity in the thalamocortical pathway travels to nascent S1 and is responsible for forming columnar territories in S1, and ultimately the S1 barrel fields (Anton-Bolanos et al. 2018). When calcium waves are disrupted by extreme hyperpolarization of thalamic neurons, the barrel fields fail to develop, even when the mice are allowed to grow up and use their whiskers (Anton-Bolanos et al. 2019). These observations raise the possibility that spontaneous activity in the embryo pre-patterns the barrel fields, although barrels are not clearly visible for a few days after birth. Nonetheless, blocking glutamatergic transmission also prevents barrel formation (Li et al. 2013), so either both types of activity are needed sequentially for barrel-field development, or experience-driven activity is required to maintain the barrel pattern. The roles of spontaneous activity in the developing somatosensory system clearly deserves closer study.

22.2.5 Transcription Factor *Lhx2* Allows S1 Cortex to Respond to Thalamic Input

In addition to the critical need for activity in generating the S1 barrel fields, two studies indicate an initial requirement for a factor intrinsic to neocortex. The transcription factor gene, *Lhx2*, identified as a "selector gene" for the cerebral cortex (Mangale et al. 2008) serves several functions in cortical development. When *Lhx2* is selectively removed from the cerebral cortex in either progenitor cells or postmitotic neurons, S1 barrel fields are, respectively, absent (Shetty et al. 2013), or abnormal (Wang et al. 2017), indicating that activity dependent patterning of S1 depends on the presence of *Lhx2*. When *Lhx2* is deleted at embryonic day 11.5 (E11.5), the barrel fields are lost. Surprisingly TCAs innervate mutant neocortex with "apparently normal regional specificity" (Shetty et al. 2013). Within this S1 region, neurons do not fire in response to individual whiskers but do fire after stimulation of multiple whiskers (Shetty et al. 2013). TCAs have not segregated into barrels despite synaptic activity.

TCAs normally synapse with layer 4 neurons in S1 barrel walls. When *Lhx2* is deleted in postmitotic neurons TCAs gather into small barrel-like shapes, but cell walls do not form correctly, and individual neurons do not orient their dendrites towards TCAs. *Lhx2* upregulates expression of several activity-regulated genes, including *Btbd3* (Matsui et al. 2013), required for dendrite orientation. The conclusions are that (1) Lhx2 is required first to allow layer 4 neurons to respond to thalamocortical inputs, develop dendritic asymmetry, and form barrel walls, and (2) that Lhx2 induces development of some of the activity-dependent genes required for S1 differentiation. These findings indicate an interesting interplay between TCA activity and dependence on Lhx2 function that together forms the barrel fields.

22.3 Mechanisms of Area Patterning Intrinsic to Neocortex

22.3.1 Neocortex is Not a Blank Slate at Birth

The idea that perinatal neocortex is a blank state without TCA input was demolished by findings in mutant mice with little or no thalamic innervation (Miyashita-Lin et al. 1999; Nakagawa et al. 1999; Zhou et al. 2010). Early development of the thalamus requires the transcription factor Gbx2. In mice in which *Gbx2* was constitutively deleted, thalamocortical projections were virtually absent. Yet delimited regions of expression of several genes, including *Id2, Epha7, Rorb, Tbr1*, and *Cdh6*, appeared highly similar in wild-type and mutant mice at birth (Miyashita-Lin et al. 1999). *Mash1*-deficient mice with aberrant thalamocortical pathfinding also showed normal regional gene expression (Nakagawa et al. 1999).

Neither mouse line with constitutive deletion of *Gbx2* or *Mash1* lived for more than a day or two after birth. The area map, as distinguished by the expression of several genes, emerges over the first week after birth and area boundaries are clear by the end of the first week. The clear question is whether mice with deficient or no thalamic innervation would develop an area map like that of wild-type mice. Mouse neocortex lacking both thalamocortical and corticothalamic axons, the "cortex isole," showed normal region-specific gene expression as well as other typical neocortical features at P6, though not at P20 when the cortex has deteriorated (Zhou et al. 2010). Whether regional gene expression at P6 marks individual areas was not directly examined. Mice with a conditional deletion of *Gbx2* in thalamus live for several weeks after birth (Vue et al. 2013). These mice have a highly abnormal thalamus and severe loss of thalamocortical axons. Just before birth, expression of *Id2, Rorb, Lmo4*, and *Cdh8* in regions is similar in mutant mice and controls, but, at P8, no specific areas are distinct (Vue et al. 2013). A future investigation of patterned gene expression on each day through the first postnatal week may be useful. A possibility is that areas may begin to form perinatally but require TCAs for maintenance. P8 could be after an intrinsic area pattern begins to degenerate.

22.3.2 Secreted Signaling Molecules that Establish Area Position

In the embryonic vertebrate spinal cord, several morphogens determine the dorsal/ventral (D/V) axis. One of these, sonic hedgehog (SHH), generated by the ventral floorplate and notochord, disperses in a high ventral to low dorsal gradient in the spinal cord primordium. The gradient of SHH regulates expression of different transcription factors at different D/V positions in the nascent spinal cord. Next, pairs of transcription factors repress one another's expression, creating progenitor domains with distinct gene expression boundaries. These progenitor cell pools generate a range of ventral spinal cord neuron types, including motor neurons (Briscoe and Ericson 2001; Briscoe et al. 2000). In the dorsal half of the spinal cord, members of other signaling molecule families, bone morphogenetic proteins (BMPs) and wingless-related integration site (WNT) proteins regulate dorsal cell type, and the fate of neural crest cells originating in the dorsal cord (Dorsky et al. 1998; Liem et al. 1997, 1995). More immediately relevant to patterning the mammalian neocortex, patterning the telencephalon in chick is coordinately regulated by sources of BMP4, SHH, and fibroblast growth factor 8 (FGF8) (Crossley et al. 2001; Ohkubo et al. 2002). Why should mammalian neocortex, which derives from the dorsal telencephalon, be different?

Patterning molecules are characteristically located at the poles and boundaries of the tissue to be patterned. Before anterior neural tube closure, several FGF genes, including *Fgf8*, *Fgf17*, and *Fgf18*, are expressed at the anterior neural ridge (ANR) (Bachler and Neubuser 2001; Crossley and Martin 1995). Once the tube closes, *Fgf* genes continue to be expressed at the anterior pole of each developing telencephalic hemisphere (Bachler and Neubuser 2001; Cholfin and Rubenstein 2007, 2008; Crossley and Martin 1995), forming in each hemisphere, an "anterior telencephalic organizer" (ATO). At the telencephalic dorsal midline, in the early embryo, multiple *Bmp* genes are expressed; subsequently both *Bmp* and *Wnt* genes are expressed in a region that develops at the midline, the dorso-medial edge of the cortical primordium, termed the cortical hem (Furuta et al. 1997; Grove et al. 1998). The cortical hem and ATO appear in other mammals, too. The cortical hem is present in humans (Abu-Khalil et al. 2004), and both the ATO and hem in the ferret (Jones et al. 2019).

22.3.3 Fibroblast Growth Factor FGF8 Controls anterior to posterior (A/P) Area Position in the Map

The prominent role of FGF8 at the isthmic organizer, a signaling center between the midbrain and hindbrain, in A/P patterning of the midbrain (Crossley et al. 1996; Harada et al. 2016; Martinez et al. 1999), suggests that FGF8 from the ATO, potentially in concert with other FGFs, confers A/P positional values to the NP. At E9.5–10.5 in the mouse, FGF8 disperses across the NP from anterior to posterior as a gradient with an exponential decline (Toyoda et al. 2010), meeting criteria for a morphogen as described by Louis Wolpert (Wolpert 1996).

Mice strongly hypomorphic for *Fgf8* die at birth, before neocortical areas are distinct. Regulating levels of *Fgf8* gene expression in the mouse NP with in-utero microelectroporation (IUME), however, results in mouse pups that are born normally and live for several weeks (Assimacopoulos et al. 2012; Fukuchi-Shimogori and Grove 2001; Toyoda et al. 2010). Excess anterior FGF8 augments endogenous FGF8, and a dominant negative construct of an FGF8 receptor, *dnfgfr3c* sequesters FGF8, reducing available levels (Toyoda et al. 2010). At these early embryonic ages, plasmids are quickly diluted out by cell division, consequently, NP cells are effectively exposed to excess, ectopic, or decreased FGF8 for only 2–3 days, commensurate with the normal time of exposure to the endogenous source. At P6, expression of several genes and proteins marks out sensory and motor area boundaries (Figure 22.1 shows some of these). Increased anterior FGF8 at E10.5 or

E11.5 enlarges anterior areas observed at P6 and shrinks more posterior areas, pushing area boundaries posteriorly. For example, the whisker barrel fields of S1, normally centrally located in the cortical hemisphere, are shifted into the posterior half of the hemisphere. Opposite shifts follow anterior electroporation of *dnfgfr3c* into the embryonic NP (Fukuchi-Shimogori and Grove 2001). These changes suggested that FGF8 establishes A/P position in the NP. To test this definitively, *Fgf8* was electroporated into the posterior NP creating a second FGF8 source opposite the endogenous anterior source. The new FGF8 source induced a duplicate or partial duplicate of S1 barrel fields that is mirror-reversed along the A/P axis relative to the native S1 (Figure 22.2). Posterior FGF8 locally reset the A/P axis of the NP, emphasizing that FGF8 establishes position in the neocortical area map (Fukuchi-Shimogori and Grove 2001). Notably, positional values are sufficiently fine grained that a second, posterior FGF8 source induces secondary barrel fields similar in size to the endogenous fields and correctly arrayed individual barrels in each distinct barrel row (Assimacopoulos et al. 2012).

As previously mentioned, formation of the S1 barrel fields requires active innervation by TCAs. The ability of ectopic FGF8 to generate duplicate barrel fields implies that FGF8 initiates a cascade of events in neocortex that lead to duplicate and ectopic innervation by somatosensory TCAs.

Dramatically, following a mid-lateral electroporation of *Fgf8*, the hemisphere splits into two at the site of electroporation, as also occurs in chick (Assimacopoulos et al. 2012; Crossley et al. 2001). Gene expression typical of the rostral telencephalic midline appears on both sides of the gap. In the posterior half of the neocortical hemisphere, a new map forms in response to the closer FGF8 source, containing putative S1, V1, and A1 (Figure 22.2). FGF8, therefore, positions not just S1 but probably all neocortical areas along the A/P axis (Assimacopoulos et al. 2012).

Confirming the role of FGF8 in A/P patterning of the neocortex, mice mildly hypomorphic for *Fgf8* show an anterior shift in the expression boundaries of regionally expressed genes in the NP (Garel et al. 2003). That is, expression of genes with a high posterior, low anterior NP gradient shift anteriorly. Among the genes examined were those encoding the transcription factors, Emx2 and Nr2f1, directly involved in area patterning (see later). Further, FGF17 is required for normal patterning of areas in the most anterior neocortex (Cholfin and Rubenstein 2007, 2008), but has a lesser effect than FGF8 on A/P patterning of the entire neocortex (Assimacopoulos et al. 2012).

22.3.4 FGF8 Indirectly Controls Trajectories of Thalamic Axons

Axons from the somatosensory relay nucleus, the VPM, faithfully track changes in S1 area position and innervate both shifted and duplicated S1. Functional innervation in duplicated S1 is indicated by the loss of barrels in both endogenous and duplicate S1 after ablating the corresponding whisker follicles (Assimacopoulos et al. 2012). These observations indicate that shifted or duplicated areas could attract thalamic axons to ectopic targets as the axons grew in, raising the question of where in the NP ectopic guidance cues are positioned.

22.3.5 Thalamic Axon Guidance Cues in the Subplate and Neocortex

Thalamic axons interact with the SP to innervate target areas (Allendoerfer and Shatz 1994; Finney et al. 1998; Friauf et al. 1990; Ghosh et al. 1990; Ghosh and Shatz 1993; Herrmann et al. 1994). Local damage of the SP prevents the entry of axons into their target cortical area (Ghosh et al. 1990), and in reeler mutants, thalamocortical axons grow to the displaced SP near the cortical surface, before diving down to innervate the layers of the neocortex (Caviness and Frost 1983). Evidently, thalamocortical axons are required to contact the SP before synapsing with neurons in the layers of the neocortex. Additionally, active synaptic interactions between thalamic axons and

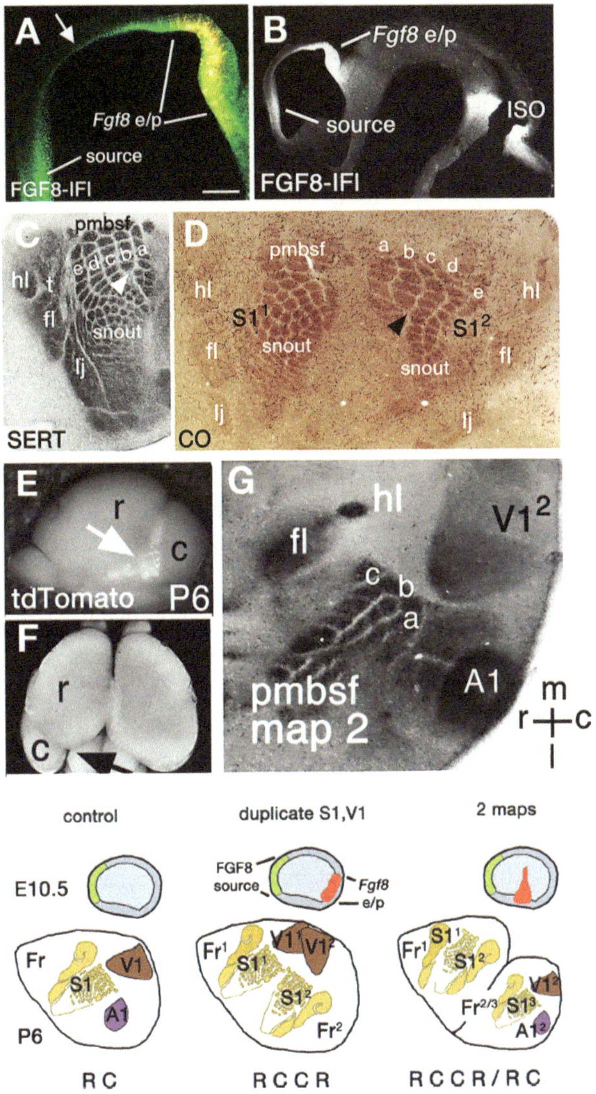

Figure 22.2 Duplicate S1 barrel fields and a secondary map generated by ectopic FGF8 sources. (A, B) Sagittal sections through an E11.5 mouse brain. Positions of the endogenous source of FGF8 and a caudal ectopic source in one mouse embryo, one day after electroporation. Rostral is to the left. (A) higher magnification of leftmost part of (B), showing double, opposing gradients of FGF8 (green). The posterior electroporation site is marked by tdTomato fluorescence (red) that when superimposed on FGF8 IFL appears yellow. An arrow indicates roughly where the FGF8 gradient begins to reverse between the two sources (B) provides a comparison of the levels of FGF8 in the electroporation site, the ATO and the isthmic organizer (ISO), which patterns the midbrain. (C, D) (C) shows the wild-type orientation and subfields of S1 (SERT-IR). In (D), a robust secondary $S1^2$ (right) faces the endogenous $S1^1$ (left) in a P6 brain in which *Fgf8* was electroporated at a posterior site at E10.5 (CO, Cytochrome oxidase). (E, F) Two views (lateral and dorsal) of a P6 mouse brain electroporated with *Fgf8* in a mid-lateral position, marked by tdTomato IFl, arrow in (E). This position of ectopic FGF8 splits the hemisphere into two parts (r, rostral and c, caudal, in E, F). (G) SERT-IR labels the "second map" that appears in the caudal half. The *Fgf8* electroporation site is rostral to the field in view. The forelimb (fl) and hindlimb (hl) and a part of the pmbsf of S1 are closer to the new FGF8 source than V1 or A1. Directions within the section shown at (G) lower right. Schematic below F, G illustrates a simple area map pattern in a control brain, a brain with a caudal electroporation site (top, red), and a brain with a mid-lateral electroporation site. Lettering below indicates the rostral (R) to caudal (C) axis changes in the two electroporated brains.

the SP are needed for neocortical target selection (Finney et al. 1998; Friauf et al. 1990; Herrmann et al. 1994). Blocking activity in SP neurons in cats, for example, greatly perturbs the density, pattern, and precision of LGN axons innervating V1 (Catalano and Shatz 1998). These authors left open, however, whether activity is instructive for growing thalamocortical axons, or permissive, allowing the axons to read target-derived molecular cues (Catalano and Shatz 1998). Experiments using timed electroporation of *Fgf8* suggests that molecular TCA guidance cues are present in both the SP and in the NP itself.

The SP and the true layers of the NP are generated in temporal order, with SP neurons born earliest. Thus, regional gene expression in the SP and putative regional identity are shifted by anterior IUME of *Fgf8* at E10.5, just as progenitor cells give rise to SP neurons. A day later, however, at E11.5, electroporation of *Fgf8*, shifts regional gene expression and regional identity in the NP but no longer in the SP where most neurons are now generated (Shimogori and Grove 2005). This serendipitous discovery allowed experiments that pulled the regional identities of the NP and SP in or out of register.

Following anterior *Fgf8* electroporation at E10.5, DiI staining from a deposit in the VPM at P5 labels axons that reach the cortex and travel posteriorly in the SP to a position beneath the shifted S1. The axons then cross the SP correctly to innervate the shifted S1 (Shimogori and Grove 2005). These observations confirm that FGF8 imparts A/P positional values to the SP (Figure 22.3). By contrast, anterior electroporation of *Fgf8* at E11.5 alters FGF8 levels after SP neurons are born, pulling the positional identity of NP and SP out of register. In this case, VPM axons cross the SP at the expected S1 location, then recognize the shifted S1 and travel posteriorly within the neocortex to innervate the shifted target area and form barrels in layer 4 (Figure 22.3) (Shimogori and Grove 2005).

The latter type of thalamocortical axon targeting is reminiscent of older experiments in which part of a presumptive area in the embryonic rat NP was dissected out and grafted into a different neocortical region in a neonatal rat (Frappe et al. 1999; Gaillard and Roger 2000). When, for example, a graft of presumptive frontal cortex was positioned in occipital cortex, thalamocortical axons first innervated the native frontal cortex in the host animal, then turned posteriorly, travelling through the NP, to innervate the graft (Frappe et al. 1999). These findings suggest both that area identity was determined in the embryonic cortical graft when it was explanted, and that the graft contained guidance cues for appropriate thalamic input. Together, results of the grafting experiments (Frappe et al. 1999; Gaillard and Roger 2000), and the effects on thalamocortical trajectories of electroporating anterior *Fgf8* or *Fgfr3c* at different ages indicate instructive, region-specific molecular cues in both the SP and NP (Shimogori and Grove 2005).

A superfluity of thalamocortical guidance cues is consistent with the complexity of the system. Thalamocortical axons do not generally exit the IC directly below the area to be innervated. Instead, the axons travel through the SP and enter the NP only when appropriate cues are available. Further, projections from thalamus to cortex do not come in a one-to-one ratio. Individual areas can receive input from several thalamic nuclei, and a single thalamic nucleus may innervate more than one area (Nauta and Feirtag 1986). Additionally, areas can be innervated by nuclei whose position in the thalamus does not correspond in a simple way to the position of the innervated areas. As examples: (1) the medio-dorsal nucleus, in the center of the thalamus, projects to prefrontal cortex; (2) the cingulate and retrosplenial areas are medial and stretch almost the whole A/P length of the mouse neocortex, yet receive input from anterior and lateral thalamic nuclei as well as the medial intralaminar nuclei and the medio-dorsal nucleus (Nauta and Feirtag 1986).

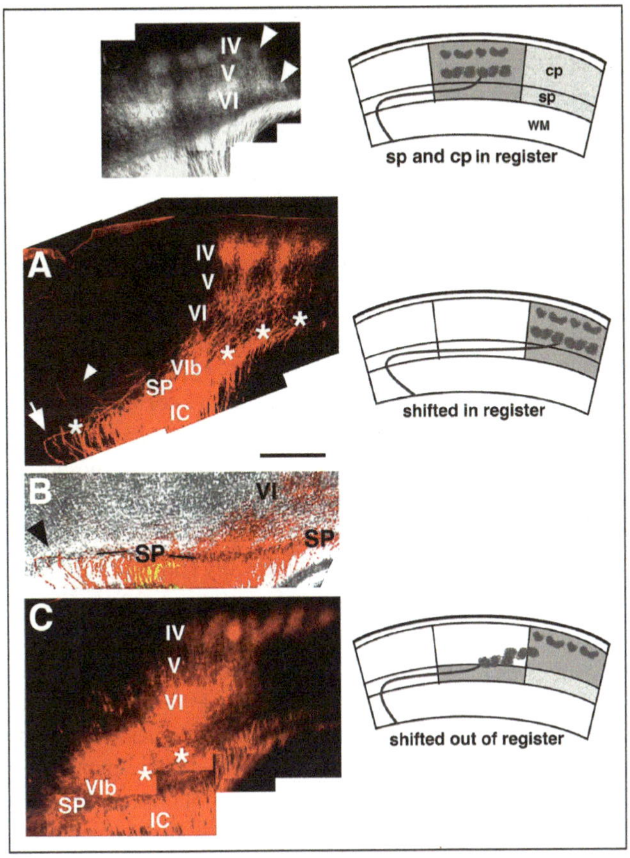

Figure 22.3 Brains with the SP and NP shifted in or out of register indicate cortical TCA guidance. Top image and schematic to right indicate the normal trajectory of TCAs in a wild-type brain and axon terminal puffs in layers 4 and 6. All brains are shown at P6, schematics at right represent TCA trajectory as TCAs enter the NP at about P0. (A, B, and schematic to right) When the SP and NP are shifted in register by an early *Fgf8* electroporation, most TCAs travel through the SP and enter the neocortical layers at the new correct site, suggesting area cues from the SP. (B and schematic to right) When the SP and NP are shifted out of register by a later *Fgf8* electroporation, when SP neurons are already generated, TCAs enter the NP at the normal site, then respond to putative cues from the shifted S1 and travel through the NP to innervate the shifted area.

22.3.6 Neocortical Patterning by the Cortical Hem

A second candidate signaling center, the cortical hem, lies along the medial edge of the cortex, next to the hippocampus, and expresses *Wnt* and *Bmp* genes (Furuta et al. 1997; Grove et al. 1998). The hem is most important as an organizer for the hippocampus (Mangale et al. 2008), and without the hem, or beta-catenin-mediated WNT signaling from the hem, only a tiny remnant hippocampus develops (Galceran et al. 2000; Lee et al. 2000). In neocortex, genetic deletion of the hem causes a reduction of dorso-medial neocortex and an expansion of ventro-lateral cortex including olfactory cortex. The greatest loss of neocortex in is in the posterior, occipital region, where primary and secondary visual areas develop.

The hem therefore influences both the A/P and M/L axes of neocortex.

22.3.7 *Emx2*, *Dmrt3* and *5*, *Nr2f1*, and Cortical Patterning

As signaling sources, both the hem and the ATO shrink and finally disappear as embryogenesis progresses and the brain grows larger. Local sources of FGF8 play other roles in cortical development, for example in the generation of anterior Cajal–Retzius cells (Zimmer et al. 2009). The germinal zone of the NP, however, becomes too large to allow widespread dispersion of FGF8 or WNT proteins. Positional information is carried on by transcription factors (TFs) expressed in gradients across the NP shaped by FGF8 and WNT3a signaling. Several TFs have been identified that regulate the position of areas in the neocortical map (O'Leary et al. 2007). The difference between neocortex and spinal cord patterning is that TFs in the VZ or subventricular zone (SVZ) (Elsen et al. 2018) of the NP do not show a sharpening of expression boundaries and remain primarily in gradients. This has been a continuing puzzle in understanding neocortical area patterning because the TF gradients do not seem to give rise to sharp boundaries as in the spinal cord. In another chapter in this book, Ypsilanti and Rubenstein systematically identify a larger panel of TFs expressed in the mouse neocortical VZ, as well as gene regulatory elements for several of these TFs. The hypothesis is that protoareas for a protomap arise from the integration of TF gradients by VZ enhancers to create sharp boundaries. This chapter will therefore focus on only a few TF genes that have been shown to regulate the area map, particularly those that reciprocally control expression of *Fgf8* and *Wnt3a*. Finally, *Nr2f1* is of particular interest because its functions in the neocortex neatly link area, layer, and cell-type development (Faedo et al. 2008)

The first TF genes shown to pattern the area map were *Emx2* (Bishop et al. 2000; Mallamaci et al. 2000), an ortholog of the *Drosophila* genes *empty spiracles* (*ems*), and *Pax6* (*small-eye*, orthologous to *Drosophila eyeless*) (Bishop et al. 2000). Both *ems* and *eyeless* have central roles in generating head structures in the fly. *Emx2* has a posteromedial-high to anterolateral-low expression gradient in the mouse NP, and accordingly, in perinatal mice lacking *Emx2* function, posteromedial NP regions shrink, and anterior frontal NP expands (Mallamaci et al. 2000). *Pax6* is expressed in high anterolateral to low posteromedial gradient in the NP, and mice lacking *Pax6* function *(sey/sey)* show opposite gene expression shifts to those in the *Emx2* mutant (Bishop et al. 2000, 2002b). Posterior shifts of gene expression at E18.5 in the *Emx2* mutant, opposed to anterior shifts in the *Pax6* mutant, were particularly striking in the case of gene pairs that are expressed in complementary patterns along the A/P axis (*Rorb* and *p75*; *Efna5* and *EphA7*) (Bishop et al. 2000, 2002a), suggesting that VZ expressed TFs may interact with one another across the neonatal NP. Mice constitutively deficient in *Emx2* die at or before birth. A transgenic mouse line carrying excess *Emx2* under the control of the Nestin promoter, however, lives past birth. Although excess *Emx2* is introduced throughout the NP expression still shows a high posterior to low anterior gradient. Excess Emx2 protein has the opposite effect of Emx2 loss, enlarging V1 and shrinking more anterior areas such as M1 (Hamasaki et al. 2004).

Emx2 not only has a direct role in patterning the neocortical area map, but also interacts with other TFs and with the morphogen genes *Fgf8*, *Fgf17*, and *Wnt3a* to modulate development of the map, with consequences that are still not fully understood (Cholfin and Rubenstein 2008; Fukuchi-Shimogori and Grove 2003). FGF8 inhibits and WNT3a increases expression of *Emx2*, consistent with the latter's high posteromedial to low anterior expression gradient (Caronia-Brown et al. 2014; Fukuchi-Shimogori and Grove 2003). Meanwhile, Emx2 maintains expression of *Wnt3a* at the hem, which is almost lost in the *Emx2* null mutant (Tole et al. 2000). Emx2 additionally suppresses *Fgf8* and *Fgf17* expression, and accordingly the expression domains of both *Fgf* genes expand in the *Emx2* null mouse (Cholfin and Rubenstein 2007; Fukuchi-Shimogori and Grove 2003). Thus, Emx2 and Wnt3a are together critical for development of caudo-medial cortex, rather as frontal cortex patterning is coordinately regulated by Emx2, Fgf8, and Fgf17 (Cholfin and Rubenstein 2008).

Dmrt3* and *Dmrt5/Dmrta2 *Dmrt* (*doublesex and mab-3 related transcription factor*) genes, often studied for their roles in sexual development, have more recently been investigated in developmental regulation and patterning of the cerebral cortex (Desmaris et al. 2018; Saulnier et al. 2012). Consistent with the latter role, in humans, *DMRTA2/DMRT5* has been associated with microcephaly and region-specific neocortical pachygyria (Urquhart et al. 2016). Both *Dmrt3* and *Dmrta2* are expressed in the mouse NP in high posterior to low anterior gradients, as is *Emx2*. FGF8 and WNT signaling regulate the gradients of *Dmrta2* and *Dmrt3* expression in the NP as for *Emx2* (Caronia-Brown et al. 2014) and reciprocally, like Emx2, Dmrt3/2a maintain expression of *Wnt3a* at the hem. Conditional deletion of *Dmrt2a* in the NP using *Nestin-Cre* or *Emx1-IRES-Cre* mice (Gorski et al. 2002; Tronche et al. 1999) reduced the size of the cortical hemisphere with a disproportionate reduction of V1 (De Clercq et al. 2018). Over-expression of *Dmrt5*, using a transgenic approach, enlarged V1 at the expense of more anterior areas, including M1 (De Clercq et al. 2018). These observations indicate a role for Dmrt5, like that of Emx2, in regulating area size and position, particularly in caudo-medial NP. These findings indicate that a small network of hem signaling proteins, Emx2, and the DMRT TFs are required for normal caudo-medial neocortex.

Couptf1/Nr2f1 Couptf1, now Nr2f1 (nuclear receptor subfamily 2, group F, member 1) is a nuclear orphan receptor that functions as a transcriptional repressor or an activator with different cofactors (Tsai and Tsai 1997). After mid-gestation in the mouse, *Nr2f1* is expressed in a steep high-posterior-to-low-anterior gradient in the NP, forming a relatively sharp boundary about two-thirds of the way along the posterior to anterior length of the hemisphere (Jones et al. 2019). Comparing across TFs with known functions in area patterning, the anterior boundary of Nr2f1 expression is probably the most distinct. The primary sensory areas, V1, A1, and S1, and secondary sensory areas arise from posterior and central progenitor cells that express *Nr2f1* strongly, whereas M1 and other areas of frontal cortex are generated by anterior progenitors that show little or no *Nr2f1* expression. In mice in which *Nr2f1* was conditionally deleted in cerebral cortex, sensory areas in postnatal neocortex were tiny and pushed to the back of the hemisphere (Armentano et al. 2007). The rest of the neocortex adopted features of motor cortex with respect to gene expression, input from VA/VL motor thalamic nuclei, and projections characteristic of motor cortex. These findings strongly suggested that Nr2f1 balances the territory allotted to motor versus sensory areas, and more specifically support a role for Nr2f1 in repressing frontal/motor area identity (Armentano et al. 2007).

Further analysis of the mutant focused on the role of Nr2f1 in differentiation of corticospinal motor neurons (CSMNs), which predominate in layer 5 of M1 (Tomassy et al. 2010). CSMN gene expression and projections were compared between M1 and S1 in wild-type mice and in comparable regions in a mutant mouse in which *Nr2f1* was conditionally deleted from the cerebral cortex. Strong expression of the transcription factor genes *Fezf2* and *Ctip2 (COUP-TF1 interacting protein 2)* is typical of CSMNs. In wild-type M1, expression of *Fezf2*, and *Ctip2* marks out a broad, dense layer 5, contrasting with a much thinner layer 5 in S1. In conditional *Nr2f1* null mutants, the NP at the normal coordinates of S1 displayed a massive increase in layer 5 neurons expressing *Fezf2* and *Ctip2* and other CSMN gene expression markers. That is, presumptive S1 had been "motorized." Consistent with this, retrograde axonal labeling revealed that neurons with atypical expression of *Fezf2* and *Ctip2* altered their axonal trajectories to project to subcerebral targets that included the spinal cord.

Nr2f1 also regulates the balance of early- and late-born neurons and the relative sizes of layer 5 cell populations (Faedo et al. 2008; Tomassy et al. 2010). These functions also come into play in mediating the apparent area shifts in mice with conditional deletion of *Nr2f1*. Corticothalamic projection neurons from layer 6 in wild-type mice are born before CSMNs at about E12.5. Loss of *Nr2f1* increased the number of E12.5 neurons that strongly express *Ctip2* in layer 6, as well as permitting neurons with a hybrid identity, suggesting that *Nr2f1* functions to repress CSMN fate during the generation of corticothalamic neurons (Tomassy et al. 2010). From a large-scale perspective, therefore, loss of Nr2f1 causes an enlarged M1 at the expense of sensory areas. At the finer scale of the neuron, abnormally large and widespread populations of neurons differentiate with CSMN or hybrid features.

Conditional loss of *Nr2f1* in postnatal neurons has also been found to cause a large expansion of M1 in P0 neocortex, with primary sensory areas again pushed back in the hemisphere and shrunken (Alfano et al. 2014). Further, over-expression of *Nr2f1* in constitutively *Nr2f1* null mice after neurogenesis rescues at least some of the deficits in the mutant cortex, suggesting *Nr2f1* is needed in postmitotic neurons to regulate sensory versus motor neuronal differentiation. This begs the question of the role of *Nr2f1* in progenitor neurons. One possibility is that proper repression of the CSMN identity requires post-mitotic cell expression of *Nr2f1*, but that *Nr2f1*-expressing progenitor cells direct this expression in their daughter neurons. The primary finding is that Nr2f1 is necessary and sufficient to repress the formation of CSMNs, a conclusion that neatly links area, layer, and cell-type development (Faedo et al. 2008).

22.3.8 Graded Expression of Transcription Factors

So far, the graded expression of patterning genes for the NP has been emphasized. If NP patterning resembled that in the ventral spinal cord, patterning genes with opposing gradients would interact to form sharply bounded domains, which would give rise to different areas. Such boundaries, however, have not been identified either among the progenitor cells in the VZ or in the subventricular zone (SVZ), where intermediate progenitor (IP) cells, generated from the VZ, are located. Gene expression in the SVZ is graded just as in the VZ (Elsen et al. 2013). A caveat here is that the overlap of expression of known patterning genes has not been as carefully examined as might be. At E9.5, for example, the expression domains of *Sp8* and *Nr2f1* along the A/P axis look distinctly complementary with minimal overlap (Borello et al. 2013). Directed exploration for genes with expression confined to distinct progenitor domains, has not been helpful so far (Donoghue and Rakic 1999; Kudo et al. 2007; Sansom et al. 2005). These searches have revealed more genes expressed in gradients in the germinal layers of the NP. Nonetheless, the distinct regions of gene expression seen in prenatal and perinatal mice without thalamic input indicates that mechanisms intrinsic to the NP can generate relatively sharp gene expression boundaries (Miyashita-Lin et al. 1999; Nakagawa et al. 1999; Zhou et al. 2010).

22.3.9 Mapping the Neocortical Primordium with Forebrain Enhancers

In contrast to the graded expression of patterning transcription factors, strikingly bounded domains of enhancer regulatory activity have been identified in the mouse NP in a series of investigations. Putative enhancers were identified in noncoding sequences of the human genome, based on the ultraconservation of these sequences across human, mouse, and rat (Pennacchio et al. 2006). Candidates were screened for spatially restricted enhancer activity by linking the human DNA fragments to a minimal promoter fused to a lacZ reporter gene and generating transgenic mice. Tissue-specific reporter gene expression was evaluated in mouse embryos at E11.5, when whole embryo staining and visualization is straightforward, and when neurogenesis is just beginning in the NP. Enhancer activity was spatially restricted, with several putative enhancers active in the mouse telencephalon (Pennacchio et al. 2006). Subsequent work provided an "enhancer atlas" of the developing mouse telencephalon showing reporter mouse lacZ expression for many reproducible forebrain enhancers. The activity patterns of several enhancers marked out clear domains in the VZ of the medial, dorsal, and lateral cortical primordium at E11.5, and subsequently in the cortical plate (Pattabiraman et al. 2014; Visel et al. 2013). Fate-mapping enhancer activity domains demonstrated that precisely positioned domains, identified at E11.5, can give rise to similarly located subdivisions of the hippocampus and neocortex in late embryonic and postnatal mice. Further assays indicated that Nr2f1 and Pax6, two of the patterning transcription factors described earlier, bound to specific sets of the dorsal telencephalic enhancers. A proposal, based on these and further findings (Pattabiraman et al. 2014), is that the graded patterning transcriptions factors interact to regulate the activity of enhancer elements. Subsequently the enhancers regulate expression of further genes, presumably in cortical protodomains, which ultimately give rise to specific areas or regions of the cerebral cortex. The Chapter 21 describes the intricate work following from these studies.

22.4 Conservation of Patterning Mechanisms among Different Mammalian Species

The protomap model was based on observations of primate neocortex (Rakic 1988), a reminder that the final goal is to discover mechanisms that pattern cerebral cortex in humans. One question is whether the processes that pattern the small lissencephalic mouse neocortex also shape the larger, gyrencephalic brains of carnivores, and primates. One reason for doubt is that patterning molecules, or morphogens, such as FGF8 and WNT3a, have limited dispersion ranges of a few hundred microns (Farin et al. 2016; Parchure et al. 2018; Scholpp and Brand 2004). Larger, more complex cortices presumably derive from larger cortical primordia whose size could prevent effective morphogen dispersion.

22.4.1 Mouse, Ferret, and Human

A way around the problem of patterning a larger brain would be to hold back growth at an early stage so that morphogen gradients can succeed in specifying brain components. This possibility was tested by examining growth of the NP in a gyrencephalic carnivore, the ferret, *Mustela putorius furo*, whose mature brain is several times the volume of the mouse brain (Jones et al. 2019). The goal was to compare the sizes of the mouse and ferret NP at an equivalent stage of whole-body embryogenesis, namely that at which FGF8 initiates NP patterning in the mouse, about E9–E9.5 (Toyoda et al. 2010). Although the NP of the ferret is ultimately much larger than that of the mouse, at this critical stage of telencephalic development, the A/P length of the NP is the same in mouse and ferret (Jones et al. 2019). Previous observations indicate that FGF8 spreads about 0.3 – 0.6 mm in an A/P gradient through the early mouse NP (Toyoda et al. 2010). The mean A/P neocortical surface length (NSL) for E9.0 and E17 ferrets was 0.4mm, well within the range of FGF8 spread, as was the mean NSL for E9.5 mice and E18 ferrets (Jones et al. 2019). Thus, FGF8 could, in principle, disperse from anterior to posterior in the ferret NP and determine the A/P axis of the ferret area map. Compatible with the hypothesis, *Fgf8* is expressed at the anterior temporal pole of the ferret. *Nr2f1* expression, downregulated by FGF8 in mice, shows similar posterior domains of expression in mice and ferrets, with fairly sharp anterior boundaries, consistent with active FGF8 signaling in the NP in both species (Jones et al. 2019).

Human embryo specimens in the Carnegie and Kyoto collections (Human Developmental Anatomy Center, Washington, DC) have been assigned to Carnegie Stages, measured, and imaged. Images, with scale bars, of first trimester embryos are available online and in e-book form (see

Jones et al. 2019 for e-book link). Initial comparisons of images of E9.5 mouse and Carnegie Stage 13 human brains suggest both the dorsal telencephalon, and NP, specifically, are close to the same size (Jones et al. 2019). A possibility therefore is that mammalian neocortices of widely varying mature sizes may be patterned in the embryo by common signaling molecules, such as FGF8 and WNT3a, if the early NP primordium is transiently kept at the same size.

A conserved function of Wnt3a in caudo-medial neocortex is supported by the juxtaposition of the cortical hem to the presumptive hippocampal primordium in ferrets (Jones et al. 2019), as in humans (Abu-Khalil et al. 2004; Jones et al. 2019). Consistent with an FGF8 gradient establishing the A/P axis in human neocortex, different concentrations of FGF8 applied to neocortical cells derived from human induced pluripotent stem cells induced appropriate, graded A/P gene expression (Imaizumi et al. 2018). Further suggesting FGF8 plays a role in neocortical area patterning, abnormalities in human cortex are linked to dysregulation of FGF8 or FGF receptor 3 signaling (Dubourg et al. 2016; Frank et al. 2002; Hevner 2005).

22.5 Conclusions

Great progress has been made in understanding how thalamocortical axons reach the NP and how axons are organized en route to exit the IC at the correct A/P and M/L coordinates. Evidence from both old and new studies further indicates that these axons are provided with final molecular guidance cues both from the SP and from within the neocortex. Other advances have identified the signaling molecules that establish position across the NP, and transcription factors downstream of Wnt3a and FGF8 that continue the area patterning process. It remains unclear what the intrinsic map of the neocortex looks like in the embryonic NP. To date no genes have been identified that are expressed in clear domains in the VZ or SVZ, marking "protoareas." Nonetheless, many studies, some cited in this chapter, indicate area specificity within the early NP, and imply that presumptive areas are at least roughly drawn out in the NP. Studies underway may show a more precise area map in the NP (Ypsilanti and Rubenstein 2016).

What the intrinsic map of the neocortex looks like through the postnatal first week in mice lacking thalamic input, is also unknown. As noted, given the clear regional expression of several genes at postnatal ages in mice lacking TCAs, a distinct possibility is that an area map at least partially develops during the first week but requires TCAs for maintenance and continued development.

An example of interplay between thalamocortical mechanisms and those intrinsic to neocortex comes from observations of S1 barrel-field development. As noted above, somatosensory TCAs are required for development of the barrel fields, but the response by neocortical neurons to TCA activity is reliant on cortical expression of the transcription factor gene, *Lhx2*. It seems likely that other examples of this type of interplay will be uncovered in future, eventually combining the two different models of area map formation into a hybrid version.

Finally, the mouse remains a vital model system for deciphering the mechanisms of basic area map formation. Keeping an open mind is suggested with respect to whether findings in mice will generalize to humans. The positions of primary areas are conserved across mammals. Additionally, the positions and timing of centers releasing signaling molecules such as FGFs and WNTs are conserved across mouse and ferret. Available data indicates that the human cerebral cortex could use the same mechanisms to establish the major axes of the neocortex.

References

Abu-Khalil, A. et al. (2004). Wnt genes define distinct boundaries in the developing human brain. *J Comp Neurol* 474: 276–288.

Ackman, J.B. et al. (2012). Retinal waves coordinate patterned activity throughout the developing visual system. *Nature* 490: 219–225.

Alfano, C. et al. (2014). Postmitotic control of sensory area specification during neocortical development. *Nat Commun* 5: 5632.

Allendoerfer, K.L. and Shatz, C.J. (1994). The subplate, a transient neocortical structure. *Ann Rev Neurosci* 17: 185–218.

Alzu'bi, A. et al. (2019). Thalamocortical afferents innervate the cortical subplate much earlier in development in primate than in rodent. *Cereb Cortex* 29: 1706–1718.

Anton-Bolanos, N. et al. (2018). Developmental interactions between thalamus and cortex. *Curr Opin Neurobiol* 52: 33–41.

Anton-Bolanos, N. et al. (2019). Prenatal activity from thalamic neurons governs the emergence of functional cortical maps in mice. *Science* 364: 987–990.

Armentano, M. et al. (2007). COUP-TFI regulates the balance of cortical patterning between frontal/motor and sensory areas. *Nat Neurosci* 10: 1277–1286.

Assimacopoulos, S. et al. (2012). Fibroblast growth factor 8 organizes the neocortical area map and regulates sensory map topography. *J Neurosci* 32: 7191–7201.

Bachler, M. and Neubuser, A. (2001). Expression of members of the Fgf family and their receptors during midfacial development. *Mech Dev* 100: 313–316.

Bishop, K.M. et al. (2000). Regulation of area identity in the mammalian neocortex by Emx2 and Pax6. *Science* 288: 344–349.

Bishop, K.M. et al. (2002a). Distinct actions of Emx1, Emx2, and Pax6 in regulating the specification of areas in the developing neocortex. *J Neurosci* 22: 7627–7638.

Bishop, K.M. et al. (2002b). Distinct actions of Emx1, Emx2, and Pax6 in regulating the specification of areas in the developing neocortex. *J Neurosci* 22: 7627–7638.

Borello, U. et al. (2013). Sp8 and COUP-TF1 reciprocally regulate patterning and Fgf signaling in cortical progenitors. *Cereb Cortex* 24: 1409–1421.

Briscoe, J. and Ericson, J. (2001). Specification of neuronal fates in the ventral neural tube. *Curr Opin Neurobiol* 11: 43–49.

Briscoe, J. et al. (2000). A homeodomain protein code specifies progenitor cell identity and neuronal fate in the ventral neural tube. *Cell* 101: 435–445.

Cadwell, C.R. et al. (2019). Development and arealization of the cerebral cortex. *Neuron* 103: 980–1004.

Caronia-Brown, G. et al. (2014). The cortical hem regulates the size and patterning of neocortex. *Development* 141: 2855–2865.

Catalano, S.M. and Shatz, C.J. (1998). Activity-dependent cortical target selection by thalamic axons. *Science* 281: 559–562.

Caviness, V.S., Jr. and Frost, D.O. (1983). Thalamocortical projections in the reeler mutant mouse. *J Comp Neurol* 219: 182–202.

Cholfin, J.A. and Rubenstein, J.L. (2007). Patterning of frontal cortex subdivisions by Fgf17. *Proc Natl Acad Sci USA* 104: 7652–7657.

Cholfin, J.A. and Rubenstein, J.L. (2008). Frontal cortex subdivision patterning is coordinately regulated by Fgf8, Fgf17, and Emx2. *J Comp Neurol* 509: 144–155.

Crossley, P.H. and Martin, G.R. (1995). The mouse Fgf 8 gene encodes a family of polypeptides and is expressed in regions that direct outgrowth and patterning in the developing embryo. *Development* 121: 439–451.

Crossley, P.H. et al. (1996). Midbrain development induced by FGF8 in the chick embryo. *Nature* 380: 66–68.

Crossley, P.H. et al. (2001). Coordinate expression of Fgf8, Otx2, Bmp4, and Shh in the rostral prosencephalon during development of the telencephalic and optic vesicles. *Neuroscience* 108: 183–206.

De Clercq, S. et al. (2018). DMRT5 together with DMRT3 directly controls hippocampus development and neocortical area map formation. *Cereb Cortex* 28: 493–509.

Deck, M. et al. (2013). Pathfinding of corticothalamic axons relies on a rendezvous with thalamic projections. *Neuron* 77: 472–484.

Dehay, C. et al. (1996). Phenotypic characterisation of respecified visual cortex subsequent to prenatal enucleation in the monkey. *J Comp Neurol* 376: 386–402.

Dehay, C. and Kennedy, H. (2007). Cell-cycle control and cortical development. *Nat Rev Neurosci* 8: 438–450.

Desmaris, E. et al. (2018). DMRT5, DMRT3, and EMX2 cooperatively repress GSX2 at the pallium-subpallium boundary to maintain cortical identity in dorsal telencephalic progenitors. *J Neurosci* 38: 9105–9121.

Donoghue, M.J. and Rakic, P. (1999). Molecular evidence for the early specification of presumptive functional domains in the embryonic primate cerebral cortex. *J Neurosci* 19: 5967–5979.

Dorsky, R.I. et al. (1998). Control of neural crest cell fate by the Wnt signalling pathway. *Nature* 396: 370–373.

Dubourg, C. et al. (2016). Mutational spectrum in holoprosencephaly shows that FGF is a new major signaling pathway. *Hum Mutat* 37: 1329–1339.

Elsen, G.E. et al. (2018). The epigenetic factor landscape of developing neocortex is regulated by transcription factors Pax6-> Tbr2-> Tbr1. *Front Neurosci* 12: 571.

Elsen, G.E. et al. (2013). The protomap is propagated to cortical plate neurons through an Eomes-dependent intermediate map. *Proc Natl Acad Sci USA* 110: 4081–4086.

Faedo, A. et al. (2008). COUP-TFI coordinates cortical patterning, neurogenesis, and laminar fate and modulates MAPK/ERK, AKT, and beta-catenin signaling. *Cereb Cortex* 18: 2117–2131.

Farin, H.F. et al. (2016). Visualization of a short-range Wnt gradient in the intestinal stem-cell niche. *Nature* 530: 340–343.

Finney, E.M. et al. (1998). Major glutamatergic projection from subplate into visual cortex during development. *J Comp Neurol* 398: 105–118.

Frank, D.U. et al. (2002). An Fgf8 mouse mutant phenocopies human 22q11 deletion syndrome. *Development* 129: 4591–4603.

Frappe, I. et al. (1999). Transplants of fetal frontal cortex grafted into the occipital cortex of newborn rats receive a substantial thalamic input from nuclei normally projecting to the frontal cortex. *Neuroscience* 89: 409–421.

Friauf, E. et al. (1990). Functional synaptic circuits in the subplate during fetal and early postnatal development of cat visual cortex. *J Neurosci* 10: 2601–2613.

Fukuchi-Shimogori, T. and Grove, E.A. (2001). Neocortex patterning by the secreted signaling molecule FGF8. *Science* 294: 1071–1074.

Fukuchi-Shimogori, T. and Grove, E.A. (2003). Emx2 patterns the neocortex by regulating FGF positional signaling. *Nat Neurosci* 6: 825–831.

Furuta, Y. et al. (1997). Bone morphogenetic proteins (BMPs) as regulators of dorsal forebrain development. *Development* 124: 2203–2212.

Gaillard, A. and Roger, M. (2000). Early commitment of embryonic neocortical cells to develop area-specific thalamic connections. *Cereb Cortex* 10: 443–453.

Galceran, J. et al. (2000). Hippocampus development and generation of dentate gyrus granule cells is regulated by LEF1. *Development* 127: 469–482.

Garel, S. et al. (2003). Molecular regionalization of the neocortex is disrupted in Fgf8 hypomorphic mutants. *Development* 130: 1903–1914.

Garel, S. and Lopez-Bendito, G. (2014). Inputs from the thalamocortical system on axon pathfinding mechanisms. *Curr Opin Neurobiol* 27: 143–150.

Garel, S. and Rubenstein, J.L. (2004). Intermediate targets in formation of topographic projections. *Trends Neurosci* 27: 533–539.

Ghosh, A. et al. (1990). Requirement for subplate neurons in the formation of thalamocortical connections. *Nature* 347: 179–181.

Ghosh, A. and Shatz, C.J. (1993). A role for subplate neurons in the patterning of connections from thalamus to neocortex. *Development* 117: 1031–1047.

Gorski, J.A. et al. (2002). Cortical excitatory neurons and glia, but not GABAergic neurons, are produced in the Emx1-expressing lineage. *J Neurosci* 22: 6309–6314.

Grove, E.A. et al. (1998). The hem of the embryonic cerebral cortex is defined by the expression of multiple Wnt genes and is compromised in Gli3-deficient mice. *Development* 125: 2315–2325.

Hamasaki, T. et al. (2004). EMX2 regulates sizes and positioning of the primary sensory and motor areas in neocortex by direct specification of cortical progenitors. *Neuron* 43: 359–372.

Harada, H. et al. (2016). Fgf8 signaling for development of the midbrain and hindbrain. *Dev Growth Diff* 58: 437–445.

Herrmann, K. et al. (1994). Ultrastructural evidence for synaptic interactions between thalamocortical axons and subplate neurons. *Eur J Neurosci* 6: 1729–1742.

Hevner, R.F. (2005). The cerebral cortex malformation in thanatophoric dysplasia. *Acta Neuropathol* 110: 208–221.

Imaizumi, K. et al. (2018). Rostrocaudal areal patterning of human PSC-derived cortical neurons by FGF8 signaling. *eNeuro* 5 (2): ENEURO.0368-17.2018.

Jones, W.D. et al. (2019). A model of neocortical area patterning in the lissencephalic mouse may hold for larger gyrencephalic brains. *J Comp Neurol* 527 (9): 1460–1477.

Krubitzer, L. and Stolzenberg, D.S. (2014). The evolutionary masquerade. *Curr Opin Neurobiol* 24: 157–165.

Kudo, L.C. et al. (2007). Genetic analysis of anterior posterior expression gradients in the developing mammalian forebrain. *Cereb Cortex* 17: 2108–2122.

LaMonica, B.E. et al. (2012). OSVZ progenitors in the human cortex. *Curr Opin Neurobiol* 22: 747–753.

Lee, S.M. et al. (2000). A local Wnt-3a signal is required for development of the mammalian hippocampus. *Development* 127: 457–467.

Li, H. et al. (2013). Laminar and columnar development of barrel cortex relies on thalamocortical neurotransmission. *Neuron* 79: 970–986.

Liem, K.F., Jr. et al. (1997). A role for the roof plate and its resident TGFbeta-related proteins in neuronal patterning in the dorsal spinal cord. *Cell* 91: 127–138.

Liem, K.F., Jr. et al. (1995). Dorsal differentiation of neural plate cells induced by BMP-mediated signals from epidermal ectoderm. *Cell* 82: 969–979.

López-Bendito, G. (2018). Development of the thalamocortical interactions. *Neuroscience* 385: 67–74.

López-Bendito, G. et al. (2006). Tangential neuronal migration controls axon guidance. *Cell* 125: 127–142.

Lui, J.H. et al. (2011). Development and evolution of the human neocortex. *Cell* 146: 18–36.
Mallamaci, A. et al. (2000). Area identity shifts in the early cerebral cortex of Emx2-/- mutant mice. *Nat Neurosci* 3: 679–686.
Mangale, V.S. et al. (2008). Lhx2 selector activity specifies cortical identity and suppresses hippocampal organizer fate. *Science* 319: 304–309.
Martinez, S. et al. (1999). FGF8 induces formation of an ectopic isthmic organizer and isthmocerebellar development via a repressive effect on Otx2 expression. *Development* 126: 1189–1200.
Matsui, A. et al. (2013). BTBD3 controls dendrite orientation toward active axons in mammalian neocortex. *Science* 342: 1114–1118.
Miyashita-Lin, E.M. et al. (1999). Early neocortical regionalization in the absence of thalamic innervation. *Science* 285: 906–909.
Moreno-Juan, V. et al. (2017). Prenatal thalamic waves regulate cortical area size prior to sensory processing. *Nat Commun* 8: 14172.
Nakagawa, Y. et al. (1999). Graded and areal expression patterns of regulatory genes and cadherins in embryonic neocortex independent of thalamocortical input. *J Neurosci* 19: 10877–10885.
Nauta, W.J.H.V. and Feirtag, M. (1986). *Fundamental Neuroanatomy*. New York: W.H.Freeman and Company.
O'Leary, D.D. (1989). Do cortical areas emerge from a protocortex? *Trends Neurosci* 12: 400–406.
O'Leary, D.D. et al. (2007). Area patterning of the mammalian cortex. *Neuron* 56: 252–269.
Ohkubo, Y. et al. (2002). Coordinate regulation and synergistic actions of BMP4, SHH and FGF8 in the rostral prosencephalon regulate morphogenesis of the telencephalic and optic vesicles. *Neuroscience* 111: 1–17.
Pallas, S.L. and Sur, M. (1993). Visual projections induced into the auditory pathway of ferrets. *J Comp Neurol* 337: 317–333.
Parchure, A. et al. (2018). Wnt and hedgehog. *Trends Cell Biol* 28: 157–170.
Pattabiraman, K. et al. (2014). Transcriptional regulation of enhancers active in protodomains of the developing cerebral cortex. *Neuron* 82: 989–1003.
Pennacchio, L.A. et al. (2006). In vivo enhancer analysis of human conserved non-coding sequences. *Nature* 444: 499–502.
Polleux, F. et al. (1997). Regulation of neuroblast cell-cycle kinetics plays a crucial role in the generation of unique features of neocortical areas. *J Neurosci* 17: 7763–7783.
Pouchelon, G. et al. (2014). Modality-specific thalamocortical inputs instruct the identity of postsynaptic L4 neurons. *Nature* 511: 471–474.
Powell, A.W. et al. (2008). Topography of thalamic projections requires attractive and repulsive functions of Netrin-1 in the ventral telencephalon. *PLoS Biol* 6: 1047–1068.
Rakic, P. (1988). Specification of cerebral cortical areas. *Science* 241: 170–176.
Rakic, P. et al. (1991). A novel cytoarchitectonic area induced experimentally within the primate visual cortex. *Proc Natl Acad Sci USA* 88: 2083–2087.
Roe, A.W.et al. (1990). A map of visual space induced in primary auditory cortex. *Science* 250: 818–820.
Roe, A.W. et al. (1992). Visual projections routed to the auditory pathway in ferrets. *J Neurosci* 12: 3651–3664.
Sansom, S.N. et al. (2005). Genomic characterisation of a Fgf-regulated gradient-based neocortical protomap. *Development* 132: 3947–3961.
Saulnier, A. et al. (2013). The doublesex homolog Dmrt5 is required for the development of the caudomedial cerebral cortex in mammals. *Cereb Cortex* 23 (11): 2552–2567.
Scholpp, S. and Brand, M. (2004). Endocytosis controls spreading and effective signaling range of Fgf8 protein. *Curr Biol* 14: 1834–1841.

Shetty, A.S. et al. (2013). Lhx2 regulates a cortex-specific mechanism for barrel formation. *Proc Natl Acad Sci USA* 110: E4913–4921.

Shimogori, T. and Grove, E.A. (2005). Fibroblast growth factor 8 regulates neocortical guidance of area-specific thalamic innervation. *J Neurosci* 25: 6550–6560.

Sur, M. (1993). Cortical specification: microcircuits, perceptual identity, and an overall perspective. *Perspect Dev Neurobiol* 1: 109–113.

Sur, M. et al. (1988). Experimentally induced visual projections into auditory thalamus and cortex. *Science* 242: 1437–1441.

Sur, M. et al. (1990). Cross-modal plasticity in cortical development. *Trends Neurosci* 13: 227–233.

Sur, M. and Rubenstein, J.L. (2005). Patterning and plasticity of the cerebral cortex. *Science* 310: 805–810.

Tole, S. et al. (2000). Emx2 is required for growth of the hippocampus but not for hippocampal field specification. *J Neurosci* 20: 2618–2625.

Tomassy, G.S. et al. (2010). Area-specific temporal control of corticospinal motor neuron differentiation by COUP-TFI. *Proc Natl Acad Sci USA* 107: 3576–3581.

Toyoda, R. et al. (2010). FGF8 acts as a classic diffusible morphogen to pattern the neocortex. *Development* 137: 3439–3448.

Tronche, F. et al. (1999). Disruption of the glucocorticoid receptor gene in the nervous system results in reduced anxiety. *Nat Genet* 23: 99–103.

Tsai, S.Y. and Tsai, M.J. (1997). Chick ovalbumin upstream promoter-transcription factors (COUP-TFs). *Endocr Rev* 18: 229–240.

Urquhart, J.E. et al. (2016). DMRTA2 (DMRT5) is mutated in a novel cortical brain malformation. *Clin Genet* 89 (6): 724–727.

Vanderhaeghen, P. and Polleux, F. (2004). Developmental mechanisms patterning thalamocortical projections. *Trends Neurosci* 27: 384–391.

Visel, A. et al. (2013). A high-resolution enhancer atlas of the developing telencephalon. *Cell* 152 (4): 895–908.

Vue, T.Y. et al. (2013). Thalamic control of neocortical area formation in mice. *J Neurosci* 33: 8442–8453.

Wang, C.F. et al. (2017). Lhx2 expression in postmitotic cortical neurons initiates assembly of the thalamocortical somatosensory circuit. *Cell Rep* 18: 849–856.

Wolpert, L. (1996). One hundred years of positional information. *Trends Genet* 12: 359–364.

Ypsilanti, A.R. and Rubenstein, J.L. (2016). Transcriptional and epigenetic mechanisms of early cortical development. *J Comp Neurol* 524: 609–629.

Zhou, L. et al. (2010). Maturation of "neocortex isole" in vivo in mice. *J Neurosci* 30: 7928–7939.

Zimmer, C. et al. (2009). Role of Fgf8 signalling in the specification of rostral Cajal-Retzius cells. *Development* 137: 293–302.

Part 6

Cortical Folding

23

Old Models Know Wrinkles Best

A Critical Review on the Mechanisms of Cortical Gyrification

Jon I. Arellano[1] *and Pasko Rakic*[1,2,*]

[1] *Department of Neuroscience*
[2] *Kavli Institute for Neuroscience at Yale, Yale University, New Haven, CT, USA*
[*] *Corresponding author*

23.1 The Early Studies on Gyrification

The presence of intricate convolutions in the human brain and other large mammals has always captivated and intrigued brain researchers. This interest is already documented in Classic Greece, where Erasistratus of Ceos in the third century BCE described the comparative anatomy of the surface of the brain and conjectured that the complexity of the convolutions of the brain was related to the intelligence of the species (Finger 2001), a motif that appears consistently through history. Interestingly, Aristotle thought that the brain was a cold and fluid organ that served to temper the heat of the heart, where the mind and soul resided. Thus, humans exhibit the largest brain because their heart is the hottest and richest in emotion and thought, and needs to be tempered to achieve the greatest intelligence of the animal kingdom (Gross 1995). The Middle Ages were not prolific on anatomical studies, but The Renaissance brought a new interest on the study of the brain, in part because the ban on cadaver dissection was lifted in the Christian world. Representation of the surface of the brain became more accurate (Ribas 2010), and the sylvian fissure is described in 1610 (Finger 2001), however, depictions of the surface of the brain frequently "resembled more a plate of macaroni than the organ of the human mind" (Bailey and Bonin 1951). More realistic drawings and detailed descriptions of sulci and gyri are documented in the late eighteenth century (D'azyr 1786; von Soemmerring 1791) and in the early nineteenth century, the studies of Gall on phrenology proposing a speculative scheme of functional localization in the surface of the brain fueled interest on the study of cortical surface. As a result, the study of gyrification flourished in the nineteenth century, describing in detail the ontogenesis of sulci and gyri in the human and other primates, and comparing in minute detail the gyrification patterns across species, families, and orders of mammals (Broca 2015; Cunningham 1892; Dareste 1855; Gratiolet 1854; Owen 1868; Pozzi 1887; Turner 1890). Connectivity of the different areas was also studied by means of fiber dissection techniques that allowed description of fiber tracts and the major connections in the brain (Türe et al. 2000). Combining both approaches, inferring functional meaning from their location and connectivity, allowed description of functional systems like the limbic lobe by Broca (Broca 2015).

Neocortical Neurogenesis in Development and Evolution, First Edition. Edited by Wieland B. Huttner.

Through these detailed studies it was appreciated, early on, that the degree of gyrification is correlated to brain size, with large mammalian brains exhibiting more gyrified cortices (Dareste 1855). Owen coined the terms lissencephalic and gyrencephalic, although originally, he proposed them as a zoologic classification of mammals that was complemented with other groups: lyencephala (marsupials and monotremes) and archencephala, a separate category just for humans, following the anthropocentric views of the time (Owen 1868). Owen was possibly influenced by the observation that mammalian orders tend to be populated by either lissencephalic (e.g., rodents) or gyrencephalic species (e.g., carnivores). However, at the time it was already clear that it was mostly due to the similarity in size of the species in a given order, instead of phylogenetic relations or zoological characteristics, as discussed by Broca (2015). Indeed, several authors (Dareste 1855) noted that in a given order, small species might exhibit lissencephalic brains, while large species tend to show gyrencephalic brains (e.g., rodents, primates). However, the terms gyrencephalic and lissencephalic survived and are commonly used as anatomical brain descriptors for species with or without convolutions, respectively.

At this time, few attempts to explain the origin of gyrification can be found in the literature, but according to Hilgetag and Barbas (2005), His (1874) studied the morphology of the brain using rubber tubes and ceramic plates as models, and proposed that the convolutions of the cortex might be due to differential growth of cortical areas competing for space, a familiar theme in contemporary theories to explain gyrification (e.g., Welker (1990), our own proposal, see Section 23.11).

23.2 Quantification of Gyrification: The Gyrification Index

An early approach of assessing gyrification was calculating the ratio between cortical surface area and exposed cortical area, an index that nowadays is known as the gyrification index (GI; Zilles et al. 1988). The first studies assessing the GI used gold or silk paper to painstakingly cover the surface area of the brain (see for example, Brodmann 1913; Donaldson 1891; Henneberg 1910). Later, Elias and Schwartz (1969) described a much simpler method based on stereology that obtained the cortical surface area from measurements in sections, which was later updated to a simpler ratio of total surface area to exposed surface area per section (Zilles et al. 1988). Several other methods to estimate gyrification have been proposed, such as measuring the ratio of cortex hidden from view (Haug 1987) obtaining a folding index after dividing cortical volume by outer (exposed) surface area (Hofman 1989), or calculating the isomorphic factor, by raising cortical surface area to the 3/2 power and dividing it by the volume (Mayhew et al. 1996). However, these methods had important limitations (Henery and Mayhew 1989) and did not gain widespread use. The GI has become the standard method for estimating gyrification as it is easy to use and is independent of brain size (Zilles et al. 2013).

23.3 The Reason for Gyrification

The most obvious answer to why gyrification occurs is to pack an enlarged cerebral cortex into a reasonable volume that is adaptive for birth and survival. Although traditional views on mammalian evolution presented a mammalian ancestor as a small animal that evolved in size (Dawkins and Wong 2005; Feldhamer et al. 2007), there is evidence that the first placental mammal was not a small but a medium-sized animal (Romiguier et al. 2013) with a slightly gyrified brain (O'Leary et al. 2013). This is an important consideration, as it implies that lissencephaly is secondary and probably comes naturally as less surface area is required in the cortex. However, aside from secondary lissencephaly in species that reduced body and brain size, in most mammalian clades the evolution of the group showed an increase in body size, as is the case for carnivores or primates (Northcutt 1981, 1985; Striedter 2005). Importantly, the increase in brain size has been propelled mostly by the growth of the neocortex, that represents about 25 percent of the mouse brain (Badea et al. 2007) but about 80 percent of the human brain (Holm et al. 2018). Since the cortex is a laminar structure, it grows mostly by increasing surface area, while only increasing modestly cortical thickness (from about 1 mm in mouse to 2–4 mm in human). These evolutionary changes in cortical surface area can be explained through changes in the mammalian developmental program in the context of the radial unit hypothesis (Rakic 1988, 1995). This model explains how lengthening of the proliferative period of neuroepithelial cells in the ventricular zone will generate more cortical radial units resulting in expansion of the cortical surface without necessarily increasing cortical thickness, while changes in the proliferative dynamics of radial glial cells, the cortical progenitors, could modify cortical thickness (Rakic 1995).

23.4 Gyrification Features

In order to discuss the possible mechanisms that produce gyrification, is necessary to consider the specific features of convoluted brains:

- Gyrification correlates strongly with brain size: small brains are always lissencephalic, while larger brains are generally convoluted, with few exceptions (e.g., manatee).
- Gyrification, when present, does not proceed at random, but follows species-specific patterns that show high similarity between closely related species, and diverges in distantly related species. Furthermore, species of the same order tend to share a basic gyrification pattern and show distinct scaling of GI with brain weight. Conversely, different mammalian orders show different layouts of gyrification and different scaling of GI with brain weight.
- Gyrification often correlates with functional maps, with sulci often acting as borders between areas.

23.5 Gyrification and Brain Size

As mentioned earlier, gyrification is strongly correlated to brain size, and the enlargement of the brain in large mammals seems to be the main reason behind the gyrification of the cortex. Extensive comparison of GIs between multiple mammalian species illustrates some interesting features of gyrification. Lissencephalic brains show GIs between 1 and 1.25, low values that reflect the absence of sulci, or the presence of few shallow sulci or the sylvian fissure as in the common Marmoset or Galago (Zilles et al. 1989, 2013) (Figure 23.1). Orders like rodents contain mostly small species and will show small GIs, typically below 2 while orders with bigger species (carnivores) will show a wider GI range between 1.5 and 2.5 (Lyras et al. 2016; Zilles et al. 2013), and large-brained, highly gyrified cetaceans reach GI values of over 5 (O'Leary et al. 2013). Interestingly, different orders show different scaling of GI values with brain size (Pillay and Manger 2007; Zilles et al. 2013). For example, cetaceans show a larger increase of gyrification as the brain enlarges than other orders such as artiodactyls (Zilles et al. 2013). This difference also applies within orders, such as prosimians vs. apes and monkeys in the primate order (Zilles et al. 1989) or felids vs. canids or mustelids

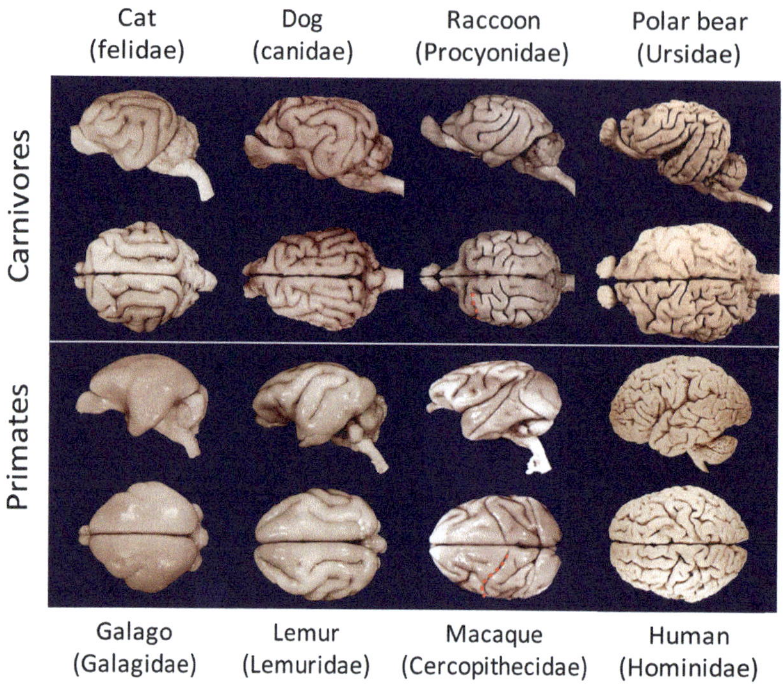

Figure 23.1 Phylogenetic similitudes and differences in gyrification between mammalian orders. Different species of *Carnivores* exhibit a similar bauplan of gyrification, as species of primates also do. Comparison between carnivores and primates reveal the differences in the general pattern of gyrification between the two orders. Red dashed lines in raccoon and macaque illustrate the location of the central sulcus, dividing motor, and sensory areas. Brain images from BrainMuseum.org.

in the carnivore order (Lyras et al. 2016). These differences are likely to reflect the different cortical organization adopted by the early ancestor of each order at the time of segregation, likely the product of changes in the developmental program, but also consequences of brain adaptations to the specific ecologic niche and mode of life of groups and species. Among the structural factors that can contribute to this variability, cortical thickness has been consistently found to be inversely correlated with gyrification, such that high convoluted brains tend to exhibit thinner cortices (Hofman 1985; Mota and Herculano-Houzel 2015; Pillay and Manger 2007; Zilles et al. 2013).

23.6 Patterns of Cortical Gyrification

Since the early studies of gyrification, it is clear that the majority of species show conserved patterns of gyrification, and the pattern is symmetrical in the cerebral hemispheres. Individual variations can always be observed, but in general the overall pattern is clearly recognizable (Welker 1990). This intra-species consistency suggests that folding of the cortex follows a stereotyped sequence during development that will likely reflect cytoarchitectonic, hodological, and functional divisions in a given species. In agreement with this logic, closely related species tend to show more similar patterns than distantly related species, And it has been consistently recognized that each mammalian order exhibits some similitude in the general "bauplan" of gyrification, as can be observed in primates (Connolly 1950) or carnivores (Welker 1990; Welker and Campos 1963) (Figure 23.1).

Differences in the general layout of gyrification between orders can be readily observed regarding the central sulcus, a conspicuous and well-delimitated sulcus that occupies a central (rostro-caudal) position in most gyrified primates, and separates motor and sensory territories, frontal and parietal lobes (Figure 23.1). The postcruciate/central sulcus has been acknowledged as the homologous sulcus in carnivores (Duque and McCormick 2010; Lockard 1985; Welker 1990; Welker and Campos 1963), although its location and orientation changes compared to primates, with a more rostral position likely due to the much smaller prefrontal cortex in carnivores (Duque and McCormick 2010) (Figures 23.1 and 23.2). In this regard, when different mammalian orders are considered, functional cortical areas tend to conserve their relative positions, but their location in the cortical mantle varies greatly (Figure 23.3), a factor that will necessarily contribute to change in the pattern of gyrification.

Historically, the study of gyrification has been largely influenced by the specifics of the human brain, and studies on human development introduced the concept of primary, secondary, and tertiary sulci/gyri, based on the time of appearance, the depth of the sulcus, and the consistency of their location and morphology between individuals (Bayley and Bonin, 1951). Gyral development in humans is quite stereotyped until the eighth gestational month, with emerging primary sulci that appear in consistent locations, sometimes delimiting cerebral lobes such as the sylvian fissure, central sulcus, parieto-occipital, calcarine, or cingulate sulcus. After that, gyrification accelerates and randomizes, adding secondary sulci/gyri that are identifiable but not consistent between individuals. A third wave of gyrification after birth will add further folding of existing gyri (Bailey and Bonin 1951; Chi et al. 1977). As a result, the human brain exhibits large heterogeny in gyrification

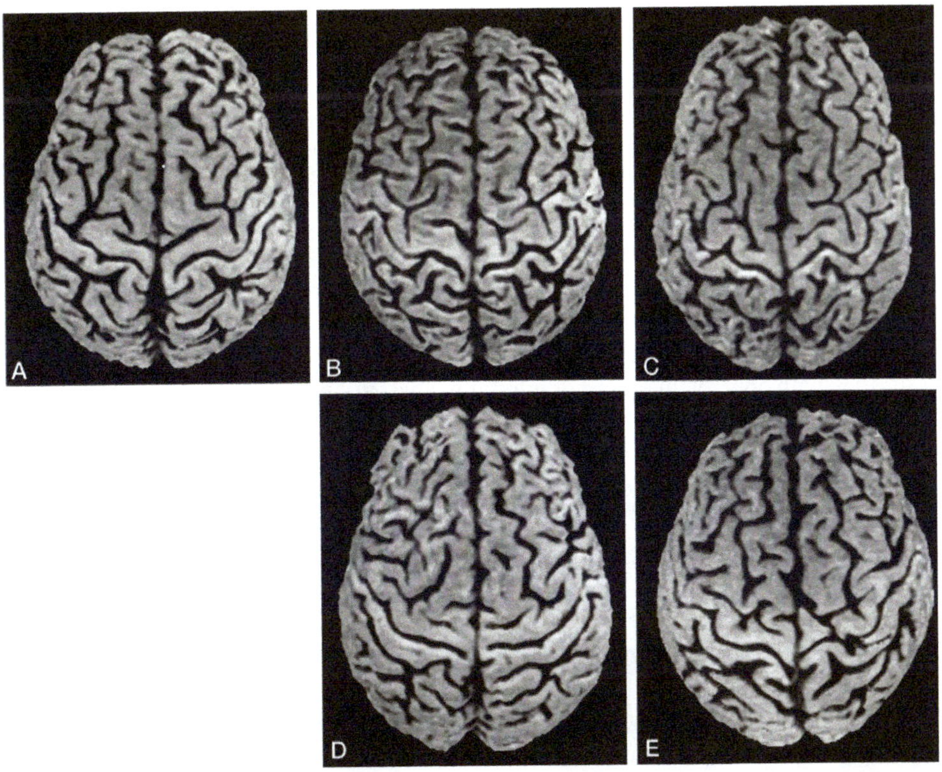

Figure 23.2 Variation in gyrification patterns in monozygotic twins. (A–E) 3D surface renderings from magnetic resonance images of five individuals. A is one monozygotic twin, and the other twin is one of B–E. Can the reader identify it? The solution is randomly located in the main text, so the reader is invited to read it all to find the answer.

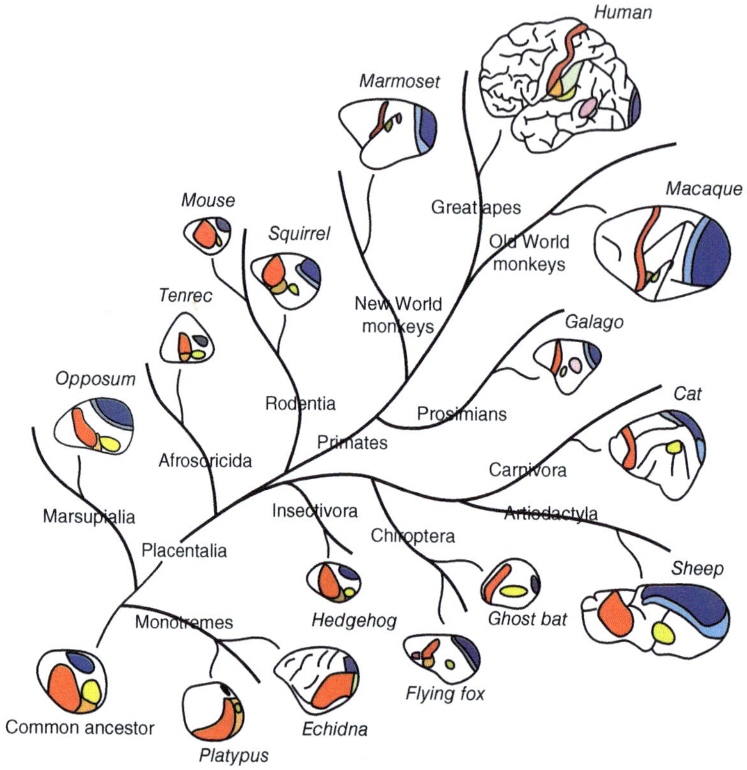

Figure 23.3 Variability in the location/extension of brain functional areas. Phylogenetic tree showing the distribution of sensory areas in different mammalian lineages, including a hypothetical common ancestor. Dark blue: primary visual cortex; light blue: secondary visual area; red: primary somatosensory area; orange: secondary somatosensory area; yellow: primary auditory area; pink; middle temporal visual area. Reproduced with permission from Krubitzer and Hunt (2010).

between individuals, even between monozygotic twins (Bartley et al. 1997; Biondi et al. 1998; Thompson et al. 2001; White et al. 2002) (Figure 23.2).

This classification is difficult to apply to most mammalian species that exhibit a consistent pattern of gyrification with only relatively minor interindividual variations (Welker 1990; Welker and Seidenstein 1959), but is expected to be present in highly gyrified groups (e.g., seals, artiodactyls like sheep or horse and cetaceans) that exhibit asymmetric gyrification between hemispheres, strongly suggesting the presence of secondary and tertiary gyrification.

23.6.1 Correlation between Gyral Morphology and Cortical Function

As mentioned earlier, there is in general a good correlation between sulcal location and functional cortical borders, particularly between cortical regions that exhibit marked differences in their cyto-, myeloarchitecture, and connectivity (Maudgil et al. 1998). Citing (Welker 1990), examples of sulci separating functional areas are the arcuate, central, and lunate sulci in primates, the ansate, lateral, suprasylvian, postcruciate, and cruciate sulci in carnivores, and the cingulate, rhinal, and Sylvian sulci in most mammals. The central sulcus in primates, the postcruciate/central sulcal complex in carnivores, or the fronto-lateral sulcus in large rodents are considered homologous sulci that separate motor and sensory cortices (Duque and McCormick 2010; Lockard 1985; Welker 1990; Welker and Seidenstein 1959) (Figures 23.1, 23.4). Specifically, it has been shown in primates

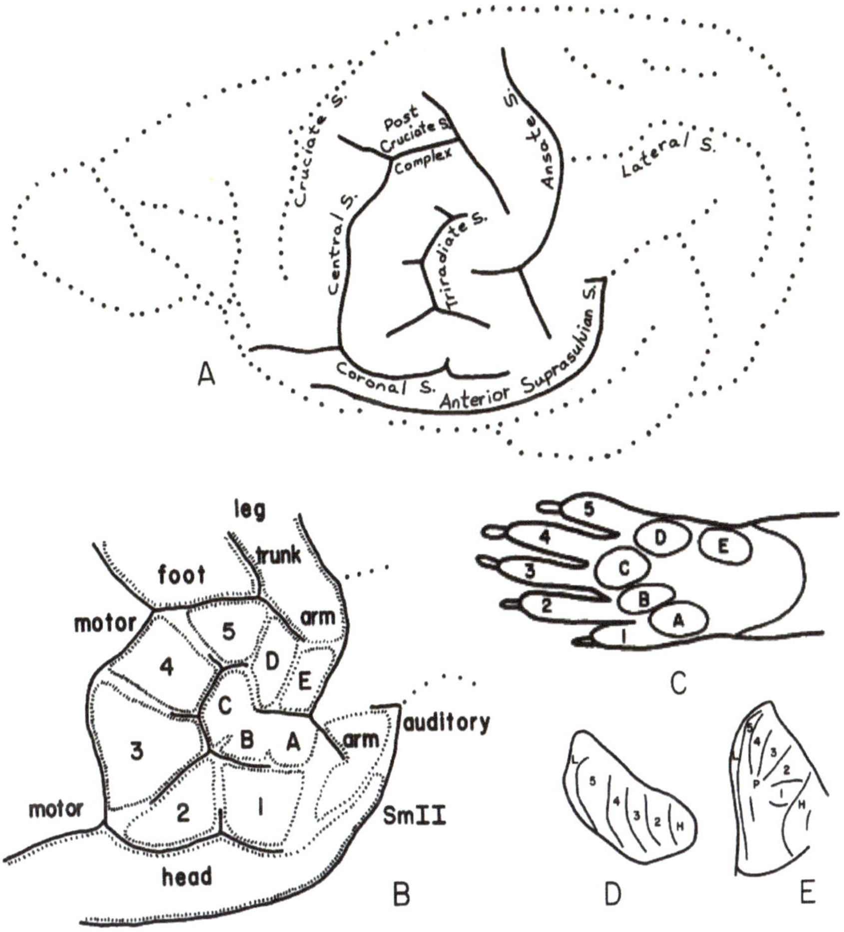

Figure 23.4 Correlation between gyrification and cortical function. (A) Lateral view of an adult raccoon brain illustrating the sulcal pattern corresponding to somatosensory areas. (B) Dorso-lateral view of the primary somatosensory cortex (left hemisphere) of an adult raccoon showing receptive fields. Note the correspondence between gyrification and sensory areas, and how sulci tend to separate relatively more distal territories. (C) Paw of an adult raccoon with labeled sensory territories. (D) coronal and (E) horizontal sections through the ventro-basal nucleus of thalamus, illustrating the subdivisions corresponding to different peripheric territories. Reproduced with permission from Welker (1990) and Welker and Campos (1963).

that the border between primary motor area 4 and somatosensory area 3 is usually located in the fundus of the sulcus, although not necessarily in the middle of it (White et al. 1997). Other sulci do not divide functional areas, but different sources of information in a given area, as is the case of the calcarine sulcus, whose fundus divides the superior from the inferior visual fields regions (Holmes 1918, 1945). Other examples include the superior and inferior precentral sulci in primates, the triradiate sulcus in raccoons, and the caudal portions of the coronal sulcus in carnivores (Welker 1990). Although it seems an obvious observation considering the brain of lissencephalic mammals, it needs to be noted that in gyrified species, many different cortical areas are not separated by sulci, implying that a gyrus can contain several cortical regions, like somatosensory areas 1, 2, and 3 in the postcentral gyrus in primates.

Welker and Campos (1963) and Welker and Seidenstein (1959) mapped functionally the brain of various species of carnivores (procyonids), and they found an exquisite correspondence between gyri and somatosensory fields (Figure 23.4). Most sulci within the somatosensory primary area occurred between the areas corresponding to representations of body regions anatomically separate, such that there were sulci between representations of forepaw and hindpaw, forepaw and head, or between the tips of two adjacent digits (Figure 23.2). In this line, major sulci did not typically separate the representations of peripherally contiguous body regions such as upper and lower arm, face and neck, or trunk and upper arm. Following the logic that sulci would appear between functionally diverse areas or regions that receive markedly different input, there would be no reason to expect sulci separating those functionally close areas. A possible speculation is that thalamic axons from adjacent peripheric fields might be bundled closer than more distant fields, due to somatotopy in the thalamus (Figure 23.4D, E). Axons from more distant peripheric fields might arrive more separated in the subplate/cortical plate and create "athalamic" spots with more sparse input that might develop into sulci (Welker 1990). In agreement with this idea, the authors described that the middle of the gyri exhibits the most activity in response to stimulation of the ventral (most sensitive) aspect of the fingers, while the lateral of the fingers was found mostly in the sulcal banks and the dorsal, hairy aspect of the finger, the less sensitive region, corresponded typically to the sulcal fundus (Welker 1990; Welker and Seidenstein 1959).

It needs to be stressed that this specific example of correlation between gyri and function is by no means the norm, since it is relatively common that a gyrus contains two different functional territories, or sulci extend across sensory and motor domains (for example, Woolsey 1960) as can be observed comparing gyri and functional/cytoarchitectonic areas in a Brodmann map (Brodmann 1913). However, this example shows convincingly that gyrification can be strongly affected by thalamocortical afferents, at least in somatosensory areas. Other factors (cortical thickness, extrathalamic afferents, efferents, underlying nuclei, or fiber tracts) might influence further the formation and morphology of gyri, diluting the apparent influence of thalamic inputs. Also, other regions of the brain such as association areas are expected to receive a larger cortico-cortical component that could also be influential in the morphology and extension of gyri, but in a much more unpredictable way. In addition, the further elaboration of gyrification of larger brains like in the human, adding secondary and tertiary convolutions is expected to introduce much more interindividual variability in the distribution and location of functional areas, making it more difficult to establish correlations with gyral morphology. As mentioned previously, we know from studies on monozygotic twins that the pattern of gyrification varies substantially (Figure 23.3) even when it starts with identical genetic information, indicating that the contribution of small stochastic developmental differences is not negligible in the final morphology of highly gyrified species like the human.

23.7 Mechanisms Underlying Gyrification

23.7.1 Gyrification as a Consequence of Space Constrains

The initial thought when one observes the elaborated convolutions of the brain in large mammals is that they might be the product of space constrains inside the cranium. That was indeed the dominant explanation that anatomists produced for most of the nineteenth and twentieth centuries. The main idea was that convolutions would arise as the cortex expanded in surface area and was confined between the cranium and subcortical structures such as the basal ganglia (Clark and Medawar 1945; Turner 1890). Other factors such as blood vessels priming sulci were also mentioned as possible contributors (Turner 1890), but the main focus was on mechanical pressure. This explanation, however, was challenged by the experiments of Barron (1950) who showed that removing large parts of the subcortical structures or significant portions of the cortex and subjacent white matter after neuronal migration in developing sheep did not prevent the normal formation of sulci and gyri in the remaining cortex. Similar findings have been observed in cases of cortical dysgenesis in humans, in which the space freed by missing cortex is filled by liquid instead of being occupied by relaxed, non-convoluted remaining cortex (see figures in Raybaud 2019 and Spreafico and Tassi 2012). In addition, an overall look at brain and skull development suggests that the expanding brain dictates the growth of the skull, whose sutures will not ossify until brain development is completed. In fact, pathologies in which sutures ossify prematurely conduct to elevated intracranial pressure and head deformities due to impeded brain growth, instead of leading to increased gyrification. Therefore, gyrification evolved in mammals as their cortex acquired enlarged surface areas, and became an intrinsic feature of cortical growth, governed by internal developmental mechanisms and independent from space constrains.

23.8 Cortical Expansion and Differential Growth of Cortical Layers

This model groups different hypotheses that share in common the idea that lateral expansion of the cortex causes lateral tension that would be released through gyrification. The initial hypothesis by Richman et al. (1975) proposed that differential growth of cortical laminae would lie behind the origin of the buckling. They indicated that upper layers 2 to 4 expand more than deep layers 5 to 6, and such differential growth will create laminar tension that would resolve through buckling of the cortex. The main support for their view was their findings of poorly developed cortical lower layers in cases of overly convoluted microgyral brains and, conversely, a decrease in upper layer neurons in lissencephalic brains. This hypothesis has received support from other groups (Armstrong et al. 1995; Hilgetag and Barbas 2005).

In the past two decades, several models have been proposed to simulate the process of gyrification (for review see Bayly et al. 2014; Kroenke and Bayly 2018; and Tallinen et al. 2016). These include numerical and also physical models using layered hydrogels with different expansion properties when immersed in a solvent that produces surprisingly realistic replicas of the process of gyrification (Tallinen et al. 2016) (Figure 23.5). There are differences in the various parameters that each model uses, but all of them require differential lateral expansion of an external layer against the subjacent structure. In addition, models allow simulation of the effect of changes in parameters such as cortical thickness, showing how thinner cortices tend to have more and smaller convolutions (cetaceans), while thick cortices exhibit less convolutions (Figure 23.5). Interestingly, the physical model depicted in Figure 23.5 only requires cortical lateral expansion to reproduce with striking realism what is observed in real brains. The numerical model adds the ratio between brain size and cortical thickness to produce different sulcation patterns (Tallinen et al. 2014, 2016).

23.9 Gyrogenesis Hypothesis

Observations in the development of the carnivore brain have indicated that before gyrification, shallow dimples appear that will be buried by adjacent cortex that would expand radially. Those dimples will become sulcal fundi while the adjacent growing cortex will become gyri (Smart and McSherry 1986a, 1986b; Welker 1990) (Figure 23.6). In support of this hypothesis is the observation

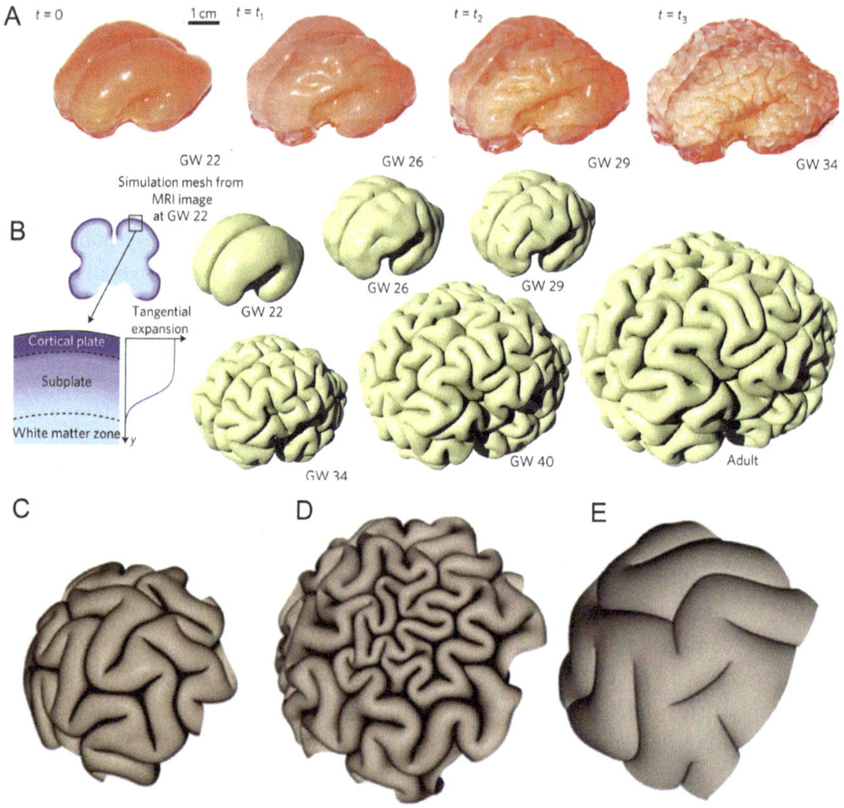

Figure 23.5 Physical and numerical models of gyrification based on cortical expansion. (A) MRI-based gestational week 20 gel-brain representing white matter is coated with a thin layer of gel (cortex) that swells by absorbing a solvent (hexanes) over time *t* (*t*1 = 4 min, *t*2 = 9 min, *t*3 = 16 min). The layered gel progressively evolves into a complex pattern of sulci and gyri during the swelling process. (B) simulation starting from a smooth fetal brain shows gyrification as a result of uniform tangential expansion of the cortical layer. The brain is modelled as a soft elastic solid and a relative tangential expansion is imposed on the cortical layer as shown at left, and the system allowed to relax to its elastic equilibrium. B–D illustrate different patterns of gyrification obtained after changing the parameters of the model. (C) Simulation with standard parameters to mimic the meninges and skull. (D) Simulation after changing the gray matter thickness in a small patch of the growing cortex leads to morphologies similar to polymicrogyria. (E) Simulation of same size as C but with thickened cortex and reduced tangential expansion displays wide gyri and shallow sulci reminiscent of pachygyric brains. A and B reproduced with permission from Tallinen et al. (2016). C to E reproduced with permission from Tallinen et al. (2014).

that the deepest sulci in the adult are typically the first to form. Similar observations were noted in primates (Connolly 1950) and a more refined hypothesis was proposed by Rose and Woolsey (1949), indicating that thalamic afferents will have discontinuities ("athalamic" cortex) that will remain as sulci, while the regions rich in thalamic afferents will grow to become gyri. The mechanisms that might produce the differential expansion of the cortex have been explained in detail by Welker (1990). Welker (1990) proposed that gyri form as the cortical plate expands in a process initiated by the invasion of axons from the thalamus and other sources, and continues with the subsequent development of the cortical circuits, involving neuronal maturation, dendritogenesis, synaptogenesis, glial population, and differentiation. Support for this model comes from Welker's studies on receptive fields in mammals, and one particularly illustrative example is the correlation

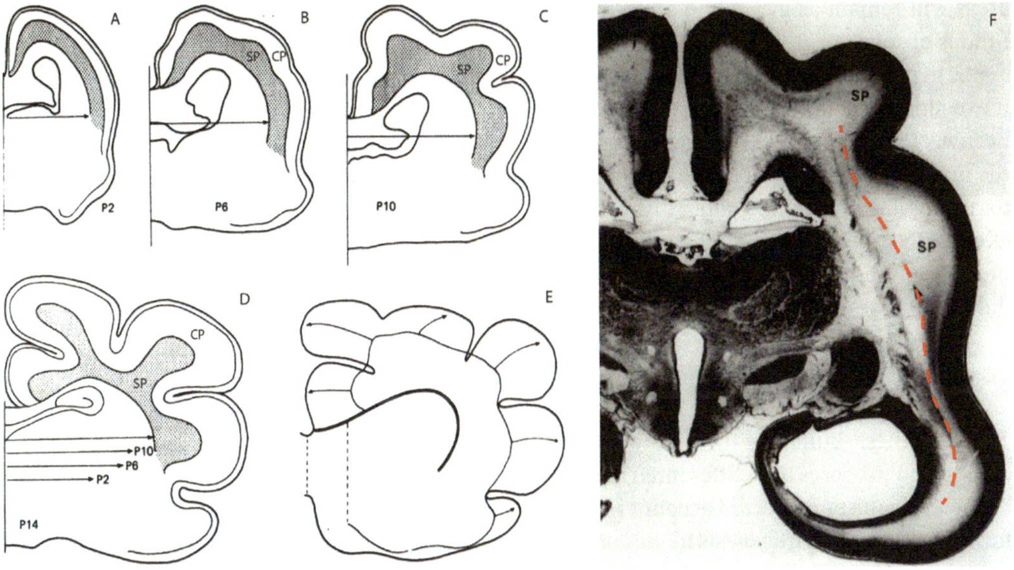

Figure 23.6 Subplate and gyrogenesis hypothesis. Diagram modified with permission from Smart and McSherry (1986b) showing how gyrification in the cortical plate (CP) seems to be driven by the growth of gyri between apparently static sulcal fundi, and enlargement of the subplate (SP) that might play a role in the radial expansion of gyri. (A–C) schematic tracing of ferret brain sections at postnatal (P) day 2, 6, and 10 respectively, taken at the level of the interventricular foramen. The shaded area indicates the subplate (note the progressive thickening of the subplate below the forming gyri) and the arrows indicate the distance from the midline to the deep surface of the subplate. (D) Coronal section of a P14 ferret brain. Arrows indicate the distance of the deep surface of the subplate from the midline at the stated postnatal ages, suggesting that the cortex moves laterally as the core of the hemisphere enlarges. (E) overlap of a P14 brain on a P6 brain with the deep subplate borders in register, illustrating sulcal fundi that remain close to the deep surface of the subplate whereas the sulcal crowns move centrifugally (arrows) from the boundary between the SP and the white matter (thick line). (F) Coronal section (Nissl stain) through the cortex of an E97 macaque fetus showing variations in the thickness of the SP zone along the extent of the CP. The dashed red line marks the border between the external capsule and the SP. Note how the SP is thickest in the lateral cortex but is reduced in the limbic cortex and below prospective sulci. Modified with permission from Kostovic and Rakic (1990). The answer to question in Figure 23.2 is D according to Biondi et al. (1998) (with permission).

between thalamo-cortical somatosensory input from the Raccoon paw, and the gyrification of the corresponding cortical receptive areas as discussed in Section 23.6.1 (Figure 23.4). As mentioned earlier, even when this exquisite correlation between thalamic input and gyral formation might not be the most prevalent scenario, this example suggest that, at least in the somatosensory cortex, the distribution of thalamic afferents might be the prime factor determining the formation and delimitation of sulci and gyri.

23.10 Axon Tension Hypothesis

A very different mechanism was proposed by Van Essen (1997) involving differential axonal tension between adjacent cortical areas. This was based on earlier studies indicating that neurites can produce tension through forced elongation, and can release it when retracting (Bray 1987; Lamoureux et al. 1989). He proposed that nearby cortical areas with strong connections will generate tangential forces that will deform the cortex producing convolutions. Strongly connected areas will remain as gyri while areas more loosely connected could drift apart or remain as the fundus of sulci.

The hypothesis of axonal tension has been very influential in the field and has the advantage that it explains the patterning of gyrification based on the specific organization of the underlying connectivity (Sporns et al. 2004). However, detailed analysis revealed some important caveats. Perhaps the most important is that axons do not follow the pattern required by the hypothesis, as they tend to run parallel to the sulcal sides, instead of perpendicular to them to draw the walls of gyri together (Xu et al. 2010). In addition, when the hypothesis was tested by physically cutting the axon bundles underneath the cortex in sections obtained at different time points during development, the cortex did not change its morphology, and kept the convolutions (Xu et al. 2010).

23.10.1 Differential Neurogenic Hypothesis

This hypothesis builds on the differential laminar expansion and gyral growth models explained earlier, and proposes that differential neurogenesis between upper and lower cortical layers might be the mechanism that could account for both phenomena. The idea is that under prospective gyri, focal increases of neurogenesis in the cortical germinal niches would produce supernumerary neurons destined to upper layers of the cortex that would cause the upper layers to expand and produce buckling of the cortex. This idea was initially proposed by Kriegstein and colleagues (Kriegstein et al. 2006) based on two main points: the growing evidence that intermediate progenitors in the subventricular zone (SVZ) would contribute to expand the population of cortical neurons in species with enlarged and gyrified neocortex such as primates and specifically humans (Lukaszewicz et al. 2005; Martínez-Cerdeño et al. 2006; Sidman and Rakic 1973; Smart et al. 2002), and the observation that the SVZ was particularly prominent in gyrified species, and it showed thickening in regions of prospective gyri.

This hypothesis was refined with the characterization of proliferative radial glia-like cells in the outer SVZ (oSVZ) lacking apical processes to the ventricle. These cells, named intermediate radial glia (Reillo et al. 2011), outer radial glia or basal radial glia (bRG), were initially described in gyrencephalic species such as ferret or human, leading to the hypothesis that they were responsible for the expansion of the cortex and gyrification (Fietz et al. 2010; Hansen et al. 2010; Reillo and Borrell 2012). Subsequent studies also described these cells in mouse, although in lower proportions (Shitamukai et al. 2011; Wang et al. 2011). And a comparative study of several species including guinea pig, ferret, sheep, cat, and human showed correlation between the number of bRG and gyrification (expressed as GI) (Reillo et al. 2011).

However, analysis of marmosets, an almost lissencephalic primate, showed high levels of bRGs, similar to those found in ferrets or human (García-Moreno et al. 2012; Kelava et al. 2012). This hypothesis has been further elaborated to include a role for the bRG cells basal process as an essential component for achieving cortical expansion and gyrification. The rationale is that the basal process of bRG cells will occupy the space between ventricular RG cells, allowing fanning out and lateral expansion producing potential guides for migration in radial directions that will increase surface area without an increase in cortical thickness (Lui et al. 2011; Reillo et al. 2011; Stahl et al. 2013). Gain or loss of function of certain genes in the germinal zones of mice induced the presence of gyral and/or sulcal formations (Del Toro et al. 2017; Florio et al. 2015; Ju et al. 2016; Rash et al. 2013; Stahl et al. 2013; Wang et al. 2016) although some of those structures do not look like bona fide gyri (Florio et al. 2015; Stahl et al. 2013). In some cases such effects are minor sulcations in the cortex with inconsistent distribution and low prevalence (Del Toro et al. 2017). Also, in the case of ARHGAP11B, a human-specific gene that has been related to increased number and proliferation of bRG (Florio et al. 2015), gain of function induced in ferrets saw both an increase of gliogenesis and a three-to-five-fold increase in upper layer neurons, consistent with the initial hypothesis. However, such large increases in neurogenesis resulted only in a 10 percent increase in surface area and a 24 percent increase in layer thickness, without changing gyrification. As a result, upper layers acquired a higher neuronal density without creating further lateral expansion and gyrification, as measured by the GI (Kalebic et al. 2018). Similarly, when expression of ARHGAP11B was induced in the lissencephalic marmoset, an increase in bRG and upper layer neurons was detected, accompanied by a slight increase in size of the cortex, but only a "bump" in the lateral aspect of the cortex was induced, that cannot be considered a bona fide gyrus (Heide et al. 2020). Another case of a hominoid-specific gene whose expression was induced in mouse progenitors is TBC1D3 (Ju et al. 2016). When the gene expression was induced by electroporation, a slight sulcation of the cortical surface could be observed in some cases. However, when expression was induced in the transgenic, sulcation could not be observed, and disruption of the lamination and distribution of upper cortical layer neurons was the main effect (Ju et al. 2016). In summary, these results have to be interpreted with caution, since some of the observed effects might not represent real gyrification but disruptions and deformations of the cortical surface and upper layer neurons.

Overall, this model of enlarged populations of basal progenitors in the oSVZ producing focal increased neurogenesis to upper cortical layers, local cortical expansion and gyrification has been widely accepted and incorporated in models to explain gyrification (e.g., Hevner 2016; Striedter et al. 2015). However, there has been also controversy over the major tenants of this hypothesis (García-Moreno et al. 2012; Hevner and Haydar 2012; Kroenke and Bayly 2018; Rash et al. 2019, 2023).

There are two main lines of criticism of this hypothesis. The most consequential is that neurogenesis and neuronal migration is basically complete before gyrification starts. Indeed, gyrification in the monkey starts around embryonic day (E) 90, when cortical neurogenesis and neuronal migration is basically complete in all cortical areas analyzed except in the primary visual cortex, which shows a protracted developmental window since it is endowed with about 2.5 times more neurons than the other cortical areas (Granger et al. 1995; Kroenke and Bayly 2018; Rakic 1974, 2002a; Rockel et al. 1980). Indeed, studies in our lab have shown that at the beginning of the period of active gyrification in the macaque embryo, between E92 and E97, only a few intermediate progenitors could be found expressing low levels of Tbr2, that are absent later at E125 when gyrification is still ongoing (Wang et al. 2017). These findings were supported by transcriptional analysis (PsychENCODE project) that confirmed that Tbr2 expression decreases dramatically from E60 and E80 to almost adult levels by E110 in the majority of cortical regions, or data from the NIH Blueprint NHP Atlas showing a clear decrease of Tbr2 RNAm between E80 and E90 and almost lack of expression at E120 in the germinal zones of the macaque cingulate cortex, including the oSVZ (Rash et al. 2023). In agreement with these data Betizeau et al. (2013) showed a low number of oRG in the oSVZ of the macaque at E94, likely reflecting the decline of the population.

The same sequence of events occurs in other species analyzed, including ferret or human (Bayer and Altman 2005; Gilardi and Kalebic 2021; Sidman and Rakic 1973; Smart and McSherry 1986b), further indicating a lack of correlation between differential neurogenesis (or simply neurogenesis) and gyrification. For the same reasons, the concept of bRG basal processes fanning out and helping the lateral dispersion of neurons described previously (Reillo et al. 2011) does not fit the timeline of gyral development.

This mismatch has been acknowledged, arguing that differences in early neurogenic processes, included an increased number of bRG progenitors in the oSVZ or the presence of a protomap revealed by differential gene expression in the germinal areas correlates with the future presence of gyri (Borrell 2018; de Juan Romero et al. 2015). However, it can be argued that such a protomap lacks enough resolution to produce individual gyri and sulci. The protomap might be responsible for the regionalization of sensory and motor areas and delimitate territories of primary, secondary, or tertiary sensory/motor areas, but it seems very unlikely that it might be able to specify the somatosensory subdomains in those areas, as shown in Figure 23.4, or to determine the configuration of gyri and sulci. It seems however more likely that thalamic and non-thalamic axonal input and signaling cues might have more influence on the differentiation of those territories into specific somatosensory/motor subdomains like those shown in Figure 23.4 (Welker and Seidenstein 1959).

The second point of criticism has been raised after showing that most bRG might not be neurogenic, but instead gliogenic at the beginning of gyrification. Voigt (1989) described the capacity of bRG cells to produce glia, and proliferation analysis of the germinal niches and cortex of the macaque at E97 has shown large numbers of cycling cells, the vast majority of which were glial precursors or endothelial cells around blood vessels (Rash et al. 2019). These results suggest that at the beginning of gyrification the oSVZ is producing mostly glia that will populate the developing cortex. These findings are in agreement with the established notion that gliogenesis starts at the peak of neurogenesis and proceeds after neurogenesis is completed in primates (Schmechel and Rakic 1979; Zecevic et al. 2005) and ferrets (Gilardi and Kalebic 2021; Voigt 1989).

23.11 Our Proposal: Gyrification is Produced by Explosive Cortical Expansion Dominated by Axonal and Glial Invasion and Cortical Differentiation

We agree with previous authors (Striedter et al. 2015; Welker 1990; White and Hilgetag 2011) that the most likely scenario is that not a single, but several mechanisms, act at different time points, and are additively responsible for gyrification of the cortex. Lateral expansion of the cortical plate seems to be the defining factor contributing to form gyri and sulci, and the results of modeling show that it is essential for producing convolutions (Bayly et al. 2014; Tallinen et al. 2014, 2016; Toro and Burnod 2005; Xu et al. 2010) (Figure 23.5). Since, as discussed previously, neurogenesis cannot be a major factor in the expansion of the cortex, other processes might be at play. We agree with previous models (Goldman-Rakic et al. 1984; Kostovic and Rakic 1990; Welker 1990) that put emphasis on the expansion of the cortical plate due to incoming axons and glia and the differentiation of the cortex to form the internal circuitry and cortical connections. These processes will produce a massive increase in neuropil that results in augmented cortical thickness and lateral expansion inducing gyrification, while the specific patterning of sulci and gyri will result from the interplay between cytoarchitectonic features (such as thickness), incorporation and differentiation of glial cells, and afferent and efferent systems.

23.12 The Subplate and Axonal Afferents, Cortical Maturation, and Gyrification

During development, incoming axons directed to the cortical plate arrive at the subplate, a transient compartment situated below the cortical plate, where they will wait for the maturation of cortical neurons before entering the cortical plate and establishing synaptic contacts (Kostovic and Rakic 1990). The subplate is poorly developed in lissencephalic species and is larger in gyrencephalic ones, especially in primates and human, where it has been more extensively studied. The subplate differentiates below the nascent cortical plate after E50 in the macaque, as a layer of disperse cells, and will grow at a fast pace by incorporating incoming axons from different systems (brain stem, basal forebrain, thalamus, callosal, and association fibers) that arrive sequentially and will remain in this compartment until they enter the cortical plate or find their subcortical targets. Interestingly, incoming axons establish synaptic contacts with differentiated subplate neurons, although the specific function of these contacts is not totally clear (Kostović 2020). By E80, the subplate reaches its maximum thickness in the somatosensory cortex of the macaque, representing about three times the thickness of the cortical plate (four times in the human at its maximum thickness at the 18th gestational week). From E80 to about E120, the subplate will remain stable in size, although with possible changes in the ratio of different axonal populations (Kostovic and Rakic 1990). Interestingly, as convolutions start to form in the cortical surface, the subplate becomes thicker where convolutions start appearing, similar to what was described in the developing ferret (Smart and McSherry 1986b) (Figure 23.6). This observation led to the hypothesis that the differential amount of incoming axons might be related to the nascent pattern of gyrification (Kostovic and Rakic 1990; Welker 1990). The timing of gyrification coincides with the influx of thalamic input (Goldman and Galkin 1978; Goldman-Rakic 1981; Rakic 1976, 1977, 1979). Therefore, the invasion of the cortex by thalamocortical axons from the subjacent subplate might be the main factor inducing the initial development of gyri, propelling the lateral expansion of the cortex. At the same time, excitatory and inhibitory cortical neurons are differentiating, extending dendrites and dendritic spines, and establishing synapses with incoming axons and with other cortical neurons to form the cortical circuitry (Bourgeois et al. 1994; Rash et al. 2023; Zecevic et al. 1989; Zecevic and Rakic 1991). In addition, glial cells invade the cortical plate and differentiate into mature astrocytes and oligos (Rash et al. 2019, 2022,; Schmechel and Rakic 1979), extending processes around the neuronal circuits. It can be predicted that all these processes will increase the proportion of neuropil in the cortical plate, produce cortical expansion, and decrease neuronal density. Indeed, a recent study from our lab, has shown that neuronal density in the cortical plate starts decreasing drastically at some point between E70 and E92, implying an increase in neuropil volume. Between E92 and E125, corresponding to the initial wave of gyrification in the monkey, neuronal density continues decreasing, indicating further increases of neuropil (Figure 23.7) (Rash et al. 2023). After this initial development, intrahemispheric and callosal cortico-cortical input enter the macaque cortex between E124 and E150, when the cortex is still expanding at a rapid pace (Wang et al. 2017), and convolutions are still growing, reaching their mature pattern (Goldman-Rakic 1981; Goldman-Rakic and Schwartz 1982). The percentage of neuropil will reach adult levels (80%) at E150 (Bourgeois et al. 1994). Similarly Wang et al. (2017) using MRI, showed that the surface area of the rhesus macaque cortex expands from 8.2 to 59 cm^2 from E75 to E137. Parallel findings have been shown in ferret (Knutsen et al. 2013). Interestingly, Wang et al. (2017) showed that the rate of cortical surface area growth changes drastically at E102, from 0.4 cm^2 per day before E102 to 1.2 cm^2 per day after. That represents a three-fold increase after E102. This timing matches the developmental processes described, and supports the hypothesis that the establishing of cortical circuits is the main driver of cortical expansion and gyrification.

Once the phase of fast growth and gyrification slows, the cortical gray matter will grow three-fold to achieve adult size (Hill et al. 2010), but the GI will remain stable (Wang et al. 2017) a finding also described in cynomolgus monkey (Sawada et al. 2012) and in human (Armstrong et al. 1995), suggesting that ongoing cortical expansion is matched with the growth of other structures including white matter, that is expected to expand noticeably due to axonal myelination, a process that

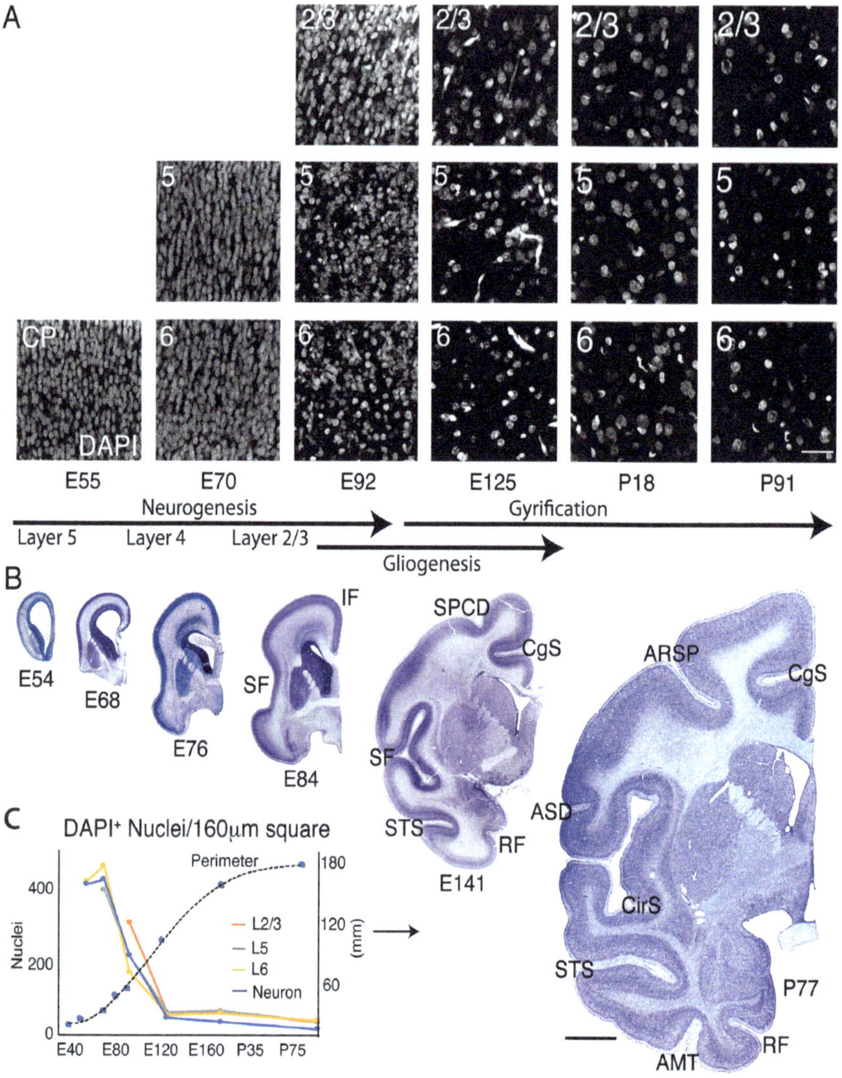

Figure 23.7 Cortical plate surface area expansion is accompanied by neuropil growth and elaboration paralleled by decrease in cellular and neuronal density. (A) Insets of DAPI-stained coronal sections of dorsal parietal macaque cortical plate (CP) from E55–P91. Numbers indicate cortical layers. Notice moderate expansion of the neuropil inducing decrease in cellular density between E70 and E92, and the large expansion of the neuropil between E92 and E125, during the time of gyral development (see also panel C). (B) Scaled Nissl-stained coronal sections of macaque from E76 to P77 illustrating cortical surface area growth and gyrification, particularly after E90, when neurogenesis is already completed. (C) Quantification of cellular density in layers 2/3, 5, and 6 and for all neurons (left axis) and cortical perimeter measured in coronal sections from the corpus callosum to the latero-ventral edge of the cortical plate at the level of the anterior commissure (right axis) from E40 to P75. Error bars represent SEM. AMT: Anterior middle temporal sulcus; ASD: Anterior subcentral dimple; ARSP: Arcuate sulcus spur; CgS: Cingulate sulcus; CirS: Circular sulcus; IF: interhemispheric fissure; RF: Rhinal fissure; SF: sylvian fissure; STS: Superior temporal sulcus. From Rash et al. (2023).

occurs mostly at later stages of development (Armstrong et al. 1995; Bayly et al. 2014; Knutsen et al. 2013; Neal et al. 2007; Wang et al. 2017). In addition, as mentioned earlier, glial cells continue populating and differentiating in the cortical plate (Rash et al. 2019).

This notion of differential cortical innervation suggests that axonal input/output might be one important factor determining the pattern of gyrification. Analogously, it could be argued that these somatosensory hotspots might be endowed with a larger number of neurons to account for an enhanced receptive field that will attract a larger number of axons, resulting in buckling of the cortex. However, there are some points that seem to favor the axonal input mechanisms over the neurogenesis mechanism. As reasoned already, the induction of such somatosensory hotspots with increased neurogenesis implies an extremely refined differential gene expression in the germinal zones. It seems more likely that neurogenesis is more or less homogeneous along the germinal niches (except in some exceptional sites like the primary visual germinal zones) and is instead the pattern of connectivity influenced by the protomap and competition from incoming afferents that contributes to the determination of the patterns of cortical expansion, connectivity, and subsequent neuron elimination.

23.13 Loss of Axonal Input and Gyrification

The importance of axonal input in determining gyrification was evidenced through lesion studies that removed cortical regions during development, altered subcortical structures, or deprived somatic input areas (Goldman and Galkin 1978; Goldman-Rakic and Rakic 1984; Rakic 1988; Welker 1990). Lesions to the prefrontal cortex of developing macaques between E102 and E106 produced changes in the pattern of gyrification, with the appearance of ectopic sulci in the surface of the cortex around the lesion but also in distant regions such as temporal and occipital cortical areas (Goldman and Galkin 1978). Remarkably, the ectopic sulci did not distribute randomly, but their location was consistent between animals and they were present in both hemispheres irrespective of the lesion being uni- or bilateral. Another important detail is that the ectopic sulci only appeared in animals at E102–E106, but not in animals at E119, when gyrification is more advanced (Goldman and Galkin 1978). As the authors consider, it is not likely that pure mechanical factors related to the lesion and creation of a cortical void are responsible for the changes in gyrification observed as this would likely produce changes around the lesion, but no changes would be expected in distant cortical regions or in the contralateral, non-lesioned hemisphere. Although highly speculative, a potential explanation for the appearance of ectopic sulci is that lack of specific input from ablated regions would reduce the number of axons invading the cortical plate in target areas, creating potential "athalamic" areas, altering the balance of forces inducing expansion of the cortex that might be translated into the appearance of ectopic sulci. Although this is hard to prove experimentally, this model would explain the appearance of ectopic sulci in distant and contralateral regions of the cortex from the damaged area, as distant and contralateral projections are expected from cortical areas. Furthermore, it would explain the consistent location of the ectopic sulci, since the connectivity of a particular cortical area is expected to show only minor variations between animals.

Subsequent studies in macaques revealed that enucleation at E60 resulted in reduction of the surface area of the primary visual cortex, while the thickness, lamination, and neuronal density were preserved. Strikingly, the remaining cortex exhibited convolutions that are not present in the normally smooth occipital lobe (Figure 23.8) (Rakic 1988; Rakic et al. 1991); It could be argued that

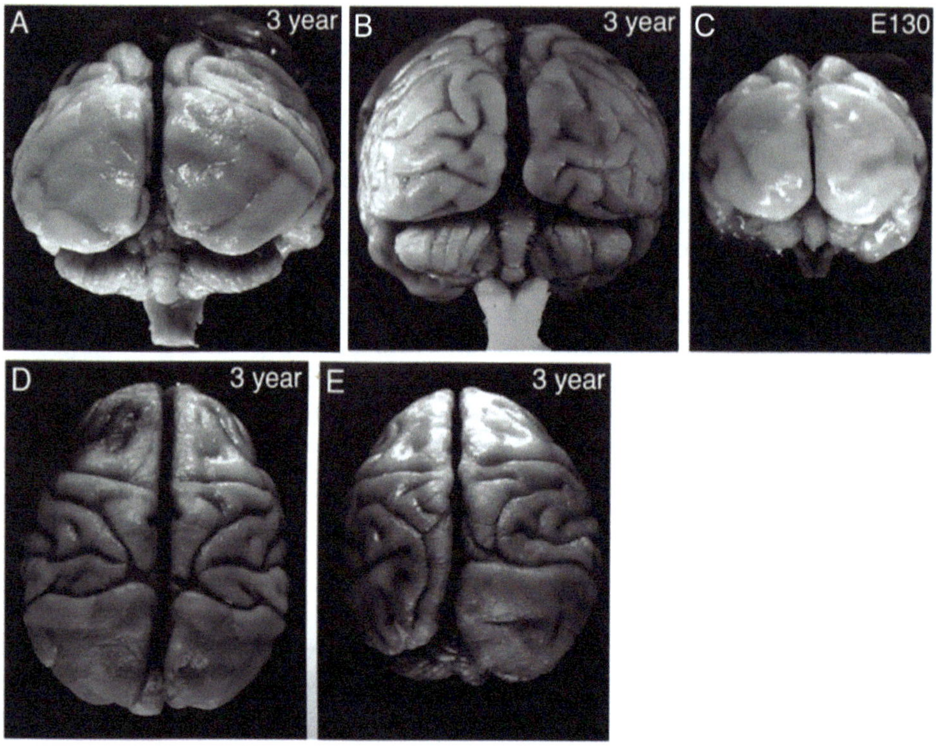

Figure 23.8 Changes in gyral pattern induced by enucleation in fetal macaque. (A) Normal occipital lobe of a 3-year-old macaque. (B) Convoluted occipital lobe of a 3-year-old macaque enucleated at E60. (C) Occipital lobe of E130 macaque embryo enucleated at E66. Note that the occipital lobe is still relatively smooth at E130, when neurogenesis is complete but thalamo-cortical input is invading the visual cortex. (D) Top view of normal 3-year-old macaque brain. (E) Top view of brain of macaque that underwent resection of the left occipital lobe at E91 shows large changes to parietal lobe gyral pattern and expansion of parietal lobe into occipital territory, with additional encroachment across the interhemispheric fissure by the contralateral occipital lobe. Images A and B reproduced with permission from Rakic (1988). C, D, and E from MacBrain Resource at Yale University.

changes in the thalamic input to the visual cortex (subplate) induced by the enucleation might produce an increase in subsequent neurogenesis and induce the formation of gyri (Gerstmann et al. 2015). However, unpublished data from our lab show that this is not the case. In fact, after enucleation at a similar time (E66), analysis of the brain at E130, about three weeks after neurogenesis is already over in the primary visual cortex (Rakic 2002b), shows a much smaller lateral geniculate nucleus and much reduced cortical projections, but a lack of ectopic convolutions. These results suggest that neurogenesis is not responsible for the effect, and instead, the altered thalamic input that will invade the visual cortex around and after this time (E130) is likely to be the factor inducing such changes (Figure 23.8C). Although the presence of ectopic sulci and gyri after deafferentation seems counterintuitive and opposing the proposed model of thalamic induction of gyrification, there is one possible explanation that complies with both. One interesting feature of the occipital primary visual cortex in macaques is that it is basically lissencephalic. This feature might be due to the homogeneous visual input received from the geniculate. If that input is depleted, the cortical surface will be reduced, as indeed is observed, but the remaining cortex might be invaded by competing axons from other sources. Those incoming axons might be diverse in origin and densities, and such heterogeneities in the input might induce gyri and sulci, similarly as the model proposed in other cortical areas (see Figure 23.4).

Other experimental manipulations, such as unilateral occipital resection performed at E91, results in notable alteration of the gyrification pattern, with changes in the parietal convolutions and expansion of the contralateral occipital cortex (Figure 23.8). Since neurogenesis in the parietal lobe was complete by the age of surgery (Rakic 1988, 2002b), it implies that changes in white matter tracts, a removal of other physical barriers such as a contralateral hemisphere, have pronounced effects on the formation and configuration of cerebral convolutions.

23.14 Conclusion

The mechanics of gyrification have seen an enormous interest in the past two decades. Innovative hypotheses relating differential neurogenesis have been proposed and extensively explored both in descriptive and experimental studies, and have gained large popularity and reputation. In this brief review we have presented the most relevant features of gyrification that can help us to understand and also test possible underlying mechanisms inducing convolutions in the cortex. Based on some of those features, particularly the timing of neurogenesis vs. gyrification, it is unlikely that differential neurogenesis might play a defining role in gyrification. We reason instead that the basic principles of the gyrogenesis hypothesis of differential growth of gyri and sulci, as proposed more than 30 years ago (Goldman-Rakic and Rakic 1984; Kostovic and Rakic 1990; Welker 1990), are the most likely mechanisms to explain cortical tangential expansion and gyrification, in agreement with some available models. The main drivers of gyral formation would be incoming axonal afferents and glial cells and differentiation and maturation of the cortical elements after neurogenesis is complete. We base our case on the timing of such processes and the agreement with the main features of gyrification, such as the general correlation between sulci and gyri and functional domains in the cortex.

Acknowledgments

We want to thank Brian Rash and Alvaro Duque for fruitful discussions on the subject. And Alvaro Duque, Director of the MacBrain resource at Yale University, for gently providing images for Figure 23.8. MacBrain Resource is supported by NIH MH113257 (To Dr. Alvaro Duque).

References

Armstrong, E. et al. (1995). The ontogeny of human gyrification. *Cereb Cortex* 5 (1): 56–63. doi: 10.1093/cercor/5.1.56.

Badea, A. et al. (2007). Morphometric analysis of the C57BL/6J mouse brain. *NeuroImage* 37 (3): 683–693. doi: 10.1016/j.neuroimage.2007.05.046.

Bailey, P. and von Bonin, G. (1951). *The Isocortex of Man*. Urbana, University of Illinois Press.

Barron, D. (1950). An experimental analysis of some factors involved in the development of the fissure pattern of the cerebral cortex. *J Exp Zool* 113 (3): 553–581.

Bartley, A.J. et al. (1997). Genetic variability of human brain size and cortical gyral patterns. *Brain* 120 (Pt 2): 257–269. doi: 10.1093/brain/120.2.257.

Bayer, S.A. and Altman, J. (2005). *The Human Brain during the Second Trimester*. Boca Raton, FL: CRC Press.

Bayly, P.V. et al. (2014). Mechanical forces in cerebral cortical folding. *J Mech Behav Biomed Mater* 29: 568–581. doi: 10.1016/j.jmbbm.2013.02.018.

Betizeau, M. et al. (2013). Precursor diversity and complexity of lineage relationships in the outer subventricular zone of the primate. *Neuron* 80 (2): 442–457. doi: 10.1016/j.neuron.2013.09.032.

Biondi, A. et al. (1998). Are the brains of monozygotic twins similar? A three-dimensional MR study. *Am J Neuroradiol* 19 (7): 1361–1367.

Borrell, V. (2018). How cells fold the cerebral cortex. *J Neurosci* 38 (4): 776–783. doi: 10.1523/JNEUROSCI.1106-17.2017.

Bourgeois, J.P. et al. (1994). Synaptogenesis in the prefrontal cortex of rhesus monkeys. *Cereb Cortex* 4 (1): 78–96. doi: 10.1093/cercor/4.1.78.

Bray, D. (1987). Growth cones. *Trends Neurosci* 10 (10): 431–434. doi: 10.1016/0166-2236(87)90015-4.

Broca, P. (2015). Comparative anatomy of the cerebral convolutions. *J Comp Neurol* 523 (17): 2501–2554. doi: 10.1002/cne.23856.

Brodmann, K. (1913). Neue Forschungsergebnisse der Grosshirn- rindenanatomie mit besonderer Berücksichtigung anthropologischer Fragen. *Verh Ges Dtsch Naturforsch Ärzte* 85: 200–240.

Chi, J.G. et al. (1977). Gyral development of the human brain. *Ann Neurol* 1 (1): 86–93. doi: 10.1002/ana.410010109.

Clark, W.E.L.G. and Medawar, P.B. (1945). *Essays on Growth and Form Presented to D'Arcy Wentworth Thompson*. Oxford: Clarendon Press.

Connolly, C.J. (1950). *External Morphology of the Primate Brain*. Springfield, IL: C. C. Thomas.

Cunningham, D.J. (1892). *Contribution to the Surface Anatomy of the Cerebral Hemispheres*. Academy House.

Dareste, C. (1855). *Troisième mémoire sur les circonvolutions du cerveau chez les mammifères*. V. Masson.

Dawkins, R. and Wong, Y. (2005). *The Ancestor's Tale: A Pilgrimage to the Dawn of Evolution*. Houghton Mifflin Harcourt.

D'azyr, V. (1786). *Traité d'anatomie et de physiologie, avec des planches coloriées représentant au naturel les divers organes de l'homme et des animaux*, vol. 1. Paris: Didot.

de Juan Romero, C. et al. (2015). Discrete domains of gene expression in germinal layers distinguish the development of gyrencephaly. *EMBO J* 34 (14): 1859–1874. doi: 10.15252/embj.201591176.

Del Toro, D. et al. (2017). Regulation of cerebral cortex folding by controlling neuronal migration via FLRT adhesion molecules. *Cell* 169 (4): 621–635.e16. doi: 10.1016/j.cell.2017.04.012.

Donaldson, H.H. (1891). Anatomical observations on the brain and several sense-organs of the blind deaf-mute, Laura Dewey Bridgman. *Am J Psychol* 4 (2): 248–294. doi: 10.2307/1411270.

Duque, A. and McCormick, D.A. (2010). Circuit-based localization of ferret prefrontal cortex. *Cereb Cortex* 20 (5): 1020–1036. doi: 10.1093/cercor/bhp164.

Elias, H. and Schwartz, D. (1969). Surface areas of the cerebral cortex of mammals determined by stereological methods. *Science* 166 (3901): 111–113. doi: 10.1126/science.166.3901.111.

Feldhamer, G.A. et al. (2007). *Mammalogy: Adaptation, Diversity, Ecology*. Baltimore, MD: JHU Press.

Fietz, S.A. et al. (2010). OSVZ progenitors of human and ferret neocortex are epithelial-like and expand by integrin signaling. *Nat Neurosci* 13 (6): 690–699. doi: 10.1038/nn.2553.

Finger, S. (2001). *Origins of Neuroscience: A History of Explorations into Brain Function*. New York: Oxford University Press.

Florio, M. et al. (2015). Human-specific gene ARHGAP11B promotes basal progenitor amplification and neocortex expansion. *Science* 347 (6229): 1465–1470. doi: 10.1126/science.aaa1975.

García-Moreno, F. et al. (2012). Compartmentalization of cerebral cortical germinal zones in a lissencephalic primate and gyrencephalic rodent. *Cereb Cortex* 22 (2): 482–492. doi: 10.1093/cercor/bhr312.

Gerstmann, K. et al. (2015). Thalamic afferents influence cortical progenitors via ephrin A5-EphA4 interactions. *Development* 142 (1): 140–150. doi: 10.1242/dev.104927.

Gilardi, C. and Kalebic, N. (2021). The ferret as a model system for neocortex development and evolution. *Front Cell Dev Biol* 9: 661759. doi: 10.3389/fcell.2021.661759.

Goldman, P.S. and Galkin, T.W. (1978). Prenatal removal of frontal association cortex in the fetal rhesus monkey. *Brain Res* 152 (3): 451–485. doi: 10.1016/0006-8993(78)91103-4.

Goldman-Rakic, P.S. (1981). Prenatal formation of cortical input and development of cytoarchitectonic compartments in the neostriatum of the rhesus monkey. *J Neurosci* 1 (7): 721–735.

Goldman-Rakic, P.S. and Rakic, P. (1984). Experimental modification of gyral patterns. In: *Cerebral Dominance: The Biological Foundations* (ed. N. Geschwind and A.M. Galaburda). Cambridge, MA: Harvard University Press.

Goldman-Rakic, P.S. and Schwartz, M.L. (1982). Interdigitation of contralateral and ipsilateral columnar projections to frontal association cortex in primates. *Science* 216 (4547): 755–757. doi: 10.1126/science.6177037.

Goldman-Rakic, P.S. et al. (1984). Dual pathways connecting the dorsolateral prefrontal cortex with the hippocampal formation and parahippocampal cortex in the rhesus monkey. *Neuroscience* 12 (3): 719–743. doi: 10.1016/0306-4522(84)90166-0.

Granger, B. et al. (1995). Tempo of neurogenesis and synaptogenesis in the primate cingulate mesocortex. *J Comp Neurol* 360 (2): 363–376. doi: 10.1002/cne.903600212.

Gratiolet, P.-L. (1854). *Mémoire sur les plis cérébraux de l'homme et des primatès*. Paris: Arthus Bertrand.

Gross, C.G. (1995). Aristotle on the brain. *The Neuroscientist* 1 (4): 245–250. doi: 10.1177/107385849500100408.

Hansen, D.V. et al. (2010). Neurogenic radial glia in the outer subventricular zone of human neocortex. *Nature* 464 (7288): 554–561. doi: 10.1038/nature08845.

Haug, H. (1987). Brain sizes, surfaces, and neuronal sizes of the cortex cerebri: a stereological investigation of man and his variability and a comparison with some mammals (primates, whales, marsupials, insectivores, and one elephant). *Am J Anat* 180 (2): 126–142. doi: 10.1002/aja.1001800203.

Heide, M. et al. (2020). Human-specific ARHGAP11B increases size and folding of primate neocortex in the fetal marmoset. *Science* 369 (6503): 546–550. doi: 10.1126/science.abb2401.

Henery, C.C. and Mayhew, T.M. (1989). The cerebrum and cerebellum of the fixed human brain. *J Anat* 167: 167–180.

Henneberg, R. (1910). Messung der Oberfläche der Grosshirnrinde. *Journal für Psychologie und Neurologie* 17: 144–158.

Hevner, R.F. (2016). Evolution of the mammalian dentate gyrus. *J Comp Neurol* 524 (3): 578–594. doi: 10.1002/cne.23851.

Hevner, R.F. and Haydar, T.F. (2012). The (not necessarily) convoluted role of basal radial glia in cortical neurogenesis. *Cereb Cortex* 22 (2): 465–468. doi: 10.1093/cercor/bhr336.

Hilgetag, C.C. and Barbas, H. (2005). Developmental mechanics of the primate cerebral cortex. *Anat Embryol* 210 (5–6): 411–417. doi: 10.1007/s00429-005-0041-5.

Hill, J. et al. (2010). A surface-based analysis of hemispheric asymmetries and folding of cerebral cortex in term-born human infants. *J Neurosci* 30 (6): 2268–2276. doi: 10.1523/JNEUROSCI.4682-09.2010.

His, W. (1874). *Unsere Körperform und das physiologische Problem ihrer Entstehung Briefe an einen befreundeten Naturforscher*. F.C.W. Vogel, 1–246. doi: 10.5962/bhl.title.28860.
Hofman, M.A. (1985). Size and shape of the cerebral cortex in mammals. I. The cortical surface. *Brain, Behav Evol* 27 (1): 28–40. doi: 10.1159/000118718.
Hofman, M.A. (1989). On the evolution and geometry of the brain in mammals. *Prog Neurobiol* 32 (2): 137–158. doi: 10.1016/0301-0082(89)90013-0.
Holm, S.K. et al. (2018). Total brain, cortical, and white matter volumes in children previously treated with glucocorticoids. *Pediatr Res* 83 (4): 804–812. doi: 10.1038/pr.2017.312.
Holmes, G. (1918). Disturbances of vision by cerebral lesions. *Br J Ophthalmol* 2 (7): 353–384.
Holmes, G. (1945). Ferrier Lecture—the organization of the visual cortex in man. *Proc R Soc London. Series B – Biol Sci* 132 (869): 348–361. doi: 10.1098/rspb.1945.0002.
Ju, X.-C. et al. (2016). The hominoid-specific gene TBC1D3 promotes generation of basal neural progenitors and induces cortical folding in mice. *eLife* 5: e18197. doi: 10.7554/eLife.18197.
Kalebic, N. et al. (2018). Human-specific ARHGAP11B induces hallmarks of neocortical expansion in developing ferret neocortex. *Elife* 7: e41241. doi: 10.7554/eLife.41241.
Kelava, I. et al. (2012). Abundant occurrence of basal radial glia in the subventricular zone of embryonic neocortex of a lissencephalic primate, the common marmoset Callithrix jacchus. *Cereb Cortex* 22 (2): 469–481. doi: 10.1093/cercor/bhr301.
Knutsen, A.K. et al. (2013). Spatial and temporal variations of cortical growth during gyrogenesis in the developing ferret brain. *Cereb Cortex* 23 (2): 488–498. doi: 10.1093/cercor/bhs042.
Kostović, I. (2020). The enigmatic fetal subplate compartment forms an early tangential cortical nexus and provides the framework for construction of cortical connectivity. *Prog Neurobiol* 194: 101883. doi: 10.1016/j.pneurobio.2020.101883.
Kostovic, I. and Rakic, P. (1990). Developmental history of the transient subplate zone in the visual and somatosensory cortex of the macaque monkey and human brain. *J Comp Neurol* 297 (3): 441–470. doi: 10.1002/cne.902970309.
Kriegstein, A. et al. (2006). Patterns of neural stem and progenitor cell division may underlie evolutionary cortical expansion. *Nat Rev Neurosci* 7 (11): 883–890. doi: 10.1038/nrn2008.
Kroenke, C.D. and Bayly, P.V. (2018). How forces fold the cerebral cortex. *J Neurosci* 38 (4): 767–775. doi: 10.1523/JNEUROSCI.1105-17.2017.
Krubitzer, L.A. and Hunt, D.L. (2010). Captured in the net of space and time. *Evol Nervous Sys* 3: 49–72. doi: 10.1016/B0-12-370878-8/00058-6.
Lamoureux, P. et al. (1989). Direct evidence that growth cones pull. *Nature* 340 (6229): 159–162. doi: 10.1038/340159a0.
Lockard, B.I. (1985). The forebrain of the ferret. *Lab Anim Sci* 35 (3): 216–228.
Lui, J.H. et al. (2011). Development and evolution of the human neocortex. *Cell* 146 (1): 18–36. doi: 10.1016/j.cell.2011.06.030.
Lukaszewicz, A. et al. (2005). G1 phase regulation, area-specific cell cycle control, and cytoarchitectonics in the primate cortex. *Neuron* 47 (3): 353–364. doi: 10.1016/j.neuron.2005.06.032.
Lyras, G.A. et al. (2016). Evolution of gyrification in carnivores. *Brain, Behav Evol* 88 (3–4): 187–203. doi: 10.1159/000453104.
Martínez-Cerdeño, V. et al. (2006). The role of intermediate progenitor cells in the evolutionary expansion of the cerebral cortex. *Cereb Cortex* 16 (Suppl 1): i152–161. doi: 10.1093/cercor/bhk017.
Maudgil, D.D. et al. (1998). Identifying homologous anatomical landmarks on reconstructed magnetic resonance images of the human cerebral cortical surface. *J Anat* 193 (Pt 4): 559–571. doi: 10.1046/j.1469-7580.1998.19340559.x.
Mayhew, T.M. et al. (1996). The gyrification of mammalian cerebral cortex. *J Anat* 188 (Pt 1): 53–58.

Mota, B. and Herculano-Houzel, S. (2015). Brain Structure. Cortical folding scales universally with surface area and thickness, not number of neurons. *Science* 349 (6243): 74–77. doi: 10.1126/science.aaa9101.

Neal, J. et al. (2007). Insights into the gyrification of developing ferret brain by magnetic resonance imaging. *J Anat* 210 (1): 66–77. doi: 10.1111/j.1469-7580.2006.00674.x.

Northcutt, R.G. (1981). Evolution of the telencephalon in nonmammals. *Ann Rev Neurosci* 4 (1): 301–350. doi: 10.1146/annurev.ne.04.030181.001505.

Northcutt, R.G. (1985). The brain and sense organs of the earliest vertebrates: reconstruction of a morphotype. In: *Evolutionary Biology of Primitive Fishes* (ed. R.E. Foreman, A. Gorbman, J.M. Dodd, and R. Olsson), 81–112. Springer US. doi: 10.1007/978-1-4615-9453-6_6.

O'Leary, M.A. et al. (2013). The placental mammal ancestor and the post-K-Pg radiation of placentals. *Science* 339 (6120): 662–667. doi: 10.1126/science.1229237.

Owen, R. (1868). *On the Anatomy of Vertebrates, Vol 3: Mammals*, vol. 3. Spottiswood and Co.

Pillay, P. and Manger, P.R. (2007). Order-specific quantitative patterns of cortical gyrification. *Eur J Neurosci* 25 (9): 2705–2712. doi: 10.1111/j.1460-9568.2007.05524.x.

Pozzi, S. (1887). Les caractères distinctifs du cerveau de l'homme au point de vue morphologique (3e conférence Broca, 1885). *Bulletins de la Société d'anthropologie de Paris* 10: 784–802.

Rakic, P. (1974). Neurons in rhesus monkey visual cortex. *Science* 183 (4123): 425–427. doi: 10.1126/science.183.4123.425.

Rakic, P. (1976). Prenatal genesis of connections subserving ocular dominance in the rhesus monkey. *Nature* 261 (5560): 467–471. doi: 10.1038/261467a0.

Rakic, P. (1977). Prenatal development of the visual system in rhesus monkey. *Philos Trans R Soc London. Series B, Biol Sci* 278 (961): 245–260. doi: 10.1098/rstb.1977.0040.

Rakic, P. (1979). Genesis of visual connections in the rhesus monkey. In: *Developmental Neurobiology of Vision* (ed. R.D. Freeman), 249–260. Springer US. doi: 10.1007/978-1-4684-3605-1_21.

Rakic, P. (1988). Specification of cerebral cortical areas. *Science* 241 (4862): 170–176. doi: 10.1126/science.3291116.

Rakic, P. (1995). A small step for the cell, a giant leap for mankind. *Trends Neurosci* 18 (9): 383–388. doi: 10.1016/0166-2236(95).

Rakic, P. (2002a). Neurogenesis in adult primates. *Progr Brain Res* 138: 3–14. doi: 10.1016/S0079-6123(02)38067-1.

Rakic, P. (2002b). Pre- and post-developmental neurogenesis in primates. *Clin Neurosci Res* 2: 29–39. doi: 10.1016/S1566-2772(02)00005-1.

Rakic, P. et al. (1991). A novel cytoarchitectonic area induced experimentally within the primate visual cortex. *Proc Natl Acad Sci USA* 88 (6): 2083–2087. doi: 10.1073/pnas.88.6.2083.

Rash, B.G. et al. (2023). Neuropil growth and gliogenesis as primary drivers of gyrification in primates. *Proc Natl Acad Sci USA* 120 (1): e2210967120. doi: 10.1073/pnas.2210967120.

Rash, B.G. et al. (2019). Gliogenesis in the outer subventricular zone promotes enlargement and gyrification of the primate cerebrum. *Proc Natl Acad Sci USA* 116 (14): 7089–7094. doi: 10.1073/pnas.1822169116.

Rash, B.G. et al. (2013). Cortical gyrification induced by fibroblast growth factor 2 in the mouse brain. *J Neurosci* 33 (26): 10802–10814. doi: 10.1523/JNEUROSCI.3621-12.2013.

Raybaud, C. (2019). Corpus callosum: molecular pathways in mice and human dysgeneses. *Neuroimaging Clin N Am* 29 (3): 445–459. doi: 10.1016/j.nic.2019.03.006.

Reillo, I. and Borrell, V. (2012). Germinal zones in the developing cerebral cortex of ferret: ontogeny, cell cycle kinetics, and diversity of progenitors. *Cereb Cortex* 22 (9): 2039–2054. doi: 10.1093/cercor/bhr284.

Reillo, I. et al. (2011). A role for intermediate radial glia in the tangential expansion of the mammalian cerebral cortex. *Cereb Cortex* 21 (7): 1674–1694. doi: 10.1093/cercor/bhq238.

Ribas, G.C. (2010). The cerebral sulci and gyri. *Neurosurg Focus* 28 (2): E2. doi: 10.3171/2009.11.FOCUS09245.

Richman, D.P. et al. (1975). Mechanical model of brain convolutional development. *Science* 189 (4196): 18–21. doi: 10.1126/science.1135626.

Rockel, A.J. et al. (1980). The basic uniformity in structure of the neocortex. *Brain* 103 (2): 221–244. doi: 10.1093/brain/103.2.221.

Romiguier, J. et al. (2013). Genomic evidence for large, long-lived ancestors to placental mammals. *Mol Biol Evol* 30 (1): 5–13. doi: 10.1093/molbev/mss211.

Rose, J.E. and Woolsey, C.N. (1949). Organization of the mammalian thalamus and its relationships to the cerebral cortex. *Electroencephalogr Clin Neurophysiol* 1: 391–404. doi: 10.1016/0013-4694(49)90212-6.

Sawada, K. et al. (2012). Fetal gyrification in cynomolgus monkeys. *Anat Rec* 295 (7): 1065–1074. doi: 10.1002/ar.22478.

Schmechel, D.E. and Rakic, P. (1979). A Golgi study of radial glial cells in developing monkey telencephalon. *Anat Embryol* 156 (2): 115–152. doi: 10.1007/BF00300010.

Shitamukai, A. et al. (2011). Oblique radial glial divisions in the developing mouse neocortex induce self-renewing progenitors outside the germinal zone that resemble primate outer subventricular zone progenitors. *J Neurosci* 31 (10): 3683–3695. doi: 10.1523/JNEUROSCI.4773-10.2011.

Sidman, R.L. and Rakic, P. (1973). Neuronal migration, with special reference to developing human brain. *Brain Res* 62 (1): 1–35. doi: 10.1016/0006-8993(73)90617-3.

Smart, I.H. and McSherry, G.M. (1986a). Gyrus formation in the cerebral cortex in the ferret. I. Description of the external changes. *J Anat* 146: 141–152.

Smart, I.H. and McSherry, G.M. (1986b). Gyrus formation in the cerebral cortex of the ferret. II. Description of the internal histological changes. *J Anat* 147: 27–43.

Smart, I.H.M. et al. (2002). Unique morphological features of the proliferative zones and postmitotic compartments of the neural epithelium giving rise to striate and extrastriate cortex in the monkey. *Cereb Cortex* 12 (1): 37–53. doi: 10.1093/cercor/12.1.37.

Sporns, O. et al. (2004). Organization, development and function of complex brain networks. *Trends Cogn Sci* 8 (9): 418–425. doi: 10.1016/j.tics.2004.07.008.

Spreafico, R. and Tassi, L. (2012). Cortical malformations. *Handb Clin Neurol* 108: 535–557. doi: 10.1016/B978-0-444-52899-5.00047-2.

Stahl, R. et al. (2013). Trnp1 regulates expansion and folding of the mammalian cerebral cortex by control of radial glial fate. *Cell* 153 (3): 535–549. doi: 10.1016/j.cell.2013.03.027.

Striedter, G.F. (2005). *Principles of Brain Evolution*. Sinauer Associates, xii, 436.

Striedter, G.F. et al. (2015). Cortical folding. *Ann Rev Neurosci* 38: 291–307. doi: 10.1146/annurev-neuro-071714-034128.

Tallinen, T. et al. (2014). Gyrification from constrained cortical expansion. *Proc Natl Acad Sci USA* 111 (35): 12667–12672. doi: 10.1073/pnas.1406015111.

Tallinen, T. et al. (2016). On the growth and form of cortical convolutions. *Nat Phys* 12 (6): Article 6. doi: 10.1038/nphys3632.

Thompson, P.M. et al. (2001). Genetic influences on brain structure. *Nat Neurosci* 4 (12): 1253–1258. doi: 10.1038/nn758.

Toro, R. and Burnod, Y. (2005). A morphogenetic model for the development of cortical convolutions. *Cereb Cortex* 15 (12): 1900–1913. doi: 10.1093/cercor/bhi068.

Türe, U. et al. (2000). Fiber dissection technique: lateral aspect of the brain. *Neurosurgery* 47 (2): 417–426. doi: 10.1097/00006123-200008000-00028.

Turner, W. (1890). The convolutions of the brain. *J Anat Physiol* 25 (Pt 1): 105–153.

Van Essen, D.C. (1997). A tension-based theory of morphogenesis and compact wiring in the central nervous system. *Nature* 385 (6614): 313–318. doi: 10.1038/385313a0.

Voigt, T. (1989). Development of glial cells in the cerebral wall of ferrets. *J Comp Neurol* 289 (1): 74–88. doi: 10.1002/cne.902890106.

von Soemmerring, S. (1791). Hirnlehre und Nervenlehre. In: *Vom Bau des Menschlichen Körpers*, vol. 5. Frankfurt: Varrentrap & Wenner.

Wang, L. et al. (2016). Hedgehog signaling promotes basal progenitor expansion and the growth and folding of the neocortex. *Nat Neurosci* 19 (7): 888–896. doi: 10.1038/nn.4307.

Wang, X. et al. (2017). Folding, but not surface area expansion, is associated with cellular morphological maturation in the fetal cerebral cortex. *J Neurosci* 37 (8): 1971–1983. doi: 10.1523/JNEUROSCI.3157-16.2017.

Wang, X. et al. (2011). A new subtype of progenitor cell in the mouse embryonic neocortex. *Nat Neurosci* 14 (5): 555–561. doi: 10.1038/nn.2807.

Welker, W. (1990). Why does cerebral cortex fissure and fold? In: *Cerebral Cortex Book Series*, vol. 88.

Welker, W.I. and Campos, G.B. (1963). Physiological significance of sulci in somatic sensory cerebral cortex in mammals of the family procyonidae. *J Comp Neurol* 120: 19–36. doi: 10.1002/cne.901200103.

Welker, W.I. and Seidenstein, S. (1959). Somatic sensory representation in the cerebral cortex of the racoon (Procyon lotor). *J Comp Neurol* 111: 469–501. doi: 10.1002/cne.901110306.

White, L.E. et al. (1997). Structure of the human sensorimotor system. *Cereb Cortex* 7 (1): 18–30. doi: 10.1093/cercor/7.1.18.

White, T. et al. (2002). Brain volumes and surface morphology in monozygotic twins. *Cereb Cortex* 12 (5): 486–493. doi: 10.1093/cercor/12.5.486.

White, T. and Hilgetag, C.C. (2011). Gyrification and neural connectivity in schizophrenia. *Dev Psychopathol* 23 (1): 339–352. doi: 10.1017/S0954579410000842.

Woolsey, C.N. (1960). Some observations on brain fissuration in relation to cortical localization of function. In: *Structure and Function if the Cerebral Cortex* (ed. D.B. Tower and J.P. Schade), 64–68. Elsevier.

Xu, G. et al. (2010). Axons pull on the brain, but tension does not drive cortical folding. *J Biomech Eng* 132 (7): 071013. doi: 10.1115/1.4001683.

Zecevic, N. et al. (1989). Changes in synaptic density in motor cortex of rhesus monkey during fetal and postnatal life. *Brain Res Dev Brain Res* 50 (1): 11–32. doi: 10.1016/0165-3806(89).

Zecevic, N. et al. (2005). Contributions of cortical subventricular zone to the development of the human cerebral cortex. *J Comp Neurol* 491 (2): 109–122. doi: 10.1002/cne.20714.

Zecevic, N. and Rakic, P. (1991). Synaptogenesis in monkey somatosensory cortex. *Cereb Cortex* 1 (6): 510–523. doi: 10.1093/cercor/1.6.510.

Zilles, K. et al. (1989). Gyrification in the cerebral cortex of primates. *Brain, Behav Evol* 34 (3): 143–150. doi: 10.1159/000116500.

Zilles, K. et al. (1988). The human pattern of gyrification in the cerebral cortex. *Anat Embryol* 179 (2): 173–179. doi: 10.1007/BF00304699.

Zilles, K. et al. (2013). Development of cortical folding during evolution and ontogeny. *Trends Neurosci* 36 (5): 275–284. doi: 10.1016/j.tins.2013.01.006.

24

Investigation of the Mechanisms Underlying the Development and Evolution of the Cerebral Cortex Using Gyrencephalic Ferrets

Yohei Shinmyo and Hiroshi Kawasaki

Department of Medical Neuroscience, Graduate School of Medical Sciences, Kanazawa University, Kanazawa, Ishikawa 920-8640, Japan

24.1 Introduction

The cerebral cortex has undergone major changes during the long history of mammalian evolution (Borrell and Gotz 2014; Fietz and Huttner 2011; Florio and Huttner 2014; Gilardi and Kalebic 2021; Hatakeyama et al. 2017; Kawasaki 2014, 2017; Kriegstein et al. 2006; Llinares-Benadero and Borrell 2019; Lui et al. 2011; Molnar et al. 2006; Poluch and Juliano 2015; Rakic 1995, 2009; Sun and Hevner 2014; Zilles et al. 2013). The numbers of neurons and glial cells in the cerebral cortex have increased, resulting in a marked expansion of the cerebral cortex. During evolution, the cerebral cortex has developed various structures, including cortical folds on its surface (i.e., gyri and sulci), and its neural circuits have increased in complexity. These changes are thought to have been important for the acquisition of higher brain functions during evolution, but the mechanisms of the development and evolution of the cerebral cortex are not fully understood.

One factor that has hindered our understanding is that mice, which are widely used for genetic analyses, have relatively small brains and do not have cortical folds. Thus, it is difficult to investigate the mechanisms of cortical folding and expansion using mice alone. It is important to analyze the molecular mechanisms using a well-developed cerebral cortex that shares similar characteristics with the human cerebral cortex. To this end, several research groups, including us, have utilized ferrets (*Mustela putorius furo*), medium-sized carnivorous mammals that have relatively large, well-developed folded cerebral cortices (Figure 24.1A–C) (Borrell et al. 2006; Fietz et al. 2010; Kawasaki et al. 2004; Neal et al. 2007; Noctor et al. 1999; Rowell et al. 2010; Smart and McSherry 1986). In addition, recent advances in genetic manipulation techniques for the ferret cerebral cortex have made it possible to analyze the molecular mechanisms of the development and evolution of the cerebral cortex (Borrell 2010; Johnson et al. 2018; Kawasaki et al. 2012, 2013; Kou et al. 2015; Nonaka-Kinoshita et al. 2013; Shinmyo et al. 2017; Tsunekawa et al. 2016; Yu et al. 2019). This review presents recent findings, revealed using ferrets, on the mechanisms of cortical folding, neural progenitor proliferation and differentiation, and astrocyte proliferation, as well as the relationships between them. By comparing these results with those previously obtained using other animal species, we further discuss the mechanisms of cortical folding that are conserved among different animal species. Our recent studies also revealed that ferrets have developed axon fiber layers in the cerebral cortex that are also present in monkeys and humans (Saito et al. 2019). Therefore, we also discuss the developmental processes and evolution of axon fiber layers in the mammalian cerebral cortex.

Neocortical Neurogenesis in Development and Evolution, First Edition. Edited by Wieland B. Huttner.

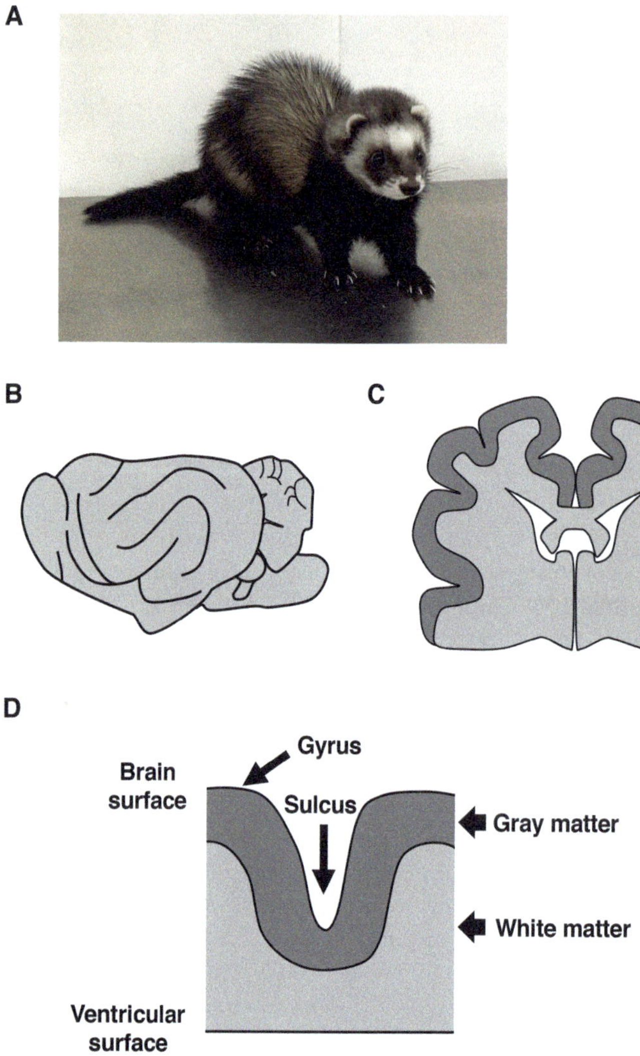

Figure 24.1 A ferret and its brain structures. (A) An adult ferret. Ferrets are medium-sized carnivorous mammals and have gyrencephalic brains. (B, C) Illustrations of a side view (B) and a coronal section (C) of the adult ferret brain. The ferret brain has folds on the surface of the cerebral cortex. (D) A schema of a cross section of cortical folds. Both the surface of gray matter and the boundary between gray matter and white matter are curved. In contrast, the surface of white matter at the lateral ventricle does not show curvature.

24.2 Developmental Processes of the Cerebral Cortex

Neurons in the cerebral cortex are produced from neuroepithelial cells (NE cells) that surround the lateral ventricle (Taverna et al. 2014). NE cells become radial glial cells (RG cells, also known as apical progenitor cells, ventricular RG cells, and apical RG cells). RG cells are located in the ventricular zone (VZ) and have bipolar radial processes that connect the ventricular and pial surfaces of the cerebral cortex (Figure 24.2) (Taverna et al. 2014). The asymmetric cell division of RG cells produces basal progenitors containing intermediate progenitor cells (IP cells) and outer radial glial cells (oRG cells, also known as OSVZ RG cells, basal RG cells, intermediate RG cells,

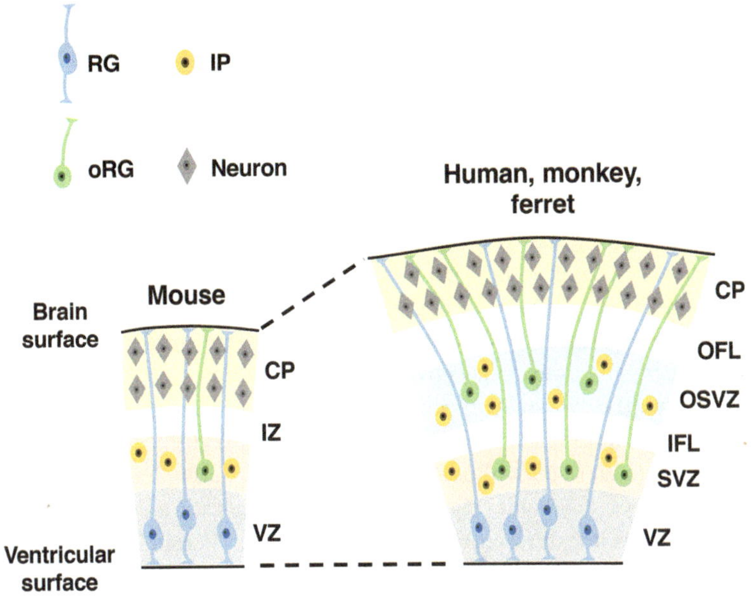

Figure 24.2 Neural progenitors in the developing cerebral cortices of lissencephalic and gyrencephalic brains. Cross sections of the developing cerebral cortices of lissencephalic and gyrencephalic brains, containing three types of neural progenitors: radial glial (RG) cells, intermediate progenitor (IP) cells, and outer radial glial (oRG) cells. In addition to the ventricular zone (VZ) and the subventricular zone (SVZ), the gyrencephalic cortex has another germinal zone, the outer subventricular zone (OSVZ). CP, cortical plate; IZ, intermediate zone; OFL, outer fiber layer; IFL, inner fiber layer.

and translocating RG cells) in the subventricular zone (SVZ) (Figure 24.2) (Taverna et al. 2014). In addition to the VZ and the SVZ, the developing cerebral cortices of gyrencephalic animal species such as humans, monkeys, and ferrets have another region called the outer SVZ (OSVZ), which contains abundant oRG cells (Figure 24.2) (Smart et al. 2002). Only a small number of oRG cells are present in mice, and it is thought that the increase in oRG cells during evolution resulted in expanded cerebral cortices containing a large number of neurons. Cortical neurons generated from these progenitors migrate toward the cortical plate using the radial processes of RG cells and oRG cells, and newly generated neurons overtake existing neurons to form the layered structure of the cerebral cortex (Silva et al. 2019). The neurons making up each layer are generated in chronological order, with lower-layer neurons being generated before upper-layer neurons. The axons of cortical neurons extend to form neural circuits, and the evolution of the gyrencephalic cerebral cortex included the development of axonal fiber layers, as described later (Molnar and Clowry 2012; Saito et al. 2019). It is known that the ratio of the number of upper-layer neurons to lower-layer neurons is much larger in humans than in rodents (DeFelipe et al. 2002), and this increase in upper-layer neurons was an important step in the evolution of the cerebral cortex.

24.3 Structural and Developmental Features of Cortical Folds

One of the salient structural features of the human cerebral cortex is numerous folds on its surface (Florio and Huttner 2014; Kawasaki 2017; Llinares-Benadero and Borrell 2019; Lui et al. 2011; Sun and Hevner 2014). Folds of the cerebral cortex are composed of ridges called gyri and furrows called sulci (Figure 24.1D). The acquisition of these folds during evolution is thought to have led to an increase in the surface area of the cerebral cortex, allowing many more neurons to be accommodated within the limited capacity of the skull. Therefore, cortical folds are considered to be an important structural basis for the development of brain functions. In fact, patients with abnormal cortical folds such as polymicrogyria and lissencephaly show severe intellectual disability (Fernandez et al. 2016; Ross and Walsh 2001). Therefore, it is important to elucidate the molecular mechanisms of the development and evolution of cortical folds and the pathophysiology of neurological disorders associated with cortical folds.

The cerebral cortex is composed of six-layered gray matter, where neurons are concentrated, and white matter, which mainly consists of axons and myelin. Cortical folds are found in animals with relatively large brains such as humans, monkeys, cats, and ferrets, but tend not to be found in animals with small brains such as rats and mice. Gyrencephalic and lissencephalic refer to the presence and absence of folds in the cerebral cortex, respectively. It is of great interest to uncover the mechanisms that determine whether the cerebral cortex becomes gyrencephalic or lissencephalic.

Cortical folds have the following structural features (Borrell 2018). Both the surface of gray matter and the boundary between gray matter and white matter are curved, resulting in all six layers of gray matter being curved along the cortical folds (Figure 24.1D). In contrast, the surface of white matter along the lateral ventricles does not show curvature (Figure 24.1D). Therefore, white matter is thicker at the gyri than at the sulci. When conducting experiments, it is important to investigate whether these physiological features of cortical folds can be observed.

Even in animals with a gyrencephalic cerebral cortex, cortical folds do not exist in the early stages of development, and folds gradually appear as the development of the cerebral cortex progresses. Cortical folds form in the fetuses (i.e., before birth) of cynomolgus monkeys, whereas cortical folds develop after birth in ferrets (Welker 1990). Sulci formed in the early stages of development are called primary sulci, and sulci formed later during development are called secondary and higher sulci (Welker 1990). In other words, during early development, the cerebral cortex exhibits a simple fold pattern with only primary sulci. As the formation of cortical folds progresses, secondary and higher sulci are added, resulting in the final pattern of folds. Interestingly, the locations of the primary sulci are well conserved among identical twins, but those of the secondary and higher sulci are less conserved. Thus, it seems that the locations of the primary sulci are determined by genetic factors, whereas additional factors are involved in the determination of the locations of the secondary and higher sulci (Lohmann et al. 1999).

24.4 Hypotheses on the Mechanisms of Cortical Folding

Several hypotheses have been proposed regarding the mechanisms of folding of the cerebral cortex (Borrell 2018; Florio and Huttner 2014; Gilardi and Kalebic 2021; Kawasaki 2014, 2017; Llinares-Benadero and Borrell 2019; Lui et al. 2011; Sun and Hevner 2014). One hypothesis was that because folds tend to be observed in animals with a large cerebral cortex, but not in animals with a small cerebral cortex, it was proposed that increased intracranial pressure leads to folding of the cerebral cortex (Welker 1990). According to this hypothesis, when the cerebral cortex expands within the limited volume of the skull, the increased intracranial pressure causes cortical folding. However, this hypothesis is now considered unlikely because lowering intracranial pressure experimentally did not eliminate folds in the cerebral cortex. The second hypothesis is that an increase in oRG cells is important for cortical folding. Indeed, the gyrencephalic cerebral cortex has a large number of oRG cells in the OSVZ during development (Figure 24.2) (Smart et al. 2002). In the brains of some animal species, such as marmosets, the OSVZ is present, but few folds are found on the cerebral cortex (Kelava et al. 2012). However, the number of neural progenitors in the OSVZ is positively correlated with the degree of cortical folding, suggesting that oRG cells are important for cortical folding (Reillo et al. 2011). The third hypothesis is that the ratio of the superficial regions to the deep regions of the cerebral cortex is important for the formation of cortical folds (Kriegstein et al. 2006; Richman et al. 1975). It is supposed that when the superficial regions expand preferentially over the deep regions, an outward protrusion is created. Consistent with this hypothesis, experiments with expandable materials successfully reproduced the fold-like structure of the mammalian cerebral cortex (Tallinen et al. 2016). The fourth hypothesis is that the tension created by axons connecting adjacent cortical regions produces folds (Van Essen 1997). This hypothesis supposes that axons connecting adjacent cortical regions bind these regions together, with the cerebral cortex between them protruding outward. Finally, in animals with cortical folds, the morphology and gene expression patterns of neural progenitors in the SVZ and the OSVZ are diverse, and this diversity may also be associated with cortical folding (Betizeau et al. 2013; de Juan Romero et al. 2015; Johnson et al. 2015; Reillo and Borrell 2012). Cortical folding is also associated with the proliferation and gene expression patterns of neural progenitors (de Juan Romero et al. 2015; Matsumoto et al. 2017; Reillo et al. 2011; Toda et al. 2016). Although many hypotheses have been proposed so far, experimental testing of these hypotheses had been delayed due to the difficulty of genetic manipulation in the gyrencephalic cerebral cortex.

24.5 Investigations of the Mechanisms of Cortical Folding using Mice

Although mice do not have cortical folds, attempts have been made to elucidate the molecular mechanisms that control the formation of folds using mice. This is primarily due to the availability of many genetic techniques for mice, such as knockout mice and transgenic mice. Early pioneering studies reported that promoting the proliferation of neural progenitors resulted in fold-like curvature on the surface of the mouse cerebral cortex (Chenn and Walsh 2002). Other studies have also reported that suppression of cell death causes curvature of the surface of the mouse cerebral cortex (Depaepe et al. 2005; Haydar et al. 1999). Since then, it has been reported that the introduction or knockout of various genes resulted in fold-like structures on the surface of the mouse cerebral cortex (Chizhikov et al. 2019; del Toro et al. 2017; Depaepe et al. 2005; Florio et al. 2015; Han et al. 2021; Ju et al. 2016; Kerimoglu et al. 2021; Kyrousi et al. 2021; Liu et al. 2017; Martinez-Martinez et al. 2016; Rash et al. 2013; Shao et al. 2020; Shqirat et al. 2021; Stahl et al. 2013; Wang et al. 2016, 2022). These results are important, as they experimentally show that curvature of the cerebral cortex can be generated by manipulating neural progenitors. In the future, it will be important to analyze the roles of these genes in animals with cortical folds, and ferrets would be an important option for this purpose.

24.6 Ferrets as a Model Animal for Investigating the Development and Evolution of the Cerebral Cortex

Ferrets are medium-sized carnivorous mammals that are approximately 50 cm long, weigh 1–2 kg, and have an average lifespan of 6–10 years (Figure 24.1A). They are thought to be descendants of the European polecat and have been domesticated by humans. Ferrets have several advantages for analyzing the mechanisms of development and evolution of the cerebral cortex.

First, ferrets can be used to analyze the molecular mechanisms that control the expansion and folding of the cerebral cortex, as well as the proliferation and differentiation of oRG cells, as described later. It would be important to combine in vivo studies using ferrets and in vitro studies using human induced pluripotent stem cell/embryonic stem cell (iPS cell/ES cell) organoids to elucidate the molecular mechanisms that caused changes in the cerebral cortex during evolution. Second, because ferrets have been used in electrophysiological and neuroanatomical studies, electrophysiological and anatomical information about the ferret brain is available (Borrell and Callaway 2002; Callaway and Katz 1993; Crowley and Katz 2000; Cucchiaro and Guillery 1984; Hahm et al. 1991; Huberman et al. 2003; Kawasaki et al. 2004; Law et al. 1988; Meister et al. 1991; Mooney et al. 1993; Sur et al. 1988). For example, many fundamental discoveries about neural plasticity and its critical period have been made in studies using ocular dominance columns of the visual cortex and the eye-specific segregation of retinal axons in the lateral geniculate nucleus of the ferret visual system. This electrophysiological and anatomical information provides important bases for interpreting the experimental results of genetic studies. Third, when ferret babies are born, their brains are at a relatively early stage of development, making them suitable for analyses of molecular mechanisms and developmental processes. Cortical folding is largely completed before birth in cynomolgus monkeys, but it progresses after birth in ferrets. Therefore, newborn ferrets, rather than fetuses, can be used for the investigation of cortical folding. Fourth, in addition to being used for neuroscience research, ferrets have also been widely used in research in other fields, including research on infectious diseases such as the influenza virus and the mechanisms of vomiting and antiemetics. As a result, ferrets are readily available, and many scientists already have at least some knowledge of ferrets. Knowledge of breeding and mating has been accumulated, and ferrets are easy to breed. Despite these advantages, genetic manipulation techniques for ferrets, which are needed to analyze the molecular mechanisms of development and evolution, had been poorly available.

24.7 Development of Genetic Manipulation Techniques for the Ferret Brain

In order to take advantage of ferrets as model animals, the development of rapid and simple genetic manipulation techniques that can be used in ferret brains had been eagerly anticipated. Because one technique that was needed was gene screening, we made a custom microarray for ferrets to identify genes that show characteristic expression patterns in the ferret brain (Kawasaki et al. 2004). Using this microarray, we identified genes that are selectively expressed in magnocellular or parvocellular neurons, which are characteristic of the developed visual system of higher mammals (Iwai et al. 2013; Kawasaki et al. 2004; Sato et al. 2017). Similarly, genes strongly expressed in future gyral regions and future sulcal regions were identified using ferret microarrays (de Juan Romero et al. 2015). Recently, RNA-seq analysis was applied to ferrets and found that ferret RG cells and human RG cells show similar gene expression (Johnson et al. 2015). In addition, the ferret genome has been sequenced, and annotated DNA sequence data are now partially available (Peng et al. 2014). As these examples show, various gene screening methods are now available for ferrets.

Another important technique for investigating the ferret brain is genetic manipulation. Previous pioneering studies reported that postnatal electroporation and in vivo injection of viral vectors can be used to transfect genes into the ferret brain (Borrell 2010; Nonaka-Kinoshita et al. 2013). Recently, we established an in utero electroporation technique for the ferret cerebral cortex with the aim of creating a simple and convenient gene manipulation technique that can be applied to most cortical neurons in the ferret cerebral cortex (Figure 24.3) (Kawasaki et al. 2012, 2013). This technique can be used to transfect not only most cortical neurons but also neural progenitors such as RG cells, IP cells, and oRG cells. It takes only one hour to perform in

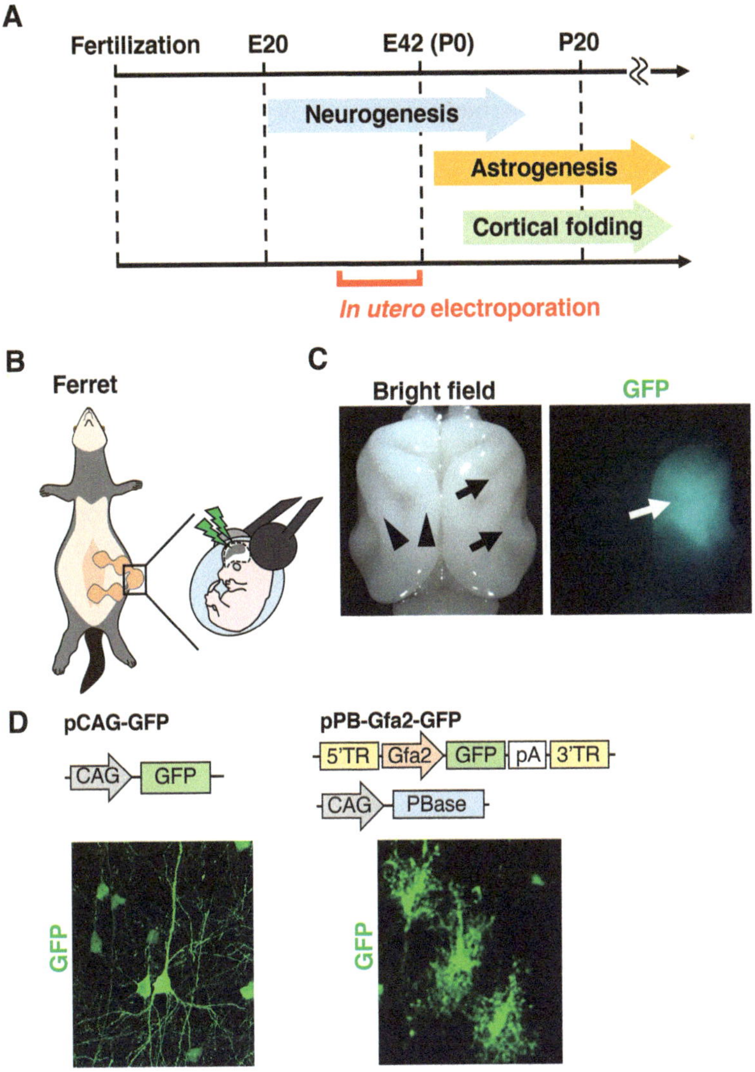

Figure 24.3 In vivo genetic manipulation for neurons and astrocytes in the ferret cerebral cortex using in utero electroporation. (A) The developmental time course of neurogenesis, astrogenesis, and cortical folding. The stages when in utero electroporation can be performed are also shown. Neurogenesis in the ferret cerebral cortex starts around embryonic day 20 (E20), and astrogenesis proceeds later than neurogenesis. Cortical folding of the ferret cerebral cortex starts around postnatal day 4 (P4). In utero electroporation of the ferret cerebral cortex can be performed from around E30, when layer 5/6 neurons are generated. (B) An illustration of an in utero electroporation procedure. (C) Dorsal views of a ferret brain in which GFP was expressed by in utero electroporation. Cortical folds, that is, gyri (black arrowheads) and sulci (black arrows), are present on the cerebral cortex. GFP signals are observed on the right side of the cerebral cortex (white arrow). (D) Selective transgene induction into neurons or astrocytes. In utero electroporation of CAG-GFP induces GFP expression in cortical neurons only (left), whereas astrocyte-specific transgene expression was achieved by the combination of in utero electroporation, the piggyBac system, and an astrocyte-specific promoter (right). Plasmids used for electroporation and GFP images taken from coronal sections are shown.

utero electroporation on one pregnant ferret mother, and transfected ferret babies can be obtained a few days later, making experiments easy and quick. In addition, multiple kinds of plasmids can be simultaneously transfected by simply mixing them, and different plasmids can be applied to different embryos in one ferret mother. As a result, experiments under various conditions can be performed simultaneously using one ferret mother. We also succeeded in gene knockout in the ferret cerebral cortex by combining in utero electroporation with the genome editing technology CRISPR/Cas9 (Shinmyo et al. 2017). Furthermore, we showed that astrocyte-specific transgene expression in the ferret cerebral cortex can be achieved by combining in utero electroporation, the piggyBac system, and cell-type specific promoters (Figure 24.3D) (Shinmyo et al. 2022). A knockin method for ferret cortical neurons using in utero electroporation and the CRISPR/Cas9 system was also reported (Tsunekawa et al. 2016). Another genetic manipulation method is genetically modifying ferrets. Knockout ferrets were created using genome editing techniques, and the roles of Aspm and Disc1 were uncovered in the ferret brain (Johnson et al. 2018; Kou et al. 2015). Transgenic ferrets were also created by inserting a transgene at the ROSA26 locus using the CRISPR/Cas9 system (Yu et al. 2019). Moreover, ferret iPS cells have been generated (Gao et al. 2020; Yoshimatsu et al. 2021), making organoid research using ferret iPS cells possible. With these technological developments, research using the ferret brain is becoming increasingly popular.

24.8 Investigation of the Mechanisms Underlying the Development and Evolution of the Cerebral Cortex using Ferrets

24.8.1 The Roles of Neural Progenitors in Cortical Folding

An increasing number of laboratories are using ferrets to analyze the molecular mechanisms of cortical folding in the cerebral cortex. Pioneering studies have reported the importance of neural progenitors in the formation of cortical folds. Pharmacological suppression of neural progenitor proliferation in the developing ferret cerebral cortex inhibited cortical folding (Haddad et al. 1979). Conversely, in the developing ferret cerebral cortex, enhancement of neural progenitor proliferation promoted cortical folding (Masuda et al. 2015; Nonaka-Kinoshita et al. 2013). Importantly, even before the formation of folds in the developing ferret cerebral cortex, the number of neural progenitors is high in future gyral regions and conversely low in future sulcal regions (Reillo et al. 2011). Similarly, in the developing cerebral cortex of monkeys, neural progenitors are more abundant in future gyral regions than in future sulcal regions (Smart et al. 2002). These results suggest that the increase in neural progenitors in future gyral regions is important for cortical folding. However, experimental enhancement of neural progenitor proliferation in the developing mouse cerebral cortex was not sufficient to cause folds (Nonaka-Kinoshita et al. 2013). Therefore, in addition to the increase in neural progenitors, there may be additional factors that are important for cortical folding.

To clarify which types of neural progenitors are important for cortical folding, the distribution patterns of oRG cells and IP cells in the developing ferret cerebral cortex were analyzed. oRG cells and IP cells were unevenly distributed and were abundant in future gyral regions, but not less so in future sulcal regions. The result raised the possibility that the higher numbers of neurons derived from oRG cells and IP cells in future gyral regions form the outward protrusions that eventually become gyri. We recently found that oRG cells in the developing ferret cerebral cortex can be divided into two groups, HOPX-positive and HOPX-negative, depending on the presence or absence of the transcription factor HOPX (Matsumoto et al. 2020). Furthermore, HOPX-positive oRG cells, rather than HOPX-negative oRG cells, were preferentially abundant in future gyral regions, and manipulation of the number of HOPX-positive oRG cells was found to affect cortical folding. These results suggest that HOPX-positive oRG cells are likely to be involved in cortical folding. In the developing mouse cerebral cortex, there are only a small number of oRG-like cells (Shitamukai et al. 2011). Interestingly, the medial regions of the mouse cerebral cortex contain relatively many oRG-like cells, and this region of the mouse cerebral cortex may resemble the ferret cerebral cortex (Vaid et al. 2018). In addition, HOPX has been shown to be important for increasing the number of oRG cells in the mouse cerebral cortex (Vaid et al. 2018). Therefore, HOPX may also be an important regulator of oRG cell production in the gyrencephalic cerebral cortex.

24.8.2 Mechanisms Regulating the Abundance of Neural Progenitors

The upstream regulatory mechanisms of neural progenitor proliferation are also an important issue. To identify genes involved in the proliferation of neural progenitors, we focused on human diseases that show abnormal cortical folds.

Thanatophoric dysplasia is a congenital disorder exhibiting abnormalities in bones and the brain including polymicrogyria, which presents with many additional cortical folds. Pioneering studies have identified a mutation in the fibroblast growth factor (FGF) receptor 3 gene in patients with thanatophoric dysplasia and have shown that this mutation produced an activated form of FGF receptor 3. It seemed likely that signal transduction downstream of the FGF receptors is involved in the proliferation of neural precursors and cortical folding (Shiang et al. 1994). To directly test whether FGF signaling causes the proliferation of neural progenitors, in utero electroporation was used to express an FGF ligand in the developing ferret cerebral cortex (Masuda et al. 2015). We found that activation of FGF signaling promoted the proliferation of oRG cells and increased the number of oRG cells. Furthermore, inhibition of FGF signaling by expressing dominant-negative FGF receptor 3 in the ferret cerebral cortex suppressed oRG cell proliferation and reduced the number of oRG cells (Matsumoto et al. 2017). These results indicate that FGF signaling regulates the proliferation of oRG cells.

PALMDELPHIN(PALMD) was reported to increase the processes of basal progenitors and stimulate their proliferation via integrin signaling (Kalebic et al. 2019). When PALMD-Caax was electroporated into the developing ferret cerebral cortex, the numbers of oRG cell processes and the proliferation of oRG cells were significantly increased. PALMD-Caax electroporated into the mouse cerebral cortex was shown to activate ß1 integrin in the SVZ, and as a result, the MAPK pathway and the PI3K pathway were activated. These results highlighted the importance of the morphology of basal progenitors and of pro-proliferative signals from the extracellular environment. Another study showed that serotonin signaling also regulates the proliferation of basal progenitors (Xing et al. 2020). The serotonin receptor 2A (HTR2A) is more highly expressed in the developing cerebral cortex of ferrets and humans than that of mice. Ectopic expression of HTR2A increased the proliferation of basal progenitors in mice, and knockout of HTR2A reduced the proliferation of basal progenitors in ferrets. These results suggest that serotonin works as an important extrinsic pro-proliferative signal for basal progenitors.

It was shown that the Hippo pathway is also involved in the regulation of the abundance and proliferation of basal progenitors (Kostic et al. 2019). The expression and activity of YAP, which is a downstream effector of the Hippo pathway, were higher in basal progenitors of ferrets and humans than in those of mice. Constitutively active YAP enhanced the proliferation of basal progenitors in the mouse cerebral cortex. Pharmacological and genetic inhibition of YAP function decreased the abundance of cycling basal progenitors in ferrets. These results suggest that an increase in YAP activity resulted in the expansion of the cerebral cortex during evolution.

Abnormalities in sonic hedgehog (Shh) signaling have also been reported in human patients with abnormal folds in the cerebral cortex. Therefore, we analyzed the roles of Shh signaling in the regulation of oRG cell proliferation and differentiation. Introducing a Shh ligand into the developing ferret cerebral cortex using in utero electroporation promoted oRG cell self-renewal and increased the number of oRG cells (Matsumoto et al. 2020). Similarly, Smoothened Agonist (SAG), a specific activator of Shh signaling, promoted the self-renewal of oRG cells in cultured ferret brain slices (Hou et al. 2021). Furthermore, suppressing Shh signaling by introducing HhipΔC22, a dominant-negative form of the Shh signaling pathway, reduced the self-renewal of oRG cells, resulting in a reduction in the number of oRG cells. These results suggest that various signaling pathways coordinately increase the number of oRG cells by promoting proliferation and self-renewal (Figure 24.4A).

In addition to elucidating the mechanisms of neural progenitor proliferation and self-renewal, it is also important to investigate the mechanisms of neural progenitor translocation. A study comparing mice and ferrets reported differences in cell motility among these animal species (Okamoto et al. 2014). Lzts1, which is associated with microtubules, was reported to regulate the production of oRG-like cells (Kawaue et al. 2019). Since oRG cells are rarely observed in mice, ferrets should be useful for investigating the mechanisms of oRG cell translocation and morphological changes. In the future, it would be important to investigate the interactions between the signaling pathways that have been identified so far to give an overall picture of the mechanisms that regulate oRG cell proliferation, self-renewal, and translocation.

24.8.3 Investigation of the Mechanisms Underlying Cortical Folding using Ferrets

Since both FGF signaling and Shh signaling increase numbers of oRG cells, we investigated whether FGF signaling and Shh signaling are involved in the formation of folds in the cerebral cortex (Masuda et al. 2015; Matsumoto et al. 2017, 2020). Activating FGF signaling by introducing an FGF ligand into the developing ferret cerebral cortex increased the number of cortical folds, resulting in a polymicrogyria-like phenotype. Importantly, these folds had the characteristics of normal folds of the cerebral cortex. That is, they contained all cortical layers (i.e., layers 1–6). In addition, although the cortical surface exhibited increased folds, the ventricular surface was smooth and did not show curvature. Furthermore, inhibiting FGF signaling by expressing dominant-negative FGF receptors in the developing ferret cerebral cortex inhibited cortical folding. Similarly, activating Shh signaling by introducing Shh ligands into the developing ferret cerebral cortex increased the number of cortical folds. Suppression of Shh signaling using HhipΔC22 inhibited the formation of folds in the cerebral cortex. These results indicate that FGF signaling and Shh signaling work together to regulate the number of oRG cells, thereby inducing the formation of folds in the cerebral cortex (Figure 24.4A) (Masuda et al. 2015; Matsumoto et al. 2017, 2020).

Interestingly, when comparing mice and ferrets, we found that the amount of Shh protein in the cerebral cortex was higher in ferrets (Matsumoto et al. 2020). In addition, Gli1 expression levels, which reflect activation of Shh signaling, were found to be higher in the ferret cerebral cortex. These results suggest that Shh signaling is more strongly activated in the ferret cerebral cortex than in the mouse cerebral cortex. It seems plausible that an increase in Shh signaling activity during evolution led to an increase in oRG cells and the acquisition of folds in the cerebral cortex (Matsumoto et al. 2020).

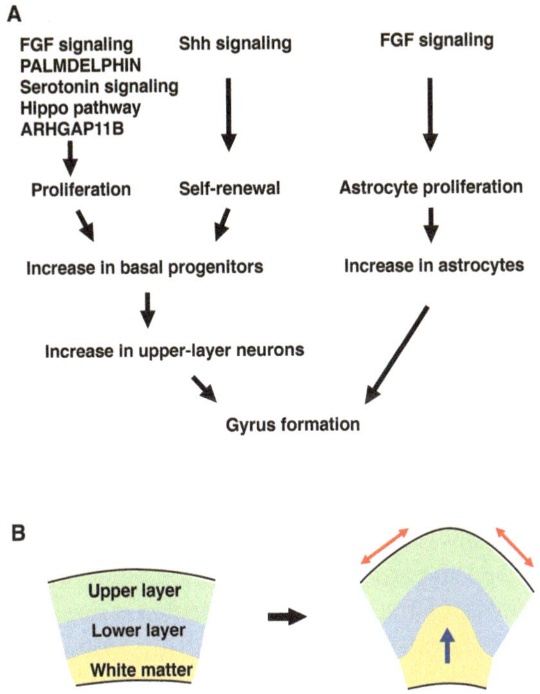

Figure 24.4 A working model of the mechanisms of cortical folding. (A) FGF signaling, PALMDELPHIN, serotonin signaling, the Hippo pathway, and ARHGAP11B promote the proliferation of basal progenitors, while Shh signaling stimulates the self-renewal of basal progenitors. These molecular pathways act to increase basal progenitors that preferentially produce upper-layer neurons, resulting in gyrus formation. Subsequently, astrogenesis enhances cortical folding. (B) Gyrus formation requires tangential expansion of the cortical surface (red arrows), which is achieved by a preferential increase in upper-layer neurons, and radial expansion induced by astrogenesis (blue arrow).

Next, we investigated the mechanisms that connect the increase in oRG cells with the morphological changes of fold formation in the cerebral cortex. A detailed analysis of the cerebral cortex, in which FGF signaling or Shh signaling was activated to promote cortical folding, showed a selective increase in the thickness of upper layers of the cerebral cortex relative to lower layers (Masuda et al. 2015; Matsumoto et al. 2017, 2020). These results were consistent with the previous hypothesis that the ratio of superficial to deep regions of the cerebral cortex is important for cortical folding (Kriegstein et al. 2006; Richman et al. 1975). To test this hypothesis, we used Cdk5 to selectively reduce the number of neurons in upper layers of the cerebral cortex. Cdk5 is a gene reported to be responsible for human lissencephaly (Magen et al. 2015) and is therefore thought to be important for cortical folding. Knocking out the Cdk5 gene in pyramidal neurons of the developing ferret cerebral cortex by using in utero electroporation and the CRISPR/Cas9 system suppressed cortical folding, consistent with reports from human patients with lissencephaly. This result suggests that Cdk5 in pyramidal neurons is important for folding of the cerebral cortex (Shinmyo et al. 2017). Since Cdk5 is required for radial migration of cortical neurons from the ventricular surface to the pial surface of the brain, it was suggested that radial migration of cortical neurons is important for cortical folding. Similarly, mutant SCN3A/Nav1.3 sodium channels suppressed both radial migration and cortical folding (Smith et al. 2018). Next, we examined to which layer of the cerebral cortex it is important for neurons to migrate. We selectively introduced dominant-negative Cdk5 into either layer 2/3 neurons or layer 5–6 neurons, and selectively inhibited the radial migration of layer 2/3 neurons or layer 5–6 neurons. As a result, inhibition of the radial migration of layer 2/3 neurons suppressed cortical folding, but that of layer 5/6 neurons did not. This result supports the hypothesis that cortical folding is induced by a preferential increase in superficial regions of the cerebral cortex compared to deep regions (Figure 24.4A, B). In the developing ferret cerebral cortex, cortical neurons have been reported to move tangentially without following strict radial paths (Gertz and Kriegstein 2015; Reillo et al. 2011). Therefore, it should also be considered that cortical folding may also require tangential dispersion of superficial regions of the cerebral cortex.

Detailed observation of the developmental processes of cortical folding over time showed that cortical folding progresses even after neurogenesis and radial migration of neurons are completed. Therefore, it seemed plausible that there are additional factors that promote cortical folding. Since astrocytes are generated after neurogenesis during development (Figure 24.3A), we speculated that astrocytes are also involved in cortical folding. In fact, it is known that when the cerebrum expanded and obtained cortical folds during evolution, the number of glial cells markedly increased (Herculano-Houzel 2014). First, we compared astrocyte gene expression in mice and ferrets to investigate the molecular mechanisms controlling the increase in astrocytes that occurred during evolution (Shinmyo et al. 2022). We found higher FGF1 expression in ferret astrocytes than in mouse astrocytes. Since FGF receptor 2 and FGF receptor 3 were also expressed in ferret astrocytes, these results raised the possibility that ferret astrocyte proliferation is governed by a positive feedback loop of autocrine/paracrine FGF signaling. Consistent with this hypothesis, the addition of the FGF receptor inhibitor BGJ398 to a primary culture of ferret astrocytes suppressed astrocyte proliferation. These results suggest that astrocyte proliferation resulting from high FGF1 expression and positive feedback was important for the increase in astrocytes that occurred during evolution. Subsequently, we investigated whether an increase in astrocytes is involved in cortical folding. Because it has been reported that in utero electroporation introduces plasmids only into neurons (Kawasaki et al. 2012, 2013), we examined the conditions that would enable selective transgene expression into glial cells. We found that astrocyte-specific and oligodendrocyte-specific transgene expression in the cerebral cortex can be achieved by combining in utero electroporation, the piggyBac system, and cell-type specific promoters (Figure 24.3D) (Hamabe-Horiike et al. 2021; Shinmyo et al. 2022). Using this system, we selectively reduced the number of astrocytes and found that cortical folding was impaired in the ferret cerebral cortex (Shinmyo et al. 2022). These results suggest that not only neurons but also astrocytes are important for cortical folding. Because a preferential increase in neurons in superficial regions causes tangential expansion of the cerebral cortex, and an increase in astrocytes causes vertical expansion, tangential expansion and vertical expansion may work together to make complete cortical folds (Figure 24.4A, B) (Shinmyo et al. 2022).

24.8.4 Common and Species-specific Mechanisms of Cortical Folding

It is important to determine whether the mechanisms of cortical folding found in ferrets are conserved in other gyrencephalic mammals including primates. Cortical folds are present in many mammals, including humans, monkeys, and ferrets, but not in some animal species, including mice. The reason why folds do not exist in the mouse cerebral cortex is an important issue to be examined. Although carnivores such as ferrets are phylogenetically farther from primates than rodents, humans and ferrets, at least in part, share some common mechanisms of cortical folding. In fact, FGF signaling and Shh signaling are involved in cortical folding in both humans and ferrets, and therefore, cortical folding induced by FGF signaling and Shh signaling seems to be an important conserved mechanism among gyrencephalic animal species. This idea is also supported by many previous studies showing that neural progenitors in gyrencephalic animals share common features. For example, the OSVZ in gyrencephalic animals have large numbers of neural progenitors (Dehay et al. 2015; Hansen et al. 2010; Hatakeyama et al. 2017; Kriegstein et al. 2006; Martinez-Cerdeno et al. 2006; Reillo and Borrell 2012). Furthermore, genes whose expression levels in neural progenitors differ between future gyral regions and future sulcal regions in ferrets show similar expression patterns in humans (de Juan Romero et al. 2015). Recently, it was reported that the microRNA miR-3607 plays an important role in the amplification of RG cells by acting as a regulator of Wnt/ß-catenin signaling in both ferrets and humans (Chinnappa et al. 2022). Interestingly, loss of miR-3607 expression reduced neural progenitors in the mouse cerebral cortex (Chinnappa et al. 2022). The common ancestor of mammals might have had folds of the cerebral cortex, and mice may have lost these folds (Kelava et al. 2013). Although ferrets share various brain structures with humans, it should be noted that these structures are often more developed in humans than in ferrets. In addition to the size of the brain, folds and upper-layer thickness are more developed in the human cerebral cortex (Hutsler et al. 2005; Zilles et al. 2013). These facts may suggest the existence of primate-specific mechanisms that further enhance the growth and folding of the cerebral cortex. Indeed, recent studies have identified primate-specific and human-specific genes that promote the amplification of neural progenitors (Arcila et al. 2014; Fiddes et al. 2018; Florio et al. 2015, 2018; Nowakowski et al. 2018; Suzuki et al. 2018). Introducing the human-specific gene ARHGAP11B into ferrets resulted in further expansion of the cerebral cortex (Kalebic et al. 2018). Therefore, ferrets should be a useful model animal for analyzing the roles of primate-specific and human-specific genes in the evolution of the cerebral cortex.

24.9 Developmental Processes and Evolution of Fiber Layers in the Cerebral Cortex

In addition to the cortical plate and the germinal zone, the developing cerebral cortices of humans and monkeys have two fiber layers, the inner fiber layer (IFL) and the outer fiber layer (OFL) (Figure 24.5A) (Molnar and Clowry 2012). However, because these two fiber layers were not identified in the mouse cerebral cortex, little was known about their developmental and evolutionary processes. Interestingly, when green florescent protein (GFP) was expressed in excitatory neurons of the ferret cerebral cortex using in utero electroporation, GFP-positive axons were found to be accumulated at locations corresponding to where the IFL and the OFL are observed in humans and monkeys (Figure 24.5A) (Saito et al. 2019). These results suggest that ferrets, like humans and monkeys, also have the IFL and the OFL in the developing cerebral cortex, and that the IFL and the OFL contain axons derived from excitatory neurons in the cerebral cortex (Saito et al. 2019).

To investigate which neural circuits the OFL and the IFL become after development progresses, we expressed GFP in cortical neurons and examined the projection of GFP-positive axons corresponding to the IFL and the OFL. We found that IFL axons predominantly became commissural and subcortical projecting axons, whereas the OFL gave rise to U-fibers (Figure 24.5B) (Yoshino et al. 2020). U-fibers are short association fibers located just below gray matter and are found in humans and monkeys (Catani et al. 2012; Meynert 1885; Nieuwenhuys et al. 1988; Ouyang et al. 2017; Schuz and Braitenberg 2002). U-fibers are thought to be important for functional

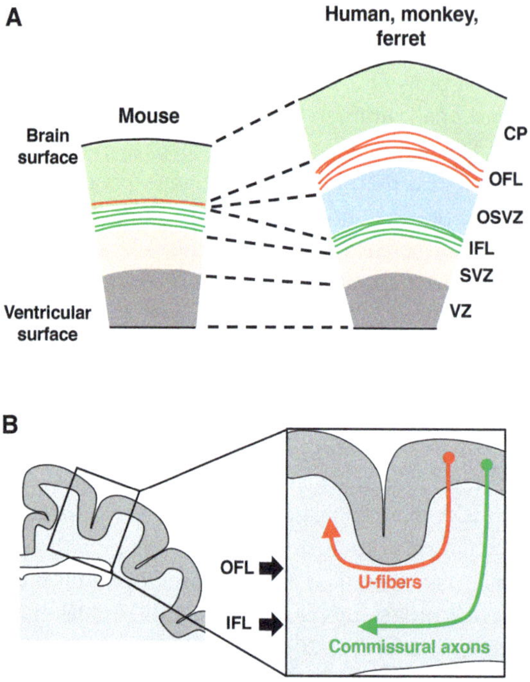

Figure 24.5 A working model of the evolution of fiber layers in the developing cerebral cortex. (A) Schemas of cross sections of the developing cerebral cortices of mice, ferrets, monkeys, and humans. Fibers in the outer fiber layers (OFL, red) increased during evolution. (B) A schema of a cross section of the adult ferret cerebral cortex. Axons in the OFL become subcortical U-fibers (red), while the IFL gives rise to commissural axons (green) and subcortical projecting axons. CP, cortical plate; OSVZ, outer subventricular zone; SVZ, subventricular zone; VZ, ventricular zone.

association among adjacent cortical areas, and their abnormalities have been reported in neurodevelopmental and psychiatric disorders. MRI and histological analyses of U-fibers have been performed using human and monkey brains, but genetic analyses of U-fibers had been difficult because the IFL and the OFL had not been reported in mice. Taken together, these results suggest that ferrets are a useful model animal for analyzing the developmental processes and functions of U-fibers (Yoshino et al. 2020).

Because U-fibers can be visualized in ferrets by expressing GFP using in utero electroporation, we expressed GFP in the mouse cortex using the same method. Interestingly, we found a small number of GFP-positive axons projecting to adjacent cortical areas in the mouse cerebral cortex (Saito et al. 2019; Yoshino et al. 2020). This result suggests that a small number of axons corresponding to U-fibers in humans, monkeys, and ferrets are also present in mice, and that an increase in these axons resulted in the formation of the OFL (Figure 24.5A, red) (Saito et al. 2019; Yoshino et al. 2020). Although these results have revealed some aspects of the developmental processes and evolution of U-fibers, many points still remain unclear. It will be important to elucidate the molecular mechanisms underlying the formation of U-fibers and their physiological and disease-related importance. Furthermore, since U-fibers are mainly observed in gyrencephalic mammal brains, it is also important to investigate the roles of U-fibers in cortical folding.

24.10 Future Prospects

The mammalian cerebral cortex is an important area of research. Our understanding of the developmental processes, functions, and pathophysiological changes of the cerebral cortex has progressed mainly using mice as model animals. Recently, the use of new animal models such as ferrets and marmosets, and the development of various genetic technologies such as in utero electroporation, genome editing, and iPS/ES cell organoids have expanded the scope of research that can be conducted on the cerebral cortex. The use of new animal models is expected to accelerate our understanding of the mechanisms underlying the development and evolution of the brain, and ferrets provide an important platform for in vivo analyses of these mechanisms.

Acknowledgments

We thank Prof. Wieland Huttner for giving us this opportunity to write this chapter. We are grateful to Zachary Blalock and the Kawasaki lab members for their helpful support. This work was supported by Grants-in-Aid for Scientific Research from the Ministry of Education, Culture, Sports, Science and Technology (MEXT), Japan Agency for Medical Research and Development (AMED), Takeda Science Foundation, the Uehara Memorial Foundation, the Kanazawa University SAKIGAKE project 2018 and the Kanazawa University CHOZEN project.

References

Arcila, M.L. et al. (2014). Novel primate miRNAs coevolved with ancient target genes in germinal zone-specific expression patterns. *Neuron* 81: 1255–1262.

Betizeau, M. et al. (2013). Precursor diversity and complexity of lineage relationships in the outer subventricular zone of the primate. *Neuron* 80: 442–457.

Borrell, V. (2010). In vivo gene delivery to the postnatal ferret cerebral cortex by DNA electroporation. *J Neurosci Methods* 186: 186–195.

Borrell, V. (2018). How cells fold the cerebral cortex. *J Neurosci* 38: 776–783.

Borrell, V. and Callaway, E.M. (2002). Reorganization of exuberant axonal arbors contributes to the development of laminar specificity in ferret visual cortex. *J Neurosci* 22: 6682–6695.

Borrell, V. and Gotz, M. (2014). Role of radial glial cells in cerebral cortex folding. *Curr Opin Neurobiol* 27: 39–46.

Borrell, V. et al. (2006). In vivo evidence for radial migration of neurons by long-distance somal translocation in the developing ferret visual cortex. *Cereb Cortex* 16: 1571–1583.

Callaway, E.M. and Katz, L.C. (1993). Photostimulation using caged glutamate reveals functional circuitry in living brain slices. *Proc Natl Acad Sci USA* 90: 7661–7665.

Catani, M. et al. (2012). Short frontal lobe connections of the human brain. *Cortex* 48: 273–291.

Chenn, A. and Walsh, C.A. (2002). Regulation of cerebral cortical size by control of cell cycle exit in neural precursors. *Science* 297: 365–369.

Chinnappa, K. et al. (2022). Secondary loss of miR-3607 reduced cortical progenitor amplification during rodent evolution. *Sci Adv* 8: eabj4010.

Chizhikov, V.V. et al. (2019). Early dorsomedial tissue interactions regulate gyrification of distal neocortex. *Nat Commun* 10: 5192.

Crowley, J.C. and Katz, L.C. (2000). Early development of ocular dominance columns. *Science* 290: 1321–1324.

Cucchiaro, J. and Guillery, R.W. (1984). The development of the retinogeniculate pathways in normal and albino ferrets. *Proc R Soc London. Series B. Biol Sci* 223: 141–164.

de Juan Romero, C. et al. (2015). Discrete domains of gene expression in germinal layers distinguish the development of gyrencephaly. *EMBO J* 34: 1859–1874.

DeFelipe, J. et al. (2002). Microstructure of the neocortex: comparative aspects. *J Neurocytol* 31: 299–316.

Dehay, C. et al. (2015). The outer subventricular zone and primate-specific cortical complexification. *Neuron* 85: 683–694.

del Toro, D. et al. (2017). Regulation of cerebral cortex folding by controlling neuronal migration via FLRT adhesion molecules. *Cell* 169: 621–635.

Depaepe, V. et al. (2005). Ephrin signalling controls brain size by regulating apoptosis of neural progenitors. *Nature* 435: 1244–1250.

Fernandez, V. et al. (2016). Cerebral cortex expansion and folding: what have we learned? *EMBO J* 35: 1021–1044.

Fiddes, I.T. et al. (2018). Human-specific NOTCH2NL genes affect Notch signaling and cortical neurogenesis. *Cell* 173: 1356–1369.e1322.

Fietz, S.A. and Huttner, W.B. (2011). Cortical progenitor expansion, self-renewal and neurogenesis-a polarized perspective. *Curr Opin Neurobiol* 21: 23–35.

Fietz, S.A. et al. (2010). OSVZ progenitors of human and ferret neocortex are epithelial-like and expand by integrin signaling. *Nat Neurosci* 13: 690–699.

Florio, M. et al. (2015). Human-specific gene ARHGAP11B promotes basal progenitor amplification and neocortex expansion. *Science* 347: 1465–1470.

Florio, M. et al. (2018). Evolution and cell-type specificity of human-specific genes preferentially expressed in progenitors of fetal neocortex. *Elife* 7: e32332.

Florio, M. and Huttner, W.B. (2014). Neural progenitors, neurogenesis and the evolution of the neocortex. *Development* 141: 2182–2194.

Gao, J. et al. (2020). Derivation of induced pluripotent stem cells from ferret somatic cells. *Am J Physiol Lung Cell Mol Physiol* 318: L671–L683.

Gertz, C.C. and Kriegstein, A.R. (2015). Neuronal migration dynamics in the developing ferret cortex. *J Neurosci* 35: 14307–14315.

Gilardi, C. and Kalebic, N. (2021). The ferret as a model system for neocortex development and evolution. *Front Cell Dev Biol* 9: 661759.

Haddad, R. et al. (1979). Neuroteratogenicity of methylazoxymethanol acetate. *Neurotoxicology* 1: 171–189.

Hahm, J.O. et al. (1991). Disruption of retinogeniculate afferent segregation by antagonists to NMDA receptors. *Nature* 351: 568–570.

Hamabe-Horiike, T. et al. (2021). Glial cell type-specific gene expression in the mouse cerebrum using the piggyBac system and in utero electroporation. *Sci Rep* 11: 4864.

Han, S. et al. (2021). Proneural genes define ground-state rules to regulate neurogenic patterning and cortical folding. *Neuron* 109: 2847–2863.

Hansen, D.V. et al. (2010). Neurogenic radial glia in the outer subventricular zone of human neocortex. *Nature* 464: 554–561.

Hatakeyama, J. et al. (2017). Developing guinea pig brain as a model for cortical folding. *Dev Growth Diff* 59: 286–301.

Haydar, T.F. et al. (1999). The role of cell death in regulating the size and shape of the mammalian forebrain. *Cereb Cortex* 9: 621–626.

Herculano-Houzel, S. (2014). The glia/neuron ratio. *Glia* 62: 1377–1391.

Hou, S. et al. (2021). Biphasic roles of hedgehog signaling in the production and self-renewal of outer radial glia in the ferret cerebral cortex. *Cereb Cortex* 31: 4730–4741.

Huberman, A.D. et al. (2003). Eye-specific retinogeniculate segregation independent of normal neuronal activity. *Science* 300: 994–998.

Hutsler, J.J. et al. (2005). Comparative analysis of cortical layering and supragranular layer enlargement in rodent carnivore and primate species. *Brain Res* 1052: 71–81.

Iwai, L. et al. (2013). FoxP2 is a parvocellular-specific transcription factor in the visual thalamus of monkeys and ferrets. *Cereb Cortex* 23: 2204–2212.

Johnson, M.B. et al. (2018). Aspm knockout ferret reveals an evolutionary mechanism governing cerebral cortical size. *Nature* 556: 370–375.

Johnson, M.B. et al. (2015). Single-cell analysis reveals transcriptional heterogeneity of neural progenitors in human cortex. *Nat Neurosci* 18: 637–646.

Ju, X.C. et al. (2016). The hominoid-specific gene TBC1D3 promotes generation of basal neural progenitors and induces cortical folding in mice. *Elife* 5: e18197.

Kalebic, N. et al. (2018). Human-specific ARHGAP11B induces hallmarks of neocortical expansion in developing ferret neocortex. *Elife* 7: e41241.

Kalebic, N. et al. (2019). Neocortical expansion due to increased proliferation of basal progenitors is linked to changes in their morphology. *Cell Stem Cell* 24: 535–550.

Kawasaki, H. (2014). Molecular investigations of the brain of higher mammals using gyrencephalic carnivore ferrets. *Neurosci Res* 86: 59–65.

Kawasaki, H. (2017). Molecular investigations of development and diseases of the brain of higher mammals using the ferret. *Proc Jpn Acad Series B: Phy Biol Sci* 93: 259–269.

Kawasaki, H. et al. (2004). Molecular organization of the ferret visual thalamus. *J Neurosci* 24: 9962–9970.

Kawasaki, H. et al. (2012). Rapid and efficient genetic manipulation of gyrencephalic carnivores using *in utero* electroporation. *Mol Brain* 5: 24.

Kawasaki, H. et al. (2013). *In vivo* genetic manipulation of cortical progenitors in gyrencephalic carnivores using *in utero* electroporation. *Biol Open* 2: 95–100.

Kawaue, T. et al. (2019). Lzts1 controls both neuronal delamination and outer radial glial-like cell generation during mammalian cerebral development. *Nat Commun* 10: 2780.

Kelava, I. et al. (2013). The secondary loss of gyrencephaly as an example of evolutionary phenotypical reversal. *Front Neuroanat* 7: 16.

Kelava, I. et al. (2012). Abundant occurrence of basal radial glia in the subventricular zone of embryonic neocortex of a lissencephalic primate, the common marmoset *Callithrix jacchus*. *Cereb Cortex* 22: 469–481.

Kerimoglu, C. et al. (2021). H3 acetylation selectively promotes basal progenitor proliferation and neocortex expansion. *Sci Adv* 7: eabc6792.

Kostic, M. et al. (2019). YAP activity is necessary and sufficient for basal progenitor abundance and proliferation in the developing neocortex. *Cell Reports* 27: 1103–1118.

Kou, Z. et al. (2015). CRISPR/Cas9-mediated genome engineering of the ferret. *Cell Rep* 25: 1372–1375.

Kriegstein, A. et al. (2006). Patterns of neural stem and progenitor cell division may underlie evolutionary cortical expansion. *Nat Rev Neurosci* 7: 883–890.

Kyrousi, C. et al. (2021). Extracellular LGALS3BP regulates neural progenitor position and relates to human cortical complexity. *Nat Commun* 12: 6298.

Law, M.I. et al. (1988). Organization of primary visual cortex (area 17) in the ferret. *J Comp Neurol* 278: 157–180.

Liu, J. et al. (2017). The primate-specific gene TMEM14B marks outer radial glia cells and promotes cortical expansion and folding. *Cell Stem Cell* 21: 635–649.

Llinares-Benadero, C. and Borrell, V. (2019). Deconstructing cortical folding: genetic, cellular and mechanical determinants. *Nat Rev Neurosci* 20: 161–176.

Lohmann, G. et al. (1999). Sulcal variability of twins. *Cereb Cortex* 9: 754–763.

Lui, J.H. et al. (2011). Development and evolution of the human neocortex. *Cell* 146: 18–36.

Magen, D. et al. (2015). Autosomal recessive lissencephaly with cerebellar hypoplasia is associated with a loss-of-function mutation in CDK5. *Hum Genet* 134: 305–314.

Martinez-Cerdeno, V. et al. (2006). The role of intermediate progenitor cells in the evolutionary expansion of the cerebral cortex. *Cereb Cortex* 16 (Suppl 1): i152–161.

Martinez-Martinez, M.A. et al. (2016). A restricted period for formation of outer subventricular zone defined by Cdh1 and Trnp1 levels. *Nat Commun* 7: 11812.

Masuda, K. et al. (2015). Pathophysiological analyses of cortical malformation using gyrencephalic mammals. *Sci Rep* 5: 15370.

Matsumoto, N. et al. (2017). Gyrification of the cerebral cortex requires FGF signaling in the mammalian brain. *Elife* 6: e29285.

Matsumoto, N. et al. (2020). A discrete subtype of neural progenitor crucial for cortical folding in the gyrencephalic mammalian brain. *Elife* 9: e54873.

Meister, M. et al. (1991). Synchronous bursts of action potentials in ganglion cells of the developing mammalian retina. *Science* 252: 939–943.

Meynert, T. (1885). *A Clinical Treatise on Diseases of the Fore-brain Based upon a Study of Its Structure, Functions, and Nutrition*. New York: G.P. Putnam's Sons.

Molnar, Z. and Clowry, G. (2012). Cerebral cortical development in rodents and primates. *Prog Brain Res* 195: 45–70.

Molnar, Z. et al. (2006). Comparative aspects of cerebral cortical development. *Eur J Neurosci* 23: 921–934.

Mooney, R. et al. (1993). Enhancement of transmission at the developing retinogeniculate synapse. *Neuron* 10: 815–825.

Neal, J. et al. (2007). Insights into the gyrification of developing ferret brain by magnetic resonance imaging. *J Anat* 210: 66–77.

Nieuwenhuys, R. et al. (1988). Long association and commissural connections. In: *The Human Central Nervous System* (ed. R. Nieuwenhuys, J. Voogd, and C. van Huijzen), 365–375. Berlin: Springer-Verlag.

Noctor, S.C. et al. (1999). Interference with the development of early generated neocortex results in disruption of radial glia and abnormal formation of neocortical layers. *Cereb Cortex* 9: 121–136.

Nonaka-Kinoshita, M. et al. (2013). Regulation of cerebral cortex size and folding by expansion of basal progenitors. *EMBO J* 32: 1817–1828.

Nowakowski, T.J. et al. (2018). Regulation of cell-type-specific transcriptomes by microRNA networks during human brain development. *Nat Neurosci* 21: 1784–1792.

Okamoto, M. et al. (2014). Ferret-mouse differences in interkinetic nuclear migration and cellular densification in the neocortical ventricular zone. *Neurosci Res* 86: 88–95.

Ouyang, M. et al. (2017). Short-range connections in the developmental connectome during typical and atypical brain maturation. *Neurosci Biobehav Rev* 83: 109–122.

Peng, X. et al. (2014). The draft genome sequence of the ferret (*Mustela putorius furo*) facilitates study of human respiratory disease. *Nat Biotechnol* 32: 1250–1255.

Poluch, S. and Juliano, S.L. (2015). Fine-tuning of neurogenesis is essential for the evolutionary expansion of the cerebral cortex. *Cereb Cortex* 25: 346–364.

Rakic, P. (1995). A small step for the cell, a giant leap for mankind. *Trends Neurosci* 18: 383–388.

Rakic, P. (2009). Evolution of the neocortex: a perspective from developmental biology. *Nat Rev Neurosci* 10: 724–735.

Rash, B.G. et al. (2013). Cortical gyrification induced by fibroblast growth factor 2 in the mouse brain. *J Neurosci* 33: 10802–10814.

Reillo, I. and Borrell, V. (2012). Germinal zones in the developing cerebral cortex of ferret: ontogeny, cell cycle kinetics, and diversity of progenitors. *Cereb Cortex* 22: 2039–2054.

Reillo, I. et al. (2011). A role for intermediate radial glia in the tangential expansion of the mammalian cerebral cortex. *Cereb Cortex* 21: 1674–1694.

Richman, D.P. et al. (1975). Mechanical model of brain convolutional development. *Science* 189: 18–21.

Ross, M.E. and Walsh, C.A. (2001). Human brain malformations and their lessons for neuronal migration. *Ann Rev Neurosci* 24: 1041–1070.

Rowell, J.J. et al. (2010). Molecular analysis of neocortical layer structure in the ferret. *J Comp Neurol* 518: 3272–3289.

Saito, K. et al. (2019). Characterization of the inner and outer fiber layers in the developing cerebral cortex of gyrencephalic ferrets. *Cereb Cortex* 29: 4303–4311.

Sato, C. et al. (2017). Cell type-specific expression of FoxP2 in the ferret and mouse retina. *Neurosci Res* 117: 1–13.

Schuz, A. and Braitenberg, V. (2002). The human cortical white matter: quantitative aspects of cortico-cortical long-range connectivity. In: *Cortical Areas: Unity and Diversity Conceptional Advances in Brain Research* (ed. A. Schuz and R. Miller), 377–385. London: Taylor & Francis.

Shao, W. et al. (2020). Centrosome anchoring regulates progenitor properties and cortical formation. *Nature* 580: 106–112.

Shiang, R. et al. (1994). Mutations in the transmembrane domain of FGFR3 cause the most common genetic form of dwarfism, achondroplasia. *Cell* 78: 335–342.

Shinmyo, Y. et al. (2022). Localized astrogenesis regulates gyrification of the cerebral cortex. *Sci Adv* 8: eabi5209.

Shinmyo, Y. et al. (2017). Folding of the cerebral cortex requires Cdk5 in upper-layer neurons in gyrencephalic mammals. *Cell Rep* 20: 2131–2143.

Shitamukai, A. et al. (2011). Oblique radial glial divisions in the developing mouse neocortex induce self-renewing progenitors outside the germinal zone that resemble primate outer subventricular zone progenitors. *J Neurosci* 31: 3683–3695.

Shqirat, M. et al. (2021). Sonic hedgehog expands neural stem cells in the neocortical region leading to an expanded and wrinkled neocortical surface. *Genes Cells* 26: 399–410.

Silva, C.G. et al. (2019). Cell migration promotes dynamic cellular interactions to control cerebral cortex morphogenesis. *Nat Rev Neurosci* 20: 318–329.

Smart, I.H. et al. (2002). Unique morphological features of the proliferative zones and postmitotic compartments of the neural epithelium giving rise to striate and extrastriate cortex in the monkey. *Cereb Cortex* 12: 37–53.

Smart, I.H. and McSherry, G.M. (1986). Gyrus formation in the cerebral cortex in the ferret. I. Description of the external changes. *J Anat* 146: 141–152.

Smith, R.S. et al. (2018). Sodium channel SCN3A (NaV1.3) regulation of human cerebral cortical folding and oral motor development. *Neuron* 99: 905–913.

Stahl, R. et al. (2013). Trnp1 regulates expansion and folding of the mammalian cerebral cortex by control of radial glial fate. *Cell* 153: 535–549.

Sun, T. and Hevner, R.F. (2014). Growth and folding of the mammalian cerebral cortex. *Nat Rev Neurosci* 15: 217–232.

Sur, M. et al. (1988). Experimentally induced visual projections into auditory thalamus and cortex. *Science* 242: 1437–1441.

Suzuki, I.K. et al. (2018). Human-specific NOTCH2NL genes expand cortical neurogenesis through Delta/Notch regulation. *Cell* 173: 1370–1384.

Tallinen, T. et al. (2016). On the growth and form of cortical convolutions. *Nat Phys* 12: 588–593.

Taverna, E. et al. (2014). The cell biology of neurogenesis. *Ann Rev Cell Dev Biol* 30: 465–502.

Toda, T. et al. (2016). An essential role of SVZ progenitors in cortical folding in gyrencephalic mammals. *Sci Rep* 6: 29578.

Tsunekawa, Y. et al. (2016). Developing a *de novo* targeted knock-in method based on *in utero* electroporation into the mammalian brain. *Development* 143: 3216–3222.

Vaid, S. et al. (2018). A novel population of Hopx-dependent basal radial glial cells in the developing mouse neocortex. *Development* 145: dev169276.

Van Essen, D.C. (1997). A tension-based theory of morphogenesis and compact wiring in the central nervous system. *Nature* 385: 313–318.

Wang, L. et al. (2016). Hedgehog signaling promotes basal progenitor expansion and the growth and folding of the neocortex. *Nat Neurosci* 19: 888–896.

Wang, W. et al. (2022). The human FOXM1 homolog promotes basal progenitor cell proliferation and cortical folding in mouse. *EMBO Rep* 23 (3): e53602.

Welker, W. (1990). Why does cerebral cortex fissure and fold? In: *Cerebral Cortex* (ed. E.G. Jones and A. Peters), 3–136. Boston, MA: Springer.

Xing, L. et al. (2020). Serotonin receptor 2A activation promotes evolutionarily relevant basal progenitor proliferation in the developing neocortex. *Neuron* 108: 1113–1129.

Yoshimatsu, S. et al. (2021). Establishment of an induced pluripotent stem cell line from a female domestic ferret (*Mustela putorius furo*) with an X chromosome instability. *Stem Cell Res* 53: 102385.

Yoshino, M. et al. (2020). The origin and development of subcortical U-fibers in gyrencephalic ferrets. *Mol Brain* 13: 37.

Yu, M. et al. (2019). Highly efficient transgenesis in ferrets using CRISPR/Cas9-mediated homology-independent insertion at the ROSA26 locus. *Sci Rep* 9: 1971.

Zilles, K. et al. (2013). Development of cortical folding during evolution and ontogeny. *Trends Neurosci* 36: 275–284.

Part 7

Cortical Development: Variations, Disorders, and Malformations

25

Genetic Variation Altering Cortical Progenitor Function Leads to Human Brain Evolution and Interindividual Differences in Human Brain Structure

Madison Rose Glass[1,2], Jason L. Stein[1,2,], and E.S. Anton[1,3,*]*

[1] *UNC Neuroscience Center, University of North Carolina at Chapel Hill, USA*
[2] *Department of Genetics, University of North Carolina at Chapel Hill, USA*
[3] *Department of Cell Biology and Physiology, University of North Carolina at Chapel Hill, USA*
* *Corresponding authors*

25.1 Introduction

The expansion of the neocortex across human evolution is thought to contribute to advanced human cognitive and social abilities (Geschwind and Rakic 2013; Pääbo 2014). Endocranial volume has greatly increased since our most recent common ancestor with chimpanzees, likely driven by expansions of neocortical surface area, which now comprises 75–84 percent of brain mass (Herculano-Houzel 2012; Lee and Wolpoff 2003). Many hypotheses about what has led to expanded cortical surface area in modern humans have centered around the functions of the cortical progenitors (Lui et al. 2011; Rakic 1988, 2009). Cortical progenitors influence cortical structure through differences in their cell cycle rate and fate decisions, which affects the total cells produced, and scaffolding the migration of neurons, which affects the placement of cells in the cortex. The radial unit hypothesis provides a framework for understanding how cortical progenitor proliferation and survival in fetal development influences adult cortical surface area (Figure 25.1). According to this hypothesis, cortical progenitors produce ontogenetic columns whose size and area form a protomap of the adult cortex. Expanding the total progenitor pool through increased progenitor self-renewal or survival will ultimately lead to more total neurons or astrocytes produced in ontogenetic columns and larger cortical surface area. On the other hand, increased cell death of cortical progenitors and their progeny, or precocious differentiation into non-mitotic cell types, will decrease total cell count and surface area in the adult brain (Rakic 1988, 2005, 2009). Recent studies, driven by association of genetic variation within human populations with brain size differences, have provided evidence that a similar mechanism that led to expansion of the human cortex across evolution also influences interindividual differences in cortical structure within human populations. In this chapter, we will discuss how both common and rare genetic variation impacts cortical progenitor cellular and molecular functions leading to individual differences in cortical structure across humans.

Neocortical Neurogenesis in Development and Evolution, First Edition. Edited by Wieland B. Huttner.

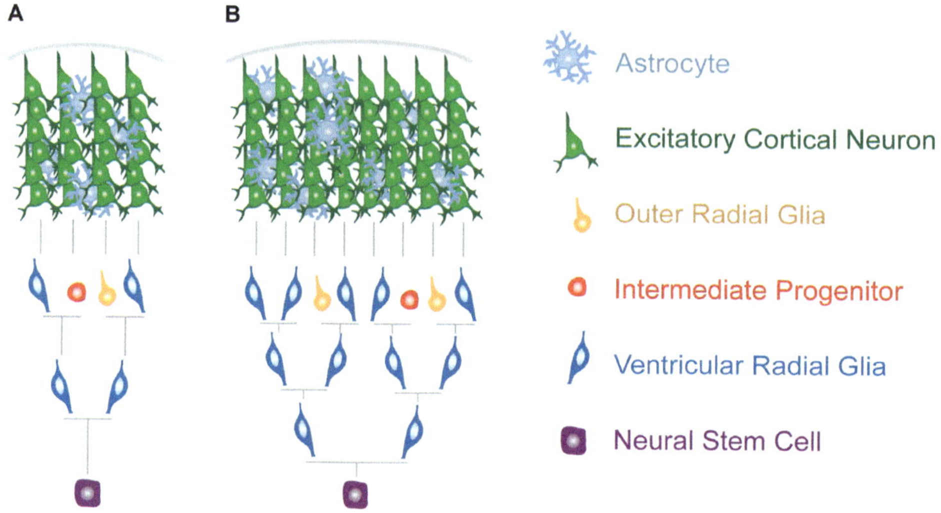

Figure 25.1 Radial unit hypothesis. Example of a smaller (A) or larger (B) progenitor pool producing excitatory neurons and astrocytes in the cortex, leading to changes in cortical surface area.

25.2 Cellular Processes Occurring during Human Corticogenesis

First, we provide a brief review of the cellular processes occurring during human corticogenesis to set the stage for how genetic variation can modulate these processes (Figure 25.2). Rapid developmental changes occur in the cortex in utero and during infancy at gross anatomical, histological, and transcriptomic levels (Kang et al. 2011; Kostović et al. 2019; Silbereis et al. 2016). Corticogenesis begins in the telencephalon during the seventh post-conception week with a layer of polarized ventricular radial glia (vRG) derived from neuroepithelial cells (Kriegstein and Götz 2003; Zhong et al. 2018). vRG surround the ventricle with their apical domain, creating a densely packed lamina called the ventricular zone (Howard et al. 2008). vRG divide through interkinetic nuclear migration, translocating the nucleus in time with the cell cycle to undergo mitosis at the ventricular surface (Lui et al. 2011; Rakic 2007). vRG divide symmetrically to proliferate into more progenitors or asymmetrically to form neurons (Noctor et al. 2004). The first produced neurons somally translocate or migrate along radial glia fibers that anchor to the basal surface to form the preplate (Kriegstein and Götz 2003; Rakic 1972, 1978). The preplate is split into the marginal zone and subplate as neurons migrate in between to form the cortical plate (Bystron et al. 2008). Cortical neurons form the cortical plate beginning with lower-layer neurons and end with upper-layer neurons, proceeding in an inside-out fashion to generate cortical columns (Rakic 1988). Starting around post-conception week 13, the ventricular zone expands through vRG proliferation to include an inner and outer subventricular zone, collectively called the germinal zone, which contains additional progenitor cell types: intermediate progenitors and outer radial glia (oRG) that lack apical domains but have processes extending to the basal surface (Hansen et al. 2010; Pollen et al. 2015). oRG are mostly located in the outer subventricular zone and produce more upper-layer neurons to help guide their migration (Nowakowski et al. 2016; Rash et al. 2019). The vRG pool expands 2 weeks before angiogenesis begins whereas the oRG and intermediate progenitors expand mostly after angiogenesis, suggesting potential different metabolic needs for these highly proliferative cell types (Marín-Padilla 2012). Further studies in mice suggest vRG can proliferate

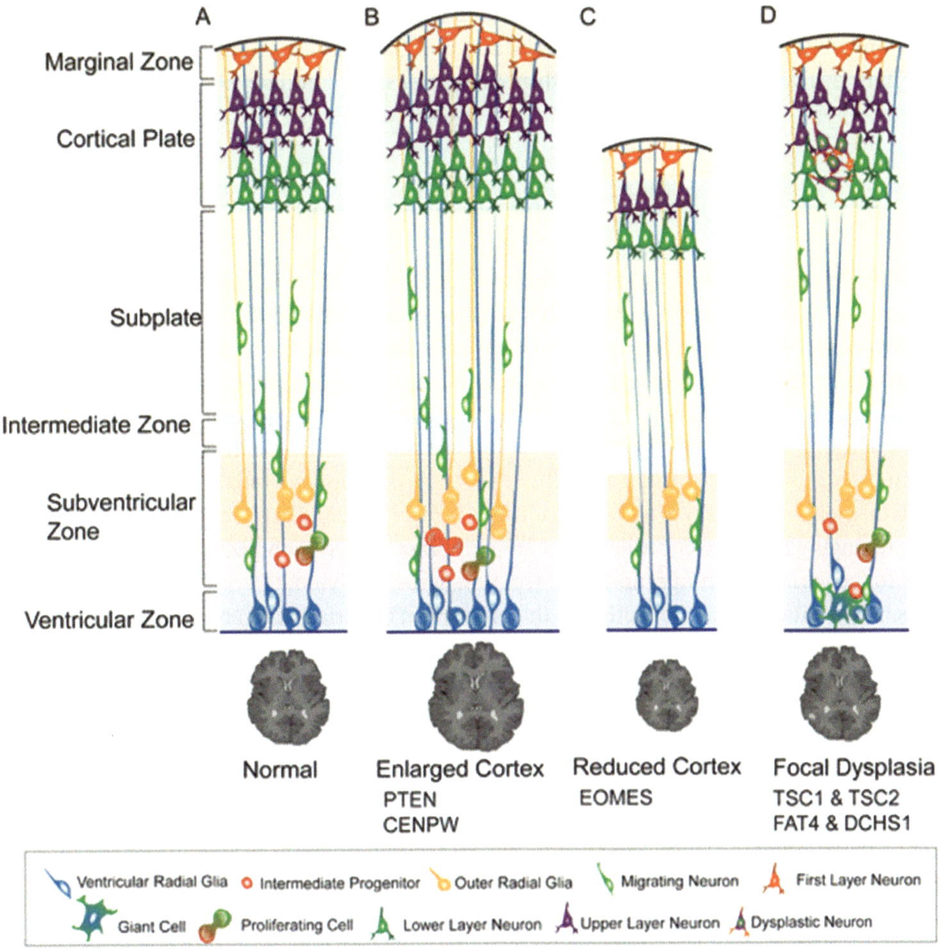

Figure 25.2 Proposed cellular mechanisms and select implicated genes in cortical alterations. (A) A neurotypical developing cortical wall with a balance of dividing progenitor cells producing neurons that can migrate into the cortical plate. (B) A disrupted cortical wall resulting in an enlarged cortex. Cortical progenitor types have increased proliferation rate, resulting in increased neuron production and additional radial units. (C) A thinner, less-complicated cortical wall resulting in reduced cortical size due to the presumed loss of intermediate progenitor subtype. (D) A cortical wall with disrupted cortical architecture. vRG with no apical contacts inhibit migration of normal cell types. Abnormal giant cells also displace other cell types in the ventricular zone. vRG with disorganized fiber perturbs typical neuronal migration and dysplastic neurons show atypical orientation and placement. MRI images adapted from Oegema et al. (2020).

under hypoxic conditions and favor glycolysis and have reduced oxidative phosphorylation more than other cortical progenitors (Namba et al. 2021). Migrating neurons and ascending axons from other brain regions form the intermediate zone, which eventually contribute to white matter in the adult cortex (Krsnik et al. 2017). The subplate forms directly below the cortical plate and also contains a milieu of tangentially migrating interneurons, radially migrating excitatory neurons, invading axons, and descending cortical projections. Interstitial neurons in the white matter originate in the subplate (Hadders-Algra 2018; Molnár et al. 2019). Lastly, when vRG self-renewing capacity is exhausted around birth, vRG differentiate into astrocytes, which retain their proliferative abilities but are distributed throughout the cortical wall and the progenitor rich germinal zone is no longer separable from white matter (Holst et al. 2019; Miller and Gauthier 2007; Rakic 2007). Changes in cell cycle, fate decisions, or migration within these transient laminae alter cortical size and structure.

25.3 Genetic Variation Shaping the Human Cortex

Human cortical surface area, cortical thickness, and gyral depth can be quantified in large populations using magnetic resonance imaging (MRI) (Desikan et al. 2006; Fischl and Dale 2000). Though MRI measurements (~1 mm^3 voxel size) do not have sufficient resolution or contrast to identify the cellular basis of the gross brain structural measures, the segmentation of the cortical gray matter is reliably achieved. Total cerebrum volume and total cortical surface area reach peak levels around 11–12 years of age. Cortical surface area reaches 186,000 mm^2 [2.5th–97.5th percentiles: 154,000–219,000 mm^2] in males and 168,000 mm^2 [2.5th–97.5th percentiles: 140,000–198,000 mm^2] in females (Bethlehem et al. 2022) (Figure 25.3). There is large variability in human cortical surface area though, ranging from the equivalent of a 16-inch pizza to a 20-inch pizza. A clear question is what leads to the variability in human brain structure across individuals?

To assess this, heritability studies estimate the proportion of variation of gross brain structure in a population that is explained by genetic differences. Heritability is often estimated by comparing monozygotic (identical) and dizygotic (fraternal) twins, with the assumption that a stronger genetic influence on a trait would result in more similarity between monozygotic twins as compared to dizygotic twins. These studies have found that brain structure is highly heritable. Total cerebral volume has heritability of 83.5 percent and cortical surface area has heritability of 91 percent (Blokland et al. 2012; Grasby et al. 2020). Heritability alone does not describe which specific variants in the genome are associated with interindividual differences in brain structure, how commonly these variants occur in populations (allele frequency), these variants' effect sizes, and what developmental age and cell type these genetic variations act through.

Work over the past 20 years has identified many variants that change the structure of the human brain along with their properties such as allele frequency and effect size (Bae et al. 2015). There are two broad classes of genetic variation: common and rare. Variants at >1 percent frequency in the population are generally considered common (McCarthy et al. 2008; Visscher et al. 2017). Common variants

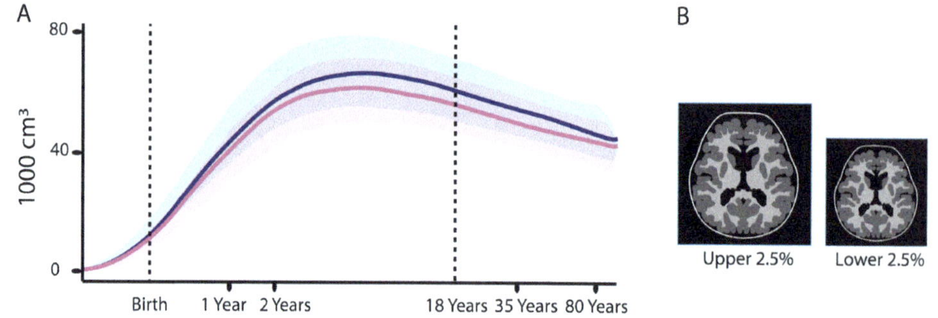

Figure 25.3 Brain structure population variability. (A) Normative growth trajectories for cortical gray matter volume for males (blue) and females (pink) with 95 percent confidence interval shaded (Bethlehem et al. 2022). Age is in log scale, showing the fastest changes early in infancy. (B) MRI images showing the differences in size of the upper and lower 2.5 percentile of cortical surface area.

arose long ago and are spread throughout a population. Though in aggregate common variants explain much of the interindividual differences in brain size, individual common variants have small effects on brain structure (Le and Stein 2019). Therefore, genome-wide association studies (GWAS) in large unrelated populations are necessary to sufficiently power studies with the goal of identifying common variants associated with differences in brain structure (Bis et al. 2012; Stein et al. 2012; Taal et al. 2012). On the other hand, many rare variants arose recently in the population through de novo mutations, which are present in the child but not the parents. These rare variants can have large impacts on the structure of the brain because they have been under less selective pressure (Chakravarti 1999). Linkage and whole exome sequencing studies have been used to identify large effect rare variants leading to changes in brain structure, mostly in families (Bae et al. 2015). Studies of rare genetic variations with large effects have led to an understanding of the cell types and biological processes altering cortical structure, and will be reviewed first along with model systems used to understand their effects.

25.4 Model Systems for Studying Rare Variation

Single gene mutations affecting brain structure have been modeled in both non-human animals and human cell lines to understand the mechanism by which the genetic changes lead to differences in brain structure (Figure 25.4). Here, we describe the strengths and limitations of frequently

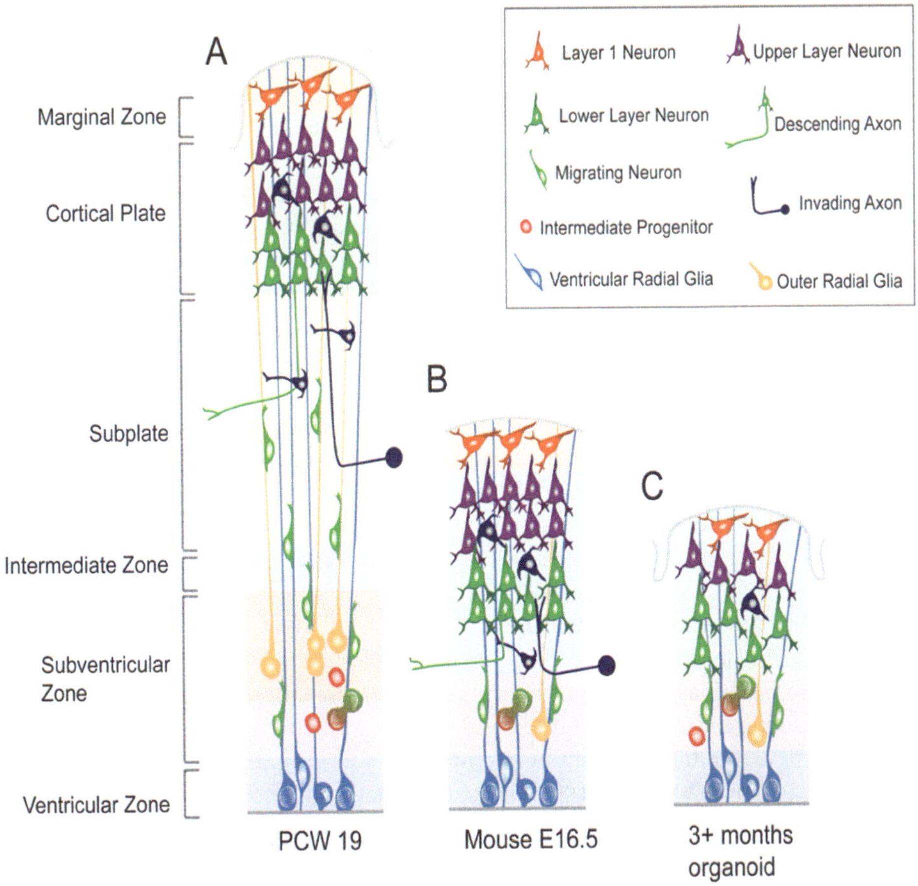

Figure 25.4 Developing cortical wall in (A) humans (B) mice, and (C) human cerebral organoids. PCW – post conception week. E – embryonic day. This figure is modified from Di Lullo and Kriegstein 2017.

used models. Mice (*mus musculus*) are a common experimental system because of their relatively quick development, large litter sizes, and genetic tractability. Mice also have relatively high conservation within exons relative to humans making them a good model system to study protein-coding mutations, though noncoding regions are in general poorly conserved (Guénet 2005). Though mice broadly mimic the laminar structure of the germinal zone, subplate, and cortical plate during development, there are notable differences between mouse and human corticogenesis. Mice have a smaller subventricular zone, which is not divided into inner and outer layers, and no outer proliferative zone because oRG and intermediate progenitors are underrepresented compared to humans (Chini and Hanganu-Opatz 2021). Additionally, mouse cortical progenitors proliferate fewer times and are more transcriptionally homogeneous, leading to a lissencephalic cortex (Calegari et al. 2005; Johnson et al. 2015; Pollen et al. 2015). However, mice share conserved transcription factors essential to excitatory neuron lineage diversification, making mouse models suitable to understand gene functions in cell fate decisions (Di Bella et al. 2021). Though genetic and brain structural differences during development and in adulthood limit the interpretation of some studies, mice remain a good model for understanding how protein-coding genetic variation alters the function of shared cell types between mice and humans.

Stem cell models, either from embryonic human stem cells or induced pluripotent stem cells, can be differentiated to model human cortical development (Hansen et al. 2011; Takahashi et al. 2007; Thomson et al. 1998; Yu et al. 2007). Importantly, human stem cell models have a human genome so conservation is not a concern, and can be derived from an individual harboring a brain-structure associated rare variant or genome edited to carry the brain-structure associated allele (Dolmetsch and Geschwind 2011; Urresti et al. 2021). Radial glia can be produced through adherent cultures, which form "rosettes" that mimic the structure of the closed neural tube and can be propagated or differentiated into neurons (Wilson and Stice 2006). Alternatively, differentiating stem cells as spheres in suspension can lead to self-organized neuroepithelial buds, which mimic the developing cortical wall (Eiraku et al. 2008; Lancaster et al. 2013). Stem cell derived human radial glia are polarized, undergo interkinetic nuclear migration, mimic the architecture of the cortical wall, and can produce astrocytes after extended differentiation periods (Lancaster et al. 2013; Qian et al. 2020; Sloan et al. 2017). Additionally, organoids modeling different brain regions can be fused together to improve understanding of cell migration and integration of each component of cortical circuits (Birey et al. 2017; Kelley and Paşca 2022). However, organoid cell types are not transcriptionally identical to primary cells of the same type, only mature to mimic mid-fetal development unless cultured for a year or more, and are under increased metabolic stress (Bhaduri et al. 2020; Gordon et al. 2021). Even with these limitations, stem cell derived models provide unparalleled access to human cortical progenitor cells and the genetic mechanisms driving their development and differentiation.

25.5 Rare Genetic Variation Impacting Cortical Progenitor Function

Rare human genetic variations with large impacts on either progenitor cell cycle, cell fate, and/or radial glia scaffolding have been identified and studied in model systems. There are many known genes where rare mutations result in microcephaly (a 2–3 standard deviation reduction in head circumference) or macrocephaly (a 2–3 standard deviation increase in head circumference), and new genes continue to be discovered (Alcantara and O'Driscoll 2014; Pirozzi et al. 2018). The radial unit hypothesis describes how mutations affecting progenitor function can drastically alter the number of mature cells leading to microcephaly and macrocephaly. Here we review six genes with known mutations that alter cortical size through impacts on distinct aspects of progenitor function.

EOMES is an example of a well-studied gene where mutations are associated with microcephaly (Figure 25.5). In a consanguineous family, several members were found to exhibit microcephaly, polymicrogyria, and agenesis of the corpus callosum. A homozygous chromosomal translocation in all affected family members was identified near, but not directly disrupting the sequence of, the gene EOMES. EOMES expression levels were absent in homozygous chromosomal translocation carriers implying that missing regulatory elements beyond the translocation breakpoint caused the lack of expression (Baala et al. 2007). Subsequent work identified regulatory elements with stronger chromatin accessibility in the developing human germinal zone that were beyond the microcephaly breakpoint (de la Torre-Ubieta et al. 2018). These elements had strong and specific chromatin interaction with the promoter region of EOMES in the germinal zone (Won et al. 2016). The impact of one of the regulatory elements beyond the translocation breakpoint on EOMES

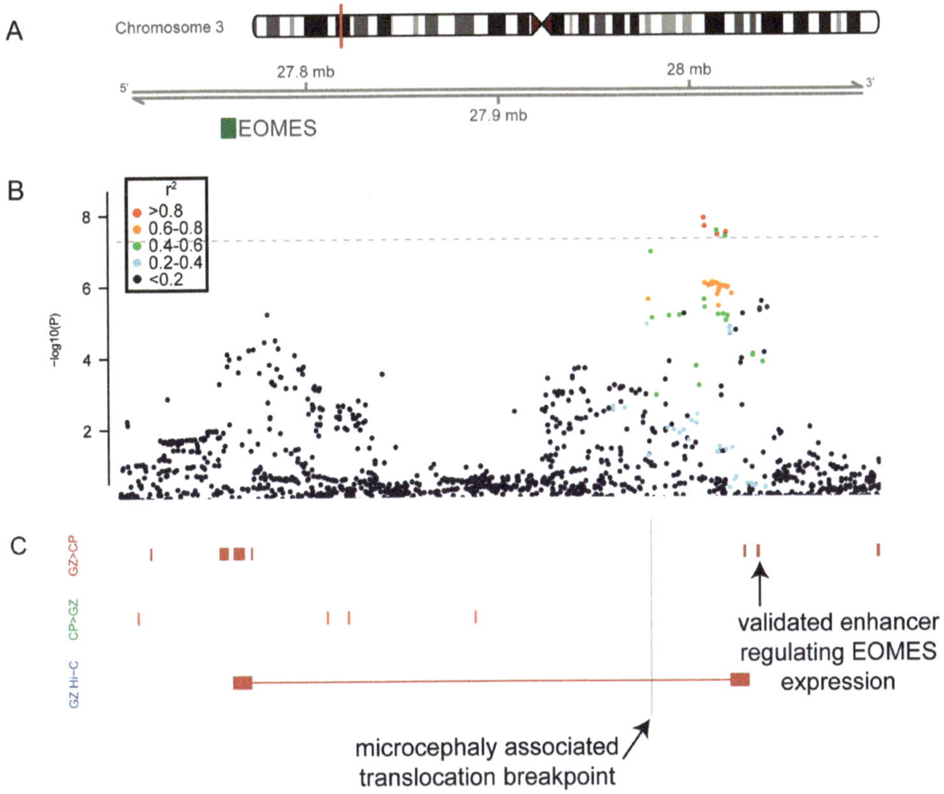

Figure 25.5 Genome annotation showing rare and common variants impacting the EOMES gene. (A) The red box shows the locus of interest on chromosome 3 including the EOMES gene. (B) The results from global cortical surface area GWAS, where several single nucleotide polymorphisms (SNPs) in linkage disequilibrium are significantly associated with cortical surface area. The dotted line represents the p-value threshold for genome wide significance. R^2 values represent correlation of the index SNP alleles to other SNP alleles in the same locus within a European population. (C) GZ > CP is chromatin accessibility higher in the progenitor-rich germinal zone than in neuron-rich cortical plate of the developing human brain. CP > GZ is chromatin accessibility higher in the neuron-rich cortical plate than in the progenitor-rich germinal zone. GZ Hi-C shows regions of the genome in contact with each other in the progenitor-rich germinal zone. CP – cortical plate, GZ – germinal zone.

expression was validated through CRISPR/Cas9 excision in human neural progenitor cells that caused decreased EOMES expression. This enhancer sequence is conserved between mouse and human, and when inserted into a lacZ construct to measure its regulatory activity in different regions of the embryonic mouse brain (Visel et al. 2007), it has forebrain specificity. That spatial expression pattern matches the expression of EOMES itself during embryonic development of the mouse brain. EOMES, also known as TBR2, is a marker and regulator of intermediate progenitors and knockout of EOMES leads to smaller brains in mice (Arnold et al. 2008). All of this evidence shows how a rare noncoding genetic variant alters cortical structure by changing the expression of a gene critical to cortical progenitor function.

Pathogenic heterozygous germline PTEN (phosphatase tensin homolog) mutations are associated with multiple hamartoma syndromes, though there is variable penetrance and no correlation between the kind of mutation and cancer predisposition or macrocephaly (Macken et al. 2019). PTEN is a tumor suppressor gene that regulates cell proliferation through the PI3K-AKT pathway (Lee et al. 2018). Loss of function PTEN mutations in cortical progenitors of mouse models lead to increased brain weight (Chen et al. 2015; Kwon et al. 2001). PTEN mutations increase total cell number in affected brain regions, due to an increase in progenitor proliferation (Chen et al. 2015). Upon homozygous deletion of PTEN, cell size also increases, though this is more notable in when PTEN is constitutively knocked out in cerebellar and hippocampal granule neurons in mice (Backman et al. 2001; Chen et al. 2015; Kwon et al. 2001). Homozygous *PTEN* deletion in human cortical organoids show enlargement of neuroepithelial buds due to an extended time of progenitor self-renewal before any asymmetric divisions. Mouse-derived organoids with the same mutations also had an expanded progenitor pool, but to a lesser degree and did not produce visibly larger neuroepithelial buds (Li et al. 2017). These models demonstrate progenitor proliferation can be regulated by proteins directly involved in the cell cycle or upstream pathways. Convergence across multiple PTEN model systems demonstrates the powerful influence that progenitor self-renewal and cell production have on cortical size.

Radial glia are multipotent and alterations to the cell fate decisions made in these progenitors can impact the overall composition and organization of the cortex. For example, 88 percent of Tuberous Sclerosis Complex (TSC) patients have cortical tubers that contain giant cells, dysmorphic neurons, astrocytes, and oligodendrocytes in different amounts (Mühlebner et al. 2016; Rosset et al. 2017). TSC is an autosomal dominant disorder with 70 percent de novo cases with mutations in either *TSC1* or *TSC2* (Rosset et al. 2017). Several mouse models with mutations *TSC1* and *TSC2* in cortical progenitors suggest the heterogeneous populations of cells in TSC cortical tubers are an incompletely differentiated glia-neuronal cell type originating from radial glia, but no individual mouse model captures the full range of cortical tuber cell types (Zimmer et al. 2020). *TSC2* deletion in cortical progenitors produced more intermediate progenitors than early born neurons during development and resulted in a thicker cortical wall with larger neurons in mice (Way et al. 2009). Mouse models of *TSC1* also report atypical cells types, including enlarged multinucleate neurons (Feliciano et al. 2011), cells with organelle dysfunction and oversize vacuoles (Goto et al. 2011), and cells expressing both neuronal and astrocyte markers (Onda et al. 2002), and subependymal nodules (Magri et al. 2011). Generally, these studies in mice suggest that mutations in TSC genes can result in altered cell fate decisions for typical cell types and the production of abnormal cells. Cortical tubers are likely caused by the inability of these abnormal cell types to migrate properly along radial glia fibers (Evsyukova et al. 2013; Mühlebner et al. 2016). Mouse models incompletely phenocopy TSC patient presentations because the abnormal cell types in the models do not form tubers, but an organoid model of both *TSC1* and *TSC2* heterozygous mutations followed by virally mediated biallelic knockdown, generated cortical tuber like masses containing giant cells, dysplastic neurons, and glia (Blair et al. 2018). Phenocopying cortical tubers in a human stem cell model systems only when a secondary insult results in biallelic knockdown may indicate a role for somatic mutations in at least some TSC patient presentations (Blair et al. 2018; Qin et al. 2010).

Genetic variants leading to disruptions of the radial glia scaffolding can result in heterotopia, a kind of focal cortical dysplasia (groups of brain cells in abnormal locations) (Gleeson et al. 1998; Severino et al. 2020). Van Maldergem syndrome is a recessive disorder linked to biallelic mutations in protocadherin components of an apical adhesive complex, *FAT4* and *DCHS1*, that often includes periventricular heterotopia with simplified cortical layers above the nodules (Mansour et al. 2012). Though germline biallelic knockout of *FAT4* and *DCHS1* in mice do not show heterotopias prenatally and do not survive past birth, transient reduction using in utero electroporation of either gene in mice shows increased proliferation coupled with a loss of cell migration (Cappello et al. 2013). Deletion in human brain organoids of both genes show heterotopia-like nodules of neurons in the ventricular-like zones. vRG in these organoids are displaced from the apical membrane and show disorganized radial fibers (Klaus et al. 2019). Together, these results suggest that the integrity of vRG polarization and fiber orientation is critical to proper cortex formation.

Collectively, these examples demonstrate how large effect variants in protein-coding regions alter cortical progenitor proliferation and cell fate decisions to change cortical size and effect radial glia scaffolding to impact cortical structure. These studies support the radial unit hypothesis and suggest that changes in gene expression level in cortical progenitors during fetal development explains variation in cortical size.

25.6 Model Systems for Studying Common Genetic Variants

Studies of common genetic variants also support the radial unit hypothesis as the guiding principle in determining cortical size, even when the changes are within the normal range of variation. Common genetic variants in the human populations act as natural experiments for determining which genetic variation impacts cortical size. Though current genetic association results do not explain all the heritability of cortical structure, as they are limited by current sample sizes, they offer a first genome-wide description of variants impacting cortical size (Grasby et al. 2020; Hofer et al. 2020). GWAS in large unrelated populations have been used to identify common variants associated with interindividual differences in gross brain structure, as measured through MRI (Bis et al. 2012; Stein et al. 2012; Taal et al. 2012). Several consortia exist to collect genotyping and MRI scans to grow GWAS sample sizes (Smith et al. 2021; Thompson et al. 2014). The ENIGMA consortium aggregated data from 60 cohorts across the world comprising almost 34,000 individuals with replication in an additional 17,000 individuals (Grasby et al. 2020). Common variants were found to explain about one-third of cortical surface area heritability. In addition, this study identified 369 loci after replication associated with interindividual differences in size of cortical region at genome-wide significant levels, providing a comprehensive understanding of common genetic variants leading to differences in human cortical size. We expect that increasing statistical power through increased sample sizes and types of variation studied through more comprehensive sequencing approaches will lead to discovery of most variants associated with differences in brain structure (Matoba et al. 2022).

Though hundreds of common variant loci impacting brain structure have been discovered (Grasby et al. 2020; Matoba and Stein 2021; Smith et al. 2021), GWAS alone does not provide insights into developmental time periods or cell types that influence a trait. When combined with regulatory activity maps GWAS can inform mechanistic hypotheses. Partitioned heritability was employed to determine whether a genetic association signal is enriched in defined regions of the genome active in a given cell type or developmental time period (Finucane et al. 2015). Using chromatin marks indicative of enhancer regions, the strongest enrichment for cortical surface area GWAS was identified in brain-specific putative enhancers (Grasby et al. 2020; Roadmap Epigenomics Consortium et al. 2015). Further studies identified fetal specific regulatory elements mapped to cell-type specific genes were enriched for cortical surface area heritability (de la Torre-Ubieta et al. 2018; Polioudakis et al. 2019). The strongest partitioned heritability enrichments for cortical surface area were detected in progenitor cell regulatory elements, implying that common genetic variation tunes progenitor regulatory element activity during fetal development leading to differences in cortical surface area in adulthood (Grasby et al. 2020; Liang et al. 2021). This finding is highly consistent with both predictions of the radial unit hypothesis and the known mechanism of rare variant associations described earlier.

Variants identified by GWAS are difficult to interpret in isolation. Because DNA is inherited in chunks during meiosis, genetic variants close to each other are correlated in a population (called linkage disequilibrium), which makes identification of the causal variant within a locus difficult (Slatkin 2008). Common variant loci rarely change the protein coding sequence of a gene and instead are found in noncoding regions of the genome, where functionality is poorly understood (Lappalainen and MacArthur 2021). Noncoding variants presumably have gene regulatory potential, but the causal gene is not always the closest gene and needs to be identified by other means (Albert and Kruglyak 2015). Also, genetic variants may exert their effects only within specific cell types or states, which are generally unknown. Another experimental system is needed to study how individual variants in the genome have specific consequences on molecular biology during cortical development to impact brain structure.

Molecular quantitative trait loci (QTL) studies offer a solution for studying how genotype influences molecular phenotypes in cortical progenitors. In these studies, cells or tissue from a population of genotyped donors enable associations to be conducted between genetic variants and molecular phenotypes to determine the downstream impacts of brain-structure associated variants. Bulk sequencing of thousands of adult postmortem brains (Sieberts et al. 2020; Zeng et al. 2022) and hundreds of postmortem fetal brains (O'Brien et al. 2018) have identified molecular QTLs. These studies have statistical power to detect associations, but lack cell type specificity and the ability to conduct validation experiments for their findings. More recently, research groups have performed molecular QTLs in human neural progenitor cells grown in vitro, which provide a unique opportunity for testing how cell type specific gene expression is associated with genotype (Aygün et al. 2021; Liang et al. 2021; Zhang et al. 2020). Testing how genotype affects cell behavior or protein levels remains difficult and is only starting to be accomplished for neural cell types in culture (Wolter et al. 2022). However, large populations of induced pluripotent stem cells or primary human neural progenitor cells that continue to be developed make this study design feasible and future studies will likely find genotype associations with neural progenitor cellular phenotypes and protein levels (Cuomo et al. 2020; Kilpinen et al. 2017; Mirauta et al. 2020).

25.7 Common Genetic Variants Influencing Cortical Size

Integrating molecular QTLs from cultured neural progenitors and neurons with GWAS enables the interpretation of individual loci's gene regulatory mechanism underlying differences in cortical surface area (Figure 25.6) (Aygün et al. 2021). A common variant locus was identified on chromosome 6 containing many noncoding single nucleotide polymorphisms associated with cortical

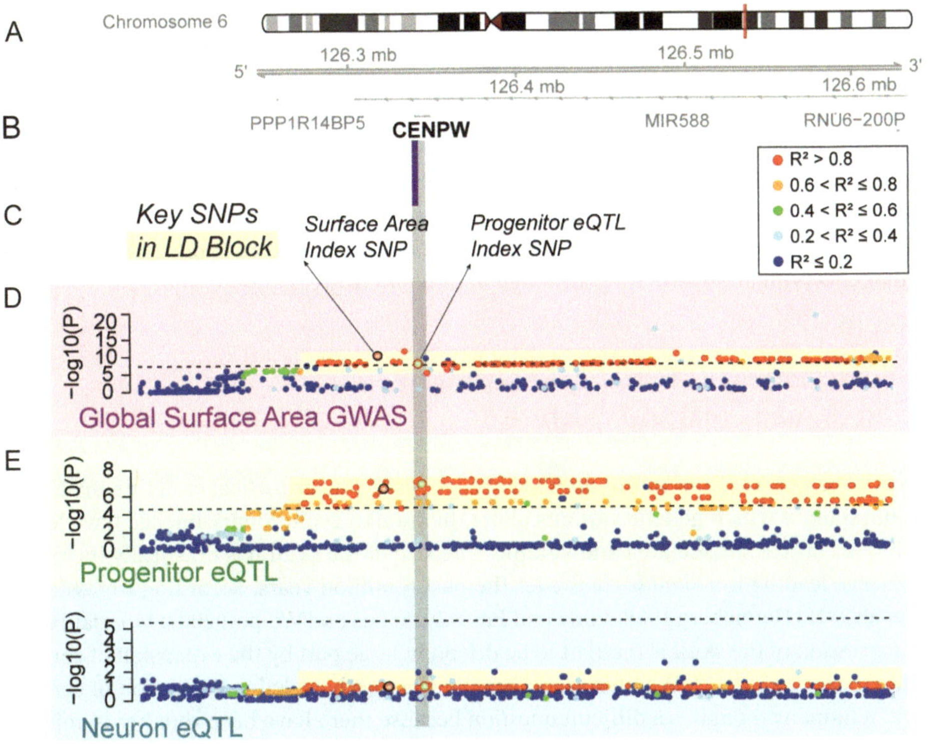

Figure 25.6 Example annotated plot showing colocalization of a single nucleotide polymorphism (SNP) identified in a global surface area GWAS with a progenitor eQTL, but not a neuron eQTL (Aygün et al. 2021). (A) The locus is on chromosome 6 in the red boxed region. (B) Annotations of the locus show genes, including CENPW, and a chromatin accessibility peak at the promoter of this gene are shown in purple. (C) Indicates SNPs important for the interpretation of the locus found in linkage disequilibrium (LD). R^2 values represent correlation of SNP alleles to other SNP alleles in the same locus. The LD block is highlighted in yellow. (D) Shows the global surface area GWAS in pink. The dotted line represents the p-value threshold for genome wide significance. (E) Shows expression QTLs (eQTLs) performed in progenitor cultures in green and eQTLs performed in neuronal cultures in blue. The LD block is present in both eQTLs and the GWAS. A chromatin accessibility peak at the promoter of CENPW contains SNPs associated with both increased global cortical surface area and increased CENPW expression in progenitors.

surface area (Grasby et al. 2020). The brain-structure associated locus shared causal variants (colocalized) with an expression QTL in progenitors affecting the nearby gene *CENPW*. In addition, a chromatin accessibility QTL in both progenitors and neurons at the promoter region of *CENPW* also colocalized with the brain structure associated locus. One variant, among the many at the locus, associated with chromatin accessibility, gene expression, and cortical surface area. This variant fell within the chromatin accessibility peak and disrupted several transcription-factor binding motifs, providing strong evidence that this is the causal variant in the region. In all, using multiple molecular QTLs in a cell-type specific system, this study found a molecular mechanism including variant, regulatory element, cell type, and gene that leads to differences in cortical surface area across humans (Aygün et al. 2021). Though the impact of altered levels of CENPW expression on progenitor proliferation or fate decisions has not yet been measured, given the known roles of CENPW in mitosis (Lee et al. 2010; McKinley and Cheeseman 2017) we presume that this variant alters neurogenesis or apoptosis in progenitor cells.

Rare and common variants affecting brain structure can also impact the same locus. One of the loci associated with global cortical surface area was in the region distal to the EOMES gene separated from the chromosomal translocation breakpoint previously described to cause microcephaly (Figure 25.5). The GWAS locus overlaps, but no individual variant directly alters, the same enhancer regions previously validated to regulate EOMES expression. Common variants at the same region have a detectable effect on cortical surface area, providing further evidence that non-coding regulation of a gene critical to progenitor function, EOMES, alters cortical size, possibly through altering cell fate decisions. This also shows that rare variants and common variants can lead to similar effects on brain structure, although to different degrees.

25.8 Uncovering Evolutionarily Relevant Genetic Variants Influencing Human Cortical Structure

The discovery of genetic variants within human populations that alter cortical structure invites an alternative question of which genetic variants along the human evolutionary lineage have led to the expansion of cortical surface area and volume. The size of the skull has drastically increased along the lineage leading to *Homo sapiens* over the past 6 million years, according to fossil evidence (Du et al. 2018; Henneberg 1988; Jantz and Jantz 2016; Lee and Wolpoff 2003; Moorjani et al. 2016). The expansion of the skull is thought to be driven in large part by the expansion of cortical surface area (Sousa et al. 2017). Which specific genetic changes have led to expansion of cortical surface area in humans though is a difficult question because there have been roughly 16 million fixed genetic changes after humans diverged from chimpanzees approximately 5–10 million years ago (Enard 2016; Mallick et al. 2016; Pääbo 2014). There have been 31,000 fixed genetic changes between modern humans and archaic humans like Neanderthal and Denisovan, where divergence occurred 200–300 thousand years ago (Mallick et al. 2016; Pääbo 2014; Prüfer et al. 2014). Identifying which of those evolutionarily relevant genetic changes impact brain features, rather than other tissues, or have neutral effects, is quite difficult (Enard 2016). Careful study of gene expression during human development and cross-species genomic comparisons can provide strong candidates for uniquely human genomic changes impacting cortical size. For example, a human accelerated region, which is a highly conserved sequence of the genome up to chimpanzees but is mutated in humans, was found to encode a novel RNA gene expressed in the marginal zone of the human fetal cortex, implying but not directly demonstrating, that this alters cortical development (Pollard et al. 2006). Human gained enhancers are regulatory elements with evidence for stronger activity in human cortical tissue as compared to macaque or mice, so likely contribute to differences in human brain structure and function (Reilly et al. 2015). It was shown that human gained enhancers were enriched with common variants associated with inferior frontal cortex structure, a brain region critical for speech and language functions (Tilot et al. 2021). A human specific gene ARHGAP11B has been shown to induce cortical folding when expressed in marmoset embryos (Heide et al. 2020) or increase cortical length in ferrets (Kalebic et al. 2018). ARHGAP11B localizes in the mitochondria and increases calcium concentration, which alters cellular metabolism and increases progenitor proliferation (Namba et al. 2020). Finally, of the 87 non-synonymous fixed genetic differences between archaic and modern human, there was a slight enrichment of these genes as being expressed in the ventricular zone of the developing cortex, implying that these variants may have led to differences in brain structure along human evolution (Prüfer et al. 2014). Determining which genetic changes have led to human brain expansion is still a new field but will likely greatly benefit from using genetically manipulable organoid models from both humans and chimpanzees (Benito-Kwiecinski et al. 2021; Pollen et al. 2019) as well as better in utero imaging of radial progenitor organization (Casingal et al. 2022).

25.9 Discussion and Future Perspectives

Though great progress has been made in identifying common and rare genetic variations that alter brain structure across the human population, additional studies will likely identify new variants as well as their molecular and cellular mechanisms. A sample size of up to 8 million may be necessary to describe all heritability of brain structure phenotypes, which is more than 100 times larger than current sample sizes, and may be possible by tapping into electronic medical records and biobanks (Matoba et al. 2022). Whole exome and whole genome sequencing of large populations of individuals with MRI will likely yield new rare coding and noncoding variants associated with differences in cortical structure as well. While sample sizes are increased to identify new brain-structure associated variants in GWAS and to include more diverse ancestries (Peterson et al. 2019), other work will help interpret already known brain-structure associated common genetic variants. We have reviewed how gene expression and chromatin accessibility QTLs from relevant cell types and developmental periods can be used to interpret trait associated variants. Expression QTLs have only been identified for 47 percent of GWAS loci from 87 traits by Genotype-tissue Expression Consortium, suggesting that QTLs from adult postmortem tissue may be insufficient to describe the function of all noncoding variations impacting gene expression (Barbeira et al. 2020; Connally et al. 2021). We expect that QTLs performed with single cell type resolution, or under different experimental stimuli, or from different developmental time points may identify more QTLs and result in a functional explanation of a greater number of brain-structure associated loci (Bryois et al. 2022 Umans et al. 2021). Other methods can be used to demonstrate the effects of common variants on gene expression, like massively parallel reporter assays, which use exogenous expression of short DNA fragments to identify regulatory activity (Townsley et al. 2020). Identifying this "missing regulation" will allow a mechanistic understanding of how genetic variation alters progenitor behavior and leads to differences in brain structure and function.

Additional mechanisms of brain-structure associated loci may be revealed by using animal models other than mice that recapitulate more aspects of human cortical development. For example, macaques (*macaca fascicularis*) have gyrencephalic brains with an increase in upper-layer neurons and larger outer subventricular zone and subplate in fetal development relative to mice (Heuer et al. 2019; Rash et al. 2019). Recent macaques studies have used gene editing techniques like TALENS to study microcephaly (Ke et al. 2016), CRISPR-Cas9 to study Phelan–McDermid syndrome (Zhou et al. 2019), and have now undergone base editing (Zhang et al. 2020). However, macaques have a protracted development of 165 days which decreases experimental efficiency and may be preferred only when simpler model systems like induced pluripotent stem cells and mice do not provide a satisfactory explanation.

Collectively, these studies on rare large-effect variants, common small-effect variants, and fixed genetic features demonstrate the multiple avenues through which genetic variation in humans impact cortical size and structure. Genetic variation can dynamically modulate how human radial glial cells function, including the regulation of gene expression, chromatin interaction, generation of the cells of the cortex, and as a migratory guide, thus fine tuning the number and placement of cortical cells underlying cortical size and structure. As such, the radial unit hypothesis remains a powerful explanatory tool for relating cortical development to cellular phenotypes that are influenced by genomic variation.

References

Albert, F.W. and Kruglyak, L. (2015). The role of regulatory variation in complex traits and disease. *Nat Rev Genet* 16 (4): 197–212.

Alcantara, D. and O'Driscoll, M. (2014). Congenital microcephaly. *Am J Med Genet Part C, Semin Med Genet* 166C (2): 124–139.

Arnold, S.J. et al. (2008). The T-box transcription factor eomes/Tbr2 regulates neurogenesis in the cortical subventricular zone. *Genes Dev* 22 (18): 2479–2484.

Aygün, N. et al. (2021). Brain-trait-associated variants impact cell-type-specific gene regulation during neurogenesis. *Am J Hum Genet* 108 (9): 1647–1668.

Baala, L. et al. (2007). Homozygous silencing of T-box transcription factor EOMES leads to microcephaly with polymicrogyria and corpus callosum agenesis. *Nat Genet* 39 (4): 454–456.

Backman, S.A. et al. (2001). Deletion of Pten in mouse brain causes seizures, ataxia and defects in soma size resembling Lhermitte-Duclos disease. *Nat Genet* 29 (4): 396–403.

Bae, B.-I. et al. (2015). Genetic changes shaping the human brain. *Dev Cell* 32 (4): 423–434.

Barbeira, A.N. et al. (2020). Exploiting the GTEx resources to decipher the mechanisms at GWAS loci. *BioRxiv*. doi: 10.1101/814350.

Benito-Kwiecinski, S. et al. (2021). An early cell shape transition drives evolutionary expansion of the human forebrain. *Cell* 184 (8): 2084–2102.e19.

Bethlehem, R.A.I. et al. (2022). Brain charts for the human lifespan. *Nature* 604 (7906): 525–533.

Bhaduri, A. et al. (2020). Cell stress in cortical organoids impairs molecular subtype specification. *Nature* 578 (7793): 142–148.

Birey, F. et al. (2017). Assembly of functionally integrated human forebrain spheroids. *Nature* 545 (7652): 54–59.

Bis, J.C. et al. (2012). Common variants at 12q14 and 12q24 are associated with hippocampal volume. *Nat Genet* 44 (5): 545–551.

Blair, J.D. et al. (2018). Genetically engineered human cortical spheroid models of tuberous sclerosis. *Nat Med* 24 (10): 1568–1578.

Blokland, G.A.M. et al. (2012). Genetic and environmental influences on neuroimaging phenotypes. *Twin Res Hum Genet* 15 (3): 351–371.

Bryois, J. et al. (2022). Cell-type specific cis-eQTLs in eight human brain cell types identify novel risk genes for psychiatric and neurological disorders. *Nat Neurosci* 25 (8): 1104–1112.

Bystron, I. et al. (2008). Development of the human cerebral cortex. *Nat Rev Neurosci* 9 (2): 110–122.

Calegari, F. et al. (2005). Selective lengthening of the cell cycle in the neurogenic subpopulation of neural progenitor cells during mouse brain development. *J Neurosci* 25 (28): 6533–6538.

Cappello, S. et al. (2013). Mutations in genes encoding the cadherin receptor-ligand pair DCHS1 and FAT4 disrupt cerebral cortical development. *Nat Genet* 45 (11): 1300–1308.

Casingal, C. et al. (2022). Coordinating cerebral cortical construction and connectivity. *Neuron* 110 (7): 1100–1115.

Chakravarti, A. (1999). Population genetics–making sense out of sequence. *Nat Genet* 21 (1 Suppl): 56–60.

Chen, Y. et al. (2015). Pten mutations alter brain growth trajectory and allocation of cell types through elevated β-catenin signaling. *J Neurosci* 35 (28): 10252–10267.

Chini, M. and Hanganu-Opatz, I.L. (2021). Prefrontal cortex development in health and disease. *Trends Neurosci* 44 (3): 227–240.

Connally, N. et al. (2021). The missing link between genetic association and regulatory function. *medRxiv*. doi: 10.1101/2021.06.08.21258515.

Cuomo, A. et al. (2020). Single-cell RNA-sequencing of differentiating iPS cells reveals dynamic genetic effects on gene expression. *Nat Commun* 11 (1): 810.

de la Torre-Ubieta, L. et al. (2018). The dynamic landscape of open chromatin during human cortical neurogenesis. *Cell* 172 (1–2): 289–304.e18.

Desikan, R.S. et al. (2006). An automated labeling system for subdividing the human cerebral cortex on MRI scans into gyral based regions of interest. *NeuroImage* 31 (3): 968–980.

Di Bella, D.J. et al. (2021). Molecular logic of cellular diversification in the mouse cerebral cortex. *Nature* 595 (7868): 554–559.

Di Lullo, E. and Kriegstein, A.R. (2017). The use of brain organoids to investigate neural development and disease. *Nat Rev Neurosci* 18 (10): 573–584. doi: 10.1038/nrn.2017.107. Epub 2017 Sep 7. PMID: 28878372; PMCID: PMC5667942.

Dolmetsch, R. and Geschwind, D.H. (2011). The human brain in a dish. *Cell* 145 (6): 831–834.

Du, A. et al. (2018). Pattern and process in hominin brain size evolution are scale-dependent. *Proc Biol Sci* 285 (1873): 20172738. doi: 10.1098/rspb.2017.2738.

Eiraku, M. et al. (2008). Self-organized formation of polarized cortical tissues from ESCs and its active manipulation by extrinsic signals. *Cell Stem Cell* 3 (5): 519–532.

Enard, W. (2016). The molecular basis of human brain evolution. *Curr Biol* 26 (20): R1109–17.

Evsyukova, I. et al. (2013). Integrative mechanisms of oriented neuronal migration in the developing brain. *Ann Rev Cell Dev Biol* 29: 299–353.

Feliciano, D.M. et al. (2011). Single-cell Tsc1 knockout during corticogenesis generates tuber-like lesions and reduces seizure threshold in mice. *J Clin Investig* 121 (4): 1596–1607.

Finucane, H.K. et al. (2015). Partitioning heritability by functional annotation using genome-wide association summary statistics. *Nat Gen* 47 (11): 1228–1235.

Fischl, B. and Dale, A.M. (2000). Measuring the thickness of the human cerebral cortex from magnetic resonance images. *Proc Natl Acad Sci USA* 97 (20): 11050–11055.

Geschwind, D.H. and Rakic, P. (2013). Cortical evolution. *Neuron* 80 (3): 633–647.

Gleeson, J.G. et al. (1998). Doublecortin, a brain-specific gene mutated in human X-linked lissencephaly and double cortex syndrome, encodes a putative signaling protein. *Cell* 92 (1): 63–72.

Gordon, A. et al. (2021). Long-term maturation of human cortical organoids matches key early postnatal transitions. *Nat Neurosci* 24 (3): 331–342.

Goto, J. et al. (2011). Regulable neural progenitor-specific Tsc1 loss yields giant cells with organellar dysfunction in a model of tuberous sclerosis complex. *Proc Natl Acad Sci USA* 108 (45): E1070–79.

Grasby, K.L. et al. (2020). The genetic architecture of the human cerebral cortex. *Science* 367 (6484): 399402.

Guénet, J.L. (2005). The mouse genome. *Genome Res* 15 (12): 1729–1740.

Hadders-Algra, M. (2018). Early human brain development. *Neurosci Biobehav Rev* 92: 276–290.

Hansen, D.V. et al. (2010). Neurogenic radial glia in the outer subventricular zone of human neocortex. *Nature* 464 (7288): 554–561.

Hansen, D.V. et al. (2011). Deriving excitatory neurons of the neocortex from pluripotent stem cells. *Neuron* 70 (4): 645–660.

Heide, M. et al. (2020). Human-specific ARHGAP11B increases size and folding of primate neocortex in the fetal marmoset. *Science* 369 (6503): 546–550.

Henneberg, M. (1988). Decrease of human skull size in the holocene. *Hum Biol* 60 (3): 395–405.

Herculano-Houzel, S. (2012). The remarkable, yet not extraordinary, human brain as a scaled-up primate brain and its associated cost. *Proc Natl Acad Sci USA* 109 (Suppl 1): 10661–10668.

Heuer, K. et al. (2019). Evolution of neocortical folding. *Cortex* 118: 275–291.

Hofer, E. et al. (2020). Genetic correlations and genome-wide associations of cortical structure in general population samples of 22,824 adults. *Nat Commun* 11 (1): 4796.

Holst, C.B. et al. (2019). Astrogliogenesis in human fetal brain. *J Anat* 235 (3): 590–615.

Howard, B.M. et al. (2008). Radial glia cells in the developing human brain. *Neurosci* 14 (5): 459–473.

Jantz, R.L. and Jantz, L.M. (2016). The remarkable change in Euro-American cranial shape and size. *Hum Biol* 88 (1): 56–64.

Johnson, M.B. et al. (2015). Single-cell analysis reveals transcriptional heterogeneity of neural progenitors in human cortex. *Nat Neurosci* 18 (5): 637–646.

Kalebic, N. et al. (2018). Human-specific ARHGAP11B induces hallmarks of neocortical expansion in developing ferret neocortex. *Elife* 7: e41241. doi: 10.7554/eLife.41241.

Kang, H.J. et al. (2011). Spatio-temporal transcriptome of the human brain. *Nature* 478 (7370): 483–489.

Ke, Q. et al. (2016). TALEN-based generation of a cynomolgus monkey disease model for human microcephaly. *Cell Res* 26 (9): 1048–1061.

Kelley, K.W. and Paşca, S.P. (2022). Human brain organogenesis. *Cell* 185 (1): 42–61.

Kilpinen, H. et al. (2017). Common genetic variation drives molecular heterogenity in human iPSCs. *Nature* 546 (7658): 370–375.

Klaus, J. et al. (2019). Altered neuronal migratory trajectories in human cerebral organoids derived from individuals with neuronal heterotopia. *Nat Med* 25 (4): 561–568.

Kostović, I. et al. (2019). Neural histology and neurogenesis of the human fetal and infant brain. *Neuroimage* 188: 743–773.

Kriegstein, A.R. and Götz, M. (2003). Radial glia diversity. *Glia* 43 (1): 37–43.

Krsnik, Ž. et al. (2017). Growth of thalamocortical fibers to the somatosensory cortex in the human fetal brain. *Front Neurosci* 11: 233.

Kwon, C.H. et al. (2001). Pten regulates neuronal soma size. *Nat Genet* 29 (4): 404–411.

Lancaster, M.A. et al. (2013). Cerebral organoids model human brain development and microcephaly. *Nature* 501 (7467): 373–379.

Lappalainen, T. and MacArthur, D.G. (2021). From variant to function in human disease genetics. *Science* 373 (6562): 1464–1468.

Le, B.D. and Stein, J.L. (2019). Mapping causal pathways from genetics to neuropsychiatric disorders using genome-wide imaging genetics: current status and future directions. *Psychiatry Clin Neurosci* 73 (7): 357–369. doi: 10.1111/pcn.12839.

Lee, S.-H. and Wolpoff, M.H. (2003). The pattern of evolution in pleistocene human brain size. *Paleobiology* 29 (2): 186–196.

Lee, S. et al. (2010). Cancer-Upregulated Gene 2 (CUG2) overexpression induces apoptosis in SKOV-3 cells. *Cell Biochem Funct* 28 (6): 461–468.

Lee, Y.-R. et al. (2018). The functions and regulation of the PTEN tumour suppressor. *Nat Rev Mol Cell Biol* 19 (9): 547–562.

Li, Y. et al. (2017). Induction of expansion and folding in human cerebral organoids. *Cell Stem Cell* 20 (3): 385–96.e3.

Liang, D. et al. (2021). Cell-type-specific effects of genetic variation on chromatin accessibility during human neuronal differentiation. *Nat Neurosci* 24 (7): 941–953.

Lui, J.H. et al. (2011). Development and evolution of the human neocortex. *Cell* 146 (1): 18–36.

Macken, W.L. et al. (2019). PTEN hamartoma tumor syndrome in childhood. *Am J Med Genet Part C, Semin Med Genet* 181 (4): 591–610.

Magri, L. et al. (2011). Sustained activation of mTOR pathway in embryonic neural stem cells leads to development of tuberous sclerosis complex-associated lesions. *Cell Stem Cell* 9 (5): 447–462.

Mallick, S. et al. (2016). The simons genome diversity project. *Nature* 538 (7624): 201–206.

Mansour, S. et al. (2012). Van Maldergem syndrome. *Eur J Hum Genet* 20 (10): 1024–1031.

Marín-Padilla, M. (2012). The human brain intracerebral microvascular system: development and structure. *Front Neuroanat* 6: 38.

Matoba, N. et al. (2022). Evaluating brain structure traits as endophenotypes using polygenicity and discoverability. *Hum Brain Mapp* 43 (1): 329–340.

Matoba, N. and Stein, J.L. (2021). From base pair to brain. *Nat Neurosci* 24 (5): 619–621.

McCarthy, M.I. et al. (2008). Genome-wide association studies for complex traits: consensus, uncertainty and challenges. *Nat Rev Genet* 9 (5): 356–369.

McKinley, K.L. and Cheeseman, I.M. (2017). Large-scale analysis of CRISPR/Cas9 cell-cycle knockouts reveals the diversity of p53-dependent responses to cell-cycle defects. *Dev Cell* 40 (4): 405–20.e2.

Miller, F.D. and Gauthier, A.S. (2007). Timing is everything. *Neuron* 54 (3): 357–369.

Mirauta, B. et al. (2020). Population-scale proteome variation in human induced pluripotent stem cells. *Elife* 9: e57390.

Molnár, Z. et al. (2019). New insights into the development of the human cerebral cortex. *J Anat* 235 (3): 432–451.

Moorjani, P. et al. (2016). Variation in the molecular clock of primates. *Proc Natl Acad Sci USA* 113 (38): 10607–10612.

Mühlebner, A. et al. (2016). Novel histopathological patterns in cortical tubers of epilepsy surgery patients with tuberous sclerosis complex. *PloS One* 11 (6): e0157396.

Namba, T. et al. (2020). Human-Specific ARHGAP11B acts in mitochondria to expand neocortical progenitors by glutaminolysis. *Neuron* 105 (5): 867–881.e9.

Namba, T. et al. (2021). Metabolic regulation of neocortical expansion in development and evolution. *Neuron* 109 (3): 408–419.

Noctor, S.C. et al. (2004). Cortical neurons arise in symmetric and asymmetric division zones and migrate through specific phases. *Nat Neurosci* 7 (2): 136–144.

Nowakowski, T.J. et al. (2016). Transformation of the radial glia scaffold demarcates two stages of human cerebral cortex development. *Neuron* 91 (6): 1219–1227.

O'Brein, H. et al. (2018). Expression quantitative trait loci in the developing humanbrain and their enrichment in neuropsychiatric disorders. *Genome Biol* 19 (1): 194.

Oegema, R. et al. (2020). International consensus recommendations on the diagnostic work-up for malformations of cortical development. *Nat Rev Neurol* 16 (11): 618–635.

Onda, H. et al. (2002). Tsc2 null murine neuroepithelial cells are a model for human tuber giant cells, and show activation of an mTOR pathway. *Mol Cell Neurosci* 21 (4): 561–574.

Pääbo, S. (2014). The human condition-a molecular approach. *Cell* 157 (1): 216–226.

Peterson, R.E. et al. (2019). Genome-wide association studies in ancestrally diverse populations. *Cell* 179 (3): 589–603.

Pirozzi, F. et al. (2018). From microcephaly to megalencephaly. *Dialogues Clin Neurosci* 20 (4): 267–282.

Polioudakis, D. et al. (2019). A single-cell transcriptomic atlas of human neocortical development during mid-gestation. *Neuron* 103 (5): 785–801.e8.

Pollard, K.S. et al. (2006). An RNA gene expressed during cortical development evolved rapidly in humans. *Nature* 443 (7108): 167–172.

Pollen, A.A. et al. (2019). Establishing cerebral organoids as models of human-specific brain evolution. *Cell* 176 (4): 743–56.e17.

Pollen, A.A. et al. (2015). Molecular identity of human outer radial glia during cortical development. *Cell* 163 (1): 55–67.

Prüfer, K. et al. (2014). The complete genome sequence of a Neanderthal from the Altai Mountains. *Nature* 505 (7481): 43–49.

Qian, X. et al. (2020). Sliced human cortical organoids for modeling distinct cortical layer formation. *Cell Stem Cell* 26 (5): 766–81.e9.

Qin, W. et al. (2010). Analysis of TSC cortical tubers by deep sequencing of TSC1, TSC2 and KRAS demonstrates that small second-hit mutations in these genes are rare events. *Brain Pathol* 20 (6): 1096–1105.

Rakic, P. (1972). Mode of cell migration to the superficial layers of fetal monkey neocortex. *J Comp Neurol* 145 (1): 61–83.

Rakic, P. (1978). Neuronal migration and contact guidance in the primate telencephalon. *Postgrad Med J* 54 (Suppl 1): 25–40.

Rakic, P. (1988). Specification of cerebral cortical areas. *Science* 241 (4862): 170–176.

Rakic, P. (2005). Less is more. *Nat Neurosci* 8 (8): 981.

Rakic, P. (2007). The radial edifice of cortical architecture. *Brain Res Rev* 55 (2): 204–219.

Rakic, P. (2009). Evolution of the neocortex. *Nat Rev Neurosci* 10 (10): 724–735.

Rash, B.G. et al. (2019). Gliogenesis in the outer subventricular zone promotes enlargement and gyrification of the primate cerebrum. *Proc Natl Acad Sci USA* 116 (14): 7089–7094.

Reilly, S.K. et al. (2015). Evolutionary genomics. Evolutionary changes in promoter and enhancer activity during human corticogenesis. *Science* 347 (6226): 1155–1159.

Roadmap Epigenomics Consortium et al. (2015). Integrative analysis of 111 reference human epigenomes. *Nature* 518 (7539): 317–330.

Rosset, C. et al. (2017). TSC1 and TSC2 gene mutations and their implications for treatment in tuberous sclerosis complex. *Genet Mol Biol* 40 (1): 69–79.

Severino, M. et al. (2020). Definitions and classification of malformations of cortical development. *Brain* 143 (10): 2874–2894.

Sieberts, S.K. et al. (2020). Large eQTL meta-analysis reveals differing patterns between cerebral cortical and cerebellar brain regions. *Sci Data* 7 (1): 340.

Silbereis, J.C. et al. (2016). The cellular and molecular landscapes of the developing human central nervous system. *Neuron* 89 (2): 248–268.

Slatkin, M. (2008). Linkage disequilibrium–understanding the evolutionary past and mapping the medical future. *Nat Rev Genet* 9 (6): 477–485.

Sloan, S.A. et al. (2017). Human astrocyte maturation captured in 3D cerebral cortical spheroids derived from pluripotent stem cells. *Neuron* 95 (4): 779–90.e6.

Smith, S.M. et al. (2021). An expanded set of genome-wide association studies of brain imaging phenotypes in UK biobank. *Nat Neurosci* 24 (5): 737–745.

Sousa, A.M.M. et al. (2017). Evolution of the human nervous system function, structure, and development. *Cell* 170 (2): 226–247.

Stein, J.L. et al. (2012). Identification of common variants associated with human hippocampal and intracranial volumes. *Nat Genet* 44 (5): 552–561.

Taal, H.R. et al. (2012). Common variants at 12q15 and 12q24 are associated with infant head circumference. *Nat Genet* 44 (5): 532–538.

Takahashi, K. et al. (2007). Induction of pluripotent stem cells from adult human fibroblasts by defined factors. *Cell* 131 (5): 861–872.

Thompson, P.M. et al. (2014). The ENIGMA consortium. *Brain Imag Behav* 8 (2): 153–182.

Thomson, J.A. et al. (1998). Embryonic stem cell lines derived from human blastocysts. *Science* 282 (5391): 1145–1147.

Tilot, A.K. et al. (2021). The evolutionary history of common genetic variants influencing human cortical surface area. *Cereb Cortex* 31 (4): 1873–1887.

Townsley, K.G. et al. (2020). Massively parallel techniques for cataloguing the regulome of the human brain. *Nat Neurosci* 23 (12): 1509–1521.

Umans, B.D. et al. (2021). Where are the disease-associated eQTLs? *Trends Genet* 37 (2): 109–124.

Urresti, J. et al. (2021). Cortical organoids model early brain development disrupted by 16p11.2 copy number variants in Autism. *Mol Psychiatry* 26 (12): 7560–7580. doi: 10.1038/s41380-021-01243-6.

Visel, A. et al. (2007). VISTA enhancer browser–a database of tissue-specific human enhancers. *Nucleic Acids Res* 35 (Database issue): D88–92.

Visscher, P.M. et al. (2017). 10 years of GWAS discovery. *Am J Hum Genet* 101 (1): 5–22.

Way, S.W. et al. (2009). Loss of Tsc2 in radial glia models the brain pathology of tuberous sclerosis complex in the mouse. *Hum Mol Genet* 18 (7): 1252–1265.

Wilson, P.G. and Stice, S.S. (2006). Development and differentiation of neural rosettes derived from human embryonic stem cells. *Stem Cell Rev* 2 (1): 67–77.

Wolter, J. et al. (2022). Cellular Genome-wide association stud identifies common genetic variation influencing lithium-induced neural progenitor proliferation. *Biol Psychiatry* 93 (1): 8–17.

Won, H. et al. (2016). Chromosome conformation elucidates regulatory relationships in developing human brain. *Nature* 538 (7626): 523–527.

Yu, J. et al. (2007). Induced pluripotent stem cell lines derived from human somatic cells. *Science* 318 (5858): 1917–1920.

Zeng, B. et al. (2022). Multi-ancestry eQTL meta-analysis of human brain identifies candidate causal variants for brain-related traits. *Nat Genet* 54 (2): 161–169.

Zhang, W. et al. (2020). Multiplex precise base editing in cynomolgus monkeys. *Nat Commun* 11 (1): 2325.

Zhong, S. et al. (2018). A single-cell RNA-seq survey of the developmental landscape of the human prefrontal cortex. *Nature* 555 (7697): 524–528.

Zhou, Y. et al. (2019). Atypical behaviour and connectivity in SHANK3-mutant macaques. *Nature* 570 (7761): 326–331.

Zimmer, T.S. et al. (2020). Tuberous sclerosis complex as disease model for investigating mTOR-related gliopathy during epileptogenesis. *Front Neurol* 11: 1028.

26

Human Neocortical Evolution and Neurological Disorders

Robert SeanHill[1,3] *and Christopher A. Walsh*[1,2,3,4,5]

[1] *Division of Genetics and Genomics, Department of Pediatrics, Manton Center for Orphan Disease Research, Allen Discovery Center for Human Brain Evolution, Boston Children's Hospital, Boston, MA, USA*
[2] *Howard Hughes Medical Institute, Boston Children's Hospital, Boston, MA, USA*
[3] *Department of Pediatrics, Harvard Medical School, Boston, MA, USA*
[4] *Department of Neurology, Harvard Medical School, Boston, MA, USA*
[5] *Broad Institute of MIT and Harvard, Cambridge, MA, USA*

26.1 Introduction

The human neocortex is one of the most complex structures ever to evolve, it endows us with the ability to use complex representational language, join complex societies, pursue science, and create art. It is the product of a genetic program that is unique to our species, and which has appeared in the blink of an eye in evolutionary time. From its origins in mammalian ancestors to the advent of *Homo sapiens*, around 200,000 years ago, the human neocortex has increased in surface area enormously, folding to form gyri and sulci in order to fit the expanded cortex into a limited size skull (Franchini 2021; Kaas 2019). It tripled in size during the *Australopithecus* to *Homo* transition ~ 2 million years ago (MYA) (Montgomery 2018), is six times larger than what would be expected from a typical placental mammal of similar size (Martin 1981), and has acquired many human specific features (Molnar et al. 2019; Mora-Bermudez and Huttner 2022; Rakic 2009). At the heart of neocortical expansion in humans is the regulation of neural stem and progenitor cells, and many of the genes involved in this regulation are thought to be targets of evolution (Pinson and Huttner 2021; Vaid and Huttner 2022; Xing et al. 2021). Because of the widespread interconnectivity of neurons through thousands of synapses, the increase in cortical size came with an exponential relative increase in synaptic interconnectivity (Schmidt and Polleux 2021). In a carefully self-orchestrated spatiotemporal dance that generates the cerebral cortex, roughly 80 billion neurons are created, migrate to the correct location, and connect with each other through ~ 100 trillion synapses to give rise to a structure that is the source of all conscious thought.

This process, though seemingly miraculous, is not a miracle, nor part of a master plan, but is an end result of selective pressure responding to random events to maximize the fitness of a population. The same processes that gave rise to the human neocortex also allowed plants to become master biochemists and Archaea to live in the most extreme environments. Evolution works on traits that are controlled by the genome, and thus genotypes that increase the probability of having viable offspring (fitness) are selected for. In the human lineage, there must have been strong selective pressure to increase the size and complexity of the neocortex, as it comes at a very high price: it accounts for 20–25 percent of the body's resting metabolic rate (Leonard et al. 2007); its long developmental time delays maturation, requiring extended parental care (Powell et al. 2019); and the large head size increases difficulty with childbirth causing increased in infant mortality (Trevathan 2015), likely representing a balancing evolutionary force. Selection for a large complex neocortex is not universal: throughout the mammalian clade there are many examples of selection for smaller brains

Neocortical Neurogenesis in Development and Evolution, First Edition. Edited by Wieland B. Huttner.

as well as for larger brains. Indeed, complex gyrated brains and simple lissencephalic brains intermingle in the mammalian phylogenetic tree (Franchini 2021). In primates, a large reduction in brain size is seen among callitrichids, including marmosets and tamarins (Montgomery and Mundy 2012). Even our close relatives, *Homo floresiensis* and *Homo naledi*, had brains that either did not grow, or shrank (Du et al. 2018; Montgomery 2018) relative to their likely forebears.

One important question is exactly which trait or traits drove selection towards a large neocortex in humans? Most certainly, humans did not evolve a large neocortex just so they could ponder why they have a large neocortex. Our ancestors with larger neocortices must have had a selective advantage that made it more likely that they would have offspring, and that those offspring would survive to generate more descendants. There are three competing theories: the ecological-intelligence hypothesis, which suggest that nonsocial challenges like acquiring food were most important; the social-intelligence hypothesis, which focuses on social challenges like cooperating with or manipulating others or forming alliances to outcompete other groups; and the cultural-intelligence hypothesis that emphasizes learning and teaching accumulated cultural knowledge (Gonzalez-Forero and Gardner 2018). Through a metabolic approach, Gonzalez-Forero and Gardner (2018) suggested that the ecological-intelligence hypothesis carried the most weight, but there is still much to be learned.

Whereas understanding the neurological phenotypes that distinguish humans from our relatives – living and extinct – seems like a problem of limitless complexity, focusing on the genome in relation to evolution makes this problem more tractable. After all, the genome is large, but is finite in size, and has recently been sequenced essentially in its entirety (Gershman et al. 2022; Nurk et al. 2022; Vollger et al. 2022). It is also essentially linear and digital (with four values, A, C, T, G at each location) in its organization, and we understand many basic principles of genetics, genomics, and evolution, which enables mathematical and statistical tools that provide durable data. Even without knowing the exact traits that drove an increase in cortical size and complexity in humans, it is clear that it is quantitative in nature and likely influenced by many hundreds to thousands of genetic factors. Studies into human height have implicated hundreds of genomic regions (Guo et al. 2018), and, more recently, large numbers of loci have been shown to affect many aspects of human brain morphology (Grasby et al. 2020; Tilot et al. 2021).

At its purist, evolution is the change in allele frequencies over time in a population of interbreeding individuals. The main forces of evolution are: natural selection, positive selection of alleles responsible for traits that increase fitness; genetic drift, random genetic changes that do not impact fitness; and purifying selection, negative selection of alleles responsible for traits that decrease fitness. The only source material for evolution to act upon is mutations or changes to the genome, occurring at the chromosomal level (duplications, deletions, transpositions, and inversions), or at the gene level (point mutations, insertions, and deletions). Evolution that brings about large changes or introduces new traits usually functions through one of three mechanisms: addition of new genes through duplication events; modification of the coding or transcribed region of an existing gene to alter its function; or modification of noncoding elements to add or change expression patterns of a gene. We will explore examples of all three of these mechanisms as they relate to neocortical development and evolution later.

There are four basic approaches that are used to identify genes or genetic factors that are important to evolution and development. The first is comparative genomics, aligning the human genome sequences to one or more closely related species and looking for regions that are unique to humans (Heide and Huttner 2021; Vollger et al. 2022; Yousaf et al. 2021; Zimmer-Bensch 2019). Such human-specific features include segmental duplications, duplicated or deleted genes, and human-specific enhancers, methylation sites, and other genomic changes. The second approach is to screen the human genome for particular features or patterns that are suspected a priori of being important (Liu et al. 2021; Mathieson 2020). These might include specific transcription factor binding sites, variations in regulatory sequences, or patters of recent selective sweeps. The third technique is to compare levels of genes or proteins expressed in particular tissues or cell types at specific developmental times between closely related species (Florio et al. 2018). The fourth method is to identify the genetic causes of diseases related to the trait of interest. For the study of the neocortex, this would include neurological disorders resulting in abnormal neocortical morphology or size (brain malformations) or disorders affecting social behaviors (autism), psychiatric disorders (schizophrenia), or intellectual disability (ID). This last method exploits the fact that, with a population size of over 7 billion individuals, the human population represents a "saturation mutation" screen for mutations in every gene, and potentially at every codon and many or most noncoding elements as well (Walsh and Engle 2010). This is to say that if a mutation anywhere in the genome is not fatal, then it is likely carried by multiple people, and if a region of the genome is essential for human brain development, a mutation within that region will result in a neurological phenotype (Walsh and Engle 2010). We continue by describing specific examples of genes involved in the development and evolution of the human neocortex, providing details on how they were identified, what their function is, and evidence that they have been subjected to natural selection.

26.2 *SRGAP2C*

26.2.1 Overview

Gene duplication events, which leave one fully functional copy of a gene intact and a second copy theoretically free of selective constraint, have long been hypothesized to be an important component of genomic evolution (Ohno et al. 1968). Genome wide scans in primates have revealed that humans and great apes are enriched for segmental duplications that arose in several waves over the past 10 million years. Along the human lineage in particular, these regions tend to contain genes involved in neurodevelopment (Bailey and Eichler 2006; Fortna et al. 2004; Heide and Huttner 2021; Pinson and Huttner 2021; Vollger et al. 2022). The Slit-Robo Rho GTPase-activating protein 2 (*SPGAP2*) and its inhibitor, encoded by *SRGAP2C*, arose from a human-specific segmental duplication (HSD) events at an opportune time along the human lineage. In a series of elegant papers over the past decade, Franck Polleux and his collogues have described the function, interaction, and evolution of *SPGAP2* and *SPGAP2C*, and the role they play in the development and working of the human neocortex.

26.2.2 Functional Analysis

SPGAP2 is one of three known Slit-Robo GTPase activating protein (SRGAP) genes. It was first studied because of its suspected role in membrane dynamics during neuronal migration and morphogenesis. Early in situ expression studies in mice found that srGAP2 was expressed in the cortical preplate and ventricular and subventricular zones during early development, in the cortical plate during radial migration, and in layers II–V of the developed brain. srGAP2 protein was found to be expressed throughout cortical development with maximum expression during the peak of neuronal migration in the cortex, and with reduced levels in the adult cortex (Bacon et al. 2009; Guerrier et al. 2009). Knockdown of srGAP2 in mice resulted in an increased rate of cortical pyramidal neuronal migration with significantly reduced branching of the leading process (LP) while over-expression resulted in slower migration and increased LP branching (Guerrier et al. 2009; Guo and Bao 2010). Later studies focused on the phenotype of dendritic spines in knock-down studies. In wild-type mice, the spines mature relatively quickly and tend to be sparse with short stems and small heads. When srGAP2 is knocked down, delayed maturation and increased density of spines with longer necks and larger heads are observed. This morphology resembles the dendritic spines of human cortical pyramidal neurons (Charrier et al. 2012). It is thought that SRGAP2 achieves its functions in neuronal migration, axon guidance and branching, and dendritic spine maturation through binding with the plasma membrane to remodel the actin cytoskeleton. The protein functions as a homodimer, and has an extended F-BAR (F-BARx) domain at its amino terminal, a central RhoGAP domain, and a c-terminal SH3 domain. The RhoGAP has been found to be a RAC1 specific GTPase activating protein (GAP) involved in cytoskeleton remodeling and limiting the density of spines (Sporny et al. 2017). The F-BARx domain, in addition to being involved in dimerization, has been shown to bind HOMER1 in the formation of excitatory synapses at the spine while the SH3 domain binds GEPHYRIN in the formation of inhibitory synapses (Fossati et al. 2016).

26.2.3 Evolution

Roughly 3.4 MYA a human-specific segmental duplication occurred that replicated the ancestral copy of *SRGAP2* (designated *SRGAP2A* to distinguish it from the other copies) located on chromosome 1q32.1 to chromosome 1q21.1. The new copy, *SRGAP2B*, contains the promoter region and first nine exons of *SRGAP2A*, but is missing 49 amino acids of the R-BARx domain, and the RhoGAP and SH3 domains, which have been replaced by a unique seven amino acid c-terminus. Another segmental duplication occurred ~ 2.4 MYA that copied *SRGAP2B* to chromosome 1p12 creating *SRGAP2C*. *SRGAP2C* is identical to *SRGAP2B* except for five nonsynonymous mutations that occurred after the duplication event that changed arginine residues to other amino acids. A final segmental duplication occurred about ~ 1 MYA, which again duplicated *SRGAP2B*, this time to chromosome 1q21.1 creating *SRGAP2D*. Genomic analysis has shown that the duplication events are present in humans and Neanderthal, but absent in chimpanzees (Sudmant et al. 2010). It is also of note that the timing of the segmental duplications occurs at the same time that our ancestors were transitioning from *Australopithecus* to *Homo* (2–3 MYA).

Among the new paralogs, *SRGAP2D* is severely truncated and thought to be a nonfunctioning pseudogene (Dennis et al. 2012). In situ and immunohistochemical analysis show that *SRGAP2A*, *SRGAP2B*, and *SRGAP2C* and their proteins are expressed in the ventricular zone, subventricular zone, and cortical plate of developing human fetal brain, as well as in the adult brain, with high levels in neural progenitor cells and immature and mature neurons. Indeed, *SRGAP2B* and *SRGAP2C* follow the expression pattern of *SRGAP2A* closely. However, *SRGAP2B* has much lower expression levels than *SRGAP2C*, has variable genomic copy number across the human population, and is hemizygously deleted in some neurotypical individuals, suggesting that it is not an essential gene (Charrier et al. 2012; Dennis et al. 2012). *SRGAP2C* on the other hand, shows strong expression and has a fixed genomic copy number. In mice, expression of SRGAP2C results in slower migration and reduced LP branching of cortical pyramidal neurons during radial expansion, and dendritic spines that are slow to mature, present in higher density, and that have long necks and large heads. This phenotype is very similar to the phenotype observed in SRGAP2 knockdown mice, and in both cases, the resulting cortical pyramidal neurons more closely resemble those normally seen in humans rather than mice. In cell lines SRGAP2A's ability to induce filopodia was abolished when it was co-expressed with SRGAP2C. These studies suggest that

SRGAP2C inhibits *SRGAP2A*. It has now been shown that SRGAP2C and SRGAP2B form a heterodimer with SRGAP2A via their truncated F-BARx domain that leads to proteasome-mediated decay (Schmidt et al. 2019). The five nonsynonymous mutations acquired by SRGAP2C after its separation from SRGAP2B are thought to increase its binding strength to SRGAP2A (Sporny et al. 2017) and perhaps contribute to its ability to suppress SRGAP2A in other ways, as SRGAP2C is more effective at inhibiting synaptic maturation and maintaining increased spine density throughout adulthood than SRGAP2B (Schmidt et al. 2019).

In an intriguing study designed to determine the extent to which SRGAP2C can humanize the mouse brain, Schmidt et al. (2021) generated transgenic mice that express SRGAP2C in all cortical glutamatergic neurons. The mice showed an increase in the number of local and long-range synapses received by layer 2/3 pyramidal neurons and a higher reliability of sensory-evoked responses by layer 2/3 pyramidal neurons. The transgenic mice also outperformed wild-type mice in a cortex-dependent texture-discrimination task. It is unclear if the improved learning was a result of increased cortico-cortical connectivity, increased local connectivity, higher reliability of sensory coding, or other factors. However, it shows that neurological changes evoked by SRGAP2C can increase the ability to solve complex cognitive task. Thus, in *SRPGA2C*, we have a gene that was created at the birth of the *Homo* genius that has been shown to improve a cognitive task when expressed in mice. While absolute proof will be difficult to obtain, it is fascinating to consider the possibility of a single gene having such a large impact on modifying the structure and function of the brain into a more human form, providing a valuable window into the inner workings of brain evolution.

26.2.4 Other Segmental Duplications

Several other human-specific genes that arose from segmental duplication in the human lineage, and are implicated in neurodevelopment, have been well studied (Heide and Huttner 2021; Pinson and Huttner 2021; Vollger et al. 2022). NOTCH2 is a cell surface receptor that is part of the conserved Notch signaling pathway, and is a critical factor in many developmental processes. In neocortical development, it controls the timing and duration of proliferation and differentiation of neural progenitor cells (NPC) (Nian and Hou 2022). Segmental duplications of the *NOTCH2* region on chromosome 1p12 prior to the human, chimpanzee, gorilla split generated truncated, likely nonfunctioning, copies of *NOTCH2* in all three species. Subsequent repair and further duplication and complex rearrangements of the copied gene in the human lineage, 4-3MYA, has resulted in four truncated copies, the pseudogene *NOTCH2NLR*, and the functional *NOTCH2NLA*, *NOTCH2NLB*, and *NOTCH2NLC* (Suzuki et al. 2018; Vollger et al. 2022). The four paralogs all have the promoter and first four exons from *NOTCH2*, which includes six N-terminal epidermal growth factor (EGF)-like domains, but have a unique fifth exon, and lack the c-terminal transmembrane and cytoplasmic domains (Fiddes et al. 2018; Suzuki et al. 2018). Copy number variation in *NOTCH2NLC* and *NOTCH2NLR* have been observed in neurotypical individuals, but deletions or duplications of the genomic region containing *NOTCH2NLA* and *NOTCH2NLB* (1q21.1 distal deletion/duplication syndrome) are associated with microcephaly and macrocephaly, respectively (Suzuki et al. 2018). Curiously, studies suggest that Neanderthal and Denisovans had two copies of *NOTCH2NLA* and *NOTCH2NLB* (Lodewijk et al. 2020). The NOTCH2NL genes are expressed in apical and basal progenitor cells during cortical development. Over-expression of *NOTCH2NLA* in embryonic mice results in an increased cycling of basal progenitors in the subventricular zone (Florio et al. 2018) while over-expression of *NOTCH2NLB* results in extended proliferation of apical progenitors in the ventricular zone (Suzuki et al. 2018) of mice. Ectopic expression of

NOTCH2NL genes in mouse cortical organoids appears to delay neuronal differentiation while deletion of the genes from human cortical organoids resulted in smaller organoids due to accelerated neuronal differentiation (Fiddes et al. 2018). The NOTCH2NL proteins are believed to function by interacting with NOTCH2 and interfering with the activity of notch ligand Delta-like 1 (DLL1) (Suzuki et al. 2018), a cis-inhibitor of NOTCH2 (Nian and Hou 2022), leading to NPC expansion (Heide and Huttner 2021).

TBC1D3 is hominid specific gene that has also undergone human-specific expansion. Over-expression of TBC1D3 in mice causes delamination of ventricular radial glia cells (vRG) and self-renewing of basal progenitors that show the morphology of outer radial glia (oRG). Further, in areas of localized oRG proliferation, cortical folding is observed in the mouse cortex (Ju et al. 2016). Downregulation of TBC1D3 in cultured human fetal brain slices results in a reduction of oRGs (Ju et al. 2016), while upregulation of TBC1D3 in human cortical organoids produced organoids that were larger than controls (Hou et al. 2021). While TBC1D3 has been shown to be involved in signaling and trafficking of epidermal growth factor receptors (Wainszelbaum et al. 2008) newer work suggest that its involvement in production of cortical neuro progenitor cells stems from its suppression of G9a (euchromatic histone-lysine *N*-methyltransferase 2), which controls dimethylation of histone 3 in lysine 9 (H3K9me2) (Hou et al. 2021). Experimental blocking of G9a activity in human cortical organoids results in an increase in neuro progenitor proliferation, similar to the over-expression of TBC1D3, while preventing TBC1D3/G9a interaction causes reduced neuro progenitor proliferation (Hou et al. 2021). The recent complete sequencing of the human genome has added new insight into the *TBC1D3* duplications (Vollger et al. 2022). It has revealed two large expansions of the genomic region where *TBC1D3* is located, which occurred along the human lineage after 2–2.62 MYA. The region remains highly variable in humans, with 3 to 14 copies of *TBC1D3* in the first expansion site and two to nine copies in the second (Vollger et al. 2022). It is unclear how this variation in copy number impacts the genes' function.

Additional well-established human specific genes resulting from segmental duplications are known to have crucial rolls in neocortical development, such as *ARHGAP11B* (Heide and Huttner 2021; Pinson and Huttner 2021), which is covered elsewhere in this book. Further, as the gaps in the human genome sequence have been filled in (segmental duplications are notoriously difficult to sequence and assemble), the list of candidate genes continues to grow (Florio et al. 2018; Vollger et al. 2022).

26.3 *ASPM*

26.3.1 Overview

Abnormal spindle-like microcephaly-associated (*ASPM*) is a prime example of a single gene that has a strong influence on neocortical size and which has been implicated in selective evolution. Mutations in *ASPM* in humans result in severe microcephaly, but notably, most of the reduction in brain volume is a result of reduced cortical surface area, with no significant change in cortical thickness (Desir et al. 2008; Passemard et al. 2016). Other brain regions are impacted, but to a lesser extent, and overall brain morphology is preserved as is overall body size in most cases. Animal and molecular studies, described later, suggest that ASPM functions by regulating the transition of ventricular radial glia cells from symmetric to asymmetric divisions, thus controlling the overall number of neurons produced during cortical neurogenesis. Evolutionary changes influencing the timing of this shift could potentially select for a larger neocortex (Johnson et al. 2018).

26.3.2 Primary Microcephaly

Primary microcephaly is a congenital neurological disorder that results in a head circumference greater than 2 (microcephaly) or 3 (severe microcephaly) standard deviations below the mean accounting for age, sex, and ethnicity (Zaqout and Kaindl 2022). Although MCPH can be caused by in utero infections, exposure to toxins, as well as inherited disorders (Jayaraman et al. 2018), autosomal recessive microcephaly (microcephaly primary hereditary (MCPH)) is characterized by greatly reduced brain volume with a simplified neocortical gyration pattern, but little change in cortical organization. The neocortex is disproportionately reduced in size compared with other brain regions (Zaqout and Kaindl 2022). The brain will typically continue to grow with age, but will always be smaller than normal. Most individuals with MCPH have mild to moderate ID and will be delayed in reaching major speech milestones. Seizures have also been reported but are unusual (Shen et al. 2005). Birth rates for MCPH are 1:250,000, but can increase to 1:10,000 in consanguineous populations.

According to OMIM (Online Mendelian Inheritance in Man; Microcephaly, primary – PS251200, May 2022), there are 28 genes associated with MCPH, with the loci sequentially labeled MCPH1 – MCPH28. The majority of these genes encode centrosomal proteins, but genes involved in microtubule dynamics, mitotic spindle formation, DNA damage responses, Wnt signaling, transcriptional regulation, and cell cycle checkpoint control are also represented. These functions are vital to neuronal progenitor proliferation, differentiation, and survival and are key factors needed to achieve a large brain size during neocortical neurogenesis (Jayaraman et al. 2018; Zaqout and Kaindl 2022).

ASPM was identified as the gene associated with the MCPH5 locus through the use of linkage mapping and Sanger sequencing in 51 individuals with MCPH from 23 consanguineous families (Bond et al. 2002, 2003; Pattison et al. 2000). While virtually all mutations appear to cause complete loss of function, there is no correlation between the position of truncating mutations and severity of the condition (Bond et al. 2003). Mutations in *ASPM* are currently the major cause of MCPH with 217 distinct mutations associated with primary microcephaly reported (HGMD v2022.1).

26.3.3 Functional Analysis

ASPM encodes the human ortholog of the *Drosophila melanogaster* asp (abnormal spindle) gene. Full-length *ASPM* consist of 28 exons and encodes a 3477 amino-acid protein. Three additional isoforms might also be expressed, varying in the number of IQ domains. The gene is ubiquitously expressed during embryonic development with a much lower expression in adult tissue. It has also been found to be upregulated in malignant cells (Kouprina et al. 2005).

The ASPM protein contains an N-terminal ASPM-SPD-2-Hydin (ASH) domain, two calponin homology (CH) domains, a series of calmodulin-binding IQ repeats, and an armadillo-like domain. The ASH domain is typically found in proteins associated with cilia, flagella, the centrosome, and the Golgi complex. The CH domains is involved in actin binding. The armadillo-like domain is believed to be involved in Wnt signaling. In humans, ASMP has 81 IQ domains, however this number is highly variable between species, and might be an important factor in determining the size of the neocortex (see Section 26.3.4) (Letard et al. 2018).

ASPM is essential for proper proliferation of neuronal progenitor cells, and an important factor in cell cycling and conversion from symmetric to asymmetric neurogenic divisions. In *Drosophila melanogaster*, flics with homozygous mutations in asp show late larval-pupal lethality due to metaphase arrest in larval neuroblasts (do Carmo Avides and Glover 1999). Studies have shown that the

Asp protein in flies is localized to the polar regions of the spindle, surrounding the centrosome, during prometaphase, metaphase, and anaphase of mitosis, but moves to the central region of the spindle microtubules during telophase (Saunders et al. 1997). Immunostaining in human HT1080 cultured cells during mitosis showed very similar results with ASPM localized to the spindle pole during prometaphase through anaphase (Kouprina et al. 2005). GFP-tagging studies have determined that the N-terminus of ASPM is required for localization to the centrosomes and spindle poles and the C-terminus is required for localization to midbodies (Paramasivam et al. 2007). Small interfering RNA (siRNA) experiments have shown that ASPM is associated with the mother centriole during S-phase, and is involved in centriole duplication (Jayaraman et al. 2016).

Fish et al. (2006) performed immunostaining on neuroepithelial cells (NE) from embryonic day (E) 12.5 mouse telencephalon to determine the subcellular localization of ASPM. Similar to flies and humans, they determined that ASPM was associated with the spindle poles during all phases of mitosis, dropping off during telophase, and showed no association with centrosomes during interphase. They used in situ hybridization to study the expression and localization of *Aspm* mRNA in the ventricular zone of the murine embryonic forebrain. They found that *Aspm* expression was highest in NE cells undergoing proliferative division, but was low in earlier developmental stages, and was gradually reduced as the cells switched to neurogenic divisions (Fish et al. 2006). These observations suggest that ASPM might be an important factor in switching from proliferative to neurogenic divisions. During neurogenesis, NE cells (the precursors of radial glial cells) undergo symmetric proliferative divisions to increase their numbers along the ventricular surface of the neuroepithelium. At a given point, the NE cells switch to asymmetric neurogenic divisions and start producing neuronal precursor cells. The longer NE cells undergo proliferative divisions before shifting to neurogenic divisions, the more neurons that will ultimately be produced, and the larger the cerebral cortex will be.

To test the role of ASPM in NE proliferation, RNA interference (RNAi) was used to knock down *Aspm* expression in the telencephalon of E10.5 – E12.2 mice. The resulting NE cells had reduced *Aspm* mRNA levels and no ASPM associated with the spindle pole. They observed a significant increase in NC cells with abnormal cleavage plane orientation and an increase in the proportion of NE cell progeny found in the neuronal layer. These results suggest that Aspm prolongs NE cell proliferative divisions (Fish et al. 2006).

At least six *Aspm* knockout mouse lines have been reported (Capecchi and Pozner 2015; Fujimori et al. 2014; Jayaraman et al, 2016; Pulvers et al. 2010; Williams et al. 2015), but their phenotypes poorly recapitulate the human phenotype. The mice show only mild microcephaly with an approximately 10 percent reduction in brain size. Further, some of the knockout mice show reduction in body weight and cortical thinning not observed in humans. At the cellular level, the mice show restricted alterations in NP cell identity and organization. While there is evidence of a reduction in the ventricular radial glial cells resulting in an increase in intermediate progenitors, no ectopic progenitor cells are observed.

It should perhaps be no surprise that the phenotype of the *Aspm* mutant mice did not precisely mirror that of the human phenotype. The mouse cortex is lissencephalic and 1,000 times smaller than the human cortex. Further, as discussed later, there are significant difference in the sequences of the human and mouse gene. To address these issues, Li et al. (2017) generated cortical organoids from three induced pluripotent stem cells lines (iPSCs) carrying different *ASPM* mutations derived from individual cases. These organoids showed reduced size, loss of lumen structure, and reduced progenitor cells compared to controls.

To study the function of ASPM in an animal model with a larger, gyrated cortex, Johnson et al. (2018) generated an *Aspm* knockout ferret. Ferrets have a gyrified cortex that is larger than mice with a greater neural progenitor cell diversity (Reillo et al. 2011; Shinmyo et al. 2022), and despite being a more distant relative to humans, they have closer ASPM protein sequence homology than do mice. The Aspm knockout ferrets were generated using genome editing constructs targeting exon 15, which results in severe microcephaly when mutated in humans. Three stable *Aspm* germline knockout ferret lines were created that were confirmed to lack ASPM. Similar phenotypes were observed in all three lines. The knockout ferrets showed microcephaly with up to a 40 percent reduction in brain weight with no reduction in body weight. The loss of volume was greatest in the frontal cortex while cortical thickness and cytoarchitecture and lamination of neurons was preserved. All phenotypes that were observed in humans with *ASPM* mutations (Johnson et al. 2018).

During normal ferret cortical neurogenesis, undifferentiated ventricular radial glial cells (VRG) can divide symmetrically to generate more VRGs, or can divide asymmetrically to generate intermediate progenitors and outer radial glia (ORG). Intermediate progenitors are neuronally fated cells that tend to migrate to the inner subventricular zone (ISVZ) while ORGs are multipotent progenitors mostly found in the outer subventricular zone (OSVZ). Close analysis of the knockout ferrets during cortical neurogenesis through immunostaining, in situ hybridization, and single-cell RNA-sequencing revealed that the loss of ASPM resulted in premature detachment of VRG cells from the ventricular zone. These displaced VRG cells migrated to the OSVZ where they exhibit ORG morphology, molecular profiles, and neurogenic potential. These results show a clear role for ASPM in the regulation of transitioning from symmetric to asymmetric VRG division, and thus the ratio of VRGs to ORGs during development which is an important factor in determining the size of the cerebral cortex (Johnson et al. 2018).

26.3.4 Evolution

Since the discovery that mutations in *ASPM* cause microcephaly, its structure has suggested an evolutionary role associated with brain size (Bond et al, 2002; Bond et al. 2003). Overall, the ASPM protein is conserved between a wide range of species, including humas, mice, flies, and worms with the exception of the number of IQ domains. It has been noted that the number of IQ domains tends to correlate with brain complexity (Bond et al. 2002). However, most mammals show similar numbers of IQ repeats, with rodents representing outliers with a smaller number of IQ repeats.

A number of groups have run computational analysis of *ASPM* sequence data to look for signs of selective evolution in humans. Most of the analysis performed rely on some variation of the d_N/d_S ration (also known as the K_a/K_s ration or ω). This is the ratio of the number nonsynonymous substitutions per nonsynonymous sites (d_N) to the number of synonymous substitutions per synonymous sites (d_S) in a given sequence. Low d_N/d_S ratios indicate a lack of nonsynonymous variations, suggesting purifying selection; higher d_N/d_S values suggest that nonsynonymous variants are favored, indicating positive selection. At least one study also implemented the McDonald–Kreitman test, a statistical test designed to determine if selective evolution has occurred in a gene within a species, and the strength of that selection. This test compares the number of nonsynonymous (P_n) to synonymous (P_s) polymorphism within a species to the number of nonsynonymous (D_n) to synonymous (D_s) substitutions fixed between two species ($D_n/D_s \leq \geq P_n/P_s$). A D_n/D_s ratio significantly lower than the P_n/P_s ratio indicates negative selection, while a D_n/D_s ratio significantly higher than the P_n/P_s ratio indicates positive selection. One caveat of the McDonald–Kreitman test is that it requires having enough sequencing data from individuals of the same species to calculate within species variation.

The first analysis was run using full-length coding sequence from just one human, one chimpanzee, and one orangutang and showed a clear signal of positive selection along both the human and chimpanzee lineages, with a stronger signal in the human lineage (Zhang 2003). As data from additional species gradually because available, the analysis was repeated. Analysis that added gorilla and rhesus macaque (Kouprina et al. 2004) as well as gibbon, macaque, and owl monkey (Evans et al. 2004) showed similar results, strong positive selection on *ASPM* with increased rates of evolution along the human lineage. One study found evidence of accelerated evolution in the African hominoid clade, which precedes hominid brain expansion by several million years. They also noted that the human and gorilla lineages showed accelerated evolution in the IQ domain, and that the strongest selection in *ASPM* among primates correlated with the most divergent gene regions between primates and non-primate mammals (Kouprina et al. 2004).

A more recent analysis that included 21 species of anthropoid primates found robust evidence for selection across primates but no increase in intensity along the human lineage (Montgomery et al. 2011). They also directly tested for selection in *ASPM* with regard to neonatal and adult brain mass and found a positive relation between *ASPM* and neonatal brain mass and somewhat weaker relationships between *ASPM* and adult brain size (Montgomery et al, 2011).

An analysis of *ASPM* among 12 species of callitrichids (a family of New World monkeys that including marmosets and tamarins) found that *ASPM* evolution is significantly negatively correlated with callitrichid brain size. This is interesting as the callitrichids are a branch of primates where a large reduction in brain mass is observed (Montgomery and Mundy 2012). It would thus appear that *ASPM* is associated with both increase and decrease in brain size. ASPM has also been found be under positive selection outside of primates. Montgomery and Mundy (2014) found evidence of *ASPM* selection across all mammals, and positive selection of *ASPM* for neonatal brain mass in Glires and Euungulata. A separate study also found strong evidence of *ASPM* selection in cetaceans (Xu et al. 2012, 2017).

Taken together, these studies provide strong evidence that *ASPM* is an important gene in the evolution of large brain size in humans. This correlates well with the role of ASPM in regulating the transition of symmetric to nonsymmetric divisions during cerebral cortical neurogenesis. However, the degree to which *ASPM* evolution alone has impacted neocortical brain size in humans is unclear. There is good evidence that other genes associated with microcephaly are also under positive selection, such as *CDK5RAP2* and some of the humans-specific genes discussed earlier (Heide and Huttner 2021; Montgomery et al. 2011). So, it is likely that *ASPM* coevolved in concert with numerous other genes, to generate the large complex neocortex present in modern humans. However, while it is tempting to suggest that genes that can cause microcephaly in humans when mutated are likely to be under positive evolutionary selection along the human lineage, evidence suggests this is not the case for most of the known MCPH genes, though they might have been under selection at some point (Montgomery and Mundy 2012, 2014; Pervaiz et al. 2021).

26.4 *GPR56*

26.4.1 Overview

G-protein-coupled receptor 56 (*GPR56/ADGRG1*) is an adhesion G-protein coupled receptor (aGPCR) that causes bilateral frontoparietal polymicrogyria (PMG) when mutated in humans. The protein itself is a membrane receptor that has been shown to play a role in a number of diverse systems. As described later, in the brain it influences neuro progenitor migration and proliferation, synaptic pruning, and neuronal myelination. *GPR56* is thus an important component of neocortical development, especially with regards to gyral patterning. Its evolutionary importance derives not from changes to its coding sequence like *ASPM*, but rather to the formation of new cis-acting regulatory elements and noncoding exons.

26.4.2 Bilateral Frontoparietal Polymicrogyria

PMG is a congenital neurological disorder that disrupts the normal gyrification pattern of the cerebral cortex resulting in many small gyri. It can occur in one (unilateral) or both (bilateral) hemispheres, and can be generalized or limited to a particular region of the brain. Its severity depends on how much of the brain is affected. Bilateral frontoparietal PMG (BFPP) is a recessively inherited form of bilateral PMG that primarily impacts the frontal and parietal lobes. White matter defects and brainstem and cerebellar hypoplasia is also usually seen on brain MRI of affected individuals. Other symptoms include severe to moderate ID, global motor delays, seizures, cerebellar signs, and dysconjugate gaze (Jin et al. 2009). Linkage mapping and Sanger sequencing in consanguineous and non-consanguineous families with children showing symptoms of BFPP was used to identify *GPR56* as the first gene discovered to cause PMG when mutated (Chang et al. 2003; Piao et al. 2002, 2004).

26.4.3 Functional Analysis

Adhesion G protein-coupled receptors (aGPCRs) are a member of a diverse group of GPCRs (G protein-coupled receptors) that includes over 800 genes in humans and are involved in a wide range of biological functions. Ligands have yet to be discovered for most of these receptors (Ganesh et al. 2020). However, known binding partners are quite diverse and include photons, ions, lipids, neurotransmitters, peptides, hormones, and proteins (Singh and Lin 2021). Structurally, all GPCRs consist of a characteristic seven transmembrane (7TM) domain and are bound to heterotrimeric G proteins consisting of three subunits (Gα, Gβ, and Gγ) that are held inactive by a guanosine diphosphate (GDP) bound to Gα, when the receptor is activated, the G proteins are disassociated from the GPCR, the Gα is activated by conversion of the GDP to GTP, and the Gβ, and Gγ subunits form a dimer. These released subunits then trigger downstream signaling or metabolic pathways. aGPCRs are noted for their large extracellular region (ECR) that contain a GPCR autoproteolysis inducing (GAIN) domain. This domain autocatalytically cleaves the receptor into two subunits that remain associated with each other, but are no longer covalently bound. The N-terminal fragment (NTF) makes up the majority of the ECR while the C-terminal fragment (CTF) consist of the transmembrane region. They are referred to as adhesion GPCRs because their NTF often contains domains associated with adhesion proteins, such as cadherin, lectin, immunoglobulin, and thrombospondin domains.

In humans, GPR56 has been shown to be expressed in brain, heart, thyroid, kidney, testis, pancreas, and skeletal muscle through Northern blot analysis (Liu et al. 1999). GPR56 plays an important role in brain development and malignancy, but has also been shown to be involved in the peripheral nervous systems, hematopoietic stem cell generation, reproductive system, muscle hypertrophy, and immune regulation (Ganesh et al. 2020). It expresses at least four different isoforms, and has 17 alternative translation start sites in the first exon (see Section 26.4.4) (Bae et al. 2014). In addition to the GAIN domain, GPR56 also has a unique 133-amino acid long laminin/neurexin/sex-hormone-binding (PLL) domain on the ECR, this domain is absent in one of the commonly expressed isoforms (Salzman et al. 2016). The ECR can also undergo N-glycosylation at seven sites, which is thought to influence protein trafficking, cell surface expression, and ligand-binding affinity (Singh and Lin 2021). A number of GPR56 ligands have been identified, and the mechanism by which the receptor responds is ligand and cell/tissue-type specific (Singh and Lin 2021), here we will only focus on those impacting neocortical development (Jeong et al. 2012). Loss of the Gpr56 gene results in neurons migrating outside of the brain, giving a cobblestone lissencephaly like phenotype. Detailed observation of the process leading to this phenotype suggest it involves breaching of the pial basement membrane causing disrupted anchorage of the radial glial endfeet, mislocalization of Cajal–Retzius cells, and neuronal over-migration (Li et al. 2008). Later studies also showed disruption of cortical organization and reduced thickness due to defective progenitor proliferation (Bae et al. 2014).

In humans, GPR56 is expressed in Tuj1b migrating neurons (including Cajal–Retzius cells), radial glial cells, as well as some interneurons in the marginal zone. The receptor is activated by collagen-type III alpha-1 (*COL3A1*), which binds to a region in the PLL domain on the ECR. COL3A1 is expressed by meningeal fibroblasts at the pia surface, and phenotypes caused by null mutation in *CDOL3A1* are similar to phenotype resulting from *GPR56* mutations (Luo et al. 2011). Upon binding to collagen, the N-terminal region ($GPR56_{N}$) separates from the C-terminal region ($GPR56_{C}$) exposing a tethered agonist that activates $GPR56_{C}$. The activated $GPR56_{C}$ couples to $G\alpha 12/13$ family of G proteins within a lipid island and activates the RhoA pathway (Iguchi et al. 2008; Luo et al. 2014). Many of the BFPP causing mutations in *GPR56* can be linked directly to the functional domains of the genes, with known mutations that prevent the protein from leaving the endoplasmic reticulum (ER) or Golgi, abolish the proteolytic cleave site, block collagen binding, or prevent RhoA activation (Jin et al. 2007). Integrin-a3 (Itga3), which binds to laminin-511 and co-localizes in radial glial cells and rostral preplate neurons, has also been implicated in the pathway, and shows an increased effect on over-migration when co-mutated with *GPR56* (Jeong et al. 2013). In the current functional model, GPR56, which is highly expressed in the basal process of neural progenitors, activates the RhoA pathway upon binding to extracellular proteins at the pial basement membrane, which not only terminates migration, but also promotes proliferation of apical and basal radial glia cells (Luo et al. 2014; Singer et al. 2013). *GPR56*, as well as other genes that disrupt the basal process of radial glia cells have been shown to reduce progenitor proliferation (Bae et al, 2014; Bizzotto and Francis 2015; Ossola and Kalebic 2021).

Mutations in *GPR56* can also result in reduction of myelination and myelin repair of axons in the central nervous system. This has been linked to reduced proliferation of oligodendrocyte precursor cells (OPC), and thus a reduction of myelin producing oligodendrocytes (Ackerman et al. 2015; Chiou et al. 2021). In OPCs, microglia-derived transglutaminase-2 (TG2) in the presence of extracellular matrix (ECM) laminin-111 activate GPR56 by binding to and disassociating $GPR56_{N}$ from $GPR56_{C}$ exposing the tethered agonist and initiating G-protein signaling. This activates the RhoA pathway that promotes OPC proliferation (Giera et al. 2018).

GPR56 has also recently been shown to play a role in synaptic pruning by microglia. In this case, an alternatively spliced isoform of GPR56 that lacks the PLL domain is expressed on the cell surface of yolk sac-derived microglia. When it is bound by externalized phosphatidylserine (PS) (which in this context is thought to flag synapses for removal), GPR56 signals to microglia to engulf the synapse. It is unclear if GPR56 functions alone or in concert with other receptors in its role of synaptic refinement (Li et al. 2020).

26.4.4 Evolution

While *GPR56* clearly plays a crucial role in brain development, its widespread involvement in multiple systems, both inside and outside the brain, suggest it would be a poor target for selective neocortical evolution, as coding changes that improved one process might disrupt another. However, Bae et al. (2014) identified a cohort of individuals with polymicrogyria that was limited to a very restricted region surrounding the Sylvian fissure. These individuals had ID, language difficulty, and seizures, but no motor disability. Brain MRI showed that Broca's area (motor speech area) in the left hemisphere, and the corresponding region in the right hemisphere, were most severely affected. The phenotype was surprisingly linked to the *GPR56* locus. Exon sequencing revealed no coding mutations, but a homozygous deletion of one copy of a 15 bp repeat was discovered in all affected individuals in the 5′-upstream regulatory region of *GPR56*. The deletion was located less than 150 bp upstream of the noncoding exon 1m (e1m) (Bae et al. 2014). *GPR56* has at least 17 alternative transcription start sites, each with its own noncoding first exon and expression profile, but all encoding for the same protein.

To determine if the 15 bp deletion disrupts GPR56 expression, Bae et al. (2014) generated transgenic mice with a construct containing 16 of the human transcription start sites driving expression of green fluorescent protein (GFP), and a second construct carrying the 15 bp deletion. The full construct showed GFP expression over the entire central nervous system, while the mutant construct showed GFP expression in the medial cortex, but not in the lateral cortex, or lateral ganglionic eminence, thus confirming that the deletion is causative of the perisylvian malformation. They further confirmed the role of GPR56 in neuro progenitors through analysis of *Gpr56* knockout mice, which showed fewer progenitors in the developing neocortex than wild-type mice, and mice that over-express human *GPR56*, which showed an increase in progenitors in the developing neocortex (Bae et al, 2014).

The *GPR56* coding sequence first arose when vertebrates and invertebrates diverged. The upstream noncoding exons and promotor regions have evolved at various points along the human lineage. Interestingly, sequence analysis reveals the remnants of transposable element insertions, that appear to be responsible for the presence of most of the upstream elements, including e1m (LINE) and the noncoding exon 2 (Alu). When placental and nonplacental mammals separated, 85 to 100 MYA, the number of noncoding elements dramatically increased. For instance, the regulatory element upstream of e1m, associated with the perisylvian phenotype, is found in all placental mammals, but is absent in monotremes, marsupials, and non-mammals. GPR56 continued to acquire new noncoding elements, alternative promoters, and untranslated exons in the primate lineage, including the noncoding exon 2 which is found only in primates. Indeed, humans and mice only share three transcriptional start sites, indicating that 14 have emerged along the human lineage, and 2 along the mouse lineage, since their last common ancestor (Bae et al. 2015, 2014).

To test GPR56 expression patterns associated with isolated promotor sequences, transgenic mice, which used a minimal 300pb e1m promotor sequence from human, mouse, marmoset, dolphin, and cat to drive b-galactosidase (b-gal) gene, were generated. While the mouse sequence showed broad expression in the nervous system, the human, marmoset, dolphin, and cat sequence all showed a similar, more restricted expression pattern (Bae et al. 2014). These results suggest that the formation of gyrencephalic brains with a Sylvian fissure (like humans, marmosets, dolphins, and cats), requires fine control over the expression of GPR56, which is afforded by multiple regulatory elements subjected to independent evolution.

This data shows that *GPR56* was important to the evolutionary expansion of the perisylvian neocortex. It further suggests a mechanism to control neuro proliferation, and perhaps synaptic pruning, in restricted regions of the neocortex that would allow for independent evolution, and possibly specialization of these regions.

26.5 Human Accelerated Regions

26.5.1 Overview

Human accelerated regions (HARs) are regions of the genome that are highly conserved in almost all mammals except humans, where they show accelerated rates of substitutions. Thousands of HARs have been identified, and they are interesting not because they are linked to strong signals of selection, but because they are highly diverse elements that might be associated with subtler levels of selection that might account for the lion's share of evolutionary change responsible for the development of the human neocortex. Other methods for detecting evidence of positive selection from genomic sequence data either rely on being able to compare the ratio of synonymous to non-synonymous changes, and are thus restricted to coding regions, or search for evidence of selective sweeps, which require the event to have occurred relatively recently. HARs are free from both of these constraints and can be detected in coding or noncoding regions, and long after the signal of a selective sweep has decayed. Researchers have been able to identify HARs that are likely essential for human cognition and social behavior, and a few that are directly associated with genes involved in neocortical evolution.

26.5.2 Definition and Discovery

The discovery of HARs was made possible by the availability of high-quality complete genomic sequences of sufficient numbers mammals for detailed comparisons. The first genome-wide screen for HARs was conducted by initially identifying orthologous regions of the chimpanzee, mouse, and rat genomes that had at least 96 percent identity over 100 bp, which yielded ~ 35,000 regions with a median length of 140 bp. The remainder of the available amniote genomes were then added to the analysis, and regions that maintained high identity in nonhuman species but showed elevated substitution rates in humans were designated HARs. Forty-nine statistically significant regions were identified and ranked. These initial HARs were overwhelmingly noncoding and tended to neighbor genes with Gene Ontology terms indicating involvement in DNA binding and transcriptional regulation. Interestingly, 24 percent of the HARs flanked genes involved in neurodevelopment. Indeed, HAR1F, the gene associated with HAR1, was shown to be co-expressed in Cajal–Retzius cells with reelin (Pollard et al. 2006a). Since this initial study, a number of groups have developed a variety of algorithms and applied them to different datasets to collectively identify over 3,000 HARs (Bird et al. 2007; Bush and Lahn 2008; Gittelman et al. 2015; Hubisz and Pollard 2014; Lindblad-Toh et al. 2011; Pollard et al. 2006b; Prabhakar et al. 2008). The expanded set of HARs however has not changed the basic findings of the initial study, that HARs are mostly noncoding (though tend to be within 1Mb of a gene) and are enriched for transcription factor binding motifs (Capra et al. 2013; Doan et al. 2016). This strongly suggests a role for some HARs as regulatory elements controlling the expression of genes whose function has been modified, through evolutionary selection, along the human lineage. Of particular interest to this review, several studies have indicated a role for HARs in human brain evolution (Boyd et al. 2015; Capra et al, 2013; Doan et al, 2016; Franchini and Pollard 2017; Girskis et al. 2021; Kamm et al. 2013a; Uebbing et al. 2021).

Purely computational analysis of HARs suffer from two major issues. First, the genomic features that define HARs, recent substitutions in humans in an otherwise conserved region are presumed to have arisen due to positive selection, however, they could also be the result of genetic drift on a region that is no longer under selective constraint or be due to GC-biased gene conversion events.

Second, it is often assumed that HARs that are part of a regulatory element, regulate the gene nearest to them. While this might often be a good bet, the functioning genome is three dimensional, and linear proximity does not guarantee interaction between control elements. Several functional studies have addressed these issues.

To definitively determine which genes HARs were associated with Doan et al. (2016) mapped 576 HARs to the promotors of more than 700 target genes using existing ChIA-PET and HiC data, and their own 4C-sequencing data. These are all high-throughput methods for determining which regions of the chromatin are in physical contact with each other. They found that 42 percent of HARs interacted with flanking genes.

To analyze the impact of HARs directly on gene expression, and thus determine if the HAR sequence is the result of drift, biased gene conversion, or evolution, Capra et al. (2013) analyzed 2649 non-coding HARs. Based on a computational analysis that accounted for sequence, evolutionary history, histone modifications, chromatin state, and transcription factor binding, they determined that 30 percent of the HARs were developmental enhancers. They tested 29 of the top-candidate HARs and their chimpanzee orthologs using a reporter assay in transgenic mice. Twenty-four showed human and chimpanzee enhancer activity, and five showed different expression between human and chimpanzees, indicating that at least some HARs are the result of selective evolution (Capra et al. 2013).

Higher throughput approaches rely on the massively parallel reporter assay (MPRA). In this method, a cell line is transfected with a library of plasmids that consists of the test enhancer sequence (HARs in this cases), a minimal promoter and reporter gene to be expressed, a barcode sequence to label the expressed mRNA, and next generation sequencing adapters. The transfected cells are allowed to transcribe the reporter gene and barcode sequence. Enhancer activity is then determined by using next generation sequencing techniques to measure the abundance of each mRNA (which is linked to the enhancer by the barcode) and the number of copies of each plasmid. Thus, enhancer activity is calculated as the ratio of the level of mRNA and count of plasmids for each enhancer. The power of this assay is that thousands of enhancers can be assayed simultaneously. One limitation is that the level of enhancer activity is only tested for the type of cell used. Two studies, using different MPRA assays, recently described the enhancer activity of HARs and their chimpanzee orthologs in neural cells. Girskis et al. (2021), reporting results from two different neural cell lines that gave similar outcomes, found that 49 percent of HARs showed enhancer activity in neurons, and of those 39 percent showed similar level of activity, 19 percent showed recued activity, and 42 percent showed increased activity when compared to the enhancer level of their chimpanzee orthologs. Uebbing et al. (2021) reported much lower levels of neuronal enhancer activity in HARs, though the difference could be a result of the Ubbing et al. study using a more restrictive MPRA assay that was unable to capture the full length of most HAR sequences. Girskis et al. (2021) compared the HARs to data from the Roadmap Epigenomics Consortium and found that 78 percent of HARs demonstrated chromatin accessibility (an indication that the gene is able to be transcribed) in at least one of the human cell or tissue types tested, and 56 percent demonstrating chromatin accessibility in human brain tissue. They also conducted DNaseI hypersensitivity mapping (DNaseI-seq), to find regions of chromatin accessibility, and chromatin immunoprecipitation followed by high-throughput sequencing (ChIP-seq) using H3K4me1 and H3K27ac, chromatin markers known to be associated with enhancer activity, on chromatin derived from neural progenitor cells (NPC) and maturing neurons from 18–19 gestational week human fetal prefrontal cortex. Five-hundred-and-four HARs overlapped with either the DNaseI hypersensitivity sites (DHSs) or the ChIP-seq peaks in either NPC or neurons. In total, 210 HARs showed neuro enhancer activity and overlapped fetal brain DHSs and enhancer ChIP-seq signals.

Of these, 63 also had long-range chromatin interactions with target genes expressed in the fetal cortex as determined by chromatin conformation data (HiC) (Girskis et al. 2021). This report provides strong evidence that some HARs are important factors in the evolution of the human neocortex.

26.5.3 Genes and Neurological Disorders Associated with Human Accelerated Regions

A few studies have linked HARs to specific genes involved in neocortical development, or to neurological disorders, and have shown that the altered HAR sequence drives differential gene expression compared to the chimpanzee ortholog. The experiments provide strong evidence that HARs are a key factor in the evolution of the human neocortex. The gene *NPAS3* (neuronal PAS domain-containing protein 3) is expressed in the developing and adult brain of mice and humans, and loss-of-function mutations in the gene have recently been associated with neurodevelopmental disorders (Rossi et al. 2021). The *NPAS3* locus shows 14 HARs, 11 of which were shown to drive expression of a reporter gene in transgenic zebrafish. One of the HARs, 2xHAR142, was shown to have a different expression pattern from its chimpanzee and mouse ortholog in a transgenic mouse enhancer assay (Kamm et al. 2013a; Kamm et al. 2013b).

FZD8 (Frizzled Class Receptor 8), a receptor of the Wnt pathway, is expressed in neural progenitors in the developing neocortex and has been implicated in brain development and size. A chromosome conformation capture assays (3C) has shown that HAR *HARE5* contacts the core *Fzd8* promoter in the mouse neocortex. Boyd et al. (2015) generated transgenic mice with Fzd8 expression under the control of either human or chimpanzee *HARE5*. The mice with the human HARE5 showed accelerated neuronal progenitor cell cycling and a 12 percent increase in cortical area compared to the mice with the chimpanzee *HARE5*.

HAR2635 showed strong fetal brain chromatin interaction with the promoter of *PPP1R17*, a gene highly expressed in the NPC of the developing human cortex which acts as a repressor of protein phosphatase complex 1 and 2A, and which was shown to regulate G1 to S transition and NPC cell cycle progression through mouse neurosphere studies. *PPP1R17* expression is absent from the developing cortex of mice and ferrets, put present in the fetal cortical NPC in humans and macaques, however, expression in humans is restricted to fetal development, while it continues into adulthood in macaques, suggestive of unique human HAR-controlled expression (Girskis et al. 2021).

Doan et al. (2016) theorized that mutations in HARs would negatively impact behavioral and cognitive functions. They analyzed large cohorts of individuals with autism spectrum disorder (ASD). First, they performed copy number variant (CNV) analysis on 2,100 sibling-matched ASD proband from the Simons Simplex Collection and found a 6.5-fold increase in de novo CNVs in the probands compared to the unaffected siblings. While many of the CNVs were large and encompassed other genes complicating the interpretation of the data, two CNVs were identified in probands that impacted just the HAR. A HAR that interacts with the promotor of NR2F2 (nuclear receptor subfamily 2, group F, member 2) was found to be duplicated in one individual. NR2F2 is highly expressed in the caudal ganglionic eminence and migrating interneurons, and CNVs of NR2F2 have been associated with ASD and ID. This analysis suggests that de novo CNVs of HAR could account for up to 1.9 percent of simplex ASD cases. A second cohort of 218 families with one or more children with ASD that was enriched for consanguineous families was analyzed for biallelic HAR mutations. They found that ASD cases from consanguineous families showed about 70 percent higher rates of rare, homozygous HAR mutations compared to unaffected siblings, with this elevation attributable to HARs that showed marks of neural enhancers (Doan et al. 2016).

In scanning ASD cohorts for HAR mutations, Doan et al. (2016) also identified several homozygous mutations in HARs that physically connect to the promoters of dose sensitive genes that are known to be involved in neocortical development. Three individuals from two families with ASD and ID had mutations in HAR426, which connects with the promoter of *CUX1*. *CUX1* shows both a gain and loss of function phenotype on neuron morphology and regulation of synaptic spine density. Luciferase reporter assay and eGFP transgenic mouse analysis both revealed that the mutant form of HAR426 boosted expression levels of CUX1 compared to the non-mutant HAR426. Similarly, two brothers with ADS and ID were identified with homozygous 5 bp INDEL that was connected with the promotor region of *PTBP2*. *PTBP2* is involved in neuronal differentiation, and deletions of the gene have been associated with ASD and ID. Luciferase reporter assay and MPRA analysis showed a 40 percent reduction in activity in the mutant form of the HAR comparted to the non-mutant form. Two different homozygous mutations were also identified in two families with ASD in an intronic HAR of *GPC4*. *GPC4* is essential for excitatory synapse development in mice, and together with *GPC3*, has been associated with Simpson-Golabi-Behmel syndrome in humans, which includes ID. Both of the mutant forms of the HAR reduced its regulatory activity by 20–25 percent in a luciferase reporter assay.

Xu et al. (2015), under the hypothesis that schizophrenia is so prevalent in the human population despite strong negative pressure against it because it is tied in with the evolutionary trajectory of humans, corelated genome-wide association study results with HARs. They found that schizophrenia-associated loci were enriched for genes near HARs. They concluded that HARs play a potentially important role in the genetic architecture of schizophrenia.

26.6 Conclusions

Evolution not only unifies biology, but also captures the imagination of biologists like no other discipline. When research leads to the discovery of a new gene or mechanism, one of the fist questions asked is "what are the evolutionary consequences of this discovery?" This is especially true when studying the human neocortex, and is often a fair question to ask. Whether the gene or mechanism is highly conserved, under recent selective pressure, or somewhere in-between, the answer is likely to provide insight into the function, development, and evolution of the neocortex.

Understanding the evolution and development of the human neocortex is a daunting task, but within a problem of seemingly celestial complexity lie at least several potentially solvable problems. We understand the basic principles by which evolution works, we now have a complete sequence of the human genome, and we are continually learning how to read and interpret it. Regions of the genome that were once popularly referred to as junk DNA, are now know to be vital to the evolution and development of the cerebral cortex (Pratt and Price 2016) thanks to new tools and methods. We have access to whole genome sequencing data and tissue samples from individuals with a range of neurological conditions and from healthy individuals and a wide array of primates and other mammals, as well as a growing collection of sequences from ancient and archaic humans. Modern sequencing techniques make it possible to obtain massive amounts of sequencing data almost instantaneously, this not only makes obtaining genome sequencing data easy, but also a whole range of data, including RNA and methylation sequencing from bulk tissue or individual cells, and an expanding set of targeted methods such as ChIA-PET, HiC, 3C, 4C,

DNaseI-seq, and ChIP-seq mentioned in this review. These sequencing techniques as well as increased automation, have allowed for the generation species-specific, tissues-specific, or cell type-specific data on gene expression, chromatin interactions, DHSs, and other epigenetic factors. New methods like CRISPR greatly reduce the burden of gene editing, and make the creation of mutant cell lines or transgenic mice easier, but have also been combined with other techniques that has allowed for the generation of transgenic ferrets and marmoset and cortical organoids, allowing for a more accurate study of gene mutation on the human brain. So we might be at the beginning of the road, "with ten miles behind me and ten thousand more to go," but we are on the road and accelerating.

Understanding human neocortical development and evolution is intimately tied to human medical genetics. Not only do genes required for cortical development identify important causes of neurological disability, but the type, location, and nature of these mutations of clinical importance identify those spots in the human genome sequence that are essential for normal brain function. Thus, our understanding of human brain evolution will continue to develop hand in hand with our understanding of human neurological disorders.

Acknowledgments

C.A. Walsh was supported by NINDS grant R01NS35129, the Allen Discovery Center Program through the Paul G. Allen Frontiers Group, and The Hock E. Tan and K. Lisa Yang Center for Autism Research at Harvard University. C.A. Walsh is an Investigator of the Howard Hughes Medical Institute.

References

Ackerman, S.D. et al. (2015). The adhesion GPCR Gpr56 regulates oligodendrocyte development via interactions with Galpha12/13 and RhoA. *Nat Commun* 6: 6122. Epub 20150121. doi: 10.1038/ncomms7122. PubMed PMID: 25607772; PubMed Central PMCID: PMC4302765.

Bacon, C. et al. (2009). Dynamic expression of the slit-robo GTPase activating protein genes during development of the murine nervous system. *J Comp Neurol* 513 (2): 224–236. doi: 10.1002/cne.21955. PubMed PMID: 19137586.

Bae, B.I. et al. (2014). Genetic changes shaping the human brain. *Dev Cell* 32 (4): 423–434. doi: 10.1016/j.devcel.2015.01.035. PubMed PMID: 25710529; PubMed Central PMCID: PMC4429600.

Bae, B.I. et al. (2014). Evolutionarily dynamic alternative splicing of GPR56 regulates regional cerebral cortical patterning. *Science* 343 (6172): 764–768. doi: 10.1126/science.1244392. PubMed PMID: 24531968; PubMed Central PMCID: PMC4480613.

Bailey, J.A. and Eichler, E.E. (2006). Primate segmental duplications. *Nat Rev Genet* 7 (7): 552–564. Epub 20060613. doi: 10.1038/nrg1895. PubMed PMID: 16770338.

Bird, C.P. et al. (2007). Fast-evolving noncoding sequences in the human genome. *Genome Biol* 8 (6): R118. doi: 10.1186/gb-2007-8-6-r118. PubMed PMID: 17578567; PubMed Central PMCID: PMC2394770.

Bizzotto, S. and Francis, F. (2015). Morphological and functional aspects of progenitors perturbed in cortical malformations. *Front Cell Neurosci* 9: 30. Epub 20150212. doi: 10.3389/fncel.2015.00030. PubMed PMID: 25729350; PubMed Central PMCID: PMC4325918.

Bond, J. et al. (2002). ASPM is a major determinant of cerebral cortical size. *Nat Genet* 32 (2): 316–320. Epub 20020923. doi: 10.1038/ng995. PubMed PMID: 12355089.

Bond, J. et al. (2003). Protein-truncating mutations in ASPM cause variable reduction in brain size. *Am J Hum Genet* 73 (5): 1170–1177. Epub 20031021. doi: 10.1086/379085. PubMed PMID: 14574646; PubMed Central PMCID: PMC1180496.

Boyd, J.L. et al. (2015). Human-chimpanzee differences in a FZD8 enhancer alter cell-cycle dynamics in the developing neocortex. *Curr Biol* 25 (6): 772–779. Epub 20150219. doi: 10.1016/j.cub.2015.01.041. PubMed PMID: 25702574; PubMed Central PMCID: PMC4366288.

Bush, E.C. and Lahn, B.T. (2008). A genome-wide screen for noncoding elements important in primate evolution. *BMC Evol Biol* 8: 17. Epub 20080123. doi: 10.1186/1471-2148-8-17. PubMed PMID: 18215302; PubMed Central PMCID: PMC2242780.

Capecchi, M.R. and Pozner, A. (2015). ASPM regulates symmetric stem cell division by tuning Cyclin E ubiquitination. *Nat Commun* 6: 8763. Epub 20151119. doi: 10.1038/ncomms9763. PubMed PMID: 26581405; PubMed Central PMCID: PMC5025044.

Capra, J.A. et al. (2013). Many human accelerated regions are developmental enhancers. *Phil Trans R Soc London Series B, Biol Sci* 368 (1632): 20130025. Epub 20131111. doi: 10.1098/rstb.2013.0025. PubMed PMID: 24218637; PubMed Central PMCID: PMC3826498.

Chang, B.S. et al. (2003). Bilateral frontoparietal polymicrogyria. *Ann Neurol* 53 (5): 596–606. doi: 10.1002/ana.10520. PubMed PMID: 12730993.

Charrier, C. et al. (2012). Inhibition of SRGAP2 function by its human-specific paralogs induces neoteny during spine maturation. *Cell* 149 (4): 923–935. Epub 20120503. doi: 10.1016/j.cell.2012.03.034. PubMed PMID: 22559944; PubMed Central PMCID: PMC3357949.

Chiou, B. et al. (2021). Cell type-specific evaluation of ADGRG1/GPR56 function in developmental central nervous system myelination. *Glia* 69 (2): 413–423. Epub 20200909. doi: 10.1002/glia.23906. PubMed PMID: 32902916.

Dennis, M.Y. et al. (2012). Evolution of human-specific neural SRGAP2 genes by incomplete segmental duplication. *Cell* 149 (4): 912–922. Epub 20120503. doi: 10.1016/j.cell.2012.03.033. PubMed PMID: 22559943; PubMed Central PMCID: PMC3365555.

Desir, J. et al. (2008). Primary microcephaly with ASPM mutation shows simplified cortical gyration with antero-posterior gradient pre- and post-natally. *Am J Med Genet Part A* 146A (11): 1439–1443. doi: 10.1002/ajmg.a.32312. PubMed PMID: 18452193.

do Carmo Avides, M. and Glover, D.M. (1999). Abnormal spindle protein, Asp, and the integrity of mitotic centrosomal microtubule organizing centers. *Science* 283 (5408): 1733–1735. doi: 10.1126/science.283.5408.1733. PubMed PMID: 10073938.

Doan, R.N. et al. (2016). Mutations in human accelerated regions disrupt cognition and social behavior. *Cell* 167 (2): 341–54e12. Epub 20160922. doi: 10.1016/j.cell.2016.08.071. PubMed PMID: 27667684; PubMed Central PMCID: PMC5063026.

Du, A. et al. (2018). Pattern and process in hominin brain size evolution are scale-dependent. *Proc Biol Sci* 285 (1873): 20172738. doi: 10.1098/rspb.2017.2738. PubMed PMID: 29467267; PubMed Central PMCID: PMC5832710.

Evans, P.D. et al. (2004). Adaptive evolution of ASPM, a major determinant of cerebral cortical size in humans. *Hum Mol Genet* 13 (5): 489–494. Epub 20040113. doi: 10.1093/hmg/ddh055. PubMed PMID: 14722158.

Fiddes, I.T. et al. (2018). Human-specific NOTCH2NL genes affect notch signaling and cortical neurogenesis. *Cell* 173 (6): 1356–69e22. Epub 20180531. doi: 10.1016/j.cell.2018.03.051. PubMed PMID: 29856954; PubMed Central PMCID: PMC5986104.

Fish, J.L. et al. (2006). Aspm specifically maintains symmetric proliferative divisions of neuroepithelial cells. *Proc Natl Acad Sci USA* 103 (27): 10438–10443. Epub 20060623. doi: 10.1073/pnas.0604066103. PubMed PMID: 16798874; PubMed Central PMCID: PMC1502476.

Florio, M. et al. (2018). Evolution and cell-type specificity of human-specific genes preferentially expressed in progenitors of fetal neocortex. *Elife* 7: e32332. Epub 20180321. doi: 10.7554/eLife.32332. PubMed PMID: 29561261; PubMed Central PMCID: PMC5898914.

Fortna, A. et al. (2004). Lineage-specific gene duplication and loss in human and great ape evolution. *PloS Biol* 2 (7). E207. Epub 20040713. doi: 10.1371/journal.pbio.0020207. PubMed PMID: 15252450; PubMed Central PMCID: PMC449870.

Fossati, M. et al. (2016). SRGAP2 and its human-specific paralog co-regulate the development of excitatory and inhibitory synapses. *Neuron* 91 (2): 356–369. Epub 20160630. doi: 10.1016/j.neuron.2016.06.013. PubMed PMID: 27373832; PubMed Central PMCID: PMC5385270.

Franchini, L.F. (2021). Genetic mechanisms underlying cortical evolution in mammals. *Front Cell Dev Biol* 9: 591017. Epub 20210215. doi: 10.3389/fcell.2021.591017. PubMed PMID: 33659245; PubMed Central PMCID: PMC7917222.

Franchini, L.F. and Pollard, K.S. (2017). Human evolution. *BMC Biol* 15 (1): 89. Epub 20171002. doi: 10.1186/s12915-017-0428-9. PubMed PMID: 28969617; PubMed Central PMCID: PMC5625771.

Fujimori, A. et al. (2014). Disruption of Aspm causes microcephaly with abnormal neuronal differentiation. *Brain Dev* 36 (8): 661–669. Epub 20131109. doi: 10.1016/j.braindev.2013.10.006. PubMed PMID: 24220505.

Ganesh, R.A. et al. (2020). GPR56. *Brain Res* 1747: 147055. Epub 20200814. doi: 10.1016/j.brainres.2020.147055. PubMed PMID: 32798453.

Gershman, A. et al. (2022). Epigenetic patterns in a complete human genome. *Science* 376 (6588): eabj5089. Epub 20220401. doi: 10.1126/science.abj5089. PubMed PMID: 35357915.

Giera, S. et al. (2018). Microglial transglutaminase-2 drives myelination and myelin repair via GPR56/ADGRG1 in oligodendrocyte precursor cells. *Elife* 7: e33385. Epub 20180529. doi: 10.7554/eLife.33385. PubMed PMID: 29809138; PubMed Central PMCID: PMC5980231.

Girskis, K.M. et al. (2021). Rewiring of human neurodevelopmental gene regulatory programs by human accelerated regions. *Neuron* 109 (20): 3239–51e7. Epub 20210902. doi: 10.1016/j.neuron.2021.08.005. PubMed PMID: 34478631; PubMed Central PMCID: PMC8542612.

Gittelman, R.M. et al. (2015). Comprehensive identification and analysis of human accelerated regulatory DNA. *Genome Res* 25 (9): 1245–1255. Epub 20150623. doi: 10.1101/gr.192591.115. PubMed PMID: 26104583; PubMed Central PMCID: PMC4561485.

Gonzalez-Forero, M. and Gardner, A. (2018). Inference of ecological and social drivers of human brain-size evolution. *Nature* 557 (7706): 554–557. Epub 20180523. doi: 10.1038/s41586-018-0127-x. PubMed PMID: 29795254.

Grasby, K.L. et al. (2020). The genetic architecture of the human cerebral cortex. *Science* 367 (6484): eaay6690. doi: 10.1126/science.aay6690. PubMed PMID: 32193296; PubMed Central PMCID: PMC7295264.

Guerrier, S. et al. (2009). The F-BAR domain of srGAP2 induces membrane protrusions required for neuronal migration and morphogenesis. *Cell* 138 (5): 990–1004. doi: 10.1016/j.cell.2009.06.047. PubMed PMID: 19737524; PubMed Central PMCID: PMC2797480.

Guo, M.H. et al. (2018). Insights and implications of genome-wide association studies of height. *J Clin Endocrinol Metab* 103 (9): 3155–3168. doi: 10.1210/jc.2018-01126. PubMed PMID: 29982553; PubMed Central PMCID: PMC7263788.

Guo, S. and Bao, S. (2010). srGAP2 arginine methylation regulates cell migration and cell spreading through promoting dimerization. *J Biol Chem* 285 (45): 35133–35141. Epub 20100901. doi: 10.1074/jbc.M110.153429. PubMed PMID: 20810653; PubMed Central PMCID: PMC2966127.

Heide, M. and Huttner, W.B. (2021). Human-specific genes, cortical progenitor cells, and microcephaly. *Cells* 10 (5): 1209. Epub 20210515. doi: 10.3390/cells10051209. PubMed PMID: 34063381; PubMed Central PMCID: PMC8156310.

Hou, Q.Q. et al. (2021). TBC1D3 promotes neural progenitor proliferation by suppressing the histone methyltransferase G9a. *Sci Adv* 7 (3): eaba8053. Epub 20210115. doi: 10.1126/sciadv.aba8053. PubMed PMID: 33523893; PubMed Central PMCID: PMC7810367.

Hubisz, M.J. and Pollard, K.S. (2014). Exploring the genesis and functions of human accelerated regions sheds light on their role in human evolution. *Curr Opin Genet Dev* 29: 15–21. Epub 20140823. doi: 10.1016/j.gde.2014.07.005. PubMed PMID: 25156517.

Iguchi, T. et al. (2008). Orphan G protein-coupled receptor GPR56 regulates neural progenitor cell migration via a G alpha 12/13 and Rho pathway. *J Biol Chem* 283 (21): 14469–14478. Epub 20080331. doi: 10.1074/jbc.M708919200. PubMed PMID: 18378689.

Jayaraman, D. et al. (2018). The genetics of primary microcephaly. *Ann Rev Genomics Hum Genet* 19: 177–200. Epub 20180523. doi: 10.1146/annurev-genom-083117-021441. PubMed PMID: 29799801.

Jayaraman, D. et al. (2016). Microcephaly proteins Wdr62 and Aspm define a mother centriole complex regulating centriole biogenesis, apical complex, and cell fate. *Neuron* 92 (4): 813–828. Epub 20161027. doi: 10.1016/j.neuron.2016.09.056. PubMed PMID: 27974163; PubMed Central PMCID: PMC5199216.

Jeong, S.J. et al. (2012). Characterization of G protein-coupled receptor 56 protein expression in the mouse developing neocortex. *J Comp Neurol* 520 (13): 2930–2940. doi: 10.1002/cne.23076. PubMed PMID: 22351047; PubMed Central PMCID: PMC3908671.

Jeong, S.J. et al. (2013). GPR56 functions together with alpha3beta1 integrin in regulating cerebral cortical development. *PloS One* 8 (7): e68781. Epub 20130709. doi: 10.1371/journal.pone.0068781. PubMed PMID: 23874761; PubMed Central PMCID: PMC3706371.

Jin, Z. (2009). GPR56 and its related diseases. *Prog Mol Biol Transl Sci* 89: 1–13. Epub 20091007. doi: 10.1016/S1877-1173(09)89001-7. PubMed PMID: 20374731.

Jin, Z. et al. (2007). Disease-associated mutations affect GPR56 protein trafficking and cell surface expression. *Hum Mol Genet* 16 (16): 1972–1985. Epub 20070618. doi: 10.1093/hmg/ddm144. PubMed PMID: 17576745.

Johnson, M.B. et al. (2018). Aspm knockout ferret reveals an evolutionary mechanism governing cerebral cortical size. *Nature* 556 (7701): 370–375. Epub 20180411. doi: 10.1038/s41586-018-0035-0. PubMed PMID: 29643508; PubMed Central PMCID: PMC6095461.

Ju, X.C. et al. (2016). The hominoid-specific gene TBC1D3 promotes generation of basal neural progenitors and induces cortical folding in mice. *Elife* 5: e18197. Epub 20160809. doi: 10.7554/eLife.18197. PubMed PMID: 27504805; PubMed Central PMCID: PMC5028191.

Kaas, J.H. (2019). The origin and evolution of neocortex. *Prog Brain Res* 250: 61–81. Epub 20190405. doi: 10.1016/bs.pbr.2019.03.017. PubMed PMID: 31703909.

Kamm, G.B. et al. (2013a). A fast-evolving human NPAS3 enhancer gained reporter expression in the developing forebrain of transgenic mice. *Phil Trans R Soc London Series B, Biol Sci* 368 (1632): 20130019. Epub 20131111. doi: 10.1098/rstb.2013.0019. PubMed PMID: 24218632; PubMed Central PMCID: PMC3826493.

Kamm, G.B. et al. (2013b). The developmental brain gene NPAS3 contains the largest number of accelerated regulatory sequences in the human genome. *Mol Biol Evol* 30 (5): 1088–1102. Epub 20130213. doi: 10.1093/molbev/mst023. PubMed PMID: 23408798; PubMed Central PMCID: PMC3670734.

Kouprina, N. et al. (2005). The microcephaly ASPM gene is expressed in proliferating tissues and encodes for a mitotic spindle protein. *Hum Mol Genet* 14 (15): 2155–2165. Epub 20050622. doi: 10.1093/hmg/ddi220. PubMed PMID: 15972725.

Kouprina, N. et al. (2004). Accelerated evolution of the ASPM gene controlling brain size begins prior to human brain expansion. *PloS Biol* 2 (5): E126. Epub 20040323. doi: 10.1371/journal.pbio.0020126. PubMed PMID: 15045028; PubMed Central PMCID: PMC374243.

Leonard, W.R. et al. (2007). Effects of brain evolution on human nutrition and metabolism. *Ann Rev Nutr* 27: 311–327. doi: 10.1146/annurev.nutr.27.061406.093659. PubMed PMID: 17439362.

Letard, P. et al. (2018). Autosomal recessive primary microcephaly due to ASPM mutations. *Hum Mutat* 39 (3): 319–332. Epub 20180116. doi: 10.1002/humu.23381. PubMed PMID: 29243349.

Li, R. et al. (2017). Recapitulating cortical development with organoid culture in vitro and modeling abnormal spindle-like (ASPM related primary) microcephaly disease. *Protein Cell* 8 (11): 823–833. Epub 20171023. doi: 10.1007/s13238-017-0479-2. PubMed PMID: 29058117; PubMed Central PMCID: PMC5676597.

Li, S. et al. (2008). GPR56 regulates pial basement membrane integrity and cortical lamination. *J Neurosci* 28 (22): 5817–5826. doi: 10.1523/JNEUROSCI.0853-08.2008. PubMed PMID: 18509043; PubMed Central PMCID: PMC2504715.

Li, T. et al. (2020). A splicing isoform of GPR56 mediates microglial synaptic refinement via phosphatidylserine binding. *EMBO J* 39 (16): e104136. Epub 20200525. doi: 10.15252/embj.2019104136. PubMed PMID: 32452062; PubMed Central PMCID: PMC7429740.

Lindblad-Toh, K. et al. (2011). A high-resolution map of human evolutionary constraint using 29 mammals. *Nature* 478 (7370): 476–482. Epub 20111012. doi: 10.1038/nature10530. PubMed PMID: 21993624; PubMed Central PMCID: PMC3207357.

Liu, J. et al. (2021). Human brain evolution: emerging roles for regulatory DNA and RNA. *Curr Opin Neurobiol* 71: 170–177. Epub 20211130. doi: 10.1016/j.conb.2021.11.005. PubMed PMID: 34861533; PubMed Central PMCID: PMC8756680.

Liu, M. et al. (1999). GPR56, a novel secretin-like human G-protein-coupled receptor gene. *Genomics* 55 (3): 296–305. doi: 10.1006/geno.1998.5644. PubMed PMID: 10049584.

Lodewijk, G.A. et al. (2020). Evolution of human brain size-associated NOTCH2NL genes proceeds toward reduced protein levels. *Mol Biol Evol* 37 (9): 2531–2548. doi: 10.1093/molbev/msaa104. PubMed PMID: 32330268; PubMed Central PMCID: PMC7475042.

Luo, R. et al. (2011). Protein-coupled receptor 56 and collagen III, a receptor-ligand pair, regulates cortical development and lamination. *Proc Natl Acad Sci USA* 108 (31): 12925–12930. Epub 20110718. doi: 10.1073/pnas.1104821108. PubMed PMID: 21768377; PubMed Central PMCID: PMC3150909.

Luo, R. et al. (2014). Mechanism for adhesion G protein-coupled receptor GPR56-mediated RhoA activation induced by collagen III stimulation. *PloS One* 9 (6): e100043. Epub 20140620. doi: 10.1371/journal.pone.0100043. PubMed PMID: 24949629; PubMed Central PMCID: PMC4065004.

Martin, R.D. (1981). Relative brain size and basal metabolic rate in terrestrial vertebrates. *Nature* 293 (5827): 57–60. doi: 10.1038/293057a0. PubMed PMID: 7266659.

Mathieson, I. (2020). Human adaptation over the past 40,000 years. *Curr Opin Genet Dev* 62: 97–104. Epub 20200801. doi: 10.1016/j.gde.2020.06.003. PubMed PMID: 32745952; PubMed Central PMCID: PMC7484260.

Molnar, Z. et al. (2019). New insights into the development of the human cerebral cortex. *J Anat* 235 (3): 432–451. Epub 20190802. doi: 10.1111/joa.13055. PubMed PMID: 31373394; PubMed Central PMCID: PMC6704245.

Montgomery, S. (2018). Hominin brain evolution. *Curr Biol* 28 (14): R788–R90. doi: 10.1016/j.cub.2018.06.021. PubMed PMID: 30040939.

Montgomery, S.H. et al. (2011). Adaptive evolution of four microcephaly genes and the evolution of brain size in anthropoid primates. *Mol Biol Evol* 28 (1): 625–638. Epub 20101020. doi: 10.1093/molbev/msq237. PubMed PMID: 20961963.

Montgomery, S.H. and Mundy, N.I. (2012). Evolution of ASPM is associated with both increases and decreases in brain size in primates. *Evolution* 66 (3): 927–932. Epub 20111201. doi: 10.1111/j.1558-5646.2011.01487.x. PubMed PMID: 22380452.

Montgomery, S.H. and Mundy, N.I. (2014). Microcephaly genes evolved adaptively throughout the evolution of eutherian mammals. *BMC Evol Biol* 14: 120. Epub 20140605. doi: 10.1186/1471-2148-14-120. PubMed PMID: 24898820; PubMed Central PMCID: PMC4055943.

Mora-Bermudez, F. and Huttner, W.B. (2022). What are the human-specific aspects of neocortex development? *Front Neurosci* 16: 878950. Epub 20220414. doi: 10.3389/fnins.2022.878950. PubMed PMID: 35495057; PubMed Central PMCID: PMC9047014.

Nian, F.S. and Hou, P.S. (2022). Evolving roles of notch signaling in cortical development. *Front Neurosci* 16: 844410. Epub 20220329. doi: 10.3389/fnins.2022.844410. PubMed PMID: 35422684; PubMed Central PMCID: PMC9001970.

Nurk, S. et al. (2022). The complete sequence of a human genome. *Science* 376 (6588): 44–53. Epub 20220331. doi: 10.1126/science.abj6987. PubMed PMID: 35357919.

Ohno, S. et al. (1968). Evolution from fish to mammals by gene duplication. *Hereditas* 59 (1): 169–187. doi: 10.1111/j.1601-5223.1968.tb02169.x. PubMed PMID: 5662632.

Ossola, C. and Kalebic, N. (2021). Roots of the malformations of cortical development in the cell biology of neural progenitor cells. *Front Neurosci* 15: 817218. Epub 20220105. doi: 10.3389/fnins.2021.817218. PubMed PMID: 35069108; PubMed Central PMCID: PMC8766818.

Paramasivam, M. et al. (2007). ASPM and citron kinase co-localize to the midbody ring during cytokinesis. *Cell Cycle* 6 (13): 1605–1612. Epub 20070427. doi: 10.4161/cc.6.13.4356. PubMed PMID: 17534152.

Passemard, S. et al. (2016). Abnormal spindle-like microcephaly-associated (ASPM) mutations strongly disrupt neocortical structure but spare the hippocampus and long-term memory. *Cortex* 74: 158–176. Epub 20151031. doi: 10.1016/j.cortex.2015.10.010. PubMed PMID: 26691732.

Pattison, L. et al. (2000). A fifth locus for primary autosomal recessive microcephaly maps to chromosome 1q31. *Am J Hum Genet* 67 (6): 1578–1580. Epub 20001107. doi: 10.1086/316910. PubMed PMID: 11078481; PubMed Central PMCID: PMC1287934.

Pervaiz, N. et al. (2021). Molecular evolutionary analysis of human primary microcephaly genes. *BMC Evol Biol* 21 (1): 76. Epub 20210503. doi: 10.1186/s12862-021-01801-0. PubMed PMID: 33941077; PubMed Central PMCID: PMC8091745.

Piao, X. et al. (2002). An autosomal recessive form of bilateral frontoparietal polymicrogyria maps to chromosome 16q12.2-21. *Am J Hum Genet* 70 (4): 1028–1033. Epub 20020213. doi: 10.1086/339552. PubMed PMID: 11845408; PubMed Central PMCID: PMC379097.

Piao, X. et al. (2004). G protein-coupled receptor-dependent development of human frontal cortex. *Science* 303 (5666): 2033–2036. doi: 10.1126/science.1092780. PubMed PMID: 15044805.

Pinson, A. and Huttner, W.B. (2021). Neocortex expansion in development and evolution-from genes to progenitor cell biology. *Curr Opin Cell Biol* 73: 9–18. Epub 20210604. doi: 10.1016/j.ceb.2021.04.008. PubMed PMID: 34098196.

Pollard, K.S. et al. (2006a). Forces shaping the fastest evolving regions in the human genome. *PLoS Genet* 2 (10): e168.Epub 20060823. doi: 10.1371/journal.pgen.0020168. PubMed PMID: 17040131; PubMed Central PMCID: PMC1599772.

Pollard, K.S. et al. (2006b). An RNA gene expressed during cortical development evolved rapidly in humans. *Nature* 443 (7108): 167–172. Epub 20060816. doi: 10.1038/nature05113. PubMed PMID: 16915236.

Powell, L.E. et al. (2019). Maternal investment, life histories and the evolution of brain structure in primates. *Proc Biol Sci* 286 (1911): 20191608. Epub 20190918. doi: 10.1098/rspb.2019.1608. PubMed PMID: 31530145; PubMed Central PMCID: PMC6784728.

Prabhakar, S. et al. (2008). Human-specific gain of function in a developmental enhancer. *Science* 321 (5894): 1346–1350. doi: 10.1126/science.1159974. PubMed PMID: 18772437; PubMed Central PMCID: PMC2658639.

Pratt, T. and Price, D.J. (2016). Junk DNA used in cerebral cortical evolution. *Neuron* 90 (6): 1141–1143. doi: 10.1016/j.neuron.2016.06.007. PubMed PMID: 27311076.

Pulvers, J.N. et al. (2010). Mutations in mouse Aspm (abnormal spindle-like microcephaly associated) cause not only microcephaly but also major defects in the germline. *Proc Natl Acad Sci USA* 107 (38): 16595–16600. Epub 20100907. doi: 10.1073/pnas.1010494107. PubMed PMID: 20823249; PubMed Central PMCID: PMC2944708.

Rakic, P. (2009). Evolution of the neocortex: a perspective from developmental biology. *Nat Rev Neurosci* 10 (10): 724–735. doi: 10.1038/nrn2719. PubMed PMID: 19763105; PubMed Central PMCID: PMC2913577.

Reillo, I. et al. (2011). A role for intermediate radial glia in the tangential expansion of the mammalian cerebral cortex. *Cereb Cortex* 21 (7): 1674–1694. Epub 20101202. doi: 10.1093/cercor/bhq238. PubMed PMID: 21127018.

Rossi, J.J. et al. (2021). Molecular characterisation of rare loss-of-function NPAS3 and NPAS4 variants identified in individuals with neurodevelopmental disorders. *Sci Rep* 11 (1): 6602. Epub 20210323. doi: 10.1038/s41598-021-86041-4. PubMed PMID: 33758288; PubMed Central PMCID: PMC7987981.

Salzman, G.S. et al. (2016). Structural basis for regulation of GPR56/ADGRG1 by its alternatively spliced extracellular domains. *Neuron* 91 (6): 1292–1304. doi: 10.1016/j.neuron.2016.08.022. PubMed PMID: 27657451; PubMed Central PMCID: PMC5036532.

Saunders, R.D. et al. (1997). The Drosophila gene abnormal spindle encodes a novel microtubule-associated protein that associates with the polar regions of the mitotic spindle. *J Cell Biol* 137 (4): 881–890. doi: 10.1083/jcb.137.4.881. PubMed PMID: 9151690; PubMed Central PMCID: PMC2139842.

Schmidt, E.R.E. et al. (2019). The human-specific paralogs SRGAP2B and SRGAP2C differentially modulate SRGAP2A-dependent synaptic development. *Sci Rep* 9 (1): 18692. Epub 20191210. doi: 10.1038/s41598-019-54887-4. PubMed PMID: 31822692; PubMed Central PMCID: PMC6904453.

Schmidt, E.R.E. and Polleux, F. (2021). Genetic mechanisms underlying the evolution of connectivity in the human cortex. *Front Neural Circuits* 15: 787164. Epub 20220107. doi: 10.3389/fncir.2021.787164. PubMed PMID: 35069126; PubMed Central PMCID: PMC8777274.

Schmidt, E.R.E. et al. (2021). A human-specific modifier of cortical connectivity and circuit function. *Nature* 599 (7886): 640–644. Epub 20211027. doi: 10.1038/s41586-021-04039-4. PubMed PMID: 34707291.

Shen, J. et al. (2005). ASPM mutations identified in patients with primary microcephaly and seizures. *J Med Genet* 42 (9): 725–729. doi: 10.1136/jmg.2004.027706. PubMed PMID: 16141009; PubMed Central PMCID: PMC1736131.

Shinmyo, Y. et al. (2022). Investigation of the mechanisms underlying the development and evolution of the cerebral cortex using gyrencephalic ferrets. *Front Cell Dev Biol* 10: 847159. Epub 20220321. doi: 10.3389/fcell.2022.847159. PubMed PMID: 35386196; PubMed Central PMCID: PMC8977464.

Singer, K. et al. (2013). GPR56 and the developing cerebral cortex: cells, matrix, and neuronal migration. *Mol Neurobiol* 47 (1): 186–196. Epub 20120922. doi: 10.1007/s12035-012-8343-0. PubMed PMID: 23001883; PubMed Central PMCID: PMC3538897.

Singh, A.K. and Lin, H.H. (2021). The role of GPR56/ADGRG1 in health and disease. *Biomed J* 44 (5): 534–547. Epub 20210504. doi: 10.1016/j.bj.2021.04.012. PubMed PMID: 34654683; PubMed Central PMCID: PMC8640549.

Sporny, M. et al. (2017). Structural history of human SRGAP2 proteins. *Mol Biol Evol* 34 (6): 1463–1478. doi: 10.1093/molbev/msx094. PubMed PMID: 28333212; PubMed Central PMCID: PMC5435084.

Sudmant, P.H. et al. (2010). Diversity of human copy number variation and multicopy genes. *Science* 330 (6004): 641–646. doi: 10.1126/science.1197005. PubMed PMID: 21030649; PubMed Central PMCID: PMC3020103.

Suzuki, I.K. et al. (2018). Human-specific NOTCH2NL genes expand cortical neurogenesis through delta/notch regulation. *Cell* 173 (6): 1370–84e16. Epub 20180531. doi: 10.1016/j.cell.2018.03.067. PubMed PMID: 29856955; PubMed Central PMCID: PMC6092419.

Tilot, A.K. et al. (2021). The evolutionary history of common genetic variants influencing human cortical surface area. *Cereb Cortex* 31 (4): 1873–1887. doi: 10.1093/cercor/bhaa327. PubMed PMID: 33290510; PubMed Central PMCID: PMC7945014.

Trevathan, W. (2015). Primate pelvic anatomy and implications for birth. *Philos Trans R Soc London Series B, Biol Sci* 370 (1663): 20140065. doi: 10.1098/rstb.2014.0065. PubMed PMID: 25602069; PubMed Central PMCID: PMC4305166.

Uebbing, S. et al. (2021). Massively parallel discovery of human-specific substitutions that alter enhancer activity. *Proc Natl Acad Sci USA* 118 (2): e2007049118. doi: 10.1073/pnas.2007049118. PubMed PMID: 33372131; PubMed Central PMCID: PMC7812811.

Vaid, S. and Huttner, W.B. (2022). Progenitor-based cell biological aspects of neocortex development and evolution. *Front Cell Dev Biol* 10: 892922. Epub 20220502. doi: 10.3389/fcell.2022.892922. PubMed PMID: 35602606; PubMed Central PMCID: PMC9119302.

Vollger, M.R. et al. (2022). Segmental duplications and their variation in a complete human genome. *Science* 376 (6588): eabj6965. Epub 20220401. doi: 10.1126/science.abj6965. PubMed PMID: 35357917; PubMed Central PMCID: PMC8979283.

Wainszelbaum, M.J. et al. (2008). The hominoid-specific oncogene TBC1D3 activates Ras and modulates epidermal growth factor receptor signaling and trafficking. *J Biol Chem* 283 (19): 13233–13242. Epub 20080304. doi: 10.1074/jbc.M800234200. PubMed PMID: 18319245; PubMed Central PMCID: PMC2442359.

Walsh, C.A. and Engle, E.C. (2010). Allelic diversity in human developmental neurogenetics: insights into biology and disease. *Neuron* 68 (2): 245–253. doi: 10.1016/j.neuron.2010.09.042. PubMed PMID: 20955932; PubMed Central PMCID: PMC3010396.

Williams, S.E. et al. (2015). Aspm sustains postnatal cerebellar neurogenesis and medulloblastoma growth in mice. *Development* 142 (22): 3921–3932. Epub 20151008. doi: 10.1242/dev.124271. PubMed PMID: 26450969; PubMed Central PMCID: PMC4712878.

Xing, L. et al. (2021). How neural stem cells contribute to neocortex development. *Biochem Soc Trans* 49 (5): 1997–2006. doi: 10.1042/BST20200923. PubMed PMID: 34397081; PubMed Central PMCID: PMC8589419.

Xu, K. et al. (2015). Genomic and network patterns of schizophrenia genetic variation in human evolutionary accelerated regions. *Mol Biol Evol* 32 (5): 1148–1160. Epub 20150212. doi: 10.1093/molbev/msv031. PubMed PMID: 25681384; PubMed Central PMCID: PMC4408416.

Xu, S. et al. (2012). Positive selection at the ASPM gene coincides with brain size enlargements in cetaceans. *Proc Biol Sci* 279 (1746): 4433–4440. Epub 20120912. doi: 10.1098/rspb.2012.1729. PubMed PMID: 22977148; PubMed Central PMCID: PMC3479811.

Xu, S. et al. (2017). Genetic basis of brain size evolution in cetaceans: insights from adaptive evolution of seven primary microcephaly (MCPH) genes. *BMC Evol Biol* 17 (1): 206. Epub 20170829. doi: 10.1186/s12862-017-1051-7. PubMed PMID: 28851290; PubMed Central PMCID: PMC5576371.

Yousaf, A. et al. (2021). Current progress in evolutionary comparative genomics of great apes. *Front Genet* 12: 657468. Epub 20210811. doi: 10.3389/fgene.2021.657468. PubMed PMID: 34456962; PubMed Central PMCID: PMC8385753.

Zaqout, S. and Kaindl, A.M. (2022). Autosomal recessive primary microcephaly. *Front Cell Dev Biol* 9: 784700. Epub 20220117. doi: 10.3389/fcell.2021.784700. PubMed PMID: 35111754; PubMed Central PMCID: PMC8802810.

Zhang, J. (2003). Evolution of the human ASPM gene, a major determinant of brain size. *Genetics* 165 (4): 2063–2070. doi: 10.1093/genetics/165.4.2063. PubMed PMID: 14704186; PubMed Central PMCID: PMC1462882.

Zimmer-Bensch, G. (2019). Emerging roles of long non-coding RNAs as drivers of brain evolution. *Cells* 8 (11): 1399. Epub 20191106. doi: 10.3390/cells8111399. PubMed PMID: 31698782; PubMed Central PMCID: PMC6912723.

27

Clinical and Molecular Overview of Cortical Malformations

Pravata M.V.[1,2], *Gressens P.*[3], *and Cappello S.*[1,2]

[1] *Max Planck Institute of Psychiatry, 80804 Munich, Germany*
[2] *Biomedical Center, Ludwig-Maximilians-Universitaet, Munich, Germany*
[3] *Université Paris Cité, INSERM, NeuroDiderot, Paris, France*

27.1 Concept of Cortical Malformations and Clinical Features

The meticulous orchestration of the formation of the cerebral cortex requires the precise regulation of progenitor proliferation, cell type specification, and migration. Additionally, extrinsic cues must work together to allow proper cortical organizations (Figure 27.1A). Seemingly subtle alternation of this process, such as inborn errors or environmental effects, can cause long-lasting consequences on adult brain complexity and function, leading to cortical malformations (CMs). CMs can be linked to a wide variety of neurological features, such as epilepsy, developmental delay, intellectual disabilities, and motor abnormalities of tone, movement, and postures. The main manifestation in CMs is abnormal cortical structure or the presence of heterotopic gray matter, often associated with abnormal brain size (i.e., microcephaly or macrocephaly). Even onsets of clinical manifestations highly vary, ranging from early childhood to adult age. CMs represent a major cause of intellectual disability, autism, cerebral palsy, and epilepsy. As for the latter, it is estimated that ~50 percent of drug resistant epilepsies treated by surgery in children are caused by CMs. The timing of mutation is often associated with the severity of the phenotype. As such, mutations causing CMs are often *de novo* during gametogenesis or postzygotic development. However, somatic mutations still exert an important contribution to CMs with focal insult, such as focal heterotopia or focal dysplasia.

The heterogeneous genetic causes of CMs are mirrored by the heterogeneous cellular phenotypes and functional outcomes that characterize these disorders. The genes that are implicated in CMs encode proteins involved in various aspects of brain development and are differentially expressed in different cellular types (Klingler et al. 2021). hemimegalencephaly

As common presentations of CMs highly vary across patients, mainly due to the high heterogeneity in genetic etiology, different classifications for CMs have been introduced in the literature over the years. Each CM type can be further classified based on morphology, topography, severity gradient, and involvement of other brain structures.

The most recent vision upholds the pivotal concept that CMs derive from disruption during three major stages of cortical development: cell proliferation and apoptosis at the progenitor level, cell migration, and post-migration development/maturation. Moreover, recent studies demonstrated that several other "extrinsic" mechanisms can overall lead to CMs.

Neocortical Neurogenesis in Development and Evolution, First Edition. Edited by Wieland B. Huttner.

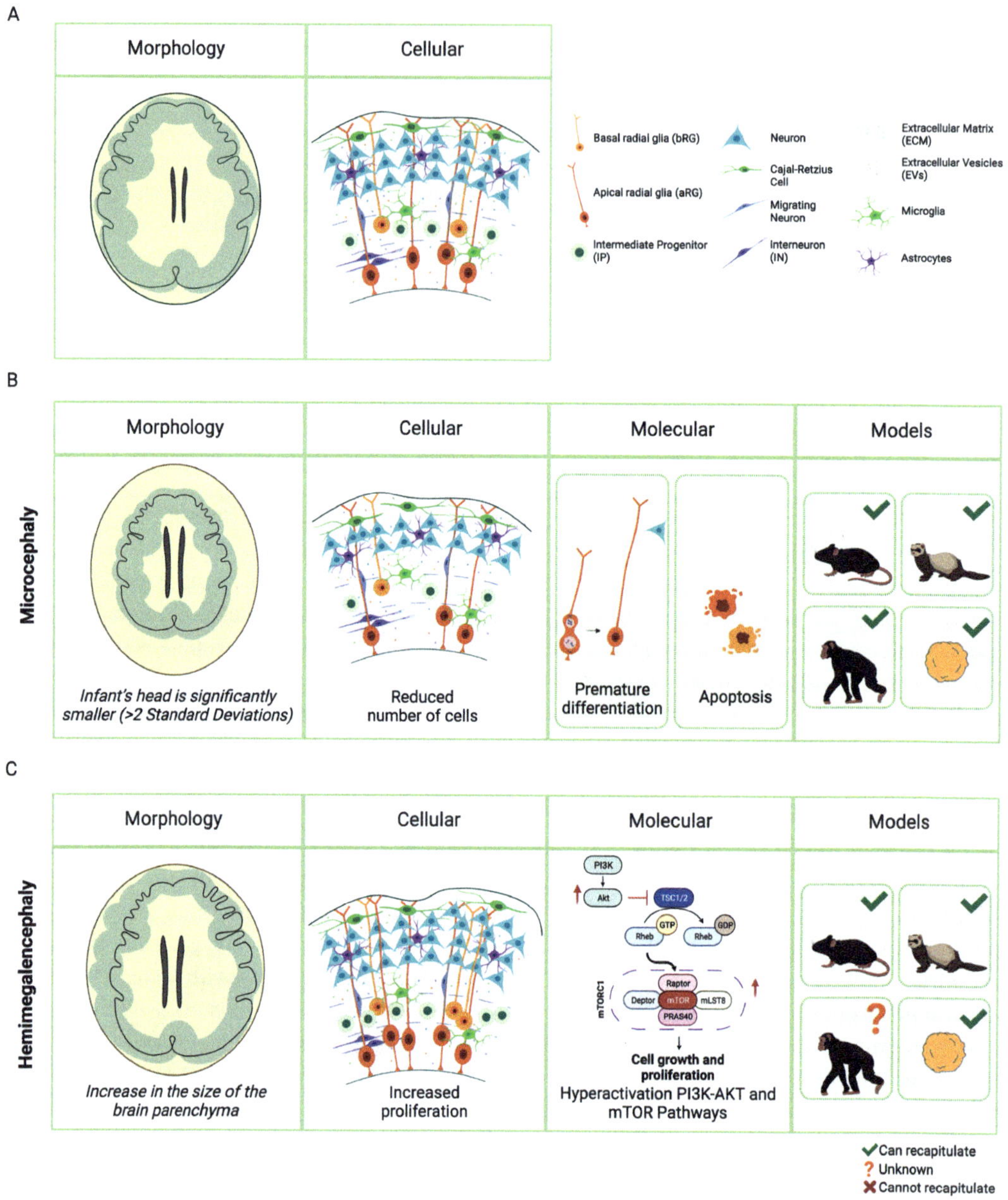

Figure 27.1 Schematic overview of cortical malformation and the models used to recapitulate different subtypes. (A) Representation of healthy conditions, both at the morphological and cellular level. (B) Summary of microcephaly at the morphological, cellular, and molecular level and overview of the model organisms that can recapitulate it. (C) Summary of hemimegalencephaly. Created with BioRender.com.

In this chapter, we provide an overview of the most common types of CMs and their etiologies by developmental stage and introduce how other extrinsic cues can affect CM clinical presentation. However, it is important to bear in mind that the classification of CMs subtypes is not as strict, as very often the same gene can give rise to different forms of CMs and have multiples molecular outcomes (Severino et al. 2020).

27.2 Progenitors: Proliferation and Apoptosis

Several cases of CMs have been linked to flaws at the level of progenitor cell types. The laminar organization of the neocortex heavily relies on the radial polarity of progenitors, which is necessary to guide the migration of daughter neurons, and their proliferation. Reduction in progenitor proliferation or survival leads to changes in brain volume and **microcephaly**, *a rare neurological condition in which an infant's head is significantly smaller (>2 Standard Deviations) than the heads of other children of the same age and sex* (Figure 27.1B**)**. In a similar fashion, localized increase in the number of proliferating neurons and/or glial cells leads to **megalencephaly**, which is caused by an *increase in the size of the brain parenchyma*.

27.2.1 Microcephaly

Several mitotic spindle-related genes participate in the microcephalic phenotype (Abdullah et al. 2017; Cueto-González et al. 2020). The most common cause of primary microcephaly is the *abnormal spindle-like microcephaly-associated protein* (*ASPM*, also known as *MCPH5*), which encodes for a mitotic spindle protein with a preferential role in regulating neurogenesis. Abrogation of the *ASPM* gene in the mouse cortex results in reduction of vertical symmetric proliferative division of apical progenitors, which causes a reduction in the progenitor pool (Fish et al. 2006). Additionally, knockout of *ASPM* in the gyrified ferret neocortex causes a premature detachment of apical radial glia (aRG) and generation of bRG, which triggered severe microcephaly (Johnson et al. 2018).

A second leading cause for primary microcephaly in humans is linked to mutations in *WDR62 (WD repeat domain 62)*, also known as *MCPH2* (Naseer et al. 2017). The gene encodes for a scaffold protein that is associated with the spindle pole. Mechanistically, WDR6 interacts with JNK1/2 (c-Jun N-terminal kinase) and AURKA/AURKB (Aurora kinase A and B), which are likely to regulate its localization to the spindle pole and cell cycle progression in neocortical progenitors (Sgourdou et al. 2017). WDR62 mutants fail to localize to the spindle pole and cells transiently arrest mitosis, causing spindle instabilities, abnormalities in centrosome inheritance, and overall reduced proliferation of neural progenitors. For a more exhaustive review of the known 28 MCPH genes, please refer to Zaqout and Kaindl (2022).

During cytokinesis, the final step of mitosis, cleavage furrow of aRG starts on the basal side and ingresses toward the apical membrane, a process which is mediated by actin-based cortex and anillin. Among the proteins involved in cytokinetic abscission are members of kinesin family member (KIF) genes. Several members of these family were linked to microcephaly, such as KIF14, KIF2A, KIF5C, and KIF11 (Malvezzi et al. 2018; Moawia et al. 2017; Poirier et al. 2013). Interestingly, the "magoo" mouse, which exhibits a fully penetrated microcephaly, carries a splice mutation in the *Kif20b* (Janisch et al. 2013). *Kif20b* mutants show changes in the midbody number, shape, and position resulting in the disruption of the abscission step, resulting in apoptosis of neural progenitors and microcephaly.

In neural progenitor cells, polarity has a prominent impact on the development and later functionality of neuronal circuits. Maintaining correct cell polarity is a fundamental cell biological feature that enables both the exposure to extrinsic signals and the neuronal migration. Several proteins selectively working in both the apical and the basal endfeet of aRG and bRG have been implicated in CMs.

Apical progenitors contain a specialized apical polarity complex, composed by Par3 (Partitioning defective protein 3), Par 6, and aPKC (atypical protein kinase C) (Bultje et al. 2009; Costa et al. 2009; Kalebic and Namba 2021), which regulates aRG proliferation and differentiation in the neocortex. The Par complex is essential for maintaining high levels of Notch on the plasma membrane of daughter cells, thus perpetuating stemness (Bultje et al. 2009; Kandachar and Roegiers 2012). Over-expression of both Par 3 and 6 promotes generation of proliferative progenitors in the developing mouse cortex (Costa et al. 2008). Conversely, loss of Par3 causes severe CMs including megalencephaly and massive ribbon-like heterotopia (which will be discussed later) (Liu et al. 2018). The molecular causes can be redirected to temporally different progenitors' behaviors in response to HIPPO and NOTCH signaling. In fact, the megalencephaly and the heterotopia phenotypes were rescued by a simultaneous removal of the HIPPO pathways effectors YAP and TAZ (Liu et al. 2018).

Cell polarity is highly reliant on traffic through the secretory pathway. Interestingly, endoplasmic reticulum (ER) stress and Golgi stress could significantly contribute to cortical impairments eliciting microcephaly (Passemard et al. 2019). As such, mutations in the ARFGEF2 (ADP-ribosylation factor guanine nucleotide-exchange factor-2), encoding for the large (>200 kDa) brefeldin A (BFA)-inhibited GEF2 protein (BIG2), are a leading cause of microcephaly. BIG2 promotes the activation of ARF (ADP-ribosylation factor) proteins by guanine-nucleotide exchange, regulating Golgi vesicular budding and uncoating. Inhibition of BIG2 decreases cell proliferation of mouse neural progenitors in vitro and disturbed the intracellular localization of molecules as E-cadherin and β-catenin by preventing their transport from the Golgi apparatus to the cell surface (Sheen et al. 2003).

Neocortical progenitor metabolism and mitochondrial activity are emerging as important players for progenitor proliferation and cortical expansion, as their dysregulation can lead to microcephaly (Namba et al. 2021). Among the microcephaly-associated and human-specific genes, *MCPH1*, *SLC25A19*, and *ARGHGAP11B* have been linked to mitochondrial function and NPC (neural progenitor cells) metabolism (Pulvers et al. 2015). Despite being preferentially localized in the centrosome, MCPH1 was recently found to localize in association with mitochondria, interacting with the mitochondrial ion channel VDAC1. Interestingly, MHCP1 is preferentially expressed in aRG of mouse and aRG and bRG of humans (Journiac et al. 2020). *Mcph1* knockout mouse possess fragmented mitochondria and defects in mitochondrial metabolism, as well as reduced mitochondrial calcium levels, thus making the presence of Mcph1 in NPCs required for maintaining optimal mitochondrial function. Amish lethal microcephaly is caused by a mutation of the *SLC25A19* (Solute carrier family 25 member 19) gene, coding for a mitochondrial thiamine pyrophosphate carrier, which is a coenzyme for α-ketoglutarate dehydrogenase (KGDH) that operates in the TCA (tricarboxylic acid) cycle (Bottega et al. 2019; Kelley et al. 2002). Notably, reduction in SLC25A19 protein levels results in lower KGDH activity, which has already been shown to lead to microcephaly (Yoon et al. 2017)

Of particular interest is *ARHGAP11B*, a human-specific gene that occurred after the split of the lineages leading to *Homo sapiens* and *Pan troglodytes* (Prüfer et al. 2014; Sudmant et al. 2010). The human specific ARHGAP11B is imported into the mitochondrial matrix and does stimulate BP proliferation, a hallmark of neocortical expansion (Florio et al. 2016; Namba et al. 2020). Although the mechanism is not fully understood, ARHGAP11B promotes glutaminolysis, which is a hallmark of cells with high proliferative capacity (Yang et al. 2017).

27.2.2 mTORopathies and Megalencephaly

NPC promotion of proliferation is mediated by several signaling pathways, such as Notch, Shh, Wnt, ERK, Hippo, PI3K-AKT (phosphatidylinositol-3-kinase), and mTOR (mammalian target of rapamycin) (Ferent et al. 2020; Kalebic and Huttner 2020). Notably, the PI3K-AKT and mTOR pathways are enriched in bRG, as forced proliferation of mouse basal progenitors (BPs) leads to PI3K-AKT hyperactivation (Andrews et al. 2020; Kalebic et al. 2019; Nowakowski et al. 2017).

More importantly, several studies have shown that diverse forms of megalencephaly are caused by aberrations in the PI3K-AKT signaling pathway (Jansen et al. 2015), in addition to other types of CMs such as hemimegalencephaly, dysplastic megalencephaly, heterotopia, polymicrogyria, pachygyria, and focal aggregates of small undifferentiated cells. Despite mouse mutants for *Akt3* and *Pten* (phosphatase and tensin homolog) showing significant enlargement of the brain, they could not recapitulate the cortical folding phenotype (Groszer et al. 2001; Tokuda et al. 2011). Remarkably, knockout of *PTEN* in human brain organoids leads to increased proliferation of neural progenitors, organoid size, and the onset of organoid folding (Li et al. 2017). Mechanistically, PI3K-AKT signaling inhibits the activity of GSK3 (glycogensynthase kinase 3), a central regulator of radial glia polarity. GSK3 inhibition in mouse aRG disrupts the radial organization of cell processes, thus impairing neuronal migration and affecting the progenitor (Kim and Snider 2011; Yokota et al. 2010). Likewise, inactivation of GSK3 in human cortical organoids increased the proliferation of neural progenitors (López-Tobón et al. 2019).

mTOR signaling is a central regulator of mammalian physiology and it is implicated in various diseases ranging from cancer to neurodevelopmental pathologies (Dobyns and Mirzaa 2019). Somatic mutations in genes involved in mTOR pathway occur in an early cell cycle of neocortical progenitors and lead to hemimegalencephaly, which causes part of the brain to be abnormally larger than the rest (Sarnat and Flores-Sarnat 2015). The pathological phenotype can be a consequence of either a rare disruptive event causing hyperactivation of the pathway, or through the collective effects of many common alleles (Reijnders et al. 2017). Such activation of the pathway typically leads to over-proliferation of neural progenitors and subsequent increase in brain size (Dobyns and Mirzaa 2019). Additionally, genes encoding for proteins involved in the mTOR pathway can also lead to MCs. One of such examples is the E3 ubiquitin ligase *NEDD4L*, whose mutations have been linked to periventricular nodular heterotopia (PNH), probably due to alteration of Akt activity at the post-translational level (Broix et al. 2016).

Mutations that affect mTOR are also a common cause of focal cortical dysplasia type II (which is discussed more fully later) (Kumari et al. 2019; Marsan and Baulac 2018). Focal cortical dysplasia type II is the main cause of refractory epilepsy and is often caused by brain somatic mutations leading to hyperactivation of mTOR (Lim et al. 2015). Over-expression of mutant mTOR by in utero electroporation in mice disrupts neuronal migration and causes seizures, whereas the inhibition of mTOR can suppress the seizures (Lim et al. 2015).

27.3 Neurons and Neuronal Migration

Neuronal migration is a major process that governs neuronal development. As such, neuronal migration disorders deeply contribute to the CMs pool. One of the major causes of defective neuronal migration is produced by defects in either the morphology of the radial glial cells that are the scaffold for the migrating neurons and/or motility and cytoskeletal defects.

27.3.1 Lissencephaly

Lissencephaly, which means "smooth brain," is a *rare brain malformation characterized by the absence of normal convolutions (folds) in the cerebral cortex and microcephaly* (Figure 27.2A). Mutations in *PAFAH1B1*, also known as *LIS1*, and doublecortin (*DCX*) have been attributed as a cause of type I lissencephaly (Jang et al. 2013; Sheen et al. 2006), accounting for approximately 85 percent of patients (Pilz et al. 1998).

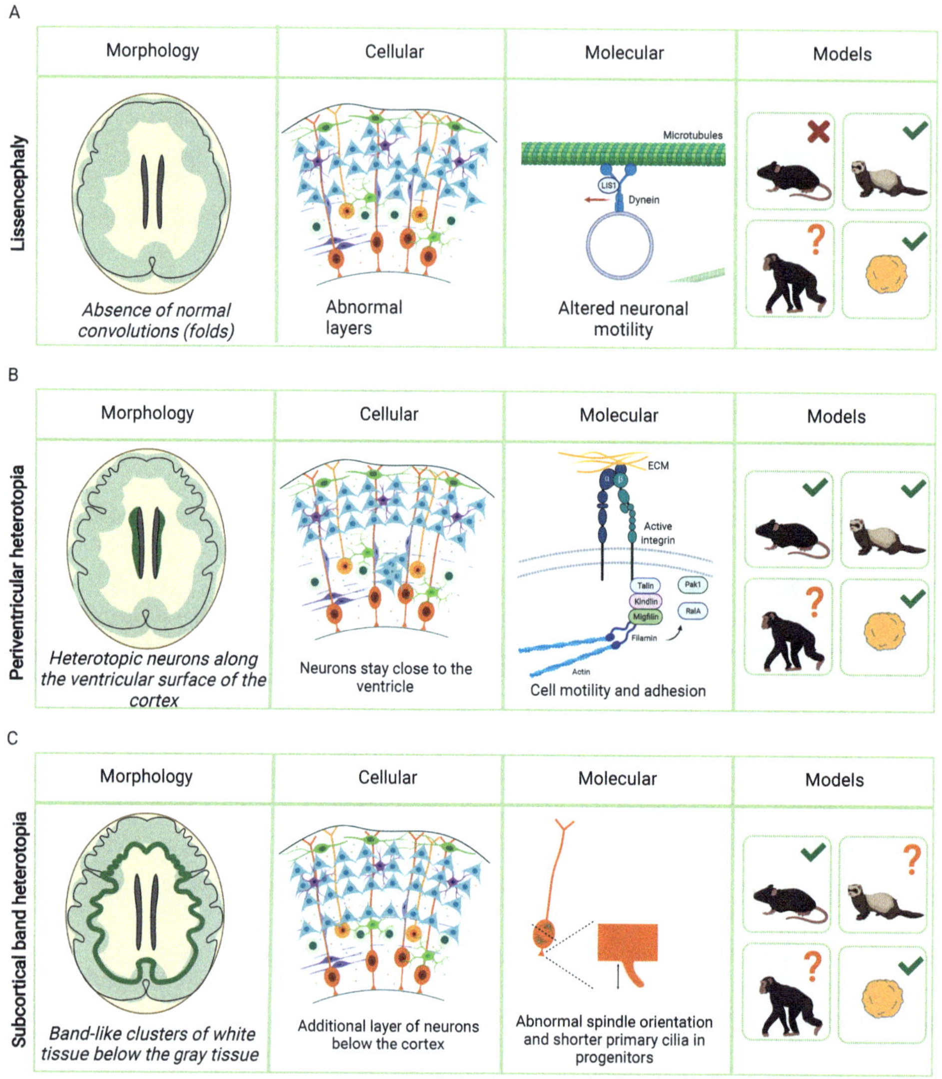

Figure 27.2 Summary of lissencephaly (A), periventricular heterotopia (B), subcortical band heterotopia (C), at the morphological, cellular, and molecular level, and model organisms capable of modelling each CM subtype. Created with BioRender.com.

This type of CMs is often associated with axon outgrowth and guidance defects such as agenesis of the corpus callosum, a rare birth defect that causes complete or partial absence of the corpus callosum (Blümcke et al. 2011). In the case of *DCX*, which is located on the X chromosome, mutations in women typically lead to heterotopia (as discussed in the next paragraph), whereas in men they are associated with lissencephaly, suggesting dose-dependent effects (Guerrini and Filippi 2005).

Another gene linked to type I lissencephaly is the *Tyrosine 3-Monooxygenase/Tryptophan 5-Monooxygenase Activation Protein, Epsilon* (*YWHAE*). YWHAE, also known as 14-3-3e, is a microtubule-associated protein that participates in the LIS1 pathway. Homozygous deletion of *Ywhae* leads to neuronal migration defects in mice. Interestingly, large deletions of the 12p13.3 regions, which contains both *YWHAE* and *LIS1*, causes Miller-Dieker Syndrome (MDS), whose patients display more severe neuronal migration defects than those possessing genetic insults in the *LIS1* gene (Moon and Wynshaw-Boris 2013).

Tubulinopathies, which results from variants in gene of the tubulin superfamily, are another leading cause of lissencephaly type 1 or polymicrogyria (Cushion et al. 2013). Mutations in tubulin genes prevent microtubule polymerization, often due to loss of Guanosine triphosphate (GTP) binding and heterodimer formation. *Tubulin Alpha 1a* (*TUBA1A*) and *Tubulin Beta 2* (*TUBB2*) are two of such examples enriched during brain development. While the former is identified in 1 percent of classic lissencephaly and 30 percent of lissencephaly with cerebellar hypoplasia (Kumar et al. 2010), *TUBB2* mutations are linked to symmetric polymicrogyria and pachygyria (Jaglin et al. 2009).

Another type of neuronal migration disorders is type II lissencephaly, in which reduction in normal sulcation is associated with a bumpy or pebbly cortical surface, thus the term cobblestone lissencephaly. Abnormal glycosylation of matrix proteins in the cerebral cortex is thought to cause such migratory defects. As matter of fact, aberrations of several O-glycosylases are linked to cobblestone lissencephaly (Herman and Siegel 2008; Yoshida et al. 2001) (discussed in more in detail in Section 27.5.4). Also, loss of function of *SNAP29* (Synaptosomal-associated protein 29) has been linked to aberrant neuronal migration and cobblestone lissencephaly (Sprecher et al. 2005). *SNAP29* encodes for a SNARE involved in autophagy through the direct control of the autophagosome membrane fusion with the lysosome membrane. Interestingly, SNAP29 loss of function impairs cell motility through defective endocytic recycling of β1-integrin, a transmembrane receptor that provides a link between the ECM and the cytoskeleton (Rapaport et al. 2010).

27.3.2 Heterotopias

27.3.2.1 Periventricular Heterotopia

Dysfunctional neuronal migration can also lead to the development of neuronal population in aberrant locations. Periventricular heterotopia (PH) is one of such disorders in which *cluster (nodular) or sheets (laminar) of neurons failed to migrate, leading to the formation of heterotopic neurons along the ventricular surface of the neocortex* (Guerrini and Filippi 2005; Guerrini and Parrini 2010) (Figure 27.2B). This type of malformation can either be found unilaterally or bilaterally. Despite affected individuals rarely having mild intellectual disability, they are usually diagnosed due to recurrent seizure symptoms and through magnetic resonance imaging (MRI). Some individuals harboring mutations in the causative genes also have microcephaly, suggestive of impaired progenitor proliferation or increased cell death (as discussed earlier). Overall, these observations suggest that genes involved in PH formation play some role in migration (heterotopia formation) and proliferation (microcephaly).

Among the most essential proteins involved in migration, cytoskeletal proteins play a major role in neuronal migration, and they are strongly correlated to PH. The most common genetic cause of PH is due to aberrations in the *Filamin A* (*FLNA*) gene, which encodes for an F-actin binding cytoplasmic protein involved in crosslinking actin filaments into the cortical cytoskeleton. Its role has been shown to be crucial in neurogenesis and neuronal migration (Zhang et al. 2013), as demonstrated by the fact that mutations in *FLNA* are linked to classical bilateral periventricular nodular heterotopia (Parrini et al. 2006; Sheen et al. 2001). Knockout of *FLNA* leads to prolongation of cell cycle length by delaying the onset and progression through mitosis due to impaired regulation of cyclin B1 deregulation which results in a decline in progenitor number and a reduction in brain size, also implicating the gene in microcephaly. Moreover, FLNA has been implicated in intracellular trafficking defects. FLNA has been shown to allow cell trafficking of b1 integrin to the cell membrane (Kim et al. 2010). Additionally, deletion of *BIG2*, an CM gene itself, promotes phosphorylation of FLNA which in turn affects FLNA-actin binding affinity and its localization, suggesting a cooperative action between actin and vesicle trafficking in the assembly of membrane proteins (Zhang et al. 2013).

Members of the cadherin superfamily have been also implicated in periventricular heterotopia. The cadherin pair DCHS1 (Dachsous cadherin-related 1) and FAT4 (FAT Atypical Cadherin4) have been associated with the Van Maldergem syndrome, which is characterized by a periventricular neuronal heterotopia (Cappello et al. 2013). Abrogation of this pair of genes in the developing mouse cortex results in increased progenitor cell number, changes in progenitors' morphology, and reduced neuronal differentiation, which causes heterotopic accumulation of cells below the neuronal layers. Cerebral organoids generated from patient-derived induced pluripotent stem cells (iPSCs), carrying mutations in *DCHS1* and *FAT4*, show the neuronal heterotopia, without an increase in progenitor proliferation, highlighting the inter-species differences (Klaus et al. 2019).

Several genes involved in PH are involved in vesicular trafficking. The microcephaly-associated gene *BIG2* causes bilateral periventricular nodular heterotopia, as well as putamina hyperintensity and microcephaly (Sheen et al. 2004; Togawa et al. 1999; Zhang et al. 2013). Via mediation of Filamin A signaling, BIG2 is involved in neuronal migration through the regulation of vesicle trafficking. Another example is given by the *low-density lipoprotein-related protein 2* (*LRP2*) that encodes megalin, a multiligand receptor. Megalin facilitates the endocytosis of sonic hedgehog (Shh) in embryonic neuroepithelium (McCarthy et al. 2002). Furthermore, megalin has been shown to bind and sequester Shh in the forebrain, and mediate Shh-Ptch endocytosis (Christ et al. 2012). Mutations to LRP2 cause Donnai-Barrow syndrome, which is associated with several neurological and cranial abnormalities, including periventricular nodular heterotopia (Kantarci et al. 2007).

Further genetic abnormalities have been associated with this disorder (Heinzen et al. 2018). Chromosomal deletion or duplication can also be linked to PH. Alterations in chromosome 5, which includes *Periventricular Nodular Heterotopia 3* (*PVNH3*) and *Periventricular Nodular Heterotopia 5* (*PVNH5*), have been identified in patients with periventricular heterotopia (Sheen et al. 2003).

27.3.2.2 Subcortical Band Heterotopia

Anomalies in progenitors can also lead to subcortical band heterotopia (SBH), a condition that occurs when *neurons migrate abnormally (heterotopia), and form abnormal areas that appear as band-like clusters of white tissue underneath the gray tissue of the cerebral cortex (subcortical), creating the appearance of a double cortex* (Figure 27.2C).

This condition is often related to mutations in genes involved in microtubule dynamics, which can also lead to abnormal spindle orientation in progenitors. As such, mutations in the *echinoderm microtubule associated protein-like 1* (*EML1*) cause perturbation of microtubule dynamics and an increase in oblique cleavage orientations of aRG, that lead to ectopic proliferation of progenitor cells in intermediate zone (IZ) and cortical plate (CP) in mice (Kielar et al. 2014). Such alteration in the progenitor niche causes complex cortical malformation characterized by megalencephaly with subcortical heterotopia (Jabali et al. 2022).

SBH is most often caused by mutations in the *DCX* gene, which encodes a microtubule associated protein that stabilizes microtubules causing bundling (Horesh et al. 1999). Accordingly, mutations in *DCX* prevent microtubule stabilization, precluding neurons from migrating into the cortical plate (Gleeson et al. 1999; Taylor et al. 2000). Some forms of SBH can be caused by a small deletion on chromosome 17, involving the *LIS1* gene. Mechanistically, LIS1 targets the cytoplasmic dynein complex in conjunction with NDE1, a microcephaly causing gene. Deletion of LIS1 leads to proliferation defects of apical progenitors due to misorientation of the mitotic spindle, reduced weakened astral microtubules and increase apoptosis.

Disruption in the physiology of adherens junctions can also lead to SBH by affecting aRG morphology and leading to detrimental consequences on the cortical lamination and neuronal migration (Veeraval et al. 2020). Adherens junctions carry out an important aspect of laminar organization, thereby recruiting transmembrane cadherins, catenins, and cytoskeletal adaptor proteins. As such, deletion of α-E-catenin in the mouse cortex causes an uncoupling of adherens junctions with the intracellular actin fibers, which results in loss of tissue polarity and formation of large subcortical heterotopia, as neurons accumulate in heterotopic positions (Schmid et al. 2014). Alteration in cadherins has a similar outcome. Abrogation of N-cadherin in mouse leads to a complete loss of cortical organization with mitotic and post-mitotic cells scattered through the cortex (Kadowaki et al. 2007). Similarly, defects in CDH2 (cadherin 2) results in disruption of adherens junctions and increase in progenitors proliferation, which again leads to subcortical band heterotopia (Gil-Sanz et al. 2014; Rakotomamonjy et al. 2017).

Rho GTPases are fundamental regulators of cytoskeleton organization and cell polarity during neocortical development. Conditional deletion of *RhoA* (Ras homolog family member A) in mouse neural progenitors leads to the disruption of apical anchoring and misorientation of aRG processes, which results in heterotopia underneath a thinner cortex, reminiscent of cobblestone lissencephaly (Cappello et al. 2012). Interestingly, a mutation in RhoA activator, *PLEKHG6* (*Pleckstrin homology and Rho GEF domain containing G6*), was found in human heterotopia and leads to the loss of a primate-specific isoform of this protein (O'Neill et al. 2018).

27.3.3 Polymicrogyria

Polymicrogyria (PMG) is a neurological disorder characterized by an *excessive number of small and fused gyri, creating a disproportionate number of brain folds* (Guerrini and Filippi 2005; Guerrini and Parrini 2010; Verrotti et al. 2010) (Figure 27.3A). Polymicrogyria develops between the late stage of neuronal migration and the early point of cortical organization (Barkovich et al. 2001; Verrotti et al. 2010). Patients with polymicrogyria show a layer of intracortical laminar necrosis and subsequent disruption of late cortical lamination.

Although its mechanism is largely unknown, a rare missense mutation in the *SRPX2* gene causes bilateral perisylvian polymicrogyria, in which the increased number of folds appear near the Sylvian fissure. *SRPX2* encodes for a secreted protein highly expressed in neurons and synapses (Sia et al. 2013). However, while human *SRPX2* is already highly expressed embryonically, measurable expression does not begin until birth in mice (Roll et al. 2006), making difficult to confirm the role of this gene in PMG (Guerrini and Filippi 2005; Guerrini and Parrini 2010).

Genetic insults in the *Rab3 GTPase-activating protein* (*RAB3GAP*) are another leading cause of polymicrogyria (Aligianis et al. 2005). RAB3GAP is a heterodimeric complex that acts as a guanine exchange factor for the RAB18 protein. Mutations in *RAB18* causes Warburg Micro syndrome, which also causes neurodevelopmental abnormalities including polymicrogyria, microcephaly, and pachygyria. Mechanistically, this could be explained by the ability of the RAB3GAP complex to recruit and stabilize the RAB18 protein (Handley et al. 2015). However, which molecular mechanism RAB18 dysfunction leads to these neurodevelopmental aberrations is still unclear.

Although PGM most often occurs as an isolated feature, it sometimes appears in multiple genetic syndromes, including 22q11.2 deletion syndrome, Adams-Oliver syndrome (genetically heterogeneous, caused by mutations in *ARHGAP31, RBPJ, DOCK6, EOGT*, and *NOTCH1*), and Zellweger spectrum (peroxisome biogenesis disorders including Zellweger syndrome, neonatal adrenoleukodystrophy, and Refsum disease) (Dobyns et al. 2008; Mohebbi et al. 2012; Robin et al. 2006).

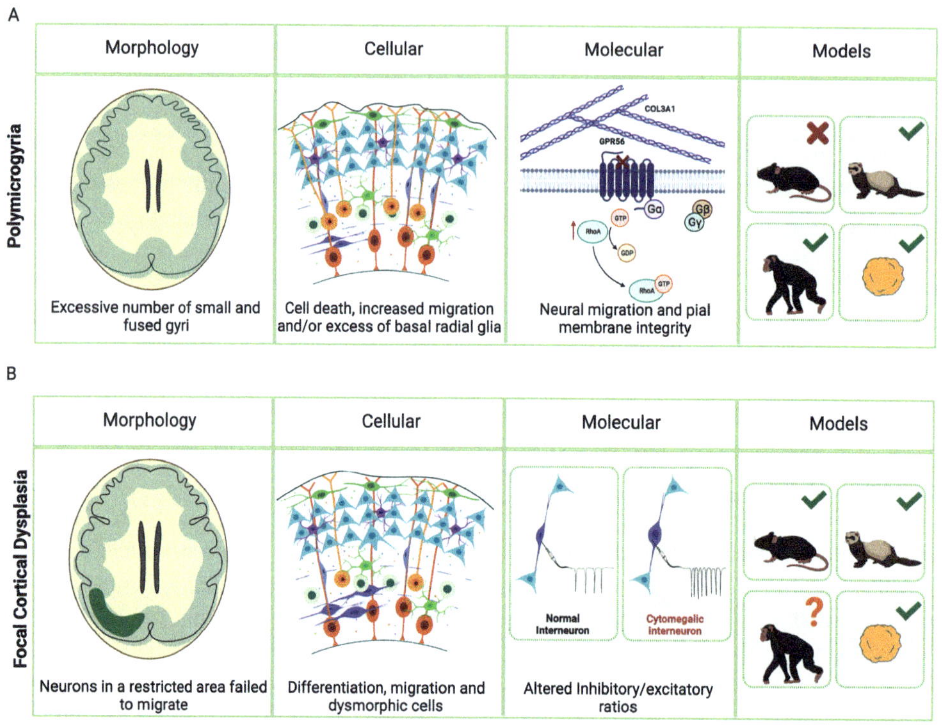

Figure 27.3 Summary of polymicrogyria (A), and focal cortical dysplasia (B) at the morphological, cellular, and molecular level, and model organisms capable of modelling each CM subtype. Created with BioRender.com.

27.4 Interneurons and Focal Cortical Dysplasia

Despite being born within the ganglionic eminence (GE), interneurons (IN) must travel over long distances into the cerebral cortex. They initially migrate tangentially in two streams; they then switch to radial migration to integrate into the various cortical layers. It is therefore foreseeable that defects in interneurons migration led to CMs. Changes in IN distribution and number have been observed in the fetal cortex of patients suffering of Focal Cortical Dysplasia (FCD), a *congenital abnormality in which neurons in a restricted area of the brain failed to migrate* (Nakagawa et al. 2017) (Figure 27.3B). Nevertheless, no differences could be seen at postnatal childhood ages when compared to healthy patients, suggesting a specific effect on migration (Pancoast et al. 2005).

Interestingly, IN seem to contribute to the seizure phenotype of FCD patients. GABA-receptor-mediated inhibition is substantially altered in regions of dysplasia, including a significant reduction in frequency and a potentially compensatory decrease in transporter-mediated GABA reuptake function (Calcagnotto et al. 2005). This suggest that alterations in GABA-mediated synaptic inhibition may play a role in the seizure phenotype in FCD patients. In addition to that, a defining feature of FCD type II is the presence of morphologically aberrant cells, including cytomegalic neurons and balloon cells, which have a single eccentric nucleus with large, homogeneous, and weakly eosinophilic cytoplasm and bear a few enlarged processes. Cytomegalic neurons possess membrane properties that could render them seizure generating, making them a hallmark of severe FCD (Mischel et al. 1995; Najm et al. 2018). Notably, cytomegalic neurons were found to be IN with more complex arborization and possess hyperexcitable properties, including the presence of spontaneous depolarization (Calcagnotto et al. 2005; Cepeda et al. 2006). Nevertheless, it is unclear whether these changes are a secondary effect to the emergence of dysplasia.

One gene that ties abnormal interneuron development to CMs is the *aristaless related homeobox* (*ARX*) gene, which encodes for a transcription factor that acts at several developmental stages including interneuron progenitor proliferation and migration (Friocourt and Parnavelas 2011). Mutations in *ARX* have been linked to lissencephalic brains with a 2–3 layered cortex with diminished neuronal populations and loss of IN (Friocourt and Parnavelas 2010; Marcorelles et al. 2010). However, it is unclear the specific role of IN in CM pathology and whether IN are directly disrupted or are secondarily affected by the abnormal development.

27.4.1 Glial Cells (Microglia, Astrocytes, and Oligodendrocytes)

The generation and expansion of non-neuronal population such as microglia, astrocytes, and oligodendrocytes are overlooked components in CMs etiology.

In the human brain, amoeboid microglial subpopulations enter the forebrain starting at 4.5 postovulatory or gestational weeks (gw) (Monier et al. 2007, 2006). They penetrate the telencephalon and diencephalon via the meninges, choroid plexus, and ventricular zone. Early colonization by amoeboid microglia–macrophages is first restricted to the white matter, where these cells migrate and accumulate in patches at the junctions of white-matter pathways, such as the three junctions that the internal capsule makes with the thalamocortical projection, external capsule, and cerebral peduncle, respectively. In the cerebral cortex anlage, migration is mainly radial and tangential towards the immature white matter, subplate layer, and cortical plate, whereas pial cells populate the prospective layer I. A second wave of microglial cells penetrates the brain via the vascular route at about 12–13 gw and remains confined to the white matter. Two main findings deserve emphasis. First, microglia accumulate at 10–12 gw at the cortical plate–subplate junction, where the first synapses are detected. Second, microglia accumulate in restricted laminar bands, most notably around 19–30 gw, at the axonal crossroads in the white matter (semiovale center) rostrally, extending caudally in the immature white matter to the visual radiations. The spatiotemporal organization of microglia in the immature white and gray matter and experimental data from rodent models support the hypothesis that these cells may play active roles in developmental processes such as axonal guidance, synaptogenesis and synaptic pruning, and neurodevelopmental apoptosis (Paolicelli and Ferretti 2017; Verney et al. 2010). In experimental models, pallium-derived microglia play several roles in neurogenesis, such as regulating the number of $Tbr2^+$ neural progenitors by phagocytosis (Barger et al. 2019; Cunningham et al. 2013) and stimulating neural stem-like cells to differentiate into $Tbr2^+$ intermediate progenitors (Arnò et al. 2014; Hattori and Miyata 2018). Interestingly, excessive exposure to microglia, which was identified in FCD patients, cause neurons in the cortical plate to differentiate abnormally, thus affecting cortical circuits. Additionally, increased numbers of activated microglia were localized around dysplastic neuronal cells, and it was correlated with the duration of the epileptic events, supporting the contribution of microglia in FCD (Boer et al. 2006; Hattori et al. 2020).

Since apical radial glial cells are likely the primary progenitor cells of a significant proportion of neocortical astrocytes (Gressens et al. 1992), mutations that affect aRGs are potentially linked to fewer astrocytes in CMs. Although this was never formally assessed, impaired elimination of extracellular debris by astrocytes may cause a chronically proinflammatory environment, possibly increasing vulnerability to disease (Kielbinski et al. 2016). Intriguingly, astrocytes were recently linked to the gyrification process (Shinmyo et al. 2022). In mice, increase in the astrocytic pool led to gyrification of the usually smooth murine brain, while reduction in the number of astrocytes in ferret lead to reduction in the gyri. Mechanistically, a positive feedback loop of FGF signaling directed by localized astrogenesis seems to be important for cortical folding in mammalian brains, highlighting the underrated importance of astrocytes in human brain development and their potential impact on CMs.

The last wave of gliogenesis in the cortex give rise to mature oligodendrocytes, which deliver structural and metabolic support to neurons through axon myelination. Defects in oligodendrocytes clustering has been very recently associated to mild malformation of cortical development with oligodendroglial hyperplasia in epilepsy (MOGHE) (Schurr et al. 2017). MOGHE is characterized by clumps of oligodendrocytes in the white matter and deep cortical layers, in addition to increased proliferative activity, hypomyelination, and superfluous heterotopic neurons in the white matter. MOGHE patients carry mutations in the *SLC35A2* gene (Bonduelle et al. 2021), which encodes for the major Golgi-localized UDP-galactose translocator (UGT), a translocator essential for glycosylation of proteins and sphingolipids. Inactivation of SLC35A2 abolishes transport of UDP-galactose from the cytosol into the Golgi vesicles, causing the synthesis of aberrant glycans lacking galactose residues (Ng et al. 2019; Sim et al. 2018). However, in what way loss of SLC35A2 function causes ectopic oligodendrocytes is still unclear and needs to be further investigated. Ventrally derived oligodendrocyte precursor cells (OPCs) travel tangentially toward the cortex together with cortical IN and it has recently been shown that these OPCs steer the migration of cortical IN away from the blood vessels to which they were both attracted, thereby allowing IN to reach their proper cortical territories (Lepiemme et al. 2022). In this context, abnormal OPCs could have a negative impact of IN migration and final location.

Thus, glial dysfunction could contribute to the pathology of CMs via creating a local proinflammatory environment driven by abnormal gliovascular interaction (Kielbinski et al. 2016) or altered glycosylation.

27.5 Other Levels of Complexity Contributing to Cortical Malformations

27.5.1 Cortical Connectivity

The complex yet organized interaction of distinct neuronal populations is essential for proper synaptic and cortical connectivity. The abnormalities in location of neuronal populations or presence of abnormal neurons may affect the subsequent developmental steps that control cortical synaptic connectivity, leading to the epileptic phenotype in CM patients. Changes in structural connectivity can also result in impaired tangential growth of the cortex and consequent white matter reduction (Budday et al. 2015). Defects in neuronal layering can rewire brain connectivity of specific circuits, leading to common CMs phenotypes such as epilepsy. As such, patients suffering from heterotopia (Shafi et al. 2015) and focal cortical dysplasia (Hong et al. 2019; Rezayev et al. 2018) often present alteration in long-range connectivity.

In a rat model for microgyria the permanent loss of all connection coming from the white matter is partly compensated by increased intracortical connectivity, with no changes in the number of cortical neurons (Jacobs et al. 1999). Nevertheless, such an area is the most probable site to cause seizures (Timofeev et al. 2014, 2000).

Altered synaptic connectivity can also lead to changes to the rhythmic electrical activity generated spontaneously and in response to stimuli, known as brain oscillations. Changes in the normal network and intrinsically bursting neurons involved in this circuit reorganization could result in either epileptiform activity or abnormal cortical oscillations that would affect the behavior (Chagnac-Amitai and Connors 1989; Chagnac-Amitai et al. 1990). One of such examples is given by FCD, where recurrent excitatory connections are enhanced, and the aberrant synaptic connectivity produces focal epileptogenic areas capable of generating epileptiform (Paz and Huguenard 2015). In both type I and II, the presence of disorganized clusters of neurons and cytomegalic neurons contributes to the increased hyperexcitability and recruitment of microcircuits in the cortex (Abdijadid et al. 2015; Blümcke et al. 2011). Although balloon cells (FCDIIB) are not claimed to be involved in epileptogenesis, they might also play a part in altered brain oscillation by interfering with neuronal connectivity. As a matter of fact, irregularities in high frequency oscillations and hyperexcitability were recorded in type II FCD, independent of the presence of balloon cells (Hu et al. 2019). Intriguingly, in both FCD I and II, the subcortical white matter neurons are disproportionate and are particularly frequent just beneath the U-fiber layer, which serve as short-range association fibers (O'Halloran et al. 2017). The U-fiber initiate from pyramidal neurons of layer 6 of the cortex, operating as short-synaptic circuits that connect neighboring cortical regions or microcircuits (Sarnat 2018). Therefore, neuronal disproportion in the U-fibers compromises the short-range network connections, increasing the microcircuit integration and subsequently altering the structure and function of local network contributing to the epileptic phenotype.

Although FCD is an example of altered connectivity, CMs are not always linked to altered cortical connectivity. Mouse models of CMs demonstrated that ectopic neurons frequently still express their proper laminar markers and possess well-preserved long-range projections (Croquelois et al. 2009; Thompson and Robertson 1987). Moreover, ectopic neurons still attract the proper subtypes of IN as if they were normally positioned in the cortex, signifying that local connectivity might likewise be preserved (Lodato et al. 2011). One of such examples is the Reeler mouse, a well-studied model for lissencephaly. Although distinct layers are no longer visible, L4-type neurons still receive proper innervation from the thalamus and somatotopic innervation of the cortex is relatively preserved (Caviness 1976; Wagener et al. 2010). Consequently, perception, learning, and memory in Reeler mutant mice are marginally affected by disrupted cortical lamination. However, patients with mutations in Reelin, rarely suffer epilepsy, strengthening the idea that improper synaptic connectivity could be one of the consequences in CM epileptic patients.

27.5.2 Extrinsic Factors (Cell Adhesion, ECM, Secreted Molecules)

Mutations in Extracellular Matrix (ECM) genes can also lead to CMs. A noteworthy example is *LAMB1* (laminin subunitβ1), whose mutations cause cobblestone lissencephaly with severe cerebellar dysplasia, brainstem hypoplasia, and occipital encephalocele (Radmanesh et al. 2013). Mechanistically, LAMB1 is a component of the pial basement membrane, and defects in this protein seem to cause defects in the anchoring of radial glial cells to the pial surface. Other proteins involved in the binding of the basal endfoot to the pia are involved in CMs. One of such proteins is *Marcks* (myristoylated alanine-rich substrate protein), a filamentous actin crosslinking protein broadly expressed in the apical membrane of radial progenitors that regulates actin cytoskeleton dynamics (Brudvig and Weimer 2015). Abrogation of *Marcks* in mice instigates disrupted basal endfeet and radial scaffold, which stems in progenitors' displacement and heterotopia (Weimer et al. 2009).

Membrane receptors can also cause CMs, such as GPR56, a receptor that mediates cell matrix adhesion in developing neurons and maintenance of the pial basement membrane integrity and cortical lamination. A deletion in the regulatory region of *GPR56* was identified in patients with polymicrogyria (Bae et al. 2014). GPR56 binds to several ECM components in the basal lamina, such as collagen COL3A1, whose interaction is disrupted by disease-associated mutations (Luo et al. 2012). Intriguingly, Col3a1 knockout in mice results in cortical dyslamination and a cobblestone-like cortical malformation (Luo et al. 2012). Mutations in the extracellular matrix gene *LGALS3BP* (galectin binding protein 3) lead to altered gyrification and neuronal heterotopia in a non-cell autonomous way (Kyrousi et al. 2021). Proteins and nucleic acids can be secreted in a soluble or vesicular manner and can contribute to modulating the extracellular space. Secretion of LGALS3BP through extracellular vesicles (EVs) proved to be crucial for gyrification, as addition of conditioned media of LGALS3BP-enriched human vesicles causes gyrification in mouse cortex, thus emphasizing the potential impact of EVs on neuronal development and MCs.

Likewise, enzymes involved in the production of ECM components have been associated with CMs. ECE2 (endothelin-converting enzyme-2), an enzyme involved in the processing of various neuroendocrine peptides, has recently been found mutated in patients with periventricular heterotopia (Buchsbaum et al. 2020). Genetic manipulation in both mouse and human models showed that ECE2 is important for apico-basal cell polarity, apical belt integrity, actin and microtubule cytoskeleton dynamics, and production of ECM components (Buchsbaum et al. 2020).

Mutations in genes required for the functional maturation of the ECM receptor α-dystroglycan are the most frequent cause of cobblestone lissencephaly (Devisme et al. 2012; LoTurco and Booker 2013; Sherr and Fernandez 2013). These genes encode for enzymes involved in glycosylation of α-dystroglycan, such as POMT1 and 2 (Protein O-mannosyltransferase 1 and 2) (Gan et al. 2021), POMGNT1 (Protein O-linked mannose N-acetylglucosaminyltransferase 1) (Xiong et al. 2006), TMEM5 (Transmembrane protein 5) (Manya et al. 2016), ISPD (Isoprenoid synthase domain containing) (Willer et al. 2012,) and others.

Probably one of the most famous ECM-associated genes involved in CMs is *Reelin*, a large, secreted glycoprotein involved in neuronal migration and proper neuronal layering. Reelin's name comes from the abnormal reeling gait of the Reeler mice, in which Reln gene is abolished (Falconer 1951). Reelin is highly expressed in Cajal–Retzius cells, the major cellular component of the marginal zone thought to have an essential role in the development of layer-specific migration of neurons (Badea et al. 2007; Falconer 1951). Mechanistically, RELN binds VLDLR and ApoER2, two members of the low-density lipoprotein receptor gene family (Hiesberger et al. 1999; Hirota et al. 2015). While VLDLR conducts the stop signal, ApoER2 is necessary for the migration of late-born neurons. Mutations in *RELN* are linked to lissencephaly with cerebellar hypoplasia as well as various neuropsychiatric disorders, such as schizophrenia and depression (Chang et al. 2007; Crino 2001; Ishii et al. 2016). Mutations in RELN linked to lissencephaly usually result in low or undetectable levels of reelin protein (Hong et al. 2000). When reeling is absent, like in the mutant Reeler mouse, the order of cortical layering becomes roughly inverted, with newly born neurons unable to pass through the older layers (Hong et al. 2000).

27.5.3 Environment

27.5.3.1 Ethanol

It is widely known that prenatal alcohol exposure, known as fetal alcohol syndrome (FAS), can trigger severe abnormalities in the developing fetus, including growth deficiency, microcephaly, heterotopias (including over-migration of ectopic neurons in meninges), and associated neurocognitive deficits. Thanks to neuroimaging, several studies have demonstrated functional connectivity disruption and a significant reduction in cortical folding amongst young children exposed to alcohol prenatally (Hendrickson et al. 2017). Rodent-derived cell culture and in vivo models have been extensively used to understand further the underpinning mechanisms behind prenatal alcohol exposure. Several laboratories have shown that part of alcohol's neurotoxicity may be caused by the induction of cell death, loss of proliferation, and cell survival, as well as changes in neuronal migration and neurotransmitters signaling (Hsiao et al. 2004; McAlhany et al. 2000; Mooney and Miller 2001; Mooney et al. 2004; Olney et al. 2002). Moreover, the state of neuronal differentiation partly determines the level of sensitivity to alcohol insult, suggesting windows of higher vulnerability in the developing fetus, although most of the developmental steps of neurons have been shown to be negatively influenced by ethanol. Exposure to ethanol can also cause enlargement of the subventricular zone (SVZ), causing premature neuronal maturation, disorganized cortical architecture, and reduction of lamina V of the rodent neocortex (Kotkoskie and Norton 1989). In addition to that, genetic susceptibility factors can increase vulnerability to in utero ethanol exposure. The identified risk factors include genes like alcohol dehydrogenase, which control the metabolism of ethanol and titrate maternal and fetal blood alcohol levels (Warren and Li 2005). Recently, FAS was modelled in vitro by treating human cerebral organoids with ethanol (Arzua et al. 2020; Zhu et al. 2017). The exposure to ethanol caused organoids to be smaller and with cortical plate disruption and ectopic neurons, which evoked cobblestone lissencephaly and PH. However, the cellular and molecular underpinnings of ethanol's action are still unclear, and further studies need to be carried out.

27.5.3.2 Inflammation

Epilepsy is often associated to phenomena such as oxidative stress (OS) and brain inflammation (Aronica and Crino 2011; Vezzani et al. 2011). Several studies support the existence of a self-sustaining cycle between OS generation and brain inflammation. Neurons are highly vulnerable to oxidative damage because of their post-mitotic stage and high metabolic demand. Expression of OS and inflammatory markers are associated to CMs, such as HME, FCD, and TSC (Arena et al. 2019). Dysmorphic neurons in HME and FCD IIa displayed higher expression of xCT, TLR4, and COX-2. Additionally, iNOS staining was enhanced in FCD IIb in both dysmorphic neurons and glia of cortical tissue of patients.

27.5.3.3 Viruses

Among nongenetic causes of CMs, *in utero* infections are among the most frequent. Several viruses can lead to microcephaly, including cytomegalovirus, HIV, and lymphocytic choriomeningitis virus. Among the most dramatic increases in in congenital microcephaly in the past decade is the recent outbreak of Zika virus (ZIKV) in Brazil. Although adult ZIKV infection was associated with neurological dysfunction such as Guillain-Barré' syndrome, and other CNS (central nervous system) complications, it was commonly assumed that the infection did not have any other side effects. Unfortunately, by the end of 2016, ZIKV infection was known to be responsible for several neurological abnormalities during infancy, such as microcephaly, lissencephaly, loss of brain volume, pachygyria, and ventriculomegaly. Organotypic brain slices from mouse brain showed that virus replication leads to increase apoptosis within the cultures through p53 regulation and impaired neuronal migration into the cortical plate (Rosenfeld et al. 2017). Additionally, ZIKV alters the DNA methylation status of neural progenitor cells, astrocytes, and differentiated neuron genes, 10 percent of which are associated with susceptibility to schizophrenia and bipolar disease. These findings suggest that brain anomalies in babies born after ZIKV infection maybe just the tip of the iceberg, and there might also be a range of neuropsychiatric complications associated with it.

While ZIKV was only recently discovered as an CM causing virus, it has been long known that cytomegalovirus infections (HCMV) are the most common cause of intrauterine and perinatal viral infections in the world (Alford et al. 1990). Mothers infected with cytomegalovirus have an increased risk of having babies with different types of CM, such as microcephaly, schizencephaly, lissencephaly-pachygyria, and polymicrogyria, as well as changes in the white matter signals, temporal cysts, and calcifications (Pascual-Castroviejo et al. 2012). Cellular studies of HCMV infection proved that the infection causes growth and structural abnormalities, probably through, among other molecular pathways, the platelet-derived growth factor receptor (PDGFR) and the epidermal growth factor receptor (EGFR) pathway (Sun et al. 2020). Neuropathological studies have also revealed a tropism of CMV for stem/progenitor cells as well as immune cells, including microglia (Cloarec et al. 2016; Teissier et al. 2014).

27.5.3.4 Radiation

Other environmental factors that might lead to CMs are X-irradiations. Studies on rats at different post-conceptional stages proved that irradiations result in malformed cortical patterns, including abnormal organization and capricious orientation of the neurons (Ferrer et al. 1984). X-irradiations can also cause blockade of proliferation of neural progenitors and/or cell death of these progenitors. In addition, X-irradiations have been shown to induce neuronal cell death, changes in dendritic morphology, decrease of synaptic proteins, and increase of IN (Puspitasari et al. 2020). Some of these disturbances might be related to irradiation-related double-strand breaks in susceptible neural cells (Sakaguchi et al. 2018).

27.5.4 Clinical Heterogeneity

In CM patients, clinical features such as seizures and neurological deficits are highly variable even within mutations in the same gene. From a clinical point of view, heterotopias can, for example, range from inapparent to severe (Barkovich and Kuzniecky 2000; Dubeau et al. 1995), and within this spectrum ~ 40 percent of NMD (neuro-muscular disease) patients present with different types of epilepsy, while the rest are seizure free. Even heterotopic patients that share mutations in the same gene, such as those with familial or sporadic *FLNA* mutations, show phenotypic heterogeneity (Parrini et al. 2006). Similarly, patients with mutations are the *DCX* gene, which is located on the X chromosome, lead to different types of CMs depending on the sex of, namely heterotopia in women and lissencephaly in men (Guerrini and Filippi 2005). Additionally, patients with insults in the *MAP1B* gene can present with a variety of seizures and cognitive impairments (Heinzen et al. 2018). Alas, there is no well-defined parallel between the severity of epileptic events and the extent of CMs (Chang et al. 2005).

The causes of the clinical heterogeneity are many, and here we touch upon a few. Genetic background is one of the most obvious causes of heterogeneity in patients. Genetic interactions between mutations and standing polymorphisms can cause mutations to show distinct phenotypic effects in different individuals (Mullis et al. 2018). Moreover, dosage-dependent gene regulation can give rise to different clinical feature, as in the case of mutations in *DCX* gene in male and females. Nonetheless, understanding of their causal genetic mechanisms remains limited, and it further requires systematic mapping of the interactions between mutations, polymorphisms, and environment that give rise to background effects.

Another important factor in clinical heterogeneity is given by locus-specific mutation. This is particularly true for missense mutations, which can translate into aminoacidic changes in the proteins. Modifications in the protein primary sequence can cause extremely different outcomes, spanning from loss/gain of function to alterations in protein–protein interactions effects. One of such examples is given by missense mutations in *RELN*, whose mutation have been associated with different patterns of lissencephaly (Crino 2001; Riva et al. 2021). Patients with missense mutations in *RELN* were associated with a spectrum of CMs, namely pachygyria or polymicrogyria. Interestingly, these mutations result in different effects on RELN physiology, spanning from changes in secretion, to aberrant cleavage (Riva et al. 2021).

Missense mutations can also alter the post-translational modification (PTM) landscape of any given CM related protein. A protein can be modified by PTM, giving rise to different proteoforms. Combinations of several PTMs are responsible for regulating and fine-tuning protein conformation and activity and can dramatically alter the function of proteins (Smith et al. 2021). It has already been hypothesized for several neurological disease that the type of PTM, their site-specific localization, and their stoichiometry can induce or mediate the severity of a disease, such as Tau aggregation and propagation in Alzheimer disease (Wesseling et al. 2020). Therefore, profiling the specific molecular characteristics of the PTM landscape of CM-associated genes could be another critical step to increasing understanding of the clinical heterogeneity in patients.

27.6 Human and Animal Models

To understand better the underpinning etiology of CMs and therapeutic targets, researchers have employed several model systems. Despite invertebrate models such as *Drosophila melanogaster* and *Danio rerio* contributing to our mechanistic understanding of CMs (Partoens et al. 2021; Rujano et al. 2013), in this section we focus on mammalian models.

Hitherto, rodent models have supported the clinical relevance of CM-associated genetic mutations. Mice knockout (KO) models of CMs associated genes were able to recapitulate basic essential mechanisms that cause CMs such as microcephaly, lissencephaly, and heterotopia. One example is given by *Eml1* KO mice, which recapitulate both the patient phenotype and genetics. Both patients and mice present neuronal heterotopia and perturbed microtubule dynamics (Bizzotto et al. 2017). Likewise, mouse models of cobblestone lissencephaly were equally valuable. Loss-of-function mutations in *Ps1*, *Ilk*, and in the basement membrane receptors such as the alpha 6 integrins, are causative of neuronal over-migration in mice as well, highlighting the value of rodent models in CM research. However, these models lack key anatomical human features that are necessary to fully recapitulate some of the phenotypes observed in the clinical condition (Wong and Roper 2016). While acute knockdown of *Dcx* in rats recapitulates the human phenotype of cortical malformations, the *Dcx* KO mice cannot (Nosten-Bertrand et al. 2008; Ramos et al. 2006). Similarly, mice KO for *Fat4* do not show periventricular heterotopia, but instead possess altered progenitor proliferation (Badouel et al. 2015; Cappello et al. 2013). Although mouse models recapitulate several neurodevelopmental features mechanistically such as the basic steps required for the generation and the migration of excitatory and inhibitory neurons, mouse and human cortex possess several structural and functional differences, including progenitor numbers, types, and expansion capacity, in the composition of the extracellular matrix (Pollen et al. 2015).

To overcome such challenges, researchers moved to models evolutionarily closer to humans, including ferret and nonhuman primates. The ferret neocortex is, for example, gyrified and possesses an outer-SVZ that contains a higher number of bRG compared to mouse (Fietz et al. 2010). Moreover, the neuronal migration dynamics are closer to human than mice, as demonstrated by their tortuous migratory pattern by using processes of multiple neighboring radial glia to scatter laterally and generate a complex cortical architecture (Del Toro et al. 2017; Gertz and Kriegstein

2015). Notably, gene expression can be manipulated in the developing ferret brain by in utero electroporation, making it an emerging model for studying cortical development (Smith et al. 2018).

Nonhuman primates have also been essential in understanding neuronal migration and CMs, due to the high similarity to the human neocortex (Aida and Feng 2020; Bauman and Schumann 2018). The developing cortex of gyrencephalic monkeys clearly possess two distinguishable inner- and outer-SVZ, as well as a higher diversity of precursor cell types compare to rodents. Nevertheless, nonhuman primates possess a smaller cortex, which highlights mechanistical differences between human and nonhuman primates. Several studies focused on such differences, demonstrating that there are differences in terms of timing of neuronal development, migration, and different metabolic rates. Moreover, the long gestation and developmental time, as well as the difficulty of the generation of transgenic animals, make the use of nonhuman primates limiting and inaccessible to most.

In the search of models that could complement in vivo models, several in vitro models have been created. The emergence of stem cell technologies in recent decades made it possible to differentiate human embryonic stem cells (hESCs) and human-induced pluripotent stem cells (iPSCs) in neuronal progenitor cells, as well as neurons and glial cells in two-dimensional (2D). A key advantage of such 2D culture is that they recapitulate the human species-specific molecular clock of development and maturation (Chandrasekaran et al. 2017; Lanjewar and Sloan 2021; Liang et al. 2020). Moreover, these cultures are extremely amenable for gene editing and manipulation, making it easier to go through high-throughput analyses, as well as several other approaches, such as single cell RNA sequencing, live imaging, and proteome wide analyses (Cota-Coronado et al. 2019; McTague et al. 2021).

The main drawback of 2D cultures is the lack of spatial organization, which makes the cellular behavior of such cultures dependent on culture conditions. To overcome that, three-dimensional (3D) cultures have recently been developed to recapitulate in vivo tissue development more closely (Kelava and Lancaster 2016; Lancaster et al. 2017; Lancaster and Knoblich 2014). Stem cells can self-organize to form 3D aggregates, namely embryoid bodies, that give rise to neuroectoderm, which will ultimately produce various CNS lineages. Although several protocols have been set up to generate patterned brain regions, all these approaches result in ventricle-like lumen from which stems a VZ/SVZ-like zone that contains aRG, bIPs, and bRG, and a CP-like zone with neurons of different layer identities, and a marginal-like zone with Cajal–Retzius neurons (Birey et al. 2022; Miura et al. 2022; Pasca 2019; Velasco et al. 2019).

Thanks to this array of 2D and 3D models, it was recently possible to investigate species-specific differences in cortical development and CMs. One of the most remarkable examples is the modelling of lissencephaly. Due to the intrinsic lack of gyrification in the mouse cortex, rodent models do not recapitulate lissencephaly, making human-derived models indispensable. Patients suffering MDS, the most severe form of lissencephaly, display several symptoms such as epilepsy and cognitive impairment. Despite mouse models of this syndrome recapitulating the molecular defects like spindle and migration, they cannot fully recapitulate the complexity of the disease. On the other hand, cerebral organoids generated using patient-derived iPSCs revealed human-specific aberrations in the aRG niche (Bershteyn et al. 2017). As matter of fact, aRG from MDS derived organoids show severe apoptosis and increased horizontal division of aRG, resulting in more neurogenic aRG divisions, overproduction of deep-layer neurons, and smaller organoid size (Bershteyn et al. 2017; Iefremova et al. 2017).

The disadvantages 3D cultures include the high variability in the efficiency of neural induction, in the brain regions generated, and between organoids and batches (Camp et al. 2015; Jabaudon and Lancaster 2018; Quadrato et al. 2017). Organoid size is also currently limited by the diffusion of oxygen and nutrients due to the absence of vascularization. However, the addition of microfilaments and scaffolding can improve neural induction efficiency, as well as the production of regions with dorsal cortical identity, and the generation of radial units (Lancaster et al. 2017).

To overcome drawbacks in 2D and 3D human cultures, in vitro neural cells, or brain organoids can be transplanted into rodents to further increase the complexity (Espuny-Camacho et al. 2013; Mansour et al. 2018). Transplanted human-derived NPCs or neurons migrate into the host tissue, where they can further maturate morphologically and electrophysiologically (Hoffmann et al. 2020; Linaro et al. 2019). Importantly, transplanted neurons show long-term survival, and they integrate into the host neural circuits (Kriks et al. 2011). Using such transplantation models, disease mechanisms can be elucidated by studying the development, migration, integration, and physiological function of neurons in an in vivo environment (Espuny-Camacho et al. 2013; Suzuki and Vanderhaeghen 2015).

Overall, as they are not representative of every possible scenario and represent the current knowledge and state of the art of the field, all models for cortical development and CMs have limitations. Nevertheless, thanks to the complementarity of such models, our understanding of CMs is continuously growing, making us closer to a better understanding of the etiologies of such a complex disorder.

References

Abdijadid, S. et al. (2015). Basic mechanisms of epileptogenesis in pediatric cortical dysplasia. *CNS Neurosci Ther* 21 (2): 92–103. doi: 10.1111/CNS.12345.

Abdullah, U. et al. (2017). A novel mutation in CDK5RAP2 gene causes primary microcephaly with speech impairment and sparse eyebrows in a consanguineous Pakistani family. *Eur J Med Genet* 60 (12): 627–630. doi: 10.1016/J.EJMG.2017.07.017.

Aida, T. and Feng, G. (2020). The dawn of non-human primate models for neurodevelopmental disorders. *Curr Opin Genet Dev* 65: 160–168. doi: 10.1016/J.GDE.2020.05.040.

Alford, C.A. et al. (1990). Congenital and perinatal cytomegalovirus infections. *Rev Infect Dis* 12 (Suppl. 7): S745–S753. doi: 10.1093/CLINIDS/12.SUPPLEMENT_7.S745.

Aligianis, I.A. et al. (2005). Mutations of the catalytic subunit of RAB3GAP cause Warburg Micro syndrome. *Nat Genet* 37 (3): 221–223. doi: 10.1038/NG1517.

Andrews, M.G. et al. (2020). mTOR signaling regulates the morphology and migration of outer radial glia in developing human cortex. *Elife* 9: 1–21. doi: 10.7554/ELIFE.58737.

Arena, A. et al. (2019). Oxidative stress and inflammation in a spectrum of epileptogenic cortical malformations. *Brain Pathol* 29 (3): 351. doi: 10.1111/BPA.12661.

Arnò, B. et al. (2014). Neural progenitor cells orchestrate microglia migration and positioning into the developing cortex. *Nat Commun* 5: 5611. doi: 10.1038/NCOMMS6611.

Aronica, E. and Crino, P.B. (2011). Inflammation in epilepsy. *Epilepsia* 52 Suppl 3 (SUPPL. 3): 26–32. doi: 10.1111/J.1528-1167.2011.03033.X.

Arzua, T. et al. (2020). Modeling alcohol-induced neurotoxicity using human induced pluripotent stem cell-derived three-dimensional cerebral organoids. *Transl Psychiatry* 10 (1): 1–21. doi: 10.1038/s41398-020-01029-4.

Badea, A. et al. (2007). Neuroanatomical phenotypes in the reeler mouse. *Neuromage* 34 (4): 1363. doi: 10.1016/J.NEUROIMAGE.2006.09.053.

Badouel, C. et al. (2015). Fat1 interacts with Fat4 to regulate neural tube closure, neural progenitor proliferation and apical constriction during mouse brain development. *Development* 142 (16): 2781–2791.

doi: 10.1242/DEV.123539/256841/AM/FAT1-INTERACTS-WITH-FAT4-TO-REGULATE-NEURAL-TUBE.

Bae, B.I. et al. (2014). Evolutionarily dynamic alternative splicing of GPR56 Regulates regional cerebral cortical patterning. *Science* 343 (6172): 764–768. doi: 10.1126/SCIENCE.1244392/SUPPL_FILE/1244392S2.MOV.

Barger, N. et al. (2019). Microglia. *Cereb Cortex* 29 (7): 2782–2796. doi: 10.1093/CERCOR/BHY145.

Barkovich, A.J. and Kuzniecky, R.I. (2000). Gray matter heterotopia. *Neurology* 55 (11): 1603–1608. doi: 10.1212/WNL.55.11.1603.

Barkovich, A.J. et al. (2001). Classification system for malformations of cortical development. *Neurology* 57 (12): 2168–2178. doi: 10.1212/WNL.57.12.2168.

Bauman, M.D. and Schumann, C.M. (2018). Advances in nonhuman primate models of autism: integrating neuroscience and behavior. *Exp Neurol* 299 (Pt A): 252. doi: 10.1016/J.EXPNEUROL.2017.07.021.

Bershteyn, M. et al. (2017). Human iPSC-derived cerebral organoids model cellular features of lissencephaly and reveal prolonged mitosis of outer radial glia. *Cell Stem Cell* 20 (4): 435–449.e4. doi: 10.1016/J.STEM.2016.12.007.

Birey, F. et al. (2022). Dissecting the molecular basis of human interneuron migration in forebrain assembloids from Timothy syndrome. *Cell Stem Cell* 29 (2): 248–264.e7. doi: 10.1016/J.STEM.2021.11.011.

Bizzotto, S. et al. (2017). Eml1 loss impairs apical progenitor spindle length and soma shape in the developing cerebral cortex. *Sci Rep* 7 (1): 1–14. doi: 10.1038/s41598-017-15253-4.

Blümcke, I. et al. (2011). The clinicopathologic spectrum of focal cortical dysplasias. *Epilepsia* 52 (1): 158–174. doi: 10.1111/J.1528-1167.2010.02777.X.

Boer, K. et al. (2006). Evidence of activated microglia in focal cortical dysplasia. *J Neuroimmunol* 173 (1): 188–195. doi: 10.1016/J.JNEUROIM.2006.01.002.

Bonduelle, T. et al. (2021). Frequent SLC35A2 brain mosaicism in mild malformation of cortical development with oligodendroglial hyperplasia in epilepsy (MOGHE). *Acta Neuropathol Commun* 9 (1): 1–13. doi: 10.1186/S40478-020-01085-3/FIGURES/4.

Bottega, R. et al. (2019). Functional analysis of the third identified SLC25A19 mutation causative for the thiamine metabolism dysfunction syndrome 4. *J Hum Genet* 64 (11): 1075–1081. doi: 10.1038/S10038-019-0666-5.

Broix, L. et al. (2016). Mutations in the HECT domain of NEDD4L lead to AKT–mTOR pathway deregulation and cause periventricular nodular heterotopia. *Nat Genet* 48 (11): 1349–1358. doi: 10.1038/ng.3676.

Brudvig, J.J. and Weimer, J.M. (2015). X MARCKS the spot. *Front Cell Neurosci* 9: 407. doi: 10.3389/FNCEL.2015.00407.

Buchsbaum, I.Y. et al. (2020). ECE2 regulates neurogenesis and neuronal migration during human cortical development. *EMBO Rep* 21 (5): e48204. doi: 10.15252/EMBR.201948204.

Budday, S. et al. (2015). Secondary instabilities modulate cortical complexity in the mammalian brain. *Philos Mag* 95 (28–30): 3244–3256. doi: 10.1080/14786435.2015.1024184.

Bultje, R.S. et al. (2009). Mammalian Par3 regulates progenitor cell asymmetric division via notch signaling in the developing neocortex. *Neuron* 63 (2): 189–202. doi: 10.1016/J.NEURON.2009.07.004.

Calcagnotto, M.E. et al. (2005). Dysfunction of synaptic inhibition in epilepsy associated with focal cortical dysplasia. *J Neurosci* 25 (42): 9649–9657. doi: 10.1523/JNEUROSCI.2687-05.2005.

Camp, J.G. et al. (2015). Human cerebral organoids recapitulate gene expression programs of fetal neocortex development. *Proc Natl Acad Sci USA* 112 (51): 15672–15677. doi: 10.1073/PNAS.1520760112.

Cappello, S. et al. (2012). A radial glia-specific role of RhoA in double cortex formation. *Neuron* 73 (5): 911–924. doi: 10.1016/J.NEURON.2011.12.030.

Cappello, S. et al. (2013). Mutations in genes encoding the cadherin receptor-ligand pair DCHS1 and FAT4 disrupt cerebral cortical development. *Nat Genet* 45 (11): 1300–1308. doi: 10.1038/ng.2765.

Caviness, V.S. (1976). Patterns of cell and fiber distribution in the neocortex of the reeler mutant mouse. *J Comp Neurol* 170 (4): 435–447. doi: 10.1002/CNE.901700404.

Cepeda, C. et al. (2006). Epileptogenesis in pediatric cortical dysplasia: the dysmature cerebral developmental hypothesis. *Epilepsy Behav* 9 (2): 219–235. doi: 10.1016/J.YEBEH.2006.05.012.

Chagnac-Amitai, Y. and Connors, B.W. (1989). Synchronized excitation and inhibition driven by intrinsically bursting neurons in neocortex. *J Neurophysiol* 62 (5): 1149–1162. 10.1152/JN.1989.62.5.1149.

Chagnac-Amitai, Y. et al. (1990). Burst generating and regular spiking layer 5 pyramidal neurons of rat neocortex have different morphological features. *J Comp Neurol* 296 (4): 598–613. doi: 10.1002/CNE.902960407.

Chandrasekaran, A. et al. (2017). Comparison of 2D and 3D neural induction methods for the generation of neural progenitor cells from human induced pluripotent stem cells. *Stem Cell Res* 25: 139–151. doi: 10.1016/J.SCR.2017.10.010.

Chang, B.S. et al. (2007). The role of RELN in lissencephaly and neuropsychiatric disease. *Am J Med Genet Part B, Neuropsychiatr Genet* 144B (1): 58–63. doi: 10.1002/AJMG.B.30392.

Chang, B.S. et al. (2005). Reading impairment in the neuronal migration disorder of periventricular nodular heterotopia. *Neurology* 64 (5): 799–803. doi: 10.1212/01.WNL.0000152874.57180.AF.

Christ, A. et al. (2012). LRP2 is an auxiliary SHH receptor required to condition the forebrain ventral midline for inductive signals. *Dev Cell* 22 (2): 268–278. doi: 10.1016/J.DEVCEL.2011.11.023.

Cloarec, R. et al. (2016). Cytomegalovirus infection of the rat developing brain in utero prominently targets immune cells and promotes early microglial activation. *PLoS One* 11 (7): e0160176. doi: 10.1371/JOURNAL.PONE.0160176.

Costa, M.R. et al. (2009). Late origin of glia-restricted progenitors in the developing mouse cerebral cortex. *Cereb Cortex* 19 (suppl_1): i135–i143. doi: 10.1093/CERCOR/BHP046.

Costa, M.R. et al. (2008). Par-complex proteins promote proliferative progenitor divisions in the developing mouse cerebral cortex. *Development* 135 (1): 11–22. doi: 10.1242/DEV.009951.

Cota-Coronado, A. et al. (2019). Editing the central nervous system through CRISPR/cas9 systems. *Front Mol Neurosci* 12: 110. doi: 10.3389/FNMOL.2019.00110/BIBTEX.

Crino, P. (2001). New RELN mutation associated with lissencephaly and epilepsy. *Epilepsy Curr* 1 (2): 72. doi: 10.1046/J.1535-7597.2001.00017.X.

Croquelois, A. et al. (2009). Characterization of the HeCo mutant mouse. *Cereb Cortex* 19 (3): 563–575. doi: 10.1093/CERCOR/BHN106.

Cueto-González, A.M. et al. (2020). Unusual context of CENPJ variants and primary microcephaly: compound heterozygosity and nonconsanguinity in an Argentinian patient. *Hum Genome Var* 7 (1): 1–5. doi: 10.1038/s41439-020-0105-3.

Cunningham, C.L. et al. (2013). Microglia regulate the number of neural precursor cells in the developing cerebral cortex. *J Neurosci* 33 (10): 4216–4233. doi: 10.1523/JNEUROSCI.3441-12.2013.

Cushion, T.D. et al. (2013). Overlapping cortical malformations and mutations in TUBB2B and TUBA1A. *Brain: A J Neurol* 136 (Pt 2): 536–548. doi: 10.1093/BRAIN/AWS338.

Del Toro, D. et al. (2017). Regulation of cerebral cortex folding by controlling neuronal migration via FLRT adhesion molecules. *Cell* 169 (4): 621–635.e16. doi: 10.1016/J.CELL.2017.04.012/ATTACHMENT/E0FB0DC8-352F-47D4-AAAF-2893DCCAC4CC/MMC2.MP4.

Devisme, L. et al. (2012). Cobblestone lissencephaly. *Brain* 135 (2): 469–482. doi: 10.1093/BRAIN/AWR357.

Dobyns, W.B. et al. (2008). Consistent chromosome abnormalities identify novel polymicrogyria loci in 1p36.3, 2p16.1-p23.1, 4q21.21-q22.1, 6q26-q27, and 21q2. *Am J Med Genet. Part A* 146A (13): 1637–1654. doi: 10.1002/AJMG.A.32293.

Dobyns, W.B. and Mirzaa, G.M. (2019). Megalencephaly syndromes associated with mutations of core components of the PI3K-AKT–MTOR pathway. *Am J Med Genet Part C: Semin Med Genet* 181 (4): 582–590. doi: 10.1002/AJMG.C.31736.

Dubeau, F. et al. (1995). Periventricular and subcortical nodular heterotopia. A study of 33 patients. *Brain: A J Neurol* 118 (Pt 5): 1273–1287. doi: 10.1093/BRAIN/118.5.1273.

Espuny-Camacho, I. et al. (2013). Pyramidal neurons derived from human pluripotent stem cells integrate efficiently into mouse brain circuits in vivo. *Neuron* 77 (3): 440–456. doi: 10.1016/J.NEURON.2012.12.011.

Falconer, D.S. (1951). Two new mutants, "trembler" and "reeler," with neurological actions in the house mouse (*Mus musculus L.*). *J Genet* 50 (2): 192–205. doi: 10.1007/BF02996215.

Ferent, J. et al. (2020). Extracellular control of radial glia proliferation and scaffolding during cortical development and pathology. *Front Cell Dev Biol* 8: 1031. doi: 10.3389/FCELL.2020.578341/BIBTEX.

Ferrer, I. et al. (1984). Cerebral malformation induced by prenatal X-irradiation. *J Anat* 138 (Pt1): 81. PMCID: PMC1164312.

Fietz, S.A. et al. (2010). OSVZ progenitors of human and ferret neocortex are epithelial-like and expand by integrin signaling. *Nat Neurosci* 13 (6): 690–699. doi: 10.1038/nn.2553.

Fish, J.L. et al. (2006). Aspm specifically maintains symmetric proliferative divisions of neuroepithelial cells. *Proc Natl Acad Sci USA* 103 (27): 10438–10443. doi: 10.1073/PNAS.0604066103/SUPPL_FILE/04066FIG8.PDF.

Florio, M. et al. (2016). A single splice site mutation in human-specific ARHGAP11B causes basal progenitor amplification. *Sci Adv* 2 (12): e1601941. doi: 10.1126/SCIADV.1601941.

Friocourt, G. and Parnavelas, J.G. (2010). Mutations in ARX result in several defects involving GABAergic neurons. *Front Cell Neurosci* 4: 4. doi: 10.3389/FNCEL.2010.00004.

Friocourt, G.M. and Parnavelas, J.G. (2011). Identification of Arx targets unveils new candidates for controlling cortical interneuron migration and differentiation. *Front Cell Neurosci* 5: 1–22. doi: 10.3389/FNCEL.2011.00028/BIBTEX.

Gan, S. et al. (2021). POMT1 and POMT2 gene mutations result in 2 cases of alpha-dystroglycanopathy. *Zhong Nan Da Xue Xue Bao. Yi Xue Ban = J Cent South Univ. Med Sci* 46 (8): 915–919. doi: 10.11817/J.ISSN.1672-7347.2021.200067.

Gertz, C.C. and Kriegstein, A.R. (2015). Neuronal migration dynamics in the developing ferret cortex. *J Neurosci* 35 (42): 14307–14315. doi: 10.1523/JNEUROSCI.2198-15.2015.

Gil-Sanz, C. et al. (2014). Proliferative defects and formation of a double cortex in mice lacking Mltt4 and Cdh2 in the dorsal telencephalon. *J Neurosci* 34 (32): 10475–10487. doi: 10.1523/JNEUROSCI.1793-14.2014.

Gleeson, J.G. et al. (1999). Doublecortin is a microtubule-associated protein and is expressed widely by migrating neurons. *Neuron* 23 (2): 257–271. doi: 10.1016/S0896-6273(00)80778-3.

Gressens, P. et al. (1992). The germinative zone produces the most cortical astrocytes after neuronal migration in the developing mammalian brain. *Neonatology* 61 (1): 4–24. doi: 10.1159/000243526.

Groszer, M. et al. (2001). Negative regulation of neural stem/progenitor cell proliferation by the Pten tumor suppressor gene in vivo. *Science* 294 (5549): 2186–2189. doi: 10.1126/SCIENCE.1065518.

Guerrini, R. and Filippi, T. (2005). Neuronal migration disorders, genetics, and epileptogenesis. *J Child Neurol* 20 (4): 287–299. doi: 10.1177/08830738050200040401.

Guerrini, R. and Parrini, E. (2010). Neuronal migration disorders. *Neurobiol Dis* 38 (2): 154–166. doi: 10.1016/J.NBD.2009.02.008.

Handley, M.T. et al. (2015). Warburg Micro syndrome is caused by RAB18 deficiency or dysregulation. *Open Biol* 5 (6): 150047. doi: 10.1098/RSOB.150047.

Hattori, Y. and Miyata, T. (2018). Microglia extensively survey the developing cortex via the CXCL12/CXCR4 system to help neural progenitors to acquire differentiated properties. *Genes to Cells: Devoted Mol Cell Mechan* 23 (10): 915–922. doi: 10.1111/GTC.12632.

Hattori, Y. et al. (2020). Transient microglial absence assists postmigratory cortical neurons in proper differentiation. *Nat Commun* 11 (1): 1–18. doi: 10.1038/s41467-020-15409-3.

Heinzen, E.L. et al. (2018). De novo and inherited private variants in MAP1B in periventricular nodular heterotopia. *PLoS Genet* 14 (5): e1007281. doi: 10.1371/JOURNAL.PGEN.1007281.

Hendrickson, T.J. et al. (2017). Cortical gyrification is abnormal in children with prenatal alcohol exposure. *Neuroimage: Clin* 15: 391–400. doi: 10.1016/J.NICL.2017.05.015.

Herman, T.E. and Siegel, M.J. (2008). Miller-Dieker syndrome, type 1 lissencephaly. *J Perinatol* 28 (4): 313–315. doi: 10.1038/SJ.JP.7211920.

Hiesberger, T. et al. (1999). Direct binding of Reelin to VLDL receptor and ApoE receptor 2 induces tyrosine phosphorylation of disabled-1 and modulates tau phosphorylation. *Neuron* 24 (2): 481–489. doi: 10.1016/S0896-6273(00)80861-2.

Hirota, Y. et al. (2015). Reelin receptors ApoER2 and VLDLR are expressed in distinct spatiotemporal patterns in developing mouse cerebral cortex. *J Comp Neurol* 523 (3): 463–478. doi: 10.1002/CNE.23691.

Hoffmann, N. et al. (2020). A xenotransplant model of human brain tumors in wild-type mice. *IScience* 23 (1): 100813. doi: 10.1016/J.ISCI.2019.100813.

Hong, S.E. et al. (2000). Autosomal recessive lissencephaly with cerebellar hypoplasia is associated with human RELN mutations. *Nat Genet* 26 (1): 93–96. doi: 10.1038/79246.

Hong, S.J. et al. (2019). A connectome-based mechanistic model of focal cortical dysplasia. *Brain* 142 (3): 688. doi: 10.1093/BRAIN/AWZ009.

Horesh, D. et al. (1999). Doublecortin, a stabilizer of microtubules. *Hum Mol Genet* 8 (9): 1599–1610. doi: 10.1093/HMG/8.9.1599.

Hsiao, S.H. et al. (2004). Critically timed ethanol exposure reduces GABAAR function on septal neurons developing in vivo but not in vitro. *Brain Res* 1008 (1): 69–80. doi: 10.1016/J.BRAINRES.2004.02.020.

Hu, W.H. et al. (2019). Focal cortical dysplasia II-related seizures originate from the bottom of the dysplastic sulcus. *Clin Neurophysiol* 130 (9): 1596–1603. doi: 10.1016/J.CLINPH.2019.05.029.

Iefremova, V. et al. (2017). An organoid-based model of cortical development identifies non-cell-autonomous defects in Wnt signaling contributing to Miller-Dieker syndrome. *Cell Rep* 19 (1): 50–59. doi: 10.1016/J.CELREP.2017.03.047.

Ishii, K. et al. (2016). Reelin and neuropsychiatric disorders. *Front Cell Neurosci* 10: 229. doi: 10.3389/FNCEL.2016.00229/BIBTEX.

Jabali, A. et al. (2022). Human cerebral organoids reveal progenitor pathology in EML1-linked cortical malformation. *EMBO Rep* 23 (5): e54027. doi: 10.15252/EMBR.202154027.

Jabaudon, D. and Lancaster, M. (2018). Exploring landscapes of brain morphogenesis with organoids. *Development* 145 (22): dev172049. doi: 10.1242/DEV.172049.

Jacobs, K.M. et al. (1999). Focal epileptogenesis in a rat model of polymicrogyria. *J Neurophysiol* 81 (1): 159–173. doi: 10.1152/JN.1999.81.1.159.

Jaglin, X.H. et al. (2009). Mutations in the beta-tubulin gene TUBB2B result in asymmetrical polymicrogyria. *Nat Genet* 41 (6): 746. doi: 10.1038/NG.380.

Jang, M.A. et al. (2013). Identification of DCX gene mutation in lissencephaly spectrum with subcortical band heterotopia using whole exome sequencing. *Pediatr Neurol* 48 (5): 411–414. doi: 10.1016/J.PEDIATRNEUROL.2012.12.033.

Janisch, K.M. et al. (2013). The vertebrate-specific Kinesin-6, Kif20b, is required for normal cytokinesis of polarized cortical stem cells and cerebral cortex size. *Development* 140 (23): 4672–4682. doi: 10.1242/DEV.093286.

Jansen, L.A. et al. (2015). PI3K/AKT pathway mutations cause a spectrum of brain malformations from megalencephaly to focal cortical dysplasia. *Brain: J Neurol* 138 (Pt 6): 1613–1628. doi: 10.1093/BRAIN/AWV045.

Johnson, M.B. et al. (2018). Aspm knockout ferret reveals an evolutionary mechanism governing cerebral cortical size. *Nature* 556 (7701): 370–375. doi: 10.1038/s41586-018-0035-0.

Journiac, N. et al. (2020). Cell metabolic alterations due to Mcph1 mutation in microcephaly. *Cell Rep* 31 (2): 107506. doi: 10.1016/J.CELREP.2020.03.070/ATTACHMENT/7C110A48-55C7-4CF2-B4F9-69406603BB88/MMC2.XLSX.

Kadowaki, M. et al. (2007). N-cadherin mediates cortical organization in the mouse brain. *Dev Biol* 304 (1): 22–33. doi: 10.1016/J.YDBIO.2006.12.014.

Kalebic, N. et al. (2019). Neocortical expansion due to increased proliferation of basal progenitors is linked to changes in their morphology. *Cell Stem Cell* 24 (4): 535–550.e9. doi: 10.1016/J.STEM.2019.02.017.

Kalebic, N. and Huttner, W.B. (2020). Basal progenitor morphology and neocortex evolution. *Trends Neurosci* 43 (11): 843–853. doi: 10.1016/J.TINS.2020.07.009.

Kalebic, N. and Namba, T. (2021). Inheritance and flexibility of cell polarity: a clue for understanding human brain development and evolution. *Development* 148 (17) : dev199417. doi: 10.1242/DEV.199417/272121.

Kandachar, V. and Roegiers, F. (2012). Endocytosis and control of Notch signaling. *Curr Opin Cell Biol* 24 (4): 534–540. doi: 10.1016/J.CEB.2012.06.006.

Kantarci, S. et al. (2007). Mutations in LRP2, which encodes the multiligand receptor megalin, cause Donnai-Barrow and facio-oculo-acoustico-renal syndromes. *Nat Genet* 39 (8): 957–959. doi: 10.1038/NG2063.

Kelava, I. and Lancaster, M.A. (2016). Dishing out mini-brains. *Dev Biol* 420 (2): 199–209. doi: 10.1016/j.ydbio.2016.06.037.

Kelley, R.I. et al. (2002). Amish lethal microcephaly: a new metabolic disorder with severe congenital microcephaly and 2-ketoglutaric aciduria. *Am J Med Genet* 112 (4): 318–326. doi: 10.1002/AJMG.10529.

Kielar, M. et al. (2014). Mutations in Eml1 lead to ectopic progenitors and neuronal heterotopia in mouse and human. *Nat Neurosci* 17 (7): 923–933. doi: 10.1038/nn.3729.

Kielbinski, M. et al. (2016). Review: roles for astrocytes in epilepsy. *Neuropathol Appl Neurobiol* 42 (7): 593–606. doi: 10.1111/NAN.12331.

Kim, H. et al. (2010). Filamin A is required for vimentin-mediated cell adhesion and spreading. *Am J Physiol - Cell Physiol* 298 (2): C221. doi: 10.1152/AJPCELL.00323.2009.

Kim, W.Y. and Snider, W.D. (2011). Functions of GSK-3 signaling in development of the nervous system. *Front Mol Neurosci* 4: 44. doi: 10.3389/FNMOL.2011.00044/BIBTEX.

Klaus, J. et al. (2019). Altered neuronal migratory trajectories in human cerebral organoids derived from individuals with neuronal heterotopia. *Nat Med* 25 (4): 561–568. doi: 10.1038/s41591-019-0371-0.

Klingler, E. et al. (2021). Mapping the molecular and cellular complexity of cortical malformations. *Science* 371 (6527): eaba4517. doi: 10.1126/SCIENCE.ABA4517/ASSET/CE42211F-95EE-4AC1-9538-7C768333C224/ASSETS/GRAPHIC/371_ABA4517_FA.JPEG.

Kotkoskie, L.A. and Norton, S. (1989). Morphometric analysis of developing rat cerebral cortex following acute prenatal ethanol exposure. *Exp Neurol* 106 (3): 283–288. doi: 10.1016/0014-4886(89)90161-1.

Kriks, S. et al. (2011). Dopamine neurons derived from human ES cells efficiently engraft in animal models of Parkinson's disease. *Nature* 480 (7378): 547–551. doi: 10.1038/nature10648.

Kumar, R.A. et al. (2010). TUBA1A mutations cause wide spectrum lissencephaly (smooth brain) and suggest that multiple neuronal migration pathways converge on alpha tubulins. *Hum Mol Genet* 19 (14): 2817–2827. doi: 10.1093/HMG/DDQ182.

Kumari, S. et al. (2019). Protein kinase D1 regulates metabolic switch in pancreatic cancer via modulation of mTORC1. *Br J Cancer* 122 (1): 121–131. doi: 10.1038/s41416-019-0629-9.

Kyrousi, C. et al. (2021). Extracellular LGALS3BP regulates neural progenitor position and relates to human cortical complexity. *Nat Commun* 12 (1): 1–22. doi: 10.1038/s41467-021-26447-w.

Lancaster, M.A. et al. (2017). Guided self-organization and cortical plate formation in human brain organoids. *Nat Biotechnol* 35 (7): 659. doi: 10.1038/NBT.3906.

Lancaster, M.A. and Knoblich, J.A. (2014). Generation of cerebral organoids from human pluripotent stem cells. *Nat Protoc* 9 (10): 2329–2340. doi: 10.1038/nprot.2014.158.

Lanjewar, S.N. and Sloan, S.A. (2021). Growing glia. *Front Cell Dev Biol* 9: 592. doi: 10.3389/FCELL.2021.649538/BIBTEX.

Lepiemme, F. et al. (2022). Oligodendrocyte precursors guide interneuron migration by unidirectional contact repulsion. *Science* 376 (6595): eabn6204. doi: 10.1126/SCIENCE.ABN6204.

Li, Y. et al. (2017). Induction of expansion and folding in human cerebral organoids. *Cell Stem Cell* 20 (3): 385–396.e3. doi: 10.1016/J.STEM.2016.11.017.

Liang, X. et al. (2020). Patient-specific neural progenitor cells derived from induced pluripotent stem cells offer a promise of good models for mitochondrial disease. *Cell Tissue Res* 380 (1): 15–30. doi: 10.1007/S00441-019-03164-X/TABLES/1.

Lim, J.S. et al. (2015). Brain somatic mutations in MTOR cause focal cortical dysplasia type II leading to intractable epilepsy. *Nat Med* 21 (4): 395–400. doi: 10.1038/nm.3824.

Linaro, D. et al. (2019). Xenotransplanted human cortical neurons reveal species-specific development and functional integration into mouse visual circuits. *Neuron* 104 (5): 972. doi: 10.1016/J.NEURON.2019.10.002.

Liu, W.A. et al. (2018). PARD3 dysfunction in conjunction with dynamic HIPPO signaling drives cortical enlargement with massive heterotopia. *Genes Dev* 32 (11–12): 763–780. doi: 10.1101/GAD.313171.118.

Lodato, S. et al. (2011). Excitatory projection neuron subtypes control the distribution of local inhibitory interneurons in the cerebral cortex. *Neuron* 69 (4): 763–779. doi: 10.1016/j.neuron.2011.01.015.

López-Tobón, A. et al. (2019). Human cortical organoids expose a differential function of GSK3 on cortical neurogenesis. *Stem Cell Rep* 13 (5): 847–861. doi: 10.1016/J.STEMCR.2019.09.005.

LoTurco, J.J. and Booker, A.B. (2013). Neuronal migration disorders. *Cell Mig Formation Neuronal Connections* 481–494. doi: 10.1016/B978-0-12-397266-8.00038-7.

Luo, R. et al. (2012). Disease-associated mutations prevent GPR56-collagen III interaction. *PloS One* 7 (1): e29818. doi: 10.1371/JOURNAL.PONE.0029818.

Malvezzi, J.V.M. et al. (2018). KIF11 microdeletion is associated with microcephaly, chorioretinopathy and intellectual disability. *Hum Genome Var* 5 (1): 1–3. doi: 10.1038/hgv.2018.10.

Mansour, A.A. et al. (2018). An in vivo model of functional and vascularized human brain organoids. *Nat Biotechnol* 36 (5): 432–441. doi: 10.1038/nbt.4127.

Manya, H. et al. (2016). The muscular dystrophy gene TMEM5 encodes a Ribitol β1,4-Xylosyltransferase required for the functional glycosylation of dystroglycan. *J Biol Chem* 291 (47): 24618. doi: 10.1074/JBC.M116.751917.

Marcorelles, P. et al. (2010). Evidence for tangential migration disturbances in human lissencephaly resulting from a defect in LIS1, DCX and ARX genes. *Acta Neuropathol* 120 (4): 503–515. doi: 10.1007/S00401-010-0692-Z/TABLES/4.

Marsan, E. and Baulac, S. (2018). Review. *Neuropathol Appl Neurobiol* 44 (1): 6–17. doi: 10.1111/NAN.12463.

McAlhany, R.E. et al. (2000). Glial-derived neurotrophic factor (GDNF) prevents ethanol-induced apoptosis and JUN kinase phosphorylation. *Dev Brain Res* 119 (2): 209–216. doi: 10.1016/S0165-3806(99)00171-6.

McCarthy, R.A. et al. (2002). Megalin functions as an endocytic sonic hedgehog receptor. *J Biol Chem* 277 (28): 25660–25667. doi: 10.1074/JBC.M201933200.

McTague, A. et al. (2021). Genome editing in iPSC-based neural systems. *Front Genome Ed* 3: 630600. doi: 10.3389/FGEED.2021.630600.

Mischel, P.S. et al. (1995). Cerebral cortical dysplasia associated with pediatric epilepsy. Review of neuropathologic features and proposal for a grading system. *J Neuropathol Exp Neurol* 54 (2): 137–153. doi: 10.1097/00005072-199503000-00001.

Miura, Y. et al. (2022). Engineering brain assembloids to interrogate human neural circuits. *Nat Protoc* 17 (1): 15–35. doi: 10.1038/s41596-021-00632-z.

Moawia, A. et al. (2017). Mutations of KIF14 cause primary microcephaly by impairing cytokinesis. *Ann Neurol* 82 (4): 562–577. doi: 10.1002/ANA.25044.

Mohebbi, M.R. et al. (2012). Zellweger syndrome and associated brain malformations. *J Child Neurol* 27 (12): 1589–1592. doi: 10.1177/0883073811435918.

Monier, A. et al. (2007). Entry and distribution of microglial cells in human embryonic and fetal cerebral cortex. *J Neuropathol Exp Neurol* 66 (5): 372–382. doi: 10.1097/NEN.0B013E3180517B46.

Monier, A. et al. (2006). Distribution and differentiation of microglia in the human encephalon during the first two trimesters of gestation. *J Comp Neurol* 499 (4): 565–582. doi: 10.1002/CNE.21123.

Moon, H.M. and Wynshaw-Boris, A. (2013). Cytoskeleton in action. *Wiley Int Rev: Dev Biol* 2 (2): 229–245. doi: 10.1002/WDEV.67.

Mooney, S.M. and Miller, M.W. (2001). Effects of prenatal exposure to ethanol on the expression of bcl-2, bax and caspase 3 in the developing rat cerebral cortex and thalamus. *Brain Res* 911 (1): 71–81. doi: 10.1016/S0006-8993(01)02718-4.

Mooney, S.M. et al. (2004). Ethanol induces heterotopias in organotypic cultures of rat cerebral cortex. *Cereb Cortex* 14 (10): 1071–1080. doi: 10.1093/CERCOR/BHH066.

Mullis, M.N. et al. (2018). The complex underpinnings of genetic background effects. *Nat Commun* 9 (1): 1–10. doi: 10.1038/s41467-018-06023-5.

Najm, I.M. et al. (2018). Review. *Neuropathol Appl Neurobiol* 44 (1): 18–31. doi: 10.1111/NAN.12462.

Nakagawa, J.M. et al. (2017). Characterization of focal cortical dysplasia with balloon cells by layer-specific markers. *Epilepsia* 58 (4): 635–645. doi: 10.1111/EPI.13690.

Namba, T. et al. (2020). Human-specific ARHGAP11B acts in mitochondria to expand neocortical progenitors by glutaminolysis. *Neuron* 105 (5): 867–881.e9. doi: 10.1016/J.NEURON.2019.11.027.

Namba, T. et al. (2021). Metabolic regulation of neocortical expansion in development and evolution. *Neuron* 109 (3): 408–419. doi: 10.1016/J.NEURON.2020.11.014.

Naseer, M.I. et al. (2017). A novel WDR62 mutation causes primary microcephaly in a large consanguineous Saudi family. *Ann Saudi Med* 37 (2): 148. doi: 10.5144/0256-4947.2017.148.

Ng, B.G. et al. (2019). SLC35A2-CDG: functional characterization, expanded molecular, clinical, and biochemical phenotypes of 30 unreported individuals. *Hum Mutat* 40 (7): 908–925. doi: 10.1002/HUMU.23731.

Nosten-Bertrand, M. et al. (2008). Epilepsy in Dcx knockout mice associated with discrete lamination defects and enhanced excitability in the hippocampus. *PLoS One* 3 (6): e2473. doi: 10.1371/JOURNAL.PONE.0002473.

Nowakowski, T.J. et al. (2017). Spatiotemporal gene expression trajectories reveal developmental hierarchies of the human cortex. *Science* 358 (6368): 1318–1323. doi: 10.1126/SCIENCE.AAP8809.

O'Halloran, R. et al. (2017). A method for U-fiber quantification from 7T diffusion-weighted MRI data tested in subjects with non-lesional focal epilepsy. *Neuroreport* 28 (8): 457. doi: 10.1097/WNR.0000000000000788.

O'Neill, A.C. et al. (2018). A primate-specific isoform of PLEKHG6 regulates neurogenesis and neuronal migration. *Cell Rep* 25: 2729–2741.e6. doi: 10.1016/j.celrep.2018.11.029.

Olney, J.W. et al. (2002). Ethanol-induced apoptotic neurodegeneration in the developing C57BL/6 mouse brain. *Brain Res. Dev Brain Res* 133 (2): 115–126. doi: 10.1016/s0165-3806(02)00279-1.

Pancoast, M. et al. (2005). Interneuron deficits in patients with the Miller-Dieker syndrome. *Acta Neuropathol* 109 (4): 400–404. doi: 10.1007/S00401-004-0979-Z/TABLES/1.

Paolicelli, R.C. and Ferretti, M.T. (2017). Function and dysfunction of microglia during brain development. *Front Synaptic Neurosci* 9: 9. doi: 10.3389/FNSYN.2017.00009/BIBTEX.

Parrini, E. et al. (2006). Periventricular heterotopia. *Brain: J Neurol* 129 (Pt 7): 1892–1906. doi: 10.1093/BRAIN/AWL125.

Partoens, M. et al. (2021). Modeling neurodevelopmental disorders and epilepsy caused by loss of function of *kif2a* in zebrafish. *eNeuro* 8 (5): 1–17. doi: 10.1523/ENEURO.0055-21.2021.

Pasca, S.P. (2019). Assembling human brain organoids. *Science* 363 (6423): 126–127. doi: 10.1126/SCIENCE.AAU5729.

Pascual-Castroviejo, I. et al. (2012). Congenital cytomegalovirus infection and cortical/subcortical malformations. *Neurologia (English Edition)* 27 (6): 336–342. doi: 10.1016/J.NRLENG.2012.07.013.

Passemard, S. et al. (2019). Endoplasmic reticulum and Golgi stress in microcephaly. *Cell Stress* 3 (12): 369–384. doi: 10.15698/CST2019.12.206.

Paz, J.T. and Huguenard, J.R. (2015). Microcircuits and their interactions in epilepsy: is the focus out of focus? *Nat Neurosci* 18 (3): 351–359. doi: 10.1038/NN.3950.

Pilz, D.T. et al. (1998). LIS1 and XLIS (DCX) mutations cause most classical lissencephaly, but different patterns of malformation. *Hum Mol Genet* 7 (13): 2029–2037. doi: 10.1093/HMG/7.13.2029.

Poirier, K. et al. (2013). Mutations in TUBG1, DYNC1H1, KIF5C and KIF2A cause malformations of cortical development and microcephaly. *Nat Genet* 45 (6): 639–647. doi: 10.1038/NG.2613.

Pollen, A.A. et al. (2015). Molecular identity of human outer radial glia during cortical development. *Cell* 163 (1): 55–67. doi: 10.1016/J.CELL.2015.09.004.

Prüfer, K. et al. (2014). The complete genome sequence of a Neanderthal from the Altai Mountains. *Nature* 505 (7481): 43–49. doi: 10.1038/NATURE12886.

Pulvers, J.N. et al. (2015). MCPH1. *Front Cell Neurosci* 9: 92. doi: 10.3389/FNCEL.2015.00092.

Puspitasari, A. et al. (2020). X-irradiation of developing hippocampal neurons causes changes in neuron population phenotypes, dendritic morphology and synaptic protein expression in surviving neurons at maturity. *Neurosci Res* 160: 11–24. doi: 10.1016/J.NEURES.2019.11.002.

Quadrato, G. et al. (2017). Cell diversity and network dynamics in photosensitive human brain organoids. *Nature* 545 (7652): 48–53. doi: 10.1038/nature22047.

Radmanesh, F. et al. (2013). Mutations in LAMB1 cause cobblestone brain malformation without muscular or ocular abnormalities. *Am J Hum Genet* 92 (3): 468–474. doi: 10.1016/J.AJHG.2013.02.005.

Rakotomamonjy, J. et al. (2017). Afadin controls cell polarization and mitotic spindle orientation in developing cortical radial glia. *Neural Dev* 12 (1): 1–10. doi: 10.1186/S13064-017-0085-2/FIGURES/5.
Ramos, R.L. et al. (2006). Heterotopia formation in rat but not mouse neocortex after RNA interference knockdown of DCX. *Cereb Cortex* 16 (9): 1323–1331. doi: 10.1093/CERCOR/BHJ074.
Rapaport, D. et al. (2010). Loss of SNAP29 impairs endocytic recycling and cell motility. *PLoS One* 5 (3): e9759. doi: 10.1371/JOURNAL.PONE.0009759.
Reijnders, M.R.F. et al. (2017). Variation in a range of mTOR-related genes associates with intracranial volume and intellectual disability. *Nat Commun* 8 (1): 1–12. doi: 10.1038/s41467-017-00933-6.
Rezayev, A. et al. (2018). Bilateral thalamocortical abnormalities in focal cortical dysplasia. *Brain Res* 1694: 38–45. doi: 10.1016/J.BRAINRES.2018.05.005.
Riva, M. et al. (2021). Functional characterization of RELN missense mutations involved in recessive and dominant forms of Neuronal Migration Disorders. *BioRxiv* 2021.05.25.445586. doi: 10.1101/2021.05.25.445586.
Robin, N.H. et al. (2006). Polymicrogyria and deletion 22q11.2 syndrome. *Am J Med Genet. Part A* 140 (22): 2416–2425. doi: 10.1002/AJMG.A.31443.
Roll, P. et al. (2006). SRPX2 mutations in disorders of language cortex and cognition. *Hum Mol Genet* 15 (7): 1195–1207. doi: 10.1093/HMG/DDL035.
Rosenfeld, A.B. et al. (2017). Replication of early and recent Zika virus isolates throughout mouse brain development. *Proc Natl Acad Sci USA* 114 (46): 12273–12278. doi: 10.1073/PNAS.1714624114/SUPPL_FILE/PNAS.201714624SI.PDF.
Rujano, M.A. et al. (2013). The microcephaly protein Asp regulates neuroepithelium morphogenesis by controlling the spatial distribution of myosin II. *Nat Cell Biol* 15 (11): 1294–1306. doi: 10.1038/ncb2858.
Sakaguchi, K. et al. (2018). High susceptibility of mouse newborns to delayed appearance of DNA double-strand breaks in neural stem/progenitor cells exposed to ionizing radiation. *J Rad Res* 59 (6): 685–691. doi: 10.1093/JRR/RRY069.
Sarnat, H.B. (2018). The 2016 Bernard Sachs Lecture. *Pediat Neurol* 83: 3–13. doi: 10.1016/J.PEDIATRNEUROL.2017.08.015.
Sarnat, H.B. and Flores-Sarnat, L. (2015). Infantile tauopathies. *Brain Dev* 37 (6): 553–562. doi: 10.1016/J.BRAINDEV.2014.08.010.
Schmid, M.T. et al. (2014). The role of α-E-catenin in cerebral cortex development: radial glia specific effect on neuronal migration. *Front Cell Neurosci* 8: 215. doi: 10.3389/FNCEL.2014.00215.
Schurr, J. et al. (2017). Mild malformation of cortical development with oligodendroglial hyperplasia in frontal lobe epilepsy. *Brain Pathol* 27 (1): 26. doi: 10.1111/BPA.12347.
Severino, M. et al. on behalf of the European Network on Brain Malformations (Neuro-MIG). (2020). Definitions and classification of malformations of cortical development. *Brain* 143 (10): 2874–2894. doi: 10.1093/BRAIN/AWAA174.
Sgourdou, P. et al. (2017). Disruptions in asymmetric centrosome inheritance and WDR62-Aurora kinase B interactions in primary microcephaly. *Sci Rep* 7: 43708. doi: 10.1038/SREP43708.
Shafi, M.M. et al. (2015). Physiological consequences of abnormal connectivity in a developmental epilepsy. *Ann Neurol* 77 (3): 487–503. doi: 10.1002/ANA.24343.
Sheen, V.L. et al. (2001). Mutations in the X-linked filamin 1 gene cause periventricular nodular heterotopia in males as well as in females. *Hum Mol Genet* 10 (17): 1775–1783. doi: 10.1093/HMG/10.17.1775.
Sheen, V.L. et al. (2006). Impaired proliferation and migration in human Miller-Dieker neural precursors. *Ann Neurol* 60 (1): 137–144. doi: 10.1002/ANA.20843.
Sheen, V.L. et al. (2004). Mutations in ARFGEF2 implicate vesicle trafficking in neural progenitor proliferation and migration in the human cerebral cortex. *Nat Genet* 36 (1): 69–76. doi: 10.1038/NG1276.

Sheen, V.L. et al. (2003). Periventricular heterotopia associated with chromosome 5p anomalies. *Neurology* 60 (6): 1033–1036. doi: 10.1212/01.WNL.0000052689.03214.61.

Sherr, E.H. and Fernandez, L. (2013). Lissencephalies and axon guidance disorders. *Neural Circuit Dev Funct Heathy Dis Brain* 573–615. doi: 10.1016/B978-0-12-397267-5.00128-X.

Shinmyo, Y. et al. (2022). Localized astrogenesis regulates gyrification of the cerebral cortex. *Sci Adv* 8 (10): 5209. doi: 10.1126/SCIADV.ABI5209/SUPPL_FILE/SCIADV.ABI5209_SM.PDF.

Sia, G.M. et al. (2013). The human language-associated gene SRPX2 regulates synapse formation and vocalization in mice. *Science* 342 (6161): 987–991. doi: 10.1126/SCIENCE.1245079.

Sim, N.S. et al. (2018). Brain somatic mutations in SLC35A2 cause intractable epilepsy with aberrant N-glycosylation. *Neurol Genet* 4 (6): e294. doi: 10.1212/NXG.0000000000000294.

Smith, L.M. et al. (2021). The human proteoform project. *Sci Adv* 7 (46): 734. doi: 10.1126/SCIADV.ABK0734/SUPPL_FILE/SCIADV.ABK0734_SM.PDF.

Smith, R.S. et al. (2018). Sodium channel SCN3A (NaV1.3) regulation of human cerebral cortical folding and oral motor development. *Neuron* 99 (5): 905–913.e7. doi: 10.1016/J.NEURON.2018.07.052/ATTACHMENT/68335E5B-393D-4D45-B118-AAD276D7538B/MMC1.PDF.

Sprecher, E. et al. (2005). A mutation in SNAP29, coding for a SNARE protein involved in intracellular trafficking, causes a novel neurocutaneous syndrome characterized by cerebral dysgenesis, neuropathy, ichthyosis, and palmoplantar keratoderma. *Am J Hum Genet* 77 (2): 242–251. doi: 10.1086/432556.

Sudmant, P.H. et al. (2010). Diversity of human copy number variation and multicopy genes. *Science* 330 (6004): 641–646. doi: 10.1126/SCIENCE.1197005.

Sun, G. et al. (2020). Modeling human cytomegalovirus-induced microcephaly in human iPSC-derived brain organoids. *Cell Rep Med* 1 (1): 100002. doi: 10.1016/J.XCRM.2020.100002.

Suzuki, I.K. and Vanderhaeghen, P. (2015). Is this a brain which I see before me? Modeling human neural development with pluripotent stem cells. *Development* 142 (18): 3138–3150. doi: 10.1242/DEV.120568.

Taylor, K.R. et al. (2000). Patient mutations in doublecortin define a repeated tubulin-binding domain. *J Biol Chem* 275 (44): 34442–34450. doi: 10.1074/JBC.M007078200.

Teissier, N. et al. (2014). Cytomegalovirus-induced brain malformations in fetuses. *J Neuropathol Exp Neurol* 73 (2): 143–158. doi: 10.1097/NEN.0000000000000038.

Thompson, S.M. and Robertson, R.T. (1987). Organisation of subcortical pathways for sensory projections to the limbic cortex. I. Subcortical projections to the medial limbic cortex in the rat. *J Comp Neurol* 265 (2): 175–188. doi: 10.1002/CNE.902650203.

Timofeev, I. et al. (2014). Neocortical focus: experimental view. *Int Rev Neurobiol* 114: 9–33. doi: 10.1016/B978-0-12-418693-4.00002-9.

Timofeev, I. et al. (2000). Origin of slow cortical oscillations in deafferented cortical slabs. *Cereb Cortex* 10 (12): 1185–1199. doi: 10.1093/CERCOR/10.12.1185.

Togawa, A. et al. (1999). Purification and cloning of a brefeldin A-inhibited guanine nucleotide-exchange protein for ADP-ribosylation factors. *J Biol Chem* 274 (18): 12308–12315. doi: 10.1074/JBC.274.18.12308.

Tokuda, S. et al. (2011). A novel Akt3 mutation associated with enhanced kinase activity and seizure susceptibility in mice. *Hum Mol Genet* 20 (5): 988. doi: 10.1093/HMG/DDQ544.

Veeraval, L. et al. (2020). Adherens junctions: guardians of cortical development. *Front Cell Dev Biol* 8: 6. doi: 10.3389/FCELL.2020.00006/BIBTEX.

Velasco, S. et al. (2019). Individual brain organoids reproducibly form cell diversity of the human cerebral cortex. *Nature* 570 (7762): 523–527. doi: 10.1038/s41586-019-1289-x.

Verney, C. et al. (2010). Early microglial colonization of the human forebrain and possible involvement in periventricular white-matter injury of preterm infants. *J Anat* 217 (4): 436–448. doi: 10.1111/J.1469-7580.2010.01245.X.

Verrotti, A. et al. (2010). New trends in neuronal migration disorders. *Eur J Paediat Neurol* 14 (1): 1–12. doi: 10.1016/J.EJPN.2009.01.005.

Vezzani, A. et al. (2011). The role of inflammation in epilepsy. *Nat Rev Neurol* 7 (1): 31–40. doi: 10.1038/NRNEUROL.2010.178.

Wagener, R. J. et al. (2010). The somatosensory cortex of reeler mutant mice shows absent layering but intact formation and behavioral activation of columnar somatotopic maps. *J Neurosci* 30 (46): 15700–15709. doi: 10.1523/JNEUROSCI.3707-10.2010.

Warren, K.R. and Li, T.K. (2005). Genetic polymorphisms: impact on the risk of fetal alcohol spectrum disorders. *Birth Defects Res Part A, Clin Mol Teratol* 73 (4): 195–203. doi: 10.1002/BDRA.20125.

Weimer, J.M. et al. (2009). MARCKS modulates radial progenitor placement, proliferation and organization in the developing cerebral cortex. *Development* 136 (17): 2965–2975. doi: 10.1242/DEV.036616.

Wesseling, H. et al. (2020). Tau PTM profiles identify patient heterogeneity and stages of Alzheimer's disease. *Cell* 183 (6): 1699–1713.e13. doi: 10.1016/J.CELL.2020.10.029.

Willer, T. et al. (2012). ISPD loss-of-function mutations disrupt dystroglycan O-mannosylation and cause Walker-Warburg syndrome. *Nat Genet* 44 (5): 575–580. doi: 10.1038/NG.2252.

Wong, M. and Roper, S.N. (2016). Genetic animal models of malformations of cortical development and epilepsy. *J Neurosci Methods* 260: 73–82. doi: 10.1016/J.JNEUMETH.2015.04.007.

Xiong, H. et al. (2006). Molecular interaction between fukutin and POMGnT1 in the glycosylation pathway of alpha-dystroglycan. *Biochem Biophys Res Commun* 350 (4): 935–941. doi: 10.1016/J.BBRC.2006.09.129.

Yang, L. et al. (2017). Glutaminolysis: a hallmark of cancer metabolism. *Ann Rev Biomed Eng* 19: 163–194. doi: 10.1146/ANNUREV-BIOENG-071516-044546.

Yokota, Y. et al. (2010). Cdc42 and Gsk3 modulate the dynamics of radial glial growth, inter-radial glial interactions and polarity in the developing cerebral cortex. *Development* 137 (23): 4101–4110. doi: 10.1242/DEV.048637.

Yoon, W.H. et al. (2017). Loss of nardilysin, a mitochondrial co-chaperone for α-ketoglutarate dehydrogenase, promotes mTORC1 activation and neurodegeneration. *Neuron* 93 (1): 115–131. doi: 10.1016/J.NEURON.2016.11.038/ATTACHMENT/D88275A2-8D92-4DEF-9336-AFAD953A2CF8/MMC1.PDF.

Yoshida, A. et al. (2001). Muscular dystrophy and neuronal migration disorder caused by mutations in a glycosyltransferase, POMGnT1. *Dev Cell* 1 (5): 717–724. doi: 10.1016/S1534-5807(01).

Zaqout, S. and Kaindl, A.M. (2022). Autosomal recessive primary microcephaly. *Front Cell Dev Biol* 9: 3635. doi: 10.3389/FCELL.2021.784700/BIBTEX.

Zhang, J. et al. (2013). Filamin a regulates neuronal migration through brefeldin a-inhibited guanine exchange factor 2-dependent Arf1 activation. *J Neurosci* 33 (40): 15735–15746. doi: 10.1523/JNEUROSCI.1939-13.2013.

Zhu, Y. et al. (2017). Probing impaired neurogenesis in human brain organoids exposed to alcohol. *Int Biol: Quant Biosci Nano to Macro* 9 (12): 968–978. doi: 10.1039/C7IB00105C.

Part 8

Overarching Topics

28

Posttranscriptional Control of Brain Development

Camila Manso Musso[1], Bianca M. Lupan[1], and Debra L. Silver[1,2]

[1] Department of Molecular Genetics and Microbiology, Duke University Medical Center, Durham, NC 27710, USA
[2] Departments of Cell Biology and Neurobiology, Duke Regeneration Center, Duke Institute for Brain Sciences, Duke University Medical Center, Durham, NC 27710, USA

28.1 Introduction

28.1.1 Cortical Development Overview

The brain is one of the most complex organs in the human body (Figure 28.1). The cerebral neocortex, the most recently evolved structure of the brain, is responsible for humans' higher cognitive abilities such as language, perception, and emotion (Defelipe 2011). It is composed of distinct neurons radially organized in six layers and tangentially divided into specialized functional areas (Greig et al. 2013). At the onset of embryonic corticogenesis, the dorsal telencephalon is composed of a neuroepithelium. Neuroepithelial precursors undergo self-renewing divisions to expand the progenitor pool. Subsequently, they generate neural progenitors termed radial glial cells (RGCs), which give rise to neurons and ultimately glial cells (Kriegstein and Alvarez-Buylla 2009). RGCs produce neurons directly, or more commonly, indirectly via basal progenitors (Malatesta et al. 2000; Noctor et al. 2001). In mice, basal progenitors are predominantly composed of intermediate progenitors (IPs) which undergo one to two self-renewing divisions before producing neurons. In contrast, the human neocortex develops from enlarged populations of basal progenitors called outer radial glial cells (oRGCs or basal radial glia, bRGCs) (Dehay et al. 2015). RGCs are bipolar, with the cell body located near the ventricle and a long basal process spanning the cortex and attached to a basement membrane at the pial surface. This RGC cellular structure provides a scaffold for new-born excitatory neurons to migrate into the cortical plate (Greig et al. 2013; Pinson and Huttner 2021). The cortical plate is formed in an inside-out fashion, whereby the deepest layers (V, VI) are generated at the onset of neurogenesis and the late-born neurons migrate past the early-born neurons to occupy the superficial layers (IV, II/III). These neurons mature and ultimately establish distinct circuits via callosal, corticofugal and corticothalamic projections.

28.1.2 *Cis* and *Trans* Control of RNA

Due to its complexity, cortical development requires tightly orchestrated control of gene expression at many levels (Figure 28.1). In particular, gene expression regulation at the level of RNA is essential for proper cortical development (Figure 28.2). Posttranscriptional control modulates RNA from the moment it is transcribed until it reaches the cytoplasm and includes alternative splicing, RNA stability, RNA modifications, subcellular localization, and translational control (Chen and Hu 2017; Corbett 2018; Lennox et al. 2018, 2020; Licatalosi and Darnell 2010; Pilaz and

Neocortical Neurogenesis in Development and Evolution, First Edition. Edited by Wieland B. Huttner.

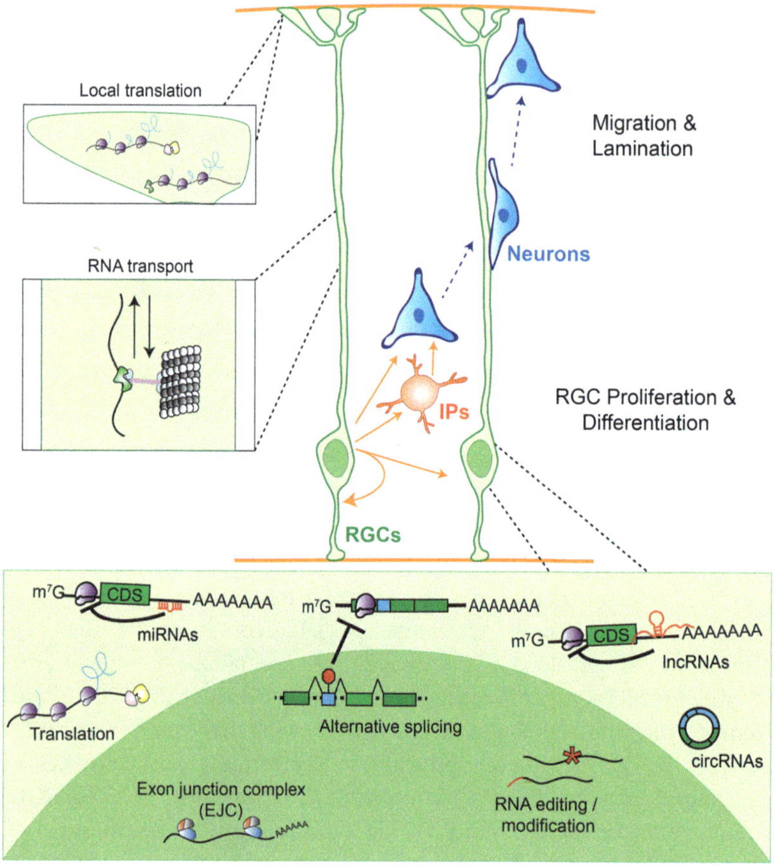

Figure 28.1 Posttranscriptional regulation of cortical development. Posttranscriptional processes collectively influence critical stages of corticogenesis: radial glial cell (RGC, green) proliferation, neuronal differentiation (excitatory neurons, blue), and migration and lamination. RGCs can undergo symmetric, self-renewing divisions or generate excitatory neurons either directly or indirectly through intermediate progenitors (IPs, orange). New-born neurons use the RGC scaffold to migrate to their final destination in the cortical plate.

Silver 2015; Ye and Blelloch 2014). These RNA fates are ultimately controlled by both *cis*- and *trans*-regulatory factors. *Trans*-factors include RNA-binding proteins (RBPs) and noncoding RNAs (ncRNAs) that recognize RNA via specific *cis* elements conferred by nucleotide sequences and/or secondary structures.

To date, more than 1,500 RBPs have been identified in humans (Gerstberger et al. 2014). Amongst these, at least 320 have been shown to be expressed throughout the developing neocortex (DeBoer et al. 2013; Gerstberger et al. 2014; McKee et al. 2005), though there are likely many more. RBPs interact with RNA to form ribonucleoprotein (RNP) complexes. The subcellular localization of an RBP within the nucleus or cytoplasm may underlie its regulatory functions including for several aspects of posttranscriptional control (Van Nostrand et al. 2021). For example, the RBP NOVA regulates both alternative splicing and poly(A)-site usage to control neuronal migration in the cortex. A large number of ncRNAs are also encoded within our genome (6 Non-coding RNA characterization 2019), including short ncRNAs (microRNAs, siRNAs, and piRNAs), long ncRNAs, and circular ncRNA. Growing evidence implicates these ncRNAs in cortical development (Salvatori et al. 2020). In this chapter we discuss the different classes of posttranscriptional control at play

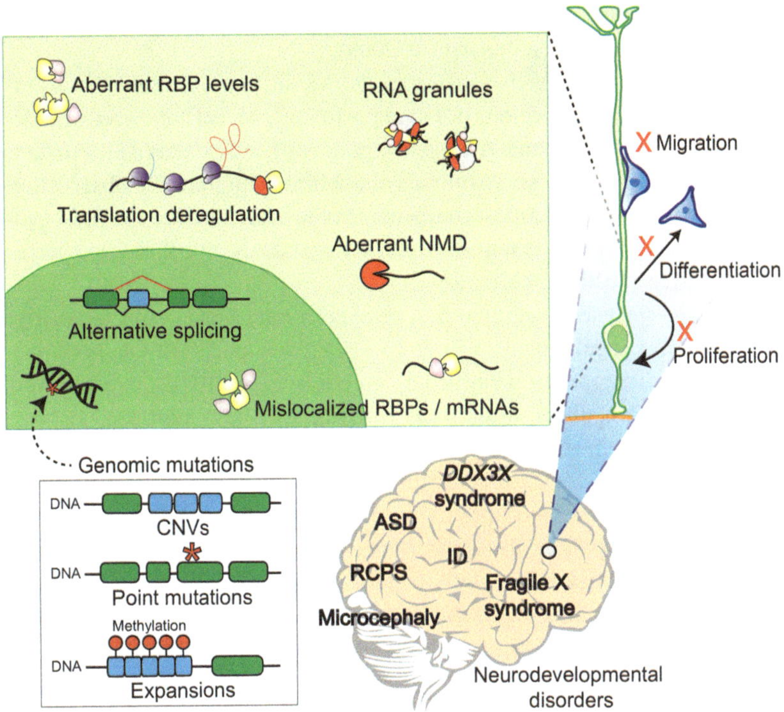

Figure 28.2 Dysregulation of posttranscriptional processes in neurodevelopmental disorders. Human mutations are associated with perturbations of posttranscriptional processes that consequently can disrupt cortical development. This may ultimately contribute to neurodevelopmental disorders such as microcephaly, intellectual disability (ID), autism spectrum disorder (ASD), Richieri-Costa-Pereira syndrome (RCPS), DDX3X syndrome, and Fragile X syndrome (FXS). RBPs – RNA-binding proteins; NMD – nonsense mediated decay; CNVs – copy number variations.

during cortical development. We further highlight selected examples of RBPs and noncoding RNAs that function during key processes of proliferation, differentiation, and neuronal migration.

28.2 Splicing

28.2.1 Alternative Splicing in the Brain

Overview: A major source of RNA diversity is alternative splicing (AS), a process that is particularly prevalent in the brain (Licatalosi and Darnell 2010). Tissue-specific splicing is highly conserved, having evolved as least 400 million years ago (Rodriguez et al. 2020). In contrast, three in four alternative exons emerged specifically in the primate lineage, implicating AS in evolution of tissues such as brain (Lin et al. 2010; Rodriguez et al. 2020).

AS is highly dynamic over the course of cortical development and across cell types. Indeed, developmentally dynamic AS events are especially frequent in the brain (Mazin et al. 2021; Rodriguez et al. 2020). Several studies have generated valuable AS atlases of cortical development in humans and mice (Dillman et al. 2013; Johnson et al. 2009; Mazin et al. 2021; Polioudakis et al. 2019; Rodriguez et al. 2020; Weyn-Vanhentenryck et al. 2018; Yan et al. 2015; Zhang et al. 2016; Zhu et al. 2018). These studies reveal a number of splicing events of interest, such as AS of the axon guidance gene *ROBO1* during human prefrontal cortex development (Johnson et al. 2009).

Single-cell comparative transcriptomes have also shed light on AS during evolution. For example, analysis of 16 human and macaque brain regions pre- and postnatally reveal concerted ontogenetic and phylogenetic cup-shaped transcriptome divergence patterns (Zhu et al. 2018). Further, analysis of pre- and postnatal development in six mammals and a bird reinforces the observation that developmentally dynamic AS events occur most frequently in the brain and are the most evolutionarily conserved (Mazin et al. 2021). The extent to which divergent AS contributes to species differences in the cortex is an active question of interest.

RBPs play key roles in AS during cortical development. A prime example is the family of polypyrimidine tract-binding (PTB) splicing regulators, PTBP1 and PTBP2. They participate in both progenitor proliferation and neuronal differentiation with complementary roles. PTBP1 expression is upregulated in progenitors and downregulated in neurons, whereas PTBP2 is expressed in both cell types (Addington et al. 2011; Kikuchi et al. 2000; Lillevali et al. 2001; Polydorides et al. 2000; Shibayama et al. 2009). Consistent with this expression pattern, PTBP1 influences the cell cycle of RGCs, and mouse models depleting *Ptbp1* exhibit premature neuronal differentiation and defective interkinetic nuclear migration. *Ptbp2* germline knockouts also show defective interkinetic nuclear migration and premature neuronal differentiation (Licatalosi et al. 2012; Shibasaki et al. 2013). A seminal study found that PTBP1 also regulates neuron-specific exons to control the neural progenitor-to-neuron cell fate transition (Zhang et al. 2016). RBP regulation of AS is also important during neuronal migration, as seen in *Nova2* knockout mice, which have defective lamination of late-born neurons (Yano et al. 2010). Together, these studies reinforce the dynamic role of RNPs in controlling AS across developmental processes of the neocortex.

How do splicing mutations influence disease? Large-scale single-cell transcriptome analyses have begun to identify candidate risk genes for neurodevelopmental and psychiatric disorders, including autism spectrum disorder (ASD), epilepsy, and schizophrenia (Parras et al. 2018; Polioudakis et al. 2019; Walker et al. 2019). For example, a study of developing ASD brains, detected a significant imbalance in isoforms of cytoplasmic polyadenylation element binding protein 4 (CPEB4), resulting in reduced CPEB4 protein levels. This is notable as cytoplasmic polyadenylation element binding protein (CPEB) was shown to bind to almost all high-confidence ASD genes revealing a new molecular signature of mRNA deadenylation for high-confidence ASD-risk genes (Parras et al. 2018). This exemplifies how high-resolution single-cell expression atlases allow the field to trace the potential etiology of neuropsychiatric diseases to splicing events.

To date, most studies of AS during neurogenesis have focused on mutations in the major splicing pathway, which excises 99 percent of introns in human cells (Jutzi et al. 2018). However, there are 700–800 introns in humans that have distinct features and are detected by different pre-mRNA machinery, termed the minor spliceosome. Mutations in minor spliceosome components also disrupt neurogenesis (Jutzi et al. 2018). For example, ablation of *Rnu11*, which encodes small nuclear RNA 11 critical for minor spliceosome function, results in microcephaly caused by the death of RGCs (Baumgartner et al. 2018). This study identified differential requirements of the minor spliceosome function in different neural cell types, which is critical for deeper understanding of neurogenesis. The emerging roles of minor intron splicing in neurological disorders was reviewed recently (Jutzi et al. 2018).

Summary: Developmentally dynamic AS events occur frequently in the developing brain and are also the most evolutionarily conserved. Human genetic studies implicate AS regulators and the process itself in neurodevelopmental disease. The RBPs discussed here, which control AS during cortical development, are just a small subset of RBPs involved in AS in the mammalian nervous system (Raj and Blencowe 2015).

28.3 Stability and Exon Junction Complex

28.3.1 The Exon Junction Complex

Overview: The exon junction complex (EJC) is composed of three core proteins – EIF4A3 (DDX48), MAGOH, and RBM8A (Y14) – which is deposited onto pre-mRNA concomitant with splicing and remains associated with the mRNA after it is exported to the cytoplasm (Ghosh et al. 2012; Kataoka et al. 2000; Le Hir et al. 2001; Shibuya et al. 2004). In the nucleus, the EJC can influence splicing of long introns. Within the cytoplasm, the EJC mediates nonsense-mediated decay (NMD), RNA localization, and translation initiation (Mao et al. 2016; Nott et al. 2004; Palacios et al. 2004). These functions are regulated by its association with transient components including PYM, SKAR, and NMD components (Diem et al. 2007; Ma et al. 2008; McMahon et al. 2016).

Use of both conditional and germline mouse mutants showed that the three core EJC components, *Eif4a3*, *Rbm8a*, and *Magoh*, are each essential for proper cortical development (Mao et al. 2015, 2016; Silver et al. 2010). Haploinsufficiency for these proteins (generated using *Emx1*-Cre) depletes the progenitor pool and induces premature neuronal differentiation as well as massive apoptosis. This disruption of neurogenesis ultimately results in severe microcephaly. These cellular defects may be partially explained by roles for the EJC in mitosis duration. *Magoh* haploinsufficient brain progenitors show delays in mitosis and these delayed cells preferentially undergo neurogenic or apoptotic divisions (Pilaz et al. 2016b). Apoptosis is also a strong contributor to the severe microcephaly caused by mutations in EJC components, as this phenotype can be rescued by genetic ablation of *p53* (Mao et al. 2015, 2016). In contrast to the core EJC components, mouse mutants in *Casc3* show relatively normal cortical development, indicating it is not an essential EJC component in brain development (Mao et al. 2017).

At both the RNA and protein levels, *Rbm8a*, *Magoh*, and *Eif4a3* mutants (embryonic day (E) 10.5 and E11.5) have alterations in common downstream molecular pathways, especially in the ribosome, proteasome, and p53 pathways (Mao et al. 2016). Consistent with data in human cell lines (Wang et al. 2014), widespread changes in AS were also present in the EJC mutants, particularly intron retention events. Notably, mis-splicing is observed for several RNA regulatory components, including ribosomes and RNA-binding proteins. Altogether, these data suggest that EJC components influence both transcript expression and splicing of RNA regulators, acting in a regulatory network that controls gene expression at the RNA level.

In humans, mutations in the EJC components cause severe neurodevelopmental disorders. Biallelic hypomorphic mutations of *EIF4A3* cause Richieri-Costa-Pereira syndrome (RCPS), a rare autosomal recessive craniofacial disorder that also presents with microcephaly and learning and language impairments (Bertola et al. 2018; Favaro et al. 2014; Hsia et al. 2018). Further, copy number variations (both gains and losses) of *EIF4A3* and *RBM8A* are linked to intellectual disability (ID) (Nguyen et al. 2013). Mutations in *RBM8A* also cause TAR syndrome, in which patients have severe microcephaly (Albers et al. 2012). Taken together, both the mouse and human data highlight the importance of proper EJC function in brain development.

Summary: Multiple studies indicate the EJC is critical for cell fate decisions during corticogenesis and when dysregulated can result in neurodevelopmental disorders. Further characterization of other EJC functions, including splicing, mRNA localization, and translational efficiency, in the cortex and their contribution to development and disease is still required. In vivo models continue to be powerful tools to interrogate the function of EJC factors in different cell types and to dissect cell autonomous versus non-cell autonomous functions. Transcriptome-wide studies of the EJC have identified binding sites in human cell culture, showing they canonically bind 24 nucleotides upstream of exon–exon junctions, and can non-canonically bind to UTRs (Sauliere et al. 2012; Singh et al. 2012). Further characterization of EJC targets in the developing cortex is still required for a better understanding of its contribution to development and disease. It remains unknown, for example, if EJC targets vary across progenitors and neuron in the developing brain.

28.3.2 RNA Decay Mechanisms

Overview: mRNA decay mechanisms are conserved in most eukaryotic organisms. Briefly, the 3′UTR poly(A) tail and 5′ cap are removed, and either end is then degraded by exonucleases (Lykke-Andersen and Jensen 2015). In certain pathways, endonucleolytic cleavage within the transcript body can also occur if the cell detects a stalled ribosome during translation (Harigaya and Parker 2010). RBPs are involved at all steps of RNA decay mechanisms and can act as either enhancers or suppressors of mRNA degradation (Lykke-Andersen and Jensen 2015).

Mutations in several mRNA stability factors are linked to perturbed neural development (Weil et al. 2020). Most in vivo studies of mRNA stability and neurogenesis have been performed by conditionally depleting the stability factors in the mouse neocortex. A recent study found that conditional deletion of *Exosc10*, which encodes a structural subunit of the RNA exosome, from mouse neural progenitors led to apoptosis and cortical agenesis (Ulmke et al. 2021). Exosc10 binds and degrades p53 signaling-related transcripts including apoptosis effectors *Aen* and *Bbc3* in order to suppress p53 signaling and apoptosis. Using *Nex*-Cre conditional depletion, Zhao et al. also found RBP HuR regulates the stability of actin regulator *Prolifin 1* mRNA (Zhao et al. 2020). Depletion of *HuR* in cortical neurons perturbs neuronal migration and proper lamination of the cortex. A seminal study in 2017 also found that loss of N^6-methyladenosine (m^6A) reader protein YTHDF2 promotes precocious neurogenesis and alters cell cycle dynamics (Yoon et al. 2017). YTHDF2 is responsible for recruiting the CCR4-NOT deadenylase complex to mRNA transcripts for their degradation (Du et al. 2016).

One of the best characterized eukaryotic RNA degradation pathways is NMD. NMD involves multiple highly coordinated steps by which NMD factors detect and degrade mRNAs that have premature termination codons (PTCs) (Lykke-Andersen and Jensen 2015). Core NMD factors include the Up-frameshift family members UPF1 (the central NMD factor), UPF2, and UPF3 (which has two mammalian paralogues, UPF3A and UPF3B). UPFs interact with one another on the mRNA transcript containing a PTC, but some pathways can proceed independently of UPF2 and/or UPF3. A small percentage of mRNAs with PTCs can escape detection and degradation. Further, NMD can exhibit variability between cells (Sato and Singer 2021). NMD also serves another critical function in mammalian cells by controlling normal homeostatic gene expression and subsequently proteomes under different conditions (Lykke-Andersen and Jensen 2015).

Given its central role in gene expression, NMD is poised to have an important role in cortical data. Indeed, loss-of-function mouse models have elucidated the roles of NMD factors in cortical development. For example, RNA sequencing of *Upf3b*-null cortices showed that UPF3B regulates transcripts implicated in neural differentiation and disease (Huang et al. 2018). In vitro differentiation of neural stem cells from *Upf3b*-null cortices at E14.5 also showed that UPF3B is required for neural stem cell differentiation in mouse neural stem cells. Loss of *Upf3b* also resulted in behavioral defects and deficient dendritic spine maturation in postnatal mice. In addition to the mouse data, human embryonic stem cells have also revealed roles of NMD factors in development, as reviewed recently (Lee et al. 2021; Lou et al. 2016).

Core NMD factors have been implicated in several neurodevelopmental diseases, including ASD, ID, and schizophrenia (Addington et al. 2011; Huang et al. 2011, 2018; Laumonnier et al. 2010; Lee et al. 2021; Lou et al. 2016; Marques et al. 2022; Tarpey et al. 2007). A study of human data found that in over 57,000 patients with neurodevelopmental disorders, core NMD genes including *UPF3A*, *UPF2*, and *SMG6*, among others, are either deleted or duplicated in the patients (Nguyen et al. 2013). Analysis of lymphoblastoid cell lines from eight patients with loss-of-function mutations in *UPF3B* also found that ~ 5 percent of the transcriptome is impacted as a result. The paralog of UPF3B, UPF3A, is stabilized in all patients' cell lines and is able to partially compensate for *UPF3B* loss-of-function (Nguyen et al. 2012).

Summary: mRNA decay factors have been implicated in fundamental aspects of cortical development, with redundant functions in some cases. Fundamental questions remain unanswered about RNA stability during cortical development, including: how much does RNA stability differ by cell type and stage, and which RBPs regulate stability in the developing cortex? Further investigations into RNA stability components and their targets, particularly in vivo, are important to address these questions.

28.4 Translational Control

Translational control is a widespread means of modulating gene expression and is particularly critical to dynamic posttranscriptional control during cortical development. Besides RBPs, translational control involves ribosomes, which are the main effectors of the translation machinery. Ribosomes are themselves key regulatory players in protein synthesis (Dalla Venezia et al. 2019). Aside from the fact that translational efficiency is linked to ribosome abundance, recent studies have demonstrated ribosome heterogeneity, giving rise to the concept of "specialized ribosomes" (Li and Wang 2020). Specific ribosome composition has the potential to modulate translation of a specific subset of mRNAs. The role of ribosome diversity in cortical progenitors is still largely unknown.

A crucial advantage conferred by translational control of gene expression is the speed of protein synthesis. Translation is at least 10 times faster than the average transcription rate, which enables rapid, highly dynamic responses to stimuli (Shamir et al. 2016). Therefore, translational control results in quick modulation of protein expression that allows cells to efficiently respond to changes in the local environment, which is especially valuable during development. On the other hand, protein synthesis is one of the most energy consuming processes in a cell, and signaling nodes such as mTOR are associated with translational regulation and energy homeostasis, reinforcing the need for precise regulation of protein synthesis in order to maintain an energetic balance (Lindqvist et al. 2018).

In the developing cortex, translational regulation has major roles in controlling the balance between self-renewing and neurogenic divisions of neural progenitors, as well as neuronal identity and lineage diversification (Hoye and Silver 2021; Saba et al. 2021). RGCs are transcriptionally prepatterned to make diverse neurons, a phenomenon termed "transcriptional priming" whereby transcripts encoding proteins that will be expressed in progeny are present, but yet not translated, in the precursor cell (Li et al. 2020; Oberst et al. 2019; Telley et al. 2019; Zahr et al. 2018). Transcriptional priming has been demonstrated in numerous transcriptomic studies showing that neural progenitors retain multipotency and self-renewal capacity while expressing mRNAs that are pro-neurogenic, such as *Neurog2*, *Cux1*, *Neurod1*, and *Neurod2* (Telley et al. 2019; Yang et al. 2014; Zahr et al. 2018). Translational repression of these transcripts is mediated by RBPs and translational machinery, until they are needed to promote neurogenesis (Park et al. 2022).

28.4.1 Translational Regulators

Overview: Translational regulators operate during diverse stages of protein synthesis, including initiation, elongation, termination, and ribosome recycling. The initiation stage, when the mRNA is engaged by translation machinery and the AUG start codon is identified, is especially subject to regulation (Sonenberg and Hinnebusch 2009). Indeed, global translation programs across cell types are often modulated by inhibition or activation of initiation factors, which ultimately determines the overall rate of protein synthesis (Gebauer and Hentze 2004). Additionally, selective regulatory mechanisms govern translation of specific mRNAs in cell type-dependent, subcellular compartment-dependent, and developmental stage-dependent manners. Such differential translation of specific mRNAs is largely mediated by the action of *trans*-acting factors such as RBPs and to a lesser extent, microRNAs (Lennox et al. 2018).

A prominent translation initiation factor important for cortical development is the eukaryotic translation initiation factor 4E (eIF4E), a 5′-cap binding protein (Amorim et al. 2018). eIF4E binds to mRNA targets and interacts with eIF4G, which in turn binds eIF4A to form the eIF4F complex allowing the recruitment of ribosomes, thereby promoting translation (Jackson et al. 2010; Sonenberg and Hinnebusch 2009). The function of eIF4E can itself be controlled by posttranslational modifications, such as phosphorylation, or by interactions with translational repressive proteins (termed eIF4E-binding proteins; 4E-BPs). In the developing cortex, eIF4E1 bound to 4E-T sequesters proneurogenic mRNAs into repressive eIF4E1/4E-T complexes in neural progenitors, which is essential for maintaining a neural stem cell state (Yang et al. 2014). 4E-T can also associate with the RBP Pumilio2 (Pum2) to inhibit translation of over 200 mRNAs, including the neurogenic transcription factors *Brn1* and *Tle4* (Zahr et al. 2018). Likewise, 4E-T together with Dcp1 inhibits neurogenesis by recruiting the RBP Smaug2 into cytoplasmic complexes, which in turn captures *Nanos1* mRNA and silences its translation in neural progenitors (Amadei et al. 2015). The absence of these repression complexes leads to aberrant expression of neuronal specifiers and compromised cortical neurogenesis.

Another RBP with major translational reprograming roles in cortical development is the cell lineage abnormal 28 (Lin28). Both paralogs, *Lin28a* and *Lin28b*, are highly abundant in neural progenitors; however, only *Lin28a* deletion causes microcephaly, while double KO of both orthologs causes severe phenotypes including neural tube defects (Herrlinger et al. 2019; Yang et al. 2015). These findings along with over-expression studies indicate that *Lin28a/b* are necessary for cell cycle progression during RGC proliferation, and also to stimulate neuronal differentiation during early neurogenesis. Polysome profiling of *Lin28a/b* KO mouse suggests that Lin28 functions activate translation of a subset of mRNAs associated with ribosome biogenesis, the mTOR pathway, and cell cycle (Herrlinger et al. 2019). In addition, Lin28 also plays important role inhibiting the progression of neuron-to-glia cell fate (Balzer et al. 2010; Luo et al. 2021).

The RNA helicase DDX3X has a prominent role in promoting translation initiation and is required for proper cortical development. Mutations in *DDX3X* cause *DDX3X* syndrome, characterized by microcephaly, corpus callosum malformation, ID, and language deficits. *DDX3X* mutations have also been identified in ASD cohorts (Tang et al. 2021). Recent *Ddx3x* loss-of-function studies in mouse models revealed that DDX3X mediates progenitor proliferation and neuronal generation via translational control of neurogenic transcripts (Hoye et al. 2022; Lennox et al. 2020). *DDX3X* mutations linked to the most severe clinical outcomes, which includes polymicrogyria, are associated with aberrant ribonucleoprotein (RNP) granule formation (Lennox et al. 2020). RNP granules serve as modulators of posttranscriptional control and are postulated to promote translational repression, or alternatively be a consequence of altered mRNA translation itself (Anderson and Kedersha 2009). Besides DDX3X, these granules have been implicated in the pathology of ID caused by *DDX6* mutations and Fragile X syndrome (FXS) (Balak et al. 2019; El Fatimy et al. 2016). A key question is whether aberrant granules are causally linked to disease or merely a biomarker.

Translational regulation has also been implicated in area-specific cytoarchitecture in the developing cortex. The RBPs Pum2 and Tar-DNA binding protein 43 (TDP-43) are involved in downstream programs controlling neuronal identity in the somatosensory area through translational modulation of *Sox5*, *Ctip2*, and *Rorβ* (Harb et al. 2022). Conditional depletion of *Pum2* or expression of a mutant TDP-43 in mice leads to perturbed layer IV/V formation of the sensory cortical area.

Summary: Considering the evidence that protein levels are explained only partially by transcriptional rates in cortical progenitors, understanding translational regulatory mechanisms is crucial to fully comprehend temporal gene regulation of neocortical development. Together these data show that translational regulation is tightly linked with self-renewing and cell fate decisions of neural progenitors, coordinating neuronal identity acquisition as development proceeds.

28.4.2 mRNA Transport, Localization, and Local Translation

Overview: An additional layer of control to fine-tune gene expression in the developing cortex is subcellular localization of mRNAs. Translational regulation can be coupled with mRNA localization mechanisms to provide spatial and temporal control of protein synthesis within subcellular compartments. RNA transport, which involves participation of RBPs and molecular motors, represents a key regulatory step in gene expression. Subcellular local gene regulation is well conserved among highly polarized cells such as neurons, which are morphologically unique and have the ability to integrate excitatory and inhibitory signals from synaptic inputs hundreds of micrometers from the site of RNA transcription in the cell nuclei (Wang et al. 2009). In the cortex, localized gene regulation has been implicated in RGCs as well as mature neurons (D'Arcy and Silver 2020).

One example of subcellular translational control in the developing cortex is the RBP CUGBP Elav-like family member 2 (CELF2). Nucleocytoplasmic transport of CELF2 coordinates self-renewal and differentiation states of RGCs (MacPherson et al. 2021). CELF2 undergoes nuclear-cytoplasmic shuffling to regulate mRNAs related to cell fate decisions such as *Neurog2*, *Neurod1*, and *Tbr2*. In self-renewing progenitors, CELF2 resides in the cytoplasm and represses mRNA translation. Once translocated back to the nucleus, CELF2 releases these mRNAs promoting neurogenesis. Perturbations in CELF2 nuclear translocation dynamics impair neuronal specification and human de novo missense mutations in this gene cause cortical malformations and neurodevelopmental defects (Itai et al. 2021; MacPherson et al. 2021).

Another RBP that influences RNA localization during cortical development is Staufen2 (Stau2). Stau2 and interacting mRNAs are apically enriched in RGCs, where it forms a complex with the translational repressor Pum2, and DDX1 (Vessey et al. 2012). Depletion of any of these components disrupts the complex and enhances neurogenesis. Knockdown of *Stau2* perturbs the localization and expression of its target mRNA *Prox1*, leading to premature neuronal differentiation at the expense of neural progenitors. Stau2 is also important for lineage progression. During progenitor divisions, it is distributed asymmetrically, segregating into the Tbr2 positive daughter, together with basal cell determinants, such as *Trim32* (Kusek et al. 2012). Taken together, these findings illustrate localization of RBPs and associated cargo mRNAs to subcellular compartments of the cell body as a pivotal portion of translation control.

RNA localization has recently been shown to occur in radial glia at the basal endfeet. The transportation and local translation of *Cyclin D2* is linked to asymmetric cell divisions of RGCs (Tsunekawa et al. 2012). A cis-acting transport element in the *Cyclin D2* 3′UTR mRNA drives its localization to the RGC basal endfeet. It is thought to be locally translated and asymmetrically inherited during mitosis by the basally positioned daughter cell, which acquires a self-renewing fate. This mechanism suggests mRNA localization has a critical role in asymmetric cell fate determination during early corticogenesis. Recent studies have revealed that the transcript, *Arhgap11a*, is subcellularly localized to basal endfeet, where its local synthesis and local RhoGAP function control endfoot morphology (Pilaz et al. 2023). This morphology non-cell autonomously dictates interneuron positioning. This suggests additional roles for localized RNAs in controlling RGC morphology and cortical organization.

The polyribosome-associated RBP Fragile X mental retardation protein (FMRP) is expressed across different cell types in the brain and broadly implicated in posttranscriptional mechanisms. In neurons, FMRP participates in dendritic and axonal mRNAs localization and acts as a key mediator of local translation (Lee et al. 2011; Wang et al. 2015). FMRP is also important for the transport of specific mRNAs through RGC basal processes and binds to over 100 mRNAs in basal endfeet (Pilaz et al. 2016b). It further controls the localization of a subset of these mRNAs. FMRP is encoded by the *FMR1* gene, in which mutations cause FXS, the most common inherited genetic cause of intellectual disability and the leading genetic contributor to autism. Understanding FMRP-mediated functions that can be targeted for therapeutic intervention is of enormous clinical interest (Wang et al. 2010).

Summary: These examples highlight roles for RNA localization, transport, and local translation within the information flow from genes to proteins of the developing neocortex. Future studies are needed to understand better the breadth of subcellular localization and translation in the cortex, including which transcripts are transported and translated in radial glia, and how this is controlled both spatially and temporally. In addition, how this layer of control contributed to cortical expansion and the diversification of neuronal types during neocortical evolution is unknown.

28.5 Noncoding RNAS: miRNAs, lncRNAs, and circRNAs

Overview: Although about 98 percent of our genome transcribes noncoding RNAs, including introns and ncRNA elements, few classes of these noncoding elements are functionally well-known (Mattick 2001). New classes have been characterized and a growing body of evidence has demonstrated their regulatory roles in neural development (Salvatori et al. 2020).

MicroRNAs (miRNAs) are a class of short ncRNAs (~22 nt) that repress translation and/or promote degradation of target mRNAs (Guo et al. 2010). About 70 percent of the miRNAs identified in humans are expressed in the nervous system (Prodromidou and Matsas 2019). Many play important roles in cortical development, including *miR-9*, *let-7*, and *miR-124*. miR-9 is particularly important in controlling the stability of *Hes1*, a Notch signaling effector, during brain development; Oscillatory gene expression of *Hes1* driven by *miR-9* is essential for neural progenitor fate decisions in vitro (Bonev et al. 2012). One of the founding members of the miRNA family, *let-7*, inhibits self-renewal and promotes cell differentiation in RGCs (Chang et al. 2012; Fairchild et al. 2019; Schwamborn et al. 2009; Zhao et al. 2013). *Let-7* is associated with cell cycle kinetics of cortical progenitors, demonstrated by the *let-7* dynamic expression profile in dividing progenitors in vivo, and manipulations of *let-7* in vitro that impact cell cycle exit and length (Fairchild et al. 2019). During cortical development, when *let-7a* is activated by TRIM32 in mouse neural progenitors, it triggers neuronal differentiation (Schwamborn et al. 2009).

miRNAs play important roles in multiple aspects of cortical evolution, including basal progenitor amplification and gyrus formation (de Juan Romero et al. 2015; Liu et al. 2021; Nowakowski et al. 2018). For example, *miR-409-3p* is an evolutionarily acquired miRNA implicated in cortical projection neuron subtype identity and promoting corticospinal motor neurons (CSMN) in vivo

(Diaz et al. 2020). In addition, a recent study based on over-expression in mouse cortices of *miR-137* and *miR-122*, which are endogenously expressed at low levels in mice, has shown their roles in processes relevant for cortical expansion. These miRNAs are implicated in maintaining the basal progenitor proliferative state and slowing down neuronal differentiation, respectively (Tomasello et al. 2022). These studies argue that miRNAs may be a strong contributor to primate specific cortical traits.

Another class of ncRNAs, long ncRNAs (lncRNAs), are at least 200 nt in length and have a broad range of functions, including posttranscriptional RNA processing, silencing and translation of mRNAs, as well as precursors of miRNAs (Briggs et al. 2015; Zhang et al. 2019). Around 40 percent of the identified lncRNAs are specifically expressed in the brain, and thousands of them arose during primate evolution (Derrien et al. 2012; Zimmer-Bensch 2019). LncRNAs show a high degree of cell-type specificity and precisely regulated temporal and spatial expression patterns in the brain (Briggs et al. 2015). To date, relatively few lncRNAs associated with cortical development have been characterized.

One exception is *Pnky*, a lncRNA expressed in embryonic and adult neural progenitors, that regulates neuronal differentiation in the embryonic and postnatal brain (Ramos et al. 2015). *Pnky* interacts with the splicing regulator PTBP1 and mediates neurogenesis through AS. Depletion of *Pnky* in the developing mouse reduces progenitors and increases neuronal differentiation. The intergenic lncRNAs *linc-brn1a* and *linc-brn1b* are also associated with neuronal differentiation (Carelli et al. 2019). Depletion of these lncRNAs, which interact with the HuR RBP, results in increased differentiation potential in vitro (Carelli et al. 2019).

LncRNAs have been linked to brain evolution. One evidence is the higher degree of genomic conservation of the landscape surrounding lncRNAs across species with large brains (Lewitus and Huttner 2015). In addition, the lncRNAs *HAR1F* and *HAR1R* are antisense transcripts of the first human accelerated region identified, *HAR1* (Pollard et al. 2006). Although its function remains to be discovered, *HAR1F* is specifically expressed from this locus in Cajal–Retzius cells and co-expressed with Reelin, an important factor during cortical development. Taken together, these studies suggest that lncRNAs are important for regulation of neurogenesis and highlight their essential functions for human brain evolution.

A recently identified class of ncRNAs is circular RNAs (circRNAs) which are mostly derived from protein-coding genes. CircRNAs are generated at the expense of canonical mRNAs, suggesting that their biogenesis *per se* is a gene expression regulatory mechanism (Rybak-Wolf et al. 2015). CircRNAs are evolutionarily conserved, abundantly expressed in neural tissue, and enriched in genes that encode synaptic proteins (You et al. 2015). Examples of circRNAs regulating cortical development include *circSlc45a4* (Suenkel et al. 2020). Knockdown of *circSlc45a4* in the developing mouse cortex leads to depletion of the basal progenitor pool and upregulation of neurogenic factors. The most abundant and well-studied mammalian circRNA is *CDR1as/ciRS-7* which harbors several binding sites for *miR-7*, acting as a miRNA sponge and ultimately posttranscriptionally regulating *miR-7* mRNA targets (Memczak et al. 2013). Expression of human/mouse *CDR1as* or downregulation of *miR-7* lead to similar neuronal defects in zebrafish. What is the role of these circRNAs in cortical development? Despite the discovery that hundreds of circRNAs are specifically expressed in mouse brain tissues, only these few examples of their functions in cortical development exist to date.

Summary: Although the ncRNA inventory has immensely expanded with innovations in RNA sequencing and single-cell sequencing technologies, functional studies on ncRNAs in nervous system development are still lagging considerably. Given the abundance of ncRNAs and their roles in neuronal regulation, it is of great importance to explore their functions and molecular mechanisms to better understand cortical development. Furthermore, lncRNA and miRNA are increasingly implicated in neurodevelopmental diseases such as ID and ASD (van de et al. 2013; Ziats and Rennert 2013). Additional investigation of their biology may help elucidate the molecular pathogenesis of these disorders. Similarly, additional research to validate and characterize ncRNAs identified in human developing cortex will continue to increase our understanding of human brain evolution.

28.6 RNA Editing and Modifications

Overview: mRNA molecules can be edited or chemically modified at the nucleotide level, which are referred to collectively as the RNA editome and epitranscriptome, respectively. Both RNA editing and modification can lead to alterations in RNA metabolism and have recently emerged as critical posttranscriptional regulators of gene expression.

RNA editing is the process of altering the sequence of an mRNA such as insertion, deletion, or, more frequently, conversion of one nucleotide (Eisenberg and Levanon 2018). The most common form of RNA editing is adenosine (A) to inosine (I) conversion, catalyzed by ADAR family members. A-to-I is particularly frequent in humans due to the presence of primate-specific repeats called Alu repeats, which recruit ADAR editing enzymes (Eisenberg et al. 2005). Editing can change a codon or modulate splice-site usage, especially when in an intron. With increasing transcriptomic studies, a large number of editing sites in diverse tissues, including adult whole mouse brains, have been identified (Li et al. 2009; Ramaswami and Li 2014), and raise questions as to how they are regulated and their functional roles in mRNA biology. A genome-wide study of the RNA editing landscape in human brain tissues spanning from fetal (<12 months) to older (≥50 years) stages suggested that editing rate patterns are associated with the temporal expression of ADAR enzymes (Hwang et al. 2016). Also, the secondary structures of RNAs affect ADAR interactions acting as a *cis*-regulatory mechanism of RNA editing.

Similar to DNA, RNA is also subjected to dynamic, reversible chemical modifications and over 100 modifications are known to date. RNA modifications can affect RNA metabolism by regulating its splicing, export, decay, or translation, representing an additional layer of gene regulation (Frye et al. 2018). Several studies have shown that the brain displays the highest degree of RNA editing and modifications (Eisenberg and Levanon 2018; Yen and Chen 2021). In mammals, N6-methyladenosine (m^6A) is the most prevalent RNA modification (Yen and Chen 2021). RNA modifications involve several proteins called writers, erasers, and readers, that install, remove, or recognize the modifications, respectively. m^6A, for example, is catalyzed by a multicomponent complex that includes the heterodimer of the writer's methyltransferase-like protein 3 and 14 (Mettl3/14).

Recent studies have reported roles for m^6A in cortical development (Livneh et al. 2020; Shafik et al. 2022; Yen and Chen 2021; Yoon et al. 2017). In mouse conditional models, m^6A depletion in neural progenitors by genetic knockout of the writer, *Mettl14*, delays cell cycle progression (Yoon et al. 2017). m^6A mediates the rapid turnover of specific mRNAs important for cell cycle and neuronal differentiation, such as *Pax6*, *Sox1*, and *Emx2*, suggesting an m^6A-dependent decay underlying temporal control of cortical neurogenesis. In addition, recent findings suggest that the decrease in progenitor proliferation and premature neuronal differentiation observed in *Mettl14* conditional knockout are driven by an increase in histone modifications (Wang et al. 2018), suggesting a potential link between RNA modification and epigenetic mechanisms. Disturbance of m^6A by *Mettl3* knockdown in mice also affects neurogenesis through modulating *Ezh2*, which encodes a histone methyltransferase (Chen et al. 2019).

m^6A readers are also linked to cortical development. FMRP reads m^6A modifications and modulates nuclear export of methylated mRNAs during neuronal differentiation. Similar to *Mettl14* depletion phenotypes, *Fmr1* knockout mice exhibit prolonged neural progenitor cell cycle (Edens et al. 2019). Another reader shown to play a role during neurogenesis is YTHDF2, which mediates degradation of specific mRNAs important for proliferation and differentiation of neural progenitors (Li et al. 2018). Altogether, these findings suggest a critical role for RNA methylation in RGC self-renewal and temporal specification during neurogenesis.

Notably, comparisons between m^6A landscapes of mouse and human cortical organoids revealed that human-specific targets are enriched for genes related to autism and schizophrenia (Yoon et al. 2017). In addition, mutations in FTO, a m^6A demethylase, are associated with neurodevelopmental disorders, including microcephaly and developmental delay (Caglayan et al. 2016).

Summary: Although RNA editing has increasingly been recognized as a molecular mechanism regulating RNA metabolism, its role in shaping cortical development remains largely understudied. Despite the identification of many RNA editing sites and its potential role in the generation of transcript diversity, their functional significance remains to be discovered. RNA modification studies are still at a relatively early stage but have progressively attracted research interest. Given the strong evidence that m^6A has essential roles in cortical development and the link between m^6A dysregulation and human neural disorders, these questions are important for future studies.

28.7 Conclusions and Future Directions

The sequential steps by which neural progenitors give rise to diverse specialized neurons that will compose the neocortex rely on exquisite regulation of gene expression in a spatial and temporal manner. Recent technological advances in sequencing have allowed for the study of mRNA levels across neocortical development. Despite a dramatically increased understanding of transcriptional control, many posttranscriptional mechanisms that fine-tune gene expression in the developing cortex remain largely unknown. While the network of transcription factors that control gene programs has been extensively characterized, posttranscriptional regulators are a more recent area of focus; many have been described, but only few are mechanistically understood. Investigating both the transcriptional and the posttranscriptional landscape at play during cortical development is pivotal to understanding corticogenesis.

Posttranscriptional events are highly organized and dynamic. Subsets of functionally related mRNAs can be co-regulated in RNP modules by one or more RBPs, a concept that gave rise to the "RNA regulon" model of gene expression (Keene 2007). RNA regulons help to physically localize and temporally coordinate processing of these mRNAs, including decay or translation. This is particularly important for rapid integration of external cues into molecular information required for biological processes, such as proliferation and differentiation, during cortical development. The role of regulons within the developing cortex needs further investigation.

Although RBPs have significant roles during brain development, how each RBP contributes to neocortical development and their specific mRNA targets at different stages remains is an area of active investigation. Indeed, some RBPs have cell type-specific functions, act in more than one aspect of mRNA metabolism, or have different functions and targets based on the subcellular localization or timing, all of which suggests their mechanisms of action are context dependent. Moreover, RBP functions and gene expression are also influenced by external cues from the surrounding microenvironment (Yuzwa et al. 2016). A number of methods have been developed for identifying RNA-protein interactions that enable discovery of RBP targets (Blue et al. 2022;

Wheeler et al. 2018), which are increasingly applied to outstanding questions in cortical development. To advance towards a more comprehensive understanding of gene regulation during cortical development, it will be crucial to understand how different RBPs and posttranscriptional processes converge and synergize.

Technological advances have facilitated an understanding of RNA regulation in the cortex. Indeed, RNA sequencing and single cell sequencing characterize transcriptomes of developing cortices across species and developmental stages (Johnson et al. 2009; Zhu et al. 2018). New technologies have also shed light on the spatial topography of gene expression during brain development (Maynard et al. 2021). Further improvement of spatial transcriptomics coupled with proteomic analyses will be invaluable for understanding local posttranscriptional mechanisms.

To date, the majority of the cortical development discoveries of posttranscriptional control has been made using mouse models. Despite limitations including the absence of some cell types and vascularization in most methods, human stem cell-derived cortical organoids have provided new opportunities to investigate posttranscriptional regulation across species as well as in normal and disease-related development (Bowles et al. 2021; Camp et al. 2015; Chan et al. 2020; Gordon et al. 2021; Jourdon et al. 2021). The development and refinement of two-dimensional and organoid models to recapitulate human brain development also has enormous potential for understanding the extent to which posttranscriptional mechanisms influenced evolution.

There is a strong link between mis-regulation of posttranscriptional processes and neurodevelopmental and neurodegenerative disorders including microcephaly, ID, ASD, FXS, and Alzheimer's and Parkinson's diseases. Identifying RBPs, ncRNAs, their targets, and understanding their molecular posttranscriptional mechanisms will therefore provide crucial insights into the etiology of neurological diseases and pave the way for potential therapeutic approaches.

References

6 Non-coding RNA characterization. *Nature* (2019). https://doi.org/10.1038/nature28175.

Addington, A.M. et al. (2011). A novel frameshift mutation in UPF3B identified in brothers affected with childhood onset schizophrenia and autism spectrum disorders. *Mol Psych* 16 (3): 238–239. doi: 10.1038/mp.2010.59.

Albers, C.A. et al. (2012). Compound inheritance of a low-frequency regulatory SNP and a rare null mutation in exon-junction complex subunit RBM8A causes TAR syndrome. *Nat Genet* 44 (4): 435–439, S431–S432. doi: 10.1038/ng.1083.

Amadei, G. et al. (2015). A Smaug2-based translational repression complex determines the balance between precursor maintenance versus differentiation during mammalian neurogenesis. *J Neurosci* 35 (47): 15666–15681. doi: 10.1523/JNEUROSCI.2172-15.2015.

Amorim, I.S. et al. (2018). The role of the eukaryotic translation initiation factor 4E (eIF4E) in neuropsychiatric disorders. *Front Genet* 9: 561. doi: 10.3389/fgene.2018.00561.

Anderson, P. and Kedersha, N. (2009). RNA granules: post-transcriptional and epigenetic modulators of gene expression. *Nat Rev Mol Cell Biol* 10 (6): 430–436. doi: 10.1038/nrm2694.

Balak, C. et al. (2019). Rare de novo missense variants in RNA helicase DDX6 cause intellectual disability and dysmorphic features and lead to P-Body defects and RNA dysregulation. *Am J Hum Genet* 105 (3): 509–525. doi: 10.1016/j.ajhg.2019.07.010.

Balzer, E. et al. (2010). LIN28 alters cell fate succession and acts independently of the let-7 microRNA during neurogliogenesis in vitro. *Development* 137 (6): 891–900. doi: 10.1242/dev.042895.

Baumgartner, M. et al. (2018). Minor spliceosome inactivation causes microcephaly, owing to cell cycle defects and death of self-amplifying radial glial cells. *Development* 145 (17): dev166322. doi: 10.1242/dev.166322.

Bertola, D.R. et al. (2018). Richieri-Costa-Pereira syndrome. *Clin Genet* 93 (4): 800–811. doi: 10.1111/cge.13169.

Blue, S.M. et al. (2022). Transcriptome-wide identification of RNA-binding protein binding sites using seCLIP-seq. *Nat Protocols* 17 (5): 1223–1265. doi: 10.1038/s41596-022-00680-z.

Bonev, B. et al. (2012). MicroRNA-9 modulates Hes1 ultradian oscillations by forming a double-negative feedback loop. *Cell Rep* 2 (1): 10–18. doi: 10.1016/j.celrep.2012.05.017.

Bowles, K.R. et al. (2021). ELAVL4, splicing, and glutamatergic dysfunction precede neuron loss in MAPT mutation cerebral organoids. *Cell* 184 (17): 4547–4563 e4517. doi: 10.1016/j.cell.2021.07.003.

Briggs, J.A. et al. (2015). Mechanisms of long non-coding RNAs in mammalian nervous system development, plasticity, disease, and evolution. *Neuron* 88 (5): 861–877. doi: 10.1016/j.neuron.2015.09.045.

Caglayan, A.O. et al. (2016). A patient with a novel homozygous missense mutation in FTO and concomitant nonsense mutation in CETP. *J Hum Genet* 61 (5): 395–403. doi: 10.1038/jhg.2015.160.

Camp, J.G. et al. (2015). Human cerebral organoids recapitulate gene expression programs of fetal neocortex development. *Proc Natl Acad Sci USA* 112 (51): 15672–15677. doi: 10.1073/pnas.1520760112.

Carelli, S. et al. (2019). HuR interacts with lincBRN1a and lincBRN1b during neuronal stem cells differentiation. *RNA Biol* 16 (10): 1471–1485. doi: 10.1080/15476286.2019.1637698.

Chan, W.K. et al. (2020). Cerebral organoids as tools to identify the developmental roots of autism. *Mol Autism* 11 (1): 58. doi: 10.1186/s13229-020-00360-3.

Chang, H.M. et al. (2012). Trim71 cooperates with microRNAs to repress Cdkn1a expression and promote embryonic stem cell proliferation. *Nat Commun* 3: 923. doi: 10.1038/ncomms1909.

Chen, J. et al. (2019). m(6)A regulates neurogenesis and neuronal development by modulating histone methyltransferase Ezh2. *Genom, Proteom & Bioinform* 17 (2): 154–168. doi: 10.1016/j.gpb.2018.12.007.

Chen, Q. and Hu, G. (2017). Post-transcriptional regulation of the pluripotent state. *Curr Opin Genet Dev* 46: 15–23. doi: 10.1016/j.gde.2017.06.010.

Corbett, A.H. (2018). Post-transcriptional regulation of gene expression and human disease. *Curr Opin Cell Biol* 52: 96–104. doi: 10.1016/j.ceb.2018.02.011.

D'Arcy, B.R. and Silver, D.L. (2020). Local gene regulation in radial glia. *Traffic* 21 (12): 737–748. doi: 10.1111/tra.12769.

Dalla Venezia, N. et al. (2019). Emerging role of eukaryote ribosomes in translational control. *Int J Mol Sci* 20 (5): 1226. doi: 10.3390/ijms20051226.

de Juan Romero, C. et al. (2015). Discrete domains of gene expression in germinal layers distinguish the development of gyrencephaly. *EMBO J* 34 (14): 1859–1874. doi: 10.15252/embj.201591176.

DeBoer, E.M. et al. (2013). Post-transcriptional regulatory elements and spatiotemporal specification of neocortical stem cells and projection neurons. *Neuroscience* 248: 499–528. doi: 10.1016/j.neuroscience.2013.05.042.

Defelipe, J. (2011). The evolution of the brain, the human nature of cortical circuits, and intellectual creativity. *Front Neuroanat* 5: 29. doi: 10.3389/fnana.2011.00029.

Dehay, C. et al. (2015). The outer subventricular zone and primate-specific cortical complexification. *Neuron* 85 (4): 683–694. doi: 10.1016/j.neuron.2014.12.060.

Derrien, T. et al. (2012). The GENCODE v7 catalog of human long noncoding RNAs. *Genome Res* 22 (9): 1775–1789. doi: 10.1101/gr.132159.111.

Diaz, J.L. et al. (2020). An evolutionarily acquired microRNA shapes development of mammalian cortical projections. *Proc Natl Acad Sci USA* 117 (46): 29113–29122. doi: 10.1073/pnas.2006700117.

Diem, M.D. et al. (2007). PYM binds the cytoplasmic exon-junction complex and ribosomes to enhance translation of spliced mRNAs. *Nat Struct Mol Biol* 14 (12): 1173–1179. doi: 10.1038/nsmb1321.

Dillman, A.A. et al. (2013). mRNA expression, splicing and editing in the embryonic and adult mouse cerebral cortex. *Nat Neurosci* 16 (4): 499–506. doi: 10.1038/nn.3332.

Du, H. et al. (2016). YTHDF2 destabilizes m(6) A-containing RNA through direct recruitment of the CCR4-NOT deadenylase complex. *Nat Commun* 7: 12626. doi: 10.1038/ncomms12626.

Edens, B.M. et al. (2019). FMRP modulates neural differentiation through m(6)A-dependent mRNA nuclear export. *Cell Rep* 28 (4): 845–854 e845. doi: 10.1016/j.celrep.2019.06.072.

Eisenberg, E. and Levanon, E.Y. (2018). A-to-I RNA editing – immune protector and transcriptome diversifier. *Nat Rev Genet* 19 (8): 473–490. doi: 10.1038/s41576-018-0006-1.

Eisenberg, E. et al. (2005). Is abundant A-to-I RNA editing primate-specific? *Trends Genet* 21 (2): 77–81. doi: 10.1016/j.tig.2004.12.005.

El Fatimy, R. et al. (2016). Tracking the Fragile X mental retardation protein in a highly ordered neuronal ribonucleoparticles population. *PLoS Genet* 12 (7): e1006192. doi: 10.1371/journal.pgen.1006192.

Fairchild, C.L.A. et al. (2019). Let-7 regulates cell cycle dynamics in the developing cerebral cortex and retina. *Sci Rep* 9 (1): 15336. doi: 10.1038/s41598-019-51703-x.

Favaro, F.P. et al. (2014). A noncoding expansion in EIF4A3 causes Richieri-Costa-Pereira syndrome, a craniofacial disorder associated with limb defects. *Am J Hum Genet* 94 (1): 120–128. doi: 10.1016/j.ajhg.2013.11.020.

Frye, M. et al. (2018). RNA modifications modulate gene expression during development. *Science* 361 (6409): 1346–1349. doi: 10.1126/science.aau1646.

Gebauer, F. and Hentze, M.W. (2004). Molecular mechanisms of translational control. *Nat Rev. Mol Cell Biol* 5 (10): 827–835. doi: 10.1038/nrm1488.

Gerstberger, S. et al. (2014). A census of human RNA-binding proteins. *Nat Rev Genet* 15 (12): 829–845. doi: 10.1038/nrg3813.

Ghosh, S. et al. (2012). Control of RNP motility and localization by a splicing-dependent structure in oskar mRNA. *Nat Struct Mol Biol* 19 (4): 441–449. doi: 10.1038/nsmb.2257.

Gordon, A. et al. (2021). Long-term maturation of human cortical organoids matches key early postnatal transitions. *Nat Neurosci* 24 (3): 331–342. doi: 10.1038/s41593-021-00802-y.

Greig, L.C. et al. (2013). Molecular logic of neocortical projection neuron specification, development and diversity. *Nat Rev Neurosci* 14 (11): 755–769. doi: 10.1038/nrn3586.

Guo, H. et al. (2010). Mammalian microRNAs predominantly act to decrease target mRNA levels. *Nature* 466 (7308): 835–840. doi: 10.1038/nature09267.

Harb, K. et al. (2022). Pum2 and TDP-43 refine area-specific cytoarchitecture post-mitotically and modulate translation of Sox5, Bcl11b, and Rorb mRNAs in developing mouse neocortex. *Elife* 11: e55199. doi: 10.7554/eLife.55199.

Harigaya, Y. and Parker, R. (2010). No-go decay. *Wiley Interdiscip Rev: RNA* 1 (1): 132–141. doi: 10.1002/wrna.17.

Herrlinger, S. et al. (2019). Lin28-mediated temporal promotion of protein synthesis is crucial for neural progenitor cell maintenance and brain development in mice. *Development* 146 (10): dev173765. doi: 10.1242/dev.173765.

Hoye, M.L. et al. (2022). Aberrant cortical development is driven by impaired cell cycle and translational control in a *DDX3X* syndrome model. *BioRxiv*. doi: 10.1101/2022.02.21.481343.

Hoye, M.L. and Silver, D.L. (2021). Decoding mixed messages in the developing cortex. *Curr Opin Neurobiol* 66: 93–102. doi: 10.1016/j.conb.2020.10.001.

Hsia, G.S.P. et al. (2018). Complexity of the 5' untranslated region of EIF4A3, a critical factor for craniofacial and neural development. *Front Genet* 9: 149. doi: 10.3389/fgene.2018.00149.

Huang, L. et al. (2011). RNA homeostasis governed by cell type-specific and branched feedback loops acting on NMD. *Mol Cell* 43 (6): 950–961. doi: 10.1016/j.molcel.2011.06.031.

Huang, L. et al. (2018). A Upf3b-mutant mouse model with behavioral and neurogenesis defects. *Mol Psychiatry* 23 (8): 1773–1786. doi: 10.1038/mp.2017.173.

Hwang, T. et al. (2016). Dynamic regulation of RNA editing in human brain development and disease. *Nat Neurosci* 19 (8): 1093–1099. doi: 10.1038/nn.4337.

Itai, T. et al. (2021). De novo variants in CELF2 that disrupt the nuclear localization signal cause developmental and epileptic encephalopathy. *Hum Mut* 42 (1): 66–76. doi: 10.1002/humu.24130.

Jackson, R.J. et al. (2010). The mechanism of eukaryotic translation initiation and principles of its regulation. *Nat Rev Mol Cell Biol* 11 (2): 113–127. doi: 10.1038/nrm2838.

Johnson, M.B. et al. (2009). Functional and evolutionary insights into human brain development through global transcriptome analysis. *Neuron* 62 (4): 494–509. doi: 10.1016/j.neuron.2009.03.027.

Jourdon, A. et al. (2021). PsychENCODE and beyond. *Neuropsychopharmacology* 46 (1): 70–85. doi: 10.1038/s41386-020-0763-3.

Jutzi, D. et al. (2018). The emerging role of minor intron splicing in neurological disorders. *Cell Stress* 2 (3): 40–54. doi: 10.15698/cst2018.03.126.

Kataoka, N. et al. (2000). Pre-mRNA splicing imprints mRNA in the nucleus with a novel RNA-binding protein that persists in the cytoplasm. *Mol Cell* 6 (3): 673–682. doi: 10.1016/s1097-2765(00)00065-4.

Keene, J.D. (2007). Biological clocks and the coordination theory of RNA operons and regulons. *Cold Spring Harb Symp Quant Biol* 72: 157–165. doi: 10.1101/sqb.2007.72.013.

Kikuchi, T. et al. (2000). Molecular cloning and characterization of a new neuron-specific homologue of rat polypyrimidine tract binding protein. *J Biochem* 128 (5): 811–821. doi: 10.1093/oxfordjournals.jbchem.a022819.

Kriegstein, A. and Alvarez-Buylla, A. (2009). The glial nature of embryonic and adult neural stem cells. *Ann Rev Neurosci* 32: 149–184. doi: 10.1146/annurev.neuro.051508.135600.

Kusek, G. et al. (2012). Asymmetric segregation of the double-stranded RNA binding protein Staufen2 during mammalian neural stem cell divisions promotes lineage progression. *Cell Stem Cell* 11 (4): 505–516. doi: 10.1016/j.stem.2012.06.006.

Laumonnier, F. et al. (2010). Mutations of the UPF3B gene, which encodes a protein widely expressed in neurons, are associated with nonspecific mental retardation with or without autism. *Mol Psychiatry* 15 (7): 767–776. doi: 10.1038/mp.2009.14.

Le Hir, H. et al. (2001). The exon-exon junction complex provides a binding platform for factors involved in mRNA export and nonsense-mediated mRNA decay. *EMBO J* 20 (17): 4987–4997. doi: 10.1093/emboj/20.17.4987.

Lee, H.Y. et al. (2011). Bidirectional regulation of dendritic voltage-gated potassium channels by the fragile X mental retardation protein. *Neuron* 72 (4): 630–642. doi: 10.1016/j.neuron.2011.09.033.

Lee, P.J. et al. (2021). Regulation of nonsense-mediated mRNA decay in neural development and disease. *J Mol Cell Biol* 13 (4): 269–281. doi: 10.1093/jmcb/mjab022.

Lennox, A.L. et al. (2020). Pathogenic DDX3X mutations impair RNA metabolism and neurogenesis during fetal cortical development. *Neuron* 106 (3): 404–420 e408. doi: 10.1016/j.neuron.2020.01.042.

Lennox, A.L. et al. (2018). RNA on the brain: emerging layers of post-transcriptional regulation in cerebral cortex development. *Wiley Interdiscip Rev Dev Biol* 7 (1): 10. doi: 10.1002/wdev.290.

Lewitus, E. and Huttner, W.B. (2015). Neurodevelopmental LincRNA microsyteny conservation and mammalian brain size evolution. *PLoS One* 10 (7): e0131818. doi: 10.1371/journal.pone.0131818.

Li, D. and Wang, J. (2020). Ribosome heterogeneity in stem cells and development. *J Cell Biol* 219 (6): e202001108. doi: 10.1083/jcb.202001108.

Li, J.B. et al. (2009). Genome-wide identification of human RNA editing sites by parallel DNA capturing and sequencing. *Science* 324 (5931): 1210–1213. doi: 10.1126/science.1170995.

Li, M. et al. (2018). Ythdf2-mediated m(6)A mRNA clearance modulates neural development in mice. *Genome Biol* 19 (1): 69. doi: 10.1186/s13059-018-1436-y.

Li, Z. et al. (2020). Transcriptional priming as a conserved mechanism of lineage diversification in the developing mouse and human neocortex. *Sci Adv* 6 (45): eabd2068. doi: 10.1126/sciadv.abd2068.

Licatalosi, D.D. and Darnell, R.B. (2010). RNA processing and its regulation. *Nat Rev Genetics* 11 (1): 75–87. doi: 10.1038/nrg2673.

Licatalosi, D.D. et al. (2012). Ptbp2 represses adult-specific splicing to regulate the generation of neuronal precursors in the embryonic brain. *Genes Dev* 26 (14): 1626–1642. doi: 10.1101/gad.191338.112.

Lillevali, K. et al. (2001). Comparative expression analysis of the genes encoding polypyrimidine tract binding protein (PTB) and its neural homologue (brPTB) in prenatal and postnatal mouse brain. *Mech Dev* 101 (1–2): 217–220. doi: 10.1016/s0925-4773(00)00566-9.

Lin, L. et al. (2010). Evolution of alternative splicing in primate brain transcriptomes. *Hum Mol Genet* 19 (15): 2958–2973. doi: 10.1093/hmg/ddq201.

Lindqvist, L.M. et al. (2018). Cross-talk between protein synthesis, energy metabolism and autophagy in cancer. *Curr Opin Genet Dev* 48: 104–111. doi: 10.1016/j.gde.2017.11.003.

Liu, J. et al. (2021). Human brain evolution: emerging roles for regulatory DNA and RNA. *Curr Opin Neurobiol* 71: 170–177. doi: 10.1016/j.conb.2021.11.005.

Livneh, I. et al. (2020). The m(6)A epitranscriptome: transcriptome plasticity in brain development and function. *Nat Rev Neurosci* 21 (1): 36–51. doi: 10.1038/s41583-019-0244-z.

Lou, C.H. et al. (2016). Nonsense-mediated RNA decay influences human embryonic stem cell fate. *Stem Cell Rep* 6 (6): 844–857. doi: 10.1016/j.stemcr.2016.05.008.

Luo, J. et al. (2021). Lin28 inhibits the differentiation from mouse embryonic stem cells to glial lineage cells through upregulation of Yap1. *Stem Cells Int* 2021: 6674283. doi: 10.1155/2021/6674283.

Lykke-Andersen, S. and Jensen, T.H. (2015). Nonsense-mediated mRNA decay. *Nat Rev Mol Cell Biol* 16 (11): 665–677. doi: 10.1038/nrm4063.

Ma, X.M. et al. (2008). SKAR links pre-mRNA splicing to mTOR/S6K1-mediated enhanced translation efficiency of spliced mRNAs. *Cell* 133 (2): 303–313. doi: 10.1016/j.cell.2008.02.031.

MacPherson, M.J. et al. (2021). Nucleocytoplasmic transport of the RNA-binding protein CELF2 regulates neural stem cell fates. *Cell Rep* 35 (10): 109226. doi: 10.1016/j.celrep.2021.109226.

Malatesta, P. et al. (2000). Isolation of radial glial cells by fluorescent-activated cell sorting reveals a neuronal lineage. *Development* 127 (24): 5253–5263. doi: 10.1242/dev.127.24.5253.

Mao, H. et al. (2017). Mouse models of Casc3 reveal developmental functions distinct from other components of the exon junction complex. *RNA* 23 (1): 23–31. doi: 10.1261/rna.058826.116.

Mao, H. et al. (2016). Haploinsufficiency for core exon junction complex components disrupts embryonic neurogenesis and causes p53-mediated microcephaly. *PLoS Genet* 12 (9): e1006282. doi: 10.1371/journal.pgen.1006282.

Mao, H. et al. (2015). Rbm8a haploinsufficiency disrupts embryonic cortical development resulting in microcephaly. *J Neurosci* 35 (18): 7003–7018. doi: 10.1523/JNEUROSCI.0018-15.2015.

Marques, A.R. et al. (2022). Gene variants involved in nonsense-mediated mRNA decay suggest a role in Autism Spectrum Disorder. *Biomedicines* 10 (3): 665. doi: 10.3390/biomedicines10030665.

Mattick, J.S. (2001). Non-coding RNAs. *EMBO Rep* 2 (11): 986–991. doi: 10.1093/embo-reports/kve230.

Maynard, K.R. et al. (2021). Transcriptome-scale spatial gene expression in the human dorsolateral prefrontal cortex. *Nat Neurosci* 24 (3): 425–436. doi: 10.1038/s41593-020-00787-0.

Mazin, P.V. et al. (2021). Alternative splicing during mammalian organ development. *Nat Genet* 53 (6): 925–934. doi: 10.1038/s41588-021-00851-w.

McKee, A.E. et al. (2005). A genome-wide in situ hybridization map of RNA-binding proteins reveals anatomically restricted expression in the developing mouse brain. *BMC Dev Biol* 5: 14. doi: 10.1186/1471-213X-5-14.

McMahon, J.J. et al. (2016). The exon junction complex in neural development and neurodevelopmental disease. *Int J Dev Neurosci* 55: 117–123. doi: 10.1016/j.ijdevneu.2016.03.006.

Memczak, S. et al. (2013). Circular RNAs are a large class of animal RNAs with regulatory potency. *Nature* 495 (7441): 333–338. doi: 10.1038/nature11928.

Nguyen, L.S. et al. (2012). Transcriptome profiling of UPF3B/NMD-deficient lymphoblastoid cells from patients with various forms of intellectual disability. *Mol Psychiatry* 17 (11): 1103–1115. doi: 10.1038/mp.2011.163.

Nguyen, L.S. et al. (2013). Contribution of copy number variants involving nonsense-mediated mRNA decay pathway genes to neuro-developmental disorders. *Hum Mol Genet* 22 (9): 1816–1825. doi: 10.1093/hmg/ddt035.

Noctor, S.C. et al. (2001). Neurons derived from radial glial cells establish radial units in neocortex. *Nature* 409 (6821): 714–720.

Nott, A. et al. (2004). Splicing enhances translation in mammalian cells. *Genes Dev* 18 (2): 210–222. doi: 10.1101/gad.1163204.

Nowakowski, T.J. et al. (2018). Regulation of cell-type-specific transcriptomes by microRNA networks during human brain development. *Nat Neurosci* 21 (12): 1784–1792. doi: 10.1038/s41593-018-0265-3.

Oberst, P. et al. (2019). Temporal plasticity of apical progenitors in the developing mouse neocortex. *Nature* 573 (7774): 370–374. doi: 10.1038/s41586-019-1515-6.

Palacios, I.M. et al. (2004). An eIF4AIII-containing complex required for mRNA localization and nonsense-mediated mRNA decay. *Nature* 427 (6976): 753–757. doi: 10.1038/nature02351.

Park, Y. et al. (2022). Making sense of mRNA landscapes. *Wiley Interdiscip Rev: RNA* 13 (1): e1674. doi: 10.1002/wrna.1674.

Parras, A. et al. (2018). Autism-like phenotype and risk gene mRNA deadenylation by CPEB4 mis-splicing. *Nature* 560 (7719): 441–446. doi: 10.1038/s41586-018-0423-5.

Pilaz, L. J. et al. (2023 March 15). Subcellular mRNA localization and local translation of Arhgap11a in radial glial cells regulates cortical development. *Neuron.* 111: 839–856.

Pilaz, L.J. et al. (2016a). Dynamic mRNA transport and local translation in radial glial progenitors of the developing brain. *Curr Biol* 26 (24): 3383–3392. doi: 10.1016/j.cub.2016.10.040.

Pilaz, L.J. et al. (2016b). Prolonged mitosis of neural progenitors alters cell fate in the developing brain. *Neuron* 89 (1): 83–99. doi: 10.1016/j.neuron.2015.12.007.

Pilaz, L.J. and Silver, D.L. (2015). Post-transcriptional regulation in corticogenesis. *Wiley Interdiscip Rev: RNA* 6 (5): 501–515. doi: 10.1002/wrna.1289.

Pinson, A. and Huttner, W.B. (2021). Neocortex expansion in development and evolution-from genes to progenitor cell biology. *Curr Opin Cell Biol* 73: 9–18.

Polioudakis, D. et al. (2019). A single-cell transcriptomic atlas of human neocortical development during mid-gestation. *Neuron* 103 (5): 785–801 e788. doi: 10.1016/j.neuron.2019.06.011.

Pollard, K.S. et al. (2006). An RNA gene expressed during cortical development evolved rapidly in humans. *Nature* 443 (7108): 167–172. doi: 10.1038/nature05113.

Polydorides, A.D. et al. (2000). A brain-enriched polypyrimidine tract-binding protein antagonizes the ability of Nova to regulate neuron-specific alternative splicing. *Proc Natl Acad Sci USA* 97 (12): 6350–6355. doi: 10.1073/pnas.110128397.

Prodromidou, K. and Matsas, R. (2019). Species-specific miRNAs in human brain development and disease. *Front Cell Neurosci* 13: 559. doi: 10.3389/fncel.2019.00559.

Raj, B. and Blencowe, B.J. (2015). Alternative splicing in the mammalian nervous system. *Neuron* 87 (1): 14–27. doi: 10.1016/j.neuron.2015.05.004.

Ramaswami, G. and Li, J.B. (2014). RADAR. *Nucleic Acids Res* 42 (Database issue): D109–D113. doi: 10.1093/nar/gkt996.

Ramos, A.D. et al. (2015). The long noncoding RNA Pnky regulates neuronal differentiation of embryonic and postnatal neural stem cells. *Cell Stem Cell* 16 (4): 439–447. doi: 10.1016/j.stem.2015.02.007.

Rodriguez, J.M. et al. (2020). An analysis of tissue-specific alternative splicing at the protein level. *PLoS Comput Biol* 16 (10): e1008287. doi: 10.1371/journal.pcbi.1008287.

Rybak-Wolf, A. et al. (2015). Circular RNAs in the mammalian brain are highly abundant, conserved, and dynamically expressed. *Mol Cell* 58 (5): 870–885. doi: 10.1016/j.molcel.2015.03.027.

Saba, J.A. et al. (2021). Translational control of stem cell function. *Nat Rev Mol Cell Biol* 22 (10): 671–690. doi: 10.1038/s41580-021-00386-2.

Salvatori, B. et al. (2020). Non-coding RNAs in nervous system development and disease. *Front Cell Dev Biol* 8: 273. doi: 10.3389/fcell.2020.00273.

Sato, H. and Singer, R.H. (2021). Cellular variability of nonsense-mediated mRNA decay. *Nat Commun* 12 (1): 7203. doi: 10.1038/s41467-021-27423-0.

Sauliere, J. et al. (2012). CLIP-seq of eIF4AIII reveals transcriptome-wide mapping of the human exon junction complex. *Nat Struct Mol Biol* 19 (11): 1124–1131. doi: 10.1038/nsmb.2420.

Schwamborn, J.C. et al. (2009). The TRIM-NHL protein TRIM32 activates microRNAs and prevents self-renewal in mouse neural progenitors. *Cell* 136 (5): 913–925. doi: 10.1016/j.cell.2008.12.024.

Shafik, A.M. et al. (2022). Epitranscriptomic dynamics in brain development and disease. *Mol Psychiatry* 27 (9): 3633–3646. doi: 10.1038/s41380-022-01570-2.

Shamir, M. et al. (2016). SnapShot. *Cell* 164 (6): 1302–1302 e1301. doi: 10.1016/j.cell.2016.02.058.

Shibasaki, T. et al. (2013). PTB deficiency causes the loss of adherens junctions in the dorsal telencephalon and leads to lethal hydrocephalus. *Cereb Cortex* 23 (8): 1824–1835. doi: 10.1093/cercor/bhs161.

Shibayama, M. et al. (2009). Polypyrimidine tract-binding protein is essential for early mouse development and embryonic stem cell proliferation. *FEBS J* 276 (22): 6658–6668. doi: 10.1111/j.1742-4658.2009.07380.x.

Shibuya, T. et al. (2004). eIF4AIII binds spliced mRNA in the exon junction complex and is essential for nonsense-mediated decay. *Nat Struct Mol Biol* 11 (4): 346–351. doi: 10.1038/nsmb750.

Silver, D.L. et al. (2010). The exon junction complex component Magoh controls brain size by regulating neural stem cell division. *Nat Neurosci* 13 (5): 551–558. doi: 10.1038/nn.2527.

Singh, G. et al. (2012). The cellular EJC interactome reveals higher-order mRNP structure and an EJC-SR protein nexus. *Cell* 151 (4): 750–764. doi: 10.1016/j.cell.2012.10.007.

Sonenberg, N. and Hinnebusch, A.G. (2009). Regulation of translation initiation in eukaryotes. *Cell* 136 (4): 731–745. doi: 10.1016/j.cell.2009.01.042.

Suenkel, C. et al. (2020). A highly conserved circular RNA is required to keep neural cells in a progenitor state in the mammalian brain. *Cell Rep* 30 (7): 2170–2179.e2175. doi: 10.1016/j.celrep.2020.01.083.

Tang, L. et al. (2021). Prospective and detailed behavioral phenotyping in DDX3X syndrome. *Mol Autism* 12 (1): 36. doi: 10.1186/s13229-021-00431-z.

Tarpey, P.S. et al. (2007). Mutations in UPF3B, a member of the nonsense-mediated mRNA decay complex, cause syndromic and nonsyndromic mental retardation. *Nat Genet* 39 (9): 1127–1133. doi: 10.1038/ng2100.

Telley, L. et al. (2019). Temporal patterning of apical progenitors and their daughter neurons in the developing neocortex. *Science* 364 (6440): eaav2522. doi: 10.1126/science.aav2522.

Tomasello, U. et al. (2022). miR-137 and miR-122, two outer subventricular zone non-coding RNAs, regulate basal progenitor expansion and neuronal differentiation. *Cell Rep* 38 (7): 110381. doi: 10.1016/j.celrep.2022.110381.

Tsunekawa, Y. et al. (2012). Cyclin D2 in the basal process of neural progenitors is linked to non-equivalent cell fates. *EMBO J* 31 (8): 1879–1892. doi: 10.1038/emboj.2012.43.

Ulmke, P.A. et al. (2021). Post-transcriptional regulation by the exosome complex is required for cell survival and forebrain development via repression of P53 signaling. *Development* 148 (3): dev188276. doi: 10.1242/dev.188276.

van de, V., II et al. (2013). Long non-coding RNAs in neurodevelopmental disorders. *Front Mol Neurosci* 6: 53. doi: 10.3389/fnmol.2013.00053.

Van Nostrand, E.L. et al. (2021). Author correction. *Nature* 589 (7842): E5. doi: 10.1038/s41586-020-03067-w.

Vessey, J.P. et al. (2012). An asymmetrically localized Staufen2-dependent RNA complex regulates maintenance of mammalian neural stem cells. *Cell Stem Cell* 11 (4): 517–528. doi: 10.1016/j.stem.2012.06.010.

Walker, R.L. et al. (2019). Genetic control of expression and splicing in developing human brain informs disease mechanisms. *Cell* 179 (3): 750–771 e722. doi: 10.1016/j.cell.2019.09.021.

Wang, B. et al. (2015). FMRP-mediated axonal delivery of miR-181d regulates axon elongation by locally targeting Map1b and Calm1. *Cell Rep* 13 (12): 2794–2807. doi: 10.1016/j.celrep.2015.11.057.

Wang, D.O. et al. (2009). Synapse- and stimulus-specific local translation during long-term neuronal plasticity. *Science* 324 (5934): 1536–1540. doi: 10.1126/science.1173205.

Wang, L.W. et al. (2010). Fragile X: leading the way for targeted treatments in autism. *Neurotherapeutics* 7 (3): 264–274. doi: 10.1016/j.nurt.2010.05.005.

Wang, Y. et al. (2018). Publisher correction. *Nat Neurosci* 21 (8): 1139. doi: 10.1038/s41593-018-0169-2.

Wang, Z. et al. (2014). Transcriptome-wide modulation of splicing by the exon junction complex. *Genome Biol* 15 (12): 551. doi: 10.1186/s13059-014-0551-7.

Weil, D. et al. (2020). Mutations in genes encoding regulators of mRNA decapping and translation initiation. *Biochem Soc Trans* 48 (3): 1199–1211. doi: 10.1042/BST20200109.

Weyn-Vanhentenryck, S.M. et al. (2018). Precise temporal regulation of alternative splicing during neural development. *Nat Commun* 9 (1): 2189. doi: 10.1038/s41467-018-04559-0.

Wheeler, E.C. et al. (2018). Advances and challenges in the detection of transcriptome-wide protein-RNA interactions. *Wiley Interdiscip Rev: RNA* 9 (1): e1436. doi: 10.1002/wrna.1436.

Yan, Q. et al. (2015). Systematic discovery of regulated and conserved alternative exons in the mammalian brain reveals NMD modulating chromatin regulators. *Proc Natl Acad Sci USA* 112 (11): 3445–3450. doi: 10.1073/pnas.1502849112.

Yang, G. et al. (2014). An eIF4E1/4E-T complex determines the genesis of neurons from precursors by translationally repressing a proneurogenic transcription program. *Neuron* 84 (4): 723–739. doi: 10.1016/j.neuron.2014.10.022.

Yang, M. et al. (2015). Lin28 promotes the proliferative capacity of neural progenitor cells in brain development. *Development* 142 (9): 1616–1627. doi: 10.1242/dev.120543.

Yano, M. et al. (2010). Nova2 regulates neuronal migration through an RNA switch in disabled-1 signaling. *Neuron* 66 (6): 848–858. doi: 10.1016/j.neuron.2010.05.007.

Ye, J. and Blelloch, R. (2014). Regulation of pluripotency by RNA binding proteins. *Cell Stem Cell* 15 (3): 271–280. doi: 10.1016/j.stem.2014.08.010.

Yen, Y.P. and Chen, J.A. (2021). The m(6)A epitranscriptome on neural development and degeneration. *J Biomed Sci* 28 (1): 40. doi: 10.1186/s12929-021-00734-6.

Yoon, K.J. et al. (2017). Temporal control of mammalian cortical neurogenesis by m(6)A methylation. *Cell* 171 (4): 877–889 e817. doi: 10.1016/j.cell.2017.09.003.

You, X. et al. (2015). Neural circular RNAs are derived from synaptic genes and regulated by development and plasticity. *Nat Neurosci* 18 (4): 603–610. doi: 10.1038/nn.3975.

Yuzwa, S.A. et al. (2016). Proneurogenic ligands defined by modeling developing cortex growth factor communication networks. *Neuron* 91 (5): 988–1004. doi: 10.1016/j.neuron.2016.07.037.

Zahr, S.K. et al. (2018). A translational repression complex in developing mammalian neural stem cells that regulates neuronal specification. *Neuron* 97 (3): 520–537.e526. doi: 10.1016/j.neuron.2017.12.045.

Zhang, X. et al. (2016). Cell-type-specific alternative splicing governs cell fate in the developing cerebral cortex. *Cell* 166 (5): 1147–1162 e1115. doi: 10.1016/j.cell.2016.07.025.

Zhang, X. et al. (2019). Mechanisms and functions of long non-coding RNAs at multiple regulatory levels. *Int J Mol Sci* 20 (22): 5573. doi: 10.3390/ijms20225573.

Zhao, C. et al. (2013). MicroRNA let-7d regulates the TLX/microRNA-9 cascade to control neural cell fate and neurogenesis. *Sci Rep* 3: 1329. doi: 10.1038/srep01329.

Zhao, Y.F. et al. (2020). Human antigen R-regulated mRNA metabolism promotes the cell motility of migrating mouse neurons. *Development* 147 (6): dev183509. doi: 10.1242/dev.183509.

Zhu, Y. et al. (2018). Spatiotemporal transcriptomic divergence across human and macaque brain development. *Science* 362 (6420): eaat8077. doi: 10.1126/science.aat8077.

Ziats, M.N. and Rennert, O.M. (2013). Aberrant expression of long noncoding RNAs in autistic brain. *J Mol Neurosci* 49 (3): 589–593. doi: 10.1007/s12031-012-9880-8.

Zimmer-Bensch, G. (2019). Emerging roles of long non-coding RNAs as drivers of brain evolution. *Cells* 8 (11): 1399. doi: 10.3390/cells8111399.

29

Regulation of mRNA Localization and Translation in Brain Development

Implications for the Mechanism Leading to the Brain Evolution and Pathogenesis

Takako Kikkawa[1], *Sharmin Naher*[2], *and Noriko Osumi*[1,2]

[1] *Department of Developmental Neuroscience, United Centers for Advanced Research and Translational Medicine (ART), Tohoku University Graduate School of Medicine, 2-1 Seiryo-Machi, Aoba-ku, Sendai, Miyagi, 980-8575, Japan*
[2] *Department of Developmental Neuroscience, Tohoku University Graduate School of Life Sciences, 2-1-1 Katahira, Aoba-ku, Sendai, Miyagi 980-8577, Japan*

29.1 Introduction

During cortical development in mammals, it is critical that a large number of neuronal and glial cells are generated at defined stages and locations in order to form the expanded cortical wall. At the early stage of development, that is, embryonic day (E) 9 to E11 in mice, neural stem cells/progenitor cells (NSPCs) are known as neuroepithelial cells. During the proliferative stage, these neuroepithelial cells undergo symmetric division, producing daughter cells with equal fates to give rise to more progenitors, resulting in a thickened pseudostratified sheet on the apical side of the neural tube (Rakic 1988). The dividing cells attached to the apical side are called apical progenitors (APs) (Gotz and Huttner 2005; Haubensak et al. 2004).

As the development proceeds, neuroepithelial cells transform into radial glial (RG) cells that extend long and thin basal processes attaching to the basal membrane at the pial surface of the cortical primordium (reviewed in Kageyama et al. 2020). At the onset of neurogenesis, RG cells start to divide asymmetrically, producing one AP cell with a self-renewing capability and the other terminally differentiating into a neuron or an intermediate progenitor (IP) cell (Gotz and Huttner 2005; Huttner and Kosodo 2005). IPs divide symmetrically in the subventricular zone (SVZ) and generate a pair of IPs or neurons. NSPCs change their cell divisional mode from symmetric to asymmetric to maintain the balance between the proliferative and neurogenic state, which is critical for establishing the architecture of the mammalian cerebral cortex (Haubensak et al. 2004; Huttner and Kosodo 2005; Miyata et al. 2004). Basal processes of the RG cells act as a scaffold for the migration of newly born neurons out of the ventricular zone (VZ) to form the cortical plate (CP) (Gotz and Huttner 2005; Noctor et al. 2001).

Cell fate determination is generally regulated by specific molecules expressed in specific cell types and developmental stages. Among various molecules, those involved in RNA localization are

Neocortical Neurogenesis in Development and Evolution, First Edition. Edited by Wieland B. Huttner.

critical for adjusting the proper timing and location of the molecules to be translated (reviewed in Martin and Ephrussi 2009). RNA molecules bind to RNA binding proteins (RBPs) to be transported to specific subcellular regions (Deshler et al. 1997). Complexes of RBP-bound mRNAs are transported in both axons and dendrites of central nervous system neurons by motor proteins (Antar et al. 2005, 2006; Dictenberg et al. 2008). Translation of mRNA is generally suppressed during transport when RBPs are bound, allowing it to be locally translated in specific subregions within the cell (Napoli et al. 2008).

The mRNA dynamics in NSPCs, particularly in highly polarized RG cells during embryonic brain development, have recently been reported (reviewed in Lennox et al. 2018; Pilaz and Silver 2017; Tsunekawa et al. 2014). Here, we focus on Fragile X mental retardation protein (FMRP, an RBP) expressed in the RG cells and mRNA transport of Cyclin D2 (Ccnd2), a cell cycle regulator. We also discuss the possible role of RNA regulation in the onset of neurodevelopmental diseases and the implications for the brain evolution.

29.2 The Roles of FMRP Target mRNAs as Responsible Factors of Fragile X Syndrome

29.2.1 FMRP Functions in the Brain

FMRP is encoded by the *Fragile X mental retardation 1* (*FMR1*) gene that is responsible for Fragile X Syndrome (FXS) included in neurodevelopmental disorders (Verkerk et al. 1991). FXS is caused by an abnormal expansion of trinucleotide (CGG) repeats in the 5′-untranslated region (5′UTR) of the *FMR1* gene located on chromosome Xq27.3 (Ashley et al. 1993). This expansion greater than 200, referred to as a full mutation, results in the hypermethylation of the *FMR1* promoter and CGG repeats, leading to the transcriptional silencing of the gene and the loss of its product FMRP (Ashley et al. 1993; Crawford et al. 2001; Garber et al. 2008; Verkerk et al. 1991).

FMRP, one of the RBPs, is widely expressed both in NSPCs and neurons in embryonic and adult brains (Darnell et al. 2011; Devys et al. 1993; Gholizadeh et al. 2015; Saffary and Xie 2011). Initially, the main functions of FMRP were investigated in the postnatal brain. FMRP localizes in the cell body, proximal dendrites, and axons of neurons in the adult brain (Antar et al. 2006; Christie et al. 2009; Price et al. 2006) and plays a profound regulatory role in synaptic plasticity (reviewed in Bassell and Warren 2008; De Rubeis and Bagni 2010). Focusing on adult neurogenesis, loss of functional FMRP in NSPCs increases their proliferation and changed specification of their fate (Luo et al. 2010). Reduction of hippocampal neurogenesis due to the ablation of FMRP impairs learning ability in mice, which is rescued in the NSPC-specific conditional FMRP restoration (Guo et al. 2011).

Later, functions of FMRP are also examined in embryonic stages. FMRP is expressed, within the developing neocortex, in NSPCs, here called RG cells, and in immature neurons (Casingal et al. 2020; Pilaz et al. 2016; Saffary and Xie 2011). Within the RG cells, FMRP is specifically accumulated at the apical and basal endfeet. It is shown in the *Fmr1* knockout (*Fmr1*-KO) that the RG cell pool is slightly decreased (Saffary and Xie 2011) and that neuronal differentiation is conversely induced (Castren et al. 2005). Regarding the maintenance of the RG cell pool, FMRP regulates the transition from the RG cells to the IPs that contribute to the indirect neurogenesis (Saffary and Xie 2011). Focusing on neurons in the embryonic cortex, *Fmr1*-KO exhibited a delayed positioning of neurons in the CP with decreased expression of N-cadherin (La Fata et al. 2014). Altogether, FMRP has multiple roles in various developmental processes, and the misregulation of FMRP in the developing brain may contribute to pathogenesis for the FXS brain (see Section 29.2.3).

29.2.2 FMRP Target mRNAs in the Central Nervous System

RBPs bind to both RNAs and proteins to control various aspects of mRNA biogenesis and metabolism (reviewed in Doyle and Kiebler 2012; Pilaz and Silver 2015). FMRP is a well-studied RBP regulating the translation, transport, and stability of its target mRNAs (Darnell et al. 2011; Korb et al. 2017; Nolze et al. 2013; Pilaz et al. 2016; Zalfa et al. 2007; Zhang et al. 2007). FMRP appears to bind to its target mRNAs via one of the two KH-type domains and the arginine-glycine rich domain (RGG box) (Ashley et al. 1993; Suhl et al. 2014). In addition, specific RNA binding motifs, that is, ACUK, WGGA, and GACR, are identified as enriched binding sequences for FMRP-target mRNAs (Ascano et al. 2012; Ray et al. 2013). These multiple binding domains and specific binding motifs thus allow FMRP to exert various functions on its specific target mRNAs.

FMRP recognizes ~4 percent of the mRNAs in the mammalian brain (Ashley et al. 1993; Bassell and Warren 2008). Recently, various mRNA targets of FMRP have been identified in a specific context due to the advancement of RNA analyzing technology. RNA immunoprecipitation (RIP) followed by microarray interrogation has previously clarified 432 candidate FMRP mRNA targets in the adult mouse brain (Brown et al. 2001). High-throughput sequencing-crosslinking immunoprecipitation (HITS-CLIP), enabling a transcriptome-wide view of RNA binding sites, has identified 842 FMRP mRNA targets in the postnatal mouse cerebrum and cerebellum (Darnell et al. 2011). Another group has utilized a photoactivatable ribonucleosides-enhanced crosslinking and immunoprecipitation (PAR-CLIP) technique that enables mapping interactions of the RBPs with mRNAs and obtaining a precise sequence resolution of the interaction finding 3,593 transcripts as targets of FMRP in HEK293 cells and specific motifs (ACUK/WGGA) with strong binding affinities to FMRP (Ascano et al. 2012). Interestingly, most of the target genes are comparably expressed in the human brain. Ribosome profiling, a whole transcriptome for analyzing the number and positions of ribosomes associated with mRNA, combined with RNA-seq, has shown a large number of mRNA targets in NSPCs isolated from the hippocampal dentate gyrus and from hippocampal tissue slices of adult mice, yielding heretofore unobtainable information on gene expression at high resolution (Liu et al. 2018; Shah et al. 2020).

We have recently identified 947 transcripts (from 865 genes) as FMRP targets in the mouse cortical primordium at E14.5 using RIP-sequencing (RIP-seq) (Figure 29.1A, Casingal et al. 2020). Among the targets, the top GO (gene ontology) terms include biological processes involved in early brain development such as "nervous system development," "generation of neurons," "neurogenesis," "neuron development," "neuron differentiation," and "neuron projection development." These results are reasonable because FMRP is localized in RG cells and maintains these cells, the main source of neuronal production during cortical development. Interestingly, our mRNA targets contain genes related to "chromatin modification" (discussed in Section 29.2.3). At the subcellular level of RG cells, RIP-Chip methodology using isolated basal endfeet of RG cells has identified 115 target mRNAs in the mouse (Pilaz et al. 2016). This finding provides novel insights into the function of FMRP control of the basal transport of specific mRNAs and the regulation of their local translation.

29.2.3 FMRP Targets with Regard to Brain Development and Diseases

Fragile X syndrome (FXS) is a designated incurable disease. Approximately 1 in 7,000 males and 1 in 11,000 females have been diagnosed with FXS (Hunter et al. 2014). Usually, males are more severely affected than females. For example, males typically show severe intellectual disability (ID) with intelligence quotient (IQ) scores of 40–50, while females are less severely affected with mild to moderate cognitive impairments with an average IQ of about 80 (Chaste et al. 2012; Dahlhaus 2018; de Vries et al. 1998, 1996; Freund et al. 1993; Huddleston et al. 2014; Lewis et al. 2006). In full

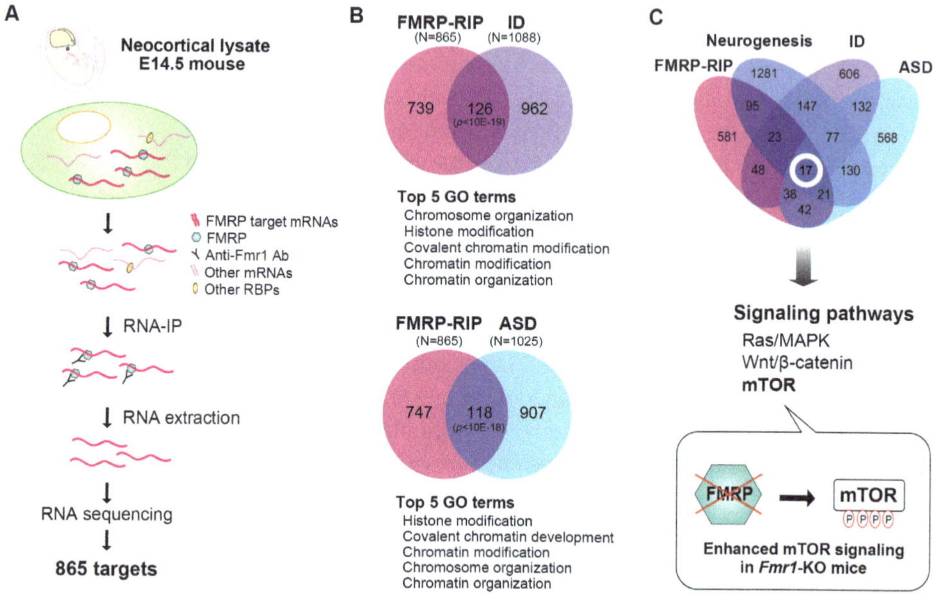

Figure 29.1 mRNA regulation by FMRP during brain development related to human Fragile X syndrome. (A) Schematic representation of RNA immunoprecipitation-sequencing (RIP-seq). Identification of 865 genes as FMRP targets in mouse neocortex at E14.5. (B) Venn diagram depicting the overlap of "FMRP target genes" and "ID genes" based on Online Mendelian Inheritance in Man (OMIM) and "ASD-associated genes" using the public database Simons Foundation Autism Research Initiative (SFARI). GO analyses show that the top five GO terms of "FMRP target genes" overlapped with "ASD/ID genes" are related to "epigenetic regulation." Hypergeometric distribution was calculated using the web tool Hypergeometric Distribution Calculator (https://keisan.casio.com/exec/system/1180573201). Values of $p < 0.05$ are considered statistically significant. (C) The four gene sets of FMRP targets (FMRP-IP), neurogenesis, ID, and ASD. Identified 17 FMRP "core" target molecules involved in Ras/MAPK, Wnt/β-catenin, and mTOR signaling pathways. Since a phosphorylated form of mTOR (p-mTOR) is elevated in the *Fmr1*-KO neocortical primordium, mTOR signaling might be enhanced in *Fmr1*-KO mice during corticogenesis. Ab: antibody; ASD: autism spectrum disorder; FMRP: Fragile X mental retardation protein; GO: Gene ontology; ID: intellectual disability; IP: immunoprecipitation; RBP: RNA binding protein.

mutation in FXS, about 96 percent of males and 64 percent of females have developmental delay or ID, and 46 percent of males and 16 percent of females are also diagnosed with autistic spectrum disorder (ASD) (Bailey et al. 2008). Autistic-like behaviors are common in FXS patients, including gaze avoidance, repetitive behavior, hand flapping/biting, and hyperarousal to sensory stimuli (Bailey et al. 2008; Kaufmann et al. 2004; McConkie-Rosell et al. 2005).

We have examined the association between our identified "FMRP target genes" with "ID genes" based on Online Mendelian Inheritance in Man (OMIM) (Amberger et al. 2019) and with "ASD-associated genes" using the public database Simons Foundation Autism Research Initiative (SFARI) (Abrahams et al. 2013). Our FMRP targets in the mouse cortical primordia significantly overlap with ID- and ASD-associated genes (Figure 29.1B, Casingal et al. 2020). Another study using the CLIP-seq in NSPCs and neurons differentiated from human pluripotent stem cells (PSCs) has identified 1,653 FMRP target genes (Li et al. 2020). These targets are also significantly associated with "ASD-associated genes" and "IQ genes" related to IQ score (Savage et al. 2018). Thus, frequent overlap of the FMRP targets in brain development with ID- and ASD-related genes in humans is reasonably suggestive of the pathogenesis of FXS, which is often co-diagnosed with ID or ASD.

What are the main target genes of FMRP that are related to the symptoms of FXS? We have further searched our FMRP targets sharing GO of "neurogenesis," "ID," and "ASD" and found 17 genes as FMRP "core" target genes (Figure 29.1C, Casingal et al. 2020). These contain not only major transcription regulators such as Pax6, Myt1l, and Tcf4 but also components of Ras/MAPK (Nf1), Wnt/β-catenin (Ahi1, Ctnna2, and Ctnnb1), and mTOR (mTOR, Ep300, Itpr1, and Synj1) signaling pathways (Figure 29.1C). It has also been reported that FMRP targets include Wnt and mTOR pathways in human PSC-derived NSPCs (Li et al. 2020), suggesting these target features are possibly common to mouse and human.

As we mentioned earlier, we found that Ctnnb1 (β-catenin, a downstream effector of Wnt signaling) is one of the targets of FMRP in the mouse cortex (Casingal et al. 2020). In the mouse cortical primordium, ablation of Wnt/β-catenin signaling induces the premature neuronal differentiation of NSPC (Draganova et al. 2015). As another aspect, *Fmr1*-KO (knockout) NSPCs derived from human PSCs also show the enhancement of the FMR1-CTNNB1-ribosome RNA network (Li et al. 2020). Enhanced ribosome biogenesis leads to increased NSPC proliferation and could cause macrocephaly (Chau et al. 2018). These molecular pathways induce the "proliferation" consistent with the macrocephaly phenotype in FXS (OMIM# 300624, Okazaki et al. 2021).

The mTOR pathway is well studied in various biological processes. The expression of a phosphorylated form of mTOR (p-mTOR) at Ser2448 is elevated in the *Fmr1*-KO neocortex, although the protein level of mTOR is not altered as shown in Figure 29.1C (Casingal et al. 2020). The result suggests that mTOR signaling might be enhanced in *Fmr1*-KO mice during corticogenesis. It remains unclear how enhanced mTOR signaling affects the corticogenesis in FXS since the function of mTOR in maintaining NSPCs or differentiating them into neurons is not consistent (reviewed in Meng et al. 2018). In a new finding regarding the role of mTOR during corticogenesis, a recent study has shown that mTOR signaling is active in human outer RG (oRG) cells and that proper activation of mTOR is essential for maintaining the basal process morphology of oRG cells and their migration behavior (Andrews et al. 2020). oRG cells are abundant in humans, therefore, dysregulation of mTOR may affect corticogenesis more in FXS patients than in FXS model mice.

Interestingly, our FMRP targets overlapped with ID- or ASD-genes are enriched with GO terms for "Chromatin/Histone modification" and "Chromosome organization" (Figure 29.1B, Casingal et al. 2020). These include chromatin-remodeling complex factors, such as Nipbl, Smarcc2, and Smarca4. In corticogenesis, Smarcc2, a chromatin remodeling complex BAF170 subunit, suppresses the expression of Pax6 target genes, for example, Tbr2 (an IP gene) as well as Cux1 and Tle (late progenitor genes), by recruiting the RE1-silencing transcription factor (REST) (Tuoc et al. 2013). Smarca4 (known as Brg1), an ATP-dependent chromatin remodeling factor, suppresses neurogenesis and promotes astrogliogenesis in the developing brain, indicating the regulation of NSPCs in neuron/glia fate specification (Matsumoto et al. 2006). FMRP could regulate the number of these epigenetic regulators and contribute to maintaining NSPCs and neural differentiation at the appropriate developmental stage. Investigation of novel epigenetic modification by FMRP during brain development may shed light on understanding of the pathogenesis of ASD.

29.3 mRNA Transport of a Cell Cycle Regulator Ccnd2

29.3.1 Functions of Cyclin D Family Members in RG Cells

During corticogenesis, asymmetric cell division and cell cycle regulation are critical for the production of new neurons while maintaining a self-renewing pool of APs (reviewed in Dehay and Kennedy 2007). The eukaryotic cell cycle is divided into four consecutive phases (Figure 29.2A), that is, G1

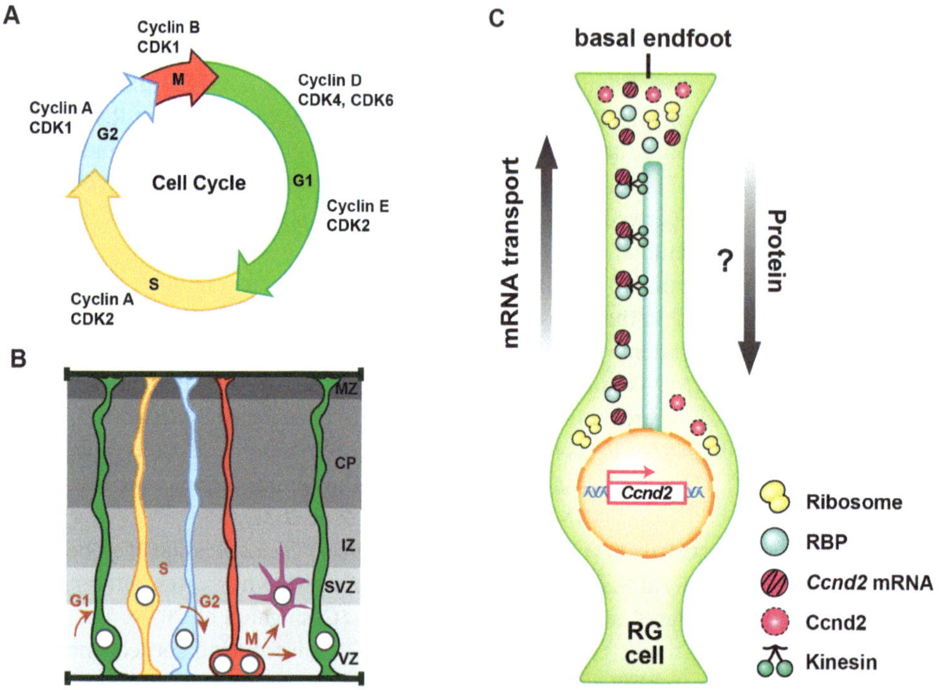

Figure 29.2 Working model of *Ccnd2* mRNA transport and its local translation in RG cells during corticogenesis. (A) The cell cycle consists of four consecutive phases (G1, S, G2, and M). Cyclin family members (i.e., cyclin A, cyclin B, cyclin D, and cyclin E) activate their respective cyclin-dependent kinases (CDKs) and promote the entry into the next phase of the cell cycle. Cyclin D forms a complex with CDK4/CDK6 to promote the transition from G1 to the S phase. Another cyclin, cyclin E associating with CDK2, also regulates progression from G1 into the S phase. cyclin A forms a complex with CDK2, and cyclin A-CDK2 complex is required to regulate the S phase. During the G2 phase, Cyclin A binds with CDK1 and promotes the entry into the M phase, which is subsequently directed by the cyclin B-CDK1 complex. (B) Interkinetic nuclear migration of radial glial (RG) cells. The nuclei of the RG cells occupy different positions along the apical–basal axis depending on the cell cycle phase. During the G1 phase, the nuclei of RG cells migrate from the apical to the basal side, and stay at the basal side within the ventricular zone (VZ) during the S phase. In the G2 phase, the nuclei undergo a basal-to-apical migration, entering the M phase upon reaching the apical surface. (C) Schematic representation of a model for *Ccnd2* mRNA transport showing that *Ccnd2* mRNA is transported from the cell soma to the basal endfoot of the RG cells along the microtubules by binding to the RNA binding proteins (RBP) and kinesin motor proteins. The identity of the RBPs and kinesins involved in *Ccnd2* mRNA transport are currently unknown. The transported mRNA is locally translated into protein via ribosomes localized at the basal endfoot. The translated protein may be transported towards the cell soma. This way, the distance for the transport from the basal endfoot to the cell soma can regulate the length of the G1 phase of the cell cycle; the longer G1 phase can eventually enhance neuronal differentiation. The question mark indicates that the Ccnd2 protein transport back to the cell soma is not yet proven. CP: cortical plate; IZ: intermediate zone; MZ: marginal zone; SVZ: subventricular zone.

phase (the longest phase and the main period of cell growth), S phase (the period when the cell duplicates its chromosomes), G2 phase (the period when the cell proceeds growing and prepares for entering the M phase), and M phase (the period for generation of two daughter cells). Depending on the phase of the cell cycle, nuclei of the NSPCs occupy different apicobasal positions within the VZ (Figure 29.2B). The nuclei of the NSPCs migrate from the apical to the basal side during G1 phase, where they stay during S phase, whereas the nuclei move toward the apical side during G2 phase and subsequently undergo mitosis at the apical surface region (Gotz and Huttner 2005; Tamai et al. 2007).

Cell cycle progression is driven by the activation of cyclin-dependent kinases (CDKs) associated with cyclins. The D-type cyclin family is composed of cyclin D1 (Ccnd1), cyclin D2 (Ccnd2), and cyclin D3 (Ccnd3) (Matsushime et al. 1991). Cyclin D-CDK4/CDK6 complexes are important for the transition from G1 to the S phase of the cell cycle through phosphorylating the retinoblastoma (Rb) protein (Ewen et al. 1993; Hinds et al. 1992; Resnitzky et al. 1994). Therefore, cyclin D family proteins can act as a positive regulator of G1 phase progression (Figure 29.2A). Cyclin D-CDK4/CDK6 activity-dependent progression in the G1 phase directly influences cell fate decisions between proliferation and differentiation (Artegiani et al. 2011; Blagosklonny and Pardee 2002; Dong et al. 2018). It has been reported that neuronal differentiation of NSPCs is increased and the pool of IPs is decreased in *Ccnd2*-deficient mice, resulting in the reduction of neuronal output and of cortical thickness (Glickstein et al. 2009). As previously reported Ccnd2 is unequally distributed into two mitotic offspring of the RG cell; one daughter cell that inherits Ccnd2 retains the self-renewing ability, while the other without Ccnd2 becomes a neuron (Tsunekawa et al. 2012; Tsunekawa and Osumi 2012). Disruption of asymmetric localization of Ccnd2 by forcing its over-expression or downregulation shows inhibition or promotion of neurogenesis, respectively (Glickstein et al. 2009; Tsunekawa et al. 2012). Therefore, Ccnd2 is a key regulator in the proper development of the brain.

The cyclin D family regulates the length of the cell cycle in NSPCs. Over-expression of the *Ccnd1* or *Ccnd1/CDK4* complex shortens the G1 phase and promotes the proliferation of the cells (Lange et al. 2009; Pilaz et al. 2009). Consistent with that result, *Ccnd2* KO mice show lengthening of the G1 phase in NSPCs at E14.5 and promotion of the differentiation to neurons, while no alteration is found in *Ccnd1* KO mice, possibly due to the compensation by *Ccnd2* (Glickstein et al. 2009). Since lengthening of the cell cycle is important for the NSPCs to switch from the proliferative stage to the neurogenic stage (Calegari et al. 2005), the cyclin D family greatly contributes to the proper production of neurons during cortical development.

29.3.2 *Ccnd2* mRNA Transport from the Cell Soma to the Basal Endfoot in RG Cells

During development of the brain, cyclin D family members are expressed in NSPCs (Glickstein et al. 2007; Tsunekawa et al. 2012). Among them, mRNA of *Ccnd2* is not only localized in the VZ but also in the cortical wall adjacent to the basal lamina (Ross et al. 1996; Ross and Risken 1994). Tsunekawa and colleagues also noticed that the *Ccnd2* mRNA is localized at the edge of the wall, and clarified its localization at the basal endfoot in the long processes of NSPCs called RG cells (Tsunekawa et al. 2012). This suggests that *Ccnd2* mRNA is localized not only in the cell soma but also in the basal endfeet of the RG cells.

The unique localization of *Ccnd2* mRNA in RG cells has posed the question of mRNA transport from the cell soma to the basal endfoot. Since 3′-untranslated region (3′UTR) is known to be essential for the transport of mRNA (reviewed in Mayr 2017), Tsunekawa et al., we have searched for the critical region within the 3′UTR of *Ccnd2*. By electroporation of the reporter construct connecting the *Ccnd2* 3′UTR to the embryonic brain, we have identified a 50-base pair (bp) *cis*-acting transport element within its 3′UTR sufficient for the basal localization of *Ccnd2* mRNA (Tsunekawa et al. 2012). Moreover, Kikkawa et al. (pers. comm.) recently generated *cis*-acting transport element-deleted mice by using the clustered regularly interspaced short palindromic repeats (CRISPR)/CRISPR-associated protein 9 (Cas9) genome editing system, and found successful inhibition of *Ccnd2* mRNA basal transport in the RG cells (Kikkawa et al. pers. comm.). These results suggest that the short *cis*-acting transport element is essential for the *Ccnd2* mRNA transport in RG cells.

Ccnd2 mRNA moves along the basal process towards the pial side during S-to-G2 phase transition by using its *cis*-acting transport element, where it is locally translated into protein (Pilaz et al. 2016; Tsunekawa et al. 2012). As mentioned earlier, Ccnd2 protein is asymmetrically inherited by one of the two daughter cells along with the basal process during mitosis. After cell division, Ccnd2 protein is accumulated in the nucleus of the basally positioned daughter cell during G1 phase, resulting in the asymmetric distribution of Ccnd2 protein between the two daughter cells, affecting the acquisition of different fates of the daughter cells (Tsunekawa et al. 2012). Thus, the regulatory process of *Ccnd2* mRNA transport system in the RG cells might be a key for appropriate corticogenesis.

29.3.3 Possible Regulation of *Ccnd2* mRNA Transport in RG Cells

From the cell soma to its final destiny, mRNA does not travel alone during the journey within the long basal process. Based on previous studies, the transport of mRNA to the distinct region within a cell is likely to be accomplished by trans-acting RBPs that bind to *cis*-acting transport elements of mRNA, as well as by cytoskeletal motor proteins as a cargo and microtubules as a rail (Brendza et al. 2000; Dictenberg et al. 2008; Palacios and St. Johnston 2001). As previously mentioned, FMRP binds to specific mRNAs and moves basally acting as a RBP in RG cells (Pilaz et al. 2016). Although a previous biochemical study shows that the *Ccnd2* mRNA binds to FMRP (Pilaz et al. 2016), localization of *Ccnd2* mRNA was not apparently altered in *Fmr1*-KO embryos (Kikkawa et al., pers. comm.). Therefore, FMRP may support specific localization of some basal molecules, yet *Ccnd2* mRNA might be transported by other RBP(s).

We consider that the kinesins, as an intracellular transporter of cargos including organelles, proteins, and mRNAs (Hirokawa et al. 1991; Kanai et al. 2004; Wu et al. 2020), might be one of the candidate motor proteins that can carry *Ccnd2* mRNA for basal transport. Among the diverse classes of kinesins, plus end-directed motor protein N-kinesins have been widely studied (reviewed in Hirokawa and Noda 2008; Hirokawa et al. 2009). In the RG, microtubules within the basal process have a mixed polarity, where two-thirds of the dynamic microtubules are plus-end out, growing toward the basal endfoot (Coquand et al. 2021). This polarity suggests that transportation in the basal process likely relies on kinesin-based movement. Interestingly, some of the N-kinesin family members are localized in the cell body and the basal endfoot of the RG cells (Naher et al. pers. comm.). It is speculated that these N-kinesin motor proteins may carry cargos containing the *Ccnd2* mRNA-protein complex along the microtubule from its minus to plus end, that is, from apical to basal side within the developing cortex. Therefore, identifying kinesin motor proteins and RBPs involved in *Ccnd2* mRNA transport and understanding the functional impact of this transport mechanism on cortical neurogenesis is an important area for future studies.

29.3.4 Hypotheses of the Role of Ccnd2 Transport System during Brain Evolution

Figure 29.2C shows a proposed working model of *Ccnd2* mRNA transport system in mouse RG cells. After transcription, *Ccnd2* mRNA is transported to the basal endfoot of RG cells via a short *cis*-acting transport element within the 3′UTR of *Ccnd2*. The mRNA of *Ccnd2* is locally translated into protein in the basal endfoot raising the question whether this phenomenon is conserved in other species.

Tsunekawa et al. have previously shown, by immunostaining, the localization of Ccnd2 protein in the human cortex (Tsunekawa et al. 2012). At 16 and 19 gestational weeks (GW), Ccnd2 is strongly detected at the marginal zone (MZ) and upper part of the CP, especially accumulating in the region of the brain surface area and not localized in the nuclei of cells in the MZ and CP. In the expanded subplate in the human brain, punctate signals are observed along with the basal process-like structure. Ccnd2 expression is also observed in the nuclei in the VZ and inner SVZ (ISVZ). These localization patterns of Ccnd2 protein in the human fetal brain are compatible with the RG cells in the mouse. Furthermore, the *cis*-acting transport element within its 3′UTR for the basal localization of *Ccnd2* mRNA is highly conserved in placental mammals, including humans, but not in other species (Kikkawa et al. pers. comm.). This raises a possibility that the system of basal transport of *Ccnd2* mRNA and its local translation may be conserved in these mammals.

Compared to the brain structure of RG cells in rodent and species with gyrencephalic brains (e.g., ferret, monkey, and human), the length of radial processes in humans has become much longer than that of mice due to the expansion of the cortical thickness due to abundant IPs in the ISVZ and to the emergence of oRG cells (reviewed in Namba and Huttner 2017). This means that, in the developing human brain, it takes a longer time for: *Ccnd2* mRNA to travel towards the basal endfoot; and for Ccnd2 protein to return to the nuclei. Since Ccnd2 protein is well-known for promoting the G1–S transition of the cell cycle by associating with Cdks in the nuclei, the transition period from G1 to S phase may be longer due to the extended trip of Ccnd2 along the basal process, eventually resulting in production of more neurons in the gyrencephalic brains.

Species with gyrencephalic brains have abundant proliferative cells in the upper layer of the SVZ called the outer SVZ (OSVZ) (Betizeau et al. 2013; Fish et al. 2008; Lukaszewicz et al. 2005; Smart et al. 2002). These cells are distinguished by their possession of basal but not apical processes (Fietz et al. 2010; Hansen et al. 2010). Ccnd2 protein is also present in the cells of the OSVZ in the human fetal brain (Tsunekawa et al. 2012). Although it remains unclear whether the *Ccnd2* mRNA is transported within oRG cells, the basal transport system in oRG cells may contribute to the expansion of the numbers of the cells in gyrencephalic brain species. Currently, we are investigating the possible role of *Ccnd2* mRNA transport and local translation in RG cells contribution to evolution.

29.3.5 Ccnd2 Functions Related to Human Diseases

Macrocephaly and microcephaly are severe malformation of the brain due to overgrowth or growth deficit, respectively. Genetic variants of *CCND2* have been identified as pathogenic causes of both malformations. To date, 12 patients with megalencephaly-polymicrogyria-polydactyly-hydrocephalus (MPPH) syndrome (Mirzaa et al. 2014) and five patients with microcephaly have been reported to have mutations in *CCND2* (Pirozzi et al. 2021). It has been previously shown in the mouse that over-expression of the *Ccnd2* gene increases proliferation of progenitor cells (i.e., RG cells and IPs) (Tsunekawa et al. 2012). Over-expression of the *Ccnd2* gene with a mutation in MPPH in the mouse increases progenitor proliferation with concomitant decreases in the fraction of cells exiting the cell cycle (Mirzaa et al. 2014). *Ccnd2* KO mice conversely exhibit microcephaly and cerebellar hypoplasia (Glickstein et al. 2009; Huard et al. 1999). The loss of Ccnd2 reduces brain volume by allowing cell cycle exit, resulting in depletion of the progenitor pool (Glickstein et al. 2009). It has also been shown that introducing siRNA for *Ccnd2* causes a reduction in the proliferation of progenitor cells (Tsunekawa et al. 2012). In both humans and mice, the gain and loss of function of Ccnd2 results in inverse brain growth phenotypes and adds *CCND2* to the growing list of the genes regulating brain growth.

CCND2 seems to be related to Alzheimer's disease (AD). A recent study has reported that *CCND2* is downregulated in both the neocortex and hippocampus of AD patients (Czapski et al. 2021). Several groups have shown dysfunction of cell cycle regulation and enhanced neurogenesis and neuronal cell death in AD patients and in the animal model of AD (Arendt et al. 1998; Busser et al. 1998; Jin et al. 2004a, 2004b). These suggest the possibility that *CCND2* is involved in the pathogenesis of AD through the regulation of neocortical and hippocampal neurogenesis.

29.4 Conclusion

It is gradually becoming clear that RNA regulation plays a role in many aspects of brain development. However, the biological functions of RNA regulation in the embryonic brain are still not fully understood. FMRP is a well-studied RBP that regulates the transport and translation of its target mRNAs. Recently, it has been revealed in neurons that FMRP regulates the expression of epigenetic regulators (Korb et al. 2017; Shah et al. 2020), which are gaining attention as a possible cause of neurodevelopmental disorders such as ASD (reviewed in Reichard and Zimmer-Bensch 2021). Further research into the regulation of FMRP-epigenetic factors in the human embryonic brain could lead to a better understanding of neurodevelopmental disorders like FXS, which is often co-diagnosed with ASD/ID. Furthermore, biological properties of transported mRNA in RG cells remain unknown. Is it necessary, for example, for *Ccnd2* mRNA to be transported outside the nuclei and locally translated in the basal endfoot? How does the RNA transport mechanism in RG cells contribute to RG cell evolution and contribute to brain size expansion? Future research will be required to explore the function of mRNA localization in the RG cells during cell cycle, such as cell fate determination.

Author contributions

Takako Kikkawa, Sharmin Naher, and Noriko Osumi drafted the manuscript and created the figures. Takako Kikkawa and Noriko Osumi discussed and polished the manuscript. All authors contributed to the study and have approved the final manuscript.

Funding

This work was supported by JSPS KAKENHI for Takako Kikkawa (#20K07237), Noriko Osumi (#19H03318), and AMED (JP21wm0425003).

References

Abrahams, B.S. et al. (2013). SFARI Gene 2.0. *Mol Autism* 4 (1): 36. doi: 10.1186/2040-2392-4-36.

Amberger, J.S. et al. (2019). OMIM.org: leveraging knowledge across phenotype-gene relationships. *Nucleic Acids Res* 47 (D1): D1038–D1043. doi: 10.1093/nar/gky1151.

Andrews, M.G. et al. (2020). mTOR signaling regulates the morphology and migration of outer radial glia in developing human cortex. *Elife* 9: e58737. doi: 10.7554/eLife.58737.

Antar, L.N. et al. (2005). Localization of FMRP-associated mRNA granules and requirement of microtubules for activity-dependent trafficking in hippocampal neurons. *Genes, Brain, Behav* 4 (6): 350–359. doi: 10.1111/j.1601-183X.2005.00128.x.

Antar, L.N. et al. (2006). Local functions for FMRP in axon growth cone motility and activity-dependent regulation of filopodia and spine synapses. *Mol Cell Neurosci* 32 (1–2): 37–48. doi: 10.1016/j.mcn.2006.02.001.

Arendt, T. et al. (1998). Neuronal expression of cycline dependent kinase inhibitors of the INK4 family in Alzheimer's disease. *J Neural Transm* 105 (8–9): 949–960. doi: 10.1007/s007020050104.

Artegiani, B. et al. (2011). Overexpression of cdk4 and cyclinD1 triggers greater expansion of neural stem cells in the adult mouse brain. *J Exp Med* 208 (5): 937–948. doi: 10.1084/jem.20102167.

Ascano, M., Jr. et al. (2012). FMRP targets distinct mRNA sequence elements to regulate protein expression. *Nature* 492 (7429): 382–386. doi: 10.1038/nature11737.

Ashley, C.T. et al. (1993). Fmr1 protein – conserved Rnp family domains and selective Rna-binding. *Science* 262 (5133): 563–566. doi: 10.1126/science.7692601.

Bailey, D.B., Jr. et al. (2008). Co-occurring conditions associated with FMR1 gene variations. *Am J Med Genet Part A* 146A (16): 2060–2069. doi: 10.1002/ajmg.a.32439.

Bassell, G.J. and Warren, S.T. (2008). Fragile X syndrome. *Neuron* 60 (2): 201–214. doi: 10.1016/j.neuron.2008.10.004.

Betizeau, M. et al. (2013). Precursor diversity and complexity of lineage relationships in the outer subventricular zone of the primate. *Neuron* 80 (2): 442–457. doi: 10.1016/j.neuron.2013.09.032.

Blagosklonny, M.V. and Pardee, A.B. (2002). The restriction point of the cell cycle. *Cell Cycle* 1 (2): 103–110. PMID: 12429916.

Brendza, R.P. et al. (2000). A function for kinesin I in the posterior transport of oskar mRNA and Staufen protein. *Science* 289 (5487): 2120–2122. doi: 10.1126/science.289.5487.2120.

Brown, V. et al. (2001). Microarray identification of FMRP-associated brain mRNAs and altered mRNA translational profiles in Fragile X syndrome. *Cell* 107 (4): 477–487. doi: 10.1016/s0092-8674(01)00568-2.

Busser, J. et al. (1998). Ectopic cell cycle proteins predict the sites of neuronal cell death in Alzheimer's disease brain. *J Neurosci* 18 (8): 2801–2807. doi: 10.1523/JNEUROSCI.18-08-02801.1998.

Calegari, F. et al. (2005). Selective lengthening of the cell cycle in the neurogenic subpopulation of neural progenitor cells during mouse brain development. *J Neurosci* 25 (28): 6533–6538. doi: 10.1523/JNEUROSCI.0778-05.2005.

Casingal, C.R. et al. (2020). Identification of FMRP target mRNAs in the developmental brain. *Mol Brain* 13 (1): 167. doi: 10.1186/s13041-020-00706-1.

Castren, M. et al. (2005). Altered differentiation of neural stem cells in Fragile X syndrome. *Proc Natl Acad Sci USA* 102 (49): 17834–17839. doi: 10.1073/pnas.0508995102.

Chaste, P. et al. (2012). High-functioning autism spectrum disorder and Fragile X syndrome. *Mol Autism* 3 (1): 5. doi: 10.1186/2040-2392-3-5.

Chau, K.F. et al. (2018). Downregulation of ribosome biogenesis during early forebrain development. *Elife* 7: e36998. doi: 10.7554/eLife.36998.

Christie, S.B. et al. (2009). The FXG. *J Neurosci* 29 (5): 1514–1524. doi: 10.1523/JNEUROSCI.3937-08.2009.

Coquand, L. et al. (2021). CAMSAPs organize an acentrosomal microtubule network from basal varicosities in radial glial cells. *J Cell Biol* 220: 8. doi: 10.1083/jcb.202003151.

Crawford, D.C. et al. (2001). FMR1 and the Fragile X syndrome. *Genet Med* 3 (5): 359–371. doi: 10.1097/00125817-200109000-00006.

Czapski, G.A. et al. (2021). Down-regulation of cyclin D2 in amyloid beta toxicity, inflammation, and Alzheimer's disease. *PLoS One* 16 (11): e0259740. doi: 10.1371/journal.pone.0259740.

Dahlhaus, R. (2018). Of men and mice. *Front Mol Neurosci* 11: 41. doi: 10.3389/fnmol.2018.00041.

Darnell, J.C. et al. (2011). FMRP stalls ribosomal translocation on mRNAs linked to synaptic function and autism. *Cell* 146 (2): 247–261. doi: 10.1016/j.cell.2011.06.013.

De Rubeis, S. and Bagni, C. (2010). Fragile X mental retardation protein control of neuronal mRNA metabolism. *Mol Cell Neurosci* 43 (1): 43–50. doi: 10.1016/j.mcn.2009.09.013.

de Vries, B.B. et al. (1998). The fragile X syndrome. *J Med Genet* 35 (7): 579–589. doi: 10.1136/jmg.35.7.579.

de Vries, B.B. et al. (1996). Mental status of females with an FMR1 gene full mutation. *Am J Hum Genet* 58 (5): 1025–1032. https://www.ncbi.nlm.nih.gov/pubmed/8651263.

Dehay, C. and Kennedy, H. (2007). Cell-cycle control and cortical development. *Nat Rev Neurosci* 8 (6): 438–450. doi: 10.1038/nrn2097.

Deshler, J.O. et al. (1997). Localization of Xenopus Vg1 mRNA by Vera protein and the endoplasmic reticulum. *Science* 276 (5315): 1128–1131. doi: 10.1126/science.276.5315.1128.

Devys, D. et al. (1993). The FMR-1 protein is cytoplasmic, most abundant in neurons and appears normal in carriers of a fragile X premutation. *Nat Genet* 4 (4): 335–340. doi: 10.1038/ng0893-335.

Dictenberg, J.B.et al. (2008). A direct role for FMRP in activity-dependent dendritic mRNA transport links filopodial-spine morphogenesis to Fragile X syndrome. *Dev Cell* 14 (6): 926–939. doi: 10.1016/j.devcel.2008.04.003.

Dong, P. et al. (2018). Cyclin D/CDK4/6 activity controls G1 length in mammalian cells. *PLoS One* 13 (1): e0185637. doi: 10.1371/journal.pone.0185637.

Doyle, M. and Kiebler, M.A. (2012). A zipcode unzipped. *Genes Dev* 26 (2): 110–113. doi: 10.1101/gad.184945.111.

Draganova, K. et al. (2015). Wnt/beta-catenin signaling regulates sequential fate decisions of murine cortical precursor cells. *Stem Cells* 33 (1): 170–182. doi: 10.1002/stem.1820.

Ewen, M.E. et al. (1993). Functional interactions of the retinoblastoma protein with mammalian D-type cyclins. *Cell* 73 (3): 487–497. doi: 10.1016/0092-8674(93)90136-e.

Fietz, S.A. et al. (2010). OSVZ progenitors of human and ferret neocortex are epithelial-like and expand by integrin signaling. *Nat Neurosci* 13 (6): 690–699. doi: 10.1038/nn.2553.

Fish, J.L. et al. (2008). Making bigger brains – the evolution of neural-progenitor-cell division. *J Cell Sci* 121 (Pt 17): 2783–2793. doi: 10.1242/jcs.023465.

Freund, L.S. et al. (1993). Psychiatric disorders associated with fragile X in the young female. *Pediatrics* 91 (2): 321–329. https://www.ncbi.nlm.nih.gov/pubmed/8380924.

Garber, K.B. et al. (2008). Fragile X syndrome. *Eur J Hum Genet* 16 (6): 666–672. doi: 10.1038/ejhg.2008.61.

Gholizadeh, S. et al. (2015). Expression of fragile X mental retardation protein in neurons and glia of the developing and adult mouse brain. *Brain Res* 1596: 22–30. doi: 10.1016/j.brainres.2014.11.023.

Glickstein, S.B. et al. (2007). Differences in cyclin D2 and D1 protein expression distinguish forebrain progenitor subsets. *Cereb Cortex* 17 (3): 632–642. doi: 10.1093/cercor/bhk008.

Glickstein, S.B. et al. (2009). Cyclin D2 is critical for intermediate progenitor cell proliferation in the embryonic cortex. *J Neurosci* 29 (30): 9614–9624. doi: 10.1523/JNEUROSCI.2284-09.2009.

Gotz, M. and Huttner, W.B. (2005). The cell biology of neurogenesis. *Nat Rev Mol Cell Biol* 6 (10): 777–788. doi: 10.1038/nrm1739.

Guo, W. et al. (2011). Ablation of Fmrp in adult neural stem cells disrupts hippocampus-dependent learning. *Nat Med* 17 (5): 559–565. doi: 10.1038/nm.2336.

Hansen, D.V. et al. (2010). Neurogenic radial glia in the outer subventricular zone of human neocortex. *Nature* 464 (7288): 554–561. doi: 10.1038/nature08845.

Haubensak, W. et al. (2004). Neurons arise in the basal neuroepithelium of the early mammalian telencephalon. *Proc Natl Acad Sci USA* 101 (9): 3196–3201. doi: 10.1073/pnas.0308600100.

Hinds, P.W. et al. (1992). Regulation of retinoblastoma protein functions by ectopic expression of human cyclins. *Cell* 70 (6): 993–1006. doi: 10.1016/0092-8674(92)90249-c.

Hirokawa, N. and Noda, Y. (2008). Intracellular transport and kinesin superfamily proteins, KIFs. *Physiol Rev* 88 (3): 1089–1118. doi: 10.1152/physrev.00023.2007.

Hirokawa, N. et al. (2009). Kinesin superfamily motor proteins and intracellular transport. *Nat Rev Mol Cell Biol* 10 (10): 682–696. doi: 10.1038/nrm2774.

Hirokawa, N. et al. (1991). Kinesin associates with anterogradely transported membranous organelles in vivo. *J Cell Biol* 114 (2): 295–302. doi: 10.1083/jcb.114.2.295.

Huard, J.M. et al. (1999). Cerebellar histogenesis is disturbed in mice lacking cyclin D2. *Development* 126 (9): 1927–1935. doi: 10.1242/dev.126.9.1927.

Huddleston, L.B. et al. (2014). Cognitive aspects of Fragile X syndrome. *Wiley Interdiscip Rev: Cogn Sci* 5 (4): 501–508. doi: 10.1002/wcs.1296.

Hunter, J. et al. (2014). Epidemiology of Fragile X syndrome. *Am J Med Genet Part A* 164A (7): 1648–1658. doi: 10.1002/ajmg.a.36511.

Huttner, W.B. and Kosodo, Y. (2005). Symmetric versus asymmetric cell division during neurogenesis in the developing vertebrate central nervous system. *Curr Opin Cell Biol* 17 (6): 648–657. doi: 10.1016/j.ceb.2005.10.005.

Jin, K. et al. (2004a). Enhanced neurogenesis in Alzheimer's disease transgenic (PDGF-APPSw, Ind) mice. *Proc Natl Acad Sci USA* 101 (36): 13363–13367. doi: 10.1073/pnas.0403678101.

Jin, K. et al. (2004b). Increased hippocampal neurogenesis in Alzheimer's disease. *Proc Natl Acad Sci USA* 101 (1): 343–347. doi: 10.1073/pnas.2634794100.

Kageyama, R. et al. (2020). The significance of gene expression dynamics in neural stem cell regulation. *Proc Jpn Acad Ser B, Phys Biol Sci* 96 (8): 351–363. doi: 10.2183/pjab.96.026.

Kanai, Y. et al. (2004). Kinesin transports RNA. *Neuron* 43 (4): 513–525. doi: 10.1016/j.neuron.2004.07.022.

Kaufmann, W.E. et al. (2004). Autism spectrum disorder in Fragile X syndrome. *Am J Med Genet Part A* 129A (3): 225–234. doi: 10.1002/ajmg.a.30229.

Korb, E. et al. (2017). Excess translation of epigenetic regulators contributes to Fragile X syndrome and is alleviated by Brd4 inhibition. *Cell* 170 (6): 1209–1223 e1220. doi: 10.1016/j.cell.2017.07.033.

La Fata, G. et al. (2014). FMRP regulates multipolar to bipolar transition affecting neuronal migration and cortical circuitry. *Nat Neurosci* 17 (12): 1693–1700. doi: 10.1038/nn.3870.

Lange, C. et al. (2009). Cdk4/cyclinD1 overexpression in neural stem cells shortens G1, delays neurogenesis, and promotes the generation and expansion of basal progenitors. *Cell Stem Cell* 5 (3): 320–331. doi: 10.1016/j.stem.2009.05.026.

Lennox, A.L. et al. (2018). RNA on the brain: emerging layers of post-transcriptional regulation in cerebral cortex development. *Wiley Interdiscip Rev: Dev Biol* 7: 1. doi: 10.1002/wdev.290.

Lewis, P. et al. (2006). Cognitive, language and social-cognitive skills of individuals with Fragile X syndrome with and without autism. *J Intellect Disabil Res* 50 (Pt 7): 532–545. doi: 10.1111/j.1365-2788.2006.00803.x.

Li, M. et al. (2020). Identification of FMR1-regulated molecular networks in human neurodevelopment. *Genome Res* 30 (3): 361–374. doi: 10.1101/gr.251405.119.

Liu, B. et al. (2018). Regulatory discrimination of mRNAs by FMRP controls mouse adult neural stem cell differentiation. *Proc Natl Acad Sci USA* 115 (48): E11397–E11405. doi: 10.1073/pnas.1809588115.

Lukaszewicz, A. et al. (2005). G1 phase regulation, area-specific cell cycle control, and cytoarchitectonics in the primate cortex. *Neuron* 47 (3): 353–364. doi: 10.1016/j.neuron.2005.06.032.

Luo, Y. et al. (2010). Fragile x mental retardation protein regulates proliferation and differentiation of adult neural stem/progenitor cells. *PLoS Genet* 6 (4): e1000898. doi: 10.1371/journal.pgen.1000898.

Martin, K.C. and Ephrussi, A. (2009). mRNA localization. *Cell* 136 (4): 719–730. doi: 10.1016/j.cell.2009.01.044.

Matsumoto, S. et al. (2006). Brg1 is required for murine neural stem cell maintenance and gliogenesis. *Dev Biol* 289 (2): 372–383. doi: 10.1016/j.ydbio.2005.10.044.

Matsushime, H. et al. (1991). Colony-stimulating factor 1 regulates novel cyclins during the G1 phase of the cell cycle. *Cell* 65 (4): 701–713. doi: 10.1016/0092-8674(91)90101-4.

Mayr, C. (2017). Regulation by 3′-untranslated regions. *Ann Rev Genet* 51: 171–194. doi: 10.1146/annurev-genet-120116-024704.

McConkie-Rosell, A. et al. (2005). Genetic counseling for Fragile x syndrome. *J Genet Couns* 14 (4): 249–270. doi: 10.1007/s10897-005-4802-x.

Meng, D. et al. (2018). mTOR signaling in stem and progenitor cells. *Development* 145 (1): dev152595. doi: 10.1242/dev.152595.

Mirzaa, G. et al. (2014). De novo CCND2 mutations leading to stabilization of cyclin D2 cause megalencephaly-polymicrogyria-polydactyly-hydrocephalus syndrome. *Nat Genet* 46 (5): 510–515. doi: 10.1038/ng.2948.

Miyata, T. et al. (2004). Asymmetric production of surface-dividing and non-surface-dividing cortical progenitor cells. *Development* 131 (13): 3133–3145. doi: 10.1242/dev.01173.

Namba, T. and Huttner, W.B. (2017). Neural progenitor cells and their role in the development and evolutionary expansion of the neocortex. *Wiley Interdiscip Rev: Dev Biol* 6: 1. doi: 10.1002/wdev.256.

Napoli, I. et al. (2008). The fragile X syndrome protein represses activity-dependent translation through CYFIP1, a new 4E-BP. *Cell* 134 (6): 1042–1054. doi: 10.1016/j.cell.2008.07.031.

Noctor, S.C. et al. (2001). Neurons derived from radial glial cells establish radial units in neocortex. *Nature* 409 (6821): 714–720. doi: 10.1038/35055553.

Nolze, A. et al. (2013). FMRP regulates actin filament organization via the armadillo protein p0071. *RNA* 19 (11): 1483–1496. doi: 10.1261/rna.037945.112.

Okazaki, T. et al. (2021). Clinical characteristics of Fragile X syndrome patients in Japan. *Yonago Acta Med* 64 (1): 30–33. doi: 10.33160/yam.2021.02.005.

Palacios, I.M. and St Johnston, D. (2001). Getting the message across. *Ann Rev Cell Dev Biol* 17: 569–614. doi: 10.1146/annurev.cellbio.17.1.569.

Pilaz, L.J. et al. (2016). Dynamic mRNA transport and local translation in radial glial progenitors of the developing brain. *Curr Biol* 26 (24): 3383–3392. doi: 10.1016/j.cub.2016.10.040.

Pilaz, L.J. et al. (2009). Forced G1-phase reduction alters mode of division, neuron number, and laminar phenotype in the cerebral cortex. *Proc Natl Acad Sci USA* 106 (51): 21924–21929. doi: 10.1073/pnas.0909894106.

Pilaz, L.J. and Silver, D.L. (2015). Post-transcriptional regulation in corticogenesis. *Wiley Interdiscip Rev: RNA* 6 (5): 501–515. doi: 10.1002/wrna.1289.

Pilaz, L.J. and Silver, D.L. (2017). Moving messages in the developing brain-emerging roles for mRNA transport and local translation in neural stem cells. *FEBS Lett* 591 (11): 1526–1539. doi: 10.1002/1873-3468.12626.

Pirozzi, F. et al. (2021). Proximal variants in CCND2 associated with microcephaly, short stature, and developmental delay. *Am J Med Genet Part A* 185 (9): 2719–2738. doi: 10.1002/ajmg.a.62362.

Price, T.J. et al. (2006). The RNA binding and transport proteins staufen and Fragile X mental retardation protein are expressed by rat primary afferent neurons and localize to peripheral and central axons. *Neuroscience* 141 (4): 2107–2116. doi: 10.1016/j.neuroscience.2006.05.047.

Rakic, P. (1988). Specification of cerebral cortical areas. *Science* 241 (4862): 170–176. doi: 10.1126/science.3291116.

Ray, D. et al. (2013). A compendium of RNA-binding motifs for decoding gene regulation. *Nature* 499 (7457): 172–177. doi: 10.1038/nature12311.

Reichard, J. and Zimmer-Bensch, G. (2021). The epigenome in neurodevelopmental disorders. *Front Neurosci* 15: 776809. doi: 10.3389/fnins.2021.776809.

Resnitzky, D. et al. (1994). Acceleration of the G1/S phase transition by expression of cyclins D1 and E with an inducible system. *Mol Cell Biol* 14 (3): 1669–1679. doi: 10.1128/mcb.14.3.1669-1679.1994.

Ross, M.E. et al. (1996). MN20, a D2 cyclin, is transiently expressed in selected neural populations during embryogenesis. *J Neurosci* 16 (1): 210–219. doi: 10.1523/JNEUROSCI.16-01-00210.1996.

Ross, M.E. and Risken, M. (1994). MN20, a D2 cyclin found in brain, is implicated in neural differentiation. *J Neurosci* 14 (11Pt 1): 6384–6391. doi: 10.1523/JNEUROSCI.14-11-06384.1994.

Saffary, R. and Xie, Z. (2011). FMRP regulates the transition from radial glial cells to intermediate progenitor cells during neocortical development. *J Neurosci* 31 (4): 1427–1439. doi: 10.1523/JNEUROSCI.4854-10.2011.

Savage, J.E. et al. (2018). Genome-wide association meta-analysis in 269,867 individuals identifies new genetic and functional links to intelligence. *Nat Genet* 50 (7): 912–919. doi: 10.1038/s41588-018-0152-6.

Shah, S. et al. (2020). FMRP control of ribosome translocation promotes chromatin modifications and alternative splicing of neuronal genes linked to Autism. *Cell Rep* 30 (13): 4459–4472. e4456. doi: 10.1016/j.celrep.2020.02.076.

Smart, I.H. et al. (2002). Unique morphological features of the proliferative zones and postmitotic compartments of the neural epithelium giving rise to striate and extrastriate cortex in the monkey. *Cereb Cortex* 12 (1): 37–53. doi: 10.1093/cercor/12.1.37.

Suhl, J.A. et al. (2014). Analysis of FMRP mRNA target datasets reveals highly associated mRNAs mediated by G-quadruplex structures formed via clustered WGGA sequences. *Hum Mol Genet* 23 (20): 5479–5491. doi: 10.1093/hmg/ddu272.

Tamai, H. et al. (2007). Pax6 transcription factor is required for the interkinetic nuclear movement of neuroepithelial cells. *Genes Cells* 12 (9): 983–996. doi: 10.1111/j.1365-2443.2007.01113.x.

Tsunekawa, Y. et al. (2012). Cyclin D2 in the basal process of neural progenitors is linked to non-equivalent cell fates. *EMBO J* 31 (8): 1879–1892. doi: 10.1038/emboj.2012.43.

Tsunekawa, Y. et al. (2014). Asymmetric inheritance of Cyclin D2 maintains proliferative neural stem/progenitor cells. *Dev Growth Diff* 56 (5): 349–357. doi: 10.1111/dgd.12135.

Tsunekawa, Y. and Osumi, N. (2012). How to keep proliferative neural stem/progenitor cells. *Cell Cycle* 11 (19): 3550–3554. doi: 10.4161/cc.21500.

Tuoc, T.C. et al. (2013). Chromatin regulation by BAF170 controls cerebral cortical size and thickness. *Dev Cell* 25 (3): 256–269. doi: 10.1016/j.devcel.2013.04.005.

Verkerk, A.J. et al. (1991). Identification of a gene (FMR-1) containing a CGG repeat coincident with a breakpoint cluster region exhibiting length variation in fragile X syndrome. *Cell* 65 (5): 905–914. doi: 10.1016/0092-8674(91)90397-h.

Wu, H. et al. (2020). A kinesin adapter directly mediates dendritic mRNA localization during neural development in mice. *J Biol Chem* 295 (19): 6605–6628. doi: 10.1074/jbc.RA118.005616.

Zalfa, F. et al. (2007). A new function for the fragile X mental retardation protein in regulation of PSD-95 mRNA stability. *Nat Neurosci* 10 (5): 578–587. doi: 10.1038/nn1893.

Zhang, M. et al. (2007). Fragile X mental retardation protein FMRP and the RNA export factor NXF2 associate with and destabilize Nxf1 mRNA in neuronal cells. *Proc Natl Acad Sci USA* 104 (24): 10057–10062. doi: 10.1073/pnas.0700169104.

30

Signal Transduction during Cortical Neurogenesis

Dan Xu[1], Yiqiang Zhi[1], and Zhiheng Xu[2]

[1] *Fujian Key Laboratory of Molecular Neurology, Institute of Neuroscience, Fujian Medical University Fuzhou 350005, China*
[2] *State Key Laboratory of Molecular Developmental Biology, Institute of Genetics and Developmental Biology, Chinese Academy of Sciences, Beijing 100101, China*

Abbreviations

Abnormal spindle-like microcephaly associated protein	ASPM	Interkinetic nuclear migration	INM
		Intermediate precursor cells	IPCs
Adenomatous polyposis coli	APC	Intermediate zone	IZ
Autism spectrum disorder	ASD	Knockout	KO
Basal neural precursor cells	BPCs	Leukemia inhibitory factor	LIF
Basal radial glia	bRG	Lipoprotein receptor related protein 5/6	LRP5/6
Basic helix-loop-helix	bHLH	Autosomal recessive primary microcephaly	MCPH
Bone morphogenetic protein	BMP	Neural progenitor cell	NPC
Cajal–Retzius	CR	Neural stem cell	NSC
Casein kinase 1	CK1	Neuroepithelial	NE
Central nervous system	CNS	Notch extracellular domain	NECD
Ciliary neurotrophic factor	CNTF	Notch intracellular domain	NICD
C-Jun N-terminal kinase	JNK	outer SVZ	oSVZ
Collapsin response mediator protein 2	CRMP2	Paired box 6	Pax6
Cortical plate zone	CP	Patched1	PTCH1
Delta-like	Dll	Radial glia	RG
Disheveled	Dvl	Retinoic acid	RA
Extracellular-signal-related kinase	ERK	Retinol dehydrogenase 10	Rdh10
Fibroblast growth factors	FGF	Serrate-like ligands	Jagged
Frizzled	Frz	Smoothened	SMO
Glioma-associated oncogene	GLI	Sonic hedgehog	SHH
Glycogen synthase kinase 3β	GSK3β	Subventricular zone	SVZ
Growth factor	GF	T cell factor/lymphoid enhancer factor	TCF/LEF
Hairy-enhancer of split	HES	Transcription factor T-brain 2	Tbr2
HES-related proteins	HERP	Transforming growth factor	TGF
Holoprosencephaly	HPE	Ventricular zone	VZ
inner SVZ	iSVZ	Vitamin A	VA

Neocortical Neurogenesis in Development and Evolution, First Edition. Edited by Wieland B. Huttner.

30.1 Introduction

During brain development, neural stem cells (NSCs) give rise to all kinds of neurons and glial cells (astrocytes and oligodendrocytes). The transition of proliferative and multipotent NSCs to fully differentiated neurons and glia cells is called neurogenesis and gliogenesis, respectively. Before neurogenesis, NSCs form a single layer of neuroepithelial (NE) cells undergoing rapid self-renewing symmetric division in the neural tube. Neurogenesis is an important developmental transition in the development of the neural progenitor cells (NPCs) with neurogenic potential and the identity of radial glial cells (RGs) (Gotz and Huttner 2005). RGs expressing paired box 6 (Pax6) are restricted to the ventricular zone (VZ). They are the primary NPCs in many regions of the developing brain (Gotz et al. 1998). RGs undergo interkinetic nuclear migration (INM) during which their nuclei undergo mitosis at the apical surface of the VZ and migrate basally for the S phase of the cell cycle (Reiner et al. 2012). They initially undergo symmetric divisions to expand their pool and switch to asymmetric neurogenic divisions at the onset of cortical neurogenesis. Subventricular zone (SVZ) is the secondary proliferative zone that appears during later stages of development. The mitotic basal neural precursor cells (BPCs)/intermediate precursor cells (IPCs) are generated in the developing brain by asymmetric division of RGs at the VZ and progressively form the SVZ to generate neurons (Haubensak et al. 2004; Noctor et al. 2004). BPCs/IPCs are generally transcription factor T-box brain 2 (Tbr2) expressing multipolar neural precursor cells (Englund et al. 2005). The SVZ in primates including monkey and human further subdivide into outer SVZ (oSVZ) and inner SVZ (iSVZ). Large amounts of RGs are present within the oSVZ/iSVZ, termed outer RGs (Hansen et al. 2010) or basal RGs (Fietz et al. 2010). They have unique features and characteristics of NPCs, which may reflect the functional adaptations of NPCs in the primate brain to promote the production of more neurons and glia required for populating larger brain structures, or they may result from the evolution of functionally unique precursor cells that are not present in other mammals.

The main neurodevelopmental processes during embryonic and postnatal periods includes the self-renewal, proliferation and differentiation of neural stem/precursor cells in VZ/SVZ and oSVZ/iSVZ, neural migration in the intermediate zone (IZ) through the oSVZ/iSVZ, subplate, and finally to the cortical plate (CP) for maturation (Gotz and Huttner 2005; Taverna et al. 2014). Intriguingly, post-mitotic neurons such as Cajal–Retzius (CR) cells and microglial also produce molecule cues that provide feedback to RGs (Paridaen and Huttner 2014). Importantly, brain development is an intricately regulated process that involves the precise spatiotemporal activation of different signaling pathways as well as environmental cues.

30.2 Wnt/β-catenin Signaling

30.2.1 Wnt/β-catenin Signaling is Essential for Neurogenesis

Wnt signaling is classically divided into canonical and noncanonical Wnt signaling pathway according to the Wnt ligands. The Wnt/β-catenin pathway is highly conserved during evolution and controls different stages of brain development. In the canonical Wnt signaling pathway, Wnt ligands are secreted glycoproteins that bind to Frizzled (Frz) receptors and then form a larger complex with low-density lipoprotein receptor related protein 5/6 (LRP5/6) on the cell surface (Figure 30.1A). β-catenin is a central and essential component of the canonical Wnt signaling pathway and acts downstream of the Frz and LRP receptors (Moon et al. 2002). In the absence of Wnt ligand, β-catenin in the cytoplasm is phosphorylated by the Axin complex/β-catenin destruction complex,

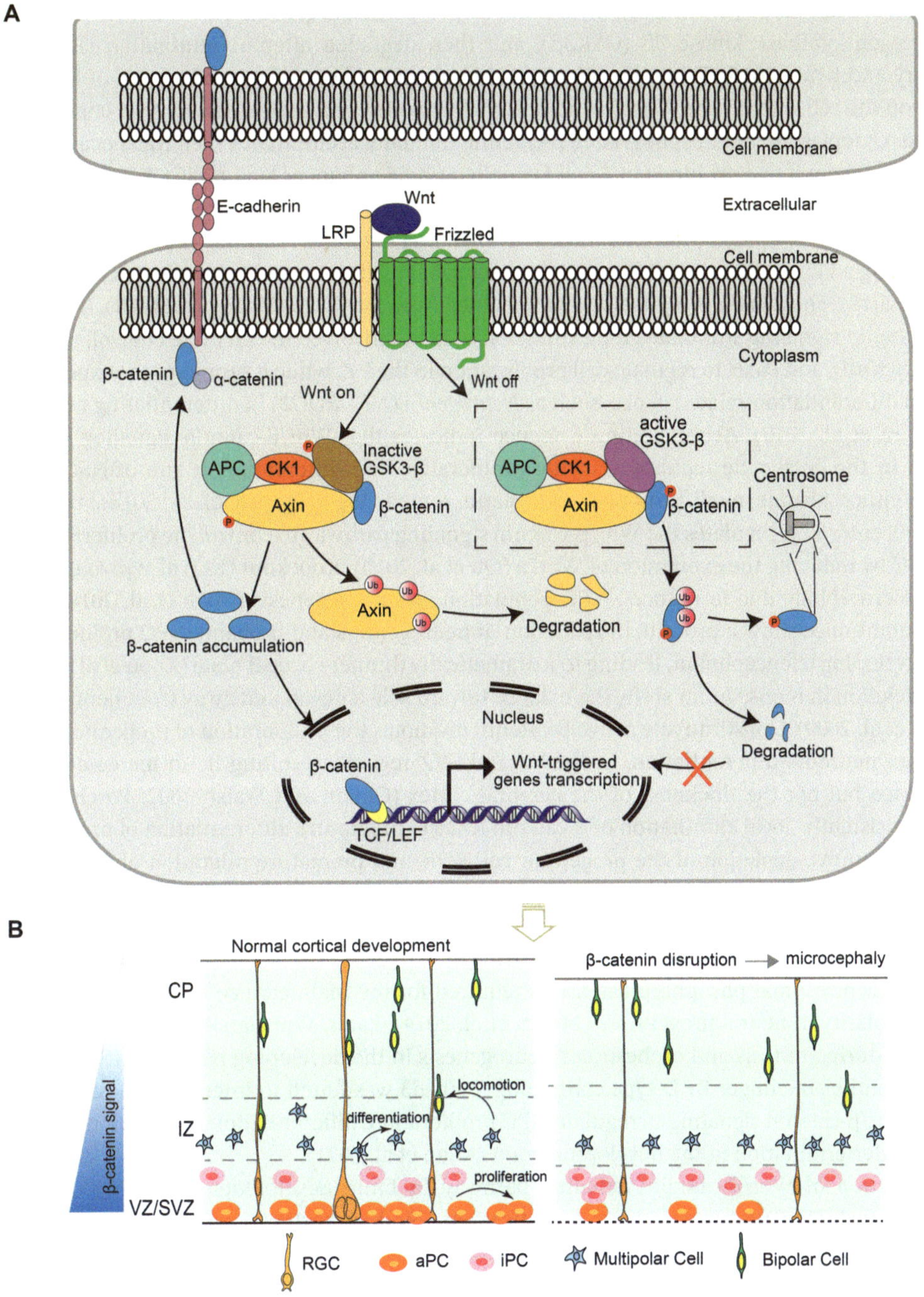

Figure 30.1 Schematic illustration of Wnt/β-catenin signaling and its roles in neurogenesis. (A) Wnts can bind to Frizzled and LRP5/6 to suppress the activity of GSK3β and the ability to degrade β-catenin. The accumulated β-catenin translocates to the nucleus and activates the transcription of target genes by interacting with TCF/LEF. In the absence of a Wnt ligand, the destruction complex of β-catenin (marked by dotted line box), a tertiary complex formed by Axin, APC, CK1α, and GSK3β, will phosphorylate β-catenin, leading to its proteasomal degradation. Phosphorylated β-catenin is also detected in the centrosome. (B) During brain development, β-catenin shows high expression in the ventricular zone (VZ) and regulates the proliferation and differentiation of neural progenitor cells (NPCs). β-catenin signal is downregulated in the CP. Mutation or disruption of β-catenin will lead to premature differentiation of NPCs and abnormal migration of neurons.

composed of scaffold protein (Axin), adenomatous polyposis coli (APC), casein kinase 1 (CK1), and glycogen synthase kinase 3β (GSK3β), and then degraded after ubiquitination (Bengoa-Vergniory and Kypta 2015). When the Wnt ligand binds to the heterodimer composed of Frz and LRP5/6 on the cell surface, the Wnt/β-catenin signaling pathway is activated and Axin complex is inhibited. Cytoplasmic unphosphorylated β-catenin gradually accumulates then translocates into the nucleus where it usually binds to T cell factor/lymphoid enhancer factor-1 (TCF/LEF) to activate the transcription of target genes (Clevers and Nusse 2012; MacDonald et al. 2009).

During brain development, the canonical Wnt signaling regulates multiple steps of neurogenesis, including NPC proliferation, differentiation, neuronal migration, and layer fate determination (Qu et al. 2013). The β-catenin signal is downregulated from the VZ to CP (Figure 30.1B). In NPCs, Wnt/β-catenin signaling stimulates the expression of genes involved in cell cycle control, such as *C-myc*, *Cyclin-D*, and *Pax6*, to regulate cell proliferation in the VZ, while it promotes the expression of neural differentiation-related genes, such as *Neurogenin* (*NEUROG2*) in differentiating neurons (Kuwahara et al. 2010). Accumulating evidence indicates that Wnt/β-catenin signaling is also involved in the epigenetic regulation of the proliferative and differentiation fate of NSC/NPC through either histone modification or chromatin remodeling (Nguyen et al. 2018). Orphan nuclear receptor TLX regulates the Wnt/β-catenin signaling pathway to control the proliferation of NSC/NPC by inducing the expression of Wnt7a (Qu et al. 2010). Knockout (KO) of *Wnt7a* in mice causes microcephaly due to reduced NPC population and neurogenesis (Miao et al. 2018). The LRP6 mutant mice show a prominent reduction of neurogenesis and probably NPC proliferation in the developing telencephalon, leading to a dramatically thinner cortical plate (Zhou et al. 2006). GSK3β deletion in mouse brain shifts the balance toward self-renewal and away from neurogenesis (Kim et al. 2009). Constitutively active β-catenin promotes the proliferation of progenitor cells, other than neuronal differentiation, in the VZ and SVZ regions, resulting in an increase in the surface area but not the thickness of the cerebral cortex (Chenn and Walsh 2002; Poschl et al. 2013). Consistently, local elimination of β-catenin leads to premature differentiation of progenitor cells into neurons, depletion of the progenitor cell pool, and premature migration of progenitor cells to the CP (Draganova et al. 2015; Woodhead et al. 2006) (Figure 30.1). Notably, several studies showed that phosphorylated β-catenin (Ser33/37/Thr41), which is predicated to be degraded quickly, also accumulated in the centrosome (Chilov et al. 2011; Huang et al. 2007; Mbom et al. 2014). The centrosomal phospho-β-catenin is required for the maintenance of symmetric cleavages and polarity in neural progenitors (Mbom et al. 2014). Later, Wnt signaling was reported to play a role during mitosis and orchestrates neurogenesis in the developing neocortex (Silva et al. 2021). Recently, zinc finger BED-type containing 3, Zbed3 was found to interact with Axin1 and activate Wnt/β-catenin signaling to regulate NPC proliferation, differentiation, as well as neuronal layer fates dertermination in the developing brain (Ruan et al. 2021).

The function of Wnt/β-catenin signaling pathway in brain development is highly context dependent including post-translational modifications, binding partners, and genomic binding regions of the target gene promoters/enhancers (Masuda and Ishitani 2017). Although β-catenin regulates the expression of many genes to exert its diverse roles, it may cooperate with different transcription factors (TCF/LEF-dependent or -independent) to activate a specific gene set from among its numerous target genes depending on the context (Masuda and Ishitani 2017). Because the processes of NPC proliferation, differentiation, neuronal migration, and layer fate determination occur sequentially, disruption of a previous one is likely to affect the subsequent processes. This may explain the discrepancy among some reports on the role of Wnt/β-catenin signaling in brain development. Nevertheless, Wnt/β-catenin signaling pathway plays a crucial role in maintaining the number of NPCs, determining the differentiation of NPC, and the cell fate of neurons.

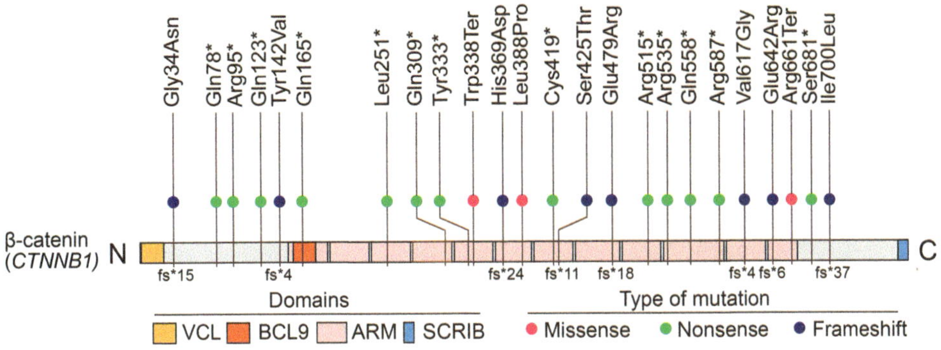

Figure 30.2 Mutations of β-catenin reported in microcephaly patients. Domains that interact with vinculin (VCL), BCL9 transcription coactivator and scribble planar cell polarity protein (SCRIB) as well as 12 armadillo repeats (ARM) are shown in different colors.

30.2.2 CTNNB1 (β-catenin Encoding Gene) and Microcephaly

Autosomal recessive primary microcephaly (MCPH) is a disease characterized by an abnormally small head circumference that manifests during prenatal development. Abnormal spindle-like microcephaly-associated protein (ASPM) is the most common cause of MCPH. It has been shown as a positive regulator of Wnt signaling and facilitates Wnt-mediated neurogenesis (Buchman et al. 2011; Major et al. 2008). β-catenin is also an integral structural component of cadherin-based adherens junction. *CTNNB1* ablation leads to loss of adhesion structure, NPC apoptosis, causing forebrain malformations (Junghans et al. 2005). Recently, mutations in *CTNNB1* have been frequently observed in patients with intellectual disability and some other clinical manifestations including motor and language delays, microcephaly, and mild visual defects (Kuechler et al. 2015; Coussa et al. 2020; Dashti et al. 2022; Kharbanda et al. 2017; Li et al. 2017; Stephanie Ho, 2021; Winczewska-Wiktor et al. 2016; Ke and Chen 2020) (Figure 30.2).

30.2.3 Wnt/β-catenin Signaling in Autism Spectrum Disorders

Autism spectrum disorder (ASD) is a heterogeneous group of neurodevelopmental disorders characterized by deficiency in social interaction and communication, as well as the presence of repetitive and stereotyped behaviors. Wnt/β-catenin transcriptional dysregulation has been consistently documented in patient-derived iPSCs and animal models for syndromic ASD (Caracci et al. 2021). Sporadic autism exomes reveal that the most severe or disruptive de novo mutations map to a highly interconnected β-catenin-linked network (O'Roak et al. 2012). In mice, *Ctnnb1* conditional knockout (cKO) in parvalbumin interneurons significantly impairs object recognition and social interactions, and enhances repetitive behaviors, mimicking the core symptoms of ASD (Dong et al., 2016). The scaffold Disheveled (Dvl) acts downstream of LRP6 co-receptor. *Dvl* KO mice exhibit sensorimotor abnormalities and abnormal social behavior (Lijam et al. 1997). More recently, excessive expression of β-catenin in mouse forebrain excitatory neurons led to reduced social interest and repetitive behaviors, effectively mimicking ASD symptoms (Alexander et al. 2020). These studies suggest that the pathogenesis of ASD may be related to the role of Wnt/β-catenin signaling in the control of excitatory/inhibitory balance and other brain developmental steps.

30.3 Notch Signaling

Notch signaling plays a critical role in animal developmental by participating in intercellular interactions. It mediates the influence and regulation of the external environment on cells, and programmatically manipulates cell fate and organ/tissue morphogenesis during early development. During brain development, Notch signaling regulates the size of the cortical progenitor pool, in part by controlling the balance between self-renewal and differentiation.

30.3.1 The Core Components of Notch Signaling

The Notch signaling pathway is composed of receptor, ligands, DNA binding proteins (mediators), other effectors, and Notch regulatory molecules. Mammals Notch has four homologues receptors (Notch1-4), Delta-like (Dll) ligands 1/3/4, and Serrate-like ligands (Jagged) 1 and 2. Unlike other receptors, Notch receptors have no enzymatic activity but undergo three proteolytic cleavage events, and their activity can be regulated by differential glycosylation during biogenesis in the endoplasmic reticulum and Golgi (Taylor et al. 2018). These cleavages are conducted by furin-like protease (S1), α-secretase (S2, ADAM17) and γ- secretase (S3). Cleavage products include Notch extracellular domain (NECD) and Notch intracellular domain (NICD).

The Notch signal is initiated by the interaction of the Notch ligand of the adjacent cell with the receptor (Zhou et al. 2010). The NICD released from the plasma membrane will translocate into the nucleus and bind transcriptional factor RBPj to regulate the downstream target genes (Honjo 2010). The Notch target genes included the hairy-enhancer of split (*HES*) and HES-related proteins (*HERP*) (Iso et al. 2003). The HES and HERP could function as classical DNA-binding repressors to antagonize the expression of proneural genes such as *Mash1*, *Math*, *NeuroD*, and *Ngn*, whereas phosphorylation of NICD-facilitated by Cdk8 kinase or ubiquitinylation of NICD via E3

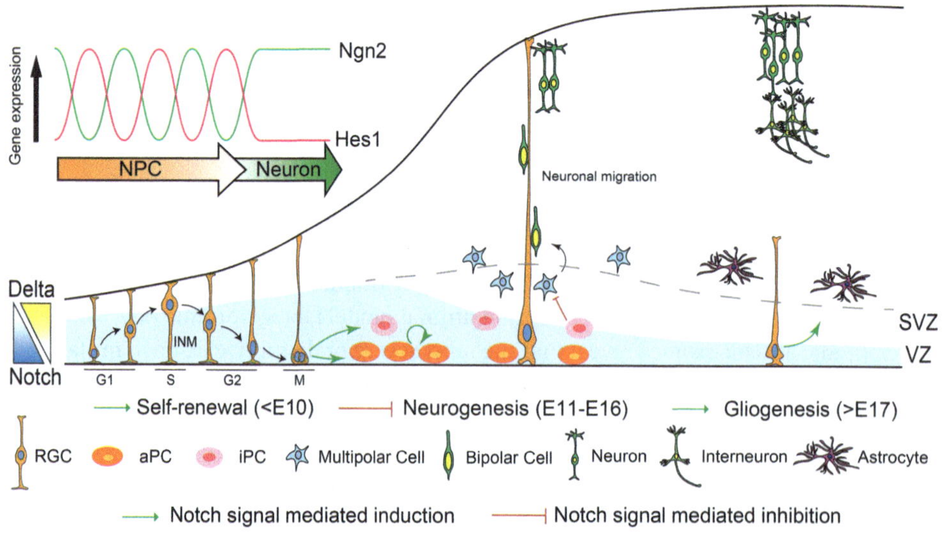

Figure 30.3 Dynamic regulation of Notch signaling modulates neurogenesis. Interkinetic nuclear migration (INM) is a key feature of cortical neurogenesis. The nuclei of progenitors move between the apical and basal surfaces of the neuroepithelium during the cell cycle. Notch expresses at higher levels at the apical side and forms the apical–basal gradient, whereas Delta expresses in a gradient with the opposite orientation. Owing to this biased distribution of Delta and Notch, the nuclear movement is important for the activation of Notch signaling and maintenance of neural progenitor cells. In the early stage of brain development, Notch promotes neural stem cell self-renewal and inhibits both neurogenesis and gliogenesis. At a later stage of differentiation, Notch selectively stimulates astrogenesis.

ubiquitin ligase F-box and WD repeat domain containing 7 (Fbw7) results in its rapid degradation and the turnover of the NICD coactivator complex. In the absence of NICD, RBPj recruits corepressor complexes to shut down the transcription of Notch target genes (Castel et al. 2013).

30.3.2 Dynamic Regulation of Notch Signaling Modulates Neurogenesis

The onset of neurogenesis and the transition from NE to RG coincides with the onset of Notch signaling (Figure 30.3). Analysis on the phenotypes of different Notch component KO mice indicates that Notch signaling affects a wide array of cellular processes including maintenance of NSC/NPC proliferation/self-renewal and differentiation, specification of cell fate, and apoptosis (Table 30.1). Repressor-type

Table 30.1 Effects of Notch signaling manipulation in neurogenesis and/or development.

Genes	Phenotypes	References
Hes1$^{-/-}$	Premature neurogenesis; Growth retardation and embryonic lethality	Hatakeyama et al. 2004; Hirata et al. 2001; Swiatek et al. 1994
Hes3$^{-/-}$	Premature neurogenesis	
Hes5$^{-/-}$	Premature neurogenesis	
Hes1$^{-/-}$; *Hes3*$^{-/-}$	Premature neurogenesis; Loss of midbrain and anterior hindbrain structures	
Hes1$^{-/-}$; *Hes5*$^{-/-}$	Premature neurogenesis; Abnormal morphology of neural tube	
RBPj$^{-/-}$	Developmental delay and embryonic lethality	Imayoshi et al. 2010; Oka et al. 1995; Son et al. 2020
RBPj$^{flox/flox}$*;Emx1-Cre*	Smaller cerebral cortex; Premature neurogenesis and disrupted radial glial structure	
RBPj-CreER^{T2}	Premature loss of neural stem cell	
Notch1$^{-/-}$	Loss of NSCs in the early embryonic brains	Basak et al. 2012; Hitoshi et al. 2002; Liu and Lobe 2010; Mason et al. 2006
Notch1$^{flox/flox}$*; Foxg1-Cre*	Increased apoptosis; Survive until birth but die within several hours	
Notch1-CreER^{T2}	Loss of mitotic progenitors in the SVZ	
IC-Notch1;pCX-Cre	Embryonic lethality; Growth arrest and various developmental defects	
Notch2-CreER^{T2}	Accelerated VZ/SVZ NSC exhaustion and an aging-like phenotype	Engler et al. 2018
Dll1$^{-/-}$	Embryonic lethality; Overproduction of neurons with an increased pace of neurogenesis	Marklund et al. 2010; Okubo et al. 2021
NC-Dll1	Increased DRG cell number and the cell proliferation rate; Increased glial differentiation and decreased neuronal differentiation	
Jagged1$^{-/-}$	Embryonic lethality and vascular defects	Nyfeler et al. 2014; Xue et al. 1999
Jagged1$^{+/-}$*;Notch1*$^{+/-}$	Decreases the number of proliferating cells in the SVZ; Majority died soon after birth and only 10% survived up to 8 days	
Jagged2$^{-/-}$	Embryonic lethality; Defects in thymic development	Jiang et al. 1998; Xu et al. 2010
Jagged2$^{flox/flox}$*; Meox2-Cre*	Cleft palate and fused tongue; Syndactyly of both forelimbs and hindlimbs	
Mash1$^{-/-}$	Morphological defects in the brain; Loss of neuronal precursors	Casarosa et al. 1999; Nieto et al. 2001
Mash1$^{-/-}$*;Ngn2*$^{-/-}$	Excessive and premature differentiation of progenitors along the astrocytic pathway	

basic helix-loop-helix (bHLH) genes *Hes1*, *Hes3*, and *Hes5* inhibit cell differentiation and keep cells in the precursor or proliferative stage. *Mash1* and *Ngn2* are activator-type bHLH transcriptional activators and drivers of neurogenesis (Castro et al. 2006). In addition to activating neural differentiation genes including members of the NeuroD family, they can activate the expression of Notch ligand genes including *Dll1*. Thus, loss of Notch activity in one daughter of a progenitor cell will result in the expression of proneural genes and Delta-like proteins in this cell and its conversion to a signaling cell to represses differentiation of its neighbors through lateral Notch signaling (Taylor et al. 2018). The NICD–RBPj transcriptional activator complex then induces *Hes1* and *Hes5* expression in the signal-receiving NSC. HES1 and HES5 proteins repress the expression of proneural genes and *Delta1* to inhibit neuronal differentiation. Accordingly, over-expression of *Hes1* in mice results in the expansion of the embryonic neural stem cell pool and stem cell reservoir in the postnatal brain (Ohtsuka and Kageyama 2021). However, sustained over-expression of *Hes1* reduced the expression of cell cycle-related proteins such as cyclin D1 and repressed both proliferation and differentiation of NPCs (Shimojo et al. 2008).

In proliferating NSCs, the Notch pathway is instrumental in sustaining the undifferentiated state and actives self-renewal in collaboration with growth factors, such as fibroblast growth factor (FGF2) and epidermal growth factor (EGF) (Yoon et al. 2004). On the other hand, Notch signaling alone can also modulate the clonal self-renewal of NSCs by inhibiting neuronal and glial cell differentiation, enhancing intercellular interactions, and regulating cell cycle progression independently of exogenous and endogenous growth factors (Nagao et al. 2007). Thus, Notch regulates multiple pivotal dimensions of the self-renewal pattern of cell division, both independently and in cooperation with growth factors.

The nuclei of RGs undergo INM between the apical and basal ends of the VZ depending on the phase of cell cycle. INM is involved in regulating the rate of neurogenesis via Notch signaling (Murciano et al. 2002). Indeed, Notch signaling activity changes according to the position of nuclei due to differential apical–basal distribution of Delta and Notch. It is likely that cells with nuclei located in the basal region (Delta-high) send Delta signals to neighboring cells with nuclei located in the apical region (Notch-high) (Figure 30.3). In the developing dorsal telencephalon of mice, Notch1 was activated in proliferating NPCs, but not in post-mitotic neurons, suggesting the spatiotemporal activation of Notch signaling during neurogenesis (Tokunaga et al. 2004).

Differentiating neurons activate Notch signaling of neighboring cells raises a question as to how NPCs are maintained during early stages before neurons are generated. Real-time imaging analysis revealed that Ngn2 expression is oscillating in NPCs but sustained in differentiating neurons (Shimojo et al. 2008) (Figure 30.3). The oscillating *Ngn2* expression is driven by *Hes1* oscillations and its negative feedback loop (Hirata et al. 2002). Intriguingly, Delta1 expression also oscillates in NPCs under the control of periodic activation by *Ngn2* and repression by *Hes1*, which seems to reciprocally activating Notch signaling and each other to maintain NPC cell fate. Notch plays different roles at distinct steps during the course of NSCs/NPCs differentiation (Ge et al. 2002; Hitoshi et al. 2002). Before the initiation of differentiation, Notch inhibits both neurogenesis and gliogenesis. Early differentiation block occurs at or before the induction of intermediate/basal progenitors such as Mash1-positive and Prox1-positive cells. In contrast, at a later stage of differentiation, Notch selectively stimulates astrogenesis. Thus, Notch signaling regulates both the transition from NSC to IPC, and subsequent lineage selection between neurons and astrocytes (Figure 30.3). How dynamic Notch signaling combined with oscillated *Ngn2/Hes1* expression to control the different processes of neurogenesis remains to be clarified.

The Notch signaling pathway plays a crucial role in the expansion of the neocortex by regulating the size of the cortical progenitor pool. Human-specific NOTCH2NL is highly expressed in RGs and may have contributed to the evolution of the larger human neocortex (Ramain et al. 2001). *NOTCH2NL* gene duplications are associated with macrocephaly and autism, and deletions with microcephaly and schizophrenia. Dysregulation of the Notch signal pathway can be found in a variety of brain disorders including cortical dysplasia and schizophrenia (Lasky and Wu 2005). On the other hand, Notch signaling could promote gliogenesis and inhibit neurogenesis directly or via crosstalk with STAT-signal pathway activated by diffusible signaling factors such as leukemia inhibitory factor (LIF), ciliary neurotrophic factor (CNTF), and bone morphogenetic proteins (BMPs) (Zhou et al. 2010). In particular, CNTF has been shown to act as a signal for differentiation of astrocytes. CNTF dependent astrogenesis was also augmented by growth factors. During early development, when NSCs actively proliferate and preferentially give rise to neurons, they act to preserve a pool of undifferentiated NSCs for later gliogenesis. Subsequently, when gliogenic signals emerge at a later stage, Notch and growth factors collaborate with such signals to promote gliogenesis actively (Nagao et al. 2007).

30.3.3 Notch Signaling and Neuronal Migration

Proper neuronal migration is orchestrated by combined membrane signal paradigms. Reelin secreted by the CR cells plays a pivotal role in radial migration. During brain development, Notch activity plays important roles in Reelin-signal-dependent neuronal migration. Reelin deficiency leads to reduced levels of the cleaved form of NICD and reduced Notch signaling in migrating neurons, resulting in migration and morphological defects (Hashimoto-Torii et al. 2008). Presenilin-1 deficiency led to loss of CR neurons and disorganization of Notch-1 on the neuronal cell membrane (Yang et al. 2017). NBS1 is a regulatory component of the NICD-RBPj-mediated transcriptional activity of Notch signaling. *Nbs1* deletion is dispensable for post-mitotic neurons, but compromises their arborization and migration due to dysregulated Notch signaling (Zhou et al. 2020). In addition, ADAM10 is required for cortical radial migration by initiating the regulated intramembrane proteolysis of Notch. The formation of NICD/RBPj complex controls microtubule structure and radial migration of cortical neurons through the transcriptional control of *Dcx* expression (Yang et al. 2017).

30.4 BMP2-SMAD Signaling

BMPs are a class of morphogens belonging to the highly conserved transforming growth factor (TGF)-β superfamily. They are critical for the development of the nervous system. BMPs secreted from the dorsal midline form a gradient that contributes to the patterning of the dorsal–ventral axis of the developing spinal cord and brain (Hebert and Fishell 2008). BMP ligands bind to either Type I or II receptors to initiate receptor complex formation between Type I and Type II receptors, which phosphorylates and activates downstream pathway-restricted transcription factors, *Smad1*, *Smad5*, and *Smad8*, which are the pivotal intracellular effectors of the BMP family of proteins.

The effects of BMP signaling on NSCs alters during different stages of development. BMP pathway components are highly expressed in both embryonic and adult neurogenic niches (Mira et al. 2010). During forebrain development, BMPs sequentially induce neurogenesis and then astrogliogenesis, and participate in neurite outgrowth from immature neurons (Bond et al. 2012). BMP7 KO in mice led to reduced proliferation, survival, and self-renewal capacity of NPCs (Segklia et al. 2012). Consistently, cKO of both SMAD1 and SMAD5 in NPCs causes microcephaly and an increased production of early-born cortical neurons at the expense of late-born ones, which correlates with the premature differentiation and depletion of NPCs (Najas et al. 2020). In adult NSC, BMPs are required to balance NSC quiescence/proliferation to maintain the NSC pool, and blocking of BMP-SMAD signaling may lead to exhaustion of NSC/NPC (Mathieu et al. 2008). Therefore, BMP signaling promotes stem cell amplification during cortical neurogenesis.

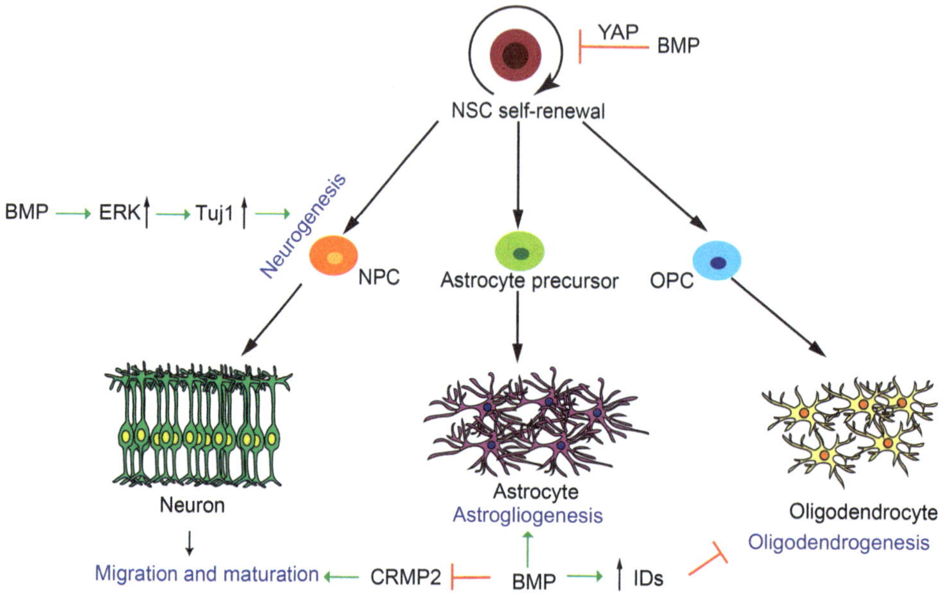

Figure 30.4 Roles of bone morphogenetic protein (BMP) signaling in neurogenesis and gliogenesis in the neocortex. BMP inhibits neural stem cell proliferation through Yes-associated protein (YAP). During neural fate specification, BMP signaling promotes neurogenesis by inducing the expression of Tuj1 through activation of the extracellular signal-related kinase pathway. BMP signaling promotes astrocyte differentiation during late embryonic and postnatal periods. In addition, BMP signaling also activates the expression of inhibitors of differentiation (IDs) that inhibit oligodendrogenesis.

Remarkably, BMP signaling is also critical for progenitor fate specification during neurogenesis and astrogliogenesis through dynamic transcriptional regulation (Figure 30.4). During neural fate specification, BMP signaling initially promotes neurogenesis by pushing progenitors toward a neuronal fate and suppressing the oligodendroglial fate. BMP signaling induces the expression of neuronal class III β-tubulin (Tuj1) through activation of the extracellular-signal-related kinase (ERK) pathway and switches from a pro-neuronal to pro-astroglial cue towards the end of neurogenesis. During the late embryonic and postnatal periods, BMP signaling promotes astrocyte differentiation. *Ngn1* is highly expressed during the peak of neurogenesis and gradually decreased with the transition to gliogenesis. *Ngn1* suppresses BMP-mediated astrocyte differentiation by sequestering downstream transcriptional regulators away from glial gene promoters, such as the glial fibrillary acidic protein (*Gfap*) promoter. LIF signaling promotes the generation of $GFAP^+$ progenitor cells, while BMP signaling promotes the generation of mature $GFAP^+$ astrocytes (Bonaguidi et al. 2005). Some microRNAs, such as miR-199a, can promote the expression of SMAD1, disrupt the differentiation process of NPC/NSC, and lead to excessive astrocyte production (Nakashima et al. 2021). In addition to promoting an astrocytic identity, BMP signaling also activates downstream signals that inhibit oligodendrogenesis (Mehler et al. 2000). Oligodendrogenesis is promoted by the bHLH transcription factors *Olig1* and *Olig2*. BMPs induce the expression of the inhibitor of differentiation (ID) gene families, *Id2* and *Id4*, in NPCs to prevent oligodendrocyte lineage commitment by sequestering *Olig1* and *Olig2* from their target promoters. Consistently, in the context of the demyelinating disease multiple sclerosis, the Wnt effector transcription factor 7-like 2 (TCF7l2) promotes oligodendroglial differentiation by repressing BMP4-mediated activity (Zhang et al. 2021).

BMP signaling regulates additional processes such as neuronal migration and dendritic morphology during the development of cortical neurons (Saxena et al. 2018). The expression of BMPs and CRMP2 correlated inversely during brain development. BMP-SMAD signaling pathway controls neuronal migration and neurite outgrowth by suppressing the transcription of CRMP2 (Sun et al. 2010). Inhibition of BMP signaling specifically affects the migration, establishment of polarity, and dendritic morphogenesis of upper-layer pyramidal neurons (Saxena et al. 2017). The noncanonical TGF-β signaling pathway has also been shown to regulate neuronal migration, axonal specification via a complex comprise of WDR62, POSH, TAK1, and C-Jun N-terminal kinase (JNK) that is involved in the activation of the JNK signaling (Zhang et al. 2016). While the canonical TGF-β signaling, on the other hand, is shown to regulate neuronal morphogenesis by suppressing the transcription of *CRMP2* as well (Nakashima et al. 2018). These studies may explain why mutations of *TGF-β receptor 1*, *SMAD4*, or TGFβ induced factor homeobox 1 (*TGIF1*) were found in patients with neurodevelopmental disorders.

30.5 Sonic Hedgehog Signaling Pathway

The morphogen protein Sonic hedgehog (SHH) signaling is well documented to be essential for the patterning and cell-fate specification of the central nervous system (CNS) (Li et al. 2020). The canonical SHH pathway primarily contains two transmembrane receptors: patched1 (PTCH1) and Smoothened (SMO, a Frizzled-class G protein–coupled receptor), and glioma-associated oncogene (GLI) transcription factors *Gli1*, *Gli2*, and *Gli3* (Stone et al. 1999). After binding to SHH, PTCH1 is inhibited and releases its inhibition of SMO, which relocates to the cilia. This activates the GLI proteins and their transfer to the nucleus. Activated nuclear *Glis* interact with the cyclic AMP response element (CRE)-binding protein (CREB) to initiate the transcription of downstream target genes (Figure 30.5).

30.5.1 SHH Signaling Coordinates the Proliferation and Differentiation of Neural and Glial Progenitor Cells

SHH plays different roles during brain development depending on its concentration, location, and timing of exposure (Agarwala et al. 2001) (Figure 30.5). Studies in SHH over-expression and *Smo*-cKO mice indicate the SHH signaling pathway regulates the proliferation of RGs and iPCs to coordinate and maintain the proliferative capacity, differentiation, and survival of neocortex neurons (Komada 2012). Disruption of *SHH* or *Gli2* gene in mice led to deficits in NPC proliferation and brain development (Palma and Altaba 2004). Activation of the SHH pathway results in increased *Gli1* expression and activation of the downstream Ras-MEK-ERK pathway to promote cell proliferation. A specific combination of FGF-2, EGF, and SHH has a potent synergistic stimulus for NSC proliferation, indicating that SHH acts as a niche factor (Martínez et al. 2013). In addition, the ligand for TLR3, polyinosinic-polycytidylic acid, negatively regulates NPC proliferation by inhibiting SHH signaling (Kavitha et al. 2011). However, factors that mediate the crosstalk between TLR3 and SHH signaling cascades are still unknown.

SHH activity is higher in the human fetal cortex than that in the mouse embryonic cortex and elevating SHH signaling is sufficient to expand basal radial glia (bRGs) to induce neocortical folding in mice. Importantly, elevating SHH signaling increases the number of both IPC and bRG, suggesting its important role in the evolutionary expansion of bRGs and neocortical growth and folding (Wang et al. 2016). The SHH pathway also orchestrates the balance between quiescent and activated NSCs during adult neurogenesis. Conditional activation of SHH signaling in adult NSCs leads to expansion of quiescent NSC and the depletion of their direct progeny by increasing symmetric divisions (Ferent et al. 2014).

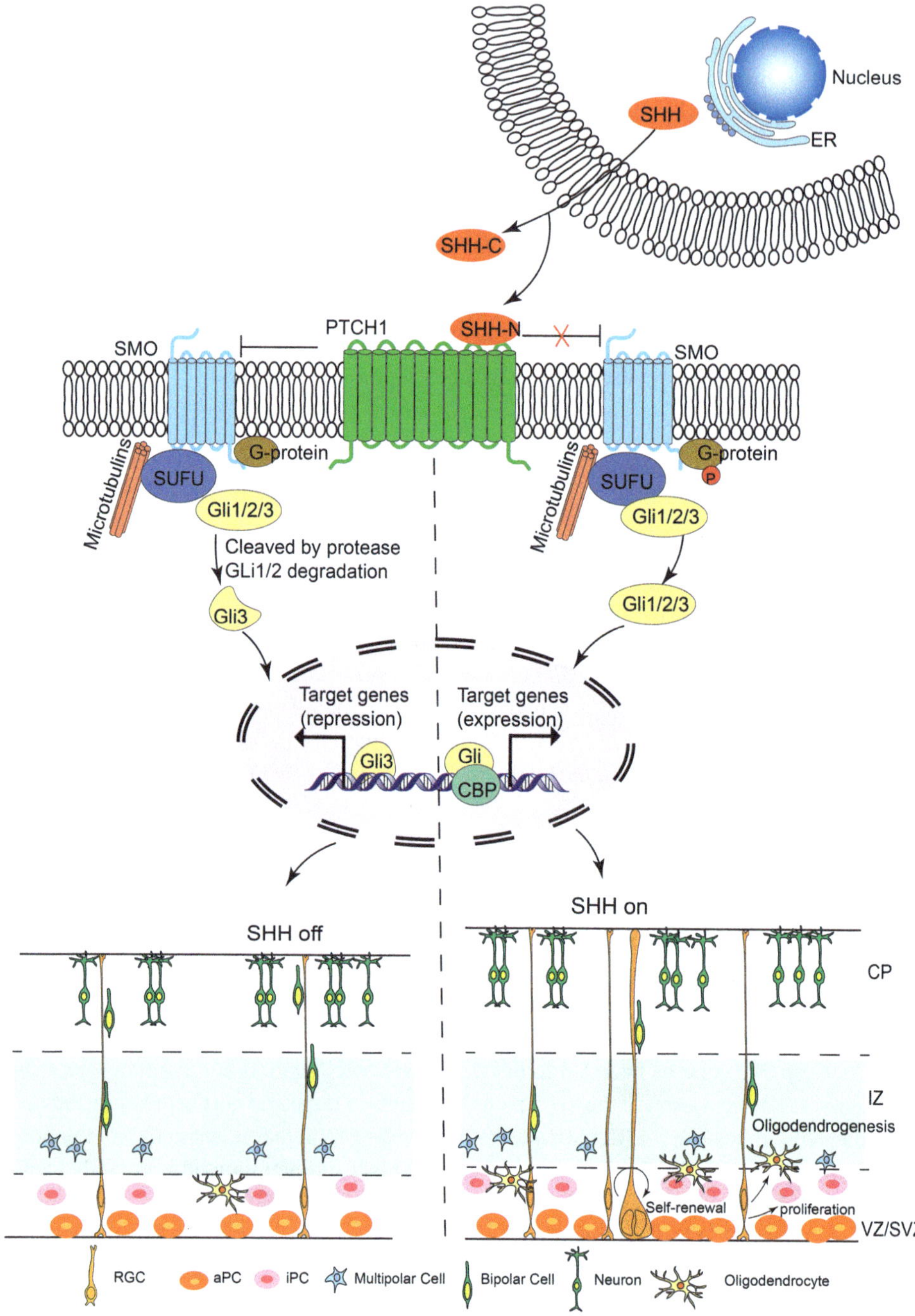

Figure 30.5 Sonic hedgehog (SHH) signaling coordinates the proliferation and differentiation of neural and glial progenitor cells, and survival of neurons in the neocortex. (A) SHH canonical signaling gets activated when it binds to its receptor patched1 (PTCH1), which relieves the inhibition of Smoothened (SMO) and then Gli proteins enter the nucleus to activate downstream target gene transcription. In the absence of SHH, PTCH1 inhibits the activity of SMO protein, thereby inhibiting the downstream pathway. (B) SHH regulates neural progenitor cell proliferation and the development of oligodendrocyte and astrocytes. Disruption of SHH leads to reduced radial glial cell (RG) and neural progenitor cells including apical progenitor cells (aPC) and intermediate progenitor cells (iPC). Activation of SHH promotes RG proliferation and self-renewal.

Oligodendrocytes also originate from neuroepithelial precursors, as do neurons and astrocytes. SHH signaling is required to generate normal numbers of neocortical oligodendrocytes during embryonic development (Figure 30.5). SHH signaling not only plays roles in oligodendrocytes lineage progression but also in differentiation after cell fate determination. Long-term inhibition of SHH signaling during oligodendrocytes differentiation by antagonist-mediated inactivation of SMO activity suppresses myelin basic protein expression, but does not completely block the expression of myelin-specific markers or differentiation in oligodendrocytes (Wang and Almazan 2016). Unique gene profiles have been identified between different astrocyte populations. Cells actively transducing SHH are identified by the expression of *Gli1*. The study that used a fate mapping approach to mark and follow a population of glial progenitor cells expressing the SHH target gene, *Gli1*, in the neonatal and postnatal brain suggests the cell-type dependent roles of the pathway in driving astrocyte development and function (Gingrich et al. 2022). SHH signaling in mature astrocytes is required for establishing structural organization and remodeling of cortical synapses in a cell type-specific manner (Hill et al. 2019). In addition, neuron-derived SHH plays roles in regulating specific populations of differentiated astrocytes (Garcia et al. 2010). In summary, SHH coordinates the proliferation and differentiation of neural and glial progenitor cells.

30.5.2 Mutations in SHH-Associated Genes Cause Holoprosencephaly

Holoprosencephaly (HPE) is a complex brain malformation caused by the inability of the brain to divide properly into the right and left hemispheres (Dubourg et al. 2007). Patients with HPE have intellectual disability, microcephaly, and epilepsy. Mutations in the *SHH* genes are the most common cause of sporadic and inherited HPE. Deletions or loss-of-function mutations of PTCH1 result in basal cell nevus syndrome (Gorlin syndrome), whereas gain-of-function mutations would cause HPE. Duplication of the *PTCH1* gene fragment also led to microcephaly without a specific mechanism being reported (Derwińska et al. 2008). In addition, mutations of *Tgif1* and *Tgif2* in mice have been shown to contribute to HPE pathogenesis by disrupting the SHH signaling pathway (Taniguchi et al. 2012).

30.6 Other Signaling Pathways: c-Jun N-terminal Kinase, Fibroblast Growth Factors, and Retinoic Acid Signaling

c-Jun N-terminal kinase: The JNK family includes three genes: *Jnk1*, *Jnk2*, and *Jnk3*. JNK signaling regulates various developmental processes including neurogenesis, neuronal differentiation, migration, and synaptogenesis (Myers et al. 2020; Westerlund et al. 2011; Xu et al. 2018; Zhang et al. 2016). Mice lacking both *Jnk1* and *Jnk2* undergo mid-gestational embryonic lethality associated with defects in neural tube closure and deregulated neural apoptosis (Kuan et al. 1999). JNK1 is likely to be the predominant isoform of JNKs that regulates neurogenesis during cortical development. Microcephaly-associated protein WDR62 specifically recruits JNK1 to the spindle pole and regulates neurogenesis via the activation of JNK signaling in the developing brain (Lim et al. 2015; Xu et al. 2014). Phenotypic and biochemical analysis of multiple KO mice revealed that MEKK3 and FBW7 bidirectionally regulate the stability of WDR62 and JNK activity, which in turn regulate the homeostasis of neural precursor cells in the cerebral cortex (Lim et al. 2015; Xu et al. 2018). JNK signaling is required for both tangential and radial migration. However, $Jnk1^{-/-}$ mice have thinner VZs suggesting the effect of neurogenesis on migration (Myers et al. 2020; Westerlund et al. 2011). Intriguingly, many signaling pathways including BMP/TGF-β, Wnt, Notch, SHH, FGF, RA, have been shown to be able to activate JNK signaling. It is possible that different isoforms of

JNKs are organized in different protein complexes in response to different stimuli in the regulation of various developmental processes (Xu et al. 2014, 2018; Zhang et al. 2016).

Fibroblast growth factors: The binding of FGFs to FGF receptors leads to enhanced receptor phosphorylation that, in turn, phosphorylates and activates different downstream pathways such as PLCγ, AKT, ERK, JNK, and STAT3. FGFs and their receptors play essential roles in the proliferation of neural stem and progenitor cell. FGF2 functions in the proliferation and differentiation of multipotent neural stem cells during brain development and in adult mouse brain (Werner et al. 2011; Yoon et al. 2004), although the neurogenic role of FGF2 can be compensated by other FGFs in the developing brain (Dono et al. 1998; Werner et al. 2011). Mice lacking FGF2, FGF17, or FGFR1 show reductions in brain volume and impairments in cognitive and social behaviors. In adult mice, activation of the FGF receptor in neural precursors can increase the number of neurons generated and reverse age-related declines in hippocampal neurogenesis (Kang and Hebert 2015).

Retinoic acid (RA): RA is a metabolite of vitamin A and an important morphogen. RA is involved in mammalian forebrain development through the regulation of homeobox genes and neurogenesis (Niederreither and Dolle 2008). RA acts as a transcriptional activating ligand by binding to the nuclear retinoic acid receptors, retinoic acid receptors (RARs) and retinoid X receptors (RXRs), to orchestrate the proliferation, differentiation, and survival of neural and glial progenitors, as well as the migration of neurons. *Foxc1* is a transcription factor expressed in the cortical meninges where it is required for the production of RA. *Foxc1* mutant mice show a dramatic increase in the number of RGs and a severe block in neuronal differentiation (Siegenthaler et al. 2009). Adequate RA production during development also depends upon the activity of retinol dehydrogenase 10 (RDH10). *Rdh10* deletion mice have less RA activity that affects the cell cycle exit of progenitor cells during corticogenesis, leading to a deficiency in projection neurons and microcephaly (Haushalter et al. 2017). Recently, single-cell epigenomics reveals that the RA signaling pathway contributes to the specification of the prefrontal cortex neuronal lineage during human cortical development (Mishra et al. 2018). RA is commonly used in vitro to induce the differentiation of stem cell populations including adult neural stem cells into neurons. Inhibition of RA synthesis or signaling significantly reduces adult neural stem and precursor cell proliferation via abrogation of cell cycle kinetics and cell cycle regulators (Mishra et al. 2018). Retinoid-sufficient and retinoid-deficient mice studied indicate RA acts as a crucial contributor in early stages of adult neurogenesis (Jacobs et al. 2006).

Although RA is essential for neurogenesis in both embryo and adult, it was demonstrated to be teratogenic (Niederreither and Dolle 2008). Both deficiency and excess of RA can disturb the neurodevelopmental process including the learning process, memory formation, cognitive function, and social memory/social communication. Retinol/ vitamin A deficiency during pregnancy increases the risk of developing schizophrenia or ASD (Cediel-Ulloa et al. 2022). Intriguingly, vitamin A supplementation in ASD children improves their symptoms. On the contrary, excess of RA and vitamin A can cause hydrocephaly, microcephaly, or a decrease in size of specific forebrain regions, together with occasional cortical heterotopias (Liu et al. 2021).

30.7 The Crosstalk between Different Signaling Pathways during Neurogenesis

Increasing evidence indicates that brain development is regulated through a complex network of signaling pathways in a developmental stage-specific manner. The combination of signals produce context-, time-, and location-dependent outcomes that fine-tune NSC/NPC expansion or self-renewal, and differentiation, thereby influencing all stages of the neurogenesis process. The biological outcome of signaling crosstalk is determined by the context of the signaling environment and the inputs of multiple signaling pathways or intracellular networks (Luo 2017; Manzari-Tavakoli et al. 2022). Signaling pathways can cooperate in a synergistic or antagonistic manner via a range of signaling crosstalk at different levels: by changing the expression and activities of ligands, antagonists, receptors, and signaling components; by incorporating transcriptional and/or chromatin modification complexes that globally influence gene expression; and by direct interactions between intracellular signaling components. The multiple signaling inputs at different levels will integrate into the core transcriptional factor network to regulate target gene expression in a cooperative manner (Luo 2017).

The BMP/TGF-β pathway, which plays an important role in stem cell self-renewal, differentiation, and astrogenesis, interacts with other signaling pathways, including Wnt/β-catenin, Notch, SHH, FGF, and cytokines, and their parallel or downstream signaling pathways such as ERK, JNK, PI3K-Akt, NF-κB, Hippo, and JAK-STAT (Luo 2017; Manzari-Tavakoli et al. 2022). Crosstalk between other signaling pathways were also reported. Wnt and FGFs direct the spatial differentiation of neurons in the midbrain through the regulation of FGF signaling by Wnt (Dyer et al. 2014). The SHH and Notch pathways cooperate to regulate the neurogenic division of neocortical progenitors. Activation of SHH signaling increases the stemness of RGs likely by upregulating downstream targets of Notch signaling such as *Hes1*. *Hes1* is not only a critical regulator of neuronal cell fate in multiple niches but also uniquely represents a molecular convergence point between SHH and Notch signaling in those niches (Dave et al. 2011). Dysfunction in Notch signaling can be complemented by promoting SHH signaling (Ohtsuka and Kageyama 2022). Because the activation of BMP/TGF-β, Wnt, Notch, SHH, FGF, RA pathways are able to activate the JNK signaling that is essential for brain development. JNK is likely to represent a unique molecular convergence point among various signaling pathways.

Through extensive interactions, different signaling pathways effectively incorporate into a complicated cellular signaling network, depending on the dosage, timing, and location of various ligand or environmental inputs, and produce an integrated output that controls neurogenesis and specifies cell-fate decisions under the physiological context.

30.8 Concluding Remarks

Brain development involves a variety of signal transduction pathways. Understanding the general properties of signal transduction processes and how these processes coordinate with each other will lead to a detailed comprehension of their specific functions in cortical neurogenesis. The unique expression patterns of the components of these signaling pathways and associated molecules largely determine their function during cortical development. Activation of signaling pathways is typically initiated by ligand binding to receptors. Most of signaling pathways regulate gene expression via transcription factors and ultimately influence cell fate determination or cell patterning. Although we have made progress in understanding the mechanisms that control brain development in the rodent cerebral cortex and other CNS regions, our understanding of human brain development is still limited. Single cell analysis of molecular diversity and epigenetic mechanisms of different cell lineages with integrated cell spatial positions may shed light on the understanding of heterogeneity, dynamics, and fate potential of NPCs during primate brain development.

To date, much of the progress in NSC research stems from studies of brain development, especially those related to signal transduction. Stem cell research has brought great promise for nerve tissue regeneration, damage repair, and neurological disease treatment. However, how this knowledge is applied for clinical treatment of neurological diseases, including developmental/degenerative disorders and brain damage, still faces great challenges.

Acknowledgments

We apologize to those researchers whose primary study is related to this topic and cannot be cited here due to space limitations.

References

Agarwala, S. et al. (2001). Sonic hedgehog control of size and shape in midbrain pattern formation. *Science* 291: 2147–2150.

Alexander, J.M. et al. (2020). Excessive beta-catenin in excitatory neurons results in reduced social and increased repetitive behaviors and altered expression of multiple genes linked to human autism. *Front Synaptic Neurosci* 12: 14.

Basak, O. et al. (2012). Neurogenic subventricular zone stem/progenitor cells are Notch1-dependent in their active but not quiescent state. *J Neurosci* 32: 5654–5666.

Bengoa-Vergniory, N. and Kypta, R.M. (2015). Canonical and noncanonical Wnt signaling in neural stem/progenitor cells. *Cell Mol Life Sci* 72: 4157–4172.

Bonaguidi, M.A. et al. (2005). LIF and BMP signaling generate separate and discrete types of GFAP-expressing cells. *Development* 132: 5503–5514.

Bond, A.M. et al. (2012). The dynamic role of bone morphogenetic proteins in neural stem cell fate and maturation. *Dev Neurobiol* 72: 1068–1084.

Buchman, J.J. et al. (2011). ASPM regulates Wnt signaling pathway activity in the developing brain. *Genes Dev* 25: 1909–1914.

Caracci, M.O. et al. (2021). Wnt/beta-catenin-dependent transcription in autism spectrum disorders. *Front Mol Neurosci* 14: 764756.

Casarosa, S. et al. (1999). Mash 1 regulates neurogenesis in the ventral telencephalon. *Development* 126: 525–534.

Castel, D. et al. (2013). Dynamic binding of RBPJ is determined by Notch signaling status. *Genes Dev* 27: 1059–1071.

Castro, D.S. et al. (2006). Proneural bHLH and Brn proteins coregulate a neurogenic program through cooperative binding to a conserved DNA motif. *Dev Cell* 11: 831–844.

Cediel-Ulloa, A. et al. (2022). Impact of endocrine disrupting chemicals on neurodevelopment. *Exp Rev Endocrinol Metabol* 17: 131–141.

Chenn, A. and Walsh, C.A. (2002). Regulation of cerebral cortical size by control of cell cycle exit in neural precursors. *Science* 297 (5580): 365–369.

Chilov, D. et al. (2011). Phosphorylated beta-catenin localizes to centrosomes of neuronal progenitors and is required for cell polarity and neurogenesis in developing midbrain. *Dev Biol* 357: 259–268.

Clevers, H. and Nusse, R. (2012). Wnt/β-catenin signaling and disease. *Cell* 149: 1192–1205.

Coussa, R.G. et al. (2020). Novel mutation in CTNNB1 causes familial exudative vitreoretinopathy (FEVR) and microcephaly. *Ophthalmic Genet* 41: 63–68.

Dashti, S. et al. (2022). Identification of a novel de novo mutation in the CTNNB1 gene in an Iranian patient with intellectual disability. *Neurol Sci* 43: 2859–2863.

Dave, R.K. et al. (2011). Sonic hedgehog and Notch signaling can cooperate to regulate neurogenic divisions of neocortical progenitors. *PloS One* 6 (2): e14680.

Derwińska, K. et al. (2008). PTCH1 duplication in a family with microcephaly and mild developmental delay. *Eur J Hum Genet* 17: 267–271.

Dong, F. et al. (2016). Deletion of CTNNB1 in inhibitory circuitry contributes to autism-associated behavioral defects. *Hum Mol Genet* 25 (13): 2738–2751.

Dono, R. et al. (1998). Impaired cerebral cortex development and blood pressure regulation in FGF-2-deficient mice. *EMBO J* 17: 4213–4225.

Draganova, K. et al. (2015). Wnt/β-catenin signaling regulates sequential fate decisions of murine cortical precursor cells. *Stem Cells* 33: 170–182.

Dubourg, C. et al. (2007). Holoprosencephaly. *Orphanet J Rare Dis* 2: 8.

Dyer, C. et al. (2014). A bi-modal function of Wnt signalling directs an FGF activity gradient to spatially regulate neuronal differentiation in the midbrain. *Development* 141: 63–72.

Engler, A. et al. (2018). Notch2 Signaling Maintains NSC Quiescence in the Murine Ventricular-Subventricular Zone. *Cell Rep* 22: 992.

Englund, C. et al. (2005). Pax6, Tbr2, and Tbr1 are expressed sequentially by radial glia, intermediate progenitor cells, and postmitotic neurons in developing neocortex. *J Neurosci* 25: 247–251.

Ferent, J. et al. (2014). Genetic activation of hedgehog signaling unbalances the rate of neural stem cell renewal by increasing symmetric divisions. *Stem Cell Rep* 3: 312–323.

Fietz, S.A. et al. (2010). OSVZ progenitors of human and ferret neocortex are epithelial-like and expand by integrin signaling. *Nat Neurosci* 13: 690–699.

Garcia, A.D. et al. (2010). Sonic hedgehog regulates discrete populations of astrocytes in the adult mouse forebrain. *J Neurosci* 30: 13597–13608.

Ge, W. et al. (2002). Notch signaling promotes astrogliogenesis via direct CSL-mediated glial gene activation. *J Neurosci Res* 69: 848.

Gingrich, E.C. et al. (2022). A subpopulation of astrocyte progenitors defined by Sonic hedgehog signaling. *Neural Dev* 17: 2.

Gotz, M. and Huttner, W.B. (2005). The cell biology of neurogenesis. *Nat Rev Mol Cell Biol* 6: 777–788.

Gotz, M. et al. (1998). Pax6 controls radial glia differentiation in the cerebral cortex. *Neuron* 21: 1031–1044.

Hansen, D.V. et al. (2010). Neurogenic radial glia in the outer subventricular zone of human neocortex. *Nature* 464: 554–561.

Hashimoto-Torii, K. et al. (2008). Interaction between reelin and Notch signaling regulates neuronal migration in the cerebral cortex. *Neuron* 60: 273–284.

Hatakeyama, J. et al. (2004). Hes genes regulate size, shape and histogenesis of the nervous system by control of the timing of neural stem cell differentiation. *Development* 131: 5539–5550.

Haubensak, W. et al. (2004). Neurons arise in the basal neuroepithelium of the early mammalian telencephalon: a major site of neurogenesis. *Proc Natl Acad Sci USA* 101: 3196–3201.

Haushalter, C. et al. (2017). Retinoic acid controls early neurogenesis in the developing mouse cerebral cortex. *Dev Biol* 430 (1): 129–41.

Hebert, J.M. and Fishell, G. (2008). The genetics of early telencephalon patterning: some assembly required. *Nat Rev Neurosci* 9: 678–685.

Hill, S.A. et al. (2019). Sonic hedgehog signaling in astrocytes mediates cell type-specific synaptic organization. *Elife* 8: e45545.

Hirata, H. et al. (2001). Hes1 and Hes3 regulate maintenance of the isthmic organizer and development of the mid/hindbrain. *EMBO J* 20: 4454–4466.

Hirata, H. et al. (2002). Oscillatory expression of the bHLH factor Hes1 regulated by a negative feedback loop. *Science* 298: 840–843.

Hitoshi, S. et al. (2002). Notch pathway molecules are essential for the maintenance, but not the generation, of mammalian neural stem cells. *Genes Dev* 16: 846–858.

Ho, S. et al. (2021). CTNNB1-related neurodevelopmental disorder in a Chinese population. *Am J Med Genet Part A* 188: 130–137.

Honjo, T. (2010). The shortest path from the surface to the nucleus: RBP-J kappa/Su(H) transcription factor. *Genes Cells* 1: 1–9.

Huang, P. et al. (2007). A novel role of phospho-beta-catenin in microtubule regrowth at centrosome. *Oncogene* 26: 4357–4371.

Imayoshi, I. et al. (2010). Essential roles of Notch signaling in maintenance of neural stem cells in developing and adult brains. *J Neurosci* 30 (9): 3489–3498.

Iso, T. et al. (2003). HES and HERP families: multiple effectors of the Notch signaling pathway. *J Cell Physiol* 194: 237–255.

Jacobs, S. et al. (2006). Retinoic acid is required early during adult neurogenesis in the dentate gyrus. *Proc Natl Acad Sci USA* 103: 3902–3907.

Jiang, R. et al. (1998). Defects in limb, craniofacial, and thymic development in Jagged2 mutant mice. *Genes Dev* 12: 1046–1057.

Junghans, D. et al. (2005). β-catenin–mediated cell-adhesion is vital for embryonic forebrain development. *Dev Dyn* 233: 528–539.

Kang, W. and Hebert, J.M. (2015). FGF signaling is necessary for neurogenesis in young mice and sufficient to reverse its decline in old mice. *J Neurosci* 35: 10217–10223.

Kavitha, Y. et al. (2011). Toll-like receptor 3 regulates neural stem cell proliferation by modulating the Sonic hedgehog pathway. *PloS One* 6: e26766.

Ke, Z. and Chen, Y. (2020). Case report. *Front Pediatr* 8: 575673.

Kharbanda, M. et al. (2017). Clinical features associated with CTNNB1 de novo loss of function mutations in ten individuals. *Eur J Med Genet* 60: 130–135.

Kim, W.Y. et al. (2009). GSK-3 is a master regulator of neural progenitor homeostasis. *Nat Neurosci* 12: 1390–1397.

Komada, M. (2012). Sonic hedgehog signaling coordinates the proliferation and differentiation of neural stem/progenitor cells by regulating cell cycle kinetics during development of the neocortex. *Congenit Anom* 52: 72–77.

Kuan, C.Y. et al. (1999). The Jnk1 and Jnk2 protein kinases are required for regional specific apoptosis during early brain development. *Neuron* 22: 667–676.

Kuechler, A. et al. (2015). De novo mutations in beta-catenin (CTNNB1) appear to be a frequent cause of intellectual disability: expanding the mutational and clinical spectrum. *Hum Genet* 134: 97–109.

Kuwahara, A. et al. (2010). Wnt signaling and its downstream target N-myc regulate basal progenitors in the developing neocortex. *Development* 137: 1035–1044.

Lasky, J.L. and Wu, H. (2005). Notch signaling, brain development, and human disease. *Pediatr Res* 57: 104R–109R.

Li, N. et al. (2017). Exome sequencing identifies a de novo mutation of CTNNB1 gene in a patient mainly presented with retinal detachment, lens and vitreous opacities, microcephaly, and developmental delay. *Medicine* 96 (20): e6914.

Li, X. et al. (2021). The role of Shh signalling pathway in central nervous system development and related diseases. *Cell Biochem Funct* 39 (2): 180–189.

Lijam, N. et al. (1997). Social interaction and sensorimotor gating abnormalities in mice lacking Dvl1. *Cell* 90: 895–905.

Lim, N.R. et al. (2015). Opposing roles for JNK and Aurora A in regulating the association of WDR62 with spindle microtubules. *J Cell Sci* 128: 527–540.

Liu, J. and Lobe, C.G. (2010). Cre-conditional expression of constitutively active Notch1 in transgenic mice. *Genesis* 45: 259–265.

Liu, Z. et al. (2021). Research progress in vitamin A and autism spectrum disorder. *Behav Neurol* 2021: 5417497.

Luo, K. (2017). Signaling cross talk between TGF-beta/Smad and other signaling pathways. *Cold Spring Harb Perspect Biol* 9 (1): a022137.

MacDonald, B.T. et al. (2009). Wnt/β-catenin signaling: components, mechanisms, and diseases. *Dev Cell* 17: 9–26.

Major, M.B. et al. (2008). New regulators of Wnt/beta-catenin signaling revealed by integrative molecular screening. *Sci Signal* 1: ra12.

Manzari-Tavakoli, A. et al. (2022). The cross-talks among bone morphogenetic protein (BMP) signaling and other prominent pathways involved in neural differentiation. *Front Mol Neurosci* 15: 827275.

Marklund, U. et al. (2010). Domain-specific control of neurogenesis achieved through patterned regulation of Notch ligand expression. *Development* 137: 437–445.

Martínez, C. et al. (2013). Proliferation of murine midbrain neural stem cells depends upon an endogenous Sonic hedgehog (Shh) source. *PloS One* 8: e65818.

Mason, H.A. et al. (2006). Loss of notch activity in the developing central nervous system leads to increased cell death. *Dev Neurosci* 28 (1–2): 49–57.

Masuda, T. and Ishitani, T. (2017). Context-dependent regulation of the beta-catenin transcriptional complex supports diverse functions of Wnt/beta-catenin signaling. *J Biochem* 161: 9–17.

Mathieu, C. et al. (2008). Endothelial cell-derived bone morphogenetic proteins control proliferation of neural stem/progenitor cells. *Mol Cell Neurosci* 38: 569–577.

Mbom, B.C. et al. (2014). Nek2 phosphorylates and stabilizes beta-catenin at mitotic centrosomes downstream of Plk1. *Mol Biol Cell* 25: 977–991.

Mehler, M.F. et al. (2000). Developmental changes in progenitor cell responsiveness to bone morphogenetic proteins differentially modulate progressive CNS lineage fate. *Dev Neurosci* 22 (1-2): 74–85.

Miao, N. et al. (2018). Opposite roles of Wnt7a and Sfrp1 in modulating proper development of neural progenitors in the mouse cerebral cortex. *Front Mol Neurosci* 11: 247.

Mira, H. et al. (2010). Signaling through BMPR-IA regulates quiescence and long-term activity of neural stem cells in the adult hippocampus. *Cell Stem Cell* 7: 78–89.

Mishra, S. et al. (2018). Retinoic acid is required for neural stem and progenitor cell proliferation in the adult hippocampus. *Stem Cell Rep* 10: 1705–1720.

Moon, R.T. et al. (2002). The promise and perils of Wnt signaling through beta-catenin. *Science* 296: 1644–1646.

Murciano, A. et al. (2002). Interkinetic nuclear movement may provide spatial clues to the regulation of neurogenesis. *Mol Cell Neurosci* 21: 285–300.

Myers, A.K. et al. (2020). JNK signaling is required for proper tangential migration and laminar allocation of cortical interneurons. *Development* 147 (2): dev180646.

Nagao, M. et al. (2007). Cross talk between Notch and growth factor/cytokine signaling pathways in neural stem cells. *Mol Cell Biol* 27: 3982–3994.

Najas, S. et al. (2020). A SMAD1/5-YAP signalling module drives radial glia self-amplification and growth of the developing cerebral cortex. *Development* 147 (13): dev187005.

Nakashima, H. et al. (2021). MeCP2 controls neural stem cell fate specification through miR-199a-mediated inhibition of BMP-Smad signaling. *Cell Rep* 35: 109124.

Nakashima, H. et al. (2018). Canonical TGF-beta signaling negatively regulates neuronal morphogenesis through TGIF/Smad complex-mediated CRMP2 suppression. *J Neurosci* 38: 4791–4810.

Nguyen, H. et al. (2018). Epigenetic regulation by BAF complexes limits neural stem cell proliferation by suppressing Wnt signaling in late embryonic development. *Stem Cell Rep* 10: 1734–1750.

Niederreither, K. and Dolle, P. (2008). Retinoic acid in development. *Nat Rev Genet* 9: 541–553.

Nieto, M. et al. (2001). Neural bHLH genescontrol the neuronal versus glial fate decision in cortical progenitors. *Neuron* 29: 401–413.

Noctor, S.C. et al. (2004). Cortical neurons arise in symmetric and asymmetric division zones and migrate through specific phases. *Nat Neurosci* 7: 136–144.

Nyfeler, Y. et al. (2014). Jagged1 signals in the postnatal subventricular zone are required for neural stem cell self-renewal. *EMBO J* 24: 3504–3515.

Oka, C. et al. (1995). Disruption of the mouse RBP-J Kappa results in early embryonic death. *Development* 121: 3291–3301.

Okubo, Y. et al. (2021). Cleaved Delta like 1 intracellular domain regulates neural development via Notch signal dependent and independent pathways. *Development* 148 (19): dev193664.

O'Roak, B.J. et al. (2012). Sporadic autism exomes reveal a highly interconnected protein network of de novo mutations. *Nature* 485: 246–250.

Ohtsuka, T. and Kageyama, R. (2021). Hes1 overexpression leads to expansion of embryonic neural stem cell pool and stem cell reservoir in the postnatal brain. *Development* 148 (4): dev189191.

Ohtsuka, T. and Kageyama, R. (2022). Dual activation of Shh and Notch signaling induces dramatic enlargement of neocortical surface area. *Neurosci Res* 176: 18–30.

Palma, V. and Altaba, A. (2004). Hedgehog-GLI signaling regulates the behavior of cells with stem cell properties in the developing neocortex. *Development* 131: 337.

Paridaen, J.T. and Huttner, W.B. (2014). Neurogenesis during development of the vertebrate central nervous system. *EMBO Rep* 15: 351–364.

Poschl, J. et al. (2013). Constitutive activation of beta-catenin in neural progenitors results in disrupted proliferation and migration of neurons within the central nervous system. *Dev Biol* 374: 319–332.

Qu, Q. et al. (2010). Orphan nuclear receptor TLX activates Wnt/β-catenin signalling to stimulate neural stem cell proliferation and self-renewal. *Nat Cell Biol* 12: 31–40.

Qu, Q. et al. (2013). Wnt7a regulates multiple steps of neurogenesis. *Mol Cell Biol* 33: 2551–2559.

Ramain, P. et al. (2001). Novel Notch alleles reveal a Deltex-dependent pathway repressing neural fate. *Curr Biol* 11: 1729–1738.

Reiner, O. et al. (2012). Interkinetic nuclear movement in the ventricular zone of the cortex. *J Mol Neurosci* 46: 516–526.

Ruan, X. et al. (2021). Zbed3 is indispensable for Wnt signaling regulation of cortical layers formation in developing brain.*Cereb Cortex* 31: 4078–4091.

Saxena, M. et al. (2018). Perturbation of canonical and non-canonical BMP signaling affects migration, polarity and dendritogenesis of mouse cortical neurons. *Development* 145 (1): dev147157.

Segklia, A. et al. (2012). Bmp7 regulates the survival, proliferation, and neurogenic properties of neural progenitor cells during corticogenesis in the mouse. *PloS One* 7: e34088.

Shimojo, H. et al. (2008). Oscillations in Notch signaling regulate maintenance of neural progenitors. *Neuron* 58: 52–64.

Siegenthaler, J.A. et al. (2009). Retinoic acid from the meninges regulates cortical neuron generation. *Cell* 139: 597–609.

Silva, F.D. et al. (2021). Mitotic WNT signalling orchestrates neurogenesis in the developing neocortex. *EMBO J* 40: e108041.

Son, A.I. et al. (2020). Dual role of Rbpj in the maintenance of neural progenitor cells and neuronal migration in cortical development. *Cereb Cortex* 30: 6444–6457.

Stone, D.M. et al. (1999). Characterization of the human suppressor of fused, a negative regulator of the zinc-finger transcription factor Gli. *J Cell Sci* 112 (Pt 23): 4437–4448.

Sun, Y. et al. (2010). The suppression of CRMP2 expression by bone morphogenetic protein (BMP)-SMAD gradient signaling controls multiple stages of neuronal development. *J Biol Chem* 285: 39039–39050.

Swiatek, P.J. et al. (1994). Notch1 is essential for postimplantation development in mice. *Genes Dev* 8 (6): 707–719.

Taniguchi, K. et al. (2012). Loss of Tgif function causes holoprosencephaly by disrupting the SHH signaling pathway. *PLoS Genetics* 8: e1002524.

Taverna, E. et al. (2014). The cell biology of neurogenesis. *Ann Rev Cell Dev Biol* 30: 465–502.

Tokunaga, A. et al. (2004). Mapping spatio-temporal activation of Notch signaling during neurogenesis and gliogenesis in the developing mouse brain. *J Neurochem* 90: 142–154.

Wang, L. et al. (2016). Hedgehog signaling promotes basal progenitor expansion and the growth and folding of the neocortex. *Nat Neurosci* 19 (8): 1115.

Wang, L.C. and Almazan, G. (2016). Role of Sonic hedgehog signaling in oligodendrocyte differentiation. *Neurochem Res* 41: 1–11.

Werner, S. et al. (2011). Fibroblast growth factor-2 deficiency causes defects in adult hippocampal neurogenesis, which are not rescued by exogenous fibroblast growth factor-2. *J Neurosci Res* 89: 1605–1617.

Westerlund, N. et al. (2011). Phosphorylation of SCG10/stathmin-2 determines multipolar stage exit and neuronal migration rate. *Nat Neurosci* 14: 305–313.

Winczewska-Wiktor, A. et al. (2016). A de novo CTNNB1 nonsense mutation associated with syndromic atypical hyperekplexia, microcephaly and intellectual disability. *BMC Neurol* 16: 35.

Woodhead, G.J. et al. (2006). Cell-autonomous β-catenin signaling regulates cortical precursor proliferation. *J Neurosci* 26: 12620–12630.

Xu, J. et al. (2010). Generation of mice with a conditional null allele of the Jagged2 gene. *Genesis* 48: 390–393.

Xu, D. et al. (2018). MEKK3 coordinates with FBW7 to regulate WDR62 stability and neurogenesis. *PLoS Biol* 16: e2006613.

Xu, D. et al. (2014). Microcephaly-associated protein WDR62 regulates neurogenesis through JNK1 in the developing neocortex. *Cell Rep* 6: 104–116.

Xue, Y. et al. (1999). Embryonic lethality and vascular defects in mice lacking the Notch ligand Jagged1. *Hum Mol Genet* 8 (5): 723–730.

Yang, Z. et al. (2017). ADAM10-initiated release of Notch intracellular domain regulates microtubule stability and radial migration of cortical neurons. *Cereb Cortex* 27: 919–932.

Yoon, K. et al. (2004). Fibroblast growth factor receptor signaling promotes radial glial identity and interacts with Notch1 signaling in telencephalic progenitors. *J Neurosci* 24: 9497–9506.

Zhang, F. et al. (2016). A novel c-Jun N-terminal Kinase (JNK) signaling complex involved in neuronal migration during brain development. *J Biol Chem* 291: 11466–11475.

Zhang, R. et al. (2018). Notch: an interactive player in neurogenesis and disease. *Cell Tissue Res* 371 (1): 73–89.

Zhang, S. et al. (2021). The Wnt effector TCF7l2 promotes oligodendroglial differentiation by repressing autocrine BMP4-mediated signaling. *J Neurosci* 41: 1650–1664.

Zhou, C.J. et al. (2006). Neuronal production and precursor proliferation defects in the neocortex of mice with loss of function in the canonical Wnt signaling pathway. *Neuroscience* 142: 1119–1131.

Zhou, Z.D. et al. (2010). Notch as a molecular switch in neural stem cells. *IUBMB Life* 62 (8): 618–23.

Zhou, Z.W. et al. (2020). NBS1 interacts with Notch signaling in neuronal homeostasis. *Nucleic Acids Research* 48 (19): 10924–10939.

31

Centrosome Regulation and Function in the Developing Neocortex

Xuan Xie[1] *and Song-Hai Shi*[1,2]

[1] *IDG/McGovern Institute for Brain Research, Tsinghua-Peking Center for Life Sciences, Beijing Frontier Center of Biological Structure, Beijing Advanced Innovation Center for Structural Biology, School of Life Sciences, Tsinghua University, Beijing 100084, China*
[2] *Chinese Institute for Brain Research, Beijing 102206, China*

The centrosome is a subcellular organelle involved in numerous cellular processes including cell division, cell migration, and sensory reception. In animal cells, it serves two primary functions, as the main microtubule-organizing center (MTOC) to organize microtubules and as the basal body to support primary ciliogenesis. As a crucial organelle ubiquitously present in nearly all cell types, the centrosome plays essential roles in the development of many organs, including the neocortex – one of the most complex and fascinating brain structures in the animal body. The neocortex is composed of a myriad of diverse neural cells that are largely produced by neural progenitor cells (NPCs) that undergo multiple rounds of division during development. Moreover, new-born neural cells often embark on extensive migration from the birthplace to their final destination and undergo complex differentiation processes to ensure highly organized structural and functional assembly of neural circuits for behavior control. Numerous mutations in genes encoding centrosome or centrosome-associated proteins have been linked to abnormal development of the neocortex and neurological diseases, such as lissencephaly, microcephaly, macrocephaly, epilepsy, and schizophrenia, indicating that the centrosome is especially important for neocortical development and function. Here we provide an overview of the recent advances in the understanding of the regulation and function of the centrosome in neocortical development, in particular, in progenitor cell division and neuronal migration and differentiation, under normal and diseases conditions.

31.1 Centrosome Structure, Biogenesis, and Function

The centrosome is a distinct cytoplasmic structure composed of two perpendicularly arranged centrioles, which are surrounded by a proteinaceous matrix called the pericentriolar material (PCM) (Figure 31.1). The centrioles are microtubule-based cylinders of defined length (~500 nm) and diameter (~250 nm) with a highly conserved nine-fold radial symmetry (Winey and O'Toole 2014). In most animal cells, the centrosome is not absolutely required, but adds to the effectiveness of cell division by facilitating the mitotic spindle assembly. Moreover, the centrosome behaves like DNA in cell division. It undergoes semi-conservative duplication, during which the existing two centrioles are used as the template to synthesize two new centrioles, once and only once with one centrosome/two centrioles inherited by each daughter cell (Figure 31.1).

Coupled with the generational difference, the centriole pair in each centrosome exhibits prominent structural and functional asymmetry. The old, fully mature mother centriole possesses two sets of

Neocortical Neurogenesis in Development and Evolution, First Edition. Edited by Wieland B. Huttner.

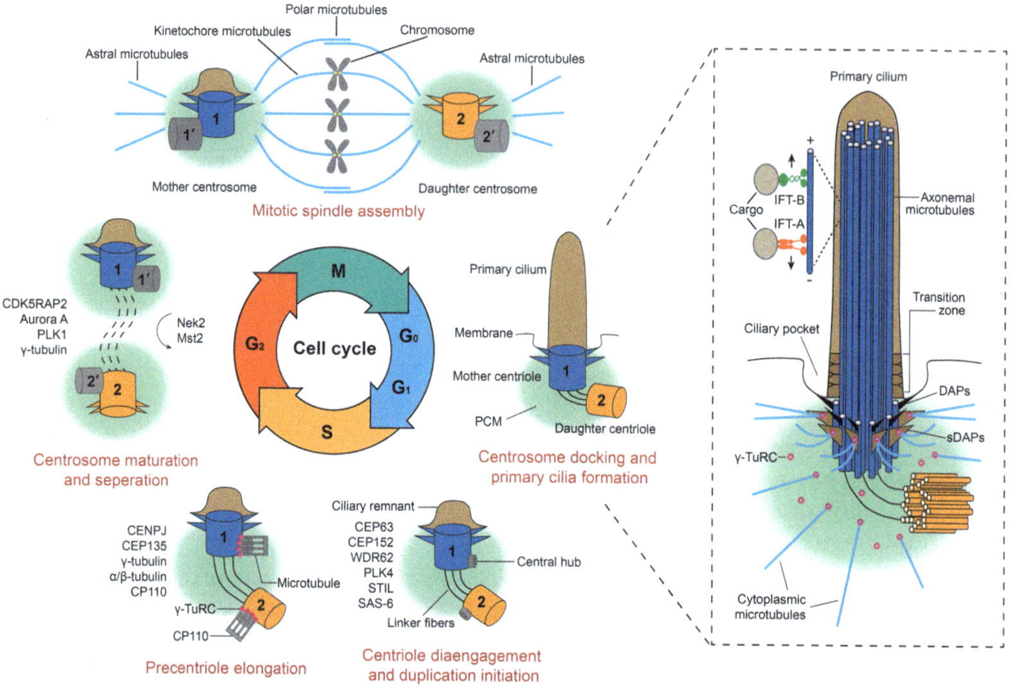

Figure 31.1 Centrosome biogenesis and primary cilium structure in animal cells. The semi-conservative centrosome biogenesis process is coupled to cell cycle progression. The centrosome duplication begins at early S phase, with the disengagement between the original mother (1) and daughter (2) centrioles that individually serve as the template for nascent procentriole formation. New-born centrioles (1′ and 2′) remain tightly engaged with their mother centrioles and elongate throughout S and G_2 phase. At G_2/M phase transition, the new centrosomes further mature by accumulating PCM and move to the opposite ends of the dividing cell, eventually forming the two poles of a mitotic spindle. Due to generational differences of their mother centrioles, the two centrosomes exhibit structural and functional differences, such as appendages. In nondividing G_1 or G_0 phase cells, the mother centriole is anchored to the cell membrane via its DAPs and serves as the basal body to support the formation of a primary cilium. The ciliary axoneme comprising nine microtubule doublets arises from a continuation of the mother centriole. At the base of the cilium, the ciliary pocket and transition zone are specialized domains to gate protein entry or exit. The IFT-A and IFT-B protein complexes are responsible for the retrograde and anterograde transport in the cilium, respectively. Besides serving as the basal body, the centrosome also acts as the main MTOC to nucleate and anchor cytoplasmic microtubules at the PCM and sDAPs.

appendages at its distal and subdistal ends, whereas the young, immature daughter centriole is shorter in length with no appendage. Both centrioles nucleate microtubules via the microtubule nucleator γ-tubulin ring complex (γ-TuRC) in the PCM associated with the proximal parts of centrioles. However, only the mother centriole is capable of anchoring microtubules at the subdistal appendages (sDAPs). In dividing cells, the centriole and centrosome actively promote mitotic spindle formation and chromosome segregation. In nondividing cells, in addition to nucleating and anchoring microtubules, the mature mother centriole can transform into a basal body by docking to the plasma membrane via the distal appendages (DAPs) and templates the assembly of a nonmotile primary cilium, a versatile cell antenna for sensation and signaling (Bornens 2012; Conduit et al. 2015; Luders and Stearns 2007).

31.1.1 The Continuous Understanding of the Centrosome

In 1876, Van Beneden first described the "polar corpuscle" structure in the mitotic eggs and later Boveri named it the "centrosome" (Lessman 2012). For nearly one-and-a-half centuries, the centrosome has attracted much research attention and continues to do so. From the start, the centrosome has been postulated to play a role in cell symmetry breaking and cell polarity maintenance. Moreover, the early experiments on centrosome activity pointed to the function of the centrosome in mitotic spindle formation and chromosome segregation underlying the chromosomal theory of heredity. The centrosome was viewed as the structure coordinating cytokinesis and karyokinesis.

Plants and fungi do not have centrosomes or centrosome-resembling organelles such as spindle pole or centriole except in flagellated male gametes. The main function of MTOC for microtubule nucleation and spindle organization appears to be taken by the nuclear envelope or surface with γ-TuRC (Luders and Stearns 2007). The centrosome in animal cells is the main MTOC, thereby orchestrating cell motility, conferring cell polarity, and facilitating mitotic spindle assembly. Nonetheless, the centrosome is dispensable for most animal cell division (Luders and Stearns 2007). Notably, the association of the centriole or basal body with flagellum is evolutionarily conserved, including in the common unicellular ancestor of eukaryotic cells. The basal body from sperm flagellum elicits centrosome assembly in zygote during fertilization. The invention of the centrosome as a cytoplasmic organelle, instead of permanently associated with an axoneme, has taken place in the Unikonta lineage. The integrated function of the centrosome as the main MTOC as well as the basal body in animal cells likely reflects the adaptive evolution of the centrosome and organisms.

Over the past two decades, with the advance of powerful genetic, biochemical, and imaging tools, the molecular composition as well as the biogenesis process of the centrosome has been dissected to a great extent. Evolutionarily conserved sets of proteins required for centriole assembly and centrosome duplication have been identified initially in worms and flies, and further characterized in mouse and human cells. The crucial components responsible for the structure and function of the centrosome have also been revealed. Hundreds of proteins are found to be localized in the centriole or the centrosome, among which many are associated with human diseases. For example, mutations of over a dozen of genes encoding centrosome or centrosome-associated proteins have been found to be linked to human primary microcephaly syndromes. In addition, the structural bases of the centriole, the γ-TuRC, and the ciliary axoneme have also been elucidated (Kiesel et al. 2020; Wieczorek et al. 2020; Winey and O'Toole 2014).

31.1.2 The Centrosome Duplication Cycle

The centrosome duplication cycle is well coupled with the cell division cycle (Figure 31.1). Cells begin with exactly one centrosome. During G_1 and early S phase, the centrosome undergoes duplication precisely once and only once in a semi-conservative fashion and then the two duplicated centrosomes move to the opposite ends of the mitotic cell to be associated with the spindle poles as G_2/M phase begins. Upon the initiation of centrosome duplication, the original mother and daughter centrioles connected with intercentriolar link become separated and each serves as a template to support the biogenesis of one procentriole adjacent to the parental centriole, which then progressively develops into a new daughter centriole pairing with the parental centriole (Bettencourt-Dias and Glover 2007).

The destabilization and fragmentation of the PCM is required for the separation of the original two centrioles and the formation of new centrioles (Enos et al. 2018; Schlaitz et al. 2007). A number of proteins, such as CEP (centrosomal protein) 63 and CEP152, are first recruited to the proximal ends of the original centrioles by the scaffold protein WDR62 (WD repeat-containing protein 62) to form a ring-like structure. Next, PLK4 (Polo-like kinase 4) is recruited to the site of nascent daughter centriole formation and subsequently autophosphorylates itself as well as recruits and phosphorylates STIL (SCL/TAL1 interrupting locus). Following this, STIL and SAS-6 (spindle assembly abnormal protein 6) oligomerize into a nine-fold symmetrical ring structure to form the central hub, then CENPJ (centromere protein J, also called SAS-4 and CPAP) and CEP135 are finally recruited to stabilize the central hub and initiate the assembly of microtubules around it (Jayaraman et al. 2016; Keller et al. 2014; Kim et al. 2013; Lin et al. 2013; Pelletier et al. 2006; Sir et al. 2011). Once the new centriole biogenesis is completed, the PCM is reformed, during which multiple coiled-coil proteins are recruited and γ-tubulin is attached to the centrosome via CDK5RAP2 (Cyclin-dependent kinase 5 regulatory subunit associated protein 2) (Dictenberg et al. 1998; Fong et al. 2008; Hamill et al. 2002). A functional PCM is essential for microtubule nucleation around the centrosome (Zheng et al. 1995).

During mitosis, the two newly formed centrosomes are disengaged by cutting the tight cohesin fiber connections between them, move to the opposite ends of the dividing cell, and accumulate PCM to nucleate microtubules (Cabral et al. 2013; Tsou and Stearns 2006). The microtubules are subsequently assembled into a spindle-like structure between the two duplicated centrosomes that drives the separation of chromosomes evenly into the two daughter cells. Mitotic microtubules can be divided into three different types according to their position and function: astral microtubules connecting the centrosome to the cell cortex, kinetochore microtubules connecting the condensed chromosomes to the centrosome, and polar microtubules connecting two spindle poles (Jean et al. 2020). Since the duplicated centrosomes nucleate most of these microtubules, they actively control the spindle polarity and orientation, and thereby the plane of cell cleavage.

During interphase, the centrosome is typically maintained near the nucleus at the center of non-ciliated cells and organizes the cytoplasmic microtubule array, or is anchored at the cell plasma membrane to function as the basal body for primary cilium formation (Burakov et al. 2003; Shao et al. 2020) (Figure 31.1). The ciliary assembly proceeds in a stepwise manner. First, the mother centriole is anchored to the plasma membrane through its DAPs to form the basal body, and microtubules are recruited to the sDAPs by dynein-based traffic. The docking site and angle of the basal body dictate the position and orientation of the resulting primary cilium. Then, TTBK2 (Tau tubulin kinase 2) acts at the distal end of the mother centriole to remove an inhibitory protein complex of axonemal growth including CP110 (centriolar coiled-coil protein of 110 KDa), CEP97, and KIF24 (kinesin family member 24) (Kobayashi et al. 2011), thereby licensing the elongation of doublet microtubules to protrude beneath an extension of membrane. The axonemal microtubules recruit intraflagellar transport (IFT) proteins to promote continuous outgrowth and maintenance of a primary cilium. Selective transport of ciliary proteins is achieved based on the structure of a ciliary pocket and transition zone at the root of the primary cilium. Upon entering the next cell division cycle, the primary cilium undergoes resorption and disassembly to release the centrosome from the plasma membrane for centrosome duplication and mitotic spindle formation (Goetz et al. 2012; Ishikawa and Marshall 2011). Therefore, the ciliary assembly and disassembly cycle is also tightly coupled to the centrosome duplication cycle and the cell division cycle.

31.1.3 Centrosome Function in Animal Cells

Since its original discovery, the centrosome has been implicated in cell division. Hundreds of proteins are preferentially localized at the centrosome, both the centrioles and the PCM, with defined functions, such as microtubule nucleators and organizers, cell cycle regulators, checkpoint proteins, and signaling molecules, indicating that the centrosome functions as the MTOC, as well as a signal coordination center. In dividing animal cells, the centrosome nucleates microtubules and drives the mitotic spindle formation for proper segregation and inheritance of chromosomes into the daughter cells. While the centrosome is dispensable for most animal cell division, centrosome loss can cause mitotic delay and elicit p53-dependent cell death (Conduit et al. 2015). Dysfunction of the centrosome has also been linked to cancer due to an increase in the level of chromosome instability or metastatic capability of cancer cells.

In nondividing animal cells, the centrosome-based primary cilium functions as a cellular antenna to sense extracellular signals, such as hormones, odorants, and growth factors, and activate diverse intracellular signal transduction pathways, such as Hedgehog, Wnt, PDGFRα, and Integrin signaling. The cytoplasmic microtubule networks emanated from the centrosome also provide the essential cytoskeletal basis for cell polarity, cell morphogenesis, cell motility, and intracellular transport (Conduit et al. 2015; Ishikawa and Marshall 2011).

31.2 Neocortical Development

The neocortex is the most recently evolved brain structure that commands higher-order brain functions, such as perception, movement, language, emotion, and cognition. It contains a vast number of diverse neurons and glial cells arranged into a six-layered structure to receive and process inputs and generate and send out outputs. The intricate architecture and organization of the neocortex is systematically and progressively built during development. Neocortical neurons and glia cells are predominantly generated through extensive progenitor cell division in the germinal zone of the developing brain and migrate from the birthplace to their final destination to establish functional neural networks, during which their production, positioning, and differentiation are precisely controlled (Sun and Hevner 2014). Notably, the centrosome, as the main MTOC for microtubule organization and mitotic spindle formation, and the basal body for primary ciliogenesis, plays crucial roles in regulating the proliferation and differentiation of NPCs, as well as in controlling the migration and differentiation of new-born neural cells. Defective centrosome behavior and function can lead to severe malformation and malfunction of the neocortex and various neurological diseases.

31.2.1 Organized Progenitor Cell Behavior and Neocortical Histogenesis

Radial glia progenitors (RGPs) are the primary type of NPCs in the developing neocortex. They originate in neural epithelial cells in the early embryonic neuroepithelium, of which an apical process and a basal process develop and remain in contact with the ventricular and pial surface, respectively. As a result, RGPs are clearly identifiable based on their distinct morphology, possessing a spindle-shaped periventricular cell body, a long and thin basal process extending to the pial surface, and a relatively short apical process (also known as the endfoot) reaching to the ventricular surface and tethered to the adjacent endfeet of nearby RGPs via junctions (Beattie and Hippenmeyer 2017) (Figure 31.2).

During neocortical development, RGPs actively divide to either amplify themselves or to produce diverse neurons and glia. The mitosis of RGPs is strictly restricted to the ventricular surface, and prior to and after that the nucleus exhibits an oscillatory behavior called interkinetic nuclear migration (INM). The S phase occurs while the nucleus is at the basal end of the ventricular zone (VZ), then the nucleus migrates apically after entering the G_2 phase. After mitosis, the nucleus migrates basally away from the ventricular surface (Bertipaglia et al. 2018). While the nucleus undergoes INM, the apical and basal processes of RGPs are always tethered at the ventricular surface via junctions and the pial basement membrane, respectively. Moreover, the centrosome

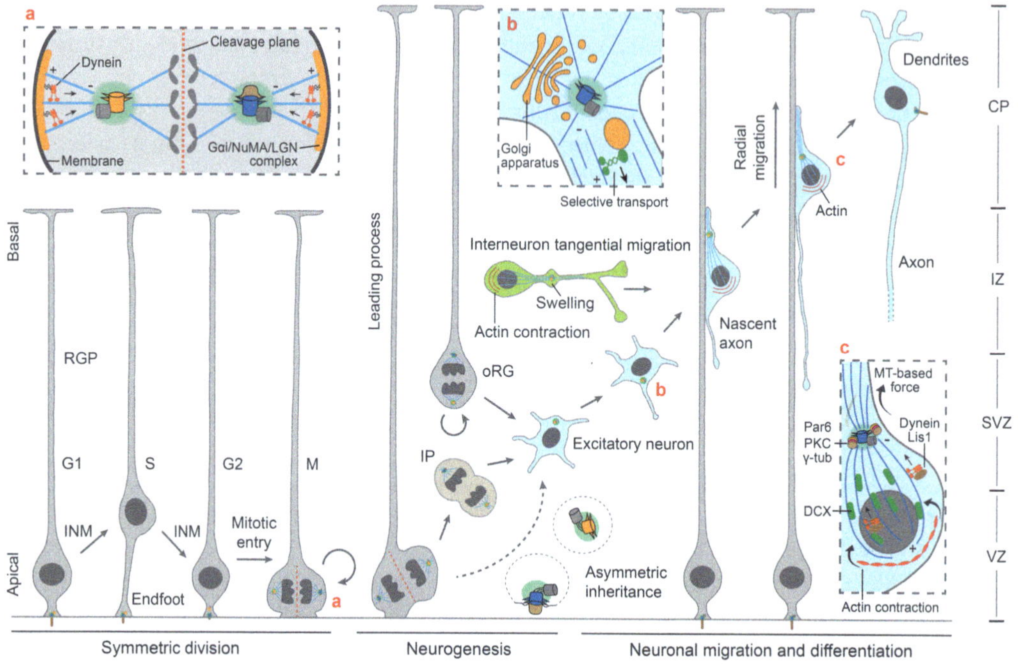

Figure 31.2 Centrosome function and regulation during neocortical development. RGPs exhibit successive INM coupled to the cell cycle progression. The nuclei of RGPs move basally during G_1 and S phases and then apically during G_2 phase, and eventually undergo mitosis at the ventricular surface. At the early embryonic stage, RGPs undergo symmetric, proliferative division to expand the progenitor pool, and then transit to the asymmetric, neurogenic division phase to produce neuron directly or indirectly via transit amplifying progenitors, such as IPs or oRGs. The change in division mode is thought to be related to the adjustment of mitotic spindle orientation, which is controlled by the interaction between astral microtubules and cell cortex (panel a). An oblique cleavage plane leads to asymmetric inheritance of the centrosome, apical membrane, and junctional complex, which likely contributes to distinct cell fate specification of daughter cells. New-born neurons ascend from the VZ to the SVZ and become polarized to develop one and only one nascent axon, during which the localization of the centrosome and Golgi apparatus appear to play critical roles (panel b). During radial migration, the coupling between the centrosome and the nucleus provides the microtubule-based force to pull the nucleus into the leading process, while the myosin-driven contraction of actin also generates an additional force to push the nucleus forward (panel c). Centrosome dislocation and actin contraction are also involved in tangential migration of neocortical interneurons.

remains anchored at the apical membrane of the apical or ventricular endfoot to support the formation of a primary cilium pointing into the lateral ventricle. The centrosome positioning and anchoring is important for the VZ integrity and proper RGP behavior and neocortical histogenesis (Jossin et al. 2017; Kadowaki et al. 2007; Kriegstein and Alvarez-Buylla 2009; Rasin et al. 2007; Shao et al. 2020). Notably, while only transiently present in the developing neocortex, RGPs play instructive roles in neocortical development. They are the major neural progenitors that produce diverse neurons and glia in an orderly fashion. In addition, the basal processes of RGPs serve as the scaffold to guide the radial migration of new-born neurons to their final destination for the formation of a layered neocortex (Beattie and Hippenmeyer 2017) (Figure 31.2). The intricate positioning and organization of the centrosome is instrumental to orderly RGP division, wave-like neurogenesis, and laminar structure formation in the developing neocortex.

During neocortical development, RGPs undergo a highly organized lineage progression program of self-proliferation, neurogenesis, and gliogenesis (Kriegstein and Alvarez-Buylla 2009; Sun and Hevner 2014). Initially, RGPs undergo symmetric, proliferative division to expand themselves. Then, they switch to asymmetric, neurogenic division to produce neurons either directly or indirectly through the generation of transit amplifying progenitors, such as intermediate progenitors (IPs) or outer subventricular zone (oSVZ) radial glial progenitors (oRGs, also called bRGs or tRGs), which can further divide in the subventricular zone (SVZ) to produce neurons (Kriegstein and Alvarez-Buylla 2009; Sun and Hevner 2014). The orientation of mitotic spindle and cleavage plane in dividing RGPs has been thought to influence the division mode and fate specification of two daughter cells, as it affects the segregation and inheritance of crucial cell fate determinants, such as Notch signaling components, by the daughter cells (Bultje et al. 2009; Morin and Bellaiche 2011).

In the developing mouse neocortex, RGPs appear at around embryonic day (E) 9.5 and predominantly undergo symmetric, proliferative division. Asymmetric neurogenic division begins at around E12.5 and reaches its peak between E13.5 and E15.5, during which individual RGPs divide to produce a self-renewing RGP and a differentiating cell, such as a neuron or an IP that further divides to generate more neurons (Figure 31.2). At approximately E16.5–E17.5, while many RGPs undergo terminal, symmetric neurogenic division to exit the cell cycle, around 15–20 percent of RGPs enter the gliogenesis phase, during which some RGPs begin to detach from the apical ventricular surface and migrate toward the pia by somal translocation. The translocating RGPs transform or divide to produce macroglia including both astrocytes and oligodendrocytes through intermediate gliogenic precursor cells (Beattie and Hippenmeyer 2017; Shen et al. 2021).

The neocortex has evolved both in size and complexity extensively in higher mammals. For example, compared with the mouse, the human neocortex is over 1,000 times larger. Structurally, the human neocortex is also highly folded, whereas the mouse neocortex is smooth. The greatly expanded and densely packed neocortex is generally considered to be the source of the remarkable cognitive capability of the human. Several hypotheses have been put forward to explain neocortical expansion and folding. One influential hypothesis is that the enhanced number and types of NPCs drive the expansion in neocortical size and regional differences in neurogenesis resulting in folding or gyrification (Kriegstein et al. 2006; Llinares-Benadero and Borrell 2019). Consistent with this, in addition to the drastic increase in RGP number, the number and types of transit amplifying progenitors arising from RGPs with different degrees of potency, such as IPs and oRGs, are also greatly enhanced in the developing primate and human neocortices to amplify the total output of RGP lineages (Beattie and Hippenmeyer 2017).

Unlike the typical RGPs in the VZ (also called the ventricular RGPs, vRGs), oRGs lack the apical endfeet contacting the ventricular surface and reside primarily in the oSVZ with a long basal process attached to the pial surface (Hansen et al. 2010) (Figure 31.2). The generation of oRGs occurs through either vRG delamination or vRG division in a cleavage plane-dependent manner. Notably, while mouse vRGs divide with a predominantly vertical cleavage plane (i.e., perpendicular to the ventricular surface) throughout neocortical development, human vRGs shift to an approximately equal number of vertical and horizontal cleavage planes at the start of oSVZ growth and oRG generation. These results indicate that the evolutionary shift in the cleavage plane may have contributed to the increase in oRGs and the formation of the oSVZ. Notably, oRGs exhibit unique mitotic somal translation (MST) through a mechanism distinct from that of INM, in which the soma ascends rapidly towards the pia before cytokinesis. The majority of human oRG division leads to oRG self-renewal with a small proportion to produce IPs. However, the spindle orientation and centrosome positioning in dividing oRGs are not well understood. In addition, while mouse IPs divide largely once to produce two neurons, human IPs appear to self-renew many times before producing neurons. Therefore, the transit amplification is a fundamental and defining feature of the evolutionary expansion of the neocortex.

31.2.2 Neuronal Migration and Differentiation

Neuronal migration is an essential process in neocortical development, as neurons are produced in specialized germinal zones that are often far away from their final destination. Neocortical excitatory neurons are generated in the VZ or the SVZ of the developing neocortex and migrate radially to constitute different layers of the neocortex in a birth date-dependent "inside-out" manner. The early-born neurons migrate to reside in the deep layers, whereas the late-born neurons migrate to pass the early-born neurons and occupy the superficial layers (Feng and Walsh 2001; He et al. 2015).

Migrating excitatory neurons go through distinct phases in their journey reflected in their morphology, migratory feature, and location (Noctor et al. 2004). Right after birth at the VZ surface upon RGP division, new-born neurons exhibit a bipolar morphology, detaching from the ventricular surface and rapidly ascending into the SVZ along the basal radial glial fiber of the mother RGP (phase 1). They then display dramatic changes in morphology to acquire a multipolar morphology and sojourn in the SVZ for up to one day (phase 2). While in a migratory pause in the radial direction, they actively extend and retract short processes, raising the possibility that they are searching or waiting for cues to proceed into the next phase. The precise role of the centrosome in this sojourn is largely unknown. In phase 3, many neurons in the SVZ exhibit a retrograde movement with the extension of an axon-like process towards the ventricular surface, suggesting a potential interaction of neurons with extrinsic signals from the ventricular end. These interplays during the second and third phases may be a prerequisite for neurons to initiate radial migration at the appropriate time, thereby reaching their correct final destination (Kriegstein and Noctor 2004; Nadarajah et al. 2002; Noctor et al. 2004; Tabata and Nakajima 2003). In phase 4, neurons undergo a morphological transition from multipolar to bipolar and embark on the glial fiber-guided radial migration towards the pia along the basal radial glial fibers of mother RGPs (Figure 31.2).

The glial fiber-guided radial migration or locomotion is achieved via a sequence of cyclical movements during which the bipolar neurons extend their leading process towards the pia, translocate their nuclei into the leading process, and retract the trailing process. Nuclear translocation is a crucial step in neuronal locomotion, as it entails the nucleus moving into the extending leading process to follow the migrating trajectory. The centrosome is always located in the leading process of migrating neurons. It is coupled to the nucleus via microtubules and provides the force to pull the nucleus forward (Ayala et al. 2007; Higginbotham and Gleeson 2007; Marin et al. 2010) (Figure 31.2). Centrosome movement into the dilated region in the leading process is commonly considered as a predictor of subsequent nuclear movement. Notably, the SVZ born neurons by IP division also undergo similar phases of radial migration (Noctor et al. 2004, 2008).

In comparison, neocortical interneurons are primarily generated in the medial ganglionic eminences (MGE) and caudal ganglionic eminences (CGE) of the developing ventral telencephalon, and undergo extensive tangential migration to reach the neocortex and then radial migration to occupy different layers (Vitalis and Rossier 2011; Wonders and Anderson 2006). During the long tangential migration phase, nascent interneurons migrate in parallel to the pia and do not tightly associate with the radial glial fibers of RGPs for locomotion or guidance. The tangential migration appears to be faster than the radial migration in speed and comprises two main steps: the formation and movement of a large swelling containing cytoplasmic organelles, such as the centrosome and the Golgi apparatus, into the leading neurite, followed by the nuclear translocation towards the displaced centrosome and Golgi apparatus (Barber and Pierani 2016; Bellion et al. 2005) (Figure 31.2). Upon arriving at their target area in the neocortex, migrating interneurons switch to radial migration to reach their final destination in the neocortex. Interestingly, interneurons also exhibit ventricle-directed movement before initiating their radial migration, suggesting a potential coordination in the migration of excitatory and inhibitory neurons by certain cues (Nadarajah et al. 2002; Yokota et al. 2007).

During radial migration, neurons switch from a multipolar to a bipolar morphology. This coincides with the neuronal polarization process, in which the apically growing neurite towards the ventricle develops into the future axon (Figure 31.2). The axon specification is a crucial early event in neuronal differentiation, as it sets the morphological and functional basis for unidirectional information flow in neurons (Noctor et al. 2004). It is driven by intricate signaling events and microtubule and actin cytoskeleton remodeling that control protein and vesicle transportation and neurite outgrowth. As the main MTOC, the centrosome has become a topic of intense research and has been suggested to play important roles in the initiation of axon development both in vitro and in vivo, as well as in neuronal morphogenesis and differentiation (Stiess and Bradke 2011; Takano et al. 2015).

31.3 Centrosome Regulation and Function in RGPs

Neocortical development begins with the formation and proliferation of RGPs in the neuroepithelium. RGPs not only serve as the major progenitor cells for the production of neocortical neurons and glial cells, but also provide the scaffold for new-born neurons to migrate to reach their final destination (Figure 31.2). The properties and behavior of RGPs fundamentally determine the structural and functional development of the neocortex, and the centrosome plays various essential roles in controlling RGP proliferation and differentiation.

31.3.1 Intricate Centrosome Organization in RGPs

The VZ of the developing neocortex is a typical pseudostratified epithelial structure and is predominantly composed of RGPs. As a broadly conserved feature of cell division in pseudostratified epithelia, RGPs undergo INM along the apicobasal axis of the VZ during interphase and ultimately undergo mitosis at the apical ventricular surface (Bertipaglia et al. 2018; Meyer et al. 2011). The subcellular localization of the centrosome is tightly regulated in coordination with RGP cell cycle progression (Figure 31.3). Throughout the process of INM, the centrosome of RGPs is constantly restricted at the apical endfeet, suggesting that the nuclear migration along the apicobasal axis is virtually centrosome-independent, but rather under the forces generated by kinesin and dynein motors associated on the nuclear envelop (Bertipaglia et al. 2018; Strzyz et al. 2015). However, the centrosome and its associated proteins, such as PCM1 (Pericentriolar material 1), CEP120, TACCs (Transforming acidic coiled-coil proteins), and DOCK7 (Dedicator of cytokinesis 7), also regulate INM indirectly through controlling microtubule organization and the centrosome–nucleus coupling (Ge et al. 2010; Xie et al. 2007; Yang et al. 2012).

In the late G_2 phase, the primary cilium axoneme is absorbed and the centrosome is detached from the plasma membrane. The centrosome then moves basally to meet with the nucleus for mitosis. In the developing mouse neocortex and chicken neural tube, the mitosis initiates when the centrosome and the nucleus meet away from the apical membrane. The mitotic cells then migrate to the ventricular surface dependent on actin filaments (Spear and Erickson 2012). However, a different scenario was observed in the rat neocortex, in which the nuclear envelop breakdown does not take place until the nucleus and the centrosome complete the apical migration and arrive at the ventricular surface (Hu et al. 2013). Where RGPs break down the nuclear envelop to initiate mitosis and whether the centrosome dislocation is associated with RGP mitotic entry remain to be the critical questions in the field (Bertipaglia et al. 2018).

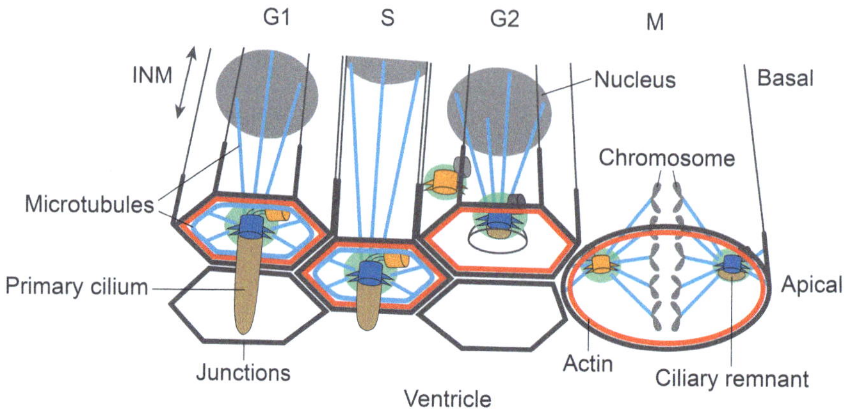

Figure 31.3 Centrosomes, primary cilia, and apical cytoskeleton organization in RGPs. Centrosomes, primary cilia, junctions, and cytoskeleton are intricately and dynamically regulated at the apical domain in RGPs as they progress through the cell cycle. The primary cilium is extended from the basal body docking at the apical membrane and protrudes into the lateral ventricle. The centrosome/basal body is also connected to the apical actin ring and junctional belt via microtubules. The nucleus undergoes INM and remain connected with the centrosome via microtubules. Prior to mitosis, the primary cilium is resorbed and a ciliary remnant appears to be attached to the old mother centriole in dividing RGPs, which may contribute to the re-formation of a primary cilium.

During mitosis, the centrosome duplicates and promotes the formation of the mitotic spindle, which is crucial for mitotic progression. After cell division is completed, the renewed RGPs enter the next round of INM and the centrosome is reanchored to the apical membrane to initiate the formation of a primary cilium (Yang et al. 2021).

31.3.2 Neocortical Neurogenesis in the Absence of the Centrosome

To uncover the essential role of the centrosome in RGP division and neocortical development, it would be imperative to eliminate the centrosome (Yang et al. 2021). Genetic studies showed that homozygous mutations of *CENPJ* lead to microcephaly in humans. The corresponding gene product CENPJ localizes at the centrosome and the spindle poles during mitosis, and is required for centriole biogenesis (Bond et al. 2005). Deletion of the *CENPJ* ortholog *Sas-4* (spindle assembly abnormal protein 4) in *Drosophila* causes a loss of centrioles and centrosomes from the embryonic to third instar larval stages, leading to slow spindle assembly and mitosis. Approximate 30 percent of asymmetrically dividing neuroblasts fail in correct cytokinesis, generating two daughter cells of equal size. Despite these defects, mutant flies develop a morphologically normal nervous system (Basto et al. 2006). The phenotypic discrepancy between *Sas-4* lacking flies and *CENPJ* mutated humans may be explained by compensatory mechanisms in flies or a more stringent temporal control of neural progenitor division and neurogenesis in mammals (Higginbotham and Gleeson 2007).

In-depth studies of forebrain-specific deletion of *CENPJ* in the developing mouse brain provide further insights. Selective removal of CENPJ/SAS-4 in RGPs leads to a progressive loss of centrioles and centrosomes, accompanied by the delocalization of RGPs from the VZ. While remaining proliferative, RGPs lacking the centrosome exhibit a delay in mitotic progression that triggers p53 upregulation and apoptosis, resulting in a strong neuronal loss and microcephaly (Insolera et al. 2014a). In addition to its role in regulating centriole biogenesis, CENPJ also acts as a scaffold for the formation of the primary cilium disassembly complex, which is recruited to the ciliary base for timely cilium disassembly and centriole release from the plasma membrane (Gabriel et al. 2016). CENPJ removal leads to a reduced cell proliferation, as well as long and thin primary cilia in RGPs, indicating that the centrosome-coupled ciliary dynamics also plays a crucial role in regulating RGP division and neocortical neurogenesis (Ding et al. 2019).

31.3.3 Asymmetric Centrosome Inheritance in Dividing RGPs

Asymmetric division of RGPs is the primary means of neocortical neurogenesis. It renews RGPs and, at the same time, generates differentiating progeny such as neurons or IPs (Miyata et al. 2004). Semi-conservative duplication of the centrosome in dividing cells produces a pair of the centrosomes with differentially aged mother centrioles, namely the mother and daughter centrosomes (Figure 31.1). Interestingly, the inheritance of the two centrosomes by two daughter cells of asymmetrically dividing RGPs is tightly regulated. The mother centrosome retaining the old mother centriole is preferentially inherited by the self-renewing RGP, whereas the daughter centrosome containing the new mother centriole is largely associated with the differentiating progeny (Wang et al. 2009).

Centrosomes with generationally different mother centrioles differ in their protein composition and biophysical properties, such as microtubule anchorage activity and the capability to mediate primary ciliogenesis (Anderson and Stearns 2009; Bornens 2002; Delattre and Gonczy 2004). The ciliary membrane is endocytosed and attached to the older mother centriole during mitosis and asymmetrically inherited by one daughter cell, which in principle permits the reestablishment of a primary cilium earlier than the non-inheriting daughter cell (Anderson and Stearns 2009; Paridaen et al. 2013) (Figure 31.3). Whether this asynchrony in primary cilium formation of two daughter cells differentially influences the response to environmental signals and thereby affects daughter cell fate specification remain to be explored. Furthermore, the mature appendages associated with the old mother centriole facilitate the anchorage of the centriole/centrosome at the VZ surface, thereby tethering the daughter cell that inherits it in the VZ. Together with differentially aged centrioles, cytoskeleton components and junctional proteins can also be asymmetrically partitioned into the two daughter cells, which confers different responses to extrinsic signals and adhesion status after mitosis (Bultje et al. 2009; Chenn et al. 1998) (Figure 31.2). Asymmetric behavior and inheritance of the centrosome has initially been observed during asymmetric division of *Drosophila* male germline stem cells and neuroblasts, suggesting that it is a conserved feature of asymmetric cell division across species (Rebollo et al. 2007; Yamashita et al. 2007).

Notably, prior to the neurogenesis phase, RGPs undergo symmetric, proliferative division to expand the progenitor pool by producing two daughter cells acquiring a similar RGP fate (Figure 31.2). While asymmetric inheritance of the centrosome fits well with RGP asymmetric division, it appears to be incompatible with RGP symmetric division. Interestingly, there are compensatory mechanisms involving active regulation of the centrosome-associated components to restore its symmetry during RGP symmetric division. Mindbomb1, a mono-ubiquitin ligase that regulates the trafficking of Notch ligands and promotes their activity, is enriched at the daughter centriole via its interaction with centriolar satellite proteins PCM1 and AZI1 (CEP131), and is preferentially inherited by the prospective neuron during asymmetric division. By contrast, during symmetric division, a supplementary pool of Mindbomb1 associated with the Golgi apparatus in interphase is released during mitosis and compensates for the asymmetry between the two centrosomes to enable similar Notch signaling and fate specification between two daughter cells

(Tozer et al. 2017). Additional compensatory mechanisms by storing and releasing other asymmetrically localized centrosomal proteins from organelles could exist and allow a reliable regulation of symmetric proliferative division and asymmetric neurogenic division (Wilsch-Brauninger and Huttner 2021).

31.3.4 Mitotic Spindle Orientation and Daughter Cell Fate Specification

The orientation of the mitotic spindle is crucial for daughter cell fate specification and tissue morphogenesis, as it influences the cleavage plane and consequently the inheritance of crucial cell fate determinants by the daughter cells. During neocortical development, RGPs switch from symmetric, proliferative division to asymmetric, neurogenic division. This switch has long been postulated to be coupled with a change in the orientation of the mitotic spindle (Haydar et al. 2003; Zhong and Chia 2008). The mitotic spindle is a microtubule-based bipolar apparatus typically with two centrosomes at its poles. It controls the axis of cell division and facilitates the segregation of chromosomes, as well as other cellular components, into the two daughter cells during mitosis.

The position and orientation of the mitotic spindle is typically regulated by astral microtubules and corresponding pulling forces between the spindle poles and cortical microtubule attachment sites. Distinct from transit amplifying progenitors that divide in the SVZ with a largely random mitotic spindle orientation (Fietz et al. 2010; Shitamukai et al. 2011), RGPs divide at the ventricular surface with a tightly regulated mitotic spindle orientation. Notably, the mitotic spindle orientation in dividing RGPs appears not set until the anaphase (Di Pietro et al. 2016; Shitamukai et al. 2011). Related to the intrinsic apicobasal polarity of RGPs and the apical domain partition and inheritance, it has long been postulated that RGPs undergo symmetric, proliferative division at the early developmental stage with a horizontal spindle orientation (i.e., a vertical cleavage plane) and asymmetric, neurogenic division at the late developmental stage with a vertical spindle orientation (i.e., a horizontal cleavage plane) (Haydar et al. 2003; Konno et al. 2008; Kosodo et al. 2004; Zhong and Chia 2008). However, it becomes clear that the mitotic spindle orientation of RGPs in the developing mouse neocortex does not switch from horizontal to vertical, but remains largely horizontal (Kawaguchi 2020), indicating that the precise link between the mitotic spindle orientation and RGP division mode being symmetric or asymmetric requires further in-depth investigation, especially in the native context.

Substantial insights have been gathered with regard to the interaction between the spindle poles and the cell cortex. During mitosis, an evolutionarily conserved molecular complex composed of Gαi (G protein subunit alpha i1), NuMA (nuclear mitotic apparatus protein), and LGN (Leu-Gly-Asn repeat enriched protein; also called Partner of Inscuteable in *Drosophila* and GRP1/2 in *C. elegans*) is localized to a particular subcortical domain and recruits microtubule minus-end-directed motor dynein, which moves along the astral microtubules and generates the force to pull the spindle poles and consequently control the position and orientation of the mitotic spindle (Hoffmann 2021; Kotak et al. 2012; Nguyen-Ngoc et al. 2007) (Figure 31.2, a). Misoriented division of neural progenitors has been linked to a number of brain developmental defects. PLK1 (Polo-like kinase 1) phosphorylates LRRK1 (Leucine rich repeat kinase 1) regulate astral microtubule nucleation and mitotic spindle orientation through CDK5RAP2-dependent centrosome maturation (Hanafusa et al. 2015; Hanafusa and Matsumoto 2015). CDK5RAP2 is one of the centrosomal proteins implicated in congenital microcephaly and mutations in human *CDK5RAP2* causes severely reduced brain size but with relatively preserved cortical patterning

(Bond et al. 2005). Neural progenitors in *CDK5RAP2* mutant mice or human patient-derived cerebral organoids exhibit impaired cell cycle progression coupled with abnormal mitotic orientation and spindle pole number, leading to proliferation and survival defects in progenitors and microcephaly (Lancaster et al. 2013; Lizarraga et al. 2010). DIAPH3 (diaphanous related formin 3), a member of the formin protein family that nucleates and elongates actin filaments, has been reported to localize at the centrosome and regulate spindle assembly and orientation. DIAPH3 deficiency causes misoriented mitotic spindle, reduced progenitor proliferation, and consequently microcephaly (Damiani et al. 2016; Lau et al. 2021). In addition, Zika virus infection also affects the centriole structure and causes spindle misorientation and premature differentiation in human iPSC-derived neural progenitors, leading to microcephaly in human newborns (Gabriel et al. 2017; Saade et al. 2020). Together, these findings emphasize the importance of the centrosome and centrosome-associated proteins in regulating the proliferation and differentiation of neural progenitors, at least partly by affecting the mitotic spindle positioning and orientation.

31.3.5 Primary Cilium Regulation and Function in RGPs

A key non-mitosis function of the centrosome in animal cells is to serve as the basal body for the formation of a primary cilium. The primary cilium is an immotile, microtubule-based antenna-like organelle extending from the cell surface and enriched with a variety of receptors and signaling molecules for receiving and transducing extrinsic signals intracellularly to the cell (Nachury and Mick 2019) (Figures 31.1 and 31.3). This "signaling hub" feature prompts the idea that primary cilia regulate RGP behavior in response to extracellular cues, in particular from the cerebrospinal fluid circulating in the lateral ventricle, with which primary cilia make direct contact. Numerous studies have been carried out to dissect the function of primary cilia in RGPs and neocortical development (Wilsch-Brauninger and Huttner 2021; Yang et al. 2021).

The primary cilia in RGPs appear to undergo incomplete disassembly prior to mitosis and the mother centriole/centrosome associated with the ciliary remnant is inherited by one daughter cell (Figure 31.3). This daughter cell could reform primary cilium earlier and preferentially retains progenitor cell character (Paridaen et al. 2013). The roles of primary cilia in RGPs have been further investigated by genetic studies. Mutations in *ARL13B* (ADP-ribosylation factor-like protein 13B) gene encoding a membrane-associated small GTPase specifically localized to primary cilia and required for axoneme assembly and maintenance lead to the classical form of Joubert syndrome, one of the ciliopathies in humans characterized by abnormal brain development (Cantagrel et al. 2008). *Foxg1-Cre* driven conditional deletion of *Arl13b* in the mouse neuroepithelium starting at ~E9.5 causes abnormal apicobasal polarity of RGPs and subsequently disrupted neuronal positioning and layer formation in the neocortex. However, neither *Nestin-Cre* nor human *GFAP-Cre* driven conditional deletion of *Arl13b* starting at ~E10.5 or ~E13.5 respectively leads to any obvious disorganization of RGPs or defects in neocortical development. These results indicate that ARL13B-mediated ciliary axoneme assembly and function play a critical role in the initial establishment of the apicobasal polarity of RGPs at the very early stage, but is dispensable for the maintenance of the polarized organization, or the majority period of neocortical development (Higginbotham et al. 2013).

Increasing evidence suggests that the developing brain interprets the loss of primary cilia in a spatiotemporally specific manner. Conditional ablation of *Ift88* (intraflagellar transport 88), *Kif3a* (kinesin family member 3a), or *Ttc21b* (tetratricopeptide repeat domain 21b) that encodes key components of the IFT complex required for primary cilium axoneme assembly and maintenance in the dorsal telencephalon by *Emx1-Cre* starting at ~E10.5 has no obvious effect on RGP behavior and cortical size (Snedeker et al. 2017). In contrast, *Foxg1-Cre* driven deletion of *Ift88* or *Kif3a* starting at ~E9.5 of the forebrain development leads to an increased cortical size. In addition, deletion of *Ift88* or *Kif3a* from the neural crest and midbrain using *Wnt1-Cre* also causes dramatic cortical malformation (Snedeker et al. 2017). These studies suggest that primary cilia play important roles in the patterning of neocortical primordium at the early stage, but are not essential for neocortical neurogenesis and lamination.

31.3.6 Other Emerging Roles of the Centrosome in RGPs

While a majority of studies focus on the canonical function of the centrosome and its associated proteins in mitosis, additional roles of the centrosome in RGPs have also been reported that collectively contribute to proper neurogenesis and neocortical size. One interesting direction is the regulation of cytoskeleton organization and apical domain properties in interphase RGPs. The apical domain of RGPs is a cytoskeleton-associated epithelial organization supported by the apical endfeet of adjacent RGPs via junctions (Kim et al. 2010; Veeraval et al. 2020) (Figure 31.3).

The subcellular localization of the centrosome in RGPs during interphase is unique. Distinct from other animal cells in which the centrosome is in close proximity to the nucleus, the centrosome in interphase RGPs is positioned away from the nucleus and anchored at the apical surface via the DAPs of the mother centriole to serve as both the MTOC and the basal body for primary cilium formation (Chenn et al. 1998; Shao et al. 2020; Wang et al. 2009). The membrane anchored centrosome supports the formation of a ring-like microtubule structure, which is juxtaposed to the apical junctional belt and generates intracellular contractile force in conjunction with the actin ring (Figure 31.3). Removal of CEP83, a root protein for DAP assembly, leads to a loss of DAPs and the detachment of the centrosome from the apical membrane. This subtle dislocation of the centrosome disrupts the microtubule ring and substantially increases the overall stiffness of the apical membrane of RGPs, resulting in the activation of YAP, excessive RGP proliferation and neurogenesis, and an enlarged neocortex with abnormal folding (Shao et al. 2020).

In addition, the period of time during which RGPs remain at the ventricular surface linked to centrosome positioning and regulation is also crucial for their mitotic control and neurogenesis. AKNA (AT-hook transcription factor), an interphase centrosome protein, localizes at the sDAPs in almost all basal progenitors at the SVZ, and is necessary and sufficient to nucleate centrosomal microtubules. It promotes the delamination of RGPs from the ventricular surface by recruiting CAMSAP3 (calmodulin-regulated spectrin associated protein 3) to the centrosome and weakening the junctional complex as well as promoting the apical endfoot constriction. Moreover, downregulation of AKNA expression drives basal progenitors to leave the SVZ and migrate basally, pointing to a bidirectional mechanism of centrosome-mediated microtubule organization for orchestrating progenitors to enter and exit the SVZ (Camargo Ortega et al. 2019). Similarly, TALPID3, another centrosome-associated protein localized at the distal end of the mother centriole, interacts with Ninein to modulate microtubule stability, and maintain the integrity of junctions to anchor RGPs (Kobayashi et al. 2014; Wang et al. 2020; Yin et al. 2009). In addition, OCCLUDIN, a junction component, localizes to the centrosome and regulates the spindle pole morphology as well as the astral and mitotic microtubule integrity. Its mutation causes prolonged M-phase and reduced RGP proliferation, and human microcephaly and neocortical malformation (Abdel-Hamid et al. 2017; Bendriem et al. 2019; Elsaid et al. 2014).

31.4 Centrosome Regulation and Function in Neuronal Migration

Neuronal migration is a fundamental process for the correct assembly and organization of the neocortex. New-born neurons migrate either radially (e.g., excitatory neurons) or tangentially (e.g., interneurons) from their birth place to the final positions in the neocortex (Kriegstein and Noctor 2004). Extensive studies on the cell biology of neuronal migration reveal that it requires drastic remodeling of the cytoskeleton and entails a complex sequence of morphogenetic and motile events typically accompanied with dynamic behavior and regulation of the centrosome (Higginbotham and Gleeson 2007; Kasioulis et al. 2017; Kuijpers and Hoogenraad 2011; Meka et al. 2020).

31.4.1 The Centrosome and Two-stroke Neuronal Locomotion

Radial glial fiber-guided radial migration of new-born excitatory neurons occurs in a "two-stroke" fashion. As bipolar neurons extend the leading process towards the pia along the mother RGP basal fiber, the centrosome first advances into the leading process, followed by the movement of the nucleus in the direction of the centrosome (Higginbotham and Gleeson 2007; Tsai and Gleeson 2005). In migrating neurons, microtubules emanated from the centrosome elongate anteriorly into the leading process and posteriorly to envelop the nucleus by forming a cage-like structure (Figure 31.2, c). The force pulling the nucleus forward is generated by the microtubules in the leading process and the centrosome is thought to be the link through which the force is transmitted (Higginbotham and Gleeson 2007; Tsai and Gleeson 2005). Over-expression of PAR6α (Par-6 family cell polarity regulator alpha), which retargets PKCζ (protein kinase C zeta) and γ-tubulin away from the centrosome and disrupts the perinuclear microtubule cage, leads to an inhibition of centrosomal motion and neuronal migration (Solecki et al. 2006, 2004). The microtubule-stabilizing protein DCX (doublecortin) also plays essential roles in maintaining the perinuclear microtubule cage and the centrosome-nucleus coupling. The microtubule-based motor protein dynein and several of its regulators, such as LIS1 (lissencephaly 1), NudE (neurodevelopment protein 1), and NudEL (neurodevelopment protein 1 like 1) have been implicated in controlling nuclear movement in migrating neurons (Figure 31.2, c). Dynein is concentrated both at the swelling region in the leading process and at the soma, pulling the captured microtubules and the attached centrosome as well as the coupled nucleus towards the swelling. Mutations in *DCX* or *LIS1* lead to lissencephaly in humans due to neuronal migration defects (Bai et al. 2003; Francis et al. 1999; Pilz et al. 1998; Tanaka et al. 2004; Tsai et al. 2005; Vallee et al. 2009; Wynshaw-Boris and Gambello 2001).

Actin cytoskeleton has also been observed both in the leading and trailing processes of migrating neurons (Tsai and Gleeson 2005). The actin-dependent myosin II motor at the rear of the soma can also generate the forward force to push the nucleus into the leading process (Schaar and McConnell 2005; Zhu et al. 2010) (Figure 31.2, c). Moreover, F-actin and myosin II motor are also found in front of the nucleus as well as in the leading process. Inhibition of myosin II causes a decrease in centrosomal and nuclear movement, indicative of a blockade of nuclear translocation without affecting centrosome positioning. On the other hand, activation of myosin II increases the coordinated centrosomal and nuclear movement, suggesting that myosin II motor in the leading process functions to pull the centrosome and nucleus forward (Solecki et al. 2009; Tsai et al. 2007). These observations suggest an important contribution of the actin cytoskeleton in centrosomal and nuclear movement during radial migration.

31.4.2 Centrosome Positioning in Migrating Neurons

The mechanism underlying centrosome positioning within the leading process of migrating neurons is hinted by a signal transduction pathway controlling the establishment of mammalian cell polarity. Scratching a confluent monolayer of primary rat astrocytes leads to a pronounced cell response in extending pseudopodium-like structures into the wound and reorienting the centrosome and the Golgi complex at the leading edge (Etienne-Manneville and Hall 2001). The centrosome reorientation depends on the local activation of integrin at the front of the cell and the activity of the small Rho-GTPase Cdc42 (cell division cycle 42), an essential regulator of cell polarity in various cell types (Allen et al. 1998; Etienne-Manneville and Hall 2001; Kroschewski et al. 1999; Nobes and Hall 1999; Raftopoulou and Hall 2004; Stowers et al. 1995). Cdc42 activity at the front edge recruits and activates the protein complex formed by PAR6 and PKCζ, both of which are required for establishing the anteroposterior cell polarity in the zygote and the apicobasal polarity of neuroepithelia and neuroblasts in *Drosophila* (Etienne-Manneville and Hall 2001; Hung and Kemphues 1999; Petronczki and Knoblich 2001). Subsequently, PKCζ phosphorylates and inactivates GSK-3β (glycogen synthase kinase 3β). Upon GSK inactivation, APC (adenomatous polyposis coli) binds and stabilizes microtubule plus-end and facilitates its association with dynein, which in turn pulls the captured microtubules and the attached centrosome towards the protrusion at the front edge via its minus-end-directed motor activity (Etienne-Manneville and Hall 2001; Higginbotham and Gleeson 2007; Palazzo et al. 2001; Zumbrunn et al. 2001).

A similar mechanism may work for centrosome positioning in migrating neurons. In addition to their localization at the centrosome to maintain the centrosome-nucleus coupling, PAR6α, PKCζ, GSK-3β, LIS1, and dynein is also found at the distal end of the leading process to regulate its outgrowth (Higginbotham and Gleeson 2007). Cdc42 also plays an important role in mediating neuronal response to SLIT, a chemorepellent signaling molecule that reverses the migration direction of neurons (Wong et al. 2001).

31.4.3 The Centrosome and Tangential Neuronal Migration

Dynamic regulation and function of the centrosome is not unique to radially migrating neurons. Proper subcellular localization of the centrosome also plays an important role during tangential migration. Tangentially migrating neocortical interneurons exhibit saltatory nucleokinesis towards a branched leading process that continuously undergoes morphological transition. The nuclear movement encompasses two successive steps. First, the cytoplasmic organelles, including the centrosome and the Golgi apparatus, undergo long-distance translocation to form a swelling in the leading process. Second, the nucleus moves forward into the leading process depending on myosin II, which transiently accumulates at the rear of the soma and periodically generates the force to push the nucleus towards the distant centrosome and Golgi apparatus (Bellion et al. 2005).

31.5 Centrosome Regulation and Function in Neuronal Polarization

Neuronal polarization, also known as axon specification, is an early neuronal developmental process that establishes distinct morphological and functional compartments of axon and dendrite for sending and receiving information, respectively. The centrosome-mediated cytoskeleton remodeling is a key regulator of neuronal polarization.

31.5.1 Centrosome Positioning and Axon Specification in Cultured Neurons

A comprehensive understanding of neuronal polarization is first achieved in the primary cultures of dissociated hippocampal pyramidal neurons and cerebellar granular neurons (Dotti et al. 1988; Powell et al. 1997). Newly dissected hippocampal pyramidal neurons appear round without any neurite shortly after dissociation and plating, followed by the outgrowth of numerous short processes and then the specification and maturation of a single axon and multiple dendrites, making it an ideal model for studying the process of neuronal polarization (Dotti et al. 1988) (Figure 31.4). Similarly, cerebellar granular neurons cultured in vitro at low density also develop in similar temporal steps to acquire their characteristic axonal and dendritic morphologies (Powell et al. 1997).

The centrosome is generally localized at the site of axon outgrowth and is identified as a robust predictor of axonal specification in cultured hippocampal neurons and cerebellar granular neurons (de Anda et al. 2005; Zmuda and Rivas 1998). It has been hypothesized that the centrosome-mediated selective stabilization of microtubules in one specific neurite guides axon specification (Witte et al. 2008) (Figure 31.4). Accordingly, neurons containing more than

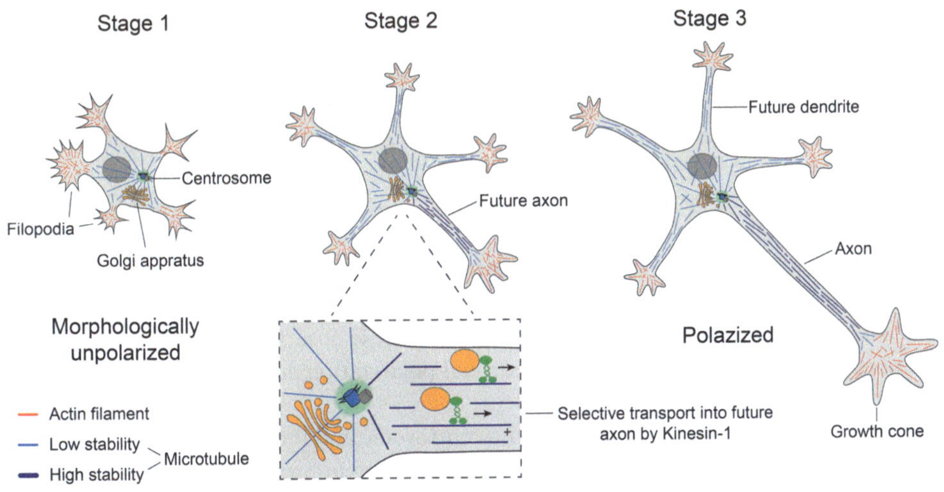

Figure 31.4 Neuronal polarization and axon specification in primary dissociated hippocampal neurons in culture. Schematic illustration of the early developmental stages (stages 1–3) of cultured hippocampal neuron in vitro. Shortly after dissociation and plating, neurons exhibit unpolarized morphology with some short actin-based protrusions called filopodia. The centrosome near the nucleus organizes microtubules in the cytoplasm and some microtubules invade into the filopodia to elongate them as neurites. Later, the centrosome and Golgi apparatus are close to the base of one neurite, supporting the formation of more stable microtubules and selective cargo transport by motor proteins to this neurite for rapid growth and development into an axon.

one centrosome generated by cytokinesis blockage develop more than one axon, suggesting that the centrosome activity is sufficient to drive axon specification (de Anda et al. 2005). Global application of Taxol, a microtubule-stabilizing drug, induces the formation of multiple axons in cultured neurons (Witte et al. 2008). In all likelihood, the centrosome position coincides with the localization of the Golgi apparatus at the base of the future axon during neuronal polarization, raising a possibility that the localization and coupling between the centrosome and the Golgi apparatus may be important for directional transport of particular proteins, such as surface receptors and signaling molecules, required for axon specification (de Anda et al. 2005; Sutterlin and Colanzi 2010) (Figure 31.4). Consistent with this, pharmacological treatments to either prevent microtubule polymerization or block protein recycling to the Golgi apparatus and the endosomes impair neuronal polarization (de Anda et al. 2005). In addition, non-centrosomal microtubule nucleation occurs at the surface of the Golgi membrane (Chabin-Brion et al. 2001; Efimov et al. 2007). These Golgi-nucleated microtubules may support the transport of Golgi-derived vesicles into the future axon. Besides vesicle transport, specific localization of motors may also play a critical role in axon specification. For example, truncated kinesin-1, a microtubule plus-end-directed motor protein, accumulates only in the emerging axon to ensure selective delivery of kinesin-1 cargoes into the axon and hence contribute to its molecular specification (Jacobson et al. 2006) (Figure 31.4). In addition, dynamic regulation of different tubulin post-translational modifications is required for sorting kinesin-1 into the future axon (Hammond et al. 2010; Konishi and Setou 2009; Reed et al. 2006). CEP120, a centrosome protein, promotes axon formation via modulating the level of microtubule acetylation and stability, revealing the centrosome-dependent selective stabilization of microtubules in future axon (Meka et al. 2022).

31.5.2 The Centrosome and Neuronal Polarization In Vivo

In the developing neocortex, neuronal migration and polarization are intertwined, indicating that axon specification and growth occur while neurons migrate (Meka et al. 2020; Noctor et al. 2004) (Figure 31.2). Consistent with the observation in vitro, the centrosome is often found at the base of the nascent axon (Tang and Marshall 2012). In situ electron microscopy analysis reveals that the centrosome in the new-born multipolar neurons of the mouse neocortex is generally located at the base of the nascent axon, which extends tangentially or towards the ventricular zone. However, as the neurons transit to a bipolar morphology and extend a pia-directed leading process to start radial migration, the centrosome is reoriented towards the pia within the leading process (Shoukimas and Hinds 1978). These observations suggest a dynamic regulation of centrosome positioning during neuronal polarization and migration in the developing neocortex.

Further live imaging experiments reveal that the centrosome and the Golgi apparatus undergo translocation in multipolar neurons in the SVZ, and that being in proximity to these organelles drives the selective and rapid outgrowth of one neurite to become the axon (de Anda et al. 2010; Sakakibara et al. 2014). The neurite that eventually develops into the axon also exhibits preferential microtubule stabilization (Witte et al. 2008). Consistently, the centrosome and the Golgi apparatus could serve as the primary source for microtubule nucleation destined for the rapidly growing neurite (Stiess and Bradke 2011), and their localization may support the preferential delivery of specific molecules and sustain the specification and outgrowth of the nascent axon

(Arimura and Kaibuchi 2007; Wiggin et al. 2005) (Figure 31.2, b). The centrosome is then translocated into the pia-directed leading process, coordinating nuclear movement during neuronal migration and the growth of apical dendrites upon the completion of migration (Meka et al. 2020; Shoukimas and Hinds 1978). These data suggest that proper localization of the centrosome and the Golgi apparatus is required for the initial step of neuronal polarization, but not for axon elongation and maturation, which appear to occur independently of centrosomal microtubule nucleation (de Anda et al. 2010; Stiess et al. 2010). In line with this, disruption of centrosomal motility via downregulation of centrosomal protein CEP120 or silencing of centriolar satellite protein PCM1 affects axon formation (de Anda et al. 2010). Downregulation of the molecules that regulate centrosome positioning and microtubule stability during neuronal migration, such as LIS1, DCX, and CDK5, also influences centrosome repositioning at the multipolar stage, affects the multipolar-to-bipolar morphological transition, and leads to impaired axon formation (Bai et al. 2003; Ohshima et al. 2007; Tsai et al. 2005).

31.5.3 Interplay of Microtubule and Actin Regulation during Neuronal Polarization

During neuronal polarization, several positive and negative feedback signals have been found to play crucial roles in driving the selection of one and only one neurite to become the axon. These signaling pathways involve dynamic modulations of cAMP, cGMP, and calcium levels in response to extracellular cues, and converge downstream at the regulation of Rho GTPase activity and cytoskeleton dynamics, including both microtubules and actin filaments (Bradke and Dotti 2000; Shelly et al. 2010; Takano et al. 2019, 2017). Recent studies suggest that radial translocation of F-actin from cell body to neurites acts as a potential inhibitory loop to promote neuronal polarization (Meka et al. 2020). In addition to its activity to nucleate and anchor microtubules, the centrosome has also been identified as a F-actin organizing center (Farina et al. 2016). Dynamic aster-like structures around the centrosome and closely associated PCM1 satellites have been observed in the soma of neurons (Meka et al. 2019). Somatic F-actin exhibits an anterograde movement to the neurites in a comet-like fashion and the intensity of F-actin signal is inversely proportional to the length of the neurites, suggesting that F-actin acts as a growth-inhibiting factor (Meka et al. 2019). Consistently, application of actin-depolymerizing drug or Rho-signaling inhibitor induces the formation of multiple axons (Bradke and Dotti 1999). These findings suggest that the centrosome preferentially moves F-actin to peripheral neurites, where the outgrowth is inhibited. On the other hand, the neurite close to the centrosome receives less F-actin but more microtubules, resulting in fast neurite outgrowth for axon specification and neuronal polarization (Meka et al. 2020, 2019).

31.6 The Centrosome and Neocortical Developmental Diseases

As discussed previously, highly orchestrated centrosomal behavior is tightly coupled with the intricate process of neocortical histogenesis, from progenitor proliferation to neurogenesis to neuronal migration and differentiation. Any mis-regulation of centrosomal behavior and function can lead to malformation and malfunction of the neocortex. Mutations of centrosome-related genes have frequently been found to be associated with various human brain developmental diseases, such as microcephaly, lissencephaly, and epilepsy.

31.6.1 Centrosomal Defects and Microcephaly

The link of the centrosome to neocortical development is best exemplified by the studies on autosomal recessive primary microcephaly (MCPH), a genetically heterogenous neurodevelopmental disorder characterized by a significantly reduced head circumference present at birth and intellectual disability. MCPH is often associated with a simplified neocortical gyration pattern due to hypoproliferation of neural progenitors and reduced neurogenesis (Higginbotham and Gleeson 2007; Saade et al. 2018). Following the discovery of the first gene linked to MCPH, a growing number of genes have been implicated in the onset of MCPH, especially with the application of whole-exome sequencing in clinical samples (Boycott et al. 2013). To date, 28 MCPH-related genes have been identified and named sequentially as MCPH1–MCPH28 (Zaqout and Kaindl 2021). Remarkably, many MCPH-related genes encode centrosomal or centrosome-associated proteins involved in centriole biogenesis, microtubule dynamics, mitotic spindle assembly, cell cycle checkpoint control, neuronal migration, and primary cilium formation (Barbelanne and Tsang 2014; Zaqout and Kaindl 2021). Additionally, some mutations of centrosome-related genes are also implicated in other developmental disorders, such as the Seckel syndrome (SCKL), microcephaly and chorioretinopathy (MCCRP), or microcephalic osteodysplastic primordial dwarfism type II (MOPDII) (Table 31.1).

ASPM (Abnormal spindle-like microcephaly associated gene; also known as *MCPH5*), is the most commonly mutated gene among MCPH patients, accounting for nearly 50 percent of cases irrespective of ethnic background (O'Neill et al. 2018; Thornton and Woods 2009). *ASPM* mRNA is particularly expressed in neural progenitors undergoing proliferative division and the level is relatively high during the early developmental stage but decreases progressively as time proceeds. ASPM protein is localized at the proximal end of the mother centriole at the mitotic spindle poles, indicating a function in regulating spindle organization and orientation (Fish et al. 2006; Jayaraman et al. 2016). The nematode orthologue ASPM-1, together with the CMD-1 (calmodulin), promotes meiotic spindle organization and regulates spindle rotation (van der Voet et al. 2009). ASPM knockdown in mouse telencephalic neuroepithelial cells alters cleavage plane orientation, leading to an increase in neuron-like progeny (Fish et al. 2006). The premature depletion of neural progenitors would explain the reduced number of neurons in human patients with MCPH. Similarly, a mouse model lacking *ASPM* exhibits premature exhaustion of neural progenitors due to defective self-renewal (Capecchi and Pozner 2015; Fujimori et al. 2014). Deletion of *ASPM* in ferrets with a gyrencephalic neocortex and greater neural progenitor cell diversity causes a drastic, premature displacement of RGPs to the oSVZ and severe microcephaly with no significant change in neocortical thickness, reflecting an evolutionary conserved role of ASPM in governing brain size (Johnson et al. 2018) (Table 31.1).

WDR62 (also known as *MCPH2*) is the second most mutated gene in human MCPH patients, which accounts for ~10 percent of cases (O'Neill et al. 2018; Thornton and Woods 2009). Recessive mutations in *WDR62* cause microcephaly and a wide spectrum of severe brain malformations (Sgourdou et al. 2017). WDR62 is concentrated at the spindle pole in a cell cycle-dependent manner from mitotic entry until metaphase-anaphase transition (Bogoyevitch et al. 2012). WDR62, together with CENPJ (also known as MCPH6), CEP63, ASPM, and Aurora A kinase, plays an essential role in maintaining the integrity of the centrosome and the mitotic spindle (Chen et al. 2014; Chou et al. 2016; Jayaraman et al. 2016). Disrupted expression of WDR62 results in defects in PCM recruitment and microtubule nucleation, mitotic spindle organization and orientation, and asymmetric centrosome inheritance abnormality. These

Table 31.1 Centrosome-related genes in neocortical developmental diseases.

Disease	Gene	Protein	Centrosome-related functions	Phenotypes in animal model and clinical cases
MCPH2	*WDR62* (WD repeat-containing protein 62)	WDR62	PCM recruitment; Centriole duplication; Spindle integrity and orientation; Primary cilia disassembly.	Spindle orientation defects (Bogoyevitch et al. 2012); Mitotic arrest (Bogoyevitch et al. 2012; Chen et al. 2014); Increased apoptosis and premature differentiation of NPCs (Bogoyevitch et al. 2012; Chen et al. 2014; Zhang et al. 2019); Increased cilium length (Zhang et al. 2019); Reduced neurogenesis and microcephaly (Chen et al. 2014; Zhang et al. 2019).
MCPH3	*CDK5RAP2* (Cyclin-dependent kinase 5 regulatory subunit associated protein 2)	CDK5RAP2	PCM recruitment; Centriole duplication; Spindle assembly and orientation.	Abnormal spindle formation and orientation (Lancaster et al. 2013; Lizarraga et al. 2010); Increased cell cycle exit (Buchman et al. 2010; Lizarraga et al. 2010); Premature differentiation of NPCs (Buchman et al. 2010; Lancaster et al. 2013); Microcephaly (Bond et al. 2005).
MCPH5	*ASPM* (Abnormal spindle-like microcephaly associated gene)	ASPM	PCM recruitment; Centrosome integrity; Spindle assembly and orientation; Restriction point progression.	Impaired cell cycle (Capecchi and Pozner 2015; Ripoll et al. 1985); Altered spindle orientation (Fish et al. 2006); Displaced and reduced NPCs (Capecchi and Pozner 2015; Johnson et al. 2018; Li et al. 2017b); Microcephaly (Capecchi and Pozner 2015; Fujimori et al. 2014; Johnson et al. 2018).
MCPH6 (SCKL4)	*CENPJ* (Centrosome protein J)	CENPJ (also known as SAS-4 or CPAP)	Centriole duplication; Centrosome integrity; Primary cilia disassembly.	Centriole loss (Basto et al. 2006; Insolera et al. 2014a); Increased apoptosis (Ding et al. 2019; Insolera et al. 2014a; McIntyre et al. 2012); Displaced and reduced NPCs (Ding et al. 2019; Insolera et al. 2014a); Increased cilium length (Ding et al. 2019); Microcephaly (Bond et al. 2005; Insolera et al. 2014a; McIntyre et al. 2012).
MCPH7	*STIL* (SCL/TAL1 interrupting locus)	STIL	Centriole duplication.	Lack of centriole and primary cilium (David et al. 2014; Pfaff et al. 2007); Disorganized mitotic spindle; Apoptosis (Novorol et al. 2013; Pfaff et al. 2007); Impaired response to SHH signaling (Izraeli et al. 1999).
MCPH8	*CEP135* (Centrosomal protein 135)	CEP135	PCM recruitment; Centriole duplication.	Abnormal basal body assembly (Hiraki et al. 2007; Jerka-Dziadosz et al. 2010); Disorganized mitotic spindles and cytoplasmic microtubules (Matsuura et al. 2004); Microcephaly (Hussain et al. 2012).
MCPH9 (SCKL5)	*CEP152* (Centrosomal protein 152)	CEP152	Centriole duplication.	Impaired PCM stabilization and reduced microtubule nucleation (Varmark et al. 2007); Lack of centrioles and ciliary defects (Blachon et al. 2008).

(Continued)

Table 31.1 (Continued)

Disease	Gene	Protein	Centrosome-related functions	Phenotypes in animal model and clinical cases
MCPH12	*CDK6* (Cyclin-dependent kinase 6)	CDK6	MTOC activity.	Microcephaly (Hussain et al. 2013).
MCPH14	*SAS-6* (Spindle assembly abnormal protein 6)	SAS-6	Centriole duplication.	Defects in centrosome duplication (Leidel et al. 2005); Impaired mitotic spindle formation (Yabe et al. 2007).
MCPH28	*RRP7A* (Ribosomal RNA processing 7 homolog A)	RRP7A	Ciliary resorption.	Ciliary resorption and cell cycle defects; Reduced brain size (Farooq et al. 2020).
SCKL6	*CEP63* (Centrosomal protein 63)	CEP63	Centriole duplication; Centrosome integrity.	P53-dependent cell death; Microcephaly (Marjanovic et al. 2015).
SCKL7	*Ninein*	Ninein	MTOC activity.	Altered microtubule organization (Goldspink et al. 2017); Microcephaly; Short stature (Dauber et al. 2012).
MCCRP1	*TUBGCP6* (Tubulin gamma complex associated protein 6)	TUBGCP6	Centriole duplication; MTOC activity.	Reduced centriole numbers (Bahtz et al. 2012); Microcephaly (Martin et al. 2014; Shurygina et al. 2020).
MCCRP2	*PLK4* (Polo-like kinase 4)	PLK4	Centriole duplication.	Microcephaly (Martin et al. 2014; Tsutsumi et al. 2016).
MCCRP3	*TUBGCP4* (Tubulin gamma complex associated protein 4)	TUBGCP4	MTOC activity.	Altered microtubule organization; Microcephaly (Da Palma et al. 2020; Scheidecker et al. 2015; Shurygina et al. 2020).
MOPD||	*PCNT* (Pericentrin)	PCNT	Centriole disengagement; PCM recruitment; MTOC activity. Cilia assembly.	Suppressed centriole disengagement (Kim et al. 2015; Lee and Rhee 2012); Altered microtubule organization (Doxsey et al. 1994; Ma and Viveiros 2014); Impaired cilia assembly (Jurczyk et al. 2004; Miyoshi et al. 2009); Abnormal interneuron migration (Endoh-Yamagami et al. 2010); Microcephaly; Short stature (Rauch et al. 2008; Waich et al. 2020).
Lissencephaly	*DCX* (Doublecortin)	DCX	Microtubule stabilization; Centrosome positioning; Centrosome-nucleus coupling.	Impaired neuronal migration; Lissencephaly (Bai et al. 2003; Francis et al. 1999; Pilz et al. 1998; Tanaka et al. 2004).
Lissencephaly	*LIS1* (Lissencephaly 1)	LIS1	Dynein regulator; Centrosome positioning; Centrosome-nucleus coupling.	Impaired neuronal migration; Lissencephaly (Pilz et al. 1998; Tanaka et al. 2004; Tsai et al. 2005; Wynshaw-Boris and Gambello 2001).

defects collectively cause failures in spindle assembly checkpoint satisfaction, mitotic arrest or delay, and apoptosis, leading to premature differentiation or loss of neural progenitors, reduced neurogenesis, and microcephaly (Bogoyevitch et al. 2012; Chen et al. 2014; Ramdas Nair et al. 2016; Sgourdou et al. 2017) (Table 31.1).

Other MCPH-associated genes encode proteins involved in centriole and mitotic spindle biogenesis, such as *CENPJ* (*MCPH6*), *STIL* (*MCPH7*), and *CDK5RAP2* (*MCPH3*). They play important roles in maintaining centrosome integrity and regulating mitotic spindle assembly and orientation during neural progenitor mitosis (Thornton and Woods 2009; Zaqout and Kaindl 2021) (Table 31.1). Various studies in animal models and human patient-derived neural progenitors have linked *CDK5RAP2* mutations with a number of mitotic defects that cause a premature differentiation of neural progenitors and reduced brain size (Buchman et al. 2010; Lancaster et al. 2013; Lizarraga et al. 2010; Yigit et al. 2015). CENPJ is required for centriole duplication and elongation. Removal of CENPJ leads to a loss of centrioles/centrosomes, mitotic delay, and p53-dependent apoptosis of neural progenitors, and consequently reduced neurogenesis and microcephaly (Insolera et al. 2014a). In addition, the conserved TCP domain of CENPJ mediates the interaction with ANA2 (Anastral spindle 2), a centrosome duplication factor, and Bld-10 (CEP135), a centriole microtubule-binding protein, essential for PCM tethering during centriole/centrosome biogenesis (Zheng et al. 2014). STIL is also a centriole duplication factor that interacts with CENPJ via the TCP domain (Tang et al. 2011).

ASPM has also been shown to regulate G_1 phase duration by modulating cyclin E ubiquitination, phosphorylation, and localization in the nucleus to control restriction point progression and stem cell maintenance (Capecchi and Pozner 2015). WDR62 also functions in post-mitotic glial cells. Glial lineage-specific WDR62 removal not only decreases the glial population, but also causes a neuroblast loss in a non-cell autonomous manner (Lim et al. 2017). Thus, the functions of MCPH-related genes in different neural lineages should be examined carefully to understand fully the underlying pathogenesis mechanisms.

31.6.2 Centrosomal Defects and Neuronal Migration Disorders

While most MCPH cases are associated with defective mitosis of neural progenitors, ectopic neurons in the periventricular region are also observed in some patients with MCPH, suggesting a neuronal migration defect (Kaindl et al. 2010). Downregulation of CENPJ in post-mitotic neurons causes a decrease in microtubule dynamics and a reduction in migration rate, accompanied by abnormal centrosome position and aberrant neuronal morphology (Garcez et al. 2015). In addition, the neuronal migration defect has also been observed in clinical cases with truncating mutations in *ASPM* (Turkyilmaz and Sager 2022).

The stable coupling between the centrosome and the nucleus in migrating neurons is pivotal for successive nucleokinesis during radial migration and requires multiple proteins such as LIS1 and DCX. In fact, *LIS1* and *DCX* mutations are strongly linked to human lissencephaly, a brain malformation characterized by the absence of normal folds in the neocortex (Pilz et al. 1998) (Table 31.1). Mechanistically, LIS1 and DCX function together with dynein to mediate centrosome–nucleus coupling during migration (Bai et al. 2003; Tsai et al. 2005). Mutations of *SDCCAG8*, another centrosomal protein highly expressed in new-born neurons, are also associated with defects in the centrosome–nucleus coupling. Knockdown of SDCCAG8 impairs centrosomal recruitment of γ-tubulin and pericentrin, interferes with microtubule organization, decouples the centrosome and the nucleus, and thereby disrupts neuronal migration (Insolera et al. 2014b).

31.6.3 Centrosomal Defects and Ciliopathies

Dysregulation of primary cilium dynamics is also found in MCPH patients. *RRP7A* (Ribosomal RNA processing 7 homolog A; also known as MCPH28) is highly expressed in neural progenitors in the developing human forebrain and localized in the centrosome and primary cilium. *RRP7A* deletion leads to impaired neurogenesis and reduced brain size in zebrafish embryos (Farooq et al. 2020). Moreover, recent studies reveal a role of cilium disassembly through the WDR62-CEP170-KIF2A pathway. WDR62 ablation in cerebral organoids causes retarded cilium disassembly and delayed cell cycle progression, resulting in premature differentiation of neural progenitors and reduced organoid size (Zhang et al. 2019). In addition, CPAP is required for primary cilium assembly in neural cells. Over-expression of wild-type CPAP promotes cilium formation and induces longer cilia, while over-expression of mutant CPAP significantly inhibits cilium biogenesis and causes cilium shortening (Wu and Tang 2012). CPAP also serves as a scaffold for the cilium disassembly complex to promote timely cilium disassembly and ensure proper cell cycle entry (Gabriel et al. 2016).

31.6.4 Centrosomal Defects and Megalencephaly

Notably, mutations in some centrosomal genes can also lead to an abnormally large brain or megalencephaly. Disruption of the DAP assembly and centrosome anchorage in RGPs via *Cep83* deletion results in the overproduction of neocortical neurons and an enlarged cortical size with abnormal folding in mice, and biallelic mutations in human *CEP83* cause infantile nephronophthisis and intellectual disability (Failler et al. 2014; Shao et al. 2020). RHAMM, a spindle-associated protein, has been shown to support the action of PLK1 at the centrosome and stabilize the astral microtubules but with no impact on the centrosome biogenesis or the spindle assembly. Neural progenitors carrying RHAMM truncation display unaffected division rate but randomized mitotic spindle orientation and division plane, resulting in megalencephaly associated with cerebral cortex thickening, as well as cerebellum enlargement and premature differentiation (Connell et al. 2017; Li et al. 2017a).

31.7 Concluding Remarks

The centrosome is a complex subcellular organelle in animal cells, comprising a large collection of proteins assembled into specialized structures with diverse functions. In general, the proximal end of the centriole/centrosome is responsible for PCM recruitment and microtubule nucleation, whereas the distal end is critical for appendage formation, membrane anchoring, and primary ciliogenesis. The behavior and regulation of the centrosome are highly orchestrated and tightly coupled with progenitor cell cycle progression and neural progeny morphogenesis and migration during neocortical development. The importance of centrosome regulation and function is further evidenced by diverse clinical symptoms and human brain malformations strongly associated with mutations in genes encoding centrosome or centrosome-related proteins. Future efforts in understanding the dynamic behavior and regulation of the centrosome as well as the associated primary cilium will not only advance our understanding the structural and functional development of the neocortex across species, but also provide new insights into the pathophysiology of many neurodevelopmental and neurobehavioral disorders.

Acknowledgments

We apologize to our colleagues whose valuable work we could not cite owing to the space limitation. We thank the Shi laboratory members, especially Jiajun Yang, for their insightful discussion and input. Our research is supported by the Ministry of Science and Technology of China (2021ZD0202300), the National Natural Science Foundation of China (32021002), Beijing Outstanding Young Scientist Program (BJJWZYJH01201910003012), Beijing Municipal Science & Technology Commission (Z20111000530000 and Z211100003321001), and the Chinese Institute for Brain Research (Beijing).

References

Abdel-Hamid, M.S. et al. (2017). Band-like calcification with simplified gyration and polymicrogyria. *J Hum Genet* 62: 553–559.

Allen, W.E. et al. (1998). A role for Cdc42 in macrophage chemotaxis. *J Cell Biol* 141: 1147–1157.

Anderson, C.T. and Stearns, T. (2009). Centriole age underlies asynchronous primary cilium growth in mammalian cells. *Curr Biol* 19: 1498–1502.

Arimura, N. and Kaibuchi, K. (2007). Neuronal polarity. *Nat Rev Neurosci* 8: 194–205.

Ayala, R. et al. (2007). Trekking across the brain. *Cell* 128: 29–43.

Bahtz, R. et al. (2012). GCP6 is a substrate of Plk4 and required for centriole duplication. *J Cell Sci* 125: 486–496.

Bai, J. et al. (2003). RNAi reveals doublecortin is required for radial migration in rat neocortex. *Nat Neurosci* 6: 1277–1283.

Barbelanne, M. and Tsang, W.Y. (2014). Molecular and cellular basis of autosomal recessive primary microcephaly. *BioMed Res Int* 2014: 547986.

Barber, M. and Pierani, A. (2016). Tangential migration of glutamatergic neurons and cortical patterning during development. *Dev Neurobiol* 76: 847–881.

Basto, R. et al. (2006). Flies without centrioles. *Cell* 125: 1375–1386.

Beattie, R. and Hippenmeyer, S. (2017). Mechanisms of radial glia progenitor cell lineage progression. *FEBS Lett* 591: 3993–4008.

Bellion, A. et al. (2005). Nucleokinesis in tangentially migrating neurons comprises two alternating phases. *J Neurosci* 25: 5691–5699.

Bendriem, R.M. et al. (2019). Tight junction protein occludin regulates progenitor self-renewal and survival in developing cortex. *Elife* 8: e49376.

Bertipaglia, C. et al. (2018). Nuclear migration in mammalian brain development. *Semin Cell Dev Biol* 82: 57–66.

Bettencourt-Dias, M. and Glover, D.M. (2007). Centrosome biogenesis and function. *Nat Rev Mol Cell Biol* 8: 451–463.

Blachon, S. et al. (2008). Drosophila asterless and vertebrate Cep152 Are orthologs essential for centriole duplication. *Genetics* 180: 2081–2094.

Bogoyevitch, M.A. et al. (2012). WD40-repeat protein 62 is a JNK-phosphorylated spindle pole protein required for spindle maintenance and timely mitotic progression. *J Cell Sci* 125: 5096–5109.

Bond, J. et al. (2005). A centrosomal mechanism involving CDK5RAP2 and CENPJ controls brain size. *Nat Genet* 37: 353–355.

Bornens, M. (2002). Centrosome composition and microtubule anchoring mechanisms. *Curr Opin Cell Biol* 14: 25–34.

Bornens, M. (2012). The centrosome in cells and organisms. *Science* 335: 422–426.

Boycott, K.M. et al. (2013). Rare-disease genetics in the era of next-generation sequencing. *Nat Rev Genet* 14: 681–691.

Bradke, F. and Dotti, C.G. (1999). The role of local actin instability in axon formation. *Science* 283: 1931–1934.

Bradke, F. and Dotti, C.G. (2000). Differentiated neurons retain the capacity to generate axons from dendrites. *Curr Biol* 10: 1467–1470.

Buchman, J.J. et al. (2010). Cdk5rap2 interacts with pericentrin to maintain the neural progenitor pool in the developing neocortex. *Neuron* 66: 386–402.

Bultje, R.S. et al. (2009). Mammalian Par3 regulates progenitor cell asymmetric division via notch signaling in the developing neocortex. *Neuron* 63: 189–202.

Burakov, A. et al. (2003). Centrosome positioning in interphase cells. *J Cell Biol* 162: 963–969.

Cabral, G. et al. (2013). Multiple mechanisms contribute to centriole separation in C. elegans. *Curr Biol* 23: 1380–1387.

Camargo Ortega, G. et al. (2019). The centrosome protein AKNA regulates neurogenesis via microtubule organization. *Nature* 567: 113–117.

Cantagrel, V. et al. (2008). Mutations in the cilia gene ARL13B lead to the classical form of Joubert syndrome. *Am J Hum Genet* 83: 170–179.

Capecchi, M.R. and Pozner, A. (2015). ASPM regulates symmetric stem cell division by tuning Cyclin E ubiquitination. *Nat Commun* 6: 8763.

Chabin-Brion, K. et al. (2001). The Golgi complex is a microtubule-organizing organelle. *Mol Biol Cell* 12: 2047–2060.

Chen, J.F. et al. (2014). Microcephaly disease gene Wdr62 regulates mitotic progression of embryonic neural stem cells and brain size. *Nat Commun* 5: 3885.

Chenn, A. et al. (1998). Intrinsic polarity of mammalian neuroepithelial cells. *Mol Cell Neurosci* 11: 183–193.

Chou, E.J. et al. (2016). Phosphorylation of CPAP by Aurora-A maintains spindle pole integrity during mitosis. *Cell Rep* 14: 2975–2987.

Conduit, P.T. et al. (2015). Centrosome function and assembly in animal cells. *Nat Rev Mol Cell Biol* 16: 611–624.

Connell, M. et al. (2017). HMMR acts in the PLK1-dependent spindle positioning pathway and supports neural development. *Elife* 6: e28672.

Da Palma, M.M. et al. (2020). TUBGCP4 – associated microcephaly and chorioretinopathy. *Ophthalmic Genet* 41: 189–193.

Damiani, D. et al. (2016). Lack of Diaph3 relaxes the spindle checkpoint causing the loss of neural progenitors. *Nat Commun* 7: 13509.

Dauber, A. et al. (2012). Novel microcephalic primordial dwarfism disorder associated with variants in the centrosomal protein ninein. *J Clin Endocrinol Metabol* 97: E2140–E2151.

David, A. et al. (2014). Lack of centrioles and primary cilia in STIL(-/-) mouse embryos. *Cell Cycle* 13: 2859–2868.

de Anda, F.C. et al. (2010). Centrosome motility is essential for initial axon formation in the neocortex. *J Neurosci* 30: 10391–10406.

de Anda, F.C. et al. (2005). Centrosome localization determines neuronal polarity. *Nature* 436: 704–708.

Delattre, M. and Gonczy, P. (2004). The arithmetic of centrosome biogenesis. *J Cell Sci* 117: 1619–1630.

Di Pietro, F. et al. (2016). Regulation of mitotic spindle orientation: an integrated view. *EMBO Rep* 17: 1106–1130.

Dictenberg, J.B. et al. (1998). Pericentrin and gamma-tubulin form a protein complex and are organized into a novel lattice at the centrosome. *J Cell Biol* 141: 163–174.

Ding, W. et al. (2019). Cenpj regulates cilia disassembly and neurogenesis in the developing mouse cortex. *J Neurosci* 39: 1994–2010.

Dotti, C.G. et al. (1988). The establishment of polarity by hippocampal neurons in culture. *J Neurosci* 8: 1454–1468.

Doxsey, S.J. et al. (1994). Pericentrin, a highly conserved centrosome protein involved in microtubule organization. *Cell* 76: 639–650.

Efimov, A. et al. (2007). Asymmetric CLASP-dependent nucleation of noncentrosomal microtubules at the trans-Golgi network. *Dev Cell* 12: 917–930.

Elsaid, M.F. et al. (2014). Whole genome sequencing identifies a novel occludin mutation in microcephaly with band-like calcification and polymicrogyria that extends the phenotypic spectrum. *Am J Med Genet A* 164A: 1614–1617.

Endoh-Yamagami, S. et al. (2010). A mutation in the pericentrin gene causes abnormal interneuron migration to the olfactory bulb in mice. *Dev Biol* 340: 41–53.

Enos, S.J. et al. (2018). Phosphatase PP2A and microtubule-mediated pulling forces disassemble centrosomes during mitotic exit. *Biol Open* 7 (1): bio029777.

Etienne-Manneville, S. and Hall, A. (2001). Integrin-mediated activation of Cdc42 controls cell polarity in migrating astrocytes through PKCzeta. *Cell* 106: 489–498.

Failler, M. et al. (2014). Mutations of CEP83 cause infantile nephronophthisis and intellectual disability. *Am J Hum Genet* 94: 905–914.

Farina, F. et al. (2016). The centrosome is an actin-organizing centre. *Nat Cell Biol* 18: 65–75.

Farooq, M. et al. (2020). RRP7A links primary microcephaly to dysfunction of ribosome biogenesis, resorption of primary cilia, and neurogenesis. *Nat Commun* 11: 5816.

Feng, Y. and Walsh, C.A. (2001). Protein-protein interactions, cytoskeletal regulation and neuronal migration. *Nat Rev Neurosci* 2: 408–416.

Fietz, S.A. et al. (2010). OSVZ progenitors of human and ferret neocortex are epithelial-like and expand by integrin signaling. *Nat Neurosci* 13: 690–699.

Fish, J.L. et al. (2006). Aspm specifically maintains symmetric proliferative divisions of neuroepithelial cells. *Proc Natl Acad Sci* 103: 10438–10443.

Fong, K.W. et al. (2008). CDK5RAP2 is a pericentriolar protein that functions in centrosomal attachment of the gamma-tubulin ring complex. *Mol Biol Cell* 19: 115–125.

Francis, F. et al. (1999). Doublecortin is a developmentally regulated, microtubule-associated protein expressed in migrating and differentiating neurons. *Neuron* 23: 247–256.

Fujimori, A. et al. (2014). Disruption of Aspm causes microcephaly with abnormal neuronal differentiation. *Brain Dev* 36: 661–669.

Gabriel, E. et al. (2017). Recent Zika virus isolates induce premature differentiation of neural progenitors in human brain organoids. *Cell Stem Cell* 20: 397–406 e395.

Gabriel, E. et al. (2016). CPAP promotes timely cilium disassembly to maintain neural progenitor pool. *EMBO J* 35: 803–819.

Garcez, P.P. et al. (2015). Cenpj/CPAP regulates progenitor divisions and neuronal migration in the cerebral cortex downstream of Ascl1. *Nat Commun* 6: 6474.

Ge, X. et al. (2010). Hook3 interacts with PCM1 to regulate pericentriolar material assembly and the timing of neurogenesis. *Neuron* 65: 191–203.

Goetz, S.C. (2012). The spinocerebellar ataxia-associated gene Tau tubulin kinase 2 controls the initiation of ciliogenesis. *Cell* 151: 847–858.

Goldspink, D.A. et al. (2017). Ninein is essential for apico-basal microtubule formation and CLIP-170 facilitates its redeployment to non-centrosomal microtubule organizing centres. *Open Biol* 7 (2): 160274.

Hamill, D.R. et al. (2002). Centrosome maturation and mitotic spindle assembly in C. elegans require SPD-5, a protein with multiple coiled-coil domains. *Dev Cell* 3: 673–684.

Hammond, J.W. et al. (2010). Posttranslational modifications of tubulin and the polarized transport of kinesin-1 in neurons. *Mol Biol Cell* 21: 572–583.

Hanafusa, H. et al. (2015). PLK1-dependent activation of LRRK1 regulates spindle orientation by phosphorylating CDK5RAP2. *Nat Cell Biol* 17: 1024–1035.

Hanafusa, H. and Matsumoto, K. (2015). LRRK1 regulates spindle orientation by phosphorylating CDK5RAP2. *Cell Cycle* 14: 3349–3350.

Hansen, D.V. et al. (2010). Neurogenic radial glia in the outer subventricular zone of human neocortex. *Nature* 464: 554–561.

Haydar, T.F. et al. (2003). Mitotic spindle rotation and mode of cell division in the developing telencephalon. *Proc Natl Acad Sci U S A* 100: 2890–2895.

He, S. et al. (2015). Inside-out radial migration facilitates lineage-dependent neocortical microcircuit assembly. *Neuron* 86: 1159–1166.

Higginbotham, H. et al. (2013). Arl13b-regulated cilia activities are essential for polarized radial glial scaffold formation. *Nat Neurosci* 16: 1000–1007.

Higginbotham, H.R. and Gleeson, J.G. (2007). The centrosome in neuronal development. *Trends Neurosci* 30: 276–283.

Hiraki, M. et al. (2007). Bld10p constitutes the cartwheel-spoke tip and stabilizes the 9-fold symmetry of the centriole. *Curr Biol* 17: 1778–1783.

Hoffmann, I. (2021). Centrosomes in mitotic spindle assembly and orientation. *Curr Opin Struct Biol* 66: 193–198.

Hu, D.J. et al. (2013). Dynein recruitment to nuclear pores activates apical nuclear migration and mitotic entry in brain progenitor cells. *Cell* 154: 1300–1313.

Hung, T.J. and Kemphues, K.J. (1999). PAR-6 is a conserved PDZ domain-containing protein that colocalizes with PAR-3 in Caenorhabditis elegans embryos. *Development* 126: 127–135.

Hussain, M.S. et al. (2012). A truncating mutation of CEP135 causes primary microcephaly and disturbed centrosomal function. *Am J Hum Genet* 90: 871–878.

Hussain, M.S. et al. (2013). CDK6 associates with the centrosome during mitosis and is mutated in a large Pakistani family with primary microcephaly. *Hum Mol Genet* 22: 5199–5214.

Insolera, R. et al. (2014a). Cortical neurogenesis in the absence of centrioles. *Nat Neurosci* 17: 1528–1535.

Insolera, R. et al. (2014b). SDCCAG8 regulates pericentriolar material recruitment and neuronal migration in the developing cortex. *Neuron* 83: 805–822.

Ishikawa, H. and Marshall, W.F. (2011). Ciliogenesis. *Nat Rev Mol Cell Biol* 12: 222–234.

Izraeli, S. et al. (1999). The SIL gene is required for mouse embryonic axial development and left-right specification. *Nature* 399: 691–694.

Jacobson, C. et al. (2006). A change in the selective translocation of the Kinesin-1 motor domain marks the initial specification of the axon. *Neuron* 49: 797–804.

Jayaraman, D. et al. (2016). Microcephaly proteins Wdr62 and Aspm define a mother centriole complex regulating centriole biogenesis, apical complex, and cell fate. *Neuron* 92: 813–828.

Jean, F. et al. (2020). Dissecting the genetic and etiological causes of primary microcephaly. *Front Neurol* 11: 570830.

Jerka-Dziadosz, M. et al. (2010). Basal body duplication in Paramecium. *Cytoskeleton* 67: 161–171.

Johnson, M.B. et al. (2018). Aspm knockout ferret reveals an evolutionary mechanism governing cerebral cortical size. *Nature* 556: 370–375.

Jossin, Y. et al. (2017). Llgl1 connects cell polarity with cell–cell adhesion in embryonic neural stem cells. *Dev Cell* 41: 481–495 e485.

Jurczyk, A. et al. (2004). Pericentrin forms a complex with intraflagellar transport proteins and polycystin-2 and is required for primary cilia assembly. *J Cell Biol* 166: 637–643.

Kadowaki, M. et al. (2007). N-cadherin mediates cortical organization in the mouse brain. *Dev Biol* 304: 22–33.
Kaindl, A.M. et al. (2010). Many roads lead to primary autosomal recessive microcephaly. *Prog Neurobiol* 90: 363–383.
Kasioulis, I. (2017). Inter-dependent apical microtubule and actin dynamics orchestrate centrosome retention and neuronal delamination. *Elife* 6: e26215.
Kawaguchi, A. (2020). Neuronal delamination and outer radial glia generation in neocortical development. *Front Cell Dev Biol* 8: 623573.
Keller, D. et al. (2014). Mechanisms of HsSAS-6 assembly promoting centriole formation in human cells. *J Cell Biol* 204: 697–712.
Kiesel, P. et al. (2020). The molecular structure of mammalian primary cilia revealed by cryo-electron tomography. *Nat Struct Mol Biol* 27: 1115–1124.
Kim, J. et al. (2015). PLK1 regulation of PCNT cleavage ensures fidelity of centriole separation during mitotic exit. *Nat Commun* 6: 10076.
Kim, S. et al. (2010). The apical complex couples cell fate and cell survival to cerebral cortical development. *Neuron* 66: 69–84.
Kim, T.S. et al. (2013). Hierarchical recruitment of Plk4 and regulation of centriole biogenesis by two centrosomal scaffolds, Cep192 and Cep152. *Proc Natl Acad Sci U S A* 110: E4849–4857.
Kobayashi, T. et al. (2014). The CP110-interacting proteins Talpid3 and Cep290 play overlapping and distinct roles in cilia assembly. *J Cell Biol* 204: 215–229.
Kobayashi, T. et al. (2011). Centriolar kinesin Kif24 interacts with CP110 to remodel microtubules and regulate ciliogenesis. *Cell* 145: 914–925.
Konishi, Y. and Setou, M. (2009). Tubulin tyrosination navigates the kinesin-1 motor domain to axons. *Nat Neurosci* 12: 559–567.
Konno, D. et al. (2008). Neuroepithelial progenitors undergo LGN-dependent planar divisions to maintain self-renewability during mammalian neurogenesis. *Nat Cell Biol* 10: 93–101.
Kosodo, Y. et al. (2004). Asymmetric distribution of the apical plasma membrane during neurogenic divisions of mammalian neuroepithelial cells. *EMBO J* 23: 2314–2324.
Kotak, S. et al. (2012). Cortical dynein is critical for proper spindle positioning in human cells. *J Cell Biol* 199: 97–110.
Kriegstein, A. and Alvarez-Buylla, A. (2009). The glial nature of embryonic and adult neural stem cells. *Ann Rev Neurosci* 32: 149–184.
Kriegstein, A. et al. (2006). Patterns of neural stem and progenitor cell division may underlie evolutionary cortical expansion. *Nat Rev Neurosci* 7: 883–890.
Kriegstein, A.R. and Noctor, S.C. (2004). Patterns of neuronal migration in the embryonic cortex. *Trends Neurosci* 27: 392–399.
Kroschewski, R. et al. (1999). Cdc42 controls secretory and endocytic transport to the basolateral plasma membrane of MDCK cells. *Nat Cell Biol* 1: 8–13.
Kuijpers, M. and Hoogenraad, C.C. (2011). Centrosomes, microtubules and neuronal development. *Mol Cell Neurosci* 48: 349–358.
Lancaster, M.A. et al. (2013). Cerebral organoids model human brain development and microcephaly. *Nature* 501: 373–379.
Lau, E.O. et al. (2021). DIAPH3 deficiency links microtubules to mitotic errors, defective neurogenesis, and brain dysfunction. *Elife* 10: e61974.
Lee, K. and Rhee, K. (2012). Separase-dependent cleavage of pericentrin B is necessary and sufficient for centriole disengagement during mitosis. *Cell Cycle* 11: 2476–2485.
Leidel, S. et al. (2005). SAS-6 defines a protein family required for centrosome duplication in C. elegans and in human cells. *Nat Cell Biol* 7: 115–125.

Lessman, C.A. (2012). Centrosomes in the zebrafish (Danio rerio). *Cilia* 1: 9.

Li, H. et al. (2017a). Spindle misorientation of cerebral and cerebellar progenitors is a mechanistic cause of megalencephaly. *Stem Cell Rep* 9: 1071–1080.

Li, R. et al. (2017b). Recapitulating cortical development with organoid culture in vitro and modeling abnormal spindle-like (ASPM related primary) microcephaly disease. *Protein Cell* 8: 823–833.

Lim, N.R. et al. (2017). Glial-specific functions of microcephaly protein WDR62 and interaction with the mitotic kinase AURKA are essential for Drosophila brain growth. *Stem Cell Rep* 9: 32–41.

Lin, Y.C. et al. (2013). Human microcephaly protein CEP135 binds to hSAS-6 and CPAP, and is required for centriole assembly. *EMBO J* 32: 1141–1154.

Lizarraga, S.B. et al. (2010). Cdk5rap2 regulates centrosome function and chromosome segregation in neuronal progenitors. *Development* 137: 1907–1917.

Llinares-Benadero, C. and Borrell, V. (2019). Deconstructing cortical folding: genetic, cellular and mechanical determinants. *Nat Rev Neurosci* 20: 161–176.

Luders, J. and Stearns, T. (2007). Microtubule-organizing centres. *Nat Rev Mol Cell Biol* 8: 161–167.

Ma, W. and Viveiros, M.M. (2014). Depletion of pericentrin in mouse oocytes disrupts microtubule organizing center function and meiotic spindle organization. *Mol Reprod Dev* 81: 1019–1029.

Marin, O. et al. (2010). Guiding neuronal cell migrations. *Cold Spring Harb Persp Biol* 2: a001834–a001834.

Marjanovic, M. et al. (2015). CEP63 deficiency promotes p53-dependent microcephaly and reveals a role for the centrosome in meiotic recombination. *Nat Commun* 6: 7676.

Martin, C.A. et al. (2014). Mutations in PLK4, encoding a master regulator of centriole biogenesis, cause microcephaly, growth failure and retinopathy. *Nat Genet* 46: 1283–1292.

Matsuura, K. et al. (2004). Bld10p, a novel protein essential for basal body assembly in Chlamydomonas. *J Cell Biol* 165: 663–671.

McIntyre, R.E. et al. (2012). Disruption of mouse Cenpj, a regulator of centriole biogenesis, phenocopies Seckel syndrome. *PLoS Genet* 8: e1003022.

Meka, D.P. et al. (2022). Centrosome-dependent microtubule modifications set the conditions for axon formation. *Cell Rep* 39: 110686.

Meka, D.P. et al. (2020). Emerging roles of the centrosome in neuronal development. *Cytoskeleton* 77: 84–96.

Meka, D.P. et al. (2019). Radial somatic F-actin organization affects growth cone dynamics during early neuronal development. *EMBO Rep* 20: e47743.

Meyer, E.J. et al. (2011). Interkinetic nuclear migration is a broadly conserved feature of cell division in pseudostratified epithelia. *Curr Biol* 21: 485–491.

Miyata, T. et al. (2004). Asymmetric production of surface-dividing and non-surface-dividing cortical progenitor cells. *Development* 131: 3133–3145.

Miyoshi, K. et al. (2009). Pericentrin, a centrosomal protein related to microcephalic primordial dwarfism, is required for olfactory cilia assembly in mice. *FASEB J* 23: 3289–3297.

Morin, X. and Bellaiche, Y. (2011). Mitotic spindle orientation in asymmetric and symmetric cell divisions during animal development. *Dev Cell* 21: 102–119.

Nachury, M.V. and Mick, D.U. (2019). Establishing and regulating the composition of cilia for signal transduction. *Nat Rev Mol Cell Biol* 20: 389–405.

Nadarajah, B. et al. (2002). Ventricle-directed migration in the developing cerebral cortex. *Nat Neurosci* 5: 218–224.

Nguyen-Ngoc, T. et al. (2007). Coupling of cortical dynein and G alpha proteins mediates spindle positioning in Caenorhabditis elegans. *Nat Cell Biol* 9: 1294–1302.

Nobes, C.D. and Hall, A. (1999). Rho GTPases control polarity, protrusion, and adhesion during cell movement. *J Cell Biol* 144: 1235–1244.

Noctor, S.C. et al. (2004). Cortical neurons arise in symmetric and asymmetric division zones and migrate through specific phases. *Nat Neurosci* 7: 136–144.

Noctor, S.C. et al. (2008). Distinct behaviors of neural stem and progenitor cells underlie cortical neurogenesis. *J Comp Neurol* 508: 28–44.

Novorol, C. et al. (2013). Microcephaly models in the developing zebrafish retinal neuroepithelium point to an underlying defect in metaphase progression. *Open Biol* 3: 130065.

O'Neill, R.S. et al. (2018). Same but different. *Mol Biol Cell* 29: 241–246.

Ohshima, T. et al. (2007). Cdk5 is required for multipolar-to-bipolar transition during radial neuronal migration and proper dendrite development of pyramidal neurons in the cerebral cortex. *Development* 134: 2273–2282.

Palazzo, A.F. et al. (2001). Cdc42, dynein, and dynactin regulate MTOC reorientation independent of Rho-regulated microtubule stabilization. *Curr Biol* 11: 1536–1541.

Paridaen, J.T. et al. (2013). Asymmetric inheritance of centrosome-associated primary cilium membrane directs ciliogenesis after cell division. *Cell* 155: 333–344.

Pelletier, L. et al. (2006). Centriole assembly in Caenorhabditis elegans. *Nature* 444: 619–623.

Petronczki, M. and Knoblich, J.A. (2001). DmPAR-6 directs epithelial polarity and asymmetric cell division of neuroblasts in Drosophila. *Nat Cell Biol* 3: 43–49.

Pfaff, K.L. et al. (2007). The zebra fish cassiopeia mutant reveals that SIL is required for mitotic spindle organization. *Mol Cell Biol* 27: 5887–5897.

Pilz, D.T. et al. (1998). LIS1 and XLIS (DCX) mutations cause most classical lissencephaly, but different patterns of malformation. *Hum Mol Genet* 7: 2029–2037.

Powell, S.K. et al. (1997). Development of polarity in cerebellar granule neurons. *J Neurobiol* 32: 223–236.

Raftopoulou, M. and Hall, A. (2004). Cell migration. *Dev Biol* 265: 23–32.

Ramdas Nair, A. et al. (2016). The microcephaly-associated protein Wdr62/CG7337 is required to maintain centrosome asymmetry in Drosophila neuroblasts. *Cell Rep* 14: 1100–1113.

Rasin, M.R. et al. (2007). Numb and Numbl are required for maintenance of cadherin-based adhesion and polarity of neural progenitors. *Nat Neurosci* 10: 819–827.

Rauch, A. et al. (2008). Mutations in the pericentrin (PCNT) gene cause primordial dwarfism. *Science* 319: 816–819.

Rebollo, E. et al. (2007). Functionally unequal centrosomes drive spindle orientation in asymmetrically dividing Drosophila neural stem cells. *Dev Cell* 12: 467–474.

Reed, N.A. et al. (2006). Microtubule acetylation promotes kinesin-1 binding and transport. *Curr Biol* 16: 2166–2172.

Ripoll, P. et al. (1985). A cell division mutant of Drosophila with a functionally abnormal spindle. *Cell* 41: 907–912.

Saade, M. et al. (2018). A centrosomal view of CNS growth. *Development* 145 (21): dev170613.

Saade, M. et al. (2020). Multimerization of Zika Virus-NS5 causes ciliopathy and forces premature neurogenesis. *Cell Stem Cell* 27: 920–936.e928.

Sakakibara, A. et al. (2014). Dynamics of centrosome translocation and microtubule organization in neocortical neurons during distinct modes of polarization. *Cereb Cortex* 24: 1301–1310.

Schaar, B.T. and McConnell, S.K. (2005). Cytoskeletal coordination during neuronal migration. *Proc Natl Acad Sci USA* 102: 13652–13657.

Scheidecker, S. et al. (2015). Mutations in TUBGCP4 alter microtubule organization via the gamma-tubulin ring complex in autosomal-recessive microcephaly with chorioretinopathy. *Am J Hum Genet* 96: 666–674.

Schlaitz, A.L. et al. (2007). The C. elegans RSA complex localizes protein phosphatase 2A to centrosomes and regulates mitotic spindle assembly. *Cell* 128: 115–127.

Sgourdou, P. et al. (2017). Disruptions in asymmetric centrosome inheritance and WDR62-Aurora kinase B interactions in primary microcephaly. *Sci Rep* 7: 43708.
Shao, W. et al. (2020). Centrosome anchoring regulates progenitor properties and cortical formation. *Nature* 580: 106–112.
Shelly, M. et al. (2010). Local and long-range reciprocal regulation of cAMP and cGMP in axon/dendrite formation. *Science* 327: 547–552.
Shen, Z. et al. (2021). Distinct progenitor behavior underlying neocortical gliogenesis related to tumorigenesis. *Cell Rep* 34: 108853.
Shitamukai, A. et al. (2011). Oblique radial glial divisions in the developing mouse neocortex induce self-renewing progenitors outside the germinal zone that resemble primate outer subventricular zone progenitors. *J Neurosci* 31: 3683–3695.
Shoukimas, G.M. and Hinds, J.W. (1978). The development of the cerebral cortex in the embryonic mouse: an electron microscopic serial section analysis. *J Comp Neurol* 179: 795–830.
Shurygina, M.F. et al. (2020). Genotype phenotype correlation and variability in microcephaly associated with chorioretinopathy or familial exudative vitreoretinopathy. *Investig Ophthalmol Vis Sci* 61: 2.
Sir, J.H. et al. (2011). A primary microcephaly protein complex forms a ring around parental centrioles. *Nat Genet* 43: 1147–1153.
Snedeker, J. et al. (2017). Unique spatiotemporal requirements for intraflagellar transport genes during forebrain development. *PLoS One* 12: e0173258.
Solecki, D.J. et al. (2006). mPar6 alpha controls neuronal migration. *J Neurosci* 26: 10624–10625.
Solecki, D.J. et al. (2004). Par6alpha signaling controls glial-guided neuronal migration. *Nat Neurosci* 7: 1195–1203.
Solecki, D.J. et al. (2009). Myosin II motors and F-actin dynamics drive the coordinated movement of the centrosome and soma during CNS glial-guided neuronal migration. *Neuron* 63: 63–80.
Spear, P.C. and Erickson, C.A. (2012). Apical movement during interkinetic nuclear migration is a two-step process. *Dev Biol* 370: 33–41.
Stiess, M. and Bradke, F. (2011). Neuronal polarization. *Dev Neurobiol* 71: 430–444.
Stiess, M. et al. (2010). Axon extension occurs independently of centrosomal microtubule nucleation. *Science* 327: 704–707.
Stowers, L. et al. (1995). Regulation of the polarization of T cells toward antigen-presenting cells by Ras-related GTPase CDC42. *Proc Natl Acad Sci U S A* 92: 5027–5031.
Strzyz, P.J. et al. (2015). Interkinetic nuclear migration is centrosome independent and ensures apical cell division to maintain tissue integrity. *Dev Cell* 32: 203–219.
Sun, T. and Hevner, R.F. (2014). Growth and folding of the mammalian cerebral cortex. *Nat Rev Neurosci* 15: 217–232.
Sutterlin, C. and Colanzi, A. (2010). The Golgi and the centrosome. *J Cell Biol* 188: 621–628.
Tabata, H. and Nakajima, K. (2003). Multipolar migration. *J Neurosci* 23: 9996–10001.
Takano, T. et al. (2019). Neuronal polarity. *Front Cell Dev Biol* 7: 69.
Takano, T. et al. (2017). Discovery of long-range inhibitory signaling to ensure single axon formation. *Nat Commun* 8: 33.
Takano, T. et al. (2015). Neuronal polarization. *Development* 142: 2088–2093.
Tanaka, T. et al. (2004). Lis1 and doublecortin function with dynein to mediate coupling of the nucleus to the centrosome in neuronal migration. *J Cell Biol* 165: 709–721.
Tang, C.J. et al. (2011). The human microcephaly protein STIL interacts with CPAP and is required for procentriole formation. *EMBO J* 30: 4790–4804.
Tang, N. and Marshall, W.F. (2012). Centrosome positioning in vertebrate development. *J Cell Sci* 125: 4951–4961.
Thornton, G.K. and Woods, C.G. (2009). Primary microcephaly *Trends Genet* 25: 501–510.

Tozer, S. et al. (2017). Differential routing of Mindbomb1 via centriolar satellites regulates asymmetric divisions of neural progenitors. *Neuron* 93: 542–551 e544.

Tsai, J.W., Bremner, K.H., and Vallee, R.B. (2007). Dual subcellular roles for LIS1 and dynein in radial neuronal migration in live brain tissue. *Nat Neurosci* 10: 970–979.

Tsai, J.W. et al. (2005). LIS1 RNA interference blocks neural stem cell division, morphogenesis, and motility at multiple stages. *J Cell Biol* 170: 935–945.

Tsai, L.H. and Gleeson, J.G. (2005). Nucleokinesis in neuronal migration. *Neuron* 46: 383–388.

Tsou, M.F. and Stearns, T. (2006). Mechanism limiting centrosome duplication to once per cell cycle. *Nature* 442: 947–951.

Tsutsumi, M. et al. (2016). Novel compound heterozygous variants in PLK4 identified in a patient with autosomal recessive microcephaly and chorioretinopathy. *Eur J Hum Genet* 24: 1702–1706.

Turkyilmaz, A. and Sager, S.G. (2022). Two new cases of primary microcephaly with neuronal migration defect caused by truncating mutations in the ASPM gene. *Mol Syndromol* 13: 56–63.

Vallee, R.B. et al. (2009). Emerging roles for myosin II and cytoplasmic dynein in migrating neurons and growth cones. *Trends Cell Biol* 19: 347–355.

van der Voet, M. et al. (2009). NuMA-related LIN-5, ASPM-1, calmodulin and dynein promote meiotic spindle rotation independently of cortical LIN-5/GPR/Galpha. *Nat Cell Biol* 11: 269–277.

Varmark, H. et al. (2007). Asterless is a centriolar protein required for centrosome function and embryo development in Drosophila. *Curr Biol* 17: 1735–1745.

Veeraval, L. et al. (2020). Adherens junctions. *Front Cell Dev Biol* 8: 6.

Vitalis, T. and Rossier, J. (2011). New insights into cortical interneurons development and classification. *Dev Neurobiol* 71: 34–44.

Waich, S. et al. (2020). Novel PCNT variants in MOPDII with attenuated growth restriction and pachygyria. *Clin Genet* 98: 282–287.

Wang, J. et al. (2020). Talpid3-mediated centrosome integrity restrains neural progenitor delamination to sustain neurogenesis by stabilizing adherens junctions. *Cell Rep* 33: 108495.

Wang, X. et al. (2009). Asymmetric centrosome inheritance maintains neural progenitors in the neocortex. *Nature* 461: 947–955.

Wieczorek, M. et al. (2020). Asymmetric molecular architecture of the human gamma-tubulin ring complex. *Cell* 180: 165–175 e116.

Wiggin, G.R. et al. (2005). Polarity proteins in axon specification and synaptogenesis. *Dev Cell* 8: 803–816.

Wilsch-Brauninger, M. and Huttner, W.B. (2021). Primary cilia and centrosomes in neocortex development. *Front Neurosci* 15: 755867.

Winey, M. and O'Toole, E. (2014). Centriole structure. *Philos Trans R Soc Lond B Biol Sci* 369 (1650): 20130457.

Witte, H. et al. (2008). Microtubule stabilization specifies initial neuronal polarization. *J Cell Biol* 180: 619–632.

Wonders, C.P. and Anderson, S.A. (2006). The origin and specification of cortical interneurons. *Nat Rev Neurosci* 7: 687–696.

Wong, K. et al. (2001). Signal transduction in neuronal migration. *Cell* 107: 209–221.

Wu, K.S. and Tang, T.K. (2012). CPAP is required for cilia formation in neuronal cells. *Biol Open* 1: 559–565.

Wynshaw-Boris, A. and Gambello, M.J. (2001). LIS1 and dynein motor function in neuronal migration and development. *Genes Dev* 15: 639–651.

Xie, Z. et al. (2007). Cep120 and TACCs control interkinetic nuclear migration and the neural progenitor pool. *Neuron* 56: 79–93.

Yabe, T. et al. (2007). The zebrafish maternal-effect gene cellular atoll encodes the centriolar component sas-6 and defects in its paternal function promote whole genome duplication. *Dev Biol* 312: 44–60.

Yamashita, Y.M. et al. (2007). Asymmetric inheritance of mother versus daughter centrosome in stem cell division. *Science* 315: 518–521.

Yang, J. et al. (2021). Centrosome regulation and function in mammalian cortical neurogenesis. *Curr Opin Neurobiol* 69: 256–266.

Yang, Y.T. et al. (2012). DOCK7 interacts with TACC3 to regulate interkinetic nuclear migration and cortical neurogenesis. *Nat Neurosci* 15: 1201–1210.

Yigit, G. et al. (2015). Mutations in CDK5RAP2 cause Seckel syndrome. *Mol Genet Genom* 3: 467–480.

Yin, Y. et al. (2009). The Talpid3 gene (KIAA0586) encodes a centrosomal protein that is essential for primary cilia formation. *Development* 136: 655–664.

Yokota, Y. et al. (2007). Radial glial dependent and independent dynamics of interneuronal migration in the developing cerebral cortex. *PLoS One* 2: e794.

Zaqout, S. and Kaindl, A.M. (2021). Autosomal recessive primary microcephaly: not just a small brain. *Front Cell Dev Biol* 9: 784700.

Zhang, W. et al. (2019). Modeling microcephaly with cerebral organoids reveals a WDR62-CEP170-KIF2A pathway promoting cilium disassembly in neural progenitors. *Nat Commun* 10: 2612.

Zheng, X. et al. (2014). Conserved TCP domain of Sas-4/CPAP is essential for pericentriolar material tethering during centrosome biogenesis. *Proc Natl Acad Sci U S A* 111: E354–363.

Zheng, Y. et al. (1995). Nucleation of microtubule assembly by a gamma-tubulin-containing ring complex. *Nature* 378: 578–583.

Zhong, W. and Chia, W. (2008). Neurogenesis and asymmetric cell division. *Curr Opin Neurobiol* 18: 4–11.

Zhu, J. et al. (2010). Finding the cell center by a balance of dynein and myosin pulling and microtubule pushing. *Mol Biol Cell* 21: 4418–4427.

Zmuda, J.F. and Rivas, R.J. (1998). The Golgi apparatus and the centrosome are localized to the sites of newly emerging axons in cerebellar granule neurons in vitro. *Cell Motil Cytoskeleton* 41: 18–38.

Zumbrunn, J. et al. (2001). Binding of the adenomatous polyposis coli protein to microtubules increases microtubule stability and is regulated by GSK3 beta phosphorylation. *Curr Biol* 11: 44–49.

32

Keeping the Cortex Afloat

Cerebrospinal Fluid Contributions to Cerebral Cortical Development

Tiara E. Lacey[1,2], *Ryann M. Fame*[1], *and Maria K. Lehtinen*[1,2]

[1] *Department of Pathology, Boston Children's Hospital, Boston, MA, 02115, USA*
[2] *Graduate Program in Biological and Biomedical Sciences, Harvard Medical School, Boston, MA, 02115, USA*

32.1 Introduction: Development of CSF-filled Ventricles

The presence of cerebrospinal fluid (CSF)-filled pockets, or ventricles, is a conserved feature across vertebrate brains. The developing mammalian brain ventricular system comprises four ventricles, the neural progenitor cells that line their walls, and the CSF within them (Figure 32.1), (Fame and Lehtinen 2020). The CSF is in continuity with the entire central nervous system from the cerebral cortex to the spinal cord. Healthy CSF is a clear and complex fluid composed of proteins, peptides, ions, and other small molecules. Of these components, CSF proteins are perhaps the best studied to date. Various components can enter the CSF by: (1) osmosis-driven ion and water transport, (2) secretion of de novo synthesized molecules from cells contacting the ventricles, and/or (3) transcytosis from systemic circulation.

Any cell in contact with the CSF can contribute to its volume and composition, but the major source of CSF is a secretory epithelial structure located in each ventricle of the brain called the choroid plexus (ChP; Figures 32.2–32.4). The neurosurgeons Harvey Cushing and Walter Dandy were the first to observe CSF secretion by the ChP and propose a model for its circulation in 1914 and 1919, respectively (Cushing 1914; Dandy 1919). For almost a century, the perceived roles of adult CSF were largely limited to serving as a fluid cushion for the brain, a sink for waste, and an ionic buffer. It is now clear that the CSF has a myriad of functions throughout life (Fame and Lehtinen 2020; Ghersi-Egea et al. 2018; Saunders et al. 2018). In this chapter, we will discuss research studies that have elucidated aspects of CSF biology relevant to cerebral cortical development. We will explain the use of model organisms, organoids, cell/ tissue culture systems, state-of-the-art microscopy, and modern genetic tools to unveil the means of production and composition of CSF in relationship to the timeline of cerebral cortical development. Finally, we will discuss how manipulating the CSF could be used therapeutically to intervene in disorders of cerebral cortical development.

Neocortical Neurogenesis in Development and Evolution, First Edition. Edited by Wieland B. Huttner.

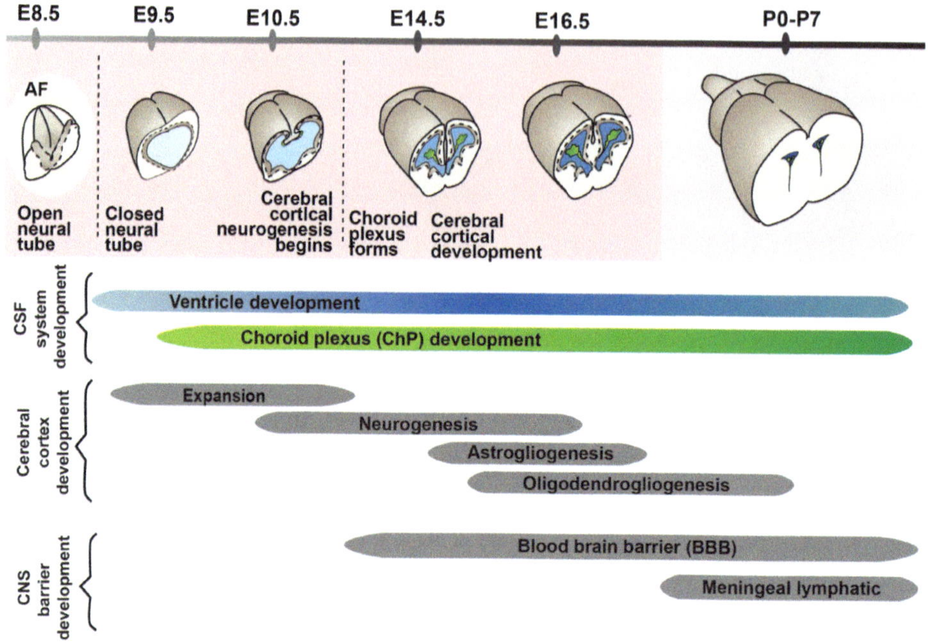

Figure 32.1 Development of the major components of the cerebrospinal fluid system and cerebral cortex occurs across central nervous system (CNS) developmental time. After neural tube closure (embryonic day (E)9 in mice; first dashed line) the brain ventricles form and expansion of the cerebral cortex begins. Around E10.5 neurogenesis commences in the cerebral cortex (second dashed line), and shortly thereafter, the choroid plexus (ChP) is visible. Perivascular components begin to arise with endothelial tight junctions appearing around E12 and maturation of barrier function beginning at E15.5. Gliogenesis of astrocytes followed by oligodendrocytes starts around E14.5. Ependymal cells are generated by radial glia beginning at E14 and then become postmitotic. Meningeal lymphatic vessels sprout from existing vessels at the base of the skull around E18 or birth in mice, and this system continues to mature throughout the first postnatal month. AF, amniotic fluid. Adapted from Fame and Lehtinen (2020).

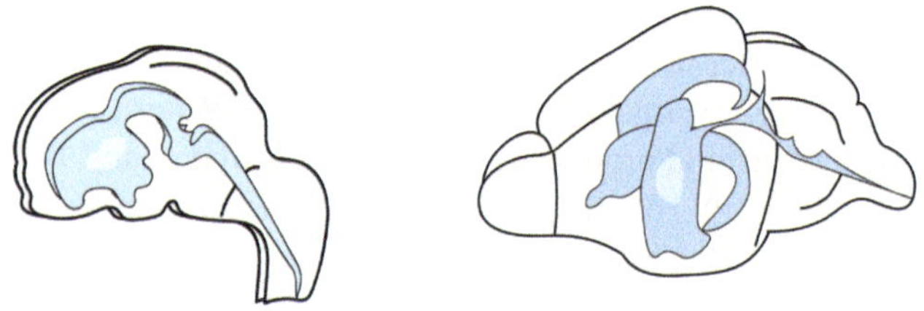

Figure 32.2 Embryonic and postnatal mouse ventricles. Schematics of three-dimensional views of embryonic (left) and postnatal (right) ventricles filled with cerebrospinal fluid (CSF; blue).

32.2 The Brain Fluid Environment during Forebrain Development

32.2.1 Generating a Brain Fluid Environment during Neurulation and Forebrain Progenitor Expansion

Prior to the formation of CSF, the developing neural plate that eventually gives rise to the mammalian brain is bathed in amniotic fluid (AF) (Figure 32.1). Throughout fetal development, AF

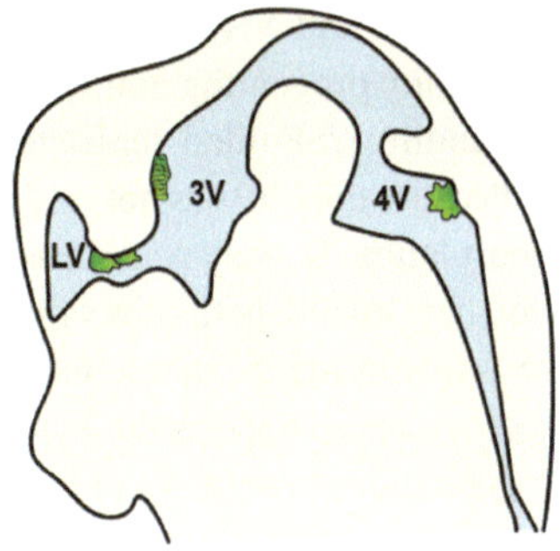

Figure 32.3 Development of the embryonic mouse ventricular system. Schematic of an oblique/lateral view of the lateral ventricles (LV), third ventricle (3V), fourth ventricle (4V), and central canal of spinal cord filled with CSF (blue) with their associated ChPs (green) at E13.5.

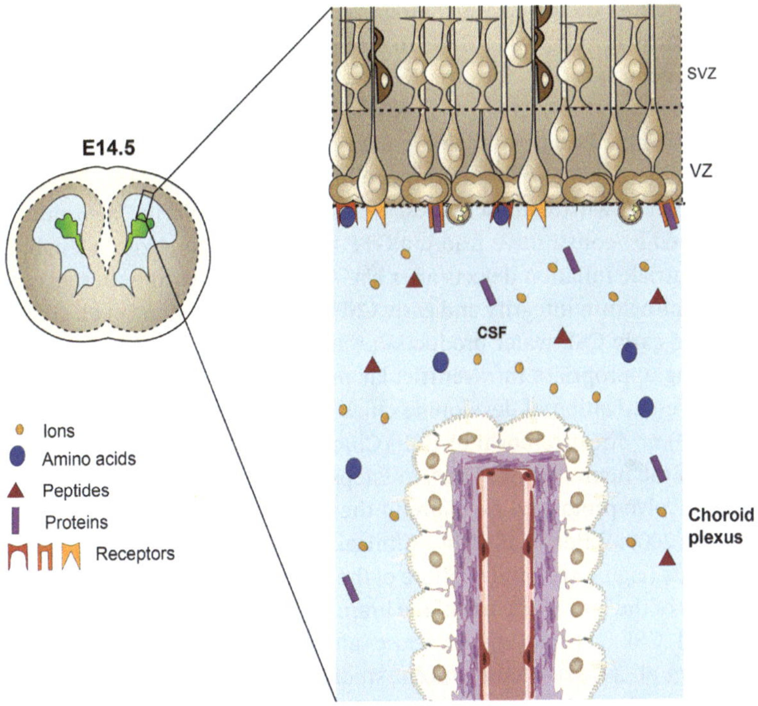

Figure 32.4 Embryonic mouse CSF and cortical environment. Left: Schematic of a coronal section of an E14.5 mouse brain showing CSF-filled lateral ventricles (blue) and ChP (green). Right: E14.5 CSF contains markers of cortical development, as well as some components, such as ions, amino acids, peptides, proteins, and receptors, that have been shown to be involved in signaling to CSF-contacting cortical neural progenitors (brown) and the ChP (tan). VZ: ventricular zone; SVZ: subventricular zone.

provides a protective fluid that surrounds the entire embryo in the amniotic sac. It provides fluid cushioning, pressure that protects against injury, and a reservoir of nutrients for the developing embryo that includes electrolytes, proteins, immunoglobulins, and vitamins (Underwood et al. 2005). At later stages, AF also accumulates waste products such as urine, following kidney maturation (Underwood et al. 2005).

Of direct relevance to the cerebral cortex, the earliest CSF is defined as AF that is captured inside the developing ventricular system following closure of the anterior and posterior neuropore (neurulation) at embryonic day (E)8.5 in developing mouse (Bueno and Garcia-Fernàndez 2016;

Massarwa and Niswander 2013) (Figures 32.1–32.3). The developing primordial brain, including forebrain progenitor zones in the neural ectoderm (neuroectoderm), rapidly grow around the expanding CSF-filled ventricles.

Because the ChP has not yet formed at this early stage, the source of early CSF, immediately following neurulation, is likely water from the AF transported via neuroepithelial progenitor cells. CSF production may involve both osmolality and ionic gradients. While the technical challenges of tracing water in real-time inside the developing brain has prevented direct experimentation to address this point, indirect evidence supports the hypothesis that osmolality of the CSF fluid environment enables the neuroepithelium to draw water from the AF and produce CSF (Alonso et al. 1999; Habgood et al. 1992).

The formation of ion gradients across cell membranes provides one mechanism for modulating osmolality and water content. A poignant example involves the sodium-potassium transporter, Na^+/K^+-ATPase, which moves three sodium ions out of a cell for every two potassium ions in, thereby regulating ion gradients across the plasma membrane. In turn, this pump also regulates cellular osmolarity. When osmolarity is high, water flows in via water channels and vice versa. In the context of ventricle development and CSF, the Na^+/K^+-ATPase has been investigated using zebrafish (Chang et al. 2012; Lowery and Sive 2005). Na^+/K^+-ATPase loss-of-function resulted in reduced ventricle volume, and disrupted neuroepithelial polarity, continuity, and barrier. These defects were accompanied by reduced neuroepithelial intracellular [Na^+] and disrupted RhoA-dependent and RhoA-independent downstream activities. Neuroepithelial polarity, continuity, and barrier could be re-established by constitutive RhoA, a GTP binding protein, expression, but RhoA could not rescue brain ventricle inflation defects after Na^+/K^+-ATPase disruption, suggesting distinct pathways for neuroepithelium integrity and early CSF production (Chang et al. 2012).

While the mechanisms driving early CSF water production remain to be fully elucidated, it is well established that maintaining appropriate intraventricular pressure is necessary for normal brain growth. For example, depressurization of developing chick brain by ventricular intubation (Desmond and Schoenwolf 1985) or direct removal of CSF (Chang et al. 2012; Gato et al. 2005) limits proliferation and health of the neural tissue. Thus, missteps in neural tube closure can disrupt pressurization as well as involve prolonged exposure of the developing neural tissue to AF instead of CSF (Lowery and Sive 2009; Wilde et al. 2014). Clinically, these consequences on brain development range from moderate (e.g., spina bifida: failure of the spinal cord to properly close) to severe (e.g., anencephaly: failure of the brain, or parts of the brain, to form).

On the other hand, elevated CSF volume and pressure are hallmarks of hydrocephalus (Bräutigam et al. 2019; Karimy et al. 2016). Notably, recent studies aimed at identifying genetic drivers of congenital hydrocephalus, a condition of excess CSF accumulation in the brain, have uncovered disease-causing mutations in *TRIM71, SMARCC1, PTCH1*, and *SHH*, all genes expressed predominantly by progenitors along the neural tube (Furey et al. 2018). While the exact mechanisms by which these specific mutations cause hydrocephalus remain to be elucidated, collectively these findings strongly implicate progenitors positioned along the neural tube as having key role(s) in establishing CSF homeostasis in addition to their classic roles in neurogenesis (Duy et al. 2023). Ventricular enlargement has also been reported in individuals with schizophrenia (Sayo et al. 2012). Elevated CSF volumes in the areas surrounding the brain (i.e., in the subarachnoid space, extra-axial CSF) in infants and young children can be predictive of later development of autism spectrum disorder (ASD) (Shen et al. 2017, 2018).

Modern neurology has leveraged CSF as a useful tool for diagnostics, and it is commonly sampled for biomarkers of neurologic diseases in the clinical setting (Bharucha et al. 2019; Deisenhammer et al. 2019; Guo et al. 2022; Harris et al. 2021; Schindler et al. 2019). In a similar approach, proteomic signatures of early CSF can be used to reveal ongoing processes of healthy forebrain development (Chau et al. 2015; Fame and Lehtinen 2019). Indeed, soon after neurulation is completed, AF and CSF begin to diverge in their proteomic composition. The embryonic CSF contains surprisingly high levels of proteins associated with ribosomes, protein translation, and metabolism, whose expression decreases in CSF as development progresses (Chau et al. 2015). Subsequent analyses demonstrated that parallel coordinated transcriptional changes take place in adjacent forebrain progenitor cells, which are a likely source of these proteins in early CSF. Concurrently, electron microscopy (EM) revealed that forebrain progenitors undergo striking changes in mitochondrial structure in the days following neural tube closure, transitioning from having glycolytic cristae at E8.5 to more mature, traditional mitochondrial structures at E10.5. Glucose usage also shifts in progenitors to match these mitochondrial changes such that E8.5 progenitors rely on glycolysis, and after neural tube closure, they increasingly use oxidative phosphorylation. The mitochondrial morphological shifts (but not the functional metabolic readout), as well as ribosome biogenesis, depend on the downregulation of the transcription factor c-MYC in forebrain progenitor cells (Figure 32.5). Unrestrained c-MYC expression at this early developmental stage increases ribosome biogenesis and delays mitochondrial maturation, ultimately resulting in a large brain phenotype (Chau et al. 2015) and the formation of rare pediatric neoplasms including ChP carcinoma (Shannon et al. 2018).

After E10.5, the processes of mitochondrial maturation and increasing oxidative capacity continue, with even further reduced glycolysis in E12.5 progenitors (Fame et al. 2019). This timing

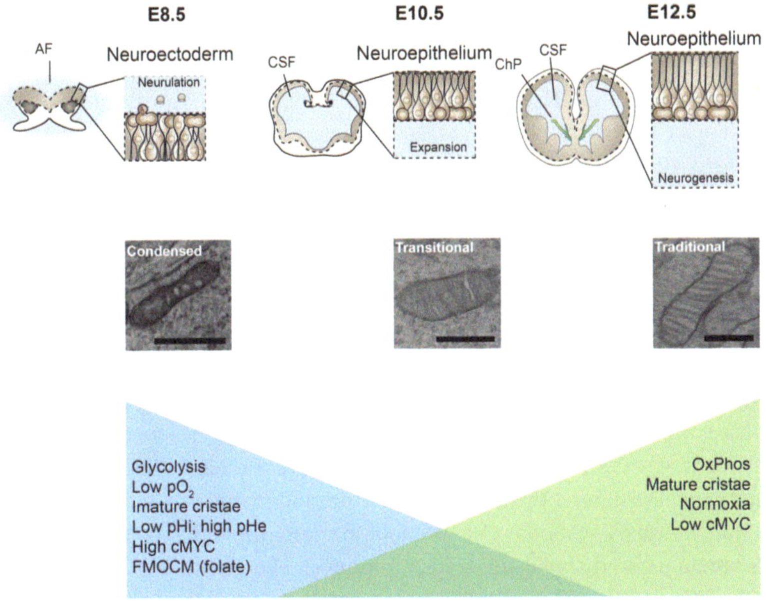

Figure 32.5 Mitochondrial changes during neurulation and early neurogenesis. Major metabolic shifts and changes in mitochondrial morphology occur during neurulation. Upper panels: Schematic of coronal sections of E8.5 mouse neuroectoderm of the open neural tube folding to generate E10.5 and E12.5 neuroepithelium. Middle Panels: Transmission electron microscopy (TEM) images of mitochondria reveal shifts from condensed to transitional and traditional morphologies at E8.5, 10.5, and 12.5, respectively. Lower Panels: Schematic indicating metabolic transitions from E8.5 (blue) to E12.5 (green). At E10.5, metabolism shifts away from glycolysis and toward oxidative phosphorylation along with changes in extracellular and intracellular pH (pHe, pHi). Concurrent with this process, chorioallantoic branching further increases the partial pressure of oxygen (pO_2) as development proceeds. FMOCM, folate-mediated one-carbon metabolism; cMYC, cellular MYC. Adapted from Fame and Lehtinen (2021).

matches the developmental stage when changes in mitochondrial function have been shown to promote differentiation through induction of maturation factor NRF2 via reactive oxygen species (ROS) (Khacho et al. 2016; Khacho and Slack 2018). Collectively, these findings demonstrate that metabolic shifting accompanies critical organelle and proteome remodeling in forebrain progenitors during early stages of cerebral cortical development and underscore CSF as a useful tool for reflecting the normal processes of brain development. In addition to providing a window into the metabolic state of the developing forebrain, the early CSF also harbors key signaling molecules that support the health, identity, and division of neural precursors (discussed later) (Chau et al. 2015; Wilde et al. 2014).

32.2.2 Production of CSF during Cerebral Cortical Development

32.2.2.1 Choroid Plexus

The ChP is a sheet of predominantly epithelial cells (but also includes mesenchymal, immune, endothelial, glial, and neuronal cells) (Dani et al. 2021), with a key function to produce CSF (Figure 32.4). CSF production entails water secretion, de novo protein synthesis and secretion, and transcytosis of peripheral factors from the blood. Newly differentiating ChP epithelial cells expand the emerging tissue into the ventricles in a "conveyor belt"-like manner (Figure 32.1), a phenomenon shown in marsupials, since their unique biology of maturing in an external pouch provides ex utero access to very early developing brain (Liddelow et al. 2010). Developmentally, ChP tissue is specified at E9.5 (Hunter and Dymecki 2007). It then begins to differentiate in mouse around E11–12 first in the hindbrain ChP (roofplate epithelium of the fourth ventricle ChP), then the telencephalic ChP (bilaterally from the dorsal midline of the telencephalon), and finally, the diencephalic ChP (anterior diencephalic roof for third ventricle ChP) (Awatramani et al. 2003; Currle et al. 2005; Hunter and Dymecki 2007; Langford et al. 2020; Liddelow et al. 2010; Monuki et al. 2001; Nielsen and Dymecki 2010; Shannon et al. 2018; Wilting and Christ 1989) (Figure 32.2). While ChP differentiation in mouse brain proceeds across all ventricles almost simultaneously at E11–12, the process can be much more protracted in other species, including sheep and humans, where weeks are reported to lapse between development of the lateral and third ventricle ChP (Dziegielewska et al. 2001; Ek et al. 2003; Ghersi-Egea et al. 2018; Jacobsen et al. 1983; O'Rahilly and Müller 1990) .

As the ChP matures, its surface area increases through microvilli and folded papillary architecture. In rat, the ChP apical surface area is estimated to increase by 550 percent from E16–P30, allowing more contact with CSF (Fame and Lehtinen 2020; Keep and Jones 1990). Additionally, the ChP proportionally increases its interaction with systemic blood through fenestrated capillaries, which is considered the source of water for ChP-secreted CSF (Keep and Jones 1990).

Despite this unique anatomical structure, the field is only beginning to understand how the ChP epithelium synthesizes and secretes proteins and metabolites into the CSF. Next generation sequencing (bulk RNA sequencing and single cell transcriptomics), along with semi-quantitative proteomics, have begun to define ChP epithelial cell secretomes. ChP tissues in each ventricle are regionally patterned, and as such, they harbor ventricle-specific transcriptional identities (Lun et al. 2015a). In turn, proteomics analyses of mouse ChP conditioned media revealed that spatial heterogeneity results in the production of ventricle-specific CSF (Lun et al. 2015a; Lun et al. 2015b), involving the secretion of many proteins implicated in brain development and health. Some of these factors (e.g., SHH and WNT5a) have specific actions on the development of hindbrain structures (Huang et al. 2009; Kaiser et al. 2019, 2021; Nielsen and Dymecki 2010). The regionalization of CSF is apparent already very early in brain development. While also studied in rodents (Lun et al. 2015b), this feature has been more precisely shown in sheep, since they have large ventricle sizes that facilitate the comparison of CSF proteomes in different ventricles during development (Cavanagh et al. 1983).

While many CSF factors with favorable effects on brain development and function can be secreted by ChP epithelial cells (e.g., IGF2, SHH, WNT5a), this is certainly not the case for all factors. Some CSF components are likely generated by neural progenitors lining the brain's ventricles. In the more mature brain, other signals, such as FGF17, may originate centrally from neurons (Iram et al. 2022), while others originate peripherally, such as leptin, a hormone produced by adipose tissue (Di Spiezio et al. 2018; Harrison et al. 2018); folate, a vitamin obtained from food (Alam et al. 2019; Grapp et al. 2013); or copper, an essential metal with an array of cellular functions (Donsante et al. 2010), which enters the brain via selective transporter systems (Fame and Lehtinen 2020).

How each tissue source contributes to CSF composition can also vary based on overall health. For example, in a mouse model of maternal inflammation, embryonic CSF acquires an inflammatory signature consisting of proinflammatory cytokines including CCL2, IFNβ, IFNγ, IL1β, and IL-6 that likely originate from central and peripheral immune cells (Cui et al. 2020) (Figure 32.6). Augmentation of CSF-CCL2 further propagates inflammation throughout the developing brain and can ultimately disrupt lamination of the cerebral cortex (Cui et al. 2020). In this manner, the CSF can also be hijacked to propagate harmful factors to the developing brain, including contributing to life-long consequences on brain function for the offspring.

ChP secretion of factors into the CSF occurs not only through direct release of proteins and vesicles, but also includes the exocytosis of nanovesicles, such as exosomes, which can ferry proteins, mRNAs, and microRNAs, representing a form of intercellular communication within the mouse CSF (Balusu et al. 2016; Feliciano et al. 2014). The embryonic CSF is estimated to contain 10^{12} nanoparticles/ml with a diameter of approximately 77nm (Feliciano et al. 2014). These nanovesicles deliver their

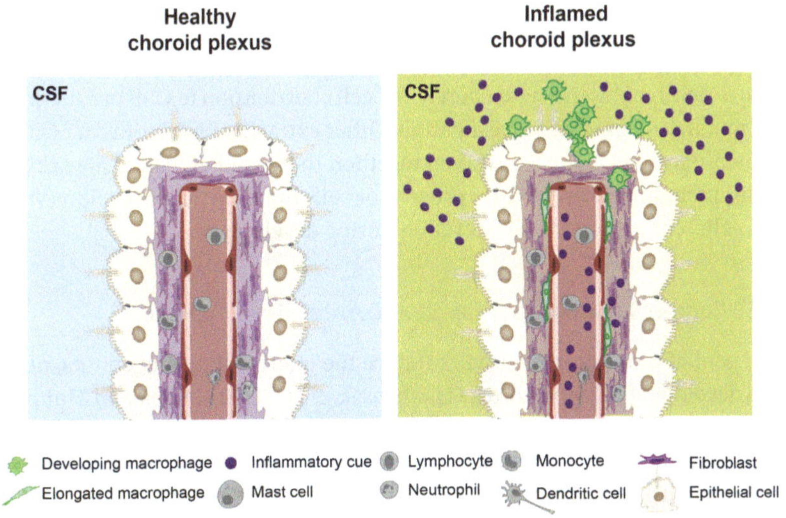

Figure 32.6 Embryonic CSF composition and choroid plexus barrier integrity is altered during maternal immune activation. Left: Healthy CSF is clear, but complex (blue). Right: During inflammatory conditions, the CSF acquires an inflammatory signature and can become xanthochromic (yellow). Also, the ChP epithelial barrier is weakened at "hotspots" located at the distal tips of ChP villi and are especially prominent in the fourth ventricle. Macrophages breach these hotspots and relocate to the epiplexus surface, the apical CSF contacting surface of the ChP. Past studies and recent single-cell transcriptomics analyses revealed that the ChP harbors a variety of immune cells including macrophages, basophils, mast cells, dendritic cells, monocytes, neutrophils, and lymphocytes.

contents, namely miRNAs and proteins (e.g., ERK, SPAK, miR for insulin and VEGF pathways, SHH, WNT5a) to neural progenitors and contain critical components of growth and proliferation pathways to further support neural stem cell amplification during corticogenesis (Feliciano et al. 2014).

Additional vesicular bodies released by the ChP include multivesicular bodies encapsulating SHH, a hydrophobic secreted factor required for embryonic development, from the ChP epithelium into the CSF (Coulter et al. 2018). WNT5A, a WNT protein expressed in the 4V ChP and key for hindbrain development, is transported long distances via lipoprotein particles in the CSF (Kaiser et al. 2019). A process of apocrine signaling has been proposed (Agnew et al. 1980; Fame and Lehtinen 2020; Gudeman et al. 1987, 1989; Hogue 1949; Tennyson and Pappas 1962) and captured in real time in adult ChP (Shipley et al. 2020). During apocrine secretion, epithelial cells accumulate cytoplasmic material in the form of blebs at their apical surface for rapid release. The composition of apocrine blebs and subsequent cargo that may be released into CSF following apocrine events remain to be elucidated. Peripheral inflammatory signals in an adult mouse model of Alzheimer's disease are also thought to trigger extracellular vesicle release into the CSF (Guha et al. 2019), and increased CSF extracellular vesicles correlate with neuronal damage in HIV patients (Vandendriessche et al. 2021).

32.2.2.2 Ependymal Cells

Postmitotic multi-ciliated ependymal cells, which line the ventricular system of the postnatal brain, have been proposed to contribute to later CSF production. Multi-ciliated ependymal cells that line the mature ventricles and spinal canal are generated by radial glia beginning at E14 in mice and then progressively become postmitotic and mature (Cañizares et al. 2020; Spassky et al. 2005) (Figure 32.7). Early work using in vitro culture of embryonic chick brains described secretory activity of ependymal cells lining the brain ventricles (Weiss 1934). Subsequent studies examining CSF production in adult dog ventricles were only able to reconcile the rate of CSF production by proposing that both the epithelial cells of the ChP and ependymal cells that line the ventricles jointly produce CSF (Bering 1959). Then further supporting this model, in 1967 Pollay and Curl deduced an approximate intraventricular rate of CSF formation of 12.67 microliters/min in the adult rabbit (Pollay and Curl 1967) consistent with ependymal cell contribution to CSF production, but the exact proportions remain under active investigation. Other extra-choroidal sources of CSF include vasculature and meninges (Li et al. 2020). Taken together, these studies lead to a working model that ventricular cells, including both the early progenitor cells that line the ventricle as well as postmitotic ependymal cells, contribute to CSF secretion during development.

32.2.3 Functions of CSF Contents during Early Cerebral Cortical Development

CSF essentially bathes the pool of progenitors that will produce the intermediate progenitors, neurons, and glial cells of the developing cerebral cortex (Haubensak et al. 2004; Namba and Huttner 2017; Stepien et al. 2021), making it a critical part of the developing stem cell niche. CSF composition appears to be tightly and spatiotemporally controlled from the initial neuropore closure up to the formation of the ChP in each ventricle of the brain (Bueno and Garcia-Fernàndez 2016; Lun et al. 2015a). Both CSF protein concentration and the CSF proteome are dynamic, changing essentially daily during the course of development (Chau et al. 2015; Lehtinen et al. 2011). Increasing evidence supports the model that age-appropriate cocktails of CSF factors help ensure that developing neural progenitors remain healthy, acquire the correct progenitor identity, and proliferate in a developmentally appropriate manner (Chau et al. 2015; Lehtinen et al. 2011; Silva-Vargas et al. 2016).

Early studies demonstrating the beneficial, niche-like role for CSF were performed in vitro where explants of developing cerebral cortex from rats were cultured in pure CSF collected from animals of different ages (embryonic to adult ages) or in artificial CSF. Artificial CSF is commonly used by electrophysiologists and is essentially an oxygenated salt solution that matches the ionic composition of

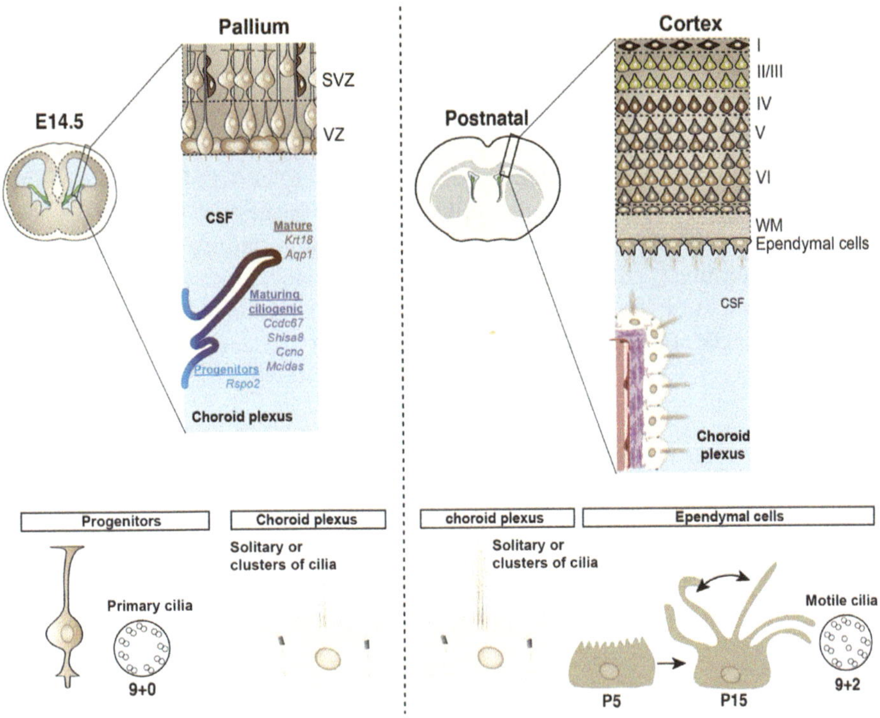

Figure 32.7 Ventricle-contacting cilia through development. Left (upper panel): Schematic of an E14.5 coronal section of a mouse brain. The pallial ventricular zone (VZ) contains CSF-contacting radial glia cell bodies and cilia whereas the subventricular zone (SVZ) comprises intermediate progenitors and immature neurons. Spatial mapping of the lateral ventricle ChP maturation regions marked by progenitors (*Rspo2*), ciliogenesis (*Ccdc67*, *Shisa8*, *Ccno*, and *Mcidas*), and mature differentiated epithelial cells (Krt18 and Aqp1). Left (lower panel): Radial glial progenitors have one primary, nonmotile cilium can detect CSF and transmit these fluid-borne signals to neural progenitors. The pallial progenitor axoneme consists of nine microtubule doublets with an absence of a central microtubule pair, often referred to as a 9 + 0 structure. Right (upper panel): Postnatal coronal section of a mouse brain. The early postnatal cortex has six distinct layers (I–VI) of cell populations that are formed in an "inside-out" manner. At this stage, underneath layer VI is a layer of white matter and postmitotic multi-ciliated ependymal cells. The epithelial cells of the lateral ventricle ChP also have cilia, which project into the CSF. Right (lower panel): Whether the lateral ventricle ChP epithelium harbors continuously motile multi-cilia, transiently motile multi-cilia, solitary primary-like cilia, or clusters of primary-like cilia is still under active investigation. Ependymal cells begin ciliogenesis around P5 in mice and have fully formed motile cilia capable of generating laminar flow by P15. The ependymal cell axoneme consists of nine microtubule doublets that surround a central microtubule pair, often referred to as a 9 + 2 structure.

native CSF but lacks all the proteins and beneficial growth factors therein. These types of experiments revealed that embryonic CSF supported the survival, polarity, and cortical progenitor cell division in cortical explants, closely approximating freshly analyzed in vivo cortex. By contrast, the CSF obtained at other ages, as well as artificial CSF, supported only limited cell division, the cortical tissue failed to thrive and lost its typical polarity. Proteomic studies of the developing CSF revealed that many protein signals in the CSF fluctuate with age. For instance, CSF-IGF2 (insulin-like growth factor 2) levels peak during late embryogenesis in rats (Lehtinen et al. 2011). CSF-IGF2 stimulates cell division by binding to receptors on the surface and primary cilia of neural stem cells. In turn, mouse genetic approaches including loss of *Igf1R* expression by cortical progenitors, or CSF collected from *Igf2*-deficient mice paired with analyses of *Igf2* knockout mouse brain have demonstrated that CSF-IGF2 regulates neurogenesis and ultimately brain size (Lehtinen et al. 2011).

Ex vivo and in vitro culture models have proven useful for testing CSF contributions to cortical development (Figures 32.8, 32.9). Pure CSF obtained from developing embryonic mouse or rat can be used for a variety of experiments ranging from cultured neural stem cells (e.g., pair cells or neurospheres) to tissue explants of the developing forebrain (Figure 32.8). As described earlier, in the explant approach, embryonic cortex dissected from the dorso-lateral cerebral cortex is placed on polycarbonate membranes and floated on defined media. For testing roles of CSF factors, explants can be cultured in 20–100 percent CSF (diluted in artificial CSF with age-specific ion concentrations) (Chau et al. 2015; Xu et al. 2021), fixed, and sectioned for immunostaining to evaluate tissue health, polarity, and proliferation (Lehtinen et al. 2011; Zappaterra et al. 2013). Age-specific effects of CSF on cortical development can be tested in this paradigm by mixing and matching developing brain tissue with different ages of CSF or even AF (Chau et al. 2015). The contributions of specific

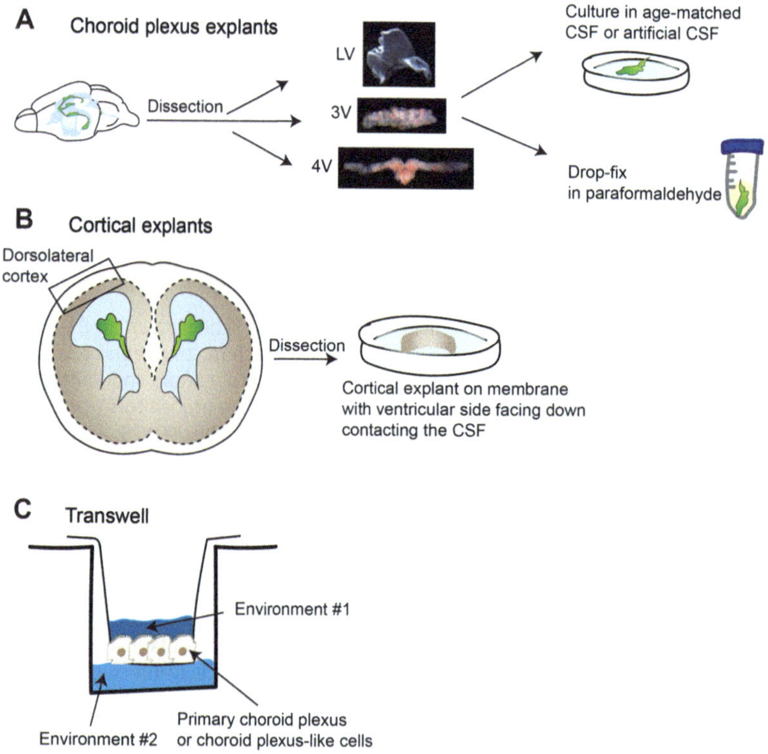

Figure 32.8 Ex vivo experimental approaches for manipulating tissues dependent on the CSF environment. (A) Whole ChP tissues from embryonic tissue are isolated as follows. LV ChP: Cerebral cortical hemispheres are separated. Following incisions into the cortical tissue at either end of the hippocampus, the hippocampus is rolled out using the flat surface of a microscalpel and the underlying LV ChP is separated from the hippocampus/fornix. 3V ChP: The dorsal midline of the midbrain is exposed and 3V ChP is isolated. Hindbrain is separated from the brain. The cisterna magna is exposed by gently guiding away the developing or mature cerebellum to expose the 4V ChP. Adapted from Dani et al. 2021. (B) The telencephalic wall is dissected onto polycarbonate membranes and cultured in artificial CSF. (C) The procedure for culturing primary cells on transwell membranes mirrors standard primary culture. Cells grown on the inner chamber membranes display the same morphology as those grown in culture dishes. The epithelial cells are connected by tight junctions and once they grow to form a confluence they form an impermeable barrier between the medium in the inner and outer chambers. Freely permeable transwell membranes sandwiched between two culture chambers facilitate transport studies of various compounds across this barrier in vitro. Adapted from Monnot and Zheng (2013).

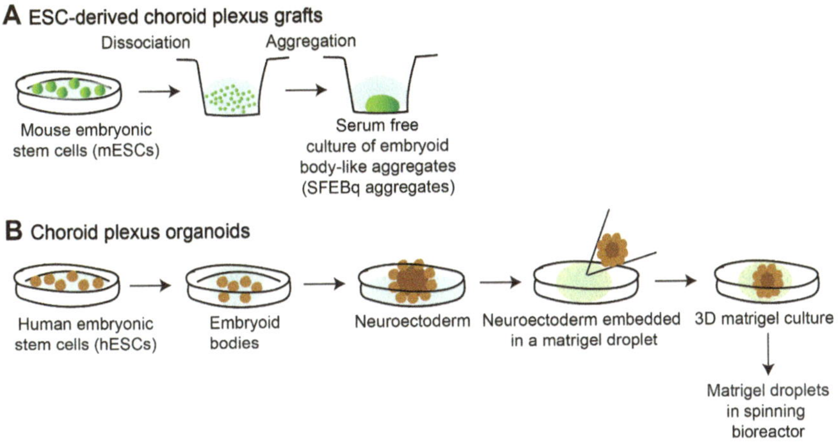

Figure 32.9 In vitro experimental approaches for CSF mediated choroid plexus grafts and organoids. (A) Mouse embryonic stem cell (mESC) derived ChP grafts are formed through a process of dissociation and aggregation to produce serum free culture embryoid body-like aggregates. SFEBqs are capable of inducing multipotential CNS progenitors that can be steered to differentiate into region-specific tissues. (B) To generate neuroectoderm from embryoid bodies, neuroectodermal tissues are maintained in 3D culture and embedded in droplets of Matrigel to provide a scaffold for more complex tissue growth. These Matrigel droplets are then transferred to a spinning bioreactor to enhance nutrient absorption. This method leads to rapid development of brain tissues, termed cerebral organoids, requiring only 8–10 days for the appearance of neural identity and 20–30 days for defined brain regions to form. Adapted from Lancaster et al. (2013).

signaling pathways can be further assayed in gain- and loss-of-function approaches using CSF collected from knockout animals (e.g., *Igf2* knockout CSF), neutralizing/depleting a factor of choice from CSF, or supplementing with a recombinant protein. The contributions of CSF factors to neural development can also be tested in parallel approaches using cultured neural stem cells (neurospheres) (Lehtinen et al. 2011) and in pair cells (Chau et al. 2015).

Collectively, the model of CSF-based signaling during stages of peak neurogenesis in the cerebral cortex has also been extended to (1) the earliest neural stem cells, when the neural tube closes and the AF captured therein forms the first CSF for the nervous system (Chau et al. 2015), and (2) adult neurogenesis in the subventricular zone (SVZ) (Doetsch 2003; Silva-Vargas et al. 2016). The developing cortex displays age and fluid-type preferences for its natural fluid environment. These developmental programs reflect the specific environmental needs of each stem cell pool. For example, the E8.5 neuroectoderm prefers its age-matched AF and the E10.5 neuroepithelium also prefers age-matched CSF as indicated by maintenance of $Sox2^{+}$ progenitors (Chau et al. 2015). A fluid preference also emerges thereafter. E10.5 forebrain progenitors thrive in E10.5 CSF while E10.5 olfactory epithelial cells strongly prefer their natural environment of E10.5 AF over E10.5 CSF (Chau et al. 2015). Thus, matching the correct fluid with age and compartment of neural stem cells is critical for promoting neural stem cell health and identity.

For cortical progenitors to receive signals from the CSF to complement their genetic programs of development, they need to maintain contact with the ventricles. In the context of cerebral cortical development, neuroepithelial cells and radial glial cells are characterized by an apical process with a primary cilium touching the CSF-filled ventricle and a basal process extending to the pial surface (Kim et al. 2010; Louvi and Grove 2011; Spassky and Meunier 2017) (Figure 32.4). When these neural stem cells lose their distinct shape including CSF contacting primary cilia, they prematurely stop dividing and die, resulting in a mouse that survives, but that lacks virtually its entire cerebral cortex (Kim et al. 2010). Nonetheless, cilia in their natural state are known to retract during cell division. In turn, neuroepithelial daughter cells that inherit the apical plasma membrane with the "mother centrioles" that induce primary cilia generation after mitosis are more likely to remain stem-like (Kosodo et al. 2004; Paridaen et al. 2013) further supporting a niche-like role for CSF.

Primary neuroepithelial cilia are signaling hubs that express cilia markers including ADCY3, ARL13b, and SSTR3 and have an axoneme of nine microtubule doublets without a central microtubule pair, referred to as 9 + 0 structure (Figure 32.7). Increasing evidence suggests that primary cilia function as essential sensors of SHH ligand and as regulators for transducing Hedgehog pathway activity, a key signaling molecule for stem cell function in the developing neuroepithelium (based on their expression of GPR161, PTCH, SMO) (Huang et al. 2010). These progenitor primary cilia also express receptors for other CSF borne signals including IGF1R (Lehtinen et al. 2011). Primary cilia are also key signaling centers for neuronal migration. Expression of ARL13b in postmitotic interneurons is required for interneuron migration into the cerebral cortex. This migration defective phenotype in *Arl13b* null interneurons cannot be rescued by Joubert syndrome associated *Arl13b* mutations suggesting that these disease-associated mutations alter *Arl13b* function during interneuron migration (Higginbotham et al. 2012). In addition to its roles on the neuroepithelium, the "hair-like protrusions" of primary cilia serve a guiding and protective role for neurons. Primary cilia on migrating immature interneurons are critical for guiding interneuron migration into the cerebral cortex (Fame et al. 2020; Higginbotham et al. 2012). These findings helped shape the model of progenitor cell morphology, with an apical surface bathed by CSF and a primary cilium that extends into the brain ventricles and allows for synchronized delivery of signals via the CSF that contribute to synchronized construction of the mammalian cerebral cortex.

In the mature brain, CSF factors also regulate adult neurogenesis in the SVZ (Doetsch 2003; Silva-Vargas et al. 2016) and have beneficial effects on hippocampal learning and memory in aging mice (Iram et al. 2022). Thus, CSF-based signaling is now appreciated to span from the earliest stages of mouse brain development, which corresponds to early second trimester of human gestation, to the aging mouse brain.

32.2.3.1 Composition of the Developing CSF

Here we highlight key regulators of gene expression and cellular function that are provided in the CSF niche to support neural development.

32.2.3.2 Proteins and Peptides

32.2.3.2.1 Insulin-like growth factors (IGF)

Insulin-like growth factors 1 and 2 (IGF1 and IGF2) are peptide hormones that regulate cell proliferation, differentiation, migration, and survival (Bergman et al. 2013). These proteins circulate bound to one of the six IGF-binding proteins (IGFBP), IGFBP-1 through IGFBP-6 (Allard and Duan 2018; Bergman et al. 2013; Holly et al. 2019). IGF2 signals through IGF1 receptor (IGF1R), localized on the apical surface survival of cortical progenitors in the ventricular zone and mediates much of the age-dependent effects of CSF has on proliferation and survival (Lehtinen et al. 2011). The presence of both IGF2 and IGF1 in the lateral ventricle CSF, and high expression in the ChP are consistent with secretion by the ChP. IGF2 expression in rat CSF peaks during periods of neurogenesis and declines in adulthood (Lehtinen et al. 2011).

32.2.3.2.2 Sonic hedgehog (SHH)

SHH is a secreted factor essential for embryonic development, serving as a morphogen (Coulter et al. 2018; Roelink et al. 1995), a mitogen (Coulter et al. 2018; Dahmane and Ruiz i Altaba 1999; Nielsen and Dymecki 2010), an axon guidance cue (Charron et al. 2003; Wilson and Stoeckli 2013), and a regulator of synapse formation (Coulter et al. 2018; Harwell et al. 2012). SHH provides instructional cues for progenitor proliferation (Coulter et al. 2018), GABAergic interneuron expansion (Huang et al. 2010), and ChP epithelial vascular outgrowth and surface area, fundamental to the functions of the ChP (Nielsen and Dymecki 2010). SHH is hydrophobic and released into the CSF encapsulated in an extracellular vesicle (Coulter et al. 2018; Huang et al. 2010). In humans, this vesicular release is dependent on the functionality of the microcephaly associated gene, *CHMP1A*, which is a part of the endosomal sorting complex required for transport and release of extracellular vesicles (Coulter et al. 2018).

32.2.3.2.3 Wingless/Integrated (WNTs)

WNTs are a family of highly conserved proteins that greatly influence cell proliferation, polarity, and fate determination of neural stem cells and progenitors through the canonical WNT/β-catenin signaling pathway. WNT4, WNT5, and the WNT modulator, TGM2, play instructive roles in brain and ChP morphogenesis (Johansson et al. 2013; Kaiser et al. 2019; Langford et al. 2020). WNT proteins are secreted and diffuse over varying ranges in the CSF to act upon β-catenin^{+} or β-catenin^{-} target cells (Borday et al. 2018). Once the WNT ligand binds to its Frizzled receptor and co-receptors on β-catenin^{+} cells, β-catenin translocates into the nucleus, and activates WNT target genes, *CyclinD1* and *Axin2* (Borday et al. 2018). Over-activation of WNT signaling increases the abundance of proliferating and neuronal-like cells, while WNT pathway inhibition does the converse (Kriska et al. 2021). Additionally, epithelial WNT5A is an important determinant of fourth ventricle ChP morphogenesis and size in the mouse (Kaiser et al. 2021), thereby likely indirectly influencing the region specific CSF secretome (Dani et al. 2021; Lun et al. 2015a).

32.2.3.2.4 Leukemia inhibitory factor (LIF)

LIF is a pleiotropic cytokine belonging to the interleukin-6 (IL-6) family, and signals via the LIF receptor, LIFRβ, and GP130 heterodimer complex, which includes ciliary neurotrophic factor (CNTR) and cytokines IL-6 and IL-11 (Bauer and Patterson 2006; Salleh and Giribabu 2014). LIF signaling promotes the self-renewal and expansion of a subpopulation of FGF responsive ventricular zone progenitors (Gregg and Weiss 2005). Chau and colleagues saw that age-matched CSF promotes SOX2^{+} neurogenic identity in developing forebrain and olfactory epithelia (Chau et al. 2015). Furthermore, they found that LIFR signaling via nascent CSF partially stimulates self-renewal of SOX2^{+} forebrain progenitor cells (Chau et al. 2015).

32.2.3.2.5 Fibroblast growth factor 2 (FGF2)

FGF2 is a mitogenic factor that signals through FGF receptors (FGFR) 1–4 (V. Kumar et al. 2021). FGF2 plays a role in triggering self-renewal and is involved in neurogenetic induction of mesencephalic neuroepithelial precursor cells during rat embryonic development (Lamus et al. 2020). Lamus et al. (2020) demonstrated that since FGF2 is localized to neuroepithelial precursors near to their CSF interface, FGF2 in the CSF could originate neuroepithelium through apical secretion from progenitors (Lamus et al. 2020). In the early stages of chick embryo development, different isoforms of FGF2 are present in the CSF and serum, and may have an extraneural origin (Martín et al. 2006). FGF2 is directly involved in both the in vivo and in vitro proliferation and neural differentiation of neuroepithelial cells in embryonic chick CSF (Martín et al. 2006).

32.2.3.2.6 Bone morphogenic protein (BMPs)

BMP5 belongs to the transforming growth factor-beta (TGFβ) superfamily that is negatively regulated by proteins noggin (Chen et al. 2004) and chordin (Stottmann et al. 2001). BMP5, along with IGF1, was identified by transcriptomic analysis as a potentially important factor in the lateral ventral

ChP secretome's recruitment of adult subventricular zone stem cells (Silva-Vargas et al. 2016). Particularly, BMP5 (Kangsamaksin and Morris 2011) and IGF1 promote a dramatic increase in epidermal stem cell clone recruitment (Silva-Vargas et al. 2016).

32.2.3.2.7 Orthodenticle homeobox 2 (OTX2)

OTX2 is a homeoprotein secreted by the ChP throughout life (Spatazza et al. 2013) that is proposed to regulate ventricular-subventricular zone neurogenesis in mice (Planques et al. 2019). Secreted OTX2 may also target cells in the visual cortex to regulate visual system plasticity at early postnatal stages (Fame and Lehtinen 2020; Spatazza et al. 2013). OTX2 can impact neuroblast migration by controlling extracellular matrix protein (THBS1, THBS4, etc.) composition and signaling produced by supporting astrocytes (Planques et al. 2019). OTX2 may also act as a key regulator of ChP development (Johansson et al. 2013).

32.2.3.3 Small Molecules and Ions

32.2.3.3.1 Retinoids

Retinoic acid (RA), a lipophilic vitamin A metabolite and morphogen found in the CSF, transforms anterior CNS neural identity to a more posterior neural fate (Alonso et al. 2011; Chang et al. 2016; Durston et al. 1989; Haskell and LaMantia 2005; Lehtinen et al. 2011; Sive et al. 1990). RA is largely synthesized from precursor molecule all-trans retinol, which is converted to all-trans retinaldehyde by retinol dehydrogenases and finally to RA by retinaldehyde dehydrogenases. RA is then carried by retinol binding protein (RBP), which is secreted by the ChP, to target cells (Alonso et al. 2011; Siegenthaler et al. 2009). After RA is internalized, it binds to nuclear retinoic acid receptors (RAR) and retinoid X receptors (RXR), which in turn regulate genes involved in differentiation and axial patterning (Alonso et al. 2011; Siegenthaler et al. 2009). In the mouse, meningeal-derived RA is required for successful corticogenesis (Siegenthaler et al. 2009) whereas in the early embryonic chick, RA is synthesized by the mesencephalic-rhombencephalic isthmus with target cells in the mesencephalic neuroepithelium (Alonso et al. 2011). By containing both RBP and all-trans retinol, the embryonic CSF can regulate RA synthesis while also serving as a potential RA delivery pathway (Alonso et al. 2011). In zebrafish larvae, RBP4 and RA synthesis in the embryonic CSF promotes embryonic neuroepithelial survival (Chang et al. 2016). In human and Rhesus macaque primates, RA responsive genes are enriched in the evolutionarily expanded prefrontal cortex (PFC) during fetal development and RA is concentrated in PFC by RA catabolism in neighboring brain regions (Shibata et al. 2021). RNA-sequencing analysis of mice lacking both components of the RAR-RXR heterodimer or RA catabolic enzyme CYP26B1 further supports critical roles for RA signaling (and its localized enrichment by catabolism) in the development and evolutionary expansion of the PFC (Shibata et al. 2021). Genome-wide association studies (GWAS) have implied overlap between ASD-risk genes and RA-target genes (Kumar et al. 2019), which future studies are needed to explore. The function of RA pathways in corticogenesis and disease processes continue to be investigated and CSF-derived RA signals are a core axis of the pathway.

32.2.3.3.2 Ions

CSF ions Na^+, K^+, Cl^-, Ca^{2+}, Mg^{2+}, and HCO_3^- serve to uphold developmentally critical ion gradients with respect to epithelia, and contribute to overall CSF osmolarity (Nabiuni et al. 2015; Xu et al. 2021). The directional fluid secretion of the ChP epithelium is dependent on an osmotic gradient regulated by the transport of ions Na^+, Cl^-, and HCO_3^- via Na^+/K^+-ATPase, carbonic anhydrase II, AQP1, and NCBE/NBCn2 (Nabiuni et al. 2015; Xu et al. 2021). Xu and colleagues show that CSF ion concentration is dynamic throughout developmental stages E14.5, P0, P7, P14, and adulthood (Table 32.1). Embryonic K^+ concentration is over two-fold higher than in the adult, ~3mM, whereas CSF Na^+ concentrations are similar inbetween the embryo and the adult (Xu et al. 2021). This observation underscores the importance of using ionically age-matched artificial CSF and/or culture media in experiments.

32.2.4 CSF Movement: Fluid Production, Dynamics, and Outflow

32.2.4.1 Fluid Production

Our understanding of CSF water content and secretion is based largely on adult studies (Damkier et al. 2013; MacAulay et al. 2022; Praetorius and Damkier 2017). In these models, the ChP is proposed to be the principal source of water for CSF, although extra-choroidal sources of CSF water (e.g., ependyma, interstitial fluid, and capillaries) are also recognized (Li et al. 2020). ChP water secretion is thought to rely on an osmotic gradient generated by ion and protein transport (Damkier et al. 2013; Praetorius and Damkier 2017). Osmolarity is defined as the difference in solute concentration that drives water movement across this gradient, which results in the production of CSF (Bueno et al. 2014; Fame et al. 2020; Orešković et al. 2017). In the ChP, CSF is produced through the transepithelial movement of ions via ion pumps and macromolecule secretion likely by osmolarity gradients (Brown et al. 2004; Damkier et al. 2013; Fame et al. 2020; Praetorius and Damkier 2017). As described earlier, one example of ion gradients that drive CSF production is the Na^+/K^+ gradient generated by the Na^+/K^+-ATPase. Ouabain, an Na^+/K^+-ATPase inhibitor, has been widely used to assess this role in ChP water and ion flux. Ex vivo preparation of a single structurally intact halved spiny dogfish shark (*Squalus acanthias*) ChP has been used to measure transport of substances across the epithelia including measuring ion flux using flux chambers to show Na^+/K^+-ATPase dependence (Villalobos et al. 2002). In vivo ouabain application in mammals reduces CSF K^+ (Smith and Johanson 1980) in support of this dependence as well. The ion gradient established by the Na^+/K^+-ATPase drives cotransport of additional ions as well (Fame and Lehtinen 2020). In turn, the osmotic pressure created promotes water secretion via Aquaporin 1 (AQP1) channels (Fame and Lehtinen 2020).

Another mechanism of ChP water movement has been proposed to partly rely on NKCC1 (*Slc12a2*), a sodium-potassium-chloride cotransporter. Although NKCC1 represents one of many ion transporters (e.g., Na^+/K^+-ATPase, Kir7.1, NBCe2, AE2) expressed by ChP epithelial cells, work on this particular cotransporter has illuminated many fundamental questions regarding how the field considers transporters of ions and water (Damkier et al. 2013; Delpire 2021; Gregoriades et al. 2019;

Table 32.1 Developmental ion concentrations in mouse CSF. Data from Xu et al. 2021. p: statistical comparison to adult values. * $p < 0.05$; ** $p < 0.01$; *** $p < 0.001$; **** $p < 0.0001$.

	E14.5	P0	P4	P7	P14	Adult
$[K^+]$ mM	7.969 ± 1.90****	9.590 ± 3.50**	4.903 ± 0.47**	4.363 ± 0.92*	3.283 ± 0.18	3.142 ± 0.61
$[Na^+]$ mM	141.1 ± 6.10	126.2 ± 11.84	131.9 ± 4.52	144.5 ± 6.65	137.3 ± 3.22	146.2 ± 14.40
$[Cl^-]$ mM	104.9 ± 5.28**	104.0 ± 3.27**	111.0 ± 2.00*	125.0 ± 2.00	115.1 ± 6.00	127.1 ± 12.01
$[Ca^{2+}]$ mM	3.42 ± 0.47*	3.70 ± 0.84*	2.63 ± 0.21	3.13 ± 0.39*	2.51 ± 0.36	2.24 ± 0.28
$[Mg^{2+}]$ mM	1.76 ± 0.07****	1.07 ± 0.04***	1.09 ± 0.01****	2.04 ± 0.19**	0.53 ± 0.05****	0.89 ± 0.04

MacAulay and Rose 2020; Praetorius and Damkier 2017; Saunders et al. 2018; Steffensen et al. 2018; Xu et al. 2021; Yang et al. 2020). For example, NKCC1 is a bidirectional cotransporter and its transport direction depends on the combined electrochemical gradients for Na^+, K^+, and Cl^-. In the developing mouse brain, CSF-K^+ levels are uniquely high, owing in part to the low expression levels of ChP-NKCC1 compared to adult, and the electrochemical gradient drives the movement of ion from the ventricles into ChP epithelial cells (Xu et al. 2021). Currently, the direction of NKCC1's electrochemical gradient in the adult brain is still under active debate. One mechanism proposes the adult brain electrochemical gradient of NKCC1 is such that ions are cotransported from ChP epithelial cells into the ventricles, and water follows the movement of the ions (MacAulay et al. 2022; Steffensen et al. 2018), whereas another mechanism hypothesizes that in the adult brain, like the developing mouse brain, electrochemical gradient of NKCC1 drives ion transport inward (Damkier et al. 2013; Praetorius and Damkier 2017). When NKCC1 expression is augmented during perinatal mouse development, such as by adeno-associated virus (AAV)-mediated over-expression (Figure 32.7), more NKCC1 is available to move ions across the ChP epithelium and CSF-K^+ levels rapidly decrease to adult levels, resulting in a mouse with unusually small brain ventricles. The resulting mouse provides a model for slit ventricle syndrome, a condition of small ventricles. Harnessing NKCC1 expression levels for the treatment of hydrocephalus in mouse models, NKCC1 over-expression was shown to prevent ventriculomegaly associated with kaolin-induced obstructive hydrocephalus (Xu et al. 2021) and post-hemorrhagic hydrocephalus (Sadegh et al., 2023). Leveraging the ChP as a tissue to remove CSF-water and ions provides a provocative new handle for the potential treatment of hydrocephalus. While exciting, many details about this process remain to be answered.

32.2.4.2 CSF Movement and Fluid Dynamics

One key role of the CSF entails transporting signaling molecules and eliminating waste. These functions implicate movement and/or flow. Fluid dynamics of CSF during the early stages of cortical development are quite different from those in adults, indicating potentially unique CSF movement during corticogenesis. CSF signaling molecules move from their source to target cells principally via volume transmission in the CSF through energy gradients (temperature, pressure, and concentration gradients) (Borroto-Escuela et al. 2015). Current data suggest that CSF movement is pulsatile, rather than purely directional, a model that is well accepted in adults (Brinker et al. 2014; Dreha-Kulaczewski et al. 2018; Fultz et al. 2019). As researchers aim to fully uncover mechanistically how this occurs, more questions arise such as: is this CSF movement a feature? In this section, we will spotlight model organisms used to explore CSF flow, and how they are used to overcome this limitation. Although the exact mechanism of CSF movement is debated (Brinker et al. 2014; Orešković and Klarica 2014; Orešković et al. 2016), this section aims to introduce developmental fluid homeostasis, the historical context of CSF circulation, the models currently used to study CSF movement, the proposed role of cilia in CSF flow, and suggested CSF outflow routes.

Historically, studying CSF movement has been difficult due to the ventricles being situated deep within the brain. Progress in understanding directionality and flow dynamics of very early CSF has been made using tracking in more accessible models like *Xenopus* (Hagenlocher et al. 2013; Miskevich 2010) and zebrafish (Fame et al. 2016; Olstad et al. 2019). The *Danio rerio* zebrafish larva is used as an in vivo model due to its tractable system with the advantage of genetics, small size, and transparency for exploring ventricular physiology and for mounting large-scale high throughput experiments (Fame et al. 2016; Olstad et al. 2019; Turner et al. 2012). While it is important to note that in zebrafish, the early formation of the ventricular system occurs through a distinct process with the opening of a solid neural keel rather than a classic neural tube closure

(Clarke 2009), their entire developmental period is external and early larvae are amenable to live imaging studies. This model organism provides evidence for a partially heart beat-dependent directional movement model of embryonic CSF during a major period of neurogenesis (Fame et al. 2016). Imaging and genetic reporters in the transparent zebrafish body also enabled striking developmental discoveries about how CSF dynamics are also tightly controlled in the spinal canal. For example at 24–30 hour post-fertilization (hpf) evidence has been presented that shows that CSF flows bidirectionally in the central canal and can affect spinal curvature (Böhm et al. 2016; Cantaut-Belarif et al. 2018; Sternberg et al. 2018). In the central canal of the spinal cord in 30 hpf zebrafish, experiments and modeling/simulations suggest that CSF flow is generated locally by caudally polarized motile cilia along the ventral wall of the central canal, and that bidirectional flow accelerates the transport of particles in the CSF via a coupled convective-diffusive transport process (Thouvenin et al. 2020).

In the African clawed frog *Xenopus laevis*, the cilia-driving gene *foxj1* is required for normal ciliogenesis and CSF flow in tadpole-stage embryos (Hagenlocher et al. 2013). Optical coherence tomography (OCT), a cross-sectional imaging modality provides evidence for a model that suggests during the developing tailbud and early tadpole stages ependymal cell cilia-driven CSF flow generates currents that are independent of cardiac pulsatile forces (Dur et al. 2020). This model also suggests that cilia-driven flow may also regulate spatial neural cell organization because the loss of cilia derived CSF circulation leads to the mispatterning of dorsal telencephalic transcription factor *Emx1* (Dur et al. 2020).

In mice, ciliated epithelia in the adult third ventricle can generate and maintain reliable yet periodically switching flow networks. Evidence from preparations of mouse, rat, and pig ventricular walls have revealed CSF flow directionality and its correlations to ciliary beating patterns and neuroblast migration (Faubel et al. 2016; Sawamoto et al. 2006), supporting the model that rats and pigs have complex, cilia-driven CSF flow patterns too (Faubel et al. 2016; Miyan et al. 2003). Adding to this model, PKD1 and PKD2, which are characterized as mechanosensory proteins in the kidney, localize to primary cilia in radial glial cells (RGCs) in mice, and their ablation disrupts the development of planar cell polarity in these cells (Ohata et al. 2015) prior to ependymal cell maturation.

In humans, CSF movement is associated with heartbeat and respiration (Dreha-Kulaczewski et al. 2018; Fultz et al. 2019; Wagshul et al. 2011) and plays a protective role in the brain by lessening the pulsatile beat-induced pressure (Mestre et al. 2018). When the heart muscle contracts and pumps blood into the arteries at systole, this results in an increase in blood flow, and cerebral blood volume. CSF outflow relieves some of this transient pressure that could otherwise be damaging (Bakshi et al. 2000). When the heart relaxes and allows blood to fill the chambers once again at diastole, the CSF is led back into the interstitial fluid and ventricles (Brinker et al. 2014). CSF movement is also coupled to neuronal function (Brinker et al. 2014). For example, neural slow waves in non-REM sleep induce hemodynamic changes that have been shown to generate wave-like CSF motion (Fultz et al. 2019). These observations suggest that early CSF movement is not solely based on directionality, but is also wave like and pulsatile (Brinker et al. 2014).

32.2.4.3 Motile Cilia Generated Flow

Cells that line the brain ventricles during development can be mono- or multi-ciliated, which temporally varies across cell type and species, and play roles in brain development and function (Fame et al. 2020) (Figure 32.7). As discussed earlier, mammalian neuroepithelial cells harbor primary cilia that regulate signaling (Fame et al. 2020). Radial glial progenitors have one primary, nonmotile cilium with mechanosensors (see earlier) that can detect CSF and transmit fluid-borne signals to neural progenitors (Ohata et al. 2015). As the brain continues to develop, progenitor zones transition to the mature ventricle lining, ependyma. Ependymal cells begin ciliogenesis around P5 in mice and have fully formed motile cilia capable of generating laminar flow by P15 (Mahuzier et al. 2018; Redmond et al. 2019) (Figure 32.7). Multi-cilia, which can be highly motile, are crucial in regulating the distribution of CSF within and across brain ventricles (Olstad et al. 2019) and often express cilia-related proteins including FOXJ1, cMYB, and GMNC. Motile cilia move via axonemal dyneins, which create sliding interactions between outer microtubules while intraflagellar transport proteins carry cargo into and out of the cilium (Ringers et al. 2020). The axoneme consists of nine microtubule doublets that surround a central microtubule pair, often referred to as a 9 + 2 structure (Ringers et al. 2020) (Figure 32.7).

ChP cilia are still the subject of ongoing investigation. In the early to late larva stage of the zebrafish ChP epithelium, the cilia are motile (D'Gama et al. 2021). In embryonic zebrafish, *foxj1a*, but not *foxj1b*, is rapidly induced in response to epithelial distension and stretch, and this expression is required for cilia motility (Hellman et al. 2010). It is proposed that during early mouse and porcine development ChP epithelium harbor motile multi-cilia, but later on lose this motility (Inoue et al. 2015; Narita et al. 2010; Narita and Takeda 2015; Nonami et al. 2013) (Figure 32.4). This hypothesis is still under active investigation. Some research groups have found solitary or clusters of primary-like cilia or cilia with 9 + 2, 9 + 0 or atypical microtubule arrangements (Banizs et al. 2005; Davenport and Yoder 2005; Swiderski et al. 2012; Yoder 2007), suggesting additional in-depth investigation is needed. The varying forms of cilia may reflect the diverse functional needs of their respective fluid environments. Mature ventricular neural stem and ependymal cells also have primary cilia, which project into the CSF of the ventricle (Mirzadeh et al. 2010; Ringers et al. 2020).

32.2.4.4 CSF Outflow Routes

CSF outflow permits CSF turnover and clearance. Historically, our understanding of CSF outflow stems from studies in adult human brain suggesting that CSF exits the subarachnoid space through specialized structures called arachnoid villi or granulations, which extend to the dura mater (Proulx 2021). However, to date, there is no definitive anatomical mechanism for how all CSF exits the brain, causing continued speculation and debate (Proulx 2021). There are several current proposed routes for CSF outflow from the brain: arachnoid projections (villi or granulations), routes through foramina in the skull along cranial nerves (including the cribriform plate), and lymphatic vessels of the dura mater that clear over half of the spinal canal CSF (Jacob et al. 2019; Pollay 2010; Proulx 2021). Recently, a new route into the skull bone marrow was also proposed (Pulous et al. 2022).

Critically, none of these proposed CSF outflow routes are mature at the time of cerebral cortical development. Arachnoid granulations have only been identified in humans, and they do not emerge until gestational week 39 and mature around 2 years of age (Gómez et al. 1982). Dural lymphatics participate in the clearance of CSF components beginning around E18 or birth and continue to mature throughout the first postnatal month in mice (Antila et al. 2017), but how these systems connect is an area of active investigation. The maturation of meningeal lymphatics depends on expression of VEGF-C and VEGFR3 by endothelial cells destined to differentiate into meningeal lymphatic vessels (Antila et al. 2017). After maturation, these developmental cues must be maintained and these vessels regress if VEGF-C and VEGFR3 are blocked postnatally (Antila et al. 2017).

The late arrival of these outflow routes raises the question of how CSF volume is modulated during earlier developmental stages. One important phenomenon is that directional CSF movement in the very early ventricular system (i.e., before ChP generation) is very slow (Fame et al. 2016; Olstad et al. 2019). This low velocity is consistent with a model of ventricular system expansion without substantial outflow. Further supporting this model, protein accumulates in the young CSF of multiple species and peaks around time of birth in rodents, before normalizing to adult levels (Saunders et al. 2018, 2023). The ChP can bidirectionally transport ions and some evidence indicates that CSF can outflow through young ChP (see earlier, Xu et al. 2021). Ultimately, the full complement of CSF routes that handle CSF production and outflow must develop to properly regulate fluid volume and solute concentrations in the CSF. However, water transport during corticogenic developmental stages remains incompletely understood.

32.2.5 Barrier Properties

The embryonic fluid and cellular environments are tightly regulated to provide a stable environment to support its normal function (Saunders et al. 2018). After neural tube closure, the neuroepithelium acts as an early brain–CSF barrier (Saunders et al. 2018). As it emerges and matures, the embryonic ChP will also perform barrier functions through tight junctions on ChP epithelial cells, expression of metabolic detoxifying enzymes, and transcytosis of signaling molecules between the blood and the CSF via the ChP epithelium (Fame and Lehtinen 2020). ChP blood–CSF barrier roles emerge prior to blood–brain barrier (BBB) development, whose key features mature during E15.5 in mice, E15 in rats, and between days 3 and 10 post-fertilization (dpf) in zebrafish (Ben-Zvi et al. 2014; O'Brown et al. 2018). This timeline highlights the possibility that the barrier mechanisms in the developing brain appropriately match each stage of its development, and change in response to the needs of its environment (Saunders et al. 2018).

The first CSF barrier to arise in development is the CSF–brain barrier, which exists at the ventricular surface before ChP or ependymal cells are present and mature (Davson and Segal 1996; Ek et al. 2001; Fossan et al. 1985; Johansson et al. 2008; Møllgård and Saunders 1986). A landmark study using sheep with horseradish peroxidase (HRP) injected into the ventricular CSF space at low volume so as to not disrupt the barrier, revealed that early (E60) HRP was restricted to the ventricular zone, but later in development (E125), HRP penetrated ~3mm further into the brain parenchyma (Fossan et al. 1985). This study indicates that a robust CSF–brain barrier exists at the neural progenitor zones early in development. This finding has also been demonstrated in rats with immuno-EM, showing localization of IGF2 to the ventricular surface without further penetration into the parenchymal space (Lehtinen et al. 2011). The CSF–brain barrier creates a unique, polarized environment for ventricularly positioned progenitors like RGCs that give rise to the neocortex, thus tightly tying these polarized progenitors to the CSF as a restricted niche-like environment.

Once the ChP emerges, it very quickly develops properties of the mature blood–CSF barrier (BCSFB) including tight junctions, efflux transporters, and selective transport via transcytosis. Fenestrated capillaries of the highly vascularized ChP enable systemic cues to reach the basal surface of ChP epithelial cells, thus the BCSFB forms at apico-laterally localized tight junctions (Figure 32.4). In humans, the early ChP emerges during gestational week 7 and expression of the tight-junction associated enzyme occludin-1 is present already during gestational week 8 (Kratzer et al. 2012). Additional barrier functions are carried out through enzymatic processing of systemic signals to limit their access to the CSF. Developmentally, expression of these enzymes changes such that the major efflux transporter *Slc22a8* (OAT3) increases expression in ChP as maturation proceeds (Strazielle and Ghersi-Egea 2015). Other sets of efflux transporters decrease in expression as the tissue reaches adult function (e.g., *Abcg2*, *Abcc9*, *Abcb1b*) (Strazielle and Ghersi-Egea 2015) suggesting life-stage specific requirements of specific enzymatic functions and thus, potentially, CSF components.

A number of technical advances have contributed to the study of the BCSFB. While primary culture of human ChP cells from embryonic or adult post-mortem tissue is possible, the cell sources remain relatively difficult to obtain and, in the case of patient samples, are highly variable between preparations. Classically, primary ChP cells or cell lines from ChP carcinoma and papilloma have been cultured on transwell filters to enable more high-throughput screening of barrier properties (Figure 32.8). This is because plating these epithelial cells on transwell membranes enables the creation of two distinct environments – one on either side of the membrane – which has been used to study transport of specific molecules from one side of the BCSFB model to the other (Blazer-Yost et al. 2011a, Blazer-Yost et al. 2011b; Hulme et al. 2022; Kratzer et al. 2018; Monnot and Zheng 2013; Preston et al. 2018; Strazielle and Ghersi-Egea 1999). However, complex three-dimensional (3-D) structures of the tissue and the complexity of cell types are lost. Additionally, polarization is often disrupted, tight junctions in these models lack functional organization, and the cells fail to recapitulate the proper monolayer "cobblestone-like" morphology of ChP epithelium (Hochstetler et al. 2022; Redzic 2013). Thus, monoculture systems are experimentally useful to study cell-type-specific barrier functions but remain limited in their ability to recapitulate whole systems. Organoids have the potential to address some of these caveats for culture-based study of the BCSFB (Figure 32.9). Directed differentiation of ChP epithelial cells has been described (Watanabe et al. 2012) and these derived epithelial cells were successfully grafted into mouse ChP, opening a path for potential cellular therapeutics (discussed more in Section 32.3). Forebrain-directed organoids have spontaneously generated variable amounts of ChP-like tissue (Lancaster et al. 2013; Quadrato and Arlotta 2017). More recently, novel methods have been developed to bias organoids to generate human ChP-like structures by treating human telencephalic organoids (Lancaster et al. 2013) with temporally restricted application of ChP-inducing signaling molecules – morphogens BMP4 and WNT prompt embryonic stem cells to adopt ChP epithelial identity (Watanabe et al. 2012) – to form a 3-D culture of ChP epithelial-like and stromal cells (Pellegrini et al. 2020b). This model produces and intra-organoid fluid that approximates elements of native CSF and may be useful in evaluating species differences, barrier properties, and susceptibility to infections like those from the SARS-CoV2 virus (Pellegrini et al. 2020a; Pellegrini et al. 2020b). These organoid models still have limitations including lack of mesenchymal, endothelial, or immune components present in vivo.

Since the 3-D structure and cellular diversity of ChP tissue is so important to understanding barrier and secretory processes, other models are required for more physiological behavior. Mouse-derived ChP explants embedded in Matrigel have been shown to form a lumen and allow study of immune cell migration in the ChP (Petersen et al. 2020) (Figure 32.9). ChP tissue explants (Figure 32.8A) better maintain relative cell type and tight junction organization compared to the culture isolated cell systems on transwells, they are usually derived from rodents and therefore unable to reflect the expanded human ChP compared to ChP with more abundant stromal tissue and some distinct transporters on the epithelial membrane (Liddelow 2015). For example, mouse and guinea pig derived ChP explants have been used as a model to study and modulate the polarized localization of some transporters (Ulloa et al. 2019). When applied with the specific caveats in mind, cell culture, organoid systems, and tissue explants together will continue to inform the current understanding of how this BCSFB regulates the developing CSF environment of the brain.

Transcytosis, a form of selective transport, is another property of the mature BCSFB. Transcytosis allows selective transport of systemic cues into the CSF through ChP. Experimental evaluation of transcytosis maturation is largely lacking, but gene expression of major molecular components including SNARE component SNAP-26 and transcripts encoding caveolar proteins CAV1 and CAV2 are already expressed by ChP epithelial cells at E16.5 at levels higher than adult values, while another caveolar protein CAV3 is expressed higher in mature ChP (Dani et al. 2021), consistent with an early higher level of transcytosis and a tighter transcytosis barrier later in life, although this remains to be experimentally validated. In sum, the ChP BCSF barrier arises quickly after the tissue emerges, but there are likely developmental time specific barrier properties that differentially support the developing CSF and brain.

32.3 Tools and Therapeutics

32.3.1 Approaches to Modulate CSF Composition

CSF provides an important fluid niche for the developing brain, and therefore, experimentally manipulating and analyzing the fluid itself is critical. CSF sampling in developmental models like mouse, sheep, opossum, and zebrafish have proven useful for understanding the changing composition of this fluid. From such sampling, it has been shown that overall protein concentrations and albumin concentration is higher in early development than in adult. Experimentally, this fluid can be subjected to polyacrylamide gel electrophoresis and silver staining or immunoblotting to identify specific components. ELISA assays (sandwich or FACS-based) enable high-sensitivity and multiplexing, which is beneficial to analyzing small volumes of fluid. CSF can be analyzed for metabolites, neurotransmitters, cells, and ions. In large enough brains, microdialysis can be employed for long-term real-time measurements of specific CSF components (Cirrito et al. 2003; Thelin et al. 2014). Bulk CSF sampling alone, however, does not discriminate between the tissue sources of specific components (Figure 32.10A). One approach for getting around this challenge is to isolate potential source tissues and sample their conditioned medium in vitro. For example, sampling ChP-conditioned medium has provided insight into differential ChP secretomes across ventricles and during development (Figure 32.8). Further technological innovation is still needed to achieve multiplexed, real-time analysis of CSF in developing and adult brains.

Targeting the ChP to express proteins provides one powerful strategy for changing the composition of the CSF. Here, we summarize some of the most-common strategies (reviewed in Jang and Lehtinen 2022). As non-inducible genetic reporters or recombination lines are systemic and temporally unrestricted, other methods are required for acute, restricted intervention. A celebrated method for targeting the developing cerebral cortex, electroporation, depends on using electrical current to directionally drive plasmids delivered into the ventricular system into progenitor zones. However, the ChP is circuitous and present throughout the brain ventricles making ChP targeted electroporation inefficient and nonspecific. Therefore, viral delivery approaches have proven to be much more useful for ChP targeting. Viruses (including AAV, adenovirus, and lentivirus) with preferred tropism to ChP over other brain tissues have been identified and can be delivered intracerebroventricularly (ICV) (Figure 32.10C). The hybrid serotype AAV2/5, which incorporates the genome of AAV2 and the capsid of AAV5, has proven tropism for ChP epithelial cells and produces robust expression (Jang and Lehtinen 2022; Jang et al. 2022). Embryonic ICV delivery of AAV2/5 is followed by ChP transduction in as soon as two days, and gene expression can be sustained for months (Cui et al. 2020; Haddad et al. 2013; Jang et al. 2022; Kaiser et al. 2021; Xu et al. 2021) (Figure 32.10C). This approach can be used to modulate CSF composition by expression of transporters (e.g., ATP7A or NKCC1), morphogens (e.g., SHH), cytokines (e.g., CCL2), and antioxidants (e.g., SOD3), all with robust impact on brain development.

Careful and innovative use of a variety of model organisms and culture systems has greatly expanded our knowledge of how the CSF and brain ventricular system develop, including the neuroepithelium and ChP. In turn, this work has informed our ability to modulate the fluid environment of the developing cortex. Additional tools like ChP specific inducible mouse lines, single-cell sequencing atlases (Dani et al. 2021), and ex utero surgical and imaging access in mouse embryos

(Cui et al. 2020) continue to move the field forward and enable unprecedented insight into how to manipulate this developing system (Figure 32.10B).

32.3.2 Therapeutic Potential for Neurodevelopmental Disorders

CSF dysregulation is well established in hydrocephalus; however, support for CSF participation in a variety of neurodevelopmental processes is growing to include ASD, schizophrenia/ schizoaffective disorder (SZ), and bipolar disorder (BD). For example, an increase in extra-axial CSF surrounding the brain (i.e., in the subarachnoid space) in infants is one pre-diagnostic predictive feature of high-risk patients who later develop ASD (Shen et al. 2017, 2018). This increase in

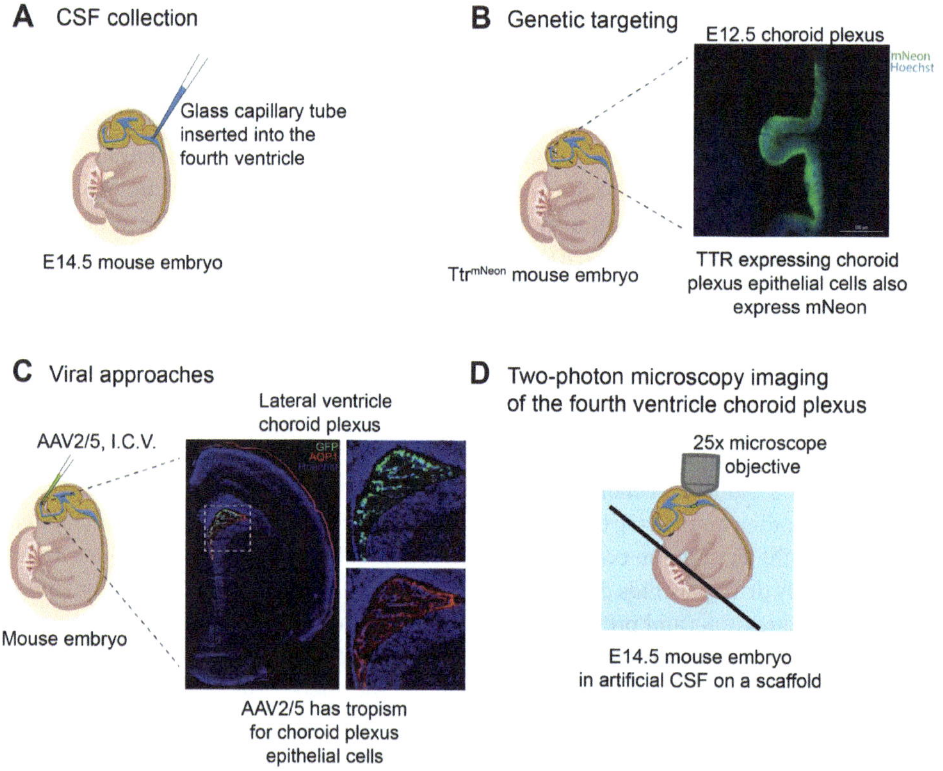

Figure 32.10 In vivo experimental approaches for sampling, manipulating, and visualizing the CSF choroid plexus interface. (A) CSF at E14.5 is collected by inserting a glass capillary into cisterna magna, and processed as described in Zappaterra et al. (2013). Location/angle of insertion varies depending on developmental stage. Samples are pooled across litters and their purity was verified under the dissection scope. Adapted from Lehtinen et al. (2011). (B) E12.5 ChP epithelial cells that express transthyretin (TTR) also express mNeon (green) in the TTR^{mNeon} mouse. Tissue was also stained with Hoechst (blue) to mark nuclei. Adapted from Fame et al. (pers. comm.). (C) GFP expression in LV ChP following in utero ICV delivery of AAV2/5-GFP. AAV2/5 delivered at E13.5 and immunostained 5 days later at E18.5 with anti-GFP (green) and anti-AQP1 (red) antibodies. Tissue stained with Hoechst (blue) to mark nuclei. Dashed line box highlights detection of AAV2/5-GFP and AQP1 expression in the ChP epithelium. Adapted from Jang and Lehtinen (2022). (D) Timed-pregnant mice (E14.5) are anesthetized with isoflurane and placed on a heating pad. A laparotomy is performed, and embryos are gently exposed. Vasculature labeling is achieved by adapting a previous liver injection protocol from Ben-Zvi et al. (2014). Texas Red-Dextran is delivered into the developing liver using a fine-tip glass capillary tube. The embryos and the placenta are carefully transferred into an imaging chamber filled with continuously circulating artificial CSF at 37°C. Adapted from Cui et al. (2020).

extra-axial CSF was not associated with people who later developed SZ, implicating that this specific CSF abnormality is preferentially associated with ASD or at least earlier-presenting neurological disorders (Murphy et al. 2020; Peterson et al. 2021). CSF abnormalities can also be associated with later-presenting neuropsychiatric diseases. Ventricular enlargement has been suggested to be an indicator for prodromal SZ presenting before the onset of psychosis (Sayo et al. 2012; Steen et al. 2006). Psychiatric diseases including depression and SZ have been reported to be associated with CSF composition changes with CSF biomarkers including higher CSF glucose and lower CSF lactate dehydrogenase when compared to BD, implicating both brain metabolism and CSF dysregulation in specific early- and long-term psychosis diagnosis (Gilmore 2010; Giné-Servén et al. 2022). Reduced corticotropin releasing hormone (CRH) in CSF and increased cortisol metabolites in urine have also been suggested as biomarkers for SZ and BD (Ishiwata et al. 2020; Steen et al. 2014), implicating CSF in reflecting the involvement of stress in the presentation of these disorders. These findings inspire future research to elucidate whether these associations are due to CSF as a primary driver of disease, or if cellular imbalance of ions, for example, is the primary driver of CSF changes during disease, with CSF phenotypes as secondary consequences.

A subset of pediatric cancers including tumors along ventricular surface, CNS metastases, and ChP tumors also present with CSF changes. Choroid plexus neoplasms (choroid plexus papilloma [CPP] and choroid plexus carcinoma [CPC]) represent rare tumors of early childhood, with median age of onset of 3.5 years (Mishra et al. 2012; Safaee et al. 2013; Shannon et al. 2018). They result in obstruction of CSF flow, and surgical resection remains the only effective therapy for these tumors. Nevertheless, they can recur and metastasize, with devastating consequences. Along the lateral ventricular surface is a common location for the spread of diffuse intrinsic pontine glioma (DIPG) in both adult and pediatric patients (Caretti et al. 2014; Qin et al. 2017). Recent studies of factors governing this selective spread implicate pleiotrophin derived from the lateral ventricle progenitors (Qin et al. 2017), which leads to the hypothesis that it could also alter CSF pleiotrophin levels. CSF has been directly implicated in metastasis as well. Specifically, CSF cytology from patients with leptomeningeal metastases of neuroblastoma or carcinomas has identified carcinogenic cells in CSF (Blatt et al. 1997; Lin et al. 2017; Martirosian et al. 2021). Interestingly these cells adapt to the nutrient poor CSF by changing gene expression to alter their metabolism including using GABA as an energy source (Martirosian et al. 2021), inspiring future studies to limit this CSF-based spread. How these tumor cells enter the CSF in the first place is also an important question and the blood-CSF barrier at the ChP has been implicated as a previously underappreciated entry site for circulating tumor cells into the brain (Vandenhaute et al. 2015).

32.4 Summary and Future Directions for the Field

32.4.1 Summary

- The developing mammalian brain ventricular system comprises four ventricles, the neural progenitor cells that line their walls, and the CSF within them.
- The CSF is known for providing a protective fluid cushion and sink for waste, but it also delivers important health and growth promoting factors for the developing brain.
- Developmentally regulated mechanisms support development of the primordial cerebral cortex also alter AF/CSF composition.
- Collectively, CSF components such as, IGFs, SHH, WNTs, LIF, OTX2, FGFs, BMPs, retinoids, ions, nanovesicles, and organelles, can modulate gene expression and cellular function to support neural development via the CSF niche.

- CSF is produced by the choroid plexus, but it is proposed that ventricular cells likely contribute to CSF secretion during development as well.
- Numerous in vivo, ex vivo, and in vitro approaches are used to modulate and study the role of CSF during corticogenesis.
- Modern neurology has leveraged CSF as a useful tool for diagnostics, and it is commonly sampled for biomarkers of neurologic diseases in the clinical setting.

32.4.2 Future Directions

32.4.2.1 Modulating CSF Composition?

Are there mechanisms in place in the ChP to sense and actively respond to CSF factors that are needed?

32.4.2.2 CSF Fluid Clearance from Developing Ventricles?

Mature CSF exits the CNS via several potential routes. None of these routes appear to be formed during the stage of cerebral cortical development. Does CSF accumulate factors, good and bad, and only turn over postnatally after clearance routes begin to form? Or, is there some CSF turnover / clearance from the embryonic mouse brain that has yet to be discovered?

32.4.2.3 Clearance of Toxic Factors from Developing CSF?

Mature ChP epithelium also clears toxic and undesirable molecules from CSF (Balusu et al. 2016). Functionally, this process involves basal surface ion transporters moving substances from the blood of the ChP fenestrated capillaries, then transcellular transport across the ChP stroma, and finally selective secretion of these components into the CSF (Fame and Lehtinen 2020). The degree to which this occurs during development is not well understood.

Acknowledgments

We apologize to investigators whose work could not be referenced owing to space limitations. We thank Dr N. Chamberlin, and members of the Lehtinen lab for helpful discussions and reading of this manuscript. This work was supported by the Bill and Melinda Gates Millennium Scholars Program (T.E.L.), NIH T32 HL110852 and OFD/BTREC/CTREC Faculty Development Fellowship Award (R.M.F.) NIH R01 NS088566, and the New York Stem Cell Foundation (M.K.L.).

References

Agnew, W.F. et al. (1980). Protein synthesis and transport by the rat choroid plexus and ependyma. *Cell Tissue Res* 208 (2): 261–281.

Alam, C. et al. (2019). Upregulation of reduced folate carrier by vitamin D enhances brain folate uptake in mice lacking folate receptor alpha. *Proc Natl Acad Sci U S A* 116 (35): 17531–17540.

Allard, J.B. and Duan, C. (2018). IGF-binding proteins *Front Endocrinol* 9: 117.

Alonso, M.I. et al. (1999). Involvement of sulfated proteoglycans in embryonic brain expansion at earliest stages of development in rat embryos. *Cells, Tissues, Organs* 165 (1): 1–9.

Alonso, M.I. et al. (2011). Cerebrospinal fluid control of neurogenesis induced by retinoic acid during early brain development. *Dev Dyn* 240 (7): 1650–1659.

Antila, S. et al. (2017). Development and plasticity of meningeal lymphatic vessels. *J Exp Med* 214 (12): 3645–3667.

Awatramani, R. et al. (2003). Cryptic boundaries in roof plate and choroid plexus identified by intersectional gene activation. *Nat Genet* 35 (1): 70–75.

Bakshi, R. et al. (2000). Intraventricular CSF pulsation artifact on fast fluid-attenuated inversion-recovery MR images. *Am J Neuroradiol* 21 (3): 503–508.

Balusu, S. et al. (2016). Identification of a novel mechanism of blood–brain communication during peripheral inflammation via choroid plexus-derived extracellular vesicles. *EMBO Mol Med* 8 (10): 1162–1183.

Banizs, B. et al. (2005). Dysfunctional cilia lead to altered ependyma and choroid plexus function, and result in the formation of hydrocephalus. *Development* 132 (23): 5329–5339.

Bauer, S. and Patterson, P.H. (2006). Leukemia inhibitory factor promotes neural stem cell self-renewal in the adult brain. *J Neurosci* 26 (46): 12089–12099.

Ben-Zvi, A. et al. (2014). Mfsd2a is critical for the formation and function of the blood-brain barrier. *Nature* 509 (7501): 507–511.

Bergman, D. et al. (2013). Insulin-like growth factor 2 in development and disease: a mini-review. *Gerontology* 59 (3): 240–249.

Bering, E.A., Jr. (1959). Cerebrospinal fluid production and its relationship to cerebral metabolism and cerebral blood flow. *Am J Physiol* 197: 825–828.

Bharucha, T. et al. (2019). Mass spectrometry-based proteomic techniques to identify cerebrospinal fluid biomarkers for diagnosing suspected central nervous system infections. A systematic review. *J Infection* 79 (5): 407–418.

Blatt, J. et al. (1997). Recognition of central nervous system metastases in children with metastatic primary extracranial neuroblastoma. *Pediatr Hematol Oncol* 14 (3): 233–241.

Blazer-Yost, B.L. et al. (2011a). Effect of carbon nanoparticles on renal epithelial cell structure, barrier function, and protein expression. *Nanotoxicology* 5 (3): 354–371.

Blazer-Yost, B.L. et al. (2011b). Lysophosphatidic acid is a modulator of cyst growth in autosomal dominant polycystic kidney disease. *Cell Physiol Biochem* 28 (6): 1255–1264.

Böhm, U.L. et al. (2016). CSF-contacting neurons regulate locomotion by relaying mechanical stimuli to spinal circuits. *Nat Commun* 7: 10866.

Borday, C. et al. (2018). An atlas of Wnt activity during embryogenesis in Xenopus tropicalis. *PloS One* 13 (4): e0193606.

Borroto-Escuela, D.O. et al. (2015). The role of transmitter diffusion and flow versus extracellular vesicles in volume transmission in the brain neural–glial networks. *Phil Trans Royal Soc London. Ser B, Biol Sci* 370 (1672): 20140183.

Bräutigam, K. et al. (2019). Pathogenesis of idiopathic normal pressure hydrocephalus. *J Clin Neurosci* 61: 10–13.

Brinker, T. et al. (2014). A new look at cerebrospinal fluid circulation. *Fluids Barriers CNS* 11 (1): 10.

Brown, C.H. et al. (2004). Phasic bursts in rat magnocellular neurosecretory cells are not intrinsically regenerative in vivo. *Eur J Neurosci* 19 (11): 2977–2983.

Bueno, D. and Garcia-Fernàndez, J. (2016). Evolutionary development of embryonic cerebrospinal fluid composition and regulation. *Fluids Barriers CNS* 13 (1): 5.

Bueno, D. et al. (2014). Embryonic blood-cerebrospinal fluid barrier formation and function. *Front Neurosci* 8: 343.

Cañizares, M.A. et al. (2020). Multiple steps characterise ventricular layer attrition to form the ependymal cell lining of the adult mouse spinal cord central canal. *J Anatomy* 236 (2): 334–350.

Cantaut-Belarif, Y. et al. (2018). The Reissner fiber in the cerebrospinal fluid controls morphogenesis of the body axis. *Curr Biol* 28 (15): 2479–2486.e4.

Caretti, V. et al. (2014). Subventricular spread of diffuse intrinsic pontine glioma. *Acta Neuropathol* 128 (4): 605–607.

Cavanagh, M.E. et al. (1983). Comparison of proteins in CSF of lateral and IVth ventricles during early development of fetal sheep. *Brain Res* 313 (2): 159–167.

Chang, J.T. et al. (2016). Zebrafish cerebrospinal fluid mediates cell survival through a retinoid signaling pathway. *Dev Neurobiol* 76 (1): 75–92.

Chang, J.T. et al. (2012). Multiple roles for the Na,K-ATPase subunits, Atp1a1 and Fxyd1, during brain ventricle development. *Dev Biol* 368 (2): 312–322.

Charron, F. et al. (2003). The morphogen sonic hedgehog is an axonal chemoattractant that collaborates with netrin-1 in midline axon guidance. *Cell* 113 (1): 11–23.

Chau, K.F. et al. (2015). Progressive differentiation and instructive capacities of amniotic fluid and cerebrospinal fluid proteomes following neural tube closure. *Dev Cell* 35 (6): 789–802.

Chen, D. et al. (2004). Bone morphogenetic proteins. *Growth Factors* 22 (4): 233–241.

Cirrito, J.R. et al. (2003). In vivo assessment of brain interstitial fluid with microdialysis reveals plaque-associated changes in amyloid-beta metabolism and half-life. *J Neurosci* 23 (26): 8844–8853.

Clarke, J. (2009). Role of polarized cell divisions in zebrafish neural tube formation. *Curr Opin Neurobiol* 19 (2): 134–138.

Coulter, M.E. et al. (2018). The ESCRT-III protein CHMP1A mediates secretion of sonic hedgehog on a distinctive subtype of extracellular vesicles. *Cell Rep* 24 (4): 973–986.e8.

Cui, J. et al. (2020). Inflammation of the embryonic choroid plexus barrier following maternal immune activation. *Dev Cell* 55 (5): 617–628.e6.

Currle, D.S. et al. (2005). Direct and indirect roles of CNS dorsal midline cells in choroid plexus epithelia formation. *Development* 132 (15): 3549–3559.

Cushing, H. (1914). Studies on the cerebro-spinal fluid: I. Introduction. *J Med Res* 31: 1–19.

Dahmane, N. and Ruiz i Altaba, A. (1999). Sonic hedgehog regulates the growth and patterning of the cerebellum. *Development* 126 (14): 3089–3100.

Damkier, H.H. et al. (2013). Cerebrospinal fluid secretion by the choroid plexus. *Physiol Rev* 93 (4): 1847–1892.

Dandy, W.E. (1919). Experimental hydrocephalus. *Ann Surg* 70 (2): 129–142.

Dani, N. et al. (2021). A cellular and spatial map of the choroid plexus across brain ventricles and ages. *Cell* 184 (11): 3056–3074.e21.

Davenport, J.R. and Yoder, B.K. (2005). An incredible decade for the primary cilium. *Am J Physiol. Renal Physiol* 289 (6): F1159–1169.

Davson, H. and Segal, M.B. (1996). *Physiology of the CSF and Blood-brain Barriers*. Boca Raton, FL: CRC Press.

Deisenhammer, F. et al. (2019). The cerebrospinal fluid in multiple sclerosis. *Front Immunol* 10: 726.

Delpire, E. (2021). Advances in the development of novel compounds targeting cation-chloride cotransporter physiology. *Am J Physiol Cell Physiol* 320 (3): C324–C340.

Desmond, M.E. and Schoenwolf, G.C. (1985). Timing and positioning of occlusion of the spinal neurocele in the chick embryo. *J Comp Neurol* 235 (4): 479–487.

D'Gama, P.P. et al. (2021). Diversity and function of motile ciliated cell types within ependymal lineages of the zebrafish brain. *Cell Rep* 37 (1): 109775.

Di Spiezio, A. et al. (2018). The LepR-mediated leptin transport across brain barriers controls food reward. *Mol Metab* 8: 13–22.

Doetsch, F. (2003). A niche for adult neural stem cells. *Curr Opin Genet Dev* 13 (5): 543–550.

Donsante, A. et al. (2010). Somatic mosaicism in Menkes disease suggests choroid plexus-mediated copper transport to the developing brain. *Am J Med Genet Part A* 152A (10): 2529–2534.

Dreha-Kulaczewski, S. et al. (2018). Respiration and the watershed of spinal CSF flow in humans. *Sci Rep* 8 (1): 5594.

Dur, A.H. et al. (2020). In Xenopus ependymal cilia drive embryonic CSF circulation and brain development independently of cardiac pulsatile forces. *Fluids Barriers CNS* 17 (1): 72.

Durston, A.J. et al. (1989). Retinoic acid causes an anteroposterior transformation in the developing central nervous system. *Nature* 340 (6229): 140–144.

Duy, P.Q. et al. (2023). A neural stem cell paradigm of pediatric hydrocephalus. *Cereb Cortex* 33 (8): 4262–4279. doi: 10.1093/cercor/bhac341.

Dziegielewska, K.M. et al. (2001). Development of the choroid plexus. *Microsc Res Tech* 52 (1): 5–20.

Ek, C.J. et al. (2001). Permeability and route of entry for lipid-insoluble molecules across brain barriers in developing Monodelphis domestica. *J Physiol* 536 (Pt 3): 841–853.

Ek, C.J. et al. (2003). Structural characteristics and barrier properties of the choroid plexuses in developing brain of the opossum (Monodelphis Domestica). *J Comp Neurol* 460 (4): 451–464.

Fame, R.M. et al. (2016). Directional cerebrospinal fluid movement between brain ventricles in larval zebrafish. *Fluids Barriers CNS* 13 (1): 11.

Fame, R.M. et al. (2020). Brain ventricular system and cerebrospinal fluid development and function: light at the end of the tube. *BioEssays: News Rev Mol Cell Dev Biol* 42 (3): e1900186.

Fame, R.M. and Lehtinen, M.K. (2019). Sister, sister. *Neuron* 102 (2): 278–279.

Fame, R.M. and Lehtinen, M.K. (2020). Emergence and developmental roles of the cerebrospinal fluid system. *Dev Cell* 52 (3): 261–275.

Fame, R.M. and Lehtinen, M.K. (2021). Mitochondria in early forebrain development. *Front Cell Dev Biol* 9: 780207. doi: 10.3389/fcell.2021.780207.

Fame, R.M. et al. (2019). A concerted metabolic shift in early forebrain alters the CSF proteome and depends on MYC downregulation for mitochondrial maturation. *Development* 146 (20): dev182857. doi: 10.1242/dev.182857.

Faubel, R. et al. (2016). Cilia-based flow network in the brain ventricles. *Science* 353 (6295): 176–178.

Feliciano, D.M. et al. (2014). Embryonic cerebrospinal fluid nanovesicles carry evolutionarily conserved molecules and promote neural stem cell amplification. *PloS One* 9 (2): e88810.

Fossan, G. et al. (1985). CSF-brain permeability in the immature sheep fetus. *Brain Res* 350 (1–2): 113–124.

Fultz, N.E. et al. (2019). Coupled electrophysiological, hemodynamic, and cerebrospinal fluid oscillations in human sleep. *Science* 366 (6465): 628–631.

Furey, C.G. et al. (2018). De novo mutation in genes regulating neural stem cell fate in human congenital hydrocephalus. *Neuron* 99 (2): 302–314.e4.

Gato, A. et al. (2005). Embryonic cerebrospinal fluid regulates neuroepithelial survival, proliferation, and neurogenesis in chick embryos. *Anat Rec Part A, Dis Mol Cell Evol Biol* 284 (1): 475–484.

Ghersi-Egea, J.-F. et al. (2018). Molecular anatomy and functions of the choroidal blood-cerebrospinal fluid barrier in health and disease. *Acta Neuropathol* 135 (3): 337–361.

Gilmore, J.H. (2010). Understanding what causes schizophrenia: a developmental perspective. *Am J Psychiatry* 167 (1): 8–10.

Giné-Servén, E. et al. (2022). Routine cerebrospinal fluid parameters as biomarkers in first-episode psychosis. *Prog Neuro-Psychopharmacol Biol Psychiatry* 112: 110424.

Gómez, D.G. et al. (1982). Development of arachnoid villi and granulations in man. *Acta Anat* 111 (3): 247–258.

Grapp, M. et al. (2013). Choroid plexus transcytosis and exosome shuttling deliver folate into brain parenchyma. *Nat Commun* 4: 2123.

Gregg, C. and Weiss, S. (2005). CNTF/LIF/gp130 receptor complex signaling maintains a VZ precursor differentiation gradient in the developing ventral fore- brain. *Development* 132: 565–578.

Gregoriades, J.M.C. et al. (2019). Genetic and pharmacological inactivation of apical Na+-K+-2Cl-cotransporter 1 in choroid plexus epithelial cells reveals the physiological function of the cotransporter. *Am J Physiol Cell Physiol* 316 (4): C525–C544.

Gudeman, D.M. et al. (1989). Release from live choroid plexus of apical fragments and electrophoretic characterization of their synthetic products. *J Neurosci Res* 24 (2): 184–191.

Gudeman, D.M. et al. (1987). Protein secretion by choroid plexus. *Tissue Cell* 19 (1): 101–109.

Guha, D. et al. (2019). Cerebrospinal fluid extracellular vesicles and neurofilament light protein as biomarkers of central nervous system injury in HIV-infected patients on antiretroviral therapy. *AIDS* 33 (4): 615–625.

Guo, Y. et al. (2022). Trends and developments in the detection of pathogens in central nervous system infections. *Front Cell Infect Microbiol* 12: 856845.

Habgood, M.D. et al. (1992). A developmentally regulated blood-cerebrospinal fluid transfer mechanism for albumin in immature rats. *J Physiol* 456 (1): 181–192.

Haddad, M.R. et al. (2013). Fetal brain-directed AAV gene therapy results in rapid, robust, and persistent transduction of mouse choroid plexus epithelia. *Mol Ther Nucleic Acids* 2: e101.

Hagenlocher, C. et al. (2013). Ciliogenesis and cerebrospinal fluid flow in the developing Xenopus brain are regulated by foxj1. *Cilia* 2 (1): 12.

Harris, C.A. et al. (2021). Cerebrospinal fluid biomarkers of neuroinflammation in children with hydrocephalus and shunt malfunction. *Fluids Barriers CNS* 18 (1): 4.

Harrison, L. et al. (2018). Fluorescent blood–brain barrier tracing shows intact leptin transport in obese mice. *Int J Obes* 43 (6): 1305–1318.

Harwell, C.C. et al. (2012). Sonic hedgehog expression in corticofugal projection neurons directs cortical microcircuit formation. *Neuron* 73 (6): 1116–1126.

Haskell, G.T. and LaMantia, A.-S. (2005). Retinoic acid signaling identifies a distinct precursor population in the developing and adult forebrain. *J Neurosci* 25 (33): 7636–7647.

Haubensak, W. et al. (2004). Neurons arise in the basal neuroepithelium of the early mammalian telencephalon. *Proc Natl Acad Sci USA* 101 (9): 3196–3201.

Hellman, N.E. et al. (2010). The zebrafish foxj1a transcription factor regulates cilia function in response to injury and epithelial stretch. *Proc Natl Acad Sci USA* 107 (43): 18499–18504.

Higginbotham, H. et al. (2012). Arl13b in primary cilia regulates the migration and placement of interneurons in the developing cerebral cortex. *Dev Cell* 23 (5): 925–938.

Hochstetler, A. et al. (2022). Hydrocephalus. *Eur J Med Res* 27 (1): 168.

Hogue, M.J. (1949). Human fetal choroid plexus cells in tissue cultures. *Anat Rec* 103 (3): 381–399.

Holly, J.M.P. et al. (2019). The neglected insulin. *Cells* 8 (10): 1207. doi: 10.3390/cells8101207.

Huang, X. et al. (2009). Sonic hedgehog signaling regulates a novel epithelial progenitor domain of the hindbrain choroid plexus. *Development* 136 (15): 2535–2543.

Huang, X. et al. (2010). Transventricular delivery of Sonic hedgehog is essential to cerebellar ventricular zone development. *Proc Natl Acad Sci USA* 107 (18): 8422–8427.

Hulme, L. et al. (2022). Functional characterization of a human choroid plexus cell line and TRPV4 stimulated transepithelial ion flux. *FASEB J* 36 (S1). doi: 10.1096/fasebj.2022.36.S1.R2144.

Hunter, N.L. and Dymecki, S.M. (2007). Molecularly and temporally separable lineages form the hindbrain roof plate and contribute differentially to the choroid plexus. *Development* 134 (19): 3449–3460.

Inoue, T. et al. (2015). Observation of the ciliary movement of choroid plexus epithelial cells ex vivo. *J Vis Exp* 101: e52991.

Iram, T. et al. (2022). Young CSF restores oligodendrogenesis and memory in aged mice via Fgf17. *Nature* 605 (7910): 509–515.

Ishiwata, S. et al. (2020). Lower cerebrospinal fluid CRH concentration in chronic schizophrenia with negative symptoms. *J Psychiatric Res* 127: 13–19.

Jacob, L. et al. (2019). Anatomy and function of the vertebral column lymphatic network in mice. *Nat Commun* 10 (1): 4594.

Jacobsen, M. et al. (1983). The choroid plexus in fetal sheep during development with special reference to intracellular plasma proteins. *Dev Brain Res* 8 (1): 77–88.

Jang, A. and Lehtinen, M.K. (2022). Experimental approaches for manipulating choroid plexus epithelial cells. *Fluids Barriers CNS* 19 (1): 36.

Jang, A. et al. (2022). Choroid plexus-CSF-targeted antioxidant therapy protects the brain from toxicity of cancer chemotherapy. *Neuron* 110 (20): 3288–3301. doi: 10.1016/j.neuron.2022.08.009.

Johansson, P.A. et al. (2008). The blood-CSF barrier explained: when development is not immaturity. *BioEssays: News Rev Mol Cell Dev Biol* 30 (3): 237–248.

Johansson, P.A. et al. (2013). The transcription factor Otx2 regulates choroid plexus development and function. *Development* 140 (5): 1055–1066.

Kaiser, K. et al. (2019). WNT5A is transported via lipoprotein particles in the cerebrospinal fluid to regulate hindbrain morphogenesis. *Nat Commun* 10 (1): 1498.

Kaiser, K. et al. (2021). MEIS-WNT5A axis regulates development of fourth ventricle choroid plexus. *Development* 148 (10): dev192054. doi: 10.1242/dev.192054.

Kangsamaksin, T. and Morris, R.J. (2011). Bone morphogenetic protein 5 regulates the number of keratinocyte stem cells from the skin of mice. *J Invest Dermatol* 131 (3): 580–585.

Karimy, J.K. et al. (2016). Cerebrospinal fluid hypersecretion in pediatric hydrocephalus. *Neurosurg Focus* 41 (5): E10.

Keep, R.F. and Jones, H.C. (1990). A morphometric study on the development of the lateral ventricle choroid plexus, choroid plexus capillaries and ventricular ependyma in the rat. *Brain Res. Dev Brain Res* 56 (1): 47–53.

Khacho, M. et al. (2016). Mitochondrial dynamics impacts stem cell identity and fate decisions by regulating a nuclear transcriptional program. *Cell Stem Cell* 19 (2): 232–247.

Khacho, M. and Slack, R.S. (2018). Mitochondrial and reactive oxygen species signaling coordinate stem cell fate decisions and life long maintenance. *Antioxid Redox Signal* 28 (11): 1090–1101.

Kim, S. et al. (2010). The apical complex couples cell fate and cell survival to cerebral cortical development. *Neuron* 66 (1): 69–84.

Kosodo, Y. et al. (2004). Asymmetric distribution of the apical plasma membrane during neurogenic divisions of mammalian neuroepithelial cells. *EMBO J* 23 (11): 2314–2324.

Kratzer, I. et al. (2018). Glutathione conjugation at the blood-CSF barrier efficiently prevents exposure of the developing brain fluid environment to blood-borne reactive electrophilic substances. *J Neurosci* 38 (14): 3466–3479.

Kratzer, I. et al. (2012). Complexity and developmental changes in the expression pattern of claudins at the blood-CSF barrier. *Histochem Cell Biol* 138 (6): 861–879.

Kriska, J. et al. (2021). On the common journey of neural cells through ischemic brain injury and Alzheimer's disease. *Int J Mol Sci* 22 (18): 9689. doi: 10.3390/ijms22189689.

Kumar, S. et al. (2019). Impaired neurodevelopmental pathways in autism spectrum disorder. *J Neurodev Disorders* 11 (1): 10.

Kumar, V. et al. (2021). Functional roles of FGF signaling in early development of vertebrate embryos. *Cells* 10 (8): 2148. doi: 10.3390/cells10082148.

Lamus, F. et al. (2020). FGF2/EGF contributes to brain neuroepithelial precursor proliferation and neurogenesis in rat embryos. *Dev Dyn* 249 (1): 141–153.
Lancaster, M.A. et al. (2013). Cerebral organoids model human brain development and microcephaly. *Nature* 501 (7467): 373–379.
Langford, M.B. et al. (2020). WNT5a regulates epithelial morphogenesis in the developing choroid plexus. *Cereb Cortex* 30 (6): 3617–3631.
Lehtinen, M.K. et al. (2011). The cerebrospinal fluid provides a proliferative niche for neural progenitor cells. *Neuron* 69 (5): 893–905.
Li, Q. et al. (2020). Aquaporin 1 and the Na+/K+/2Cl- cotransporter 1 are present in the leptomeningeal vasculature of the adult rodent central nervous system. *Fluids Barriers CNS* 17 (1): 15.
Liddelow, S.A. (2015). Development of the choroid plexus and blood-CSF barrier. *Front Neurosci* 9: 32.
Liddelow, S.A. et al. (2010). Development of the lateral ventricular choroid plexus in a marsupial, Monodelphis domestica. *Cerebrospinal Fluid Res* 7: 16.
Lin, X. et al. (2017). Cerebrospinal fluid circulating tumor cells. *Neuro-Oncol* 19 (9): 1248–1254.
Louvi, A. and Grove, E.A. (2011). Cilia in the CNS. *Neuron* 69 (6): 1046–1060.
Lowery, L.A. and Sive, H. (2005). Initial formation of zebrafish brain ventricles occurs independently of circulation and requires the nagie oko and snakehead/atp1a1a.1 gene products. *Development* 132 (9): 2057–2067.
Lowery, L.A. and Sive, H. (2009). Totally tubular. *BioEssays: News Rev Mol Cell Dev Biol* 31 (4): 446–458.
Lun, M.P. et al. (2015a). Spatially heterogeneous choroid plexus transcriptomes encode positional identity and contribute to regional CSF production. *J Neurosci* 35 (12): 4903–4916.
Lun, M.P. et al. (2015b). Development and functions of the choroid plexus-cerebrospinal fluid system. *Nat Rev Neurosci* 16 (8): 445–457.
MacAulay, N. and Rose, C.R. (2020). CrossTalk opposing view. *J Physiol* 598 (21): 4737–4739.
MacAulay, N. et al. (2022). Cerebrospinal fluid production by the choroid plexus: a century of barrier research revisited. *Fluids Barriers CNS* 19 (1): 26.
Mahuzier, A. et al. (2018). Ependymal cilia beating induces an actin network to protect centrioles against shear stress. *Nat Commun* 9 (1): 2279.
Martín, C. et al. (2006). FGF2 plays a key role in embryonic cerebrospinal fluid trophic properties over chick embryo neuroepithelial stem cells. *Dev Biol* 297 (2): 402–416.
Martirosian, V. et al. (2021). Medulloblastoma uses GABA transaminase to survive in the cerebrospinal fluid microenvironment and promote leptomeningeal dissemination. *Cell Rep* 35 (13): 109302.
Massarwa, R. and Niswander, L. (2013). In toto live imaging of mouse morphogenesis and new insights into neural tube closure. *Development* 140 (1): 226–236.
Mestre, H. et al. (2018). Flow of cerebrospinal fluid is driven by arterial pulsations and is reduced in hypertension. *Nat Commun* 9 (1): 4878.
Mirzadeh, Z. et al. (2010). Cilia organize ependymal planar polarity. *J Neurosci* 30 (7): 2600–2610.
Mishra, A. et al. (2012). Choroid plexus carcinoma. *J Pediatric Neurosci* 7 (1): 71–73.
Miskevich, F. (2010). Imaging fluid flow and cilia beating pattern in Xenopus brain ventricles. *J Neurosci Methods* 189 (1): 1–4.
Miyan, J.A. et al. (2003). Development of the brain: a vital role for cerebrospinal fluid. *Can J Physiol Pharmacol* 81 (4): 317–328.
Møllgård, K. and Saunders, N.R. (1986). The development of the human blood-brain and blood-CSF barriers. *Neuropathol Appl Neurobiol* 12 (4): 337–358. doi: 10.1111/j.1365-2990.1986.tb00146.x.
Monnot, A.D. and Zheng, W. (2013). Culture of choroid plexus epithelial cells and in vitro model of blood-CSF barrier. *Methods Mol Biol* 945: 13–29.

Monuki, E.S. et al. (2001). Patterning of the dorsal telencephalon and cerebral cortex by a roof plate-Lhx2 pathway. *Neuron* 32 (4): 591–604.

Murphy, V.A. et al. (2020). Extra-axial cerebrospinal fluid relationships to infant brain structure, cognitive development, and risk for schizophrenia. *Biol Psychiatry: Cogn Neurosci Neuroimag* 5 (7): 651–659.

Nabiuni, M. et al. (2015). CSF protein contents and their roles in brain development. *Zahedan J Res Med Sci* 17 (9): e1042. doi: 10.17795/zjrms-1042.

Namba, T. and Huttner, W.B. (2017). Neural progenitor cells and their role in the development and evolutionary expansion of the neocortex. *Wiley Interdiscip Rev: Dev Biol* 6 (1). doi: 10.1002/wdev.256.

Narita, K. et al. (2010). Multiple primary cilia modulate the fluid transcytosis in choroid plexus epithelium. *Traffic* 11 (2): 287–301.

Narita, K. and Takeda, S. (2015). Cilia in the choroid plexus. *Front Cell Neurosci* 9: 39.

Nielsen, C.M. and Dymecki, S.M. (2010). Sonic hedgehog is required for vascular outgrowth in the hindbrain choroid plexus. *Dev Biol* 340 (2): 430–437.

Nonami, Y. et al. (2013). Developmental changes in ciliary motility on choroid plexus epithelial cells during the perinatal period. *Cytoskeleton* 70 (12): 797–803.

O'Brown, N.M. et al. (2018). Bridging barriers. *Genes Dev* 32 (7–8): 466–478.

Ohata, S. et al. (2015). Mechanosensory genes Pkd1 and Pkd2 contribute to the planar polarization of brain ventricular epithelium. *J Neurosci* 35 (31): 11153–11168.

Olstad, E.W. et al. (2019). Ciliary beating compartmentalizes cerebrospinal fluid flow in the brain and regulates ventricular development. *Curr Biol* 29 (2): 229–241.e6.

O'Rahilly, R. and Müller, F. (1990). Ventricular system and choroid plexuses of the human brain during the embryonic period proper. *Am J Anat* 189 (4): 285–302.

Orešković, D. and Klarica, M. (2014). A new look at cerebrospinal fluid movement. *Fluids Barriers CNS* 11 (1): 16.

Orešković, D. et al. (2016). Cerebrospinal fluid secretion by the choroid plexus? *Physiol Rev* 96 (4): 1661–1662.

Orešković, D. et al. (2017). Role of choroid plexus in cerebrospinal fluid hydrodynamics. *Neuroscience* 354: 69–87.

Paridaen, J.T.M.L. et al. (2013). Asymmetric inheritance of centrosome-associated primary cilium membrane directs ciliogenesis after cell division. *Cell* 155 (2): 333–344.

Pellegrini, L. et al. (2020a). SARS-CoV-2 infects the brain choroid plexus and disrupts the blood-CSF barrier in human brain organoids. *Cell Stem Cell* 27 (6): 951–961.e5.

Pellegrini, L. et al. (2020b). Human CNS barrier-forming organoids with cerebrospinal fluid production. *Science* 369 (6500): eaaz5626. doi: 10.1126/science.aaz5626.

Petersen, N. et al. (2020). Three-dimensional explant platform for studies on choroid plexus epithelium. *Front Cell Neurosci* 14: 108.

Peterson, M. et al. (2021). Evidence for normal extra-axial cerebrospinal fluid volume in autistic males from middle childhood to adulthood. *NeuroImage* 240 (118387): 118387.

Planques, A. et al. (2019). OTX2 signals from the choroid plexus to regulate adult neurogenesis. *eNeuro* 6 (2): ENEURO.0262-18.2019. doi: 10.1523/ENEURO.0262-18.2019.

Pollay, M. (2010). The function and structure of the cerebrospinal fluid outflow system. *Cerebrospinal Fluid Res* 7: 9.

Pollay, M. and Curl, F. (1967). Secretion of cerebrospinal fluid by the ventricular ependyma of the rabbit. *Am J Physiol* 213 (4): 1031–1038.

Praetorius, J. and Damkier, H.H. (2017). Transport across the choroid plexus epithelium. *Am J Physiol Cell Physiol* 312 (6): C673–C686.

Preston, D. et al. (2018). Activation of TRPV4 stimulates transepithelial ion flux in a porcine choroid plexus cell line. *Am J Physiol Cell Physiol* 315 (3): C357–C366.

Proulx, S.T. (2021). Cerebrospinal fluid outflow: a review of the historical and contemporary evidence for arachnoid villi, perineural routes, and dural lymphatics. *Cell Mol Life Sci* 78 (6): 2429–2457.

Pulous, F.E. et al. (2022). Cerebrospinal fluid can exit into the skull bone marrow and instruct cranial hematopoiesis in mice with bacterial meningitis. *Nat Neurosci* 25 (5): 567–576.

Qin, E.Y. et al. (2017). Neural precursor-derived pleiotrophin mediates subventricular zone invasion by Glioma. *Cell* 170 (5): 845–859.e19.

Quadrato, G. and Arlotta, P. (2017). Present and future of modeling human brain development in 3D organoids. *Curr Opin Cell Biol* 49: 47–52.

Redmond, S.A. et al. (2019). Development of ependymal and postnatal neural stem cells and their origin from a common embryonic progenitor. *Cell Rep* 27 (2): 429–441.e3.

Redzic, Z.B. (2013). Studies on the human choroid plexus in vitro. *Fluids Barriers CNS* 10 (1): 10.

Ringers, C. et al. (2020). The role of motile cilia in the development and physiology of the nervous system. *Philos Trans Royal Soc London. Series B, Biol Sci* 375 (1792): 20190156.

Roelink, H. et al. (1995). Floor plate and motor neuron induction by different concentrations of the amino-terminal cleavage product of sonic hedgehog autoproteolysis. *Cell* 81 (3): 445–455.

Safaee, M. et al. (2013). Choroid plexus papillomas. *Neuro-Oncol* 15 (3): 255–267.

Salleh, N. and Giribabu, N. (2014). Leukemia inhibitory factor. *Sci World J* 2014: 201514.

Saunders, N.R. et al. (2023). The choroid plexus. *Physiol Rev* 103 (1): 919–956. doi: 10.1152/physrev.00060.2021.

Saunders, N.R. et al. (2018). Physiology and molecular biology of barrier mechanisms in the fetal and neonatal brain. *J Physiol* 596 (23): 5723–5756.

Sawamoto, K. et al. (2006). New neurons follow the flow of cerebrospinal fluid in the adult brain. *Science* 311 (5761): 629–632.

Sayo, A. et al. (2012). Study factors influencing ventricular enlargement in schizophrenia. *NeuroImage* 59 (1): 154–167.

Schindler, S.E. et al. (2019). Emerging cerebrospinal fluid biomarkers in autosomal dominant Alzheimer's disease. *Alzheimer's Dementia* 15 (5): 655–665.

Shannon, M.L. et al. (2018). Mice expressing Myc in neural precursors develop choroid plexus and ciliary body tumors. *Am J Pathol* 188 (6): 1334–1344.

Shen, M.D. et al. (2017). Increased extra-axial cerebrospinal fluid in high-risk infants who later develop autism. *Biol Psychiatry* 82 (3): 186–193.

Shen, M.D. et al. (2018). Extra-axial cerebrospinal fluid in high-risk and normal-risk children with autism aged 2-4 years. *Lancet Psychiatry* 5 (11): 895–904.

Shibata, M. et al. (2021). Regulation of prefrontal patterning and connectivity by retinoic acid. *Nature* 598 (7881): 483–488.

Shipley, F.B. et al. (2020). Tracking calcium dynamics and immune surveillance at the choroid plexus blood-cerebrospinal fluid interface. *Neuron* 108 (4): 623–639.e10.

Siegenthaler, J.A. et al. (2009). Retinoic acid from the meninges regulates cortical neuron generation. *Cell* 139 (3): 597–609.

Silva-Vargas, V. et al. (2016). Age-dependent niche signals from the choroid plexus regulate adult neural stem cells. *Cell Stem Cell* 19 (5): 643–652.

Sive, H.L. et al. (1990). Identification of a retinoic acid-sensitive period during primary axis formation in Xenopus laevis. *Genes Dev* 4 (6): 932–942.

Smith, Q.R. and Johanson, C.E. (1980). Effect of ouabain and potassium on ion concentrations in the choroidal epithelium. *Am J Physiol* 238 (5): F399–406.

Spassky, N. et al. (2005). Adult ependymal cells are postmitotic and are derived from radial glial cells during embryogenesis. *J Neurosci* 25 (1): 10–18.

Spassky, N. and Meunier, A. (2017). The development and functions of multiciliated epithelia. *Nat Rev Mol Cell Biol* 18 (7): 423–436.

Spatazza, J. et al. (2013). Choroid-plexus-derived Otx2 homeoprotein constrains adult cortical plasticity. *Cell Rep* 3 (6): 1815–1823.

Steen, N.E. et al. (2014). Altered systemic cortisol metabolism in bipolar disorder and schizophrenia spectrum disorders. *J Psychiatric Res* 52: 57–62.

Steen, R.G. et al. (2006). Brain volume in first-episode schizophrenia. *Br J Psychiatry: J Mental Sci* 188: 510–518.

Steffensen, A.B. et al. (2018). Cotransporter-mediated water transport underlying cerebrospinal fluid formation. *Nat Commun* 9 (1): 2167.

Stepien, B.K. et al. (2021). Length of the neurogenic period-A key determinant for the generation of upper-layer neurons during neocortex development and evolution. *Front Cell Dev Biol* 9: 676911.

Sternberg, J.R. et al. (2018). Pkd2l1 is required for mechanoception in cerebrospinal fluid-contacting neurons and maintenance of spine curvature. *Nat Commun* 9 (1): 3804.

Stottmann, R.W. et al. (2001). The BMP antagonists Chordin and Noggin have essential but redundant roles in mouse mandibular outgrowth. *Dev Biol* 240 (2): 457–473.

Strazielle, N. and Ghersi-Egea, J.F. (1999). Demonstration of a coupled metabolism-efflux process at the choroid plexus as a mechanism of brain protection toward xenobiotics. *J Neurosci* 19 (15): 6275–6289.

Strazielle, N. and Ghersi-Egea, J.-F. (2015). Efflux transporters in blood-brain interfaces of the developing brain. *Front Neurosci* 9: 21.

Swiderski, R.E. et al. (2012). Structural defects in cilia of the choroid plexus, subfornical organ and ventricular ependyma are associated with ventriculomegaly. *Fluids Barriers CNS* 9 (1): 22.

Tennyson, V.M. and Pappas, G.D. (1962). An electron microscope study of ependymal cells of the fetal, early postnatal and adult rabbit. *Zeitschrift für Zellforschung und Mikroskopische Anatomie* 56 (5): 595–618. doi: 10.1007/bf00540584.

Thelin, E.P. et al. (2014). Microdialysis monitoring of CSF parameters in severe traumatic brain injury patients. *Front Neurol* 5: 159.

Thouvenin, O. et al. (2020). Origin and role of the cerebrospinal fluid bidirectional flow in the central canal. *Elife* 9: e47699. doi: 10.7554/eLife.47699.

Turner, M.H. et al. (2012). A method for detecting molecular transport within the cerebral ventricles of live zebrafish (Danio rerio) larvae. *J Physiol* 590 (10): 2233–2240.

Ulloa, V. et al. (2019). Basal sodium-dependent vitamin C transporter 2 polarization in choroid plexus explant cells in normal or scorbutic conditions. *Sci Rep* 9 (1): 14422.

Underwood, M.A. et al. (2005). Amniotic fluid: not just fetal urine anymore. *J Perinatol* 25 (5): 341–348.

Vandendriessche, C. et al. (2021). Importance of extracellular vesicle secretion at the blood-cerebrospinal fluid interface in the pathogenesis of Alzheimer's disease. *Acta Neuropathol Commun* 9 (1): 143.

Vandenhaute, E. et al. (2015). The choroid plexus may be an underestimated site of tumor invasion to the brain. *Cancer Cell Int* 15: 102.

Villalobos, A.R.A. et al. (2002). Transepithelial organic anion transport by shark choroid plexus. *Am J Physiol Regul, Int Comp Physiol* 282 (5): R1308–16.

Wagshul, M.E. et al. (2011). The pulsating brain. *Fluids Barriers CNS* 8 (1): 5.

Watanabe, M. et al. (2012). BMP4 sufficiency to induce choroid plexus epithelial fate from embryonic stem cell-derived neuroepithelial progenitors. *J Neurosci* 32 (45): 15934–15945.

Weiss, P.A. (1934). *Secretory Activity of the Inner Layer of the Embryonic Mid-brain of the Chick, as Revealed by Tissue Culture*. Philadelphia, PA: Wistar Institute Press.

Wilde, J.J. et al. (2014). Genetic, epigenetic, and environmental contributions to neural tube closure. *Ann Rev Genet* 48: 583–611.

Wilson, N.H. and Stoeckli, E.T. (2013). Sonic hedgehog regulates its own receptor on postcrossing commissural axons in a glypican1-dependent manner. *Neuron* 79 (3): 478–491.

Wilting, J. and Christ, B. (1989). An experimental and ultrastructural study on the development of the avian choroid plexus. *Cell Tissue Res* 255 (3): 487–494.

Xu, H. et al. (2021). Choroid plexus NKCC1 mediates cerebrospinal fluid clearance during mouse early postnatal development. *Nat Commun* 12 (1): 447.

Yang, X. et al. (2020). Structure of the human cation-chloride cotransporter NKCC1 determined by single-particle electron cryo-microscopy. *Nat Commun* 11 (1): 1016.

Yoder, B.K. (2007). Role of primary cilia in the pathogenesis of polycystic kidney disease. *J Am Soc Nephrol* 18 (5): 1381–1388.

Zappaterra, M.W. et al. (2013). Isolation of cerebrospinal fluid from rodent embryos for use with dissected cerebral cortical explants. *J Vis Exp* 73: e50333.

33

Comparative Cognitive Neuroscience and Dorsal and Ventral Streams in Primates

Jon H. Kaas, Hui-Xin Qi, and Iwona Stepniewska

Department of Psychology, Vanderbilt University, Nashville, TN, USA

33.1 Introduction

One cannot resist being impressed by the differences in cognitive abilities between humans and other primates. This branch of mammalian evolution emerged as much as 80 million years ago as small nocturnal mammals that adapted to the fine branches of trees and bushes in the tropical forests (see Kaas et al. 2022). Early primates already had large forward facing eyes and good vision. By living in the small branches high above ground, and feeding at night on insects and fruit, they avoided the dangers of the dominating dinosaurs. These early primates lived longer than most mammals, who also were small and nocturnal. The potential for living longer, and possibly having dependent offspring over longer periods of development perhaps promoted the evolution of larger primates and more complex brains after the extinction of dinosaurs and diurnal life became possible.

Early primates resembled some extant primates in size and adaptations for nocturnal life with good vision. The two major branches of primate evolution are known as the strepsirrhine and haplorhine primates. Most of the strepsirrhine primates remained small and nocturnal (galagos, lemurs, and lorises), with especially mouse lemurs (Saraf et al. 2019) and galagos (Wong and Kaas 2010) resembling early primates. The haplorhine primates formed the other major branch of the initially diurnal primate radiation that divided into tarsiers and anthropoids. The ancestors of early tarsiers returned to nocturnal life, and adaptations to dim light, while the other branch, anthropoid primates, branched into platyrrhines (New World monkeys) and catarrhines (Old World monkeys, apes, and humans). Only the ancestors of present day New World owl monkeys and tarsiers became nocturnal again. Overall, there are over 200 extant species of primates (Fleagle 1999) covering a wide range of body and brain types and cognitive abilities. The closest existing relatives of primates are tree shrews and flying lemurs (that are not shrews or lemurs). Their brains do not have a number of primate cortical features, especially in their visual systems (Kaas and Preuss 2014). These relatives of primates also seem to have fewer cognitive abilities than most or all primates, as do the more studied mice and rats.

Cognitive abilities are often related to human mental states, such as those dependent on learning, imitation, language, causal reasoning, and decision making. Much has been made of humans, and perhaps others, having a "theory of mind," which means one knows what others know or do not know. This cognitive ability may be largely restricted to humans. As determining the cognitive ability of humans typically depends on interactions based on language, it is difficult to document the cognitive abilities attributed to other primates, including chimpanzees and bonobos (e.g., Premack 2007).

Neocortical Neurogenesis in Development and Evolution, First Edition. Edited by Wieland B. Huttner.

In general, it is easier to demonstrate that chimpanzees, and even macaque monkeys have similar sensory abilities as humans than to establish cognitive similarities (Povinelli 2000). Yet, differences across primates in cognition seem so great, that there are many ongoing attempts to relate cognitive differences to differences in brains. These differences include those in overall brain size, sizes of brains in relation to body size, sizes of parts of brains such as neocortex or prefrontal cortex, numbers and types of neurons, numbers and types of subdivisions of neocortex such as columns, domains and areas, and cortical systems and subsystems. Subcortical structures admittedly contribute to cognition (Janacsek et al. 2022), but are less frequently related to cognitive abilities. Cognitive abilities often depend on the functioning of multiple brain structures, including the nuclei of the thalamus, the basal ganglia, the cerebellum, and midbrain, but impairments in cognition are more directly related to neocortical damage. The neocortex is obviously most important in primates, but all information comes to the neocortex via the dorsal thalamus either directly or from the cortex to the thalamus and back to the cortex (Sherman and Guillery 2006).

As it can both be difficult to access cognition in nonhuman primates, and determine what brain structures are critical in specific aspects of cognition, the approach taken here is to consider possible neural correlates of cognition. Brain size and relative brain size have most frequently been related to cognition and intelligence, so we start with brain size, and then proceed to other brain variables.

33.2 Brain Size and Relative Brain Size

Relating cognition and intelligence to brain size has the advantage of dealing directly with the problem that these abilities are often broadly distributed in the brain. Acquiring new information requires sensory and perceptual systems that start with peripheral receptors. Memory systems depend on the hippocampus as well as the neocortex. Decisions on actions depend on motor skills and abilities, perceptions and memory, and sensory guidance. Sometimes, decisions need to be made immediately, or suddenly changed, all involving many brain parts and systems. Thus, the parts of the brain that are involved in many aspects of cognition are distributed across areas of neocortex, as well as subcortical structures. This suggests that cognitive abilities may increase with brain size. Brain size is also considered to be an important variable because it is easily measured, both in extant primates and other mammals, but also approximated from the fossil skulls of extinct primates and other mammals using endocasts of the brain cavity (e.g., Kaas and Preuss 2014). As a result, the sizes of brains of modern humans can be compared to those of early hominins (Australopithecus, Homo habilis, and Homo erectus), providing evidence that early walking ancestors had brains about the size of those of modern chimpanzees, and then brains rapidly increased from ape sized (400–500cc) to human sized (1200–1400cc) over the last two million years (Monson et al. 2022). As large human brains depend on an exceptional prenatal growth rate, we now know that a human-like growth rate was reached in our ancestors less than 1 million years ago.

An extensive early effort to relate brain size to intelligence was that of Harry Jerison (1973) in the *Evolution of the Brain and Intelligence*. The great increase in brain size from ape-like ancestors to modern humans undoubtedly relates to the threefold increase in brain size. However, there are reasons to not over-estimate the role of brain size. One should recognize that a major factor in brain sizes is that it increases with body size. Why this occurs is not completely understood, as a larger body does not appear to need a comparably larger brain. And, human females are typically smaller than males and have smaller brains, while competing very well academically and cognitively with males. In recognition of the evidence that cognition and intelligence do not correlate that well with brain size, Jerison (1973) proposed that the "proper mass" of the brain is related to body size, while concluding that the important variable is how much the brain exceeds in size that which was predicted by body size. The use of the "better than expected" increase in brain size, the encephalization quotients (EQ), reduces this problem, but does not eliminate it. While we are proud of having the largest brains for primates, and brains that are large for our body size, elephants and whales have larger brains and larger bodies. Their cognitive abilities, to the extent examined, are impressive.

Measures of brain size can be extended to consider the sizes of parts of the brain, and even neurons (Kaas 2000). As brains get bigger, neurons that make connections with different parts of the brain need longer and thicker axons to maintain these connections and conduction speeds, and typically neurons for mammals are mostly larger for larger brains. Alternatively, in many small mammals and birds, distances between and within brain parts are small, and small neurons will do. In addition, the proportion of connections that each neuron makes with all other neurons goes down with larger brains, unless the brain circuits are recognized. The changes in the sizes of parts of the brain across species of mammals are considerable. For example, the least shrew, has the smallest amount of cortex, while the neocortex in humans being over 500 times larger and more than twice as thick. Primary visual cortex in humans is nearly 700 times larger in surface area than in mice. The horizontal spread of dendritic arbors of neurons in cortex either became greater in large cortical areas, or they sample less of the total inputs. These alterations and changes with brain size suggest that small brains can be more efficient, and this explains why some birds and mammals with very small brains function as well as they do (Olkowicz et al. 2016). But, there are also ways of compensating for the problems introduced as brains get bigger. In general, mammals with larger brains reduce the number of more costly long connections, especially the thicker axons that conduct faster (Ringo 1991). This reduction especially includes the connections between the two hemispheres, including those between large primary sensory areas. In humans, cortical functions differ in the two hemispheres and this could reduce long connections. In large brains, there are more cortical areas, and this increases the proportions of processing that is done locally over short connections. In addition, increasing the number of processing steps and branches in processing systems seems to be basic to developing higher cognitive functions. The estimated number of cortical areas in humans is about 360, while those in galagos with much smaller brains may be in the order of 50 areas per hemisphere. Although measures of brain size have been useful, other measures of brains may be more predictive. This includes the numbers of neurons in neocortex.

33.3 Neuron Numbers in Neocortex

Measures of brain size have obviously been easier to obtain than accurate measures of numbers of neurons in brains and parts of brains. However, a revolution occurred with the publication of a method to rapidly obtain reliable measures of numbers of neurons in brain size by homogenizing brains or brain parts into suspensions of cell nuclei that can be identified immunocytochemically as from neurons or non-neurons, the isotropic fractionation method (Herculano-Houzel and Lent 2005). This easy-to-use method allowed rapid and accurate estimates of neuron numbers of brain and brain parts across species. The most important outcome of these many studies is that all brains are not made the same way. That is, brain size and the sizes of parts of the brain do not accurately reflect the number of neurons that are in the brains and parts of brains. This has been illustrated in several ways. First, cortex size and cortical numbers of neurons are more predictive than brain size and overall number of neurons. While elephant brains have more neurons than human brains, most of the elephant neurons are in the cerebellum, and humans have more neurons in neocortex (Herculano-Houzel et al. 2014). The numbers of neurons in neocortex is a much better predictor of cognitive abilities than overall brain size and number of neurons. Second, all cortex is not the same across species and families. Primates have more densely packed neurons in the cortex than other studied mammals (Herculano-Houzel et al. 2007). For similar sizes of cortex, primates have more neurons. Third, neuron densities, in especially primates, vary within and across cortical areas (Collins et al. 2010). The variation across areas can be as much as four times greater in some areas than others. In general, this relates to neuron size. Areas such as primary motor cortex have larger neurons overall as a portion of these neurons need to project all the way to the spinal cord, and large neurons can maintain long, thick axons that conduct spikes faster (Kaas 2000). More neurons are small in primary visual areas as most connections are short and within primary visual cortex, something done well by small neurons. As numbers of neurons correlate with cognitive abilities (Herculano-Houzel 2017) they appear to be a permissive factor in subdivisions of cortex, allowing increases in cognitive performance. One supporting example of this premise is from the brains of birds. Although the brains of birds are organized differently than in mammals, their cognitive abilities also depend on associative pallial (forebrain) regions that are enlarged in crows and other corvid species and have twice as many neurons as in non-corvid birds (Strockens et al. 2022). And, corvids have impressive cognitive abilities in comparison to other birds (Gunturkun and Bugnyar 2016).

In the human brain, several regions have expanded and increased their numbers of neurons (Chaplin et al. 2013; Hill et al. 2010). Prefrontal cortex in humans has long been considered to be important in planning and making decisions (Passingham and Wise 2012). While prefrontal cortex in humans and nonhuman primates contains about the same proportion of cortical neurons overall (Gabi et al. 2016), prefrontal cortex is not uniform in structure and function, and granular prefrontal cortex of primates, thought to be important in working memory, has more densely packed neurons (Collins et al. 2016).

An outcome of increasing cortical size over brain size in primates is the "corticalization of brain function." As more and more of the processing in the brains of primates increases with cortical size and neuron numbers, the greater the influence of the cortex on subcortical structures, and the greater the impact of removing the cortical influences. This is especially the case for motor control in humans where matching cortical lesions have much more detrimental impact than in smaller primates and other mammals (Herculano-Houzel et al. 2016). The expansion of cortex in size and number of neurons in relation to subcortical structures is a major trend in primates and other mammals, which in general, should make the behavioral and cognitive input of cortical lesions more profound. Larger primate brains have proportionally more neurons in cortical visual (Collins et al. 2013) and auditory (Wong et al. 2013) areas than in subcortical structures. Thus, as primate species with larger brains have added proportionately more neurons to cortex than subcortical structures, there is a "corticalization of function."

33.4 Increasing the Complexity of Cortical Processing: The Dorsal Stream

Mammals and especially primates, increase the complexity of their cortical processing by separating cortical areas into modules of different specialized functions, and producing cortical systems that process information that leads to actions over multiple steps. Columns or modules are best known for areas of visual cortex. All primates divide primary visual cortex into cytochrome oxidase (CO) modules that are called blobs surrounded by non-blob regions having different types of inputs from the lateral geniculate nucleus (Kaas 2012). In addition, subdivisions of layer IV get different classes of inputs from the lateral geniculate nucleus (LGN). As a result, a single area, V1, has parts of three functionally distinct streams of visual processing that project to different band-like modules in the second visual area (V2) and to the middle temporal visual area (MT) and the dorso-lateral visual area (DL or V4). These separate streams feed into two major caudal to frontal processing streams (Figure 33.1), the dorsal stream for actions and the ventral stream for object identification (see Goodale and Milner 1992).

The dorsal stream progresses over specialized higher order visual areas into adjoining posterior parietal cortex and then to more rostral domains in posterior parietal cortex where electrical stimulation evokes domain specific actions such as running or climbing, reaching, protecting the body or face, grasping, hand-to-mouth, and looking to a location (Kaas et al. 2022; Kaas and Stepniewska 2016). These domains are smaller than most sensory or motor areas, but they also have been called areas in posterior parietal cortex. They project to functionally matched domains in motor cortex and premotor cortex, and projections from functionally matched domains in all three regions converge in the basal ganglia (Stepniewska et al. 2020). Domains in posterior parietal cortex also receive variable sensory inputs from the somatosensory and auditory systems, while those in premotor cortex have inputs from prefrontal cortex. We proposed that the three matched sets of domains, in posterior parietal cortex, premotor cortex, and primary motor cortex, are parts of a decision-making process in what to do, with domains competing with each other for dominance and producing a behavior. The decision of what to do in posterior parietal cortex is based on ongoing sensory information, while premotor cortex domains evaluate information from prefrontal and

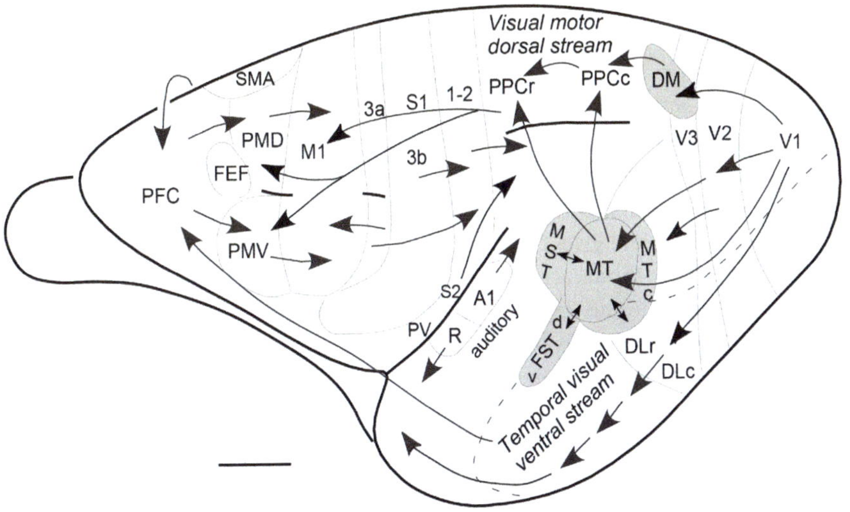

Figure 33.1 Patterns of feedforward connections in the dorsal and ventral visual streams and other streams in strepsirrhine primates (galagos). A1 – primary auditory cortex; DLr and DLc – rostral and caudal parts of dorso-lateral visual area; DM – dorso-medial visual area; FEF – frontal eye field; FST – fundal superior temporal area rostral (r) and ventral (v); M1 – primary motor cortex; MT – middle temporal area; MST – middle superior temporal area; MTc – middle temporal caudal area; PFC – prefrontal cortex; PMD and PMV – dorsal and ventral premotor cortex; PPCr and PPCc – rostral and caudal parts of posterior parietal cortex; PV – parietal ventral somatosensory area; R – rostral auditory area; SMA – supplementary motor area; S1 (3b) – primary somatosensory area; S2 – secondary somatosensory area; V1 – primary visual area; V2 – second visual area; V3 – third visual area; 3a – somatosensory area 3a; 1–2 somatosensory areas 1–2. Scale bar = 5 mm.

cingulate cortex on the payoffs of decisions based on memory and previous experience, and alternatives. Inputs to primary motor cortex complete and determine the outcome. Outcomes can suddenly change due to further processing in the basal ganglia.

While all primates have these three sets of domains in posterior parietal and frontal cortex, they can be modified by experience, and subdivided to create new action-specific sets of domains. Thus, humans appear to have additional domains for tool use (Frey 2007) and language (Rauschecker and Scott 2009). And especially small mammals would likely have domains for escape, and use vision to seek places to hide (Cisek 2007). As the roles of posterior parietal cortex and prefrontal cortex expanded, especially in humans, the increased sources of information further improved the decision-making process of dorsal stream motor behavior. Due to its major role in goal selection, all of prefrontal cortex has been seen as "premotor in nature" (Fine and Hayden 2022).

Finally, the domain sequences of posterior parietal cortex have been less fully revealed in macaques and humans than in galagos, owl monkeys, and squirrel monkeys, where the focus has been on using electrical microstimulation to evoke classes of complex movements (Kaas and Stepniewska 2021). In macaques and humans, microelectrode recordings and imaging have provided evidence for at least four domains, the anterior intraparietal area (AIP) for grasping and manipulation, the ventral intraparietal area (VIP) for defensive movements of the face and head such as eye closure; the medial intraparietal area (MIP) for reaching, and the lateral intraparietal area (LIP) for looking and focusing attention (Grefkes and Fink 2005). Comparisons between macaques and humans indicate that posterior parietal cortex in humans has greatly expanded (Chaplin et al. 2013; Hill et al. 2010) and the locations of domains relative to the intraparietal sulcus have changed somewhat in humans. Such studies suggest that more cortical domains exist in this cortex in humans and these domains are implicated in higher cognitive functions.

33.5 The Ventral Stream of Visual Processing

The ventral stream of visual processing has been mainly studied in macaques and humans, and much less is known about New World monkeys and strepsirrhine primates such as galagos. The studied domains of the ventral stream are in the temporal lobe where visual inputs are from parts of early visual areas such as the second visual area (V2), the third visual area (V3), and the dorsolateral visual area (DL or V4). These inputs are relaying information about the shapes, sizes, colors, and orientations of parts of objects to the upper temporal lobe to create a domain where neurons are selectively responsive to views and parts of faces, bodies, and other objects. There are several interacting domains for different aspects of faces that have been intensively studied in macaques (Arcaro et al. 2017, 2019; Tsao et al. 2003). These face sensitive domains are interconnected to form a face identification network (Grimaldi et al. 2016). A face domain somewhat outside that network, the middle dorsal (MD) face area, extracts information about face identity as well as face expression and direction of gaze (Yang and Freiwald 2021). Thus, face domains collectively provide critically important information in social primates about the identities of individuals and their intentions. Face recognition is very important in highly social monkeys such as macaques, and even more so in humans.

In some primates, the face-sensitive domains in temporal cortex are in slightly thicker cortex so that they can be identified anatomically in brain sections. These "bumps" of thicker cortex have been identified as face patches in macaques, and have been identified anatomically in baboons, apes, and humans (Arcaro et al. 2020). Thus, face-sensitive domains appear to be widespread features of the larger Old World primates. There is also evidence of face-sensitive neurons in the temporal cortex of New World marmoset monkeys that are social (Hung et al. 2015), but no evidence yet from strepsirrhine primates, although early visual areas are known to project to temporal cortex in galagos. However, the limited evidence in New World monkeys as well as Old World monkeys suggest that face-sensitive domains emerged in the common ancestors of the two radiations at least 35 million years ago.

Present evidence supports the conclusion that many of the connections between visual areas and domains emerge during prenatal development without direct visual experience, and are refined by visual experience after birth (Arcaro and Livingstone 2017; Arcaro et al. 2019). Thus, the newborn primates need visual experience with faces to refine the face domains and make them fully functional (Arcaro et al. 2017). Monkeys reared without seeing faces develop domains sensitive to other body parts. In humans, the face domains can be modified by additional experience as humans strive to become expert on identifying species of birds and makes of cars (Gauthier et al. 2000). Occipital and temporal areas that contribute to the ventral stream processing also contribute directly to prefrontal cortex (Kravitz et al. 2013).

The auditory (Kaas and Hackett 2000; Rauschecker 2018) and somatosensory systems (Mishkin 1979) form analogous dorsal and ventral streams, and interact with the domains in the visual dorsal and ventral streams at several levels (Renier et al. 2009). When sounds and touch were used for identifications, they activated frontal cortex and the insula, and when used for localization, regions of parietal cortex were more active in humans. Thus, parts of dorsal and ventral streams are multimodal.

33.6 Cognition in Apes and Humans

Our closest relatives are chimpanzees and bonobos. Our branch of primate evolution diverged from the one that led to these two great apes 7–8 million years ago. The common ancestors of these apes and humans were obviously more chimp like than human like. Chimps did not change much from the common ancestors and they remain adapted to the tropical rainforest lifestyle. Our ancestors spread into other environments, and developed cognitive abilities to adjust and prosper in many environments. With tools and fire, it was possible to consistently get and process more food, and evolve a larger, but more costly, brain with more cortex, more cortical areas and domains, and more neurons. The cognitive and perceptual abilities of chimps have been studied rather extensively. Comparative studies of brain organization in chimps and humans have been more limited, simply because many of the productive methods of studying brain functions cannot be applied. Nevertheless, a great deal is available from histological and fMRI imaging studies. Chimps and humans have two major differences in cognition. One is in language, which is fair to say is missing in chimps, although they can sometimes learn the meaning of a large number of words. The other is in reasoning about causes.

Povinelli and co-workers have extensively studied the abilities of chimps, compared to humans, on their understanding of causal mechanisms in tool use (Povinelli 2000). The general conclusion is that chimps are very much like humans in sensory abilities. Thus, they can judge a difference in two identical size balls when one is heavier. But they fail to use the heavier ball to displace a food object. Children immediately understand that the weighted ball is better. Chimps also fail to pick the tool that fits through a hole or is capable of retrieving an object. They also seem to have little understanding about what their caretakers know or do not know. Overall, many experiments support the conclusion that chimps do not understand unobservable causal mechanisms (Penn and Povinelli 2007), while humans do, to the extent that they also have false beliefs, such as believing that a good-luck charm brings good luck.

33.7 Language, Speech, and Reading

The spoken language has been a major factor in human cognition, so much so that it is difficult to imagine thinking without it. The human language areas are critically involved in the human specific mediation of language. Although, some chimps have been able to assign meaning to random sounds (Preuss 2011), as we do for speech, the numbers of sounds that they learn to associate with objects and actions remains small, and are acquired with difficulty. Apes communicate, as do most mammals, but they do not have anything close to human abilities. In contrast, young children rapidly come to understand the meaning of large numbers of words, and fluently use them. Language was likely shared by coexisting Neanderthals, and other related hominids, but reading emerged in humans rather recently and reading is not acquired as easily as speaking. It is not certain how these abilities evolved in the 7–8 million years since our ancestors diverged from that leading to modern day apes, but language in our ancestors goes back at least to the emergence of our species some 300,000 years ago and most likely earlier. Language in humans depends on the large regions or areas of Broca and Wernicke of the frontal and temporal lobes of the left cerebral hemisphere, as human-specific areas. However, homologues of Broca's and Wernicke's areas likely exist in the right frontal and temporal cortex of humans, where they have not been modified and specialized for language, and in frontal and temporal cortex of apes and perhaps monkeys. Homologues of language areas have been proposed for both human Wernicke's area (planum temporal) and Broca's area in monkeys and apes (Preuss 2011). Architectonic subdivisions of neocortex in general have been identified as similar in monkeys and humans, and with the main differences being in size (Petrides and Pandya 1994). However, cortical regions and subdivisions have been substantially altered and modified for producing and understanding speech in the left frontal cortex of the ancestors of our species.

As the result of learning and activity-based plasticity, regions of especially temporal cortex have been modified postnatally to function in fluent reading. This includes a region of temporal cortex between auditory and visual regions that become responsive to spoken and written words (Wilson et al. 2018). In humans, a large pathway exists between the temporal lobe and frontal cortex. This arcuate fasciculus to frontal from temporal cortex is expanded bilaterally in humans compared to chimpanzees (Sierpowska et al. 2022). The enlarged pathways in the left cerebral hemisphere are thought to be critical in language, and those in the right hemisphere in tool use and planning.

33.8 Primate Memory and Prefrontal Cortex

The evolution of memory types and the neural mechanisms of memory are described in a recent book by Murray et al. (2019). Neural systems for reinforcement learning and Pavlovian conditioning are widespread across animals and depend on various systems. Navigation, the ability to move about and return to a same home base, is important to all mammals that move from place to place, and navigation involves the hippocampus and adjoining cortical structures. As primate brains got bigger, with more cortical areas and neurons, additional types of memory were added and refined. The hippocampus remains important in memories used for navigation, but the hippocampus is also critical for memory transfer over the times it takes to establish long-term storage in areas and regions of neocortex. Thus, much or all of neocortex is involved in memories. As mentioned in considering the dorsal and ventral streams of sensory processing, decision making in posterior parietal cortex depends on a competitive analysis of ongoing sensory events. The decision outcomes next depend on the influence of prefrontal cortex on action selection in premotor cortex.

Prefrontal cortex contains the mechanisms to resolve action conflict with memories that provide the estimated values of alternative behaviors. These are parts of the executive functions of prefrontal cortex. In humans, posterior parietal cortex contains memories of how to use tools and other objects. Premotor cortex represents classes of movements and their value via prefrontal cortex. Representations of self and events, as well as facts and cultural values, are widespread. A part of prefrontal cortex with densely packed small neurons (granular prefrontal cortex) is well developed in monkeys, apes and humans, and this cortex is important in maintaining short-term memories of ongoing events (working memory).

33.9 Conclusions

Early primates were small and nocturnal. Many evolved into larger, diurnal monkeys, apes and humans, with larger brains, more neocortex, and more neurons, domains, and areas in neocortex. Much of the processing in all primates involved a dorsal stream of visual processing for guiding actions and a ventral stream for identifying objects. These streams were joined by interacting streams for auditory and somatosensory processing. These streams were part of a larger decision-making process that depended on distributed memories of past behavior and ongoing motivation. Primates with larger brains and more neocortex have the advantages of more advanced processing, and more behavioral alternatives. The dorsal and ventral streams became larger, with more subdivisions and inputs in the larger primates, and humans advanced by adding language and tool use to the dorsal and ventral streams.

References

Arcaro, M.J. and Livingstone, M.S. (2017). A hierarchical, retinotopic proto-organization of the primate visual system at birth. *Elife* 6: e26196. doi: 10.7554/eLife.26196.

Arcaro, M.J. et al. (2020). Anatomical correlates of face patches in macaque inferotemporal cortex. *Proc Natl Acad Sci USA* 117 (51): 32667–32678. doi: 10.1073/pnas.2018780117.

Arcaro, M.J. et al. (2019). Universal mechanisms and the development of the face network. *Ann Rev Vis Sci* 5: 341–372. doi: 10.1146/annurev-vision-091718-014917.

Arcaro, M.J. et al. (2017). Seeing faces is necessary for face-domain formation. *Nat Neurosci* 20 (10): 1404–1412. doi: 10.1038/nn.4635.

Chaplin, T.A. et al. (2013). A conserved pattern of differential expansion of cortical areas in simian primates. *J Neurosci* 33 (38): 15120–15125. doi: 10.1523/JNEUROSCI.2909-13.2013.

Cisek, P. (2007). Cortical mechanisms of action selection: the affordance competition hypothesis. *Philos Trans Royal Soc London. Series B, Biol Sci* 362 (1485): 1585–1599. doi: 10.1098/rstb.2007.2054.

Collins, C.E. et al. (2010). Neuron densities vary across and within cortical areas in primates. *Proc Natl Acad Sci USA* 107 (36): 15927–15932. doi: 10.1073/pnas.1010356107.

Collins C.E. et al. (2013). Faster scaling of visual neurons in cortical areas relative to subcortical structures in non-human primate brains. *Brain Struct Funct* 218 (3): 805–816. doi: 10.1007/s00429-012-0430-5.

Collins, C.E. et al. (2016). Cortical cell and neuron density estimates in one chimpanzee hemisphere. *Proc Natl Acad Sci USA* 113 (3): 740–745. doi: 10.1073/pnas.1524208113.

Fine, J.M. and Hayden, B.Y. (2022). The whole prefrontal cortex is premotor cortex. *Philos Trans Royal Soc London. Series B, Biol Sci* 377 (1844): 20200524. doi: 10.1098/rstb.2020.0524.

Fleagle, J.G. (1999). *Primate Adaption and Evolution*. New York: Academic Press.
Frey, S.H. (2007). What puts the how in where? Tool use and the divided visual streams hypothesis. *Cortex* 43 (3): 368–375. doi: 10.1016/s0010-9452(08)70462-3.
Gabi, M. et al. (2016). No relative expansion of the number of prefrontal neurons in primate and human evolution. *Proc Natl Acad Sci USA* 113 (34): 9617–9622. doi: 10.1073/pnas.1610178113.
Gauthier, I. et al. (2000). Expertise for cars and birds recruits brain areas involved in face recognition. *Nat Neurosci* 3 (2): 191–197. doi: 10.1038/72140.
Goodale, M.A. and Milner, A.D. (1992). Separate visual pathways for perception and action. *Trends Neurosci* 15 (1): 20–25. doi: 10.1016/0166-2236(92)90344-8.
Grefkes, C. and Fink, G.R. (2005). The functional organization of the intraparietal sulcus in humans and monkeys. *J Anat* 207 (1): 3–17. doi: 10.1111/j.1469-7580.2005.00426.x.
Grimaldi, P. et al. (2016). Anatomical connections of the functionally defined "face patches" in the macaque monkey. *Neuron* 90 (6): 1325–1342. doi: 10.1016/j.neuron.2016.05.009.
Gunturkun, O. and Bugnyar, T. (2016). Cognition without cortex. *Trends Cog Sci* 20 (4): 291–303. doi: 10.1016/j.tics.2016.02.001.
Herculano-Houzel, S. (2017). Numbers of neurons as biological correlates of cognitive capability. *Curr Opin Behav Sci* 16: 1–7.
Herculano-Houzel, S. et al. (2014). The elephant brain in numbers. *Front Neuroanat* 8: 46. doi: 10.3389/fnana.2014.00046.
Herculano-Houzel, S. et al. (2007). Cellular scaling rules for primate brains. *Proc Natl Acad Sci USA* 104 (9): 3562–3567. doi: 10.1073/pnas.0611396104.
Herculano-Houzel, S. et al. (2016). Corticalization of motor control in humans is a consequence of brain scaling in primate evolution. *J Comp Neurol* 524 (3): 448–455. doi: 10.1002/cne.23792.
Herculano-Houzel, S. and Lent, R. (2005). Isotropic fractionator. *J Neurosci* 25 (10): 2518–2521. doi: 10.1523/JNEUROSCI.4526-04.2005.
Hill, J. et al. (2010). Similar patterns of cortical expansion during human development and evolution. *Proc Natl Acad Sci USA* 107 (29): 13135–13140. doi: 10.1073/pnas.1001229107.
Hung, C.C. et al. (2015). Functional mapping of face-selective regions in the extrastriate visual cortex of the marmoset. *J Neurosci* 35 (3): 1160–1172. doi: 10.1523/JNEUROSCI.2659-14.2015.
Janacsek, K. et al. (2022). Subcortical cognition. *Ann Rev Neurosci* 45: 361–386. doi: 10.1146/annurev-neuro-110920-013544.
Jerison, H.J. (1973). *Evolution of the Brain and Intelligence*. Elsevier.
Kaas, J.H. (2000). Why is brain size so important. *Brain Mind* 1: 7–23.
Kaas, J.H. (2012). Evolution of columns, modules, and domains in the neocortex of primates. *Proc Natl Acad Sci USA* 109 (Suppl 1): 10655–10660. doi: 10.1073/pnas.1201892109.
Kaas, J.H. and Hackett, T.A. (2000). Subdivisions of auditory cortex and processing streams in primates. *Proc Natl Acad Sci USA* 97 (22): 11793–11799. doi: 10.1073/pnas.97.22.11793.
Kaas, J.H. and Preuss, T.M. (2014). Human brain evolution. In: *Fundamental Neuroscience*, 4e (ed. L.R. Squire), 901–918. London: Elsevier, Inc.
Kaas, J.H., Qi, H.X., and Stepniewska, I. (2022). Escaping the nocturnal bottleneck, and the evolution of the dorsal and ventral streams of visual processing in primates. *Philos Trans Royal Soc London. Series B, Biol Sci* 377 (1844): 20210293. doi: 10.1098/rstb.2021.0293.
Kaas, J.H. and Stepniewska, I. (2016). Evolution of posterior parietal cortex and parietal-frontal networks for specific actions in primates. *J Comp Neurol* 524 (3): 595–608. doi: 10.1002/cne.23838.
Kaas, J.H. and Stepniewska, I. (2021). Using electrical stimulation to explore and augment the functions of parietal-frontal cortical networks in primates. In: *Modern Approaches to Augmentation of Brain Function, Contemporary Clinical Neuroscience* (ed. I. Opris et al.), 3–18. Cham, Switzerland: Springer Nature.

Kravitz, D.J., Saleem, K.S., Baker, C.I. et al. (2013). The ventral visual pathway. *Trends Cog Sci* 17 (1): 26–49. doi: 10.1016/j.tics.2012.10.011.

Mishkin, M. (1979). Analogous neural models for tactile and visual learning. *Neuropsychologica* 17: 139–151.

Monson, T.A., Weitz, A.P., Brasil, M.F., and Hlusko, L.J. (2022). Teeth, prenatal growth rates, and the evolution of human-like pregnancy in later Homo. *Proc Natl Acad Sci USA* 119 (41): e2200689119. doi: 10.1073/pnas.2200689119.

Murray, E. et al. (2019). *The Evolutionary Road to Human Memory*. Oxford: Oxford University Press.

Olkowicz, S. et al. (2016). Birds have primate-like numbers of neurons in the forebrain. *Proc Natl Acad Sci USA* 113 (26): 7255–7260. doi: 10.1073/pnas.1517131113.

Passingham, D. and Wise, S. (2012). *The Neurobiology of Prefrontal Cortex*. Oxford: Oxford University Press.

Penn, D.C. and Povinelli, D.J. (2007). On the lack of evidence that non-human animals possess anything remotely resembling a "theory of mind". *Philos Trans Royal Soc London. Series B, Biol Sci* 362 (1480): 731–744. doi: 10.1098/rstb.2006.2023.

Petrides, M. and Pandya, D.N. (1994). Comparative architectonic analysis of the human and macaque frontal cortex. In: *Handbook of Neuropsychology* (ed. F. Booker and J. Grafman), Vol. 9, 17–58. Amsterdam: Elsevier. 1993.

Povinelli, D.J. (2000). *Folk Physics for Apes*. New York: Oxford University Press.

Premack, D. (2007). Human and animal cognition: continuity and discontinuity. *Proc Natl Acad Sci USA* 104 (35): 13861–13867. doi: 10.1073/pnas.0706147104.

Preuss, T.M. (2011). The human brain. *Ann New York Acad Sci* 1225 (Suppl 1): E182–E191. doi: 10.1111/j.1749-6632.2011.06001.x.

Rauschecker, J.P. (2018). Where did language come from? Precursor mechanisms in nonhuman primates. *Curr Opin Behav Sci* 21: 195–204. doi: 10.1016/j.cobeha.2018.06.003.

Rauschecker, J.P. and Scott, S.K. (2009). Maps and streams in the auditory cortex. *Nat Neurosci* 12 (6): 718–724. doi: 10.1038/nn.2331.

Renier, L.A. et al. (2009). Multisensory integration of sounds and vibrotactile stimuli in processing streams for "what" and "where". *J Neurosci* 29 (35): 10950–10960. doi: 10.1523/JNEUROSCI.0910-09.2009.

Ringo, J.L. (1991). Neuronal interconnection as a function of brain size. *Brain, Behav Evol* 38 (1): 1–6. doi: 10.1159/000114375.

Saraf, M.P. et al. (2019). Architectonic features and relative locations of primary sensory and related areas of neocortex in mouse lemurs. *J Comp Neurol* 527 (3): 625–639. doi: 10.1002/cne.24419.

Sherman, S.M. and Guillery, R.W. (2006). Exploring the thalamus and its role in cortical function. 2e. Cambridge: MIT Press.

Sierpowska, J. et al. (2022). Comparing human and chimpanzee temporal lobe neuroanatomy reveals modifications to human language hubs beyond the frontotemporal arcuate fasciculus. *Proc Natl Acad Sci USA* 119 (28): e2118295119. doi: 10.1073/pnas.2118295119.

Stepniewska, I. et al. (2020). Functionally matched domains in parietal-frontal cortex of monkeys project to overlapping regions of the striatum. *Prog Neurobiol* 195: 101864. doi: 10.1016/j.pneurobio.2020.101864.

Strockens, F. et al. (2022). High associative neuron numbers could drive cognitive performance in corvid species. *J Comp Neurol* 530 (10): 1588–1605. doi: 10.1002/cne.25298.

Tsao, D.Y. et al. (2003). Faces and objects in macaque cerebral cortex. *Nat Neurosci* 6 (9): 989–995. doi: 10.1038/nn1111.

Wilson, S.M. et al. (2018). Convergence of spoken and written language processing in the superior temporal sulcus. *Neuroimage* 171: 62–74. doi: 10.1016/j.neuroimage.2017.12.068.

Wong, P. and Kaas, J.H. (2010). Architectonic subdivisions of neocortex in the Galago (Otolemur garnetti). *AnatRecord* 293 (6): 1033–1069. doi: 10.1002/ar.21109.
Wong, P. et al. (2013). Faster scaling of auditory neurons in cortical areas relative to subcortical structures in primate brains. *Brain, Behav Evol* 81 (4): 209–218. doi: 10.1159/000350709.
Yang, Z. and Freiwald, W.A. (2021). Joint encoding of facial identity, orientation, gaze, and expression in the middle dorsal face area. *Proc Natl Acad Sci USA* 118 (33): e2108283118. doi: 10.1073/pnas.2108283118.

Index

Neocortical Neurogenesis in Development and Evolution, First Edition. Edited by Wieland B. Huttner.

Printed in the USA/Agawam, MA
September 16, 2026

910661.194